Pediatric Critical Care Medicine

Derek S. Wheeler • Hector R. Wong
Thomas P. Shanley

Editors

Pediatric Critical Care Medicine

Volume 1: Care of the Critically Ill or Injured Child

Second Edition

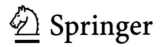

Editors
Derek S. Wheeler, MD, MMM
Division of Critical Care Medicine
Cincinnati Children's Hospital Medical Center
University of Cincinnati College of Medicine
Cincinnati, OH
USA

Thomas P. Shanley, MD
Michigan Institute for Clinical and Health
Research
University of Michigan Medical School
Ann Arbor, MI
USA

Hector R. Wong, MD
Division of Critical Care Medicine
Cincinnati Children's Hospital Medical Center
University of Cincinnati College of Medicine
Cincinnati, OH
USA

ISBN 978-1-4471-6361-9   ISBN 978-1-4471-6362-6   (eBook)
DOI 10.1007/978-1-4471-6362-6
Springer London Heidelberg New York Dordrecht

Library of Congress Control Number: 2014937450

Printed on acid-free paper

Springer is part of Springer Science+Business Media (www.springer.com)

For Cathy, Ryan, Katie, Maggie, and Molly

"You don't choose your family. They are God's gift to you..."
Desmond Tutu

Foreword to the First Edition

The practitioner of *Pediatric Critical Care Medicine* should be facile with a broad scope of knowledge from human developmental biology, to pathophysiologic dysfunction of virtually every organ system, and to complex organizational management. The practitioner should select, synthesize and apply the information in a discriminative manner. And finally and most importantly, the practitioner should constantly "listen" to the patient and the responses to interventions in order to understand the basis for the disturbances that create life-threatening or severely debilitating conditions.

Whether learning the specialty as a trainee or growing as a practitioner, the pediatric intensivist must adopt the mantle of a perpetual student. Every professional colleague, specialist and generalist alike, provides new knowledge or fresh insight on familiar subjects. Every patient presents a new combination of challenges and a new volley of important questions to the receptive and inquiring mind.

A textbook of pediatric critical care fills special niches for the discipline and the student of the discipline. As an historical document, this compilation records the progress of the specialty. Future versions will undoubtedly show advances in the basic biology that are most important to bedside care. However, the prevalence and manifestation of disease invariably will shift, driven by epidemiologic forces, and genetic factors, improvements in care and, hopefully, by successful prevention of disease. Whether the specialty will remain as broadly comprehensive as is currently practiced is not clear, or whether sub-specialties such as cardiac- and neurointensive care will warrant separate study and practice remains to be determined.

As a repository of and reference for current knowledge, textbooks face increasing and imposing limitations compared with the dynamic and virtually limitless information gateway available through the internet. Nonetheless, a central standard serves as a defining anchor from which students and their teachers can begin with a common understanding and vocabulary and thereby support their mutual professional advancement. Moreover, it permits perspective, punctuation and guidance to be superimposed by a thoughtful expert who is familiar with the expanding mass of medical information.

Pediatric intensivists owe Drs. Wheeler, Wong, and Shanley a great debt for their work in authoring and editing this volume. Their effort was enormously ambitious, but matched to the discipline itself in depth, breadth, and vigor. The scientific basis of critical care is integrally woven with the details of bedside management throughout the work, providing both a satisfying rationale for current practice, as well as a clearer picture of where we can improve. The coverage of specialized areas such as intensive care of trauma victims and patients following congenital heart surgery make this a uniquely comprehensive text. The editors have assembled an outstanding collection of expert authors for this work. The large number of international contributors is striking, but speaks to the rapid growth of this specialty throughout the world.

We hope that this volume will achieve a wide readership, thereby enhancing the exchange of current scientific and managerial knowledge for the care of critically ill children, and stimulating the student to seek answers to fill our obvious gaps in understanding.

Chicago, Illinois, USA   Thomas P. Green
New Haven, CT, USA   George Lister

Preface to the Second Edition

The specialty of pediatric critical care medicine continues to grow and evolve! The modern PICU of today is vastly different, even compared to as recently as 5 years ago. Technological innovations in monitoring, information management, and even medical documentation have seemed to change virtually overnight. We have witnessed the gradual disappearance of some time-honored, traditional devices such as the pulmonary artery catheter. At the same time, we have observed the rapid evolution and adoption of newer monitoring techniques such as continuous venous oximetry and near-infrared spectroscopy. Some PICUs are even now using telemedicine to remotely provide care for critically ill children. Many of us can recall a time when cellular phones were prohibited in the PICU – today, many of us can remotely monitor the status of our patients from these same cellular phones! Advances in molecular biology have led to the era of personalized medicine – we can now individualize our treatment approach to the unique and specific needs of a patient. We now routinely rely on a vast array of condition-specific biomarkers to initiate and titrate therapy. Some of these advances in molecular biology have uncovered new diseases and conditions altogether! At the same time, pediatric critical care medicine has become more global. We are sharing our knowledge with the world community. Through our collective efforts, we are advancing the care of our patients. Pediatric critical care medicine will continue to grow and evolve – more technological advancements and scientific achievements will surely come in the future. We will become even more global in scope. However, the human element of what pediatric critical care providers do will never change. "For all of the science inherent in the specialty of pediatric critical care medicine, there is still art in providing comfort and solace to our patients and their families. No technology will ever replace the compassion in the touch of a hand or the soothing words of a calm and gentle voice" [1]. I remain humbled by the gifts that I have received in my life. And I still remember the promise I made to myself so many years ago – the promise that I would dedicate the rest of my professional career to advancing the field of pediatric critical care medicine as payment for these gifts. It is my sincere hope that the second edition of this textbook will educate a whole new generation of critical care professionals, and in so-doing help me continue my promise.

Cincinnati, OH, USA   Derek S. Wheeler, MD, MMM

Reference

1. Wheeler DS. Care of the critically ill pediatric patient. Pediatr Clin North Am 2013;60:xv–xvi. Copied with permission by Elsevier, Inc.

Preface to the First Edition

Promises to Keep

The field of critical care medicine is growing at a tremendous pace, and tremendous advances in the understanding of critical illness have been realized in the last decade. My family has directly benefited from some of the technological and scientific advances made in the care of critically ill children. My son Ryan was born during my third year of medical school. By some peculiar happenstance, I was nearing completion of a 4-week rotation in the Newborn Intensive Care Unit. The head of the Pediatrics clerkship was kind enough to let me have a few days off around the time of the delivery – my wife Cathy was 2 weeks past her due date and had been scheduled for elective induction. Ryan was delivered through thick meconium-stained amniotic fluid and developed breathing difficulty shortly after delivery. His breathing worsened over the next few hours, so he was placed on the ventilator. I will never forget the feelings of utter helplessness my wife and I felt as the NICU Transport Team wheeled Ryan away in the transport isolette. The transport physician, one of my supervising third year pediatrics residents during my rotation the past month, told me that Ryan was more than likely going to require ECMO. I knew enough about ECMO at that time to know that I should be scared! The next 4 days were some of the most difficult moments I have ever experienced as a parent, watching the blood being pumped out of my tiny son's body through the membrane oxygenator and roller pump, slowly back into his body (Figs. 1 and 2). I remember the fear of each day when we would be told of the results of his daily head ultrasound, looking for evidence of

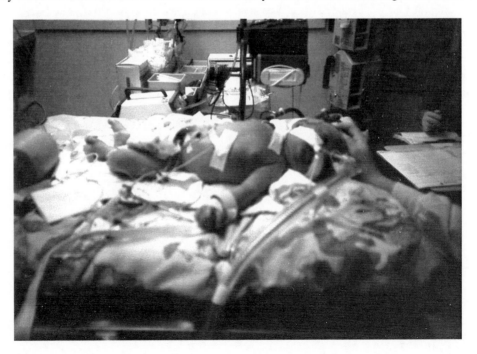

Fig. 1

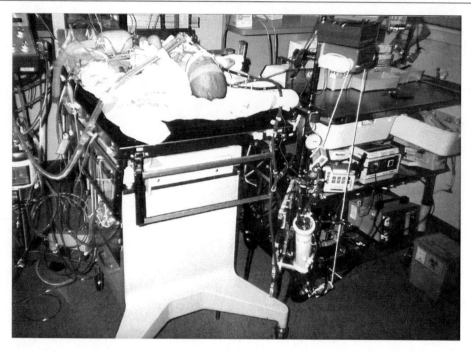

Fig. 2

intracranial hemorrhage, and then the relief when we were told that there was no bleeding. I remember the hope and excitement on the day Ryan came off ECMO, as well as the concern when he had to be sent home on supplemental oxygen. Today, Ryan is happy, healthy, and strong. We are thankful to all the doctors, nurses, respiratory therapists, and ECMO specialists who cared for Ryan and made him well. We still keep in touch with many of them. Without the technological advances and medical breakthroughs made in the fields of neonatal intensive care and pediatric critical care medicine, things very well could have been much different. I made a promise to myself long ago that I would dedicate the rest of my professional career to advancing the field of pediatric critical care medicine as payment for the gifts that we, my wife and I, have been truly blessed. It is my sincere hope that this textbook, which has truly been a labor of joy, will educate a whole new generation of critical care professionals, and in so-doing help make that first step towards keeping my promise.

Cincinnati, OH, USA   Derek S. Wheeler, MD, MMM

Acknowledgements

With any such undertaking, there are people along the way who, save for their dedication, inspiration, and assistance, a project such as this would never be completed. I am personally indebted to Michael D. Sova, our Developmental Editor, who has been a true blessing. He has kept this project going the entire way and has been an incredible help to me personally throughout the completion of this textbook. There were days when I thought that we would never finish – and he was always there to lift my spirits and keep me focused on the task at hand. I will be forever grateful to him. I am also grateful for the continued assistance of Grant Weston at Springer. Grant has been with me since the very beginning of the first edition of this textbook. He has been a tremendous advocate for our specialty, as well as a great mentor and friend. I would be remiss if I did not thank Brenda Robb for her clerical and administrative assistance during the completion of this project. Juggling my schedule and keeping me on time during this whole process was not easy! I have been extremely fortunate throughout my career to have had incredible mentors, including Jim Lemons, Brad Poss, Hector Wong, and Tom Shanley. All four are gifted and dedicated clinicians and remain passionate advocates for critically ill children, the specialties of neonatology and pediatric critical care medicine, and me! I want to personally thank both Hector and Tom for serving again as Associate Editors for the second edition of this textbook. Their guidance and advice has been immeasurable. I have been truly fortunate to work with an outstanding group of contributors. All of them are my colleagues and many have been my friends for several years. It goes without saying that writing textbook chapters is a difficult and arduous task that often comes without a lot of benefits. Their expertise and dedication to our specialty and to the care of critically ill children have made this project possible. The textbook you now hold in your hands is truly their gift to the future of our specialty. I would also like to acknowledge the spouses and families of our contributors – participating in a project such as this takes a lot of time and energy (most of which occurs outside of the hospital!). Last, but certainly not least, I would like to especially thank my family – my wife Cathy, who has been my best friend and companion, number one advocate, and sounding board for the last 22 years, as well as my four children – Ryan, Katie, Maggie, and Molly, to whom I dedicate this textbook and all that I do.

Contents

Contributors

Bokhary Abdulmohsen, MD Department of Pediatric Critical Care, Al Hada Armed Forces Hospital, Tai, Kingdom of Saudi Arabia

Nicholas S. Abend, MD Department of Neurology and Pediatrics, The Children's Hospital of Philadelphia, Philadelphia, PA, USA

Catherine K. Allan, MD Division of Cardiac Intensive Care, Department of Cardiology, Boston Children's Hospital, Boston, MA, USA

Andrew C. Argent, MB, BCh, MMed, FCPaeds, DCH School of Child and Adolescent Health, University of Cape Town, Cape Town, South Africa
Paediatric Intensive Care Unit, Red Cross War Memorial Children's Hospital, Cape Town, South Africa

Hany Bahouth, MD Department of Trauma and Emergency Surgery, Rambam Medical Center, Haifa, Israel

Paul R. Bakerman, MD Critical Care Medicine, Phoeniz Children's Hospital, Phoenix, AZ, USA

Gad Bar-Joseph, MD Department of Pediatric Intensive Care, Meyer Children's Hospital, Rambam Medical Center, Haifa, Israel

Rajit K. Basu, MD, FAAP Division of Critical Care Medicine, Cincinnati Children's Hospital Medical Center, Cincinnati, OH, USA

Michael J. Bell, MD Department of Critical Care Medicine, Children's Hospital of Pittsburgh, Pittsburgh, PA, USA

James B. Besunder, DO Department of Pediatrics, Akron Children's Hospital, Akron, OH, USA

Michael T. Bigham, MD Division of Critical Care Medicine, Department of Pediatrics, Akron Children's Hospital, Akron, OH, USA

Donald L. Boyer, MD Department of Anesthesiology and Critical Care Medicine, The Children's Hospital of Philadelphia and the Perelman School of Medicine at the University of Pennsylvania, Philadelphia, PA, USA

Susan L. Bratton, MD, MPH Department of Pediatrics, Primary Children's Medical Center, Salt Lake City, UT, USA

George Briassoulis, MD, PhD PICU, University Hospital, University of Crete, Heraklion, Crete, Greece

Richard J. Brilli, MD Division of Critical Care Medicine, Department of Pediatrics, Nationwide Children's Hospital, The Ohio State University College of Medicine, Columbus, OH, USA

Sandra D.W. Buttram, MD Critical Care Medicine, Phoenix Children's Hospital, Phoenix, AZ, USA

Charles D. Cadenhead, FAIA, FACHA, FCCM WHR Architects, Houston, TX, USA

Joseph A. Carcillo Jr., MD Pediatric Intensive Care Unit, Children's Hospital of Pittsburgh of UPMC, Pittsburgh, PA, USA

Franco A. Carnevale, RN, PhD Pediatric Critical Care, Montreal Children's Hospital, McGill University, Montreal, QC, Canada

Ira M. Cheifetz, MD, FCCM, FAARC Division of Pediatric Critical Care Medicine, Department of Pediatrics, Duke Children's Hospital, Durham, NC, USA

Ted Cieslak, MD Clinical Services Division, US Army Medical Command, Army Surgeon General, Fort Sam Houston, TX, USA

Timothy T. Cornell, MD Department of Pediatrics and Communicable Diseases, C.S. Mott Children's Hospital University of Michigan, Ann Arbor, MI, USA

Jason Coryell, MD Department of Pediatrics, Doernbecher Children's Hospital, Oregon Health and Sciences University, Portland, OR, USA

Maryse Dagenais, RN, MSc (A) Pediatric Intensive Care Unit, Montreal Children's Hospital, Montreal, QC, Canada

Mary K. Dahmer, PhD Department of Pediatrics, Critical Care Medicine, The University of Michigan, Ann Arbor, MI, USA

Girish G. Deshpande, MD Department of Pediatrics, Children's Hospital of Illinois, Peoria, IL, USA

Prasad Devarajan, MD Division of Nephrology and Hypertension, Cincinnati Children's Hospital Medical Center, Cincinnati, OH, USA

Sonny Dhanani, BSc (Pharm), MD, FRCPC Pediatric Intensive Care Unit, Children's Hospital of Eastern Ontario, Ottawa, ON, Canada

Madan Dharmar, MBBS, PhD Department of Pediatrics, UC Davis Children's Hospital, Sacramento, CA, USA

John Fiadjoe, MD Department of Anesthesiology and Critical Care Medicine, Children's Hospital of Philadelphia, Philadelphia, PA, USA

Cortney B. Foster, DO Department of Pediatric Critical Care, University of Maryland School of Medicine, Baltimore, MD, USA

W. Joshua Frazier, MD Division of Critical Care Medicine, Nationwide Children's Hospital, Columbus, OH, USA

Rani Ganesan, MD Department of Pediatrics, Rush University Medical Center, Chicago, IL, USA

John S. Giuliano Jr., MD Department of Pediatrics, Yale University School of Medicine, New Haven, CT, USA

Stuart L. Goldstein, MD Division of Nephrology and Hypertension, Center for Acute Care Nephrology, Cincinnati Children's Hospital Medical Center, Cincinnati, OH, USA

Amir Hadash, MD Department of Pediatric Intensive Care, Meyer Children's Hospital, Rambam Medical Center, Haifa, Israel

Mark W. Hall, MD Division of Critical Care Medicine, Nationwide Children's Hospital, Columbus, OH, USA

Mary Elizabeth Hartman, MD, MPH Department of Pediatric Critical Care Medicine, St. Louis Children's Hospital, Washington University in St. Louis, St. Louis, MO, USA

Michael J. Hobson, MD Division of Critical Care Medicine, Cincinnati Children's Hospital Medical Center, Cincinnati, OH, USA

K. Sarah Hoehn, MD, MBe University of Kansas Medical Center, Kansas City, KS, USA

Christopher P. Holstege, MD Department of Emergency Medicine, University of Virginia Health System, Charlottesville, VA, USA

Laura M. Ibsen, MD Department of Pediatrics, Doernbecher Children's Hospital, Oregon Health and Sciences University, Portland, OR, USA

Anat Ilivitzki, MD Department of Radiology, Rambam Medical Center, Haifa, Israel

Philippe Jouvet, MD, PhD Department of Pediatrics, Sainte-Justine, Montreal, QC, Canada

Jean Sébastien Joyal, MD, PhD Department of Pediatrics, Sainte-Justine, Montreal, QC, Canada

Jennifer Kaplan, MD, MS Division of Critical Care Medicine, Department of Pediatrics, Cincinnati Children's Hospital Medical Center, University of Cincinnati College of Medicine, Cincinnati, OH, USA

Eric J. Kasowski, DVM, MD, MPH US Centers for Disease Control and Prevention, Atlanta, GA, USA

Todd J. Kilbaugh, MD Department of Anesthesiology and Critical Care Medicine, Children's Hospital of Philadelphia, Philadelphia, PA, USA

Niranjan Kissoon, MD, FRCP(C), FAAP, FCCM, FACPE Department of Pediatrics and Emergency Medicine, The University of British Columbia, Vancouver, BC, Canada

Department of Medical Affairs, BC Children's Hospital and Sunny Hill Health Centre for Children, Vancouver, BC, Canada

Monica E. Kleinman, MD Division of Critical Care Medicine, Department of Anesthesiology, Children's Hospital Boston, Boston, MA, USA

Catherine D. Krawczeski, MD Division of Pediatric Cardiology, Stanford University School of Medicine, Palo Alto, CA, USA

Steven L. Kunkel, MS, PhD Department of Pathology, University of Michigan, Ann Arbor, MI, USA

Stéphane Leteurtre, MD, PhD Department of Pediatrics, Jeanne de Flandre, Lille, France

Gwen J. Lombard, PhD, RN Department of Neurosurgery, University of Florida, Gainesville, FL, USA

James P. Marcin, MD, MPH Department of Pediatrics, UC Davis Children's Hospital, Sacramento, CA, USA

M. Michele Mariscalco, MD Department of Pediatrics, University of Illinois College of medicine at Urbana Champaign, Urbana, IL, USA

David Markenson, MD Disaster Medicine and Regional Emergency Services, Maria Fareri Children's Hospital and Westchester Medical Center, Valhalla, NY, USA

Katherine Mason, MD Department of Pediatrics, Rainbow Babies Children's Hospital, Cleveland, OH, USA

Mark J. McDonald, MD Department of Pediatrics, University of Louisville, Louisville, KY, USA

Kathleen L. Meert, MD Department of Pediatrics, Children's Hospital of Michigan, Detroit, MI, USA

Michael T. Meyer, MD Division of Pediatric Critical Care Medicine, Medical College of Wisconsin, Children's Hospital of Wisconsin, Milwaukee, WI, USA

Kelly Nicole Michelson, MD, PhD Division of Pediatric Critical Care Medicine, Department of Pediatrics, Ann and Robert H. Lurie Children's Hospital of Chicago, Chicago, IL, USA

Jennifer A. Muszynski, MD Division of Critical Care Medicine, The Ohio State University College of Medicine, Nationwide Children's Hospital, Columbus, OH, USA

Elizabeth A. Newell, MD Department of Critical Care Medicine, Children's Hospital of Pittsburgh, Pittsburgh, PA, USA

Matthew F. Niedner, MD Pediatric Intensive Care Unit, Division of Critical Care Medicine, Department of Pediatrics, University of Michigan Medical Center, Mott Children's Hospital, Ann Arbor, MI, USA

Akira Nishisaki, MD, MSCE Department of Anesthesiology and Critical Care Medicine, The Children's Hospital of Philadelphia, Philadelphia, PA, USA

Folafoluwa Olutobi Odetola, MD, MPH Pediatrics and Communicable Diseases, University of Michigan Hospital and Health Systems, Ann Arbor, MI, USA

Waseem Ostwani, MD Department of Pediatric Critical Care Medicine, C.S. Mott Children's Hospital, Ann Arbor, MI, USA

Murray M. Pollack, MD Department of Child Health, University of Arizona College of Medicine – Phoenix, Phoenix, AZ, USA

John Pope, MD Department of Pediatrics, Akron Children's Hospital, Akron, OH, USA

W. Bradley Poss, MD Department of Pediatric Critical Care, University of Utah, Salt Lake, UT, USA

François Proulx, MD Department of Pediatrics, Sainte-Justine, Montreal, QC, Canada

Michael W. Quasney, MD, PhD Department of Pediatrics, Critical Care Medicine, The University of Michigan, Ann Arbor, MI, USA

Adrienne G. Randolph, MD, MSc Division of Critical Care Medicine, Department of Anesthesia, Perioperative and Pain Medicine, Children's Hospital Boston, Boston, MA, USA

Kyle J. Rehder, MD Division of Pediatric Critical Care Medicine, Department of Pediatrics, Duke Children's Hospital, Durham, NC, USA

Peter C. Rimensberger, MD Department of Pediatrics, Service of Neonatology and Pediatric Intensive Care, University Hospital of Geneva, Geneva, Switzerland

Ramesh C. Sachdeva, MD, PhD, JD, FAAP, FCCM Department of Pediatric Critical Care, Medical College of Wisconsin, Milwaukee, WI, USA

Candace Sadorra, BS Department of Pediatrics, UC Davis Children's Hospital, Sacramento, CA, USA

Ajit A. Sarnaik, MD Department of Pediatrics, Children's Hospital of Michigan, Detroit, MI, USA

Matthew C. Scanlon, MD Department of Pediatric Critical Care,
Medical College of Wisconsin, Children's Hospital of Wisconsin, Milwaukee, WI, USA

Thomas P. Shanley, MD Michigan Institute for Clinical and Health Research,
University of Michigan Medical School, Ann Arbor, MI, USA

David K. Shellington, MD Division of Pediatric Critical Care,
University of California, San Diego, San Diego, CA, USA

Sam D. Shemie, PhD Department of Critical Care, Montreal Children's Hospital,
Montreal, QC, Canada

Linda B. Siegel, MD, FAAP Divisions of Pediatric Critical Care Medicine and Pediatric
Palliative CareCohen, Children's Medical Center, New Hyde Park, NY, USA

Philip C. Spinella, MD, FCCM Division of Critical Care, Critical Care Translation
Research Program, Washington University in St. Louis Medical School, St. Louis, MO, USA

David C. Stockwell, MD, MBA Department of Critical Care Medicine,
Children's National, Washington, DC, USA

Jennifer S. Storch, RN, CNRN, CCRN Regional Burn Center ICU,
University of California San Diego Medical Center, San Diego, CA, USA

Paul A. Stricker, MD Department of Anesthesiology and Critical Care Medicine,
The Children's Hospital of Philadelphia and the Perelman School of Medicine at the
University of Pennsylvania, Philadelphia, PA, USA

Janice E. Sullivan, MD Department of Pediatrics and Pharmacology & Toxicology,
University of Louisville, Louisville, KY, USA

Lei Sun, PhD Department of Pediatrics and Communicable Diseases,
University of Michigan, C.S.Mott Children's Hospital, Von Voigtlander Women's hospital,
Ann Arbor, MI, USA

Jill S. Sweney, MD Department of Pediatric Critical Care, University of Utah,
Salt Lake City, UT, USA

Ravi R. Thiagarajan, MBBS, MPH Department of Cardiology,
Boston Children's Hospital, Boston, MA, USA

Cecilia D. Thompson, MD Division of Critical Care Medicine,
Mount Sinai Kravis Children's Hospital, New York, NY, USA

James Tibballs, MBBS, MEd, MBA, MD Pediatric Intensive Care Unit,
Royal Children's Hospital, Melbourne, Melbourne, VIC, Australia

Shane M. Tibby, MBChB, MRCP, MSc (appl stat) PICU Department,
Evelina London Children's Hospital, London, UK

Alexis Topjian, MD, MSCE Department of Anesthesia and Critical Care,
The Children's Hospital of Philadelphia, Philadelphia, PA, USA

Adalberto Torres Jr., MD, MS Department of Pediatrics,
University of Illinois College of Medicine at Peoria, Peoria, IL, USA

Jennifer L. Turi, MD Division of Pediatric Critical Care Medicine,
Department of Pediatrics, Duke Children's Hospital, Durham, NC, USA

Meredith G. van der Velden, MD Department of Anesthesia, Children's Hospital Boston,
Boston, MA, USA

R. Scott Watson, MD, MPH Department of Pediatric Critical Care Medicine, Children's Hospital of Pittsburgh of UPMC, Pittsburgh, PA, USA

Peter H. Weinstock, MD, PhD Division of Critical Care, Department of Anesthesia, Perioperative and Pain Medicine, Boston Children's Hospital, Boston, MA, USA

Derek S. Wheeler, MD, MMM Division of Critical Care Medicine, Cincinnati Children's Hospital Medical Center and University of Cincinnati College of Medicine, Cincinnati, OH, USA

Hector R. Wong, MD Division of Critical Care Medicine, Cincinnati Children's Hospital Medical Center, University of Cincinnati College of Medicine, Cincinnati, OH, USA

Luke A. Zabrocki, MD Division of Pediatric Critical Care, Naval Medical Center San Diego, San Diego, CA, USA

Basilia Zingarelli, MD, PhD Division of Critical Care Medicine, Cincinnati Children's Hospital Medical Center, Cincinnati, OH, USA

Andrew C. Argent and Niranjan Kissoon

Abstract

Pediatric critical care aims on saving the lives of sick and injured children, however, most children die without access to pediatric critical care. With progress towards attainment of the Millennium Development Goals across the world, there has been a significant drop in child mortality in most countries. As issues such as nutrition, immunization, access to clean water and sanitation, and access to healthcare are addressed, pediatric critical care will become an increasingly important part of any strategy to reduce childhood deaths. Critical care can only be beneficial in an integrated health system, but the time –sensitive nature of the care required by sick children poses specific challenges. As processes to recognize and treat sick children improve, the role of and need for intensive care services will increase. It is important that these services should be efficient as possible and should not develop de novo but within an integrated network for the provision of care for critically ill children.

Keywords

Critical care • Children • Developing world • Resource-limited settings • Mortality

Introduction

The ultimate aim of critical care services is to save lives and limit morbidity in the critically ill. However, globally the majority of children live in poorer countries and most childhood deaths occur in a few poor countries. Most children,

A.C. Argent, MB, BCh, MMed, FCPaeds, DCH
School of Child and Adolescent Health,
University of Cape Town, Cape Town, South Africa

Paediatric Intensive Care Unit, Red Cross War Memorial
Children's Hospital, Klipfontein Road, Rondebosch,
Cape Town 7700, South Africa
e-mail: andrew.argent@uct.ac.za

N. Kissoon, MD, FRCP(C), FAAP, FCCM, FACPE (✉)
Department of Pediatrics and Emergency Medicine,
The University of British Columbia, Vancouver, BC Canada

Acute and Critical Care – Global Child Health, BC Children's
Hospital and The University of British Columbia,
4480 Oak Street, Room B245, Vancouver, BC V6H3V4, Canada
e-mail: nkissoon@cw.bc.ca

who die, live in circumstances where they have extremely limited access to any medical services and no intensive care facilities. Indeed, there is a link between mortality among children <5 years of age and the country per capita income, as can be clearly seen in Fig. 1.1, with most childhood deaths occurring in the poorest countries of the world. However, Fig. 1.1 also demonstrates that countries with similar incomes may have widely different mortality among children <5 years (consider South Africa, Brazil, and Chile), and countries with widely divergent incomes, may have similar mortality among children <5 years (consider Cuba and the United States of America). It is thus important to focus not only the resources that are available for the care of sick children, but among a myriad of factors, also on the way in which those resources are deployed and utilized.

Frustratingly we already know how to save most of the 23,000 children who die every day [1] although the implementation of those measures are complex and vary among different locations [2]. The interventions required to save those lives have been clearly outlined by several authors in the last decade [3–7]. The financial requirements of

D.S. Wheeler et al. (eds.), *Pediatric Critical Care Medicine*,
DOI 10.1007/978-1-4471-6362-6_1, © Springer-Verlag London 2014

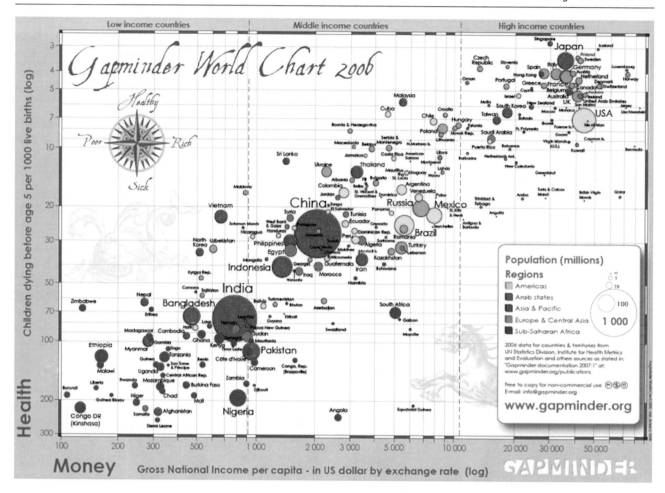

Fig. 1.1 The relationship between per capita income and under-5 mortality (Reprinted with permission from http://www.worldmapper.org © Copyright 2006 SASI Group (University of Sheffield) and Mark Newman (University of Michigan))

implementing those interventions have also been calculated, posing huge ethical challenges and dilemmas for policy makers and citizens in the small proportion of the world who control most of the international financial resources [5, 8, 9]. There can be little doubt, in countries where mortality for children <5 years exceeds 50/1,000 live births that the focus of child death prevention should be on immunization, maternal education and health, provision of clean water and adequate sanitation (together with programs to ensure personal hygiene and hand washing throughout communities), and access to basic healthcare resources [10]. There have been dramatic improvements in child survival wherever these services are implemented [3, 11].

Although the term "pediatric critical care" is often applied specifically to the care of children in the pediatric intensive care unit (PICU), the term more appropriately applies to "the treatment of any child with a life threatening illness or injury (or who requires major elective surgery) from the time of first presentation to health care services until discharge home and completion of rehabilitation" [12]. In this context, critical care services are not confined to any special unit or location

and includes interventions in a wide range of situations throughout healthcare systems, including training of villagers in basic first aid and resuscitation [13], provision of low-cost antibiotics to village healthcare workers [14], appropriate modification of the World Health Organization's (WHO) Integrated Management of Childhood Illness (IMCI) protocols (see below), development of district hospital services [15, 16] and development of other aspects of hospital services [17], reorganization of emergency services at referral hospitals [18], provision of oxygen therapy for hypoxemic children [19–21], and development of emergency medicine services.

What Is Required to Provide Critical Care?

The underlying principles intrinsic to the development of critical care services for children are outlined in Table 1.1 and highlight the need for integrated systems that provide consistent and effective therapy for sick or injured children from presentation through discharge home (Fig. 1.2) [22]. In resource poor environments, many system changes

Table 1.1 The essential components of pediatric critical care

Focus	Recognition of life-threatening injury or illness
	Rapid response (in structured format) to issues that are likely to threaten life (ABC approach)
	Rapid intervention (surgery or medical therapy or both) to try and stop the development of further problems
	Ongoing attention to basic care (Airway, Breathing, Circulation, Disability/Drug therapy, Fluids, Glucose levels, Nutrition etc.)
	Search for underlying diseases processes that are amenable to therapy and then timely provision of that therapy
Team approach	Need for continuous care that is consistent and delivery by a multidisciplinary team with complementary skills
	Concern for the overall context of the child including the family and the community
	Care that crosses the conventional boundaries of medical disciplines
Structured organization	Need for a stable organizational structure and function that ensures that all the services, consumables, staff etc. are available as and when required
	Use of evidence based protocols (preferably ones that have been developed for local conditions and implemented using the team approach)
	Development structured protocols on issues such as discharge and admission policies (preferably ones that have been developed and agreed up by the health structures)
	Integration within the health care services of the region
Accountability	Monitoring of outcomes (and ideally resource utilization)
	Accountability to all interested parties
Sustainability	An underlying premise of the development of a critical care service must be that the resources are available to maintain and sustain that service over a reasonable period of time, without undermining other services within the health care services
Equipment	The equipment required for critical care can range from very basic (provision of oxygen and intravenous fluids) through to highly complex machines that are expensive and have very high operating costs

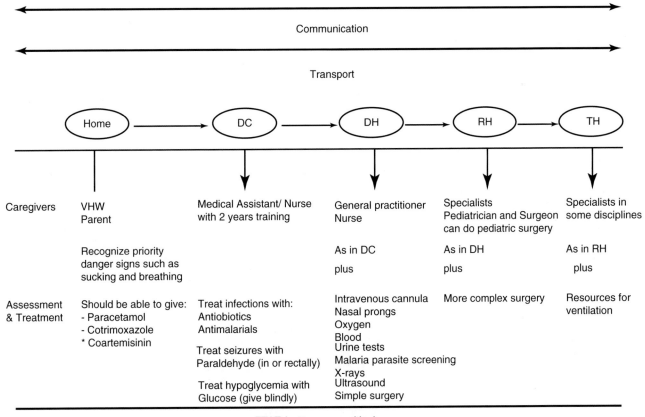

Fig. 1.2 The journey in seeking healthcare for the critically ill child. *DC* district clinic, *DH* district hospital, *RH* regional hospital, *TH* tertiary hospital, *VHW* village health worker, *IMCI* integrated management of childhood illnesses, *ETAT* emergency triage assessment and treatment

Table 1.2 Resources available for healthcare

Country	Income per capita (GDP per capita in US$)	Government health expenditure per person per annum (current US$)	Doctors per 1,000 population	Nurses per 1,000 population
USA	$39,710	$2,548	2.56	9.37
South Africa	$10,960	$114	0.77	4.08
Chile	$10,500	$137	1.09	0.63
Brazil	$8,020	$96	1.15	3.84
India	$3,100	$7	0.6	0.8
Nigeria	$930	$6	0.28	1.7

Based on data obtained from World Health Statistics 2006. World Health Organization (WHO). France; 2006

that can improve care and outcomes for the critically ill do not require major capital investments or substantial increases in resources. For example, a number of authors have described how reorganization of trauma and emergency services can significantly lower pediatric mortality from acute illness or injury [23]. In settings such as Northern Cambodia and Iraq, substantial reductions in trauma mortality were achieved by providing training to prehospital personnel [24, 25], while in Ghana innovative training programs for professional drivers reduced trauma mortality [26]. In Malawi, reorganization of pediatric emergency services at a large urban hospital substantially reduced pediatric mortality at minimal expense [18]. An important component of this particular reorganization was that pediatric trauma patients were channeled through a pediatric service, and not through an adult trauma service. Even within the developed world, there is evidence that children have better outcomes following severe trauma when managed in centers and by services that are focused on the needs of children [27–29]! At an international level, the WHO sponsored program for IMCI was developed in an attempt to standardize and improve the care quality of sick children across the world, with at least some evidence of success [2, 30–33]. The WHO program appropriately focuses on improvement in hospital care of sick children [17, 34].

Thus critical care principles can and should be applied to the provision of healthcare services for severely ill or injured children throughout the world and are not limited to intensive care units. However one of the specific requirements of critical care is the time dependency of effective therapy. In a range of settings, it has clearly been shown that early and effective therapy may substantially improve outcomes for critically ill patients. Time sensitive treatment is important in both adults [35, 36] and children [37, 38]. This may provide substantial challenges in resource limited settings, where transport services and access to surgical and anesthetic services (particularly for children) may be severely limited.

What Is Required to Provide Intensive Care?

Recently, a number of authors have suggested that intensive care services should be available to both adults and children throughout the world [39–42]. There is hardly any ethical justification for children in different parts of the world having different access to intensive care [10]. Ideally every child in the world should have ready access to appropriate medical care, however the simple reality is that in many parts of the world intensive care is unaffordable to children, as shown in Table 1.2 which highlights some of the resources available for healthcare in various parts of the world. When <$10 is available per capita per annum for healthcare expenditure, it is simply not possible to spend $100 per day on basic ventilatory facilities [40] let alone the $1,000 per day as is commonly spent in modern intensive care facilities in the rich countries. However it is perhaps possible to spend the $51 per patient required to provide oxygen therapy to children with pneumonia [20], and it is certainly possible to spend the $6 per annum required to implement most of the measures required to substantially reduce child mortality, and the very low expenditure required to provide early antibiotic therapy to sick neonates in rural communities [14, 43, 44].

In contrast to critical care, intensive care can only be provided where there is substantial infrastructure in place. Recommendations for the facilities required for intensive care in countries such as the United States of America [45, 46] and the United Kingdom include substantial requirements for services such as trained staff (in PICU, in operating rooms, surgical staff, anesthesia), laboratory services, blood bank supplies, imaging equipment, etc. For many of the poorer countries in the world such facilities are either simply not available, or access and availability is extremely limited. However, the WHO recommends that intensive care facilities should be available in all hospitals that provide for major surgery [47]. In this context, they are referring to the provision of facilities with increased capacity for monitoring and intervention, not necessarily "intensive care" as would be expected in the richer countries. This recommendation highlights the significant role that intensive care services may play in facilitating the development of surgical programs, with the capacity to perform major surgery on children.

It is also important to note that within the last decade there has been a substantial increase in the number of countries that have lowered the mortality rate among children <5 years to <20–30 per 1,000 live births, and where there has been an improvement in per capita income, and in the amount of resources available for the provision of healthcare services. In this context there is an appropriate growth in the availability of intensive care services for children. It is difficult to establish the growth in the number of PICUs across the world, but in countries such as China there have been substantial increases in the number of PICUs established and functional, as is illustrated by a recent report from 26 intensive care units with 11,521 patients over a 12 month period [48]. There is considerable variation in the reported outcomes for children from intensive care units in developing countries, with many units reporting very high mortality rates. Many reasons may contribute to the high mortality, including a high incidence of infectious disease [49] and trauma (compared to the high proportion of elective surgical patients seen in the PICUs of rich countries), late referral of patients due to difficulties in the overall delivery of critical care, inadequate PICU numbers for the patient load, poor selection of patients for PICU admission and management, high rates of nosocomial infection, low staffing ratios and infrequent presence of pediatric intensivists, and poor education of staff among others. To this end, a number of studies demonstrated that the presence of a pediatric intensivist lowers mortality in a developing world context [50, 51] with similar effects related to centralization of pediatric intensive care facilities [52].

There are considerable challenges in the provision of training programs for pediatric intensive care in the developing world, and a number of organizations such as the World Federation of Pediatric Intensive and Critical Care Societies (WFPICCS) have recently focused on programmes to provide educational materials [12]. There is also considerable debate around issues such as whether intensivists (or anesthetists) from the developing world should travel to rich countries for training, or whether it is preferable for rich countries to provide training support to developing countries [53, 54] – both options may be appropriate depending upon local circumstances.

Critical Care in Mass Disaster Situations

Complex emergencies include crisis, wars and natural disasters that adversely and acutely impact public health systems and its protective infrastructure (water, sanitation, shelter, food, health). Under these circumstances there is excess mortality, usually greater than one death per 10,000 of the population per day. These complex emergencies seem to be more common in poorer regions of the world and their adverse impact greater because of inadequate resources even under stable conditions. Complex emergencies are dynamic with variable duration of impact, need for emergency services, recovery, rehabilitation and developmental processes. Critical care has a major role to play in these emergencies. While in the developed world there are networks of care and transport systems, robust infrastructure in many cases to combat these emergencies, in many parts of the world they are sorely lacking. The challenge in these settings may well be to improve existing critical care facilities (which will improve day to day care of patients) and hence increase the capacity to cope with disaster situations. Critical care during mass disaster situations and in austere environments are covered separately elsewhere in this textbook.

Ethical Considerations

While there are no ethical grounds for limiting the access of children in poor countries to intensive care [10], the reality is that children in poorer settings have access to fewer intensive care resources. In this situation there is a significant need to focus on the appropriate allocation of limited resources. When resources are limited ethical decisions around access to intensive care are related not only to the needs of the individual child, but also to the needs of the healthcare system and the implications of access to intensive care for the development of other important health programs. Thus there is increased focus on the ethical grounds underpinning the allocation of scarce critical care resources in developing countries [55, 56], with programs such as the accountability for reasonableness showing potential as a framework for decision making [11, 57, 58]. This stands in contrast to some of the ethical issues that seem to be in the forefront in richer countries [59].

Conclusions

While pediatric critical care is focused on saving the lives of sick and injured children, most children world wide die without access to paediatric critical care. With progress towards attainment of the Millenium development goals across the world, there has been a significant drop in child mortality in most countries. As issues such as nutrition, immunization, access to clean water and sanitation, access to healthcare are addressed, pediatric critical care will become an increasingly important part of any strategy to further reduce childhood deaths. Critical care can only function in the context of an integrated health system, but the time –sensitive nature of the care required by sick children poses specific challenges to the development of these systems. As processes to recognize and treat sick children improve the role of and need for intensive care services will increase. It is fundamentally important that these services be as efficient as possible and should not develop *de novo* but within an integrated network for the provision of care for critically ill children.

References

1. Shann F, Duke T. Twenty-three thousand unnecessary deaths every day: what are you doing about it? Pediatr Crit Care Med. 2009;10(5):608–9.
2. Anand K, Patro BK, Paul E, et al. Management of sick children by health workers in Ballabgarh: lessons for implementation of IMCI in India. J Trop Pediatr. 2004;50(1):41–7.
3. Bhutta ZA, Ahmed T, Black RE, et al. What works? Interventions for maternal and child undernutrition and survival. Lancet. 2008;371(9610):417–40.
4. Victora CG, Black RE, Bryce J. Learning from new initiatives in maternal and child health. Lancet. 2007;370(9593):1113–4.
5. Bryce J, Black RE, Walker N, et al. Can the world afford to save the lives of 6 million children each year? Lancet. 2005;365(9478):2193–200.
6. Black RE, Morris SS, Bryce J. Where and why are 10 million children dying every year? Lancet. 2003;361(9376):2226–34.
7. Jones G, Steketee RW, Black RE, et al. How many child deaths can we prevent this year? Lancet. 2003;362(9377):65–71.
8. Knippenberg R, Lawn JE, Darmstadt GL, et al. Systematic scaling up of neonatal care in countries. Lancet. 2005;365(9464):1087–98.
9. Lawn JE, Cousens SN, Darmstadt GL, et al. 1 year after the Lancet Neonatal Survival Series – was the call for action heard? Lancet. 2006;367(9521):1541–7.
10. Shann F, Argent AC. In: Fuhrman BP, Zimmerman JJ, editors. Pediatric intensive care in developing countries. 3rd ed. Philadelphia: Mosby/Elsevier; 2006.
11. Kapiriri L, Martin DK. Successful priority setting in low and middle income countries: a framework for evaluation. Health Care Anal. 2009;18(2):129–47. Epub 2009 Mar 14.
12. Kissoon N, Argent A, Devictor D, et al. World Federation of Pediatric Intensive and Critical Care Societies (WFPICCS) – its global agenda. Pediatr Crit Care Med. 2009;10(5):597–600.
13. Tiska MA, Adu-Ampofo M, Boakye G, et al. A model of prehospital trauma training for lay persons devised in Africa. Emerg Med. 2004;21(2):237–9.
14. Bhutta ZA, Zaidi AK, Thaver D, et al. Management of newborn infections in primary care settings: a review of the evidence and implications for policy? Pediatr Infect Dis J. 2009;28(1 Suppl): S22–30.
15. English M, Esamai F, Wasunna A, et al. Delivery of paediatric care at the first-referral level in Kenya. Lancet. 2004;364(9445):1622–9.
16. English M, Esamai F, Wasunna A, et al. Assessment of inpatient paediatric care in first referral level hospitals in 13 districts in Kenya. Lancet. 2004;363(9425):1948–53.
17. Duke T, Kelly J, Weber M, et al. Hospital care for children in developing countries: clinical guidelines and the need for evidence. J Trop Pediatr. 2006;52(1):1–2. Epub 2006 Jan 16.
18. Molyneux E, Ahmad S, Robertson A. Improved triage and emergency care for children reduces inpatient mortality in a resource-constrained setting. Bull World Health Organ. 2006;84(4):314–9. Epub 2006 Apr 13.
19. Subhi R, Adamson M, Campbell H, et al. The prevalence of hypoxaemia among ill children in developing countries: a systematic review. Lancet Infect Dis. 2009;9(4):219–27.
20. Duke T, Wandi F, Jonathan M, et al. Improved oxygen systems for childhood pneumonia: a multihospital effectiveness study in Papua New Guinea. Lancet. 2008;372(9646):1328–33. Epub 2008 Aug 15.
21. Matai S, Peel D, Wandi F, et al. Implementing an oxygen programme in hospitals in Papua New Guinea. Ann Trop Paediatr. 2008;28(1):71–8.
22. Kissoon N. Out of Africa – a mother's journey. Pediatr Crit Care Med. 2011;12(1):73–9.
23. Molyneux E. Emergency care for children in resource-constrained countries. Trans R Soc Trop Med Hyg. 2009;103(1):11–5. Epub 2008 Sep 2.
24. Husum H, Gilbert M, Wisborg T, et al. Rural prehospital trauma systems improve trauma outcome in low-income countries: a prospective study from north Iraq and Cambodia. J Trauma. 2003;54(6): 1188–96.
25. Husum H, Gilbert M, Wisborg T. Training pre-hospital trauma care in low-income countries: the 'Village University' experience. Med Teach. 2003;25(2):142–8.
26. Mock CN, Tiska M, Adu-Ampofo M, et al. Improvements in prehospital trauma care in an African country with no formal emergency medical services. J Trauma. 2002;53(1):90–7.
27. Potoka DA, Schall LC, Ford HR. Improved functional outcome for severely injured children treated at pediatric trauma centers. J Trauma. 2001;51(5):824–32; discussion 832–4.
28. Oyetunji TA, Haider AH, Downing SR, et al. Treatment outcomes of injured children at adult level 1 trauma centers: are there benefits from added specialized care? Am J Surg. 2011;201(4):445–9.
29. Morrison W, Wright JL, Paidas CN. Pediatric trauma systems. Crit Care Med. 2002;30(11 Suppl):S448–56.
30. Adam T, Edwards SJ, Amorim DG, et al. Cost implications of improving the quality of child care using integrated clinical algorithms: evidence from northeast Brazil. Health Policy. 2009;89(1):97–106. Epub 2008 Jun 25.
31. Bryce J, Gouws E, Adam T, et al. Improving quality and efficiency of facility-based child health care through integrated management of childhood illness in Tanzania. Health Policy Plan. 2005;20 Suppl 1:i69–76.
32. Bryce J, Victora CG, Habicht JP, et al. Programmatic pathways to child survival: results of a multi-country evaluation of integrated management of childhood illness. Health Policy Plan. 2005;20 Suppl 1:i5–17.
33. Gove S, Tamburlini G, Molyneux E, et al. Development and technical basis of simplified guidelines for emergency triage assessment and treatment in developing countries. WHO Integrated Management of Childhood Illness (IMCI) referral care project. Arch Dis Child. 1999;81(6):473–7.
34. Graham SM, English M, Hazir T, et al. Challenges to improving case management of childhood pneumonia at health facilities in resource-limited settings. Bull World Health Organ. 2008;86(5): 349–55.
35. Kumar A, Roberts D, Wood KE, et al. Duration of hypotension before initiation of effective antimicrobial therapy is the critical determinant of survival in human septic shock. Crit Care Med. 2006;34(6):1589–96.
36. Rivers E, Nguyen B, Havstad S, et al. Early goal-directed therapy in the treatment of severe sepsis and septic shock. N Engl J Med. 2001;345(19):1368–77.
37. Han YY, Carcillo JA, Dragotta MA, et al. Early reversal of pediatric-neonatal septic shock by community physicians is associated with improved outcome. Pediatrics. 2003;112(4):793–9.
38. Dellinger RP, Levy MM, Carlet JM, et al. Surviving sepsis campaign: international guidelines for management of severe sepsis and septic shock: 2008. Crit Care Med. 2008;36(1):296–327.

39. Baker T. Pediatric emergency and critical care in low-income countries. Paediatr Anaesth. 2009;19(1):23–7.

40. Baker T. Critical care in low-income countries. Trop Med Int Health. 2009;14(2):143–8. Epub 2009 Jan 21.

41. Fowler RA, Adhikari NK, Bhagwanjee S. Clinical review: critical care in the global context - disparities in burden of illness, access, and economics. Crit Care. 2008;12(5):225. Epub 2008 Sep 9.

42. Walker IA, Morton NS. Pediatric healthcare – the role for anesthesia and critical care services in the developing world. Paediatr Anaesth. 2009;19(1):1–4.

43. Bhutta ZA, Memon ZA, Soofi S, et al. Implementing community-based perinatal care: results from a pilot study in rural Pakistan. Bull World Health Organ. 2008;86(6):452–9.

44. Bhutta ZA, Darmstadt GL, Hasan BS, et al. Community-based interventions for improving perinatal and neonatal health outcomes in developing countries: a review of the evidence. Pediatrics. 2005;115(2 Suppl):519–617.

45. Haupt MT, Bekes CE, Brilli RJ, et al. Guidelines on critical care services and personnel: recommendations based on a system of categorization of three levels of care. Crit Care Med. 2003;31(11):2677–83.

46. De Lange S, Van Aken H, Burchardi H, et al. European Society of Intensive Care Medicine Statement: intensive care medicine in Europe–structure, organisation and training guidelines of the Multidisciplinary Joint Committee of Intensive Care Medicine (MJCICM) of the European Union of Medical Specialists (UEMS). Intensive Care Med. 2002;28:1505–11.

47. Surgical care at the district hospital – the WHO manual. Geneva: World Health Organization; 2003. http://whqlibdoc.who.int/publications/2003/9241545755.pdf. Accessed 18 Feb 2014.

48. Hu X, Qian S, Xu F, et al. Incidence, management and mortality of acute hypoxemic respiratory failure and acute respiratory distress syndrome from a prospective study of Chinese paediatric intensive care network. Acta Paediatr. 2010;99(5):715–21. Epub 2010 Jan 21.

49. Isturiz RE, Torres J, Besso J. Global distribution of infectious diseases requiring intensive care. Crit Care Clin. 2006;22(3):469–88, ix.

50. Goh AY, Lum LC, Abdel-Latif ME. Impact of 24 hour critical care physician staffing on case-mix adjusted mortality in paediatric intensive care. Lancet. 2001;357(9254):445–6.

51. Goh AY, Abdel-Latif M, Lum LC, et al. Outcome of children with different accessibility to tertiary pediatric intensive care in a developing country – a prospective cohort study. Intensive Care Med. 2003;29(1):97–102. Epub 2002 Dec 4.

52. Goh AY, Mok Q. Centralization of paediatric intensive care: are critically ill children appropriately referred to a regional centre? Intensive Care Med. 2001;27(4):730–5.

53. Walker IA. Con: pediatric anesthesia training in developing countries is best achieved by out of country scholarships. Paediatr Anaesth. 2009;19(1):45–9.

54. Gathuya ZN. Pro: pediatric anesthesia training in developing countries is best achieved by selective out of country scholarships. Paediatr Anaesth. 2009;19(1):42–4.

55. Goh AY, Lum LC, Chan PW, et al. Withdrawal and limitation of life support in paediatric intensive care. Arch Dis Child. 1999;80(5):424–8.

56. Jeena PM, McNally LM, Stobie M, et al. Challenges in the provision of ICU services HIV infected children in resource poor settings: a South African case study. J Med Ethics. 2005;31(4):226–30.

57. Kapiriri L, Norheim OF, Martin DK. Fairness and accountability for reasonableness. Do the views of priority setting decision makers differ across health systems and levels of decision making? Soc Sci Med. 2009;68(4):766–73. Epub 2008 Dec 18.

58. Kapiriri L, Martin DK. A strategy to improve priority setting in developing countries. Health Care Anal. 2007;15(3):159–67.

59. Frey B. Overtreatment in threshold and developed countries. Arch Dis Child. 2008;93(3):260–3. Epub 2007 Sep 14.

Pediatric Critical Care and the Law: Medical Malpractice

2

Ramesh C. Sachdeva

Abstract

Although some basic concepts related to medicolegal aspects for the practicing physician have remained unchanged over several years, there is a rapid increase in case-law and new trends emerging in this field. Accordingly, this chapter is divided into three parts. First, a basic overview related to medico-legal civil liability for the practicing physician is discussed, including steps that physicians should consider to minimize this liability. Second, some of the unique legal issues in the practice of pediatric critical care are discussed. Third, several PICUs are in the midst of implementing electronic health records (EHR). The implementation of electronic health records and availability of electronic patient data creates unique challenges and legal issues previously unknown, and key concepts related to these new emerging areas are also discussed.

Keywords

Medical malpractice • Liability • Tort • Legal issues • Expert witness • Standard of care

Introduction

Given the high acuity and associated risks of patients treated in the pediatric intensive care unit (PICU), it is important that pediatric critical care physicians have a thorough understanding of the medicolegal aspects related to their practice (Fig. 2.1). Pediatric critical care physicians need to be aware of four distinct areas of civil liability (discussed below). This chapter primarily discusses the medico-legal concepts related to medical negligence, with a brief discussion of the False Claims Act. However, critical care physicians should also be aware of interactions between ethical and legal concepts

related to withdrawal of care and brain death, and also issues related to obtaining informed consent particularly in elective situations in contrast to emergency situations in the PICU. These issues are discussed in greater detail in other chapters of this textbook.

Although some basic concepts related to medicolegal aspects for the practicing physician have remained unchanged over several years, there is a rapid increase in case-law and new trends emerging in this field. Accordingly, this chapter is divided into three parts from the perspective of the physicians in the U.S. First, a basic overview related to medico-legal civil liability for the practicing physician is discussed, including steps that physicians should consider to minimize this liability. Second, some of the unique legal issues in the practice of pediatric critical care are discussed. Third, several PICUs are in the midst of implementing electronic health records (EHR). The implementation of electronic health records and availability of electronic patient data creates unique challenges and legal issues previously unknown, and key concepts related to these new emerging areas are also discussed.

R.C. Sachdeva, MD, PhD, JD, FAAP, FCCM
Department of Pediatric Critical Care,
Medical College of Wisconsin,
9000 W. Wisconsin Avenue, MS-681, Milwaukee, WI 53226, USA
e-mail: rsachdeva@aap.org

Fig. 2.1 Potential scope of civil
legal exposure

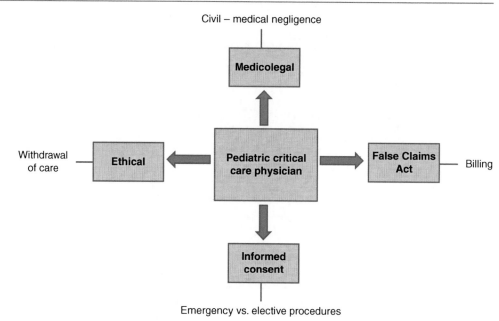

Medico-legal Civil Liability for Pediatric Critical Physicians

Typically, medico-legal civil liability for pediatric critical physicians relates to medical malpractice claims for negligence. The underlying premise is that there is no intent for the injury caused to the child. Such negligence claims require that the family of the injured child (plaintiff) affirmatively prove four key elements – *duty, breach, causation, and harm* (this is extensively discussed in many legal writings) [1]. The physician must have a *duty* to the patient. This is generally not an issue in the PICU where the physician is responsible for the children receiving medical care. *Harm* is also generally not a controversial issue with respect to proof because it typically forms a basis of initiating the claim. The two elements that become the subject of debate include *breach* and *causation*. *Breach* relates to the notation that a departure from the standard of care occurred. It is important to point out that this standard of care represents a national standard as highlighted in the case *Hall* vs. *Hilbun* [2]. In this particular case, the underlying issue was whether a surgeon breached the standard of care when he was at home and the patient suffered a complication after an exploratory laporatomy resulting in cardiorespiratory arrest. The surgeon argued that the care was consistent with the local practice (locality rule). However, the Supreme Court of Mississippi held that the surgeon be judged based upon a national standard of care. With respect to the application of this concept for the pediatric critical care physician, it is important to recognize that local practices within the PICU, although acceptable and popular locally, may be considered as departures from the standard of care if a national standard for that particular critical care condition exists.

The other element in an injury claim that is frequently subject to debate relates to the notion of *causation*. *Causation* implies that the physician's actions resulted in the alleged harm. This can have unique implications in the pediatric critical care setting, where care is provided on a successive basis by multiple physicians during the course of care. Accordingly, it is generally not an acceptable defense that a physician did not cause harm if the underlying problem was precipitated by physician care provided earlier in the course of the care. A hypothetical example would be the situation in which a critical care physician inadvertently placed a central venous catheter in an artery and the care of the child is then taken over by a second physician. The second physician fails to detect this error and the patient suffers harm. In this case, it would generally not be a defense for the second physician that the procedure was performed by someone else. This concept relates to the legal theory of multiple defendants, where several physicians may work in series or tandem and be responsible for patient injury.

Once the injured party (family) feels that the child has suffered an injury and obtains legal counsel, the first step relates to the concept of the *Statute of Limitations*. This is a predefined number of years established by state law during which time the medical malpractice claim can be initiated. This step typically is followed by a series of discovery during which interrogatories and depositions may be conducted and there is a thorough medical record review. The case can be settled by both parties anytime during the litigation period. A small number of cases proceed to a jury trial where both parties have the opportunity to provide legal arguments to the jury before making a final decision. As medical malpractice liability is based upon state laws which differ

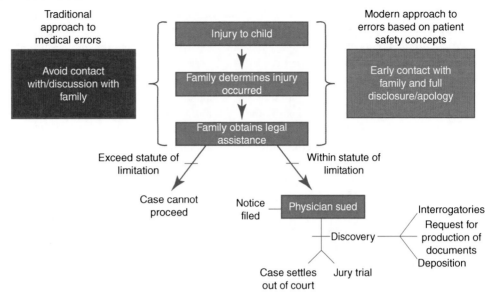

Fig. 2.2 Progression of a hypothetical medicolegal case and changing paradigm for medical ethics/disclosure

significantly across states, it is important for the pediatric critical physician to be fairly familiar with laws where they practice. Differences in state laws not only result in differences in liability but also in differences in the final payments to the injured party.

Steps to Minimize Medico-legal Liability for the Pediatric Critical Care Physician

In order to minimize the medico-legal liability, physicians must carefully keep the following considerations in mind. First, in the practice of pediatric critical care, it is important to be up-to-date on national recommendations for various clinical conditions. As mentioned earlier, it is generally not a defense that the standard of care being practiced was consistent with a local practice but inconsistent with a national standard. Second, physicians should maintain impeccable medical records and documentation of the care being provided. With the trend towards adoption of electronic health records, many of the issues related to legibility of handwriting will evaporate, but newer issues previously not addressed will emerge. Third, it is important to have open and honest communication with families. The emerging literature from patient safety supports that full disclosure of mistakes and patient safety related adverse events to the family in a timely manner in fact reduces the likelihood of subsequent lawsuits. Finally, it is important to approach the medico-legal litigation in professional manner. Typically when physicians are sued, many view this as a direct attack on their professional credibility. This is understandable. However, in order for successful resolution of the underlying lawsuit, it is important to fully cooperate with the investigation in a professional and truthful manner.

Figure 2.2 illustrates the progression of a hypothetical medico-legal case highlighting the change in approaches to medical errors and mistakes based upon the emerging quality and patient safety literature. In the past, the traditional approach to medical errors included avoiding any discussion with the family. The modern approach encourages early and full disclosure with an apology for the situation to the family. The physician should consult with their legal counsel as quickly as possible after learning of a patient safety event. Also, it is important to distinguish between an apology for a particular situation that a family is dealing with versus an admission of a mistake, and the physician should discuss this carefully with their legal counsel to ensure that the goals of full disclosure and transparency for patient safety are met without increasing the individual likelihood of incurring liability.

Legal Standards for Admissibility of Medical Evidence and Expert Testimony

A common issue emerging in medical malpractice related litigation surrounds the notion of determining the standard of care. Typically this standard of care would be established by expert testimony. There are two standards utilized in determining the admissibility of scientific evidence into legal evidence. First, the *Frye* standard which relates to the notion of general acceptance of the scientific evidence in the relevant field [3]. The role of the court is to prevent less than optimal science from being admitted into evidence. Many states have utilized the *Frye* standard for determining scientific admissibility. Subsequently, in the *Daubert* vs. *Merrell Dow* [4] case, the U.S. Supreme Court rejected the *Frye* test of general acceptance and established the *Daubert* standard, which relates to the notion that the scientific knowledge must be derived from scientifically sound methods for ensuring reliability and relevancy. Under the *Daubert* approach the court could use a broad range of criteria to establish the scientific reliability and relevance of the expert evidence. In order to determine the reliability factors using the *Daubert* standard, the court evaluates the totality of circumstances including considering factors whether the scientific theory being proposed has been empirically tested, whether there has been peer review and publication, determination of the potential error rate including the notion of Type 1 and Type 2 statistical error rates, and the need for the technique and results to be explained in simple terms. Although the *Daubert* standard typically emerged as a federal standard, it has increasingly been adopted by several states as their evidentiary standards. This has a unique application in the PICU where new research techniques are frequently leveraged in innovative new therapies and management techniques of care. Generally, the standard of care would be established by experts providing testimony for both parties. Recent decisions in the *Kumho Tire* [5] case highlighted that experts do not need to necessarily have a specific level of certification or education, and in fact, sufficient training and experience may be adequate to deem an individual an expert for establish credibility towards the expert testimony.

Unique Issues in the Pediatric Intensive Care Unit Setting

The discussion in this chapter is largely limited to civil medico-legal situations. However, it is important for the critical care physician to recognize the breath of legal issues that surround decision making in the PICU setting. Several issues span underlying ethical principles, including research and policies on medical futility, end of life decisions, withdrawal of care, and determination of brain death. The full discussion of these topics is beyond the scope of this chapter. However, an emerging area of interest for the critical care physician related to *qui tam litigation* is briefly discussed below. The concepts of *qui tam litigation* (derived from the Latin phrase, *qui tam pro domino rege quam pro se ipso in hac parte sequitur*, meaning *he who sues in this matter for the king as well as for himself*, in which an individual who assists a prosecution can receive all or part of any penalty imposed) stem from the legal provisions of the False Claims Act [6]. The False Claims Act essentially prohibits falsification of billing to government (Centers for Medicare and Medicaid) for services provided. At the superficial level, this can be viewed in terms of obvious fraudulent actions such as billing for services or procedures that were not performed. However, the False Claims Act has recently been expanded to also cover gross breaches in the quality of care provided, which may be viewed as the absence of care. For example, case law from

the nursing homes suggests that patients who developed pressure ulcers due to lack of appropriate nursing home staffing may be subject to liability under the False Claims Act [7]. Further, the False Claims Act provision includes protection and incentivization for whistleblowers. The application of the False Claims Act for combating healthcare fraud is an area of increasing interest in the U.S.

The potential implications for the PICU setting may be important. For example, recently the Centers for Medicare and Medicaid (CMS) adopted policies for nonpayment of "never" events. These complications will not be reimbursed by insurance because they should never occur if the hospital care is functioning appropriately. Examples of "never" events include wrong site surgery, hospital acquired conditions such as pressure ulcers, and more recently, hospital acquired catheter associated blood stream infections. This could create unique new problems from a billing perspective for critical care physicians and their institutions. Therefore, it is important for the pediatric critical care physician to be abreast of these new emerging rules and policies to avoid the unintentional liability that may arise because of compliance failure.

Emerging Medico-legal Issues Resulting from the Availability of Electronic Data from EHR

Most institutions in the U.S. healthcare system are in the midst of EHR implementation. Many PICUs have already adopted electronic health records. This is intended to improve the care quality of including patient safety. However, the increasing availability of electronic data can result in unintended consequences from a medico-legal standpoint. A case from the Wisconsin Supreme Court, *Johnson* vs. *Kokemoor* [8] highlights the potential implications. In this case, the plaintiff had an operation for a carotid aneurysm. Unfortunately, the plaintiff had a complication. The ensuing litigation was based on an argument of battery for the lack of obtaining informed consent utilizing available outcomes data. The plaintiff argued that the surgeon was aware of the comparative outcomes data for his performance compared to a renowned health system in the region which also had available outcomes data for the procedure. The surgeon failed to share these comparative outcomes data with the patient while obtaining informed consent for the surgical procedure. The Wisconsin State Supreme Court determined that this was material for the decision making by the patient and the failure of having this information was interpreted as failure of obtaining full informed consent. The *Johnson* vs. *Kokemoor* decision, although a landmark decision in this field, has gained limited acceptance in other jurisdictions over the past few years. This may be secondary to the lack of readily available outcomes data to perform meaningful statistical comparisons as was highlighted in this opinion. However, the availability of EHR in the future will result in this issue being magnified as physicians, hospitals, and insurance agencies rapidly acquire physician level performance data which can then be subjected to statistical comparisons with other providers [9].

The field of pediatric critical care medicine is particularly well-suited for comparative outcomes information to be used in the legal setting because of the availability of validated risk adjustment tools that have gained peer reviewed acceptance. An example of this is the Pediatric Risk of Mortality (PRISM) Score [10]. As most critical care physicians are familiar, risk adjustment tools such as the PRISM Score allows for comparison of standardized mortality that adjusts for severity of illness at the time of PICU admission. For example, mortality within PICUs can be risk adjusted to allow for comparisons across PICUs as well as over time within a PICU however, the algorithm requires periodic recalibration.

However, risk of mortality scores such as the PRISM, allow for meaningful physiologic based clinical risk adjustment among groups of patients and was never intended to be used at the individual level to predict risk of death. Therefore, such systems should not be used for prognosis for an individual patient. With the availability of large granular data sets, resulting from the adoption of electronic health records, and with the increasing sophistication of statistical and analytical techniques, it will be likely that risk adjustment can be computed at the patient level in the future. Efforts to perform quality comparisons at the regional and national level have already been successfully implemented [11]. Although this methodology is still early in its development, the rapid growth of large data sets will likely allow the continued refinement of such methodologies. The legal implications of the possibility are presently unknown but would likely be used by the legal community.

Other electronic sources are also available (including the KIDS database, PHIS, Society for Thoracic Surgeons Congenital Heart Disease registry, etc.). Some data sets can be evaluated for changes in outcome or care over time to identify trends that may not otherwise be known. Data mining may allow the identification of unique trends related to quality of care for specific physicians. These approaches are still at the level medical outcomes research and have not yet been introduced into the courtroom. However, future mediolegal litigation will very likely attempt to expand the scope of evidence to include results from such analyses using large databases and patient registries.

There has already been a growing interest and movement within the legal profession to incorporate such information to enhance the scope of evidence and the various aspects of litigation [12]. Another application of these increasing electronic patient data sources are evaluation of quality of care and the potential introduction of such results into legal evidence remains unknown at present but it would be extremely important for the pediatric critical care physician to remain aware of the growing trends in this area which will likely impact their practice in the future.

The intersection of medicine and law continues to raise new issues and challenges as both of these fields continue to evolve. In the future, the intersection of medicine and law related to electronic data, discoverability, and admissibility into evidence will continue to be intensely debated in settings such as pediatric critical care which represent the forefront of advances in medicine.

Acknowledgements The author would like to thank Caroline Hackstein and Lisa Ciesielczyk for their assistance in the preparation of this manuscript.

References

1. Sachdeva RC, D'Andrea LA. Emerging medicolegal issues in the practice of pediatric sleep medicine. Child Adolesc Psychiatr Clin N Am. 2009;18:1017–25.
2. Hall v. Hilbun, 466 So.2d 856 (Sup. Ct. Miss., 1985).
3. Frye v. United States. 293 F. 1013 (D.C. Cir 1923).
4. Daubert v. Merrell Dow Pharmaceuticals, 509 U.S. 579. 1993.
5. Kumho Tire Co. v. Carmichael, 526 U.S. 137. 1999.
6. The False Claims Act (FCA). 31 U.S.C. §§ 3729–3733.
7. United States ex rel. Aranda v. Cmty. Psychiatric Ctrs. of Oklahoma, 945 F. Supp. 1485 (W.D. Okla. 1996).
8. Johnson v. Kokemoor, 199 Wis. 2d 615,545 N.W.2d 495. 1996.
9. Sachdeva RC. Electronic healthcare data collection and pay-for-performance: translating theory into practice. Ann Health Law. 2007;16:291–311.
10. Pollack MM, Ruttimann UE, Getson PR. The pediatric risk of mortality (PRISM) score. Crit Care Med. 1988;16:1110–6.
11. Slater A, Shann F, ANZICS Paediatric Study Group. The suitability of the Pediatric Index of Mortality (PIM), PIM2, the Pediatric Risk of Mortality (PRISM), and PRISM III for monitoring the quality of pediatric intensive care in Australia and New Zealand. Pediatr Crit Care Med. 2004;5:447–54.
12. Sachdeva RC, Blinka DD. Improving the odds of success: quantitative methodology in law practice. Wis Lawyer. 2005;78:12.

Charles D. Cadenhead

Abstract

The purpose of this chapter is to develop an awareness of important elements in hospital critical care architectural design. Intended for the non-designer, focus will be on functional programmatic elements, fundamental planning concepts, physical ICU organization and future trends. The sources and references provided will lead the interested reader to extensive materials which will broaden the knowledge of both design practice and evidence-based design research.

Keywords

ICU Design • Critical Care Unit Design • ICU Design Competition • Best Practice Units • ICU Planning

Introduction

The purpose of this chapter is to develop an awareness of important elements in hospital critical care architectural design. Intended for the non-designer, the focus will be on functional programmatic elements, fundamental planning concepts, physical ICU organization and future trends. Engineering material is not discussed (mechanical, electrical and structural), although its importance should not be underestimated. The sources and references provided will lead the interested reader to extensive materials which will broaden the knowledge of both design practice and evidence-based design research.

A Little History and Statistics

For most readers intensive care units (ICU) have always existed, in the same way we of today feel that hospitals have always existed. However, it is generally accepted that the first designated ICUs were opened in Copenhagen, Denmark,

in 1953, and at Dartmouth-Hitchcock Medical Center, New Hampshire, in 1955 [1]. The first North American children's hospital was the Children's Hospital of Philadelphia (CHOP), which opened in 1855. CHOP also opened the first pediatric ICU (PICU) in the United States [2]. Without doubt, intensive care was provided to patients prior to these dates, but more likely in general wards and former recovery rooms, rather than areas and spaces specifically designed for the purpose. As of 2009, there were 5,795 licensed hospitals in the US, each with at least one critical care unit [3]. In 2007 there were 67,357 adult ICU beds and 4,044 PICU beds within 337 PICUs. To round out critical care in the US, in addition to the above, there were approximately 1,500 Neonatal ICUs, with a total of about 20,000 beds [4, 5]. In 2005, the national financial resources to support critical care medicine was approximately $81.7B, representing 13.4 % of hospital costs and 4.1 % of national health expenditures [5].

Advances in Health Design and Sources for Inspiration

The rapid improvement in healthcare design over the past four decades is truly exciting. Although not universal, the uninspired hospital designs of pre and post-WW ll are being

C.D. Cadenhead, FAIA, FACHA, FCCM
WHR Architects,
1111 Louisiana St., Floor. 26, Houston, TX 77002, USA
e-mail: ccadenhead@whrarchitects.com

D.S. Wheeler et al. (eds.), *Pediatric Critical Care Medicine*,
DOI 10.1007/978-1-4471-6362-6_3, © Springer-Verlag London 2014

Fig. 3.1 1992 ICU design
competition winner. Swedish
Medical Center. Englewood,
Colorado (Courtesy of WHR
Architects)

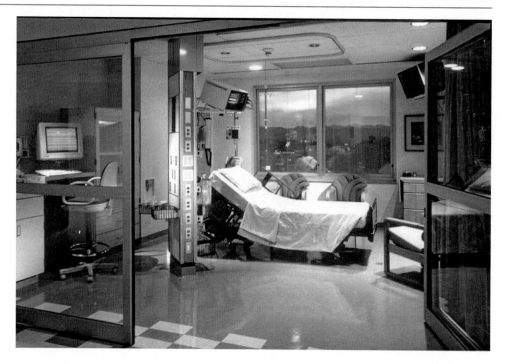

Fig. 3.2 2009 ICU design
competition winner. Memorial
Sloan-Kettering Cancer Center
New York City, New York
(Courtesy of MSKCC and Neil
Halpern, M.D., ICU Medical
Director)

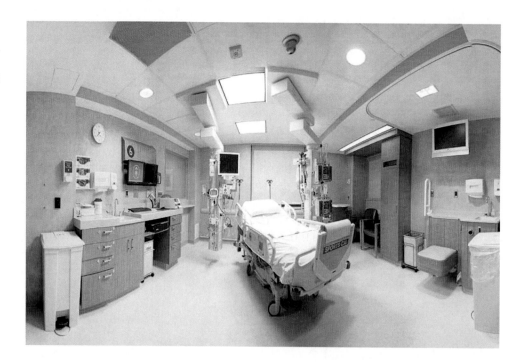

replaced by the much improved health centers of today. This chapter includes information and resources from the author's 2009 study of award winning ICU designs, beginning with a competition in 1992, and ending with the 2009 design competition winner [6, 7] (Figs. 3.1 and 3.2). Design Competition winners from 2010 to 2013 have also been reviewed by the author and, when useful, these ICU projects have been used to describe certain design features. These award-winning units have been designated as best-practice units by physicians,

nurses, other multidisciplinary ICU team members, and architects that were, or are, members of the Society of Critical Care Medicine (SCCM), the American Association of Critical Care Nurses (AACN) and the American Institute of Architects/Academy of Architecture for Health (AIA/AAH). In addition, design research by medical and architectural practitioners is discussed, and practical information related to the design process is included. Graphic illustrations are incorporated – they are truly "worth a thousand words."

Case Studies, Comparisons and Practice

An interesting way to develop ICU design knowledge is to study exemplary units. The objective of the SCCM study is twofold: (1) to discover themes that correlate with therapeutic and supportive environments, and (2) to use the rich information available from the annual SCCM design competition to identify contributions to evidence-based design data. This analysis describes program, architectural planning and trends in highly respected ICU designs.

All types of critical care units are eligible for entry into the design competition, including pediatric, neonatal, adult care units and those of various medical subspecialties. All SCCM design competition entries are accompanied by a set of forms completed by each submitting ICU. This information provides background data for those judging the entries and also includes a small scale floor plan of the unit. In addition, each ICU provides a video walk-through with a voice-over description of the unit illustrating the attributes the staff feels are especially important. This entry information was established for the first competition in 1992 and has been continually received from the submittals since.

From 1992 until 2009, the competition received only North American entries. As such, most submittals have followed the *Guidelines for Design and Construction of Healthcare Facilities*, published by the Facility Guidelines Institute and the AIA/AAH [8]. Since 2010, several entries have been international submissions, providing interesting comparisons among ICU designs worldwide. The design competition study included 12 adult ICUs built between 1990 and 2007 (Fig. 3.3).

Each of the winning units in the selected sample underwent a room-by-room and area-by-area analysis of floor plans to document the detailed functional program, net square footage/meters (NSF/NSM) of each room, departmental gross square footage/meters (DGSF/DGSM) and building gross square footage/meters (BGSF/BGSM) of each unit. Protocol for the area take-offs was based on the 2008 "Analysis of Departmental Area in Contemporary Hospitals: Calculation Methodologies & Design Factors in Major Patient Care Departments", ensuring a consistent and pre-validated method of area analysis [9]. Additional design characteristics unique to each ICU were obtained by floor plan review and from the submittal materials and video and documented in a spreadsheet format. The author has also had the opportunity to visit five of the 12 winning designs, providing interesting "lessons learned" that are not so obvious from the entry information and present the opportunity to

	Winning Year	SCCM ICU Competition Winners & Project Location	Institution Type & ICU Type	Construction Type & Architects	Hospital Beds	ICU Beds
1	1992	The Swedish Medical Center Englewood, Colorado	Community Hospital CCU/Multidisciplinary	New Construction WHR & H+L Architects	310	32
2	1993	East Jefferson General Hospital Metairie, Louisiana	Community Hospital Medical/Surgical	New Construction Blitch Knevel Architects	473	20
3	1996	Legacy Good Samaritan Hospital Portland, Oregon	Tertiary Care Center Multidisciplinary	Mixed (New & Renovation) Tom Sagerser Architect	550	28
4	1997	Southeast Missouri Hospital Cape Girardeau, Missouri	Community Hospital Cardiothoracic Surgery	New Construction Christner Partnership	281	12
5	2000	Clarian Health Group Methodist Hospital Indianapolis, Indiana	Academic Medical Center CCU/Cardio Medical	New Construction BSA LifeStructures	834	56
6	2001	St. Joseph's Health Center Kansas City, Missouri	Community Hospital Med/Surg/Cardiovascular	New Construction Hart Freeland Roberts, Inc.	300	16
7	2003	Harris Methodist Fort Worth Hospital Fort Worth, Texas	Community Hospital Adolescent/Adult	New Construction The Stichler Group, Inc.	601	20
8	2003	McGill University Health Center Montreal, Quebec, Canada	Tertiary Care & Teaching Surg/Med/Cardio/Trauma	Renovation Construction Fichten Soiferman Architects	550	26
9	2005	The Queen's Medical Center Honolulu, Hawaii	Tertiary, Level II Trauma Cardiac & Thoracic	New Construction Anbe, Aruga, Ishizu Architects	505	40
10	2006	Sharp Grossmont Hospital La Mesa, California	Acute Care Hospital Adult Medical/Surgical	Renovation Construction The Design Partnership	450	24
11	2008	Emory University Hospital Atlanta, Georgia	Academic Medical Center Neurology & Neurosurgical	Mixed (New & Renovation) HKS Architects	597	20
12	2009	Memorial Sloan-Kettering Cancer Center New York City, New York	Tertiary Center & Teaching Adult Medical/Surgical	Renovation Construction daSILVA Archtiects	435	20

Fig. 3.3 SCCM ICU design competition winning entries included in sample size

see units several years after opening and observe how they have fared. The design competition entry data, information collected through post-occupancy tours and architectural plan analysis, have yielded interesting comparisons of past SCCM ICU winning designs. The findings compare and contrast planning approach and concept, space program components and areas, social organization of the unit, architectural layout, configurations and circulation patterns.

Construction Types

Most of the design competition units, 7 of the 12, were new construction. Three were renovation and two were mixed (new construction and renovation). It is rare for an ICU project to be built in isolation and existing conditions, new or old, are always a major challenge in ICU design. These conditions could be square footage availability, the site geometry required to work around other hospital functions, and the structural pattern of columns or location of large mechanical or electrical equipment. Balancing these physical conditions with medical programmatic goals, and the administrators' budgetary demands, calls for creativity and flexibility on everyone's part. What is true is that some of the best ICUs have come from projects with the greatest limitations – new, renovation, on a rooftop or within an old building.

Functional Types

A typology of adult ICUs often includes the following medical specialties: medical ICU, surgical ICU, neurological ICU, coronary care unit (CCU), respiratory ICU, burn ICU, and mixed service ICU. In the design competition, 6 of the 12 units provide mixed critical care services. The remaining units provide specialized services. It is unusual for hospitals of a moderate size, say up to 300 beds, to have more than one ICU. The operational expense and difficulty of staffing lead to larger, single ICUs with multiple medical specialties to be provided. In designing these types of multipurpose units, there is always great debate about providing the best care environment for the various needs of patients. The neurological patients may benefit by ceiling-hung, pendent boom systems, whereas other patients may not require this expensive system for medical utilities. Flexibility in admitting patterns comes into play, and standardization is always important for supporting nursing care.

Layout Types

Rashid [10] presents an analysis of the physical design characteristics of a set of ICUs which include a number of the SCCM best-practice examples [10]. His research indicates

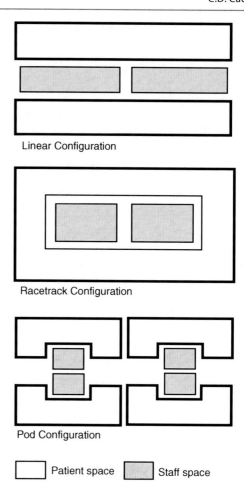

Fig. 3.4 Layout typologies of hospital units (Courtesy of WHR Architects)

that, "*the layout of an ICU is arguably the most important design feature affecting all aspects of intensive care services including patient privacy, comfort and safety, staff working condition, and family integration*" (p.285). In general terms, no single ICU geometry has been found to be clearly superior over another. A wide-ranging consensus appears to be that patient room size and unit comprehensive scale and program more effectively impact healing. Layout generally determines the location, configuration and relationship between different spaces within a unit, and possible sharing of space and functions (Fig. 3.4).

While no single plan configuration has been proven superior to others, unit layout significantly influences the important ability of the caregiver to see the patient. In all ICU designs, whether a centralized, decentralized or combination approach is taken, nurses remain vigilant about their ability to see and access patients. In an interesting 2010 research paper, *Relationship Between ICU Design and Mortality* [11], the conclusion was reached that, "severely ill patients may experience higher mortality rates when assigned to ICU rooms that are poorly visualized by nursing staff and physicians." The setting of this study was an older

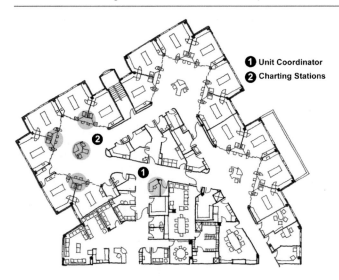

Fig. 3.5 St. Joseph's Health Center ICU, Kansas City, Missouri, 2001 winner. Pod design incorporating fully decentralized charting model (Courtesy of WHR Architects)

MICU in a large urban teaching hospital and the data of all patients admitted during 2008 was evaluated. This unit has a single nursing station and does not have decentralized documentation stations located near the beds. Not unusual in these older units, only a few patients can be clearly observed from the nurse station, some can be only partially seen, and others not at all.

In the SCCM design competition study, the largest number of units utilized the pod, or grouping, concept of decentralization, with varying bed numbers ranging from four to eight beds per pod. St. Joseph's Health Center ICU, Kansas City, Missouri, the 2001 SCCM design winner, utilizes a fully decentralized charting model, with two groups of six beds and one group of four beds (Fig. 3.5). One of the units demonstrates a more linear configuration, while three present pure racetrack configurations. "Racetrack" implies service in the center and patient beds on the perimeter with a loop corridor space connecting all the elements in between. The pod arrangement, for beds and support spaces, appears to be a frequently employed concept among winning designs, likely for ease of patient monitoring and decreased walking distances by staff. However, few of the units are purely one layout, with several including characteristics of multiple layout types.

Unit Circulation

The designation of space for circulation has moved towards an "on-stage/off-stage" model in more recent years and certainly in the past three winning entries (interestingly, this theme is taken from the Disney-World design concept of separating public from service). It must be noted that incorporating multiple circulation routes adds to the overall departmental square footage area of an ICU, thus increasing costs associated with construction of units. However, cost and space allowing, this notion of separate paths of movement and circulation will likely continue to be a tendency seen in future critical care designs. In our practice, we have found this design approach to be a beneficial circulation strategy for both patient and family and support staff.

The new Ann & Robert H. Lurie Children's Hospital of Chicago, 2013 winner of the SCCM ICU design competition, does a remarkable job of clearly separating patient and family circulation from staff and materials circulation on a complex floor (Fig. 3.6). In this vertical and very urban hospital solution, no fewer than three elevator cores support the 40-bed PICU floor. Floor plan review implies that staff and physicians can circulate the entire floor without unnecessarily crossing paths with families. The circulation path even preserves exterior views for some staff support spaces.

Departmental Areas

Departmental gross square feet (DGSF) area per bed, all the usable space, excluding that which cannot be used to directly support the ICU, shows a clear increase in the past 5 years. A number of the design competition study units, and continuing with the most recent three winners (2011–2013), are approximately 1,100 DGSF/Bed (102 DGSM/Bed), or larger. The 2011 36-bed Dutch winning unit, University Medical Center Utrecht, is approximately 1,380 DGSF per bed, the largest of any unit in the 21-year history of the competition (Fig. 3.7). This ICU project was a roof-top vertical expansion with a very comprehensive program, both of which may have contributed to size.

Overall, best-practice ICUs have a wide range of gross departmental area per bed, varying between 654 DGSF (60 sq m) and 1,380 DGSF (100 sq m). In addition, the average departmental areas consistently differ depending on construction type. Significant reasons for this size variation appear to relate to whether:
- All ICU administrative, educational, and/or research offices are included within the ICU
- Any diagnostic and/or therapeutic services have been included, e.g., pharmacy, imaging
- Dedicated spaces for families are included, e.g., sleep areas, consultation rooms, lockers
- On-stage/off-stage circulation has been included

Patient Room Design and Bed Number

The patient room is the most fundamental working module of a critical care unit. Our study of intensive care environments dates back almost two decades and 20 years ago the trend to private patient rooms appeared to be rapidly

Fig. 3.6 Ann & Robert H.
Lurie Children's Hospital of
Chicago, Chicago, Illinois,
2013 winner (Courtesy of
WHR Architects)

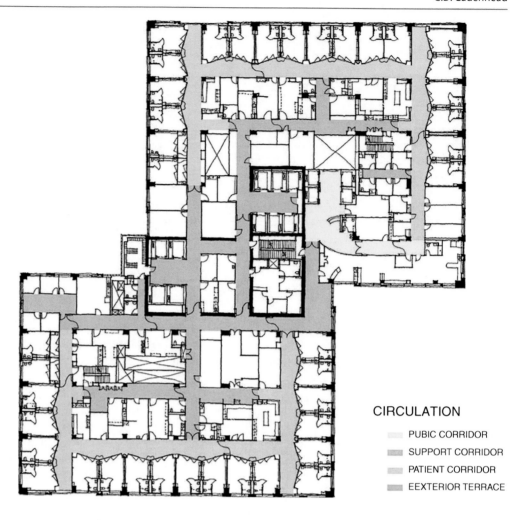

CIRCULATION

▨ PUBIC CORRIDOR
▨ SUPPORT CORRIDOR
▨ PATIENT CORRIDOR
▨ EEXTERIOR TERRACE

becoming the norm. This is further supported by the fact that no double occupancy rooms were noted in any of the adult units surveyed. Pediatric ICUs continue to include some double-occupancy rooms, citing the need for sibling utilization. Starting in 2010, largely for infection control reasons, the FGI Guidelines [3] no longer allow semi-private patient rooms in new construction. These same Guidelines, used by most States for healthcare facilities, require that all patient rooms, acute and ICU, include an exterior window for natural light and views to the outside, and a dedicated waste disposal system connected to each patient room (a toilet or soiled hopper sink).

Our SCCM study finds unit size, as measured by bed number, of adult ICUs varying between 12 and 40 patient beds, with the average number being 24, and the number of beds occurring most frequently being 20. This is higher than the 8 to 12 bed target recommended by the SCCM 2012 *Guidelines for Intensive Care Unit Design* [12]. It should be noted that in the larger units, beds are typically grouped into smaller numbers generally reflecting the eight to 12 bed target.

A comparison of net square footage areas of patient rooms shows a range of values, with the largest rooms in units from years 2000 (Clarion Health Group Methodist Hospital, 353 SF) (Fig. 3.8) and 2008 (Emory University, 352 SF) (Fig. 3.9). In both these submittals, while not universally adopted among units, significant family space has been included in or adjacent to the patient room. The Emory University patient room includes a family space of 115 SF (10.5 SM). In the majority of units, the average size of a patient room has remained at approximately 250 sq ft (SF) (23 sq m) over the last 17 years.

Space Allocation by Category

Although patient room sizes appear relatively consistent, total departmental areas per bed have steadily increased in recent years. A look at the amount of departmental gross SF for patient rooms in each unit demonstrates an average of almost 50 % (Fig. 3.10). The remaining space serves as support for the unit. Therefore, various support areas and

Fig. 3.7 University Medical Center, Utrecht, Netherlands, 2011 winner (Courtesy of WHR Architects)

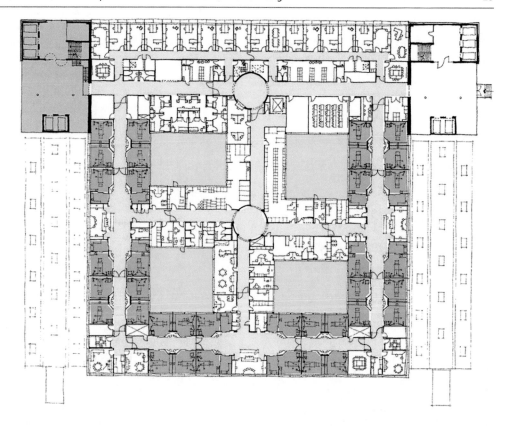

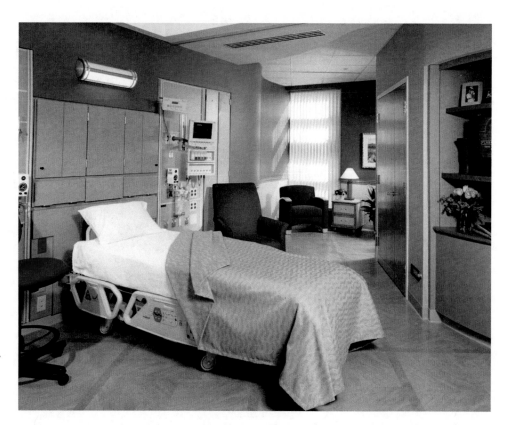

Fig. 3.8 Clarian Health Group Methodist Hospital Cardiac ICU, Indianapolis, Indiana, 2000 winner. Acuity adaptable room and headwall (Courtesy of BSA LifeStructures)

service spaces are an important, and growing, determinant of ICU gross area requirements. Recent years have also seen an increase in administrative, education and support located within units, particularly in academic teaching centers (Fig. 3.11).

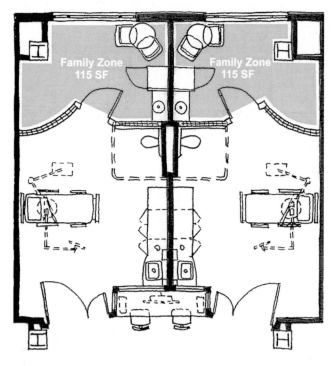

Fig. 3.9 Emory University Hospital Neurosciences ICU, Atlanta, Georgia, 2008 winner. Family zone within the patient room (Courtesy of WHR Architects)

Discussion and Exemplary Designs

The following discussion highlights examples of best-practice ICU designs in conjunction with the categories used in the area take-off analysis of the units. Figure 3.10 provides an overview of program components included in each category. Although not included in the area take-off analysis, outdoor space is included in the following section, given the growing importance of outdoor space to the well-being of patients, family and staff.

Patient Care

Patient Toilet Facilities and Waste Disposal
All of the units studied include both a modular sink and toilet within the patient room, or a toilet room directly accessible from the patient bed. Two units were found to have private enclosed toilet rooms, now required, adjoining the patient room, while three others employ a combination of private and shared toilet rooms. The remaining units employed waste disposal systems adjacent to the bed. No award winning facility built or renovated after 1998 has shared toilet rooms. The 2000 winning unit, with a full bath/toilet, was designed as an acuity-adaptable unit serving patients through the continuum of their stay (Fig. 3.8).

Patient Bed Location and Medical Utilities
Within the critical care environment, it is crucial to maintain access to the patient, making the bed placement and delivery of medical support important design considerations.

Fig. 3.10 Program categories used during area take-off analysis of best-practice ICU designs & percentages of total department area

ICU Program Components & Percentage of Departmental Area

		Percentage Range	Variance	Average
1	**Patient Care** Includes the patient room and patient toilet room	38.6 - 68.1%	29.5%	48.0%
2	**Staff & Material Support** Includes centralized & decent charting, clean & soiled, etc.	15.1 - 32.0%	16.9%	23.0%
3	**Staff Facilities** Includes staff lounge, lockers, toilets, on-call rooms, etc.	3.0 - 9.1%	6.1%	6.0%
4	**Diagnostic & Therapeutic** Includes imaging suites, dialysis, pharmacy, lab, etc.	0.0% - 8.1%	8.1%	2.0%
5	**Administration & Education** Includes classrooms, conference spaces, offices, etc.	2.8 - 24.2%	21.4%	9.0%
6	**Public & Family** Includes waiting areas, family sleep rooms, amenities, etc.	5.7 - 25.2%	19.5%	12.0%

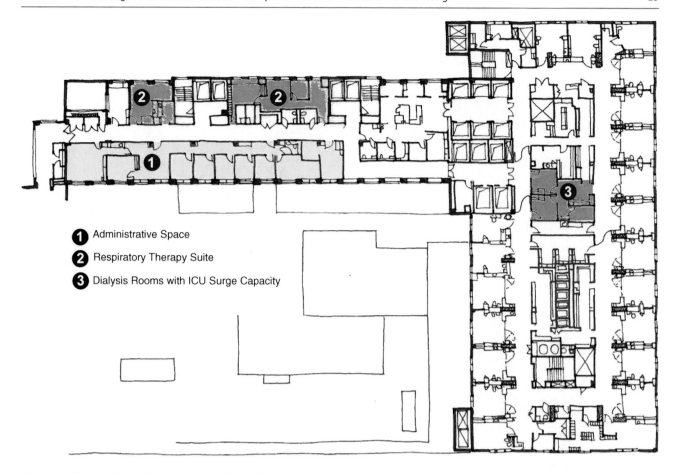

Fig. 3.11 Memorial Sloan-Kettering Cancer Center ICU, New York City, New York, 2009 winner. Administrative and support spaces within the unit (Courtesy of WHR Architects)

1 Administrative Space

2 Respiratory Therapy Suite

3 Dialysis Rooms with ICU Surge Capacity

Traditionally, medical devices have been located on a vertical surface at the head of the patient bed, the "headwall." More recently the trend has been to use an articulating ceiling-mounted arm(s) with all monitoring, outlets and gases included, known as a "boom" (Fig. 3.12). Four of the winning units have headwalls. One unit, the 1992 winner, used a single fixed power column. Ceiling mounted booms were used in the majority of units; three ICUs employed a single arm boom, while four others employed dual arm booms. The dual arm booms have added enormous flexibility by freeing the bed from the wall, and integrating technology to deliver critical utilities and monitoring. Current research demonstrates that booms have an advantage over headwalls in the case of high-acuity ICU patients, and when procedures are performed at the bedside. Booms may not provide a proportionate level of advantage, when compared with the additional cost involved in their procurement, in the case of lower-acuity ICU patients, as well as when procedures are not typically conducted in the patient room [13].

Patient Room and Technology

The most current competition winner in the study, Memorial Sloan-Kettering Cancer Center ICU, from 2009, is a good

example of a technologically advanced ICU. The included composite and annotated photograph captures the many features of this unit and patient room, including E-glass (a type of glass that when electrically charged becomes opaque) sliding doors and vision panels between rooms, in-room barcode reader and label printer, wireless IR transmitter and webcam, secure nurse server, and other features (Fig. 3.13).

Staff and Material Support

Degree of Nursing Centralization

In older units, it is common to see a central nurse station as the primary gathering and work space within the staff work area. Generally, this nurse station was located in the middle of the ICU. More recently, this centralized work and charting area, now referred to as a multidisciplinary team station [12], has often been augmented or replaced with decentralized stations. Interestingly, all ICUs surveyed had some form of decentralized charting space with none employing exclusively centralized nursing support. The 1992 Swedish Medical Center ICU allocates space for four

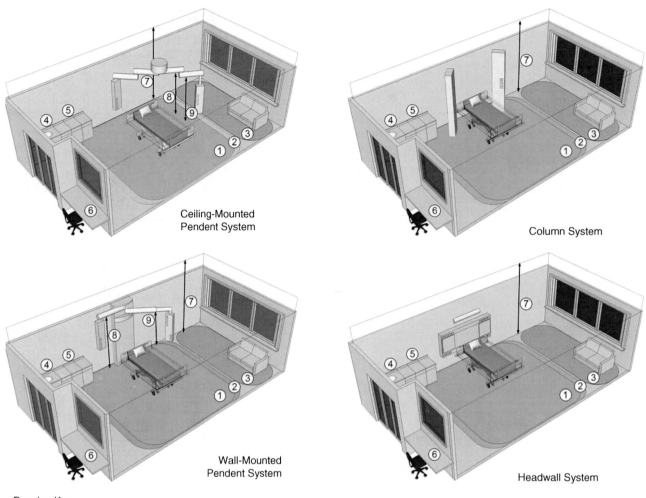

Drawing Key

1 Patient Zone: 15.4'×15.5' (W×D)
2 Bariatric Patient Zone: 15.5'×17' (W×D)
3 Family Zone
4 Hygiene Zone
5 Clinical Zone

6 Nurse Charting Station
7 Ceiling Height: 9' to 11'
8 Clearance: 8' to 10'
9 Clearance: 7' to 9'

Fig. 3.12 ICU patient support options (Courtesy of WHR Architects)

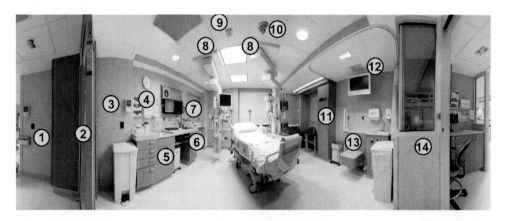

Fig. 3.13 Memorial Sloan-Kettering Cancer Center (MSKCC) ICU, New York City, New York, 2009 winner. Incorporation of advanced technology for patient care and monitoring purposes (Courtesy of MSKCC & Neil Halpern, M.D., ICU Medical Director). Features of new ICU patient rooms help improve efficiency: *1* nurse server provides supplies to ICU room and opens from outside & inside with secure ID card access reader, *2* E-glass slide and break away doors, *3* inside opening of nurse server, *4* wireless clock, *5* storage cabinets, *6* computer with double monitor, *7* barcode reader and lab label printer, *8* twin mobile articulating arms (BOOMS), *9* wireless IR transmitter, *10* web cam, *11* patient closet and DVD player, *12* flat screen TV on articulating arm, *13* toilet, *14* nursing work area with computer, sink, phone, and storage

Fig. 3.14 Swedish Medical
Center ICU, Englewood,
Colorado, 1992 winner. Proximity
of ICU to cardiac catheterization
suite (Courtesy of WHR
Architects)

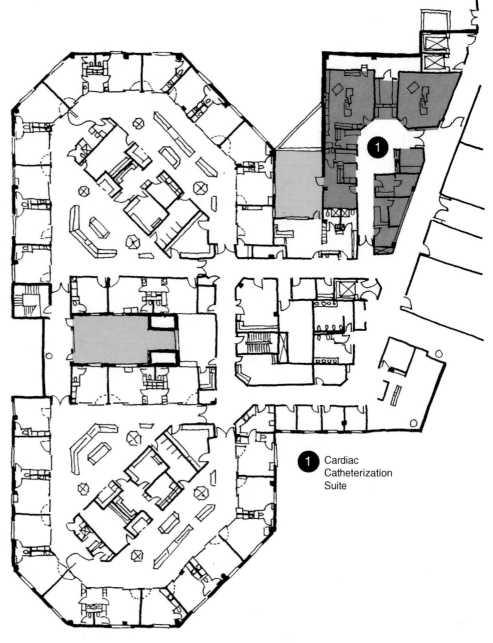

1   Cardiac
    Catheterization
    Suite

central stations, each serving an eight bed pod, and incorporating computer charting terminals inside each patient room (Fig. 3.14). St. Joseph's Health Center is unique to the group as a completely decentralized unit, stating in the submission narrative the main reason for this design shift being noise control (Fig. 3.5). Although nursing support areas do not appear to have grown in overall area during the last two decades, the notion of decentralization is seen throughout by way of charting stations within patient rooms or within corridors looking into single or pairs of patient rooms. This study demonstrates that the configuration of staff work spaces has not yet been resolved in the best-practice adult ICUs. It remains to be seen whether pure decentralization will be utilized in future designs or whether a hybrid model will continue, perhaps indicating the value of communication, training and socialization between caregivers.

Staff Facilities

Staff Access to Nature

There appears to be an increased emphasis on stress-relieving respite spaces for staff incorporating a connection to nature. The Queen's Medical Center in Honolulu, Hawaii, located a central staff lounge for views to the ocean and maintained three lanais, or outdoor patios, for both staff and family access and benefit. The 2006 winner, Sharp Grossmont

Fig. 3.15 Sharp Grossmont
Hospital ICU, La Mesa,
California, 2006 winner. Centrally
located exterior courtyard:
1,500 sq ft (approx. 140 sq m)
(Courtesy of WHR Architects)

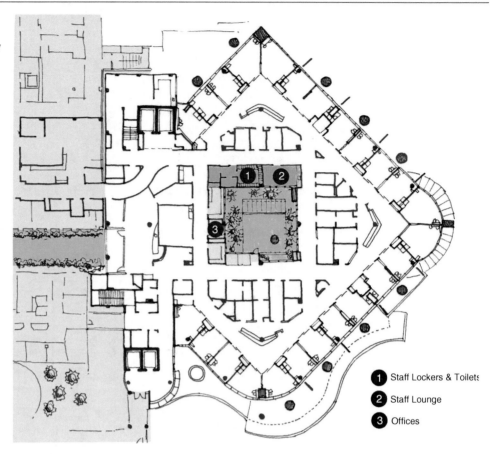

1 Staff Lockers & Toilets

2 Staff Lounge

3 Offices

Hospital ICU, has a 1,500 SF (140 SM) exterior courtyard in the center of the critical care unit. The courtyard also contains a skylight feature which allows for daylight access to the emergency department located directly below this space (Fig. 3.15). Along with dedicated staff lounge spaces seen in all units, five of the 12 ICUs provide an exterior courtyard or terrace for staff access. On call suites with sleep rooms and shower facilities located on the unit itself are seen in the majority (eight) of the ICUs surveyed, with several locating the overnight facilities just outside the unit for easy access.

Diagnostic and Therapeutic

Proximity to Diagnostic and Treatment Support

An interesting trend noted across all units is the proximity to diagnostic and treatment support spaces, located either within the actual ICU, close to the unit on the same level, or connected vertically to a location directly above or below the unit by elevator. The 1992 Swedish Medical Center ICU is located next to the cardiac catheterization suite and was placed strategically within the hospital to allow lateral access to the emergency room, operating room, recovery room, radiology, and laboratory (Fig. 3.14). At the Memorial Sloan-Kettering Cancer Center, the hospital's hemodialysis suite is incorporated within the ICU providing round-the-clock access to

renal technicians while providing two dialysis rooms for ICU surge capacity. The respiratory therapy suite is also located on the floor, serving both the ICU and the overall hospital, and the MRI suite is horizontally accessible (Fig. 3.11). An integral part of Emory University Hospital's Neurosciences ICU design was the location of a CT scanner within the unit itself, allowing critically ill patients to conveniently undergo scanning without the need for transport to the radiology department (Fig. 3.16). This trend of proximity to diagnostic and treatment facilities appears in numerous units in different forms. Interestingly, although this decision of placing the diagnostic facilities within the ICU itself can sometimes mean fewer patient rooms, proximity to D&T services has been chosen over patient rooms in several instances, indicating the importance of these spaces in the view of care providers.

Administration and Education

Proximity to Administration and Education Spaces

Space allocation for administrative and educational areas within units appears to be on an upward trend, most notably in academic medical centers where teaching and research is an integral part of daily ICU activities. All units surveyed contain some amount of offices on the unit, while others

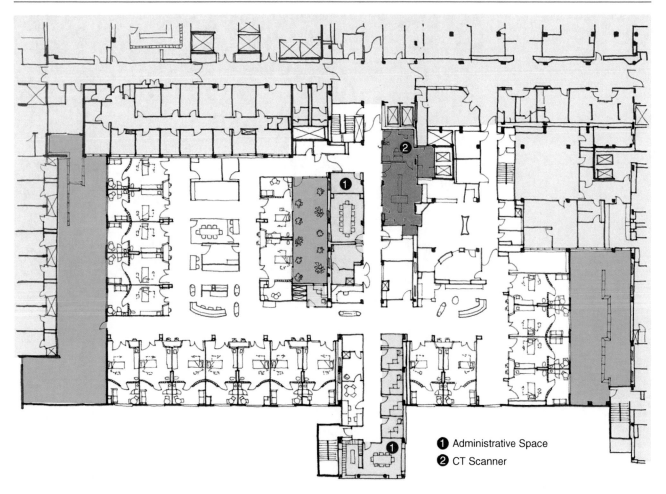

Fig. 3.16 Emory University Hospital Neurosciences ICU, Atlanta, Georgia, 2008 winner. Administrative and support spaces within the unit (Courtesy of WHR Architects)

include all departmental offices, conference and seminar rooms within the ICU itself. This tendency is illustrated by the two most recent winning entries where a significant amount of unit area is given towards administrative and teaching functions. In the case of Emory University Hospital, 9 % of the departmental gross area is dedicated space for this programmatic function, while at Memorial Sloan-Kettering Cancer Center's ICU, this number has increased to 14 %. Furthermore, there appears to be a preference for staff meeting and education spaces located on the unit itself, if this is at all feasible. At Memorial Sloan-Kettering this was determined to be important enough that a research lab was relocated to allow the administrative suite to be located adjacent to the bed unit. Conference and rounding rooms, incorporating advanced technology allowing for remote patient care planning, are being seen in recent years, specifically in the 2009 winner Memorial Sloan-Kettering Cancer Center. It is likely we will observe a continuing trend of administrative and education space incorporated into the designs of critical care environments, especially teaching facilities, given the importance placed on proximity and flexibility of these spaces with patient care areas (Figs. 3.11 and 3.16).

Public and Family

Family Space

Jastremski and Harvey [14] suggest that an ideal patient room should incorporate three zones: a patient zone, a family zone and a caregiver zone [14]. Several of the winning designs have completely re-evaluated the patient room to incorporate designated family space, including families as an integral part of the healing process. Perhaps the most distinctive in this category is the 2008 winner, Emory University Hospital's Neurosciences ICU. This unit is unique in its allocation of 115 SF (10.5 m²) of space for a family room incorporated within the patient room, separated by a glass block partition, allowing natural light to penetrate through the family room into the patient zone. This "adjacent studio apartment" acts as a private place for respite and communication (Fig. 3.17). The patient room size, including this family space, is over 350 SF. Interestingly, 18 % of the unit's departmental gross area is dedicated to family space in this ICU, including each family zone within the patient rooms, waiting areas, lounge and amenities such as a kitchen, showers, and laundry facilities.

Fig. 3.17 Emory University Hospital Neurosciences ICU, Atlanta, Georgia, 2008 winner. View of the patient room with family zone (Courtesy of Owen Samuels, M.D., ICU Medical Director)

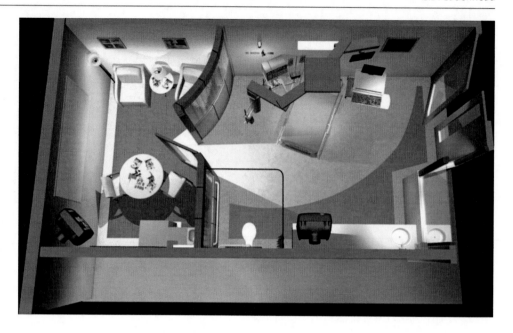

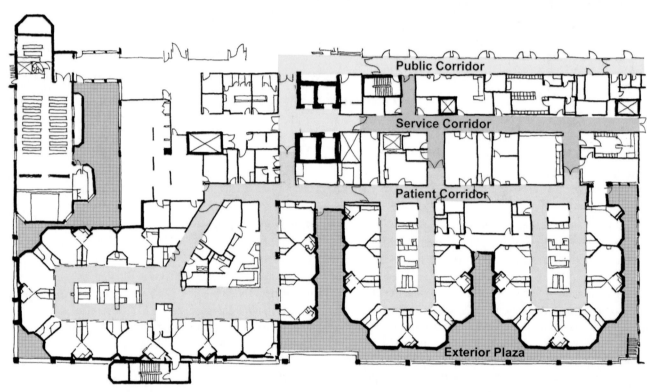

Fig. 3.18 Legacy Good Samaritan Multidisciplinary ICU, Portland, Oregon, 1996 winner. Unique geometry allowing increased unit perimeter and plaza access; on-stage/off-stage circulation (Courtesy of WHR Architects)

Outdoor Space

Green Space

With a number of studies showing the benefits of access to nature and its healing properties, it is becoming more common to see natural elements in the intensive care environment [15]. Legacy Good Samaritan Hospital is perhaps the most extreme example of this by the provision of an extensive external plaza surrounding the unit for use by all users, including staff, patients and families. This unit design is all the more impressive in that it was a vertical rooftop expansion above a garage. The design intent was to provide patients who may be clinically stable access the outdoors directly from their rooms onto the outdoor plaza (Fig. 3.18).

Best-Practice Critical Care Design Trends

1 Larger Units

More and larger units will likely be needed in the future as need grows. Area for support spaces will likely increase, given the trend observed among best-practice units.

2 The Patient Room

All-private rooms in critical care have become the design standard with a stable room size of about 250 SF (23 SM); family space will likely be in addition to this.

3 The Family Zone

Recent units, where possible, incorporate designated family and visitor space and amenities into the unit or within the patient room itself.

4 Technology & Life Support Systems

The majority of units, notably recent ones, employed ceiling mounted booms rather than the traditional headwall unit within the patient room design.

5 Design for Interdisciplinary Teams

All units showed some combination of centralized & decentralized layouts for staff work stations, while only two designs were fully decentralized.

6 Proximity to Diagnostic & Treatment

Recent units appear to be incoporating diagnostic and treatment modalities into their designs, often as shared services with the entire hospital.

7 Administrative & Support Spaces

An increase in administrative and education space within the unit has been noted over the last several years, particularly within teaching hospitals.

8 Unit Geometry

No single ICU geometry has been noted as superior to another; the pod concept is seen in recent years, along with a combination of different configurations.

9 Unit Circulation

Distinction of circulation regarding on-stage and off-stage separations are becoming more common and will likley continue to be seen in future designs.

10 Access to Nature

The importance of nature for patients, families and staff is increasingly recognized and incorporated into critical care units where possible.

Fig. 3.19 Best-practice ICU design trends observed among winning units

Several units analyzed have incorporated light courts into the designs, allowing for an increase in exterior perimeter and therefore patient room numbers. The majority of units (seven) incorporate some form of outdoor spaces into the unit design.

Conclusion and Future Trends

Intensive care units rely on the most advanced care, technology and staff hospitals can provide. Strategies for improving the work environment and positively improving patient safety and outcomes are exemplified in many of these design winning ICUs and are important to the future world of critical care medicine. This overview has identified important physical design features of some of the best-practice example ICUs in the United States, Canada and Europe. Critically observing many ICU designs has led to a certain amount of future prognostication. Below is a collection of future trends (Fig. 3.19). Thus far, these trend statements have held their value.

Acknowledgements The author would like to recognize the invaluable contributions to this study by Diana Anderson, MD, MArch; Neil Halpern, MD, Medical Director, Memorial Sloan Kettering Cancer Center ICU; Owen Samuels, MD, Medical Director, Emory University Hospital ICU; Professor D. Kirk Hamilton, FAIA, Texas A&M University; WHR Architects and the WHR Tradewell Fellows, Houston, Texas; and Lyle R. Cadenhead, PhD.

References

1. Hilberman M. The evolution of intensive care units. Crit Care Med. 1975;3(4):159–65.
2. About us: our history. The Children's Hospital of Philadelphia. 2013. http://www.chop.edu/about/our-history/. Accessed 5 Aug 2013.
3. Health Forum LLC. American Hospital Association Hospital Statistics, 2011 (2009 survey data). Chicago: American Hospital Association; 2011.
4. Carr BG, Addyson DK, Kahn JM. Variation in critical care beds per capita in the United States: implications for pandemic and disaster planning. JAMA. 2010;303:1371–2.
5. Halpern NA, Pastores SM. Critical care medicine in the United States 2000–2005: an analysis of bed numbers, occupancy rates, payer mix and costs. Crit Care Med. 2010;38:65–71.
6. Cadenhead C, Anderson D. Critical care unit design, the winners and future trends: an investigative study. World Health Des J. 2009;2:72–7.
7. Society of Critical Care Medicine (SCCM), American Association of Critical Care Nurses (AACN), and American Institute of Architects (AIA): award winning ICU designs: how to build a better facility for patients and caregivers. Society of Critical Care Medicine; 2010.
8. The Facility Guidelines Institute: guidelines for design and construction of health care facilities. Chicago: The Facility Guidelines Institute; 2010.
9. Allison D, Hamilton DK. Analysis of department area in contemporary hospitals: calculation methodologies & design factors in major patient care departments. Funded in part by the American Institute of Architects' Academy of Architecture for Health Foundation; 2008.
10. Rashid M. A decade of adult intensive care unit design: a study of the physical design features of the best-practice examples. Crit Care Nurs Q. 2006;29(4):282–311.

11. Leaf DE, Homel P, Factor PH. Relationship between ICU design and mortality. Chest. 2010;137:1022–7.

12. Thompson D, Hamilton DK, Cadenhead C. Guidelines for intensive care unit design. Crit Care Med. 2012;40:1586–600.

13. Pati D, Evans J, Waggener L, et al. An exploratory examination of medical gas booms versus traditional headwalls in intensive care unit design. Crit Care Nurs Q. 2008;31:340–56.

14. Jastremski CA, Harvey M. Making changes to improve the intensive care unit experience for patients and their families. New Horiz. 1998;6:99–109.

15. Ulrich RS. View through a window may influence recovery from surgery. Science. 1984;224:420–1.

PICU Administration

4

Cortney B. Foster and David C. Stockwell

Abstract

In the past 50 years, the pediatric intensive care unit (PICU) has evolved into a multidisciplinary organization delivering care to critically ill children with diverse diagnoses and physiological support needs. The development of pediatric critical care medicine subspecialists as the primary care team functioning within the PICU has led to vast improvements in pediatric mortality. With the increasing complexity of the PICU, the role of administration in outlining unit structure and enhancing team development and multidisciplinary care is crucial to ensuring quality care, patient safety and the best achievable patient outcomes for critically ill children.

The care team, under the leadership of a medical director, includes pediatric intensivists, subspecialists, physician extenders, nurses, respiratory therapists, pharmacists, nutritionists and other ancillary staff. A cohesive team, with strong communication and coordination, can maximize the contributions of all members toward the common goal of excellent patient care. However, the PICU must additionally provide other patient and institutional services such as a family centered approach with parental involvement in bedside rounds and throughout their children's illness. The PICU plays a resource role within the hospital, and a close working relationship with other divisions is integral for maintaining smooth patient flow and continuity of care. Additionally the unit is a research and training site for new intensivists and other clinicians.

Keywords

PICU • Administration • Team • Quality improvement • Multidisciplinary

C.B. Foster, DO
Department of Pediatric Critical Care, University of Maryland School of Medicine, 110 S. Paca Street, Suite 820, Baltimore, MD 21201, USA
e-mail: cfoster@cnmc.org

D.C. Stockwell, MD, MBA (✉)
Department of Critical Care Medicine, Children's National, 111 Michigan Avenue NW, Suite M4800, Washington, DC 20010, USA
e-mail: dstockwell@childrensnational.org

Introduction

The pediatric intensive care unit (PICU) encompasses multiple disciplines which share the care of the critically ill and medically complex child. The field of pediatric critical care medicine has developed considerably over the past three decades, and the complexity of care and involvement of specialists continues to grow [1, 2]. Extensive research has focused on the role of the PICU and of the intensivist in the care of critically ill children, and has demonstrated substantial decreases in mortality [3]. With the increasing complexity of services and care provided in the PICU, the role of administration in outlining unit structure and enhancing team development and multidisciplinary care is crucial to ensuring quality care, patient safety and the best achievable patient outcomes for critically ill children.

D.S. Wheeler et al. (eds.), *Pediatric Critical Care Medicine*,
DOI 10.1007/978-1-4471-6362-6_4, © Springer-Verlag London 2014

Pediatric Intensive Care Unit Structure

Historical Perspective

The field of pediatric critical care medicine has evolved greatly over the past several decades due to advances in the knowledge of disease pathophysiology and technology available to treat patients suffering from disease. In 1985, the American Board of Pediatrics (ABP) recognized the subspecialty of pediatric critical care medicine and determined criteria for certification in the field, and in 1990 the Residency Review Committee of the Accreditation Council for Graduate Medical Education (ACGME) accomplished the accreditation of the first pediatric critical care training programs [1].

In the early 1990s very little was written about the composition and organization of the nascent pediatric intensive care unit. However, research was beginning to demonstrate consistent associations between aspects of the organization, structure of PICUs and patient outcomes [4]. A regional study in the Northwest United States demonstrated that care in tertiary centers with intensive care units dedicated to children was associated with a lower mortality rate, adjusted for severity of illness, than care in non-tertiary centers without PICUs [5].

Subsequent investigations into the many existing PICUs revealed a wide diversity of features. A national survey of 235 hospitals published in 1993 revealed that the largest proportion of intensive care units were comprised of four to six beds, while only 6 % had greater than 18 beds. Mortality rates differed significantly between the size-based groups, with an increase in mortality coinciding with increased bed capacity. A pediatric intensivist was available to 73.2 % of intensive care units and 79.6 % of units had a full time medical director [4].

Levels of Care

The concept of Level I and Level II pediatric intensive care units was developed and outlined by the American Academy of Pediatrics (AAP) Section on Critical Care and Committee on Hospital Care in 1993, and guidelines for specifications of each were updated in 2004. A Level I PICU provides multidisciplinary, definitive care to all ages of pediatric patients with a wide range of complex and evolving illnesses. It is differentiated from a Level II PICU primarily by organizational structure, staff and resource availability, pre-hospital care, quality improvement, and training and educational programs. In order to qualify as a Level I PICU, a unit must meet many specifications, including having a physician of postgraduate year 3 level or above in house 24 h per day, a pediatric intensivist available within 30 min or less, and a wide range of pediatric subspecialists available within 1 h or

less. In addition, in contrast to a Level II PICU, a Level I PICU must have an associated emergency department with two available resuscitation areas, access to fluoroscopy and MRI, capabilities of cardiopulmonary bypass, bronchoscopy, endoscopy, and availability of a second operating room within 45 min, 24 h per day [1].

In some institutions, an intermediate care unit exists for patients requiring a higher level than routine inpatient care, but not intensive care. Such patients may require more frequent vital sign monitoring or nursing assessments, but do not require invasive monitoring. Such a unit improves flexibility in patient triage, and allows patient care to be targeted more closely to patient needs based on the severity of illness [6].

Patient Population

The Society of Critical Care Medicine (SCCM) Pediatric Section Admission Criteria Task Force created guidelines for admission and discharge policies for the PICU from a consensus opinion of nurses, physicians and associated healthcare professionals. Admission criteria include any child with severe or life threatening single organ dysfunction or multisystem disease requiring complex interventions exceeding the maximal support able to be provided on the general hospital unit. Discharge criteria are met when the disease process is reversed or the unstable condition that required admission into the PICU has resolved and the child no longer requires intervention in excess of general hospital unit capabilities [7].

Subspecialty Care

Several subspecialties exist within the realm of pediatric critical care and over the last few decades have emerged as dedicated clinical entities [8]. One such field is pediatric cardiac intensive care, which focuses on critically ill adult, pediatric, and neonatal patients with congenital and acquired heart disease [9]. Other subspecialties within pediatric critical care include neurologic intensive care, surgical intensive care and trauma intensive care.

Team Structure

Medical Director

The pediatric intensive care unit medical director must maintain certification by the ABP in general pediatrics as well as certification in either pediatric critical care medicine, anesthesiology with specialized training in pediatric critical care or in pediatric surgery with additional qualifications in surgical critical care. According to guidelines formulated by the AAP and SCCM, if the medical director is not a pediatrician, a pediatric intensivist should be appointed as co-director. The medical director of the pediatric intensive care unit has many roles and responsibilities including participation in the creation, review and implementation of multidisciplinary PICU policies. In addition, the medical director should help coordinate staff education, maintain a database describing unit statistics and performance, participate in budget planning, supervise resuscitations, and foster communication with referring clinicians and subspecialists. In conjunction with the nursing director, he or she should also implement quality improvement measures, and encourage research participation [1].

Physician Team

Currently, intensive care physician staffing models are varied, and the model that provides the best care at the greatest value remains to be determined. However there are organizations advocating for standards. A consortium of healthcare purchasers entitled the Leapfrog Group, recommends that intensivists be present in the ICU during daytime hours 7 days per week and available to discuss cases at all other times. The Leapfrog Group recommendations are based on studies demonstrating improved mortality rates and the efficiency of bed utilization when a pediatric intensivist participates as a care team member [10]. A subsequent study reported that extending intensivist staffing to 24-h coverage was associated with further reduction in mortality [11]. However, only 30 % of hospitals reported compliance with the Leapfrog recommendation in 2011 [12].

Extending attending coverage to 24 h per day resulted in no difference in mortality, but did result in decreased length of stays and increased adherence to patient care protocols when evaluated in adult medical ICUs [13]. A recent prospective study conducted at a 24 bed adult ICU in the Midwest found that 24-h intensive care unit coverage by an intensivist decreased length of stay and cost estimates for critically ill patients admitted overnight when compared to resident and fellow coverage overnight with on-call intensivist coverage [12].

A Level I PICU allows care to be transferred from the attending physician to an in-house physician at the postgraduate year three training level in pediatrics or anesthesia, but an attending physician should always be available within 30 min for assistance. Care may also be transferred to physician extenders including physician assistants (PAs) or nurse practitioners (NPs). A 1994 U.S. based survey found the use of PAs or NPs in 17 % of 69 institutions with PICUs. A 5 year study of physician assistants in a six bed unit in

New York found the PA role to be one not only of patient care, but also of resident education and support of nursing, respiratory therapy, and ancillary staff [14]. These findings were consistent with a 2008 review of the impact of NPs and PAs in ICUs which found involvement in patient care, research, reinforcement of practice guidelines as well as parent and staff education. At that time over 115,000 NPs and 63,000 PAs were practicing in the U.S., with 68 % of acute care NPs in the ICU setting. These numbers are expected to grow. The Committee on Manpower for the Pulmonary and Critical Care Societies projects increasing gaps between the intensivist workforce and patient care needs. This shortfall is expected to be 35 % by 2030, with physician extenders likely to fill the growing gap. However, at the time of review, only two randomized controlled studies had assessed the use of physician extenders in the ICU, with limited data regarding quality of care, comparative outcomes and cost of care. More research is needed in this area in the coming years [15].

In addition to the pediatric intensivist, subspecialty support is integral to patient care in the PICU. Available physicians in a Level I unit include a pediatric cardiologist, pediatric anesthesiologist, pediatric neurologist, pediatric surgeon, pediatric neurosurgeon, pediatric radiologist, a psychiatrist or psychologist, an otolaryngologist, an orthopedic surgeon, and a cardiothoracic surgeon. In addition, it is ideal to have a craniofacial surgeon, an oral surgeon, a pediatric hematologist/oncologist, a pediatric pulmonologist, a pediatric endocrinologist, a pediatric gastroenterologist, and a pediatric allergist readily available for patient care [1].

Nursing Team

A nurse manager experienced in a PICU and preferably with a master's degree in pediatric nursing or nursing administration should be available for all Level I and Level II intensive care units. The nurse manager is responsible for guaranteeing that the PICU is appropriately staffed in numbers and in skill level, as well as monitoring equipment and supplies. The nurse manager works with the medical director to prepare budgets, establish and review policies and procedures, coordinate staff education, and assist with quality assurance and nursing research. In addition to a nurse manager, an advanced practice nurse (APN) should be available in all Level I units to provide clinical leadership to the nursing staff. The role of the APN may be filled by a nurse practitioner with a master's degree in nursing, certification as a national pediatric nurse practitioner and previous preceptorship in pediatric critical care or by a clinical nurse specialist with a master's degree in nursing, and pediatric critical care certification and expertise [1].

Nurses working in a Level I or Level II PICU should complete orientation with a clinical and didactic component prior to assuming patient care responsibilities. The orientation program and a continuing education program should be created and implemented by the department, and core competencies assessed on a regular basis. Educational needs and core competencies should be determined based on the patient population and needs of a given unit [1].

Respiratory Therapy

Respiratory therapy personnel should be specifically designated to the PICU and in house 24 h per day in a Level I ICU. Therapists should have specific training in pediatric intensive care and managing pediatric respiratory failure and equipment. The department should have a supervisor responsible for staffing, monitoring performance, and ensuring adequate training of members [1].

Ancillary Staff

A pharmacist should be assigned to a Level I ICU and be in house 24 h daily. Pharmacists should attend multidisciplinary patient rounds when possible, as it has been shown that pharmacist participation in rounds is associated with fewer adverse drug events due to prescribing errors [16]. In addition, nutritionists, case managers, social workers, child life specialists, physical therapists, occupational therapists, speech therapists, and clergy must be readily accessible. Biomedical specialists must be available within 1 h, 24 h daily in all Level I and Level II PICUs, and a unit secretary assigned to all Level I PICUs [1].

Multidisciplinary Approach

A multidisciplinary approach is required to maintain status as a Level 1 ICU and also is mandatory for optimal patient outcomes. The unit must be staffed with 24 h coverage by board certified intensivists or equivalents, and the unit director ideally should be an intensivist. Nursing staff should be led by a qualified nurse manager, and all nursing staff should be trained in critical care. Respiratory therapy, laboratory service and radiographic service must be available 24 h per day. Pharmacists should ideally participate on rounds and a full array of subspecialists must be able within 30 min to provide care to patients [1]. Implementation of a multidisciplinary model of care has been shown to decrease hospital and ICU lengths of stay as well as cost of care [17]. Similarly, a recent retrospective study conducted at large academic MICU involved a multi-component reorganization of an already Leapfrog Group-compliant unit. In addition to geographic relocation and 24-h intensivist staffing, changes

included focus on a multidisciplinary approach with addition of a clinical pharmacist to the patient care team and an increased number of respiratory therapists. Results indicated that the multi-component reorganization was associated with reductions in mortality and an increase in ventilator-free days [11].

Roles of the Leadership Team

Quality and Safety Assurance

Improvement of quality and safety of care in the PICU is critical. Benefits include improvement of patient outcomes and prevention of harm, reduction of cost of care and enhanced staff satisfaction [18]. The complexity of critical care patients increases both the potential frequency and consequences of errors and standardization of care models is more difficult in units caring for a diverse array of patient ages and pathology [2]. Other challenges in the ICU setting include the need for 24 h continuity of care, balancing the prevention of staff fatigue and burnout with minimizing data loss and patient risk during transfer of care [3]. The unit leadership must also balance patient safety with the educational needs of critical care fellows and other trainees, creating an environment that is safe both for the patient and the learner [19].

Assessment of care quality in the ICU is more complex compared to other parts of the hospital [20]. In the PICU, particular attention must be paid both to diagnostic and treatment errors, especially medication errors, as well as the risk of nosocomial infection and procedural complications [21].

As in other fields of medicine, safety systems from other industries, especially aviation, have served as a model for quality improvement and the avoidance of errors [3]. Quality improvement depends on both the identification of errors and development of system changes to prevent their recurrence [3, 21]. Monitoring should include patient complications, as well as adverse events and critical incidents which can reduce patient safety, even if they do not lead directly to complications. For this reason, systems of voluntary, anonymous, non-punitive incident reporting have become widely implemented. Analysis of the context of critical incidents may lead to the development of system changes in the ICU, the hospital, or beyond. Though they must be adapted to local circumstances, interventional studies demonstrate both error reduction and improved patient outcomes in response to new standards and guidelines [3].

Voluntary reporting is the mainstay of adverse event reporting but is insufficient to provide a comprehensive spectrum of adverse events. Therefore seeking other areas of input helps provide a broader view of potential liabilities [22]. Trigger systems provide an excellent strategy for adverse event detection because more events are reported compared to entirely voluntary systems, chart reviews or administrative databases [23]. A 2011 study of hypoglycemia in children identified 198 adverse events related to hypoglycemia, but the hospital voluntary reporting system did not identify any of the 198 adverse events related to hypoglycemia [24].

In addition to continuous critical incident monitoring, the PICU may employ other strategies to improve patient safety. These may include divisional education conferences, including morbidity and mortality review, periodic internal and external audits, and specific quality improvement projects in response to safety concerns [18]. All levels of staff may initiate quality improvement, and discussion of incidents and interventions must involve the entire ICU team [3, 18]. A culture of open communication facilitated by senior physicians can aid the achievement of shared team goals including patient safety [19]. Conversely, deficient communication and teamwork increase medical errors [25]. Regularly completed multidisciplinary evaluations enhance communication and decrease emotional exhaustion among ICU staff [26].

PICU patients can be admitted from all hospital areas including the emergency department, the general pediatric ward, and the post-anesthesia care unit. Disruptions in patient flow can cause congestion in other areas of the hospital with the potential to decrease safety and hospital efficiency and increase staff stress [27]. Studies report greater variability in need for ICU admission from scheduled surgical procedures compared to admission from the emergency department. When ICU resources are limited, attempts to deflect admission after surgical procedures are more common than from the ED [28]. A prospective 2009 study implemented a system to improve flow which decreased diversions of patients from the unit and cancellations of operations due to lack of bed availability. Key strategies included creating a flow model based on anticipated needs for scheduled surgeries with a limit of five reserved bed spaces per day, scheduling of a case and a surgical bed at the same time, and a daily huddle with anesthesia, surgery, and intensive care unit representatives to verify the plan for the day and predict the schedule for the following day [27].

Team Development

The key elements involved in team performance are leadership, communication, coordination and decision making [29]. Review of data from critical incident studies in ICUs has highlighted the importance of effective team leadership in patient safety [29]. Leadership skills are also important in cardiopulmonary resuscitation. Team performance is best when the first arriving team leader to a critical incident adopts and maintains directed leadership behavior.

Additionally, good physician management and leadership skills are associated with improved efficiency of patient care as measured by completion of tasks on daily goal sheets [30]. Quality physician leadership not only improves patient care, but also positively impacts unit morale. Research in neonatal ICUs has shown that leaders listening to and encouraging participation of junior team members leads to increased involvement of team members in quality improvement programs. In addition, leadership training of physicians and senior nurses in teamwork skills leads to staff viewing leadership more positively [29].

In addition to leadership, communication is an integral part of team performance. Survey research has shown that ICUs with teams reporting high levels of trust and goal sharing and low levels of conflict have lower risk adjusted mortality rates [29]. Team oriented intensive care units have lower nursing turnover, higher quality of care, shorter length of stay, and more adequately meet the needs of family members [31]. In addition, cooperation between physicians and ICU nurses decreases reports of burnout in survey research [29], and truly collaborative care leads to unit stabilization [32]. An examination of ICU critical incident and adverse event data found persistent communication errors resulting in patient harm. The most common sources of error were communication errors during routine patient care, transfer of care to other providers, and emergencies [33]. High fidelity simulation can be used to evaluate and enhance team communication, and can improve communication and performance in the management of septic shock [29].

Team coordination centers on communication and refers to a combined team effort to reach a common goal. In a coordinated effort, each team member is aware of the actions of other members [29]. Poor coordination during training exercises in crisis management results in errors [34]. Positive perception of team coordination by ICU team members is associated with lower rates of errors [35]. Strategies including standardized patient hand off and daily goal sheets can be used to improve team coordination in ICUs. Daily goal sheets improve residents' and nurses' understanding of patient care duties and reduce length of stay [29]. In addition, daily goal sheets have been shown to enhance communication among care team members and to improve the nursing team's ability to identify the physician in charge [36].

Adequate team leadership, communication and cooperation fosters team decision making, and shared decision making in the ICU is associated with improved patient outcomes. Specifically, physician encouragement of contributions of team members during decision making on rounds is associated with a decrease in adverse events [29]. Staff cohesion regarding patient safety can be assessed on a routine basis via tools such as the Hospital Survey on Patient Safety Culture, formulated by the Agency for Healthcare Research and Quality in 2004 [37]. The Safety Attitudes Questionnaire (SAC) is an additional tool designed to measure overall safety climate within the ICU. Regular utilization of such tools can aid the administration in monitoring the pulse of the team and making adjustments when necessary. These results also allow comparative analysis against benchmarks from other institutions [38].

Family Centered Care

Parents of critically ill children view communication and information sharing by the medical team as key components of quality care [39]. Family centered care is a model that creates a partnership between providers and families in the delivery of care to children [40], and has become the standard of care in pediatrics [41]. A 2003 policy statement from the AAP states that "conducting attending physician rounds (ie, patient presentations and rounds discussions) in patients' rooms with the family present should be standard practice" [42]. A small randomized controlled trial revealed that parents felt more informed about their children when they were present on rounds and that they preferred to attend rounds [41].

A prospective observational study conducted in 2009 found that inclusion in morning rounds improves the satisfaction level of family members. In addition, it found that on the first day of admission, family members were less likely to understand the plan for the day and were less comfortable asking questions. Early studies evaluated possible negative effects of family centered care, including lengthened rounds, less time spent on teaching for residents, and possible family concerns about privacy violations. Research, however, has not shown that family centered care increases rounding time or decreases teaching time [41, 43]. Creation of a patient and family advisory council to help guide the leadership of the PICU towards patient centered care has been used in some centers.

Hospital Relations

An important role of the PICU is to serve as a support structure for other hospital divisions. The PICU admits patients from all areas of the hospital including the emergency department, hospital ward, and post-anesthesia care unit. In addition, the PICU staff is an important part of the rapid response team, the code blue team, and the trauma resuscitation team. Many hospitals are also utilizing PICU staff in the transport of critically ill children from referral centers to the PICU [44].

The PICU has an integral role during in-hospital cardiac arrests as members of code-blue and urgent-response teams.

In a 2007 assessment, the incidence of pediatric in-hospital cardiopulmonary arrests was between 0.7 % and 3 % of all hospital admissions and the survival to discharge for such patients between 15 % and 27 %. An estimated 8.5–14 % of all in-hospital cardiopulmonary arrests occurred in children outside of the ICU [45].

A 2007 survey of 181 acute-care pediatric hospitals in North America, all with PICUs, found that 96 % had formal pediatric resuscitation teams [46] and anyone, including staff and visitors, could activate the team. In addition to resuscitation or code-blue teams, 75 % of these hospitals also had organized urgent-response teams to respond to the clinically deteriorating child prior to incidence of cardiopulmonary or respiratory arrest. The purpose of an urgent-response team is to provide the necessary care to improve a patient's condition and prevent a need for escalation of care, to aid in efficient transfer to a higher level of care, or to discuss appropriate end-of-life care [46]. The implementation of these teams has been shown to decrease the risk of in-hospital cardiopulmonary or respiratory arrest outside of critical care areas [45]. The current frequency of their use within these hospitals is not known [46].

In addition to having a wide range of roles and relationships outside of the unit, critical care staff routinely interact with members of all pediatric divisions to provide comprehensive care to their patients. A close working relationship between the critical care division and all other divisions in the hospital can be fostered by the use of liaisons. Liaisons are particularly important in fields with a natural link to the ICU due to the severity of patient illness. Examples of such fields are hematology/oncology, neurosurgery, general surgery, and trauma surgery. A study of the New York State Trauma registry in 2004 found that 59 % of pediatric trauma was managed in hospitals with a PICU, and that mortality was lower in hospitals with a PICU compared to hospitals without. Intensivist involvement in patient care has been shown to be associated with better outcomes in patients following esophagectomy, abdominal aortic aneurysm surgery and intracerebral hemorrhage. A meta-analysis in 2002 found that the mandated involvement of an intensivist was associated with lower in-hospital mortality in 16 of the 17 studies [47].

Education and Training

Continuing education for PICU physicians and staff members is of paramount importance in quality patient care, as well as team morale and staff retention. Participation in local and national meetings on relevant critical care topics presents an additional opportunity for staff education and development, as well as networking and collaboration with other physicians and institutions [1]. The inclusion of a pediatric critical care training program may improve patient outcomes. A cohort study comparing adjusted mortality rates between PICUs staffed by critical care fellows and pediatric residents with PICUs staffed by residents alone showed better rates in those units with fellowship programs [48].

Education of new pediatric intensivists takes place largely in the ICU setting through pediatric critical care fellowship training programs approved by the ACGME. ICUs with training programs may be Level I or Level II but must possess adequate research experience and resources, as well as patient volume and diversity of pathology. The leadership of the PICU has a duty to help train fellows in the administrative, management and leadership skills necessary for practice as an intensivist. One survey revealed that the majority of intensivists learn such skills via role-modeling rather than formal training. These respondents felt least prepared to manage conflict and stress, a mandatory skill for senior intensive care clinicians [49]. The PICU also plays an important role in multidisciplinary education including training for nurses, respiratory therapists and local EMS providers. PICU staff may also participate in educational programs for the general public [1].

Conclusion

The PICU is a well-established entity within the field of pediatrics that encompasses multiple disciplines. As pediatric critical care increases in complexity, the administration of the ICU must adapt to ensure the highest quality of care of critically ill children and their families. Further research should focus on continued development of the multidisciplinary team approach, refinement of quality improvement and safety measures and the continued education of all levels of intensive care staff.

References

1. Rosenberg DI, Moss MM, Section on Critical Care and Committee on Hospital Care. Guidelines and levels of care for pediatric intensive care units. Pediatrics. 2004;114:1114–25.
2. Frey B, Argent A. Safe paediatric intensive care, part 1: does more medical care lead to improved outcome? Intensive Care Med. 2004;30:1041–6.
3. Frey B, Argent A. Safe paediatric intensive care, part 2: workplace organisation, critical incident monitoring and guidelines. Intensive Care Med. 2004;30:1292–7.
4. Pollack MM, Cuerdon TC, Getson PR. Pediatric intensive care units: results of a national survey. Crit Care Med. 1993;21:607–12.
5. Pollack MM, Alexander SR, Clarke BA, et al. Improved outcomes from tertiary center pediatric intensive care: a statewide comparison of tertiary and nontertiary care facilities. Crit Care Med. 1991;19:150–8.
6. Jaimovich DG, The Committee on Hospital Care and Section on Critical Care. Admission and discharge guidelines for the pediatric patient requiring intermediate care. Crit Care Med. 2004;32:1215–8.
7. American Academy of Pediatrics, Committee on Hospital Care and Section on Critical Care and Society of Critical Care Medicine, Pediatric Section Admission Criteria Task Force. Guidelines for developing admission and discharge policies for the pediatric intensive care unit. Pediatrics. 1999;103:840–2.
8. Fraisse A, Le Bel S, Mas B, Macrae D. Paediatric cardiac intensive care unit: current setting and organization in 2010. Arch Cardiovasc Disord. 2010;103:546–51.
9. Chang AC. How to start and sustain a successful pediatric cardiac intensive care program: a combined clinical and administrative strategy. Pediatr Crit Care Med. 2002;3:107–11.
10. Pollack MM, Katz RW, Ruttimann UE, Getson PR. Improving the outcome and efficiency of intensive care: the impact of an intensivist. Crit Care Med. 1988;16:11–7.
11. Netzer G, Liu X, Shanholtz C, et al. Decreased mortality resulting from a multicomponent intervention in a tertiary care medical intensive care unit. Crit Care Med. 2011;39:284–93.
12. Banerjee R, Naessens JM, Seferian EG, et al. Economic implications of nighttime attending intensivist coverage in a medical intensive care unit. Crit Care Med. 2011;39:1257–62.
13. Gajic O, Afessa B, Hanson AC, et al. Effect of 24-hour mandatory versus on-demand critical care specialist presence on quality of care and family and provider satisfaction in the intensive care unit of a teaching hospital. Crit Care Med. 2008;36:36–44.
14. Mathur M, Rampersand A. Physician assistants as physician extenders in the pediatric intensive care unit setting—a 5-year experience. Pediatr Crit Care Med. 2005;6:14–9.
15. Kleinpell RM, Ely EW, Grabenkort R. Nurse practitioners and physician assistants in the intensive care unit: an evidence-based review. Crit Care Med. 2008;36:2888–97.
16. Leape LL, Cullen DJ, Clapp MD, et al. Pharmacist participation on physician rounds and adverse drug events in the intensive care unit. JAMA. 1999;281:267–70.
17. Young MP, Gooder VJ, Oltermann MH, et al. The impact of a multidisciplinary approach on caring for ventilator-dependent patients. Int J Qual Healthc. 1998;10:15–26.
18. Gallesio AO, Ceraso D, Palizas F. Improving quality in the intensive care unit setting. Crit Care Clin. 2006;22:547–71.
19. Reader TW, Flin R, Cuthbertson BH. Team leadership in the intensive care unit: The perspective of specialists. Crit Care Med. 2011;1683–91.
20. Pollack MM, Cuerdon TT, Patel KM, et al. Impact of quality-of-care factors on pediatric intensive care unit mortality. JAMA. 1994;272:941–6.
21. Slonim AD, Pollack MM. Integrating the Institute of Medicine's six quality aims into pediatric critical care: relevance and applications. Pediatr Crit Care Med. 2005;6:264–9.
22. Levtzion-Korach O, Frankel A, Alcalai H, et al. Integrating incident data from five reporting systems to assess patient safety: making sense of the elephant. Jt Comm J Qual Patient Saf. 2010;36:402–10.
23. Agarwal S, Classen D, Larsen G, et al. Prevalence of adverse events in pediatric intensive care units in the United States. Pediatr Crit Care Med. 2010;11:568–78.
24. Dickerman MJ, Jacobs BR, Vinodrao H, Stockwell DC. Recognizing hypoglycemia in children through automated adverse-event detection. Pediatrics. 2011;127:e1035–41.
25. Allan CK, Thiagarajan RR, Beke D, et al. Simulation-based training delivered directly to the pediatric cardiac intensive care unit engenders preparedness, comfort, and decreased anxiety among multidisciplinary resuscitation teams. J Thorac Cardiovasc Surg. 2010;140:646–52.
26. Sluiter JK, Bos AP, Tol D, et al. Is staff well-being and communication enhanced by multidisciplinary work shift evaluations? Intensive Care Med. 2005;31:1409–14.
27. Ryckman FC, Yelton PA, Anneken AM, et al. Redesigning intensive care unit flow using variability management to improve access and safety. Jt Comm J Qual Patient Saf. 2009;35:535–43.

28. McManus ML, Long MC, Cooper A, et al. Variability in surgical caseload and access to intensive care services. Anesthesiology. 2003;98:1491–6.

29. Reader TW, Flin R, Mearns K, Cuthbertson BH. Developing a team performance framework for the intensive care unit. Crit Care Med. 2009;37:1787–93.

30. Stockwell DC, Slonim AD, Pollack MM. Physician team management affects goal achievement in the intensive care unit. Pediatr Crit Care Med. 2007;8:540–5.

31. Shortell SM, Zimmerman JE, Rousseau DM, et al. The performance of intensive care units: does good management make a difference? Med Care. 1994;32:508–25.

32. Ackerman AD. Retention of critical care staff. Crit Care Med. 1993;21:S394–5.

33. Provonost P, Thompson D, Holzmueller C, et al. Toward learning from patient safety reporting systems. J Crit Care. 2006;21: 305–15.

34. Lighthall GK, Barr J, Howard SK. Use of a fully simulated intensive care environment for critical care event management training for internal medicine residents. Crit Care Med. 2003;31: 2437–43.

35. van Beuzekom M, Akerboom S, Boer F. Assessing system failures in operating rooms and intensive care units. Qual Saf Health Care. 2007;16:45–50.

36. Agarwal S, Frankel L, Tourner S, et al. Improving communication in a pediatric intensive care unit using daily patient goal sheets. J Crit Care. 2008;23:227–35.

37. Agency for Healthcare Research and Quality. Hospital survey on patient safety culture. http://www.ahrq.gov/qual/patientsafetyculture/hospsurvindex.htm. Accessed 18 Aug 2011.

38. Sexton JB, Helmreich RL, Neilands TB, et al. The safety attitudes questionnaire: psychometric properties, benchmarking data, and emerging research. BMC Health Serv Res. 2006;6:44–54.

39. Kleiber C, Davenport T, Freyenberger B. Open bedside rounds for families with children in pediatric intensive care units. Am J Crit Care. 2006;15:492–6.

40. Frazier A, Frazier H, Warren NA. A discussion of family-centered care within the pediatric intensive care unit. Crit Care Nurs Q. 2010;33:82–6.

41. Aronson PL, Yau J, Helfaer MA, Morrison W. Impact of family presence during pediatric intensive care unit rounds on the family and medical team. Pediatrics. 2009;124:1119–25.

42. American Academy of Pediatrics, Committee on Hospital Care. Family centered care and the pediatrician's role. Pediatrics. 2003;112:691–7.

43. Phipps LM, Bartke CN, Spear DA, et al. Assessment of parental presence during bedside intensive care unit rounds: effect on duration, teaching and privacy. Pediatr Crit Care Med. 2007;8:220–4.

44. Borrows EL, Lutman DH, Montgomery MA. Effect of patient- and team-related factors on stabilization time during pediatric intensive care transport. Pediatr Crit Care Med. 2010;11:451–6.

45. Brilli RJ, Gibson R, Luria JW, et al. Implementation of a medical emergency team in a large pediatric teaching hospital prevents respiratory and cardiopulmonary arrests outside the intensive care unit. Pediatr Crit Care Med. 2007;8:236–46.

46. VandenBerg SD, Hutchison JS, Parshuram CS. A cross-sectional survey of levels of care and response mechanisms for evolving critical illness in hospitalized children. Pediatrics. 2007;119:e940–6.

47. Dean JM. Role of the pediatric intensivist in the management of pediatric trauma. J Trauma. 2007;63:S101–5.

48. Pollack MM, Patel KM, Ruttimann UE. Pediatric critical care training programs have a positive effect on pediatric intensive care mortality. Crit Care Med. 1997;25:1637–42.

49. Stockwell DC, Pollack MM, Turenne W, Slonim AD. Leadership and management training of pediatric intensivists: how do we gain our skills? Pediatr Crit Care Med. 2005;6:665–70.

Nursing Care in the Pediatric Intensive Care Unit

5

Franco A. Carnevale and Maryse Dagenais

Abstract

This chapter reviews several key topics in pediatric critical care nursing (PCCN). The complex role of the pediatric critical care nurse is described. First, the nurse is required to continually examine physiologic monitors and treatment devices, along with the child's body. Second, in the event of any irregularity, the nurse must instantly judge the significance of the event and initiate an appropriate response. Third, the nurse has a primary responsibility for ensuring patient safety. Fourth, the nurse is also responsible for maintaining a bedside environment that fosters the psychosocial adaptation of the child and family. Fifth, the nurse also functions as an "integrator" of patient information. Expertly practiced PCCN will help ensure optimal outcomes in terms of patient survival and morbidity, as well as child and family adaptation to the stresses of the experience. Infrastructural supports required to foster the development of PCCN are discussed. These include education programs for junior and senior staff, a medical-nursing co-management administrative structure, adequate staffing (both in terms of quantity and level of PCCN expertise), as well as the promotion and utilization of research to adapt nursing care to new understandings of the needs of critically ill children and their families. The strength of a PICU's service is directly tied to the quality and rigor of care that the nursing team can provide, in collaboration with the entire pediatric critical care team.

Keywords

Nursing administration • Nursing education • Pediatric critical care nursing • Nursing ethics • Nursing research

F.A. Carnevale, RN, PhD (✉)
Pediatric Critical Care,
Montreal Children's Hospital, McGill University,
Montreal Children's Hospital (Room A-413),
Montreal, QC H3H 1P3, Canada
e-mail: franco.carnevale@mcgill.ca

M. Dagenais, RN, MSc (A)
Pediatric Intensive Care Unit, Montreal Children's Hospital,
Montreal Children's Hospital (Room D-990),
Montreal, QC H3H 1P3, Canada
e-mail: Maryse.Dagenais@muhc.mcgill.ca

Role of the Pediatric Critical Care Nurse

The increasing complexity of pediatric critical care has required a corresponding evolution in the sophistication of pediatric critical care nursing (PCCN). The role of the nurse in this setting is multi-faceted [1]. First, the nurse serves as a form of "total systems monitor"—continually examining all the physiologic monitors and treatment devices, along with the child's body. This requires the acquisition of "peripheral vision". A skillful nurse learns to adjust settings on critical care equipment so it can serve as an extension of his/her own sensory system. The nurse has to perform routine "maintenance" activities (e.g., medication preparation, blood procurement, etc.) while remain-

D.S. Wheeler et al. (eds.), *Pediatric Critical Care Medicine*,
DOI 10.1007/978-1-4471-6362-6_5, © Springer-Verlag London 2014

ing attentive to the child's physiologic status—continually *tuned in* to the immediate recognition of any disruption in the child's condition. Second, in the event of any irregularity, the nurse must instantly judge the significance of the event and initiate an appropriate response. Such irregularities are frequently attributable to equipment artifacts or to "normal" patient functions such as movement or coughing that may trigger a variety of electronic alarms. The nurse has to immediately determine the importance of such events by "scanning" the child's body and surrounding equipment and discerning whether this implies a potential threat to the patient or not. If a significant problem is detected, then the nurse has to implement the required intervention (e.g., manual ventilation, airway suctioning). In cases of uncertainty or serious problems, the nurse will need to notify the physician. However, this notification needs to be done with discretion given the competing demands on the physician's time. Third, the nurse has a primary responsibility for ensuring patient safety [1–4], although this is not exclusively a nursing responsibility. He/she needs to prevent adverse events through the use of appropriate security measures (e.g., bedside rails, restraints, medication preparation procedures, infusion pump settings). Fourth, the nurse is also responsible for maintaining a bedside environment that fosters the psychosocial adaptation of the child and family [5]. He/she has to be attentive to the patient's psychological condition by addressing expressed needs while continually anticipating additional needs, inferred from a strong understanding of children's coping with critical illness. This involves the use of basic comforting skills, play therapies (in collaboration with child life specialists), as well as selected psychotherapeutic interventions (e.g., empathic listening, cognitive reframing), in collaboration with members of the mental health disciplines. He/she is also required to attend to the needs of the child's family, recognizing the extraordinary distress that can result from the illness and the benefit that the child will derive from the family's successful adaptation to the situation. Fifth, the nurse also functions as an "integrator" of patient information. The nurse is in continual contact with a vast body of bedside and laboratory patient information. Consequently, the nursing record serves as an integrated record of patient data that provides (a) a vital reference source for other health care professionals, (b) a log for subsequent shifts that need to compare data against prior events, and (c) a permanent record for retrospective reviews (e.g., morbidity and mortality analyses or quality improvement audits). The nurse also serves as a "live" patient data source. Given the rapid pace with which events unfold in the pediatric intensive care unit (PICU), the nurse is required to keep abreast of all that is going on with his/her assigned patient, to help ensure integrated coordinated patient care.

Turning to a *pilot in a cockpit* metaphor, PCCN typically involves highly routine surveillance functions, vigilantly attending to a multitude of cues to ensure an early recognition of *turbulence* or *system failure*. Such events must be immediately recognized and corrective interventions should be expediently and effectively implemented while ensuring the comfort and safety of the *passengers*. PCCN practiced in this manner will help ensure optimal outcomes in terms of patient survival and morbidity, as well as child and family adaptation to the stresses of the experience. This requires an education, administration, and innovation and research infrastructure that will foster and support expert nursing practice. The remainder of this chapter discusses these infrastructural elements.

Education

Orientation of New Staff

Typically, entry-level nursing education programs provide some basic exposure to general pediatric nursing, but little direct experience in critical care (neither adult nor pediatric) is offered. Academic programs in critical care nursing or PCCN are generally restricted to graduate advanced practice programs for clinical nurse specialists or nurse practitioners. Newly hired PICU nurses typically have little or no prior PCCN training. Such training is usually acquired "on the job". Given the critical condition of the PICU patient population and the need to provide no margin for "learning curve" errors, employers need to develop closely supervised education programs that expediently enable the new PICU nurse to acquire baseline knowledge and skills to manage less critical patients initially. Ultimately there is a gradual advancement in the complexity of assigned patients as expertise evolves.

New recruits, who usually have no prior PICU experience, arrive with (a) related experience such as neonatal critical care, (b) general pediatric experience, (c) adult critical care experience, (d) neither pediatric nor adult critical care experience (e.g., general adult medicine), or (e) no experience at all (i.e., a new graduate). Although the direct hiring of the latter candidates is a hotly contested point, they can successfully adapt to a PICU setting, given adequate educational, mentoring, and administrative support [6, 7]. In light of these commonly diverse backgrounds, every PICU needs to maintain an orientation program for new staff that can be readily tailored to the variable needs of new staff [8]. An orientation program should consist of (a) 1–2 weeks of introductory reviews and (b) a 3- to 4-week clinical preceptorship directly supervised by a senior PICU nurse (4–8 weeks for a new graduate). The introductory reviews should include (a) assigned readings, drawing selected chapters from seminal PCCN textbooks and recent journal publications [9–11]; (b) lectures that review basic critical care theory (e.g., evaluation of vital functions, hemodynamic evaluation, blood gas interpretation, neurologic evaluation, critical care pharmacology); (c) demonstration and practice of common procedures (e.g., airway suctioning, manual ventilation, blood procurement from arterial catheter); (d) discussion of the role of the PICU nurse; (e) overview of pertinent psychosocial issues; (f) introduction to key members of the PICU team; and (g) review of key PICU policies and procedures and other textual resources available to nurses. Such reviews can be conducted with a cohort group of new recruits [6, 7].

Clinical Preceptorship

The clinical preceptorship should enable new staff to directly care for PICU patients with direct supervision [6–8]. This implies a co-assignment with a senior nurse that serves as a clinical preceptor. Ideally, the new nurse will work with one sole preceptor throughout the preceptorship, to ensure pedagogical continuity. The preceptor–preceptee dyad should be initially counted as one sole nurse, in terms of workload assignment, to ensure that the preceptor can provide the required level of support and supervision. Patient acuity and the level of preceptee autonomy should be gradually increased at a pace where the learner is capable of safely caring for a stable patient without continuous and direct supervision by the final two to three assigned shifts of the preceptorship.

Sometimes, the learner's background and capabilities enable a rapid progression, whereas for others this process may need to be slowed to a point where the preceptorship needs to be extended. In these latter cases, performance limitations need to be explicitly stated for the learner and an additional training plan developed. The preceptorship is formally completed when the learner has fulfilled all of the required skill and knowledge objectives or, on occasion, if it is judged that the learner will not be able to continue his/her employment in the PICU. Candidates successfully completing their preceptorship may benefit from a subsequent (formal or informal) mentorship wherein they can derive ongoing clinical and professional guidance from either their original preceptors or other suitable senior staff. Such mentorships may be organized as a group program, which can foster learning and bonds among new nurses [7, 8, 12, 13].

Clinical preceptors supporting such a preceptorship program should be provided with the educational and administrative support that is necessary to fulfill this critical role. In addition to advanced expertise in PCCN, preceptorship also requires a body of knowledge and skills that are not readily acquired through clinical care. This includes an understanding of (a) adult learning principles, (b) bedside instructional techniques, (c) clinical performance appraisal, and (d) dynamics of the preceptee–preceptor relationship. This can be acquired through a combination of classroom activities and direct coaching from an experienced nursing educator. Preceptors require administrative support wherein they can readily negotiate preceptee patient assignments (*workload* as well as *type* of patient) according to the preceptee's learning needs, discuss any performance problems that arise, and review general issues that may help improve the unit's preceptorship program.

Senior Staff Development

This discussion has focused exclusively on the learning needs of newly hired staff. However, orientation and preceptorship programs provide a basic level of PCCN preparation. Additional educational programs are therefore required to ensure the ongoing development of PICU nursing staff [1, 8]. Most importantly, nurses need ready access to advanced experts in PCCN (e.g., exemplary senior nurses, clinical nurse specialists, and nurse practitioners) as well as pediatric critical care physicians and other experts (e.g., respiratory therapists) who can provide bedside coaching for the management of emerging issues in everyday practice. Structured classroom-type and simulation programs should also be developed. These can be topic specific, such as: (a) Pediatric Advanced Life Support course; (b) an intermediate level workshop examining selected PCCN functions (e.g., stabilization of a postoperative cardiac surgery patient, continuous renal-replacement therapy); (c) review session on analgesia and sedation; or (d) trauma management workshop.

Advanced senior staff development programs are also required. For example, the Montreal Children's Hospital PICU has a 10-day PCCN course for senior nursing staff (which has been running for over 25 years) that provides an advanced review of critical care topics. This includes a thorough review of recent practices, ongoing debates, and emerging trends through lectures, case reviews, assigned readings, homework exercises, and student presentations (Table 5.1). Such programs help prepare senior staff to manage the most complex PICU patients while serving as clinical leaders and mentors for junior staff. Some universities offer postgraduate programs in pediatric critical care. These include courses that aim to advance the nurse's repertoire of knowledge, skills, attitudes and professional values. It may also prepare them for formal credentialing exams such as the Canadian Nurses Association certification in pediatric critical care [14].

Table 5.1 Senior staff development course for pediatric intensive care unit nursing: principal topics

Mechanics of ventilation
Control of breathing
Gas exchange and transport
Myocardial mechanics
Cardiac electrophysiology
Hemodynamic physiology
Critical care pharmacology
Fluids, electrolytes, and nutrition
Cerebral injury
Seizures
Sepsis
Immune function
Coagulopathies
Shock
Trauma
Hepatic dysfunction
Renal dysfunction
Analgesia and sedation
Extracorporeal membrane oxygenation and ventricular assist devices
Ethics

Administration

Structure

The PICU nursing manager needs to understand the complexity of the nursing service required in a PICU [15]. The manager commonly determines (a) the number of staff required for a given mix of patients, (b) support services available to nurses, (c) access to educational programs and resources, and (d) the number and type of new staff targeted for recruitment. Thus, the manager can profoundly enable or disable the functioning of a PICU nursing team. Such a manager should ideally have a strong background in PCCN as well as nursing management. The PICU should be co-managed by the medical director and nursing manager, each holding primary responsibility for his/her respective discipline while jointly managing areas of common concern (e.g., quality improvement). This structure facilitates reciprocal problem solving and support, which have been associated with improved patient outcomes [16, 17]. The inclusion of other professionals, such as child life specialist, physiotherapist, social worker, in regular meetings will help the nursing and medical managers to establish care priorities in light of the critically ill child's many needs.

Staffing

The most prominent administrative problem raised in PCCN relates to nursing staffing levels. What nurse/patient ratios are required to provide necessary care? This problem is related to increasing concerns about cost containment and nursing shortages in the face of rising demands for PICU services [17]. Nurse/patient ratios have obvious implications for nursing staff satisfaction and morale but have also been linked to patient outcomes. Evidence emerging out of other settings indicates that low nursing staffing levels are directly related to increased patient morbidity [2–4, 15–19]. This problem has been scarcely examined within the PICU setting, although one study reported that patients are more likely to experience unplanned extubations if they are assigned to a nurse caring for two patients rather than one [18].

The American Academy of Pediatrics Section on Critical Care and the American Academy of Pediatrics Committee on Hospital Care have jointly published *Guidelines and levels of care for pediatric intensive care units* [20]. This article indicates that nurse/patient ratios should vary according to patient needs, ranging from 2:1 (2 nurses per patient) to 1:3 (1 nurse per 3 patients). However, no further detail is provided on how specific staffing determinations should be made. Likewise no international guidelines propose widely accepted PICU nursing staffing standards, and a corresponding diversity of viewpoints on how this problem ought to be managed exist [21, 22]. The British Association of Critical Care Nurses has recently published staffing guidelines. They emphasize that patient safety depends on patient access to qualified registered nurses supported by an administrative structure that allows nurses to focus on patient care. Auxiliary workers can play a key role in assisting nurses but the nurse remains responsible for patient care [23]. Findings from a study by the Canadian Health Services Research Foundation support these findings [24].

Ball has examined the utility of nursing workload measures as a means for addressing this problem in critical care in general [25]. She questions the validity of such tools for these purposes, arguing that nursing staffing requirements should be based on patient needs and on the nursing care that would meaningfully address these needs rather than a count of tasks performed. Furthermore, no accepted tool exists for the measurement of PCCN workload. Although validated PICU acuity measures are available, these do not directly correlate with nursing workload. It appears that the best available means for determining workload is the judgment of nursing managers. This further justifies the necessity that such managers possess a strong grasp of PCCN.

Innovation and Research

Although PICU nurses share numerous concerns and interests with physicians and other critical care practitioners, a number of topics have gained particular importance in PCCN. These relate to problems that more immediately concern nurses, although not exclusively. In fact, the PCCN literature has taken the lead in examining topics that are highly relevant to other critical care practitioners as well.

The PCCN literature examines physiologic, psychosocial, and ethical problems, as well as the educational and administrative issues discussed earlier. This literature is accessible through excellent PCCN textbooks [9, 10] and a number of highly respected critical care nursing journals (as well as non-nursing journals). *Pediatric Intensive Care Nursing* is an international journal exclusively devoted to PCCN. PICU nurses needing to consult colleagues about specific clinical problems can do so through the international PCCN Internet discussion group *PICU-Nurse-International* (http://health. groups.yahoo.com/group/PICU-Nurse-International/).

Nursing research on pain management and withdrawal reactions has complemented medical research. As nurses commonly assess when to administer analgesics to children who are intubated and cannot communicate, nursing research has examined the effectiveness of various pain assessment tools [26–31]. Nurses have also advanced knowledge on opioid/benzodiazepine withdrawal reactions, a frequent iatrogenic complication of PICU care [32–34]. Other topics reviewed in this literature include prone positioning [35], pressure ulcers [36], airway suctioning practices [37], environmental noise [38], and PICU ethical dilemmas [39].

Pediatric critical care nursing researchers have demonstrated a particular interest in psychosocial problems. This research has examined parental needs and stressors [40, 41], sibling experiences [41], the experience of the critically ill child [42], the experience of the entire family as a whole [41, 43], and family presence during resuscitation [44, 45]. A major finding of this psychosocial research is that *families are not visitors* [5, 41]. Family members are attempting to fulfill their respective family functions in the PICU (e.g., parenting); they are not visiting. The extent to which the experiences of individual family members can be favorably supported, these members will derive benefits that can also benefit the critically ill child. Family presence and participation in the patient's care can foster the well-being of both the patient and the family. Therefore, the PICU should ensure that families have access to essential physical comforts, as well as supportive psychosocial services. In light of the long-term psychological consequences that critical illness may entail for the child and family, these families could also benefit from integrated long-term follow-up services. Finally, the PICU setting is one of the primary sites of child deaths in pediatrics. The PICU staff should thus be sensitive to caring for the special needs of dying children and their families [46, 47].

Nursing-led research on PICU ethical concerns has highlighted that PICU staff struggle with *moral distress*; this is a malaise that results when situational constraints prevent clinicians from doing what they believe is the right thing to do

[48]. Other ethics research has examined PICU decision-making, parental roles, communication [49], as well as concerns relating to the long-term care of PICU "survivors" with complex continuing care needs [50].

Conclusion

Pediatric critical care nursing is a major component of excellent pediatric critical care. The provision of this specialized nursing requires significant educational and administrative support while continually drawing on ongoing PCCN clinical innovations and research to adapt nursing care to new understandings of the needs of critically ill children and their families. The strength of a PICU's service is inescapably tied to the quality and rigor of care that the nursing team can provide, in collaboration with the entire pediatric critical care team.

References

1. Benner P, Hooper-Kyriakidis P, Stannard D. Clinical wisdom and interventions in critical care: a thinking-in-action approach. Philadelphia: WB Saunders; 1999.
2. Aiken LH, Clarke SP, Sloane DM, Sochalski J, Silber JH. Hospital nurse staffing and patient mortality, nurse burnout, and job dissatisfaction. JAMA. 2002;288(16):1987–93.
3. Cho SH, Ketefian S, Barkauskas VH, et al. The effects of nurse staffing on adverse events, morbidity, mortality, and medical costs. Nurs Res. 2003;52:71–9.
4. Clarke SP, Aiken LH. An international hospital outcomes research agenda focused on nursing: lessons from a decade of collaboration. J Clin Nurs. 2008;17(24):3317–23.
5. Carnevale FA. The injured family. In: Moloney-Harmon PA, Czerwinski SJ, editors. Nursing care of the pediatric trauma patient. St. Louis: WB Saunders; 2003. p. 107–17.
6. Proulx DM, Bourcier BJ. Graduate nurses in the intensive care unit: an orientation model. Crit Care Nurse. 2008;4:44–52.
7. Ihlenfeld JT. Hiring and mentoring graduate nurses in the intensive care unit. Dimens Crit Care Nurs. 2005;24(4):175–8.
8. Czerwinski S, Martin ED. Facilitation of learning. In: Curley MAQ, Moloney-Harmon P, editors. Critical care nursing of infants and children. 2nd ed. Philadelphia: WB Saunders; 2001. p. 85–106.
9. Curley MAQ, Moloney-Harmon P, editors. Critical care nursing of infants and children. 2nd ed. Philadelphia: WB Saunders; 2001.
10. Slota M, editor. AACN core curriculum for pediatric critical care nursing. 2nd ed. Philadelphia: Elsevier/WB Saunders Co.; 2006.
11. Marcoux KK. Current management of status asthmaticus in the pediatric ICU. Crit Care Nurs Clin North Am. 2005;17(4):463–79.
12. Kanaskie ML. Mentoring: a staff retention tool. Crit Care Nurs Q. 2006;29(3):248–52.
13. Benner P, Sutphen M, Leonard V, Day L. Educating nurses: a call for radical transformation. San Francisco: Jossey-Bass; 2010.
14. Rose L, Goldsworthy S, O'Brien-Pallas L, Nelson S. Critical care nursing education and practice in Canada and Australia: a comparative review. Int J Nurs Stud. 2008;45(7):1103–9.
15. Fagan MJ. Leadership in pediatric critical care. In: Curley MAQ, Moloney-Harmon P, editors. Critical care nursing of infants and children. 2nd ed. Philadelphia: WB Saunders; 2001. p. 71–83.
16. Tourangeau AE, Cranley LA, Jeffs L. Impact of nursing on hospital patient mortality: a focused review and related policy implications. Qual Saf Health Care. 2006;15(1):4–8.

17. Pyykko AK, Ala-Kokko TI, Laurila JJ, Miettunen J, Finnberg M, Hentinen M. Nursing staff resources in direct patient care: comparison of TISS and ICNSS. Acta Anaesthesiol Scand. 2004;48(8):1003–5.

18. Marcin JP, Rutan E, Rapetti PM, Brown JP, Rahnamayi R, Pretzlaff RK. Nurse staffing and unplanned extubation in the pediatric intensive care unit. Pediatr Crit Care Med. 2005;6(3):254–7.

19. West E, Mays N, Rafferty AM, Rowan K, Sanderson C. Nursing resources and patient outcomes in intensive care: a systematic review of the literature. Int J Nurs Stud. 2009;46(7):993–1011.

20. Rosenberg DI, Moss MM, American Academy of Pediatrics Section on Critical Care, American Academy of Pediatrics Committee on Hospital Care. Guidelines and levels of care for pediatric intensive care units. Pediatrics. 2004;114(4):1114–25.

21. Carnevale FA. PICU nurse–patient ratios: in search of the "right" numbers. Pediatr Intensive Care Nurs. 2001;2(1):7–9.

22. Clarke T, Mackinnon E, England K, Burr G, Fowler S, Fairservice L. A review of intensive care nurse staffing practices overseas: what lessons for Australia? Intensive Crit Care Nurs. 2000;16(4):228–42.

23. Bray K, Wren I, Baldwin A, St Ledger U, Gibson V, Goodman S, Walsh D. Standards for nurse staffing in critical care units determined by: The British Association of Critical Care Nurses, The Critical Care Networks National Nurse Leads, Royal College of Nursing Critical Care and In-flight Forum. Nurs Crit Care. 2010;15:109–11.

24. Ellis J, Priest A, MacPhee M, Sanchez McCutcheon A, on behalf of CHSRF and partners. Staffing for safety: a synthesis of the evidence on nurse staffing and patient safety. Canadian Health Services Research Foundation. 2006. http://www.chsrf.ca/Migrated/PDF/ResearchReports/CommissionedResearch/staffing_for_safety_policy_synth_e.pdf. Accessed 9 Nov 2012.

25. Ball C. Patient-nurse ratios in critical care: time for some radical thinking. Intensive Crit Care Nurs. 2001;17(3):125–7.

26. Johnston CC, Stevens B, Craig KD, et al. Developmental changes in pain expression in premature, full-term, two- and four-month-old infants. Pain. 1993;52:201–8.

27. Alexander E, Carnevale FA, Razack S. Evaluation of a sedation protocol for intubated critically ill children. Intensive Crit Care Nurs. 2002;18:292–301.

28. Ista E, van Dijk M, Tibboel D, de Hoog M. Assessment of sedation levels in pediatric intensive care patients can be improved by using the COMFORT "behavior" scale. Pediatr Crit Care Med. 2005;6(1):58–63.

29. Johnston CC, Gagnon A, Rennick J, Rosmus C, Patenaude H, Ellis J, Shapiro C, Filion F, Ritchie J, Byron J. One-on-one coaching to improve pain assessment and management practices of pediatric nurses. J Pediatr Nurs. 2007;22(6):467–78.

30. Ranger M, Johnston CC, Anand KJ. Current controversies regarding pain assessment in neonates. Semin Perinatol. 2007;31(5):283–8.

31. Franck LS, Ridout D, Howard R, Peters J, Honour JW. A comparison of pain measures in newborn infants after cardiac surgery. Pain. 2011;152(8):1758–65.

32. Franck LS, Naughton I, Winter I. Opioid and benzodiazepine withdrawal symptoms in paediatric intensive care patients. Intensive Crit Care Nurs. 2004;20(6):344–51.

33. Franck LS, Harris SK, Soetenga DJ, Amling JK, Curley MAQ. The withdrawal assessment tool – version 1: an assessment instrument for monitoring opioid and benzodiazepine withdrawal symptoms in pediatric patients. Pediatr Crit Care Med. 2008;9(6):573–80.

34. Ista E, van Dijk M, de Hoog M, Tibboel D, Duivenvoorden HJ. Construction of the Sophia Observation withdrawal Symptoms-scale (SOS) for critically ill children. Intensive Care Med. 2009;35(6):1075–81.

35. Curley MA, Thompson JE, Arnold JH. The effects of early and repeated prone positioning in pediatric patients with acute lung injury. Chest. 2000;118:156–63.

36. Curley MA, Quigley SM, Lin M. Pressure ulcers in pediatric intensive care: incidence and associated factors. Pediatr Crit Care Med. 2003;3:284–90.

37. Akgul S, Akyolcu N. Effects of normal saline on endotracheal suctioning. J Clin Nurs. 2002;11(6):826–30.

38. Milette IH, Carnevale FA. I'm trying to heal: noise levels in a pediatric intensive care unit. Dynamics. 2003;14(4):14–21.

39. Carnevale FA. Ethical care of the critically ill child: a conception of a "thick" bioethics. Nurs Ethics. 2005;12(3):239–52.

40. Fisher MD. Identified needs of parents in a pediatric intensive care unit. Crit Care Nurse. 1994;14(3):82–90.

41. Carnevale FA. "Striving to recapture our previous life": the experience of families of critically ill children. Off J Can Assoc Crit Care Nurs. 1999;9(4):16–22.

42. Rennick JE, Johnston CC, Dougherty G, et al. Children's psychological responses after critical illness and exposure to invasive technology. J Dev Behav Pediatr. 2002;23:133–44.

43. Youngblut JM, Lauzon S. Family functioning following pediatric intensive care unit hospitalization. Issues Compr Pediatr Nurs. 1995;18:11–25.

44. Latour JM. Perspectives on parental presence during resuscitation: a literature review. Pediatr Intensive Care Nurs. 2002;3(1):5–8.

45. Gaudreault J, Carnevale FA. Should I stay or should I go? Parental struggles when witnessing resuscitative measures on another child in the pediatric intensive care unit. Pediatr Crit Care Med. 2012;13:146–51.

46. Widger KA, Wilkins K. What are the key components of quality perinatal and pediatric end-of-life care? A literature review. J Palliat Care. 2004;20(2):105–12.

47. Longden JV. Parental perceptions of end-of-life care on paediatric intensive care units: a literature review. Nurs Crit Care. 2011;16(3):131–9.

48. Austin W, Kelecevic J, Goble E, Mekechuk J. An overview of moral distress and the paediatric intensive care team. Nurs Ethics. 2009;16:57–68.

49. Carnevale FA, Canoui P, Cremer R, Farrell C, Doussau A, Seguin MJ, Hubert P, Leclerc F, Lacroix J. Parental involvement in treatment decisions regarding their critically ill child: a comparative study of France and Quebec. Pediatr Crit Care Med. 2007;8:337–42.

50. Carnevale FA, Alexander E, Davis M, Rennick JE, Troini R. Daily living with distress and enrichment: the moral experience of families with ventilator assisted children at home. Pediatrics. 2006;117:e48–60.

Sandra D.W. Buttram, Paul R. Bakerman,
and Murray M. Pollack

Abstract

Today's health care environment is focused on providing both high quality and error-free care. Transparency is becoming an expectation, with many outcomes reported publically. Scoring systems are an objective measure which can be used to assess quality of care, assist with the evaluation and modification of complex systems of care, improve patient outcomes and predict morbidity and mortality. Their role has become secure in critical care because physician's judgments are too subjective for quality assessment in large samples.

The development of scoring systems began as external influences in the 1960s favored the assessment of outcome. Concerns about the quality of medical care escalated following the Institute of Medicine Report in 1999 which ultimately led to the Patient Safety and Quality Improvement Act of 2005. A successful scoring system must include a model with carefully defined predictor variables and outcome. The model must be reliable and the scoring system requires both internal and external validation.

Scoring systems were developed to predict mortality in adults (APACHE: Acute Physiology and Chronic Health Evaluations Score) and children (PRISM: Pediatric Risk of Mortality Score). They have also been used to predict morbidity and functional outcome. Scoring systems that apply to specific patient populations such as trauma and congenital heart disease have been developed.

Clinical scoring systems provide a standardized method for intensive care benchmarking and have increased in number and utility over the past 30 years. They are progressively more applicable to clinicians and health services researchers and in the future may be pertinent to individual patients. It is in the intensivist's best interest to understand scoring systems, their applications and implications.

Keywords

Benchmarking • Mortality Prediction • Outcome • Pediatric Risk of Mortality • PRISM III • Prognostication • Quality • Scoring systems • Severity of Illness • Risk stratification

S.D.W. Buttram, MD (✉) • P.R. Bakerman, MD
Critical Care Medicine, Phoenix Children's Hospital,
1919 E. Thomas Road, Phoenix, AZ 85016, USA
e-mail: sbuttram@phoenixchildrens.com;
pbakerm@phoenixchildrens.com

M.M. Pollack, MD (✉)
Department of Child Health,
University of Arizona College of Medicine – Phoenix,
1919 E. Thomas Road, Phoenix, AZ 85016, USA
e-mail: mpollack@phoenixchildrens.com

Introduction

Today's health care environment is focused on providing both high quality and error-free care. Transparency is becoming an expectation, with many outcomes reported publically. Comparative data bases with case-mix adjusted outcomes are available to many children's hospitals. High-profile programs such as pediatric cardiovascular surgery and pediatric critical care have access to national and international benchmarks

D.S. Wheeler et al. (eds.), *Pediatric Critical Care Medicine*,
DOI 10.1007/978-1-4471-6362-6_6, © Springer-Verlag London 2014

for outcomes. Parallel to the movement focusing on quality, there has been a national effort to reduce errors, especially those falling into the category of "never events". This movement was sparked by the Institute of Medicine's (IOM) 1999 report highlighting the need to reduce medical errors with subsequent recommendations in 2001 to improve quality and promote evidence-based practice [1, 2].

A common adage is "you can't improve what you can't measure". Scoring systems are usually an objective measure which can assess quality of care, assist with the evaluation and modification of complex systems of care, improve patient outcomes, and predict morbidity and mortality. Their role has become secure in critical care because physician's judgments are too subjective to be used for quality assessment in large samples, as well as the fact that there is a need for severity of illness assessments in clinical studies. Physician prognostication may be inaccurate for a number of reasons [3–11]. First, there are differences in a physician's ability to predict outcome based on the stage of the practitioner's career. Second, there is a tendency to overly weigh recent experience, particularly when experience with a specific condition is limited. Third, physicians may be unable to continuously account for all relevant clinical components that are important in predicting outcome. Finally, literature supporting evidence-based medicine is ever expanding and may exceed many clinicians' ability to remain current [12–19].

History

External influences have played a significant role in stimulating an environment that favors the assessment of outcome and the development of scoring systems designed to accomplish case-mix adjustment. In the 1960s, the US federal government focused its attention on social issues, including the healthcare safety net. Medicare and Medicaid programs were developed as fee for service plans, with access to healthcare services regardless of the ability to pay. Universal access to care and the concept of patient entitlement changed the perception of healthcare from a privilege to a right. Medical advances in areas such as dialysis and mechanical ventilation led to increasingly "high-tech care" and advanced the emerging specialty of critical care medicine. The result of these changes was increased utilization and cost. As healthcare costs exploded, there was increased focus on appropriate utilization of resources, the quality of these services, and the relationship between cost and quality (e.g. the value equation). These concerns also stimulated the need for objective scoring systems.

Concerns about the quality of medical care have escalated over the last 20 years. In the 1990s, the New England Journal of Medicine published a series of articles highlighting medical errors [20, 21]. Public interest in quality became more visible following the Institute of Medicine Report in 1999 [1]. This and subsequent reports ultimately led to the Patient Safety and Quality Improvement Act of 2005, which led to the establishment of a system of patient safety organizations and a national patient safety database.

Intensive Care Units (ICUs) were early leaders in developing methods of quality assessment using accurate and reliable adjustments for case-mix differences. Prognostication in the ICU is essential to the debates about quality and cost. It is essential that the technologically advanced care provided in ICUs results in a meaningful outcome to patients and families. Mortality, morbidity and functional outcome prediction are central to these discussions. Thus, prognostic methods are a logical focus for intensive care physicians.

Early scoring systems such as the Glasgow Coma Scale and the APGAR score were developed to assess outcome in select populations. In the 1970s and 1980s, subsequent scoring systems were developed to appraise global ICU care and outcomes which allowed for evaluation of quantity of care, quality of care, and cost. The physiology-based scoring systems enabled case-mix adjustments and comparisons. Importantly, these developments led to the conclusion that there were differences in the practice patterns and quality among ICUs [22].

Physiology-based scoring systems were initially built on the concept that there is a direct relationship between mortality and the number of failing organ systems. Organ system failure results from physiologic derangements that were modeled to produce relatively accurate mortality risk estimates. Mortality prediction scores included the Acute Physiology and Chronic Health Evaluations Score (APACHE) and the Pediatric Risk of Mortality Score (PRISM). These early scoring systems have been modified and adapted, while others have been developed that evaluate morbidity or apply to select patient populations.

Use of Scoring Systems

Physicians and hospitals use internal and external benchmarking to assess quality of care. Benchmarking establishes an external standard reference to which performance levels can be compared and may be used to define "best practice". Internal benchmarking allows an organization to compare performance within itself while external benchmarking compares performance between hospitals or services such as ICUs. Scoring systems may also be incorporated into clinical pathways to remove subjective assessments and incorporate evidence based medicine. These pathways are developed to improve care quality, decrease variability between individual providers and improve the efficiency through which care is delivered. The ultimate goal is to deliver high quality care in the most cost effective manner.

Clinical trials often include scoring systems. Scoring systems can be used to control for case-mix index, control for severity of illness between treatment groups or aid in risk stratification of enrolled subjects. They can also be used to compare expected to observed outcomes. Mortality prediction scores such as APACHE and PRISM have commonly been used in this manner.

While it may seem attractive to apply probabilities to direct patient care, this practice is potentially problematic. Risk assessment is less reliable when applied to an individual patient. In particular, the real range (i.e. the 95 % confidence interval) of the computed estimate is often much larger than the user appreciates. This is especially relevant when the computed mortality risk is very high, but the confidence interval is very wide (i.e. imprecise). Perhaps most importantly, the prognostic performance of physicians is approximately equivalent to the performance of scoring systems for individual patients [7, 8, 23]. At this time, scoring systems are primarily intended to provide objective assessment of quality of care, to assess the effects of interventions provided by a healthcare system [19], and for use in severity of illness assessment for individual trials but should not be applied to individual patients.

Elements of a Scoring System

The important elements of a successful scoring system include outcome, predictor variables, and model. The outcome should be objective, clearly defined and relevant. Historically, mortality has been the primary outcome measure for ICU prognostication, with more recent interest in morbidity and functional outcomes.

Predictor (independent) variables should also be objective, clearly defined, reliably measured, mutually exclusive, applicable across institutions, and as free from lead-time bias as possible. To minimize bias associated with model development, these variables should be defined and collected a priori. Data elements may include diagnoses, physiologic status, physiologic reserve, response to therapy and intensity of interventions [24]. These elements must be logical for the intended use of the scoring system. For example, a recent effort to use Pediatric Index of Mortality (PIM2) for cardiovascular ICU patients led to poor predictor performance [25]. This was not surprising given, the paucity of acute physiological variables and cardiac diagnoses included in the score.

Model development is the next element in scoring system design. Typically, individual predictor variables are tested with a univariate analysis for statistical association to the outcome. The variables that are "loosely associated" with outcome (e.g. $p < 0.30$) from the univariate analysis are then combined in a multivariate analysis. The type of multivariate analysis is outcome specific. Logistic regression is used for dichotomous outcomes such as survival/death. Linear regression is used for continuous variables such as length of stay. Multivariate linear or quadratic discriminate function analysis is most often used for categorical outcomes such as diagnoses [26, 27]. For each independent variable included in the model, a general guideline suggests that there should be at least ten outcome events (e.g. deaths) in the analysis.

Reliability

Reliability of the data elements and the model are vital to a successful scoring system. Clearly defined data elements, precise timing of data collection and standardized training for data collectors all contribute to high quality data acquisition. Reliability of the score can be measured within (*intra-rater*) or between (*inter-rater*) observers [24, 27]. The kappa (κ) statistic can be used to measure the level of agreement with 0 representing chance and 1 representing perfect agreement. The type of data determines the most appropriate reliability measurement. Dichotomous data uses the κ statistic, ordinal data uses the weighted κ statistic, and interval data uses the intraclass correlation coefficient [27].

Validity

Validation of a scoring system is the final test to determine whether the score measures what it was designed to measure. A scoring system is often first validated internally. Internal validation can be accomplished by using subsets of the population from which the score was derived. Three common techniques for internal validation include: data-splitting, cross-validation and bootstrapping [27, 28]. Data-splitting involves randomly dividing the sample into a training set and a validation set, with the training set used for initial model development. Cross-validation generates multiple training and validation sets through repeated data-splitting. Bootstrapping tests the model's performance on a large number of randomly drawn samples from the original population. If a score has good internal validity then it can be externally validated. External validation requires application of the scoring system to a patient population separate from the initial study.

Discrimination and *calibration* are two common statistical methods that are used to assess the model performance [24]. Discrimination is the ability of a model to distinguish between outcome groups, assessed by the area under the receiver operating characteristic curve. As the area under the curve (AUC) approaches one, the discrimination of the scoring system approaches perfection. The AUC of chance performance is 0.5 and for perfect performance is 1.0.

Calibration measures the correlation between the predicted outcomes and actual outcome over the entire range of risk prediction. The most accepted method for assessing calibration is the goodness-of-fit statistic proposed by Lemeshow and Hosmer [29].

Types of Scoring Systems

Scoring systems allow objective quantification of complex clinical states. They can be categorized by the type of predictor variables used to predict outcome. Examples include intervention specific, physiology specific, disease or condition specific and functional outcome scoring systems.

Intervention Specific Scoring Systems

Conceptually, more therapies are provided to sicker patients. The number of interventions that patients receive during their hospitalization can be associated with severity of illness. The Therapeutic Intervention Scoring System (TISS) [30] is an example of this type of scoring system and has been applied to pediatric patients [31]. The initial TISS score included 76 different therapeutic and monitoring interventions scored on a scale of 1–4 based on complexity and invasiveness. Interventions increase with severity of illness, thereby increasing the TISS score which predicts the risk of mortality. However, individual and institutional practice regarding use of interventions may vary which will affect the TISS score independent of the patient's physiology.

Physiology Specific Scoring Systems

Adult Mortality Scores

The most common adult ICU mortality scores are the APACHE, Mortality Probability Model (MPM), and Simplified Acute Physiology Score (SAPS). APACHE IV uses the worst physiologic values from the first 24 h of ICU admission. Weighted variables including age, physiologic data and chronic co-morbid conditions combined with major disease categories are used to predict hospital mortality [32]. The MPM III collects information at time of ICU admission (MPM_0). Age, physiologic data and acute and chronic diagnoses are included in the MPM III. The MPM III adds a "zero factor" term for elective surgical patients that have no risk factors identified by the MPM variables to accommodate for the low mortality risk in this patient population [33]. SAPS 3 is similar to MPM III collecting data at time of ICU admission to predict the probability of hospital mortality. SAPS 3 includes variables relating to patient characteristics before ICU admission and the circumstances of ICU admission in addition to age and physiologic data [34]. Table 6.1 summarizes model characteristics for each of these adult mortality scoring systems.

Pediatric Mortality Scores

The two most common pediatric ICU mortality scores are the PRISM and the PIM. Pediatric scoring systems are similar to their adult counterparts in many respects. The most recent version, PRISM III, was developed from over 11,000 patients in 32 centers in the United States [35]. It consists of 17 physiologic variables collected within the first 12 h (PRISM III-12) or first 24 h (PRISM III-24) of ICU admission (Table 6.1). The most abnormal values at 12 and 24 h are recorded and used to predict the risk of mortality. PRISM has been externally validated [36] and is the first pediatric scoring system to be protected by site licenses.

The PIM2 was developed from over 20,000 patients in 14 centers in Australia, New Zealand and Great Britain (Table 6.1) [37]. Ten variables are collected within the period of time from initial ICU team patient contact, regardless of location, up to 1 h after ICU admission. Conceptually, data is collected early in treatment to more accurately reflect the patient's physiologic state rather than the quality of ICU treatment rendered. While lead time bias theoretically applies to all scoring systems, there is no evidence that data collected during the first 12 or 24 h of ICU admission adversely affects the validity of a model.

Pediatric Morbidity Scores

Morbidity occurs more commonly than mortality and offers an alternative method for assessment of quality of care. The Pediatric Multiple Organ Dysfunction Score (PEMOD) and Pediatric Logistic Organ Dysfunction (PELOD) were modified from previously developed adult scores [38–40] to describe complications and morbidity in pediatric ICU patients [41]. These scoring systems quantify organ system dysfunction based on objective criteria of severity. However, these scores were developed (PEMOD and PELOD) and validated (PELOD only) on relatively small patient populations [42].

Disease or Condition Specific Scoring Systems

Trauma

The most widely used and validated trauma scoring system is the Revised Trauma Score (RTS) [43]. Components of the RTS include Glasgow Coma Scale, systolic blood pressure and respiratory rate. The RTS was initially designed for use by prehospital care personnel to identify adult trauma patients that would benefit from care at a designated trauma center. Subsequently, it has been used to predict mortality from blunt and penetrating injuries and has been validated for use in pediatric trauma patients [44–46].

Table 6.1 Adult and pediatric physiology specific mortality score model design

	Adult			Pediatric	
	APACHE IV	MPM III	SAPS 3	PRISM III	PIM2
Outcome measure	Mortality	Mortality	Mortality	Mortality	Mortality
Developed/revised (year)	1980/2006	1985/2007	1984/2005	1988/1996	1997/2003
Population					
Development set	110,558	124,885	16,784	11,165	20,787
Internal validation set	40 %	40 %	20 %	10 %	7 centers
# ICU/# Hospitals	104/45	135/98	307/NA	NA/32	NA/14
Time of data collection	First 24 h ICU admission	ICU admission	ICU admission	12 h and 24 h from ICU admission	ICU admission
AUC/goodness of fit (validation set)	0.88/p=0.08	0.823/p=0.31 (MPM$_0$)	0.848/p=0.39	0.941/p=0.4168 (PRISM III-12) 0.944/p=0.5504 (PRISM III-24)	0.9/p=0.42
Comments	Worst physiologic value in 1st 24 h			Most abnormal values 1st 12 h and 2nd 12 h of ICU stay PRISM III-12 -1st 12 h of ICU stay PRISM III-24 – 1st 24 h of ICU stay	
References	Zimmerman 2006	Higgins 2007	Moreno 2005	Pollack 1996	Slater 2003

APACHE Acute Physiology and Chronic Health Evaluations, *MPM* Mortality Probability Model, *SAPS* Simplified Acute Physiology Score, *PRISM* Pediatric Risk of Mortality Score, *PIM* Pediatric Index of Mortality, *NA* not available, *ICU* intensive care unit, *AUC* area under the curve

The Abbreviated Injury Scale (AIS) was originally developed to quantify injuries sustained in motor vehicle accidents [47]. The Injury Severity Score (ISS) was adapted from the AIS [48]. The ISS categorizes injuries to six regions of the body and rates the injury severity on a scale of 1–5 (1=minor, 5=critical/survival uncertain). The Trauma Score and Injury Severity Score (TRISS) method combines the RTS and ISS to create a mortality prediction score [49]. TRISS is commonly used for trauma benchmarking and can be applied to the pediatric population [44, 45, 50].

Congenital Heart Disease

Congenital heart disease (CHD) patients are a classic example of a population that requires coordination of multiple services and care systems to achieve a good outcome. Scoring systems for congenital heart disease are based on the diagnosis rather than patient specific physiologic variables. There are three scoring systems that have been developed to assess outcome of these patients. The earliest were the Risk Assessment in Congenital Heart Surgery (RACHS-1) and the Aristotle Basic Complexity (ABC) scores. Both were developed by consensus of experts. In contrast, the most recently developed score, the Society of Thoracic Surgery and the European Association for Cardiothoracic Surgery (STS-EACTS) Congenital Heart Surgery mortality score was empirically derived by retrospective analysis of outcomes from the procedure list defined by the ABC score.

RACHS-1 was the first pediatric congenital heart surgery scoring system developed [51]. This scoring system was developed by an 11 member panel of pediatric cardiologists and cardiovascular surgeons. Data was initially analyzed from over 9,000 patients in the Pediatric Cardiac Care Consortium [52] and hospital discharge data. This score was subsequently refined utilizing multi-institutional databases [53]. Similarly, the ABC score utilized the expert opinions of 50 internationally based congenital heart surgeons to evaluate 145 surgical procedures based on potential mortality, morbidity and technical difficulty [54]. The ABC score was subsequently validated using more than 35,000 cases from the STS-EACTS database [55].

The STS-EACTS score was developed to measure mortality associated with CHD based on analysis of more than 77,000 cases in the STS-EACTS database between 2002 and 2007 [56]. In total, 148 procedures were classified in mortality risk categories from 1 to 5 (1=low mortality risk, 5=high mortality risk). The score was externally validated in 27,700 operations, and showed a higher degree of discrimination for predicting mortality than the RACHS-1 or ABC score [56]. As with previous scores, a major limitation is that the STS-EACTS score does not allow adjustment for patient-specific risk factors.

Other

There are many scoring systems for specific conditions that are potentially relevant to the management of ICU patients. Some examples include scoring systems for croup [57], asthma [58], bronchiolitis [59] and meningococcemia [60, 61]. These scores have been used for triage decision making and severity of illness measurement. However, the ability to validate these models is limited by small patient populations.

Functional Outcome Scores

Functional outcome scores such as Pediatric Cerebral Performance Category (PCPC) and Pediatric Overall Performance Category (POPC) are modified from the Glasgow Outcome Scale [62, 63]. These scores are used to assess short-term changes in cognition (PCPC) and physical disabilities (POPC). Their major drawback is the need for the observer to project a functional status. While the PCPC has been correlated to 1 and 6 month neuropsychological tests such as the Bayley and IQ testing, there is a very large distribution of the neuropsychological tests in PCPC categories. The lack of discrimination would necessitate very large sample sizes if the test were used for long term outcome [64].

The Functional Status Scale (FSS) was recently developed to objectively measure functional outcome across the entire pediatric age range [65]. FSS was developed through a consensus process of pediatric experts and measures six domains of functioning. Domains include mental status, sensory functioning, communication, motor functioning, feeding and respiratory status which are scored from 1 to 5 (1=normal, 5=very severe dysfunction). The Adaptive Behavior Assessment System II (ABAS II) was used to establish construct validity and calibration within each functional domain. The FSS showed very good discrimination with ABAS II categories.

The Future of Scoring Systems

The future of scoring systems is likely to be largely influenced by the changes occurring in the structure and organization of care. Very large databases will become available to health services researchers that will enable more accurate and reliable mortality predictions. More reliable outcome predictions with general models such as PRISM and with disease or condition specific models will be used to assess and benchmark the quality of care in individual pediatric ICUs (PICU). These databases may become large enough to build models with sufficient performance characteristics that they have applicability to the individual pediatric critical care patient. The interest in transparency may dictate public disclosure of this information.

More reliable morbidity assessment methods such as the FSS will shift the paradigm of critical care outcome measurement from mortality prediction to a more global evaluation of functional outcome and morbidity. This will focus quality assessment of PICU therapies on morbidity as well as mortality which will further stimulate advances in quality research, case-mix adjustment methods, and forecasting outcomes. PICU admission data combined with quality of care data will be used to forecast long-term pediatric disability. When the likelihood of new morbidity as well as death becomes part of the outcome prediction models, they will have much greater applicability and utility to individual patients and individual patient decisions.

Conclusion

Scoring systems in intensive care medicine have increased in number and utility over the past 30 years. They are increasingly applicable to clinicians and health services researchers and in the future may be applicable to individual patients. Clinical scoring systems provide a standardized method for ICU benchmarking and are required by governing health care bodies. Additionally, benchmarking information is used by health care payers in creating managed care contracts. Consumer demands for error-free medicine, quality improvement and transparency may lead to public scoring of hospitals and individual physicians. These forces will continue to increase the need for risk adjusted outcomes and institutional benchmarking. It is in the intensivist's best interest to understand scoring systems, their applications and implications.

References

1. Kohn LT, Corrigan JM, Donaldson MS, editors. To err is human: building a safer health system. Washington, DC: National Academy Press; 1999.
2. Institute of Medicine. Crossing the quality chasm: a new health system for the twenty-first century. Washington, DC: National Academies Press; 2001.
3. Perkins HS, Jonsen AR, Epstein WV. Providers as predictors: using outcome predictions in intensive care. Crit Care Med. 1986;14:105–10.
4. Knaus WA, Wagner DP, Lynn J. Short-term mortality predictions for critically ill hospitalized adults: science and ethics. Science. 1991;254:389–94.
5. Poses RM, Bekes C, Copare FJ, et al. The answer to "what are my chances, doctor?" Depends on whom is asked: prognostic disagreement and inaccuracy for critically ill patients. Crit Care Med. 1989;17:827–33.
6. Poses RM, Bekes C, Winkler RL, et al. Are two (inexperienced) heads better than one (experienced) head? Averaging house officers' prognostic judgments for critically ill patients. Arch Intern Med. 1990;150:1874–8.
7. Stevens SM, Richardson DK, Gray JE, et al. Estimating neonatal mortality risk: an analysis of clinicians' judgments. Pediatrics. 1994;93:945–50.
8. McClish DK, Powell SH. How well can physicians estimate mortality in a medical intensive care unit? Med Decis Making. 1989;9:125–32.
9. Dawes RM, Faust D, Meehl PE. Clinical versus actuarial judgment. Science. 1989;243:1668–74.
10. Kruse JA, Thill-Baharozian MC, Carlson RW. Comparison of clinical assessment with APACE II for predicting mortality risk in patients admitted to a medical intensive care unit. JAMA. 1988;260:1739–42.
11. Marcin JP, Pollack MM, Patel KM, et al. Prognostication and certainty in the Pediatric Intensive Care Unit. Pediatrics. 1999;104(4):868–73.

12. Hanson CW, Marshall BE. Artificial intelligence applications in the intensive care unit. Crit Care Med. 2001;29:427–35.

13. Iberti TJ, Fischer EP, Leibowitz AB, et al. A multicenter study of physicians' knowledge of the pulmonary artery catheter. JAMA. 1990;264:2928–32.

14. Levetown M, Pollack MM, Cuerdon TT, et al. Limitations and withdrawals of medical intervention in pediatric critical care. JAMA. 1994;272:1271–5.

15. Morris AH. Developing and implementing computerized protocols for standardization of clinical decisions. Ann Intern Med. 2000;132:373–83.

16. Tversky A, Kahneman D. Availability. A heuristic for judging frequency and probability. In: Kahneman D, Slovic P, Tversky A, editors. Judgment under uncertainty: heuristics and biases. New York: Cambridge University Press; 1982. p. 163–78.

17. Jennings D, Amabile T, Ross L. Informal covariation assessment: data-based versus theory-based judgments. In: Kahneman D, Slovic P, Tversky A, editors. Judgment under uncertainty: heuristics and biases. New York: Cambridge University Press; 1982. p. 211–30.

18. Miller G. The magical number seven plus or minus two: some limits on our capacity for processing information. Psychol Rev. 1956;63:81–97.

19. Pearson GA. Mathematical morbidity in paediatric intensive care. Lancet. 2003;362:180–1.

20. Brennan TA, Leape LL, Laird N, et al. Incidence of adverse events and negligence in hospitalized patients: results of the Harvard Medical Practice Study I. N Engl J Med. 1991;324:370–6.

21. Leape LL, Brennan TA, Laird N, et al. The nature of adverse events in hospitalized patients: results of the Harvard Medical Practice Study II. N Engl J Med. 1991;324:377–84.

22. Pollack MM, Ruttimann UE, Getson PR. Accurate prediction of the outcome of pediatric intensive care. A new quantitative method. N Engl J Med. 1987;316:134–9.

23. Marcin JP, Pollack MM, Patel KM, et al. Combining physician's subjective and physiology-based objective mortality risk predictions. Crit Care Med. 2000;28:2984–90.

24. Pollack MM. Prediction of outcome. In: Fuhrman BP, Zimmerman JJ, editors. Pediatric critical care. 2nd ed. St. Louis: Mosby; 1998.

25. Pollack MM. It is what it was. Pediatr Crit Care Med. 2011;12:228–9.

26. Hand DJ. Statistical methods in diagnosis. Stat Methods Med Res. 1992;1:49–67.

27. Marcin JP, Pollack MM. Review of the methodologies and applications of scoring systems in neonatal and pediatric intensive care. Pediatr Crit Care Med. 2000;1:20–7.

28. Ruttimann UE. Statistical approaches to development and validation of predictive instruments. Crit Care Clin. 1994;10:19–35.

29. Lemeshow S, Hosmer DW. A review of goodness-of-fit statistics for use in the development of logistic regression models. Am J Epidemiol. 1982;115:92–106.

30. Cullen DJ, Civetta JM, Briggs BA, Ferrara LC. Therapeutic intervention scoring system: a method for quantitative comparison of patient care. Crit Care Med. 1974;2:57–60.

31. Pollack MM, Yeh TS, Ruttimann UE, et al. Evaluation of pediatric intensive care. Crit Care Med. 1984;12:376–83.

32. Zimmerman JE, Kramer AA, McNair DS, et al. Acute Physiology and Chronic Health Evaluation (APACHE) IV: hospital mortality assessment for today's critically ill patients. Crit Care Med. 2006;34:1297–310.

33. Higgins TL, Teres D, Copes WS, et al. Assessing contemporary intensive care unit outcome: an updated Mortality Probability Admission Model (MPM$_0$-III)*. Crit Care Med. 2007;35:827–35.

34. Moreno RP, Metnitz PG, Almeida E, et al. SAPS 3-from evaluation of the patient to evaluation of the intensive care unit. Part 2: development of a prognostic model for hospital mortality at ICU admission. Intensive Care Med. 2005;31:1345–55.

35. Pollack MM, Patel KM, Ruttimann UE. PRISM III: an updated Pediatric Risk of Mortality score. Crit Care Med. 1996;24:743–52.

36. Pollack MM, Ruttimann UE, Getson PR. Pediatric risk of mortality (PRISM) score. Crit Care Med. 1988;16:1110–6.

37. Slater A, Shann F, Pearson G, et al. PIM2: a revised version of the Paediatric Index of Mortality. Intensive Care Med. 2003;29:278–85.

38. Marshall JC, Cook DJ, Christou NV, et al. Multiple organ dysfunction score: a reliable descriptor of a complex clinical outcome. Crit Care Med. 1995;23:1638–52.

39. LeGall JR, Klar J, Lemeshow S, et al. The logistic organ dysfunction system a new way to assess organ dysfunction in the intensive care unit. JAMA. 1996;276:802–10.

40. Vincent JL, Moreno R, Takala J, et al. The SOFA (Sepsis-related Organ Failure Assessment) score to describe organ dysfunction/failure on behalf of the Working Group on Sepsis-Related Problems of the European Society of Intensive Care Medicine. Intensive Care Med. 1996;22:707–10.

41. Leteurtre S, Martinot A, Duhamel A, et al. Development of a pediatric multiple organ dysfunction score: use of two strategies. Med Decis Making. 1999;19:399–410.

42. Leteurtre S, Martinot A, Duhamel A, et al. Validation of the pediatric logistic organ dysfunction score: prospective, observational, multicentre study. Lancet. 2003;362:192–7.

43. Champion HR, Sacco WJ, Copes WS, et al. A revision of the trauma score. J Trauma. 1989;29:623–9.

44. Kaufmann CR, Maier RV, Kaufmann EJ, et al. Validity of applying adult TRISS analysis to injured children. J Trauma. 1991;31:691–8.

45. Orliaguet G, Meyer P, Blanot S, et al. Validity of applying TRISS analysis to paediatric blunt trauma patients managed in a French paediatric level I trauma centre. Intensive Care Med. 2001;27:743–50.

46. Eichelberger MR, Bowman LM, Sacco WJ, et al. Trauma score versus revised trauma score in TRISS to predict outcome in children with blunt trauma. Ann Emerg Med. 1989;18:939–42.

47. Baker SP, O'Neill B, Haddon W, et al. The injury severity score: a method for describing patients with multiple injuries and evaluating emergency care. J Trauma. 1974;14:187–96.

48. Copes WS, Lawrick M, Champion HR, et al. A comparison of abbreviated injury scale 1980 and 1985 version. J Trauma. 1988;28:78–86.

49. Boyd CR, Tolson MA, Copes WS. Evaluating trauma care: the TRISS method. J Trauma. 1987;27:370–8.

50. Eichelberger MR, Mangubat EA, Sacco WS, et al. Comparative outcomes of children and adults suffering blunt trauma. J Trauma. 1988;28:430–4.

51. Jenkins KJ, Gauvreau K, Newburger JW, et al. Consensus-based method for risk adjustment for surgery for congenital heart disease. J Thorac Cardiovasc Surg. 2002;123:110–8.

52. Moller JH. Perspectives in pediatric cardiology, Surgery of congenital heart disease: pediatric cardiac care consortium 1984–1995, vol. 6. New York: Futura Publishing; 1998. p. 279–329.

53. Jenkins KJ, Gauvreau K. Center specific differences in mortality: preliminary analyses using the Risk Adjustment in Congenital Heart Surgery (RACHS-1) method. J Thorac Cardiovasc Surg. 2002;124:97–104.

54. Lacour-Gayet F, Clarke D, Jacobs J, et al. The Aristotle score for congenital heart surgery. Pediatr Card Surg Annu Sem Thorac Cardiovasc Surg. 2004;7:185–91.

55. O'Brien SM, Jacobs JP, Clarke DR, et al. Accuracy of the Aristotle basic complexity score for classifying the mortality and morbidity potential of congenital heart surgery operations. Ann Thorac Surg. 2007;84:2027–37.

56. O'Brien SM, Clarke DR, Jacobs JP, et al. An empirically based tool for analyzing mortality associated with congenital heart disease. J Thorac Cardiovasc Surg. 2009;138:1139–53.

57. Jacobs S, Shortland G, Warner J, et al. Validation of a croup score and its use in triaging children with croup. Anaesthesia. 1994; 49:903–6.

58. Wood DW, Downes JJ, Lecks HI. A clinical scoring system for the diagnosis of respiratory failure. Preliminary report on childhood status asthmaticus. Am J Dis Child. 1972;123:227–8.

59. Walsh P, Rothenberg SJ, O'Doherty S, et al. A validated clinical model to predict the need for admission and length of stay in children with acute bronchiolitis. Eur J Emerg Med. 2004;11:265–72.

60. Alistair PJT, Sillis JA, Hart CA. Validation of the Glasgow Meningococcal Septicemia Prognostic Score: a 10-year retrospective survey. Crit Care Med. 1991;19:26–30.

61. Hachimi-Idrissi S, Corne L, Ramet J. Evaluation of scoring systems in acute meningococcaemia. Eur J Emerg Med. 1998;5:225–30.

62. Fiser DH. Assessing the outcome of pediatric intensive care. J Pediatr. 1992;121:68–74.

63. Marcin JP, Pollack MP. Review of the acuity scoring systems for the pediatric intensive care unit and their use in quality improvement. J Intensive Care Med. 2007;22:131–40.

64. Fiser DH, Long N, Roberson PK, Hefley G, Zolten K, Brodie-Fowler M. Crit Care Med. 2000;28(7):2616–20.

65. Pollack MM, Holubkov R, Glass P, et al. Functional status scale: new pediatric outcome measure. Pediatrics. 2009;124:e18–28.

Pharmacology in the PICU

7

James B. Besunder and John Pope

Abstract

Rational drug therapy requires the application of pharmacologic principles to maximize efficacy while minimizing adverse reactions. In the setting of the Pediatric Intensive Care Unit (PICU), drug therapy is predicated on an understanding of the pathophysiology of the disease being treated, the pharmacology of the drug(s) selected and the expected effects (therapeutic and toxic) of the chosen agents. An understanding of how disease processes, genetics and other concurrent treatments affect the pharmacologic properties of drugs is also paramount to a rational approach to drug therapy. Two therapeutic strategies, target effect and target concentration are commonly employed when administering medications to treat specific diseases.

Pharmacokinetics describe the processes of drug absorption, distribution, biotransformation, and excretion; what the body does to a drug. Pharmacodynamics describe the relationship between a drug's concentration at its site of action and its effect; what a drug does to the body. Pharmacokinetics and Pharmacodynamics may be influenced by developmental changes, interactions with other drugs or nutrients, disease states, and genetic influences such as polymorphisms.

Drug interactions can be classified as drug-drug, drug-disease, or drug-food interactions. The mechanism can be divided into pharmaceutical, pharmacokinetic or pharmacodynamic interactions. The most serious drug interactions involve drugs with severe toxicities and a narrow therapeutic index.

Medication errors are a common cause of adverse drug reactions and have unfortunately been associated with fatalities in too many cases.

This chapter reviews basic pharmacologic principles and their bedside application to provide a guide for safe and rational drug therapy in caring for the critically ill child.

Keywords

Pharmacokinetics • Pharmacodynamics • Drug interactions • Drug safety • Pharmacogenetics • First order kinetics • Zero order kinetics • Target effect strategy • Target concentration strategy

Rational drug therapy requires the application of pharmacologic principles to maximize efficacy while minimizing adverse reactions. In the setting of the Pediatric Intensive Care Unit (PICU), rational drug therapy is predicated on an understanding of the pathophysiology of the disease being treated and the pharmacology of the drug(s) selected and their expected effects (therapeutic and toxic). An understanding

J.B. Besunder, DO (✉) • J. Pope, MD
Department of Pediatrics, Akron Children's Hospital,
1 Perkins Square, Akron, OH 44308, USA
e-mail: jbesunder@chmca.org; jpope@chmca.org

D.S. Wheeler et al. (eds.), *Pediatric Critical Care Medicine*,
DOI 10.1007/978-1-4471-6362-6_7, © Springer-Verlag London 2014

of how disease processes, genetics and other concurrent treatments affect the pharmacologic properties of drugs is also paramount to a rational approach to drug therapy. This chapter reviews basic pharmacologic principles and their application in caring for the critically ill child.

Principles of Pharmacokinetics and Pharmacodynamics

The clinical effect of a drug, whether it is a therapeutic or toxic effect, depends upon the drug's concentration at the site of action and the subsequent host response [1, 2]. Pharmacokinetics describes the processes of drug absorption, distribution, biotransformation, and excretion (i.e., what the body does to a drug). Pharmacokinetics determines a drug's concentration at its site of action. It is only the free (unbound) fraction of drug in plasma that is available for distribution into tissues to exert a therapeutic or toxic effect. It is also only the free fraction of drug that is available for biotransformation and elimination from the body. Pharmacodynamics describes the relationship between a drug's concentration at its site of action and its effect (i.e., what the drug does to the body). It encompasses the mechanism(s) of action of a drug, its therapeutic effect, and its safety profile. The pharmacokinetic and pharmacodynamic properties of an agent may be influenced by developmental changes, interactions with other drugs or nutrients, disease states, and genetics.

Pharmacokinetics

Absorption

Absorption describes the rate and extent to which a drug leaves its administration site and can be influenced by physicochemical factors, patient factors, and disease states (Table 7.1). Increased oral drug absorption is favored by small molecular size, the nonionized state, and high lipid solubility. Several aspects of oral drug absorption are pertinent to the critical care setting. An understanding of oral absorption is important in the setting of an acute ingestion in order to anticipate when toxic symptoms may commence. Second, the oral route for drug absorption should not be relied upon early in the course of an acutely ill patient, particularly if there is evidence of hypoperfusion or hypotension. Once stable, however, it is important to appreciate that there is no difference in drug effectiveness between oral and intravenous (IV) administration for many classes of drugs (e.g. H_2 blockers, nonsteroidal anti-inflammatory agents, steroids, anticonvulsants). The oral route may be less expensive and obviate IV administration when vascular access is limited. However, other factors such as level of consciousness, nothing-by-mouth status, or drug-food interactions may

Table 7.1 Factors affecting drug absorption

Physicochemical factors	Disease states
Product formulation	Shock
Disintegration and dissolution rates	Congestive heart failure
Drug release characteristics	Gastroenteritis
Ionization state	Short gut
Lipid/water solubility	**Patient factors**
Drug concentration	Gastric emptying time
Molecular weight	Intestinal motility
	Absorptive surface area
	pH at absorptive site
	Blood flow to administration site

Table 7.2 Alternative routes of drug administration

Intramuscular	Per rectum	Intranasal
Fosphenytoin	Acetaminophen	DDAVP
Midazolam	Diazepam	Midazolam[b]
Phenobarbital	Midazolam[b]	Fentanyl[b]
Succinylcholine	Lorazepam	Sufentanyl[b]
Vecuronium	Carbamazepine	Ketamine[b]
Pancuronium	Thiopental	**Sublingual**
Rocuronium	Clonazepam	Nitroglycerin
Morphine	Valproic acid	Nifedipine
Ketamine	Topiramate	**Subcutaneous**
Glucagon	**Percutaneous**	Insulin
Antibiotics[a]	Nitroglycerin	Epinephrine
Deferoxamine	Clonidine	Octreotide
	Fentanyl	Morphine(pump)
		Deferoxamine(pump)

[a]All β-lactam and cephalosporins that can be administered IV, aminoglycosides, clindamycin
[b]Administer the IV formulation

necessitate IV administration. Finally, diarrheal states are rarely associated with drug malabsorption.

Other routes besides the oral and IV routes may be utilized for drug administration in the intensive care unit (Table 7.2). These alternative routes are typically used when the patient's disease state or condition precludes oral drug administration or vascular access is limited. The intraosseous route can be utilized in an emergency for virtually all drugs, including inotropes, pressors, and anticonvulsants [3], while epinephrine, atropine, and lidocaine can be administered via an endotracheal tube. Absorption of drugs following intramuscular (IM) injection is influenced by many of the physicochemical and physiological factors that affect oral absorption. Tissue perfusion is a critical factor affecting drug absorption from the injection site. Patients with shock, congestive heart failure (CHF), or hypotension may not reliably absorb drugs administered IM. Other important factors include absorptive surface area, water solubility at physiologic pH (e.g. low water solubility of phenytoin and digoxin results in precipitation at the injection site), and muscle activity.

The rectal route is useful for administration of certain drugs when the oral route is contraindicated or when vascular access is not available. Many anticonvulsant drugs may be given per rectum (PR) including diazepam [Diastat®, Elan®]; the liquid, oral formulations of valproic acid, carbamazepine, topiramate, and clonazepam; and the IV forms of midazolam and lorazepam. The potential for hepatic first pass metabolism is less with the PR than the oral route because approximately 50 % of the absorbed drug bypasses the liver. However, rectal drug absorption may be irregular, incomplete, or cause mucosal irritation.

The intranasal route (IN) is the preferred site for administration of DDAVP in children with diabetes insipidus. This route has been used for administration of sedative agents preoperatively or in the PICU for procedural sedation over the past 15 years. IN administration has pharmacokinetic advantages over the oral and PR routes, including faster onset of action and potentially higher bioavailability and plasma concentration. Following IN administration of a 0.2 mg/kg dose of midazolam, plasma concentrations exceeding the threshold level for sedation are reached in 6 min with peak plasma concentrations observed in approximately 12 min [4]. These plasma concentrations are comparable to those obtained 30 min after IM [5] or oral administration [6] and much greater than those observed after PR administration of the same dose [4]. Chiaretti et al. reported a mean duration of sedation of 23 min (range 10–50 min) in 46 children following a 0.5 mg/kg IN dose for procedural sedation [7]. Pretreatment with IN lidocaine spray (10 mg) prevented nasal burning and bitter taste. In the home setting, IN midazolam is at least as effective as rectal diazepam for management of acute seizures, less expensive and socially, a more acceptable alternative [8]. Bhattacharyya and colleagues performed a randomized, controlled study of IN midazolam vs rectal diazepam in children presenting to their emergency department or outpatient clinic. Time to administer the drug (50.6 s vs 68.3 s) and time to cessation of seizure (116.7 s vs 178.6 s) were both significantly shorter for the midazolam group [9]. Vomiting and excessive drowsiness occurred more frequently in the diazepam group (10.4 % vs 0 %, p=0.009). IN midazolam should be considered as an alternative to PR administration of benzodiazepines in the hospitalized patient without vascular access because of its favorable pharmacokinetics, safety, and cost, in addition to obviating rectal administration.

Drug Distribution

Drug distribution describes the movement of drugs, active metabolites, and toxins from the systemic circulation to tissues or other body compartments. Drugs must distribute to their target tissues to exert a therapeutic or toxic effect. The extent and rate of distribution out of the blood compartment is influenced by binding affinity of the drug for plasma and tissue proteins, lipid/water solubility, ionization state at physiologic pH, and molecular size. Increased plasma protein binding, in general, decreases the free fraction of drug available for distribution (e.g. warfarin). An alteration in plasma or tissue protein binding is an important mechanism for drug-drug interactions. The more lipid soluble a drug is, the greater its extent and more rapid its distribution. This may have important clinical implications. For example, theophylline, being poorly lipophilic, does not distribute into adipose tissue. In obese patients, dosing should be based on ideal body weight rather than actual weight. β(beta)-Blockers, in part because of their differences in lipid/water solubility, have varying abilities to cross the blood brain barrier and cause central nervous system side effects. Diazepam, being extremely lipophilic, reaches peak brain concentrations in 60 s compared to phenytoin and phenobarbital which reach peak brain concentrations in 45–60 min. The degree of protein binding and the volume of distribution are also important factors in determining whether a drug can be removed from the body by dialysis. In general, highly protein bound drugs or drugs with a large volume of distribution are not amenable to removal by dialysis.

Drug Metabolism

The primary organ for drug metabolism is the liver, although the kidney, intestine, lung, adrenal, and skin are also capable of biotransforming certain compounds. For many drugs (i.e., lipophilic weak acids or weak bases), biotransformation to more polar, water-soluble compounds facilitates their elimination from the body via the bile, kidney, or lung. Although the biotransformation of most drugs results in pharmacologically weaker or inactive compounds, parent compounds may be transformed into active metabolites (e.g. vecuronium, procainamide, carbamazepine) or into a toxic metabolite (e.g. acetaminophen to N-acetyl-para-benzoquinoneimine). Conversely, pharmacologically inactive parent compounds or prodrugs may be converted to their active moiety (e.g. enalapril to enalaprilat).

Drug biotransformation within the hepatocyte involves two primary enzymatic processes: phase I or nonsynthetic, and phase II, or synthetic reactions. Phase I reactions, including oxidation, reduction, hydrolysis, and hydroxylation reactions, are typically catalyzed by the mixed-function oxidase enzyme systems located in the microsomes (e.g. cytochrome P450 system). Cytochrome P450 enzymes are categorized into families (e.g. CYP1, CYP2, CYP3) and subfamilies identified by a letter (e.g. CYP3A). Within a subfamily there may be different isoforms identified by an Arabic number (e.g. CYP3A4). CYP3A4 is the major metabolic pathway, being responsible for the metabolism of ~50 % of drugs, followed by CYP2D6 (31 %), and CYP2C9 (10 %) [10]. The various isoforms have characteristic inhibitors and inducers of their activity. Knowledge of which drugs are substrates for the different cytochrome P450 isoforms, as well as their selective inhibitors/inducers, allows for the understanding and prediction of drug-drug and herbal-drug interactions (see later discussion). Phase II reactions primarily involve conjugation with glycine, glucuronide, or sulfate. Conjugation reactions are also involved in drug detoxification (e.g. conjugation of N-acetyl-para-benzoquinoneimine with glutathione).

Recently, Phase III enzymes have been identified that include P-glycoprotein (PGP) and related transporters. These enzymes are located in numerous organs including the liver, intestine, and kidney. PGP can block or facilitate drug entry into cells. PGP is located in intestinal cells, renal tubular cells, biliary cannilicular cells, and the blood brain barrier. Interactions at these sites, particularly with PGP, explain some of the non-metabolic drug -drug interactions that have been described (see later discussion) [11].

Drug Elimination

Drug elimination usually occurs through the kidney or the liver. There are a few notable exceptions including the degradation of succinylcholine by plasma pseudocholinesterase and atracurium and cisatracurium by Hoffman degradation (pH and temperature dependent). The renal elimination of drugs mostly depends on glomerular filtration with tubular secretion also playing a role. The amount of drug that is filtered per unit time is influenced by the degree of protein binding of the drug; the greater the protein binding, the less the amount of filtered drug. As mentioned previously, the degree of protein binding also influences the elimination of a drug in patients undergoing hemodialysis or peritoneal dialysis; that is drugs that are highly protein bound are less easily dialyzed.

Developmental Effects on Pharmacokinetics and Pharmacodynamics

Safe and effective drug therapy for children requires an understanding of ontogenetic changes in drug disposition and action. Developmental effects on pharmacokinetics explain many of the differences in the dose-response curve among different age groups. Pharmacodynamics may also undergo developmental changes as seen with the increased risk of apnea with opiates in infants less than 6 months of age. However, because of the paucity of information describing these changes, we discuss only the developmental effects on pharmacokinetics. This topic has been extensively reviewed elsewhere [12–14]. Neonates have a relatively higher gastric pH which increases the bioavailability of basic compounds such as penicillin G, whereas weak acids such as

phenobarbital may require a higher oral dose in order to achieve therapeutic plasma levels. Gastric acid secretion appears to increase as a function of postnatal age and approaches adult values by 3 months of age [15]. The rate of gastric emptying is highly variable during the neonatal period and is influenced by a number of factors. In general, the rate at which drugs are absorbed is slower in neonates and infants. This may delay the time to and blunt the peak plasma drug concentration.

The absolute amounts of body water and fat clearly depend on the child's age and have been well characterized by Friis-Hansen [16]. The percentage of body weight composed of fat approximates 0.5 % in the young fetus, increasing to 15 % at birth, and 20 % by age 6 months, before beginning to fall gradually until adolescence [14, 16]. Highly lipid soluble agents such as inhalational anesthetic agents and lipophilic sedative/hypnotic agents (e.g. diazepam, fentanyl) exhibit a larger apparent volume of distribution (V_d) in infants because of their relatively larger proportion of body fat. Neonates and infants up to approximately 6–12 months of age also have a relatively larger percentage of total body weight as water and a larger extracellular fluid compartment compared to adults. These differences increase the V_d of water-soluble drugs (e.g. aminoglycosides) and result in lower plasma concentrations when the drugs are administered according to body weight.

Drug binding to plasma proteins depends on a number of age-related variables, most notably the amount of circulating albumin and α-1 acid glycoprotein, the number of binding sites, and their binding affinity [17]. Developmental changes in these variables can influence the distribution of highly bound drugs. In general, neonates have an increased free fraction of highly bound drugs owing to a reduced quantity of plasma proteins, decreased binding affinity of fetal albumin for weak acids, and the presence of endogenous substances (e.g. bilirubin, free fatty acids) that compete for binding sites on plasma proteins with drugs. Beyond the neonatal period, these changes do not appear to be clinically significant. However, ontogenetic changes in tissue binding can affect drug distribution beyond the neonatal period. The myocardial to plasma ratio of digoxin in children up to approximately 3 years of age is two to three times that of adults. This, along with increased erythrocyte binding, greatly increases the V_d of digoxin [18, 19].

The variability in activity of Phase I enzymes at birth and their ontological maturation can be explained by genetic variation (e.g. CYP2C9, CYP2C19, CYP2D6) in some isoforms but not others such as CYP3A4 [20] (see later discussion). The activity of many Phase I enzyme systems, particularly the oxidizing enzymes, is markedly reduced in newborns. This is reflected by the prolonged elimination time for drugs dependent on these pathways (e.g. midazolam, phenytoin). The maturation of the hepatic cytochrome P450 system appears to be a function of postnatal age with metabolic capacities for the group reaching or exceeding that of adults by 3–6 months of age [13]. For example, hepatic clearance of midazolam increases nearly eightfold from birth to 3 months of age [21]. Subsequently, clearance exceeds adult rates up to approximately 10 years of age for most drugs metabolized by Phase I enzymes (e.g. carbamazepine, theophylline, warfarin). This mandates higher drug doses adjusted for body weight to maintain therapeutic plasma levels in this age range compared to adults. Anderson and Lynn [22] reviewed the differences in activity of specific Phase 1 enzyme isoforms at birth and their maturational process. Activity of CYP3A4 (e.g. midazolam) increases to ~20 % adult values by 1 month of age and reaches 72 % by 1 year of age. CYP2C9 activity (e.g. warfarin) is ~20 % of adult values at birth and reaches 50 % by 1 month of age. CYP1A2 (e.g. caffeine) activity is negligible at birth and reaches adult values by 10–11 months of age. CYP2D6 activity increases sharply after birth until 2 weeks of age, and then does not increase further during the first year of life.

There is a paucity of data describing the ontogeny of phase II enzyme reactions, though there appears to be great variation in the maturation of the different conjugation pathways. Glucuronidation of drugs is very immature at birth and matures at a rate similar to that for GFR (see below) [23], achieving adults rates by approximately 3 years of age [24]. Examples of drugs primarily cleared by glucuronidation include acetaminophen, morphine, dexmedetomidine and propofol, The capacity to biotransform propofol matures faster than the former drugs because propofol also undergoes Phase 1 enzyme reactions [23]. On the other hand, sulfation appears to be more mature at birth. For example, acetaminophen-sulfate formation is increased in neonates and young children compared to adolescents and adults [25]. The overall increased conjugation of acetaminophen (and consequently a smaller percentage of the parent compound undergoing oxidative metabolism) in young children along with larger glutathione stores are possible explanations for the lower risk of acetaminophen-induced hepatotoxicity observed in children under 6 years of age.

A similar age-dependent increase in the functional capacity of the kidney is also observed. Most drugs, or their water-soluble metabolites, are excreted from the body by the kidneys. Glomerular filtration rate (GFR) approximates 2–4 ml/min in full-term infants, increasing to ~8–20 ml/min by 2–3 days of life, and approaches adult values by ~3–5 months of age [26]. The maturation of GFR is a function of gestational age and postconceptual age rather than postnatal age [27]. Tubular secretion is immature at birth as well and matures at a slower rate than GFR reaching adult values by ~30 weeks of life [28]. An adjustment in the dosing interval for drugs such as the aminoglycosides and vancomycin that reflects these principles is required in premature and term infants to obviate toxicity.

Pharmacogenomics

Just as ontogenetic development has a tremendous impact on drug biotransformation, it has been known for some time that certain adverse drug reactions are a consequence of inherited variations in biotransforming enzyme activity. Pharmacogenomics is the study of the role of genetic variation in drug response and uses genome wide association methodology to identify specific, individual candidate genes responsible for variation. Pharmacogenetics refers to the effect of a specific gene on drug disposition [29, 30]. Genetic polymorphisms in the cytochrome P450 enzyme system account for many of the known heritable variations in drug metabolism. For example, there are multiple variants of CYP2D6 that can be inherited resulting in poor, intermediate, extensive, or ultrarapid metabolism of target substrates [31]. Codeine is transformed to morphine by CYP2D6. Patients with poor CYP2D6 activity achieve significantly less analgesic effect from codeine than patients with higher levels of enzyme activity [32]. Patients with ultrarapid genotype are at risk for significant toxicity due to the rapid conversion of codeine to morphine, leading to increased serum concentrations of the latter, resulting in CNS and respiratory depression [33]. Breastfed infants of mothers with an ultrarapid metabolizing genotype are at risk of developing morphine toxicity when the neonate's mother is taking therapeutic doses of codeine [34]. Genetic polymorphism of CYP2C9 accounts for a portion of the interindividual variation in response to warfarin [31], and decreased activity of this enzyme has also resulted in phenytoin toxicity [35]. Genotype affects other mechanisms of drug disposition as well. Warfarin effect is also determined by mutations in the drug's target, vitamin K epoxide reductase, encoded by the vitamin K reductase complex 1 (*VCORC1*). Genotyping patients for *CYP2C9* and *VCORC1* has been shown to decrease the incidence of hospitalization for bleeding and thromboembolism when compared to standard dosing [36]. Testing for HLA-B genotype is used to decrease the risk of Stevens-Johnson syndrome in at-risk populations, such as Asians, receiving carbamazepine. Carriers of *HLAB*1502* are at higher risk for life-threatening skin reactions such as Stevens-Johnson syndrome when exposed to carbamazepine [37]. Variation in response of asthmatics to inhaled corticosteroids has been linked to glucocorticoid-induced transcript 1 gene (*GLCCI1*). Asthmatics with a *GLCCI1* variant were shown to have a significant decrease in their response to inhaled glucocorticoids [38]. Genetic determination of drug response is certainly only part of a complex system. Disease state, age, and other medications all may interact with a patient's genetic make-up leading to alterations in the expected response to a drug [39, 40]. Despite our rapidly expanding knowledge of pharmacogenomics, its clinical applicability is still limited to few medications. The clinical utility of pharmacogenomics is likely to change in the near future as more genetic markers are defined which predict both adverse and desired responses to individual medications.

Bedside Application of Pharmacokinetic Principles

There are five key parameter estimates that are useful in predicting a drug's plasma concentration and in selecting or modifying a dosing strategy. These are bioavailability (F), V_d, clearance (Cl), elimination half life ($t_{1/2}\beta(beta)$), and elimination rate constant (K_d).

Bioavailability

Bioavailablity of a drug is not synonymous with absorption. It reflects the fraction of the administered drug dose that reaches the systemic circulation as unchanged drug. For orally administered drugs, it is affected by absorption and metabolism in the gastrointestinal tract and liver. If the extraction ratio by the liver for a drug is high (see later discussion of clearance), it will exhibit a large *first pass effect*, and only a small fraction of the administered dose will reach the systemic circulation (low bioavailability). A comparison of a drug's bioavailablity following nonintravenous and IV (100 % for most drugs) administration can be used to select a dose when converting from IV therapy. For example, the bioavailability of furosemide is approximately 50 %. Therefore, the dose of the drug should be doubled when switching from IV to oral administration. On the other hand, phenobarbital, phenytoin, and valproic acid have an oral bioavailability of nearly 100 %. Therefore, the same total daily dose should be used when switching to oral therapy. However, although the total daily dose of drugs such as phenytoin and valproic acid is the same regardless of whether administered orally or IV, the dosing interval is usually shorter when given IV. This is due to the relatively long absorption curve for these drugs and the desire to minimize peak-trough fluctuations in plasma levels (e.g. IV valproic acid and phenytoin are commonly administered every 6 and 8 h, respectively vs. every 8 and 12 h, respectively with oral dosing).

Volume of Distribution

The volume of distribution (V_d) of a drug relates the amount of drug in the body to its plasma concentration. It is a hypothetical volume in which a drug is placed in order to yield the initial plasma concentration. It is useful in calculating loading doses of drugs according to the following equation:

$$\Delta C = D / V_d$$

where ΔC is the change in plasma concentration and D is the dose administered.

For example, if the average V_d of theophylline is 0.5 L/kg (95 % CI: 0.3–0.7 L/kg), then a loading dose of 6 mg/kg (equal to 7.5 mg/kg aminophylline) would achieve a post distribution plasma concentration of 12 mg/L (95 % CI: 9–20 mg/L). Obtaining a peak level 30 min after the bolus is administered allows one to calculate the patient's actual V_d using the above equation. This calculated V_d can then be used if subsequent bolus doses are required.

Clearance

Clearance (Cl) describes the rate of drug removal. It can be addressed in terms of plasma clearance (Clp), organ clearance, or total body clearance. Plasma clearance is the volume of plasma from which a drug is completely removed per unit of time. Drugs can be cleared by several mechanisms, the most important of which include metabolic biotransformation in the liver, elimination in the feces or urine, and exhalation by the lungs. Hepatic clearance can be classified as either flow limited or capacity limited, depending on the drug's extraction ratio. Flow-limited drugs (e.g. lidocaine) have a high extraction ratio and a high intrinsic metabolic clearance as compared to flow rate. Hepatic blood flow, therefore, is the rate-limiting factor regarding clearance of these drugs. Factors such as CHF, shock, and drugs (e.g. β(beta)-blockers, cimetidine) that reduce hepatic blood flow will decrease their clearance and increase the risk of toxicity. As previously mentioned, drugs whose clearance is flow limited, also demonstrate a marked first pass effect. Most drugs metabolized by the liver, however, are capacity limited – the rate-limiting step in hepatic clearance is not hepatic blood flow, rather, it is the capacity of the liver to take up and metabolize the drug.

Plasma clearance of a drug is described most frequently by the following equations:

$$Clp = (0.693)(V_d) / t_{1/2\beta(beta)} = (K_d)(V_d)$$

or Clp = IR/Cpss

Rearranged, the second equation yields the steady-state relationship for drugs obeying first order elimination kinetics (see later discussion):

$$IR = (Clp)(Cpss)$$

where IR is the amount of drug administered per unit time (e.g. $\mu g\ kg^{-1}\ min^{-1}$, mg/day, etc.), and Cpss is the steady-state plasma drug concentration. In other words, the amount of drug given per unit time equals the amount of drug removed.

Elimination Half-Life

The elimination half life ($t_{1/2}\beta_{(beta)}$) of a drug is commonly used to describe its disappearance from the blood. This pharmacokinetic parameter estimate reflects the time required for half the amount of drug present in the blood to be cleared from the blood. After one half- life, 50 % of the drug initially present remains, after two half-lives, 25 % remains, and so forth. The $t_{1/2}\beta_{(beta)}$ is described by the following equation:

$$t_{1/2\beta(beta)} = 0.693 / \left(K_d \right)$$

where K_d is the slope of the log concentration versus time curve. Most drugs are administered at intervals of one to three half-lives. A dosing interval of one half-life may be selected if it is desirable to minimize peak-trough fluctuations in concentration (with anticonvulsants) or when a certain plasma concentration must be exceeded for the majority of the dosing interval (e.g. effective β(beta)-lactam antibiotic therapy requires that the plasma concentration exceeds the MIC of the organism for most of the dosing interval). A longer dosing interval is selected for drugs requiring a low trough concentration in order to avoid toxicity (e.g. aminoglycosides). It is also a very useful clinical parameter in the selection of a dosing interval and occasionally a drug dose in patients with organ failure. For drugs exclusively eliminated by the kidneys, the increase in dosing interval is inversely proportional to the ratio of the normal to observed $t_{1/2}\beta_{(beta)}$. The $t_{1/2}\beta_{(beta)}$ is also useful in predicting when steady state is achieved. For drugs eliminated by first order kinetics (see later discussion), steady state is reached after five half lives. If the $t_{1/2}\beta_{(beta)}$ is long, the time to reach its steady state plasma concentration will also be long. For drugs with a relatively long $t_{1/2}\beta_{(beta)}$, a loading dose of the drug may be given to rapidly achieve the target concentration if an immediate effect of the drug is desired (e.g. phenytoin, phenobarbital, digitalis, theophylline, milrinone). The loading dose is based on the average V_d derived from population statistics and the desired plasma concentration. The maintenance dose and dosing interval (or continuous infusion rate) are then selected to maintain the desired plasma drug level.

Metabolism and elimination of most drugs exhibit first order or linear kinetics; a constant fraction of drug is lost per unit time. Under these conditions, $t_{1/2}\beta_{(beta)}$ and Cl are independent of drug dose and are constant. Therefore, the plasma concentration at steady state is linearly proportional to the dose per unit time. For example, if a patient's steady state

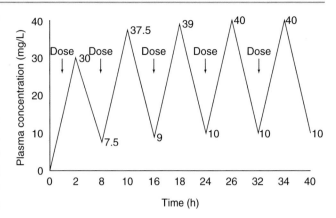

Fig. 7.1 Law of superimposition. Vancomycin plasma concentrations over time following administration of 20 mg/kg every 8 h

plasma phenobarbital concentration is 20 mg/L and a concentration of 30 mg/L is desired, then the dose should be increased by 50 %.

The law of superimposition can be applied to drugs eliminated by first order kinetics and administered as intermittent IV or oral doses. It assumes that V_d and $t_{1/2}\beta_{(beta)}$ do not change. It predicts the peak and trough plasma concentrations at steady state following the first dose of a drug. Figure 7.1 illustrates this principle. A 20 mg/kg dose of vancomycin is administered and a peak level of 30 mg/L is obtained 1 h after a 1-h infusion. A trough concentration of 7.5 mg/L is obtained 8 h after the first dose. If the dose, dosing interval, V_d and $t_{1/2}\beta_{(beta)}$ remain unchanged, steady state-peak and trough levels of ~40 mg/L and 10 mg/L, respectively, will be achieved. In this example, the V_d is 0.67 L/kg and the $t_{1/2}\beta_{(beta)}$ is 3 h (the time between peak and trough levels is 6 h, which represents two half- lives). We often use this principle to modify the dose or dosing interval prior to reaching steady state conditions in order to achieve target concentrations. For example, in a critically ill child with suspected methicillin resistant *Staphylococcal aureus* (MRSA) infection, a peak level after the first dose and a trough prior to the second can facilitate achieving the desired trough concentration (see more discussion under target concentration). Knowledge of $t_{1/2}\beta_{(beta)}$ and first order kinetics may also allow predictions of duration of symptoms following an acute overdose. For example, if a patient has a peak carbamazepine level of 40 mg/L and has received effective gastric decontamination, then the level should fall below 20 mg/L after one half-life (approximately 10–15 h).

Zero order or nonlinear kinetics describes drug elimination when the metabolic or elimination pathways are saturable. When this occurs, a constant amount rather than a constant fraction (as occurs with first order kinetics) of drug is metabolized per unit time. Clearance and $t_{1/2}\beta$, therefore, vary with the concentration of the drug. This process

Fig. 7.2 First-order vs zero-order pharmacokinetics. The figure on the *left* illustrates the relationship between rate of drug elimination and plasma concentration under first and zero order conditions. The figure on the *right* depicts the change in plasma concentration as a function of dose under first and zero-order kinetic conditions

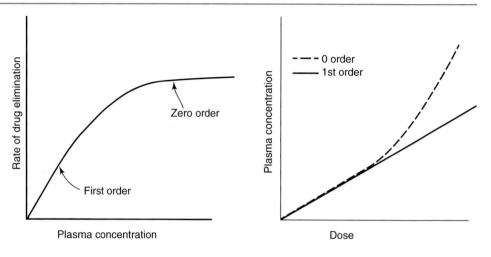

is known as Michaelis-Menten kinetics. The K_m of a drug defines the plasma concentration at which half of the maximal rate of drug elimination (V_{max}) is reached. When the plasma concentration is less than K_m, the drug is eliminated by a first order process, and when the plasma concentration exceeds K_m, the drug is eliminated by a zero order process. At high plasma concentrations, the $t_{1/2}\beta_{(beta)}$ appears very long. Dose adjustments should be made cautiously as small increases in dose may cause large increases in drug concentration since drug elimination does not increase proportionately. In general, daily dose adjustments should not exceed 10–20 % of the dose, and the plasma level should be followed closely. Common drugs or toxins that obey zero order kinetics include phenytoin, salicylates, ethanol, furosemide, and indomethacin. Also, it appears that approximately 40 % of children may eliminate theophylline according to Michaelis-Menten kinetics rather than as a first order process with the K_m being in the low to mid therapeutic range [41]. Figure 7.2 illustrates differences between first order and zero order kinetics.

Target-Effect Versus Target-Concentration Strategies

One of two therapeutic strategies is commonly employed when administering medications to treat specific diseases. Most medications are administered using a target-effect strategy, i.e., a drug is administered with a therapeutic end-point in mind. The patient is monitored for attainment of the therapeutic goal or development of toxicity related to the medication. If the therapeutic goal is not obtained and toxicity is not observed, one may consider titrating the dose of the medication. Another agent may be substituted or added if the therapeutic goal is not achieved, sequential increases in dose does not result in a heightened physiological effect, or if toxicity supervenes. For instance, in a patient with septic shock, low systemic vascular resistance and hypotension, dopamine

Table 7.3 Indications for plasma drug concentration monitoring

Significant interindividual variation in pharmacokinetics (e.g. theophylline)
Narrow therapeutic index (e.g. theophylline)
Zero-order kinetics apply (e.g. phenytoin)
Signs of toxicity may be delayed or difficult to recognize clinically (e.g. tacrolimus, aminoglycosides)
Physiologic, pathologic or developmental factors are present which may affect drug pharmacokinetics (e.g. pregnancy, organ dysfunction, prematurity; various medications)
Intercurrent illness present which may affect drug pharmacokinetics (e.g. influenza and theophylline, trauma and phenytoin)
Drugs used to treat chronic states with intermittent symptoms (e.g. anticonvulsants and seizures)
Usual dose does not produce expected results
Monitoring compliance
Suspected drug-drug or drug-food interaction

Reprinted from Reed and Blumer [43]. With permission from Elsevier

is started and the dose titrated to achieve a targeted blood pressure. If the desired blood pressure is not reached despite using 20 mcg kg⁻¹ min⁻¹ of dopamine, a second agent such as norepinephrine can be added and titrated to achieve the target blood pressure [42]. In this example, there is no reason the dose of dopamine cannot be increased above 20 mcg kg⁻¹ min⁻¹ except that the likelihood of achieving therapeutic efficacy above this dose diminishes. A more potent, direct-acting vasopressor such as norepinephrine, is more likely to achieve the targeted goal.

The target-concentration strategy uses measurement of a drug concentration, usually in serum or plasma, as an intermediate end-point to achieving the desired therapeutic effect. The drug concentration often also serves as a marker for an increased risk of developing drug toxicity. Table 7.3 [43] illustrates situations in which plasma drug monitoring may be useful. Interpretation of a serum drug concentration is no different than the interpretation of any laboratory value. The serum drug concentration needs to be evaluated in light of the overall therapeutic goal for the patient. For example, the "normal" therapeutic range for phenytoin is 10–20 mg/L. A patient who continues to seize despite a serum phenytoin concentration in the therapeutic range, may still achieve the desired goal with a higher concentration [44]. The phenytoin concentration can be pushed above the upper limit of its reported normal range because the toxicities at levels of 25–30 mg/L are benign. It is obvious that one must understand the pharmacology of the drug being used in order to interpret its serum concentration. It would be very dangerous, for instance, to push a patient's serum theophylline concentration above the upper limit of its therapeutic range. Utilizing the serum drug concentration to adjust dosing requires an understanding of the disease under treatment, the patient's current physiologic state and concurrent medications the patient is receiving. For instance, in a patient with MRSA pneumonia, the dose of vancomycin needs to be adjusted based on trough serum concentrations. The trough serum concentration is a surrogate marker for the more relevant parameter, the ratio of the area under the serum-concentration-time curve to the mean inhibitory concentration for the organism being treated (AUC/MIC). Achieving an AUC/MIC of greater than 400 is more likely to result in cure [45]. A trough serum concentration of 15–20 mg/L correlates with an AUC/MIC over 400 for most isolates. Knowledge of the resistance pattern of the isolate under treatment is important as it will not be possible to achieve an AUC/MIC of >400 in an isolate with an MIC of >2 mg/L. In this case, an alternative anti-staphlococcal agent such as linezolid should be used. Targeting a serum vancomycin concentration over 15 mg/L needs to be balanced with the patient's risk for nephrotoxicity. In patients receiving other nephrotoxic medications such as aminoglycosides, or with poor renal perfusion, as in septic shock, the risk of kidney injury with vancomycin is increased. Interpretation of serum drug concentrations also mandates that the timing of the serum sample in relation to the drug dose is well documented. Appropriate interpretation of a drug level is nearly impossible if it cannot be accurately related to the time the drug was administered. It is best to try to avoid obtaining blood for measurement of serum drug concentrations through the same line the drug was administered. The drug may remain in the catheter resulting in a falsely elevated serum concentration measurement.

Drug Interactions

Drug interactions have been associated with increased lengths of stay [46]. Because they are potentially preventable, it is important to have an understanding of the most common types encountered in the ICU. Drug interactions can be classified as drug-drug, drug-disease, or drug-food interactions. The mechanism can be divided into pharmaceutical, pharmacokinetic or pharmacodynamic interactions.

The most serious drug interactions involve drugs with severe toxicities and a narrow therapeutic index. In the PICU setting, this list includes anticonvulsants (e.g. phenytoin, valproic acid, carbamazepine, phenobarbital), antiarrhythmics (e.g. digoxin, amiodarone, lidocaine), warfarin, and chemotherapeutic or immunosuppressive agents (e.g. mercaptopurine, azathioprine, cyclosporine, tacrolimus) to name a few. The new second and third generation anticonvulsants (e.g. gabapentin, levetiracetam, oxcarbazepine, zonisamide, lacosamide) are less likely to be involved in drug interactions because they are not highly bound to plasma proteins and are either renally eliminated or biotransformed by noncytochrome P450 enzymes or are conjugated with glucuronide with the exceptions of lamotrigine and topiramate. Carbamazepine, oxcarbazepine, phenobarbital, phenytoin, and primidone induce the metabolism of lamotrigine and topiramate. Valproic acid inhibits lamotrigine metabolism but increases topiramate clearance. On the other hand, lamotrigine induces valproate metabolism, increases digoxin clearance, but decreases phenytoin clearance. Drug interactions involving the newer generation anticonvulsants have recently been reviewed by Johannessen Landmark and Patsalos [47], while Perucca has reviewed relevant interactions with all anticonvulsants [48].

Drug-Drug Interactions

One drug may diminish or potentiate the effect of another drug or create a new effect not observed with either drug alone. Pharmacokinetic interactions affect drug absorption, distribution, metabolism or excretion and result in an increase or decrease in drug concentration at the site of action. Pharmacodynamic interactions affect the response to either drug due to action at a common receptor or different sites. Critically ill children are at great risk for serious adverse reactions secondary to drug-drug interactions since they often times have multiple organ dysfunction, altered pharmacokinetics and pharmacodynamics, and are receiving multiple drugs. Further, early signs of an adverse reaction may be masked by the patient's underlying disease or condition. Table 7.4 outlines characteristics of drugs and patients at risk for clinically significant interactions. Although we will divide drug-drug interactions for the purposes of discussion by their mechanism, it is important that many drug-drug interactions arise due to concomitant pharmacokinetic and pharmacodynamic mechanisms. QT prolongation serves as an example [49]. Class IA (e.g. quinidine, procainamide) and III (e.g. sotalol) antiarrhythmic drugs can cause QT prolongation and torsades de pointes with therapeutic dosing. A pharmacodynamic interaction can occur resulting in torsades de pointes if another drug is administered which also prolongs the QT interval including such drugs as 5-HT-3

Table 7.4 Risk factors for drug-drug interactions in the ICU setting

Drug	Patient
Induce/inhibit drug metabolism	Coagulation disorder
Narrow therapeutic index	*Bleeding diathesis*
Associated with serious toxicities	*Hypercoagulable state*
Highly protein bound (>80–90 %)	Renal or hepatic impairment
Affect vital organ function	CNS disorder
CNS	*Seizure*
Cardiovascular	Metabolic disturbances
Renal/hepatic function	*Electrolyte*
Coagulation	*Glucose*
Oral complexing agents	Receiving multiple drugs
Higher drug dose	
Longer duration of therapy	

receptor antagonists (e.g. ondansitron), droperidol, antipsychotics (e.g. phenothiazines, haloperidol), atypical atipsychotics (clozapine, quetiapine, olanzapine, risperidone), tricyclic antidepressants, SSRI's (e.g. fluoxetine, citalopram), and antimicrobial agents (e.g. macrolides, fluoroquinolones, triazole antifungals). Many of the aforementioned drugs may also precipitate torsades de pointes by a pharmacokinetic mechanism as well. For example, many of the antidepressants and antipsychotics (e.g. tricyclics, haloperidol) that prolong the QT interval are metabolized by cytochrome P_{450} enzymes. Erythromycin and clarithromycin are not only the macrolides most likely to cause torsades, but they are also potent inhibitors of CYP3A4. On the other hand, azithromycin is less likely to cause torsades and is not a potent inhibitor of CYP3A4. The triazole antifungal agents also inhibit CYP3A4 with itraconazole and ketoconazole being more potent than fluconazole or voriconazole. Finally, an indirect pharmacodynamic mechanism may also result in torsades de pointes secondary to QT prolongation. This can occur with the combination of a QT prolonging drug with a diuretic agent that causes hypokalemia. Another example of combined pharmacokinetic and pharmacodynamic mechanisms for an interaction is anticonvulsant –induced resistance to neuromuscular blocking agents (see later).

Pharmacokinetic Interactions

Absorption

Drugs that delay gastric emptying (e.g. anticholinergic agents such as glycopyrrolate) decrease the rate but not the extent of absorption. Fortunately this is rarely of clinical significance. Prokinetic agents, on the other hand, may decrease the extent of absorption (e.g. metaclopramide and digoxin) [50] or increase bioavailability. For example, metaclopramide increases cyclosporine bioavailability by 30 % [51].

Drug-drug interactions affecting absorption can also occur by physicochemical complexation. Charcoal, the anion-exchange resin, cholestyramine, kaolin-pectin combinations, and the bismuth component of salicylate-bismuth mixtures should be considered capable of adsorbing most drugs and should be used cautiously and judiciously in patients receiving drugs with a narrow therapeutic index (e.g. warfarin, digoxin, etc.). Other examples include sucralfate with phenytoin or ciprofloxacin [52, 53], and antacids binding phenytoin, captopril or ciprofloxacin [54, 55]. It is recommended that the medication be administered 1 h prior to or 2–3 h after the administration of the complexing agent.

Drug effects on the gastrointestinal flora may also result in a drug-drug interaction. Digoxin is metabolized in the intestine to digoxin reducing substances that are excreted in the feces. Tetracycline, ampicillin, and the macrolide antibiotics increase digoxin bioavailability by altering its metabolism in the intestine. The impact of this interaction appears to be dependent on age. Although intestinal colonization with digoxin-reducing organisms approaches adult values by 2 years of age, excretion of reduced digoxin in stool does not reach adult levels until adolescence [56]. Based on this finding, we would anticipate that the bioavailability of digoxin in infants would exceed that observed in adults.

Valproic acid plasma concentrations decline significantly in patients receiving carbapenam antibiotics. The interaction is clinically significant in approximately 55 % of patients with a mean decline in valproate levels of 66 % within 24 h described in one study [57]. The interaction occurs by multiple mechanisms affecting absorption, distribution, and metabolism [58]. The carbapenam class of agents appear to decrease intestinal transepithelial transport of valproic acid resulting in a 57 % decrease in bioavailability [58]. The effects on distribution and metabolism will be discussed below.

Distribution

The most common type of drug interaction involving distribution is the result of an alteration in protein binding. Recall that it is the free or unbound fraction of a drug that is not only pharmacologically active, but is available for metabolism or excretion. If a drug is displaced from its protein binding site, the free drug concentration transiently increases and may result in toxicity. Because drug metabolism or elimination will also increase, the total drug concentration will be lower and the free concentration unchanged compared to their prior concentrations once a new steady state is achieved. In order for the displacement interaction to be of clinical significance, both drugs need to be at least 80–90 % protein bound, the displaced drug must demonstrate capacity limited clearance (e.g. phenytoin) or have a small V_d <0.15 L/kg (e.g. warfarin), and have a narrow therapeutic index. The most important clinical example is the displacement of warfarin by other highly protein bound drugs such as aspirin, sulfa, and amiodarone. The displacement of phenytoin by another drug rarely results in clinical toxicity, in contrast to the potential for toxicity from a displacement reaction involving accumulated organic acids in patients with renal failure (see drug-disease interactions below). Free phenytoin levels, rather than total phenytoin plasma concentration may need to be monitored in both circumstances. Valproic acid displaces phenytoin from plasma proteins. The interaction results in a lower total phenytoin plasma concentration and an increase of 35 % in the free fraction. Overall there is no significant change in the free plasma phenytoin concentration [59], therefore a patient may have a therapeutic effect from phenytoin despite a subtherapeutic total concentration.

Alterations in tissue binding may also result in clinically significant effects. For example, quinidine and amiodarone displace digoxin from its tissue binding sites. This leads to a decrease in V_d and an increase in digoxin plasma concentration. The maintenance dose of digoxin should be reduced by 50 % when concomitant administration of quinidine or amiodarone is required. The carbapenams prevent the efflux of valproate out of red blood cells by an effect on ATP-binding cassette transporters thereby increasing the V_d and decreasing the plasma concentration [58].

Metabolism

Most clinically significant drug-drug interactions involve changes in drug metabolism and are the result of enzyme inhibition or induction. Certain drugs are "generalized" inducers (e.g. phenobarbital, rifampin, carbamazepine) or inhibitors (e.g. erythromycin, triazole antifungal agents, cimetidine, amiodarone, fluoxetine, paroxitine) of the cytochrome P_{450} system, while other drugs specifically induce or inhibit the metabolism of selected drugs by preferential effects on certain P_{450} isoforms. Nafcillin therapy results in warfarin resistance. Although the exact mechanism has not been elucidated, it appears to be secondary to enzyme induction [60]. As mentioned earlier, knowledge of which drugs are substrates for the different cytochrome P_{450} isoforms as well as their selective inhibitors/inducers, allows for the understanding and prediction of drug-drug interactions (Table 7.5).

Nivoix et al. has recently reviewed drug-drug interactions involving the triazole antifungal agents [61]. Important consequences may include increased immunosupressant drug levels, prolonged INR with warfarin, and increased anticonvulsant levels. Conversely, induction of triazole metabolism could result in therapeutic failures.

Table 7.5 Substrates, inhibitors, and inducers of selected cytochrome P_{450} isoforms

Isoform	Substrate	Inhibitors		Inducers	
		Drugs	Herbals, etc[a]	Drugs	Herbals, etc[a]
1A2	Theophylline	Amiodarone	Echinacea	Rifampin	Cigarette smoke
	Acetaminophen	Triazoles[b]		Carbamazepine	St John's wort
	Propranolol	Macrolides[c]		Phenobarbital	Cruciferous vegetables
	Caffeine	Cimetidine		Omeprazole	
	Amitriptylline	Ciprofloxacin			
	Clozapine	Amlodipine			
		Fluoxetine			
		Nifedipine			
2C9	Warfarin	Amiodarone triazoles	Echinacea	Rifampin	St John's wort
	Phenytoin	Nicardipine	?Garlic	Carbamazepine	
	Amiodarone	Omeprazole		Phenobarbital	
	Carvedilol	Trimethoprim/sulfa		Phenytoin	
		Isoniazid		Nafcillin	
		Metronidazole			
2D6	Captopril	Amiodarone		Rifampin	St John's wort?
	β-blockers	Triazoles			
	Procainamide	SSRI's[e]			
	Dextromethorphan	Quinidine			
	Codeine	Cimetidine			
	Antipsychotics[d]	Isoniazid			
	SSRI's[e]				
2C19	Diazepam	Fluconazole	St John's wort[g]	Rifampin	St John's wort[g]
	PPI's[f]	Ketoconazole		Carbamazepine	
	Imipramine	PPI's[f]		Phenytoin	
	Phenytoin	Nicardipine		Phenobarbital	
	Phenobarbital	SSRI's[e]			
		Isoniazid			

(continued)

Table 7.5 (continued)

Isoform	Substrate	Inhibitors		Inducers	
		Drugs	Herbals, etc[a]	Drugs	Herbals, etc[a]
2E1	Acetaminophen	Isoniazid			Alcohol[h]
	Theophylline	Alcohol[h]			St John's wort
3A3	Amiodarone	Triazoles[b]		Rifampin	St John's wort[j]
3A4	Cyclosporine	Protease		Carbamazepine	Echinacea[l]
	Tacrolimus	Inhibitors		Phenobarbital	Gingko?
	Midazolam	Macrolides[c]		Phenytoin	
	CCB[i]	Amiodarone		Grapefruit	
		CCB[i]		Juice[k]	
		Isoniazid			

Modified from Reed and Blumer [114]. With permission from Elsevier
[a]Herbal therapies, foods, chemicals
[b]Ketoconazole, itraconazole> fluconazole, voriconazole
[c]Erythromycin, clarithromycin, but not azithromycin
[d]Tricyclic antidepressants (imipramine, nortriptyline), thioridazine, haloperidol, risperidone
[e]Serotonin reuptake inhibitors (particularly fluoxetine, paroxetine, sertraline)
[f]PPI's (omeprazole, lansoprezole, pantoprazole)
[g]Inhibits at very high doses; otherwise is an inducer
[h]Chronic alcohol use causes a modest, short lived induction in man; acute alcohol ingestion inhibits (From Prescott [115])
[i]Calcium channel blockers (particularly verapamil, nicardipine, diltiazem)
[j]Induces intestinal CYP3A4 activity(decreased bioavailability) and hepatic CYP3A4 activity
[k]Major effect on intestinal CYP3A4 activity(decreased bioavailability) rather than on hepatic CYP3A4 activity
[l]Inhibits intestinal CYP3A4 activity(increased bioavailability) but induces hepatic CYP3A4 activity

Enzyme induction may also play a role in poisonings such as acetaminophen. It appears that an induced liver is more susceptible to acetaminophen hepatotoxicity, presumably via increased formation of its toxic metabolite, N-acetyl-para-benzoquinoninime. There are insufficient data, however, to determine what acetaminophen concentration poses a risk. Therefore, it has been recommended that the treatment line should be lowered to a line that intersects 100 mg/L at 4 h and 25 mg/L at 12 h post ingestion (from 150 to 37.5 mg/L, respectively) in chronic alcohol users or in patients receiving enzyme inducing drugs such as the anticonvulsants or isoniazid [62].

Induction requires synthesis of new enzymes so that time to onset of the interaction may be delayed compared to those involving enzyme inhibition. Time to onset of and maximal induction vary with the inducing agent, dose, and duration of exposure as well as the half life of the induced drug. For example, onset of induction by rifampin is approximately 2 days whereas phenobarbital induction begins in approximately 6–7 days. Maximal induction of theophylline by rifampin and phenobarbital are observed in 4 days and 4 weeks, respectively. Following discontinuation of the inducing drug, the time course to return to the noninduced state is similar to that of induction. Most of the new generation anticonvulsants are not inducers of hepatic enzymes. However, most are eliminated, at least in part by inducible P_{450} enzymes [47, 48].

Enzyme inhibition may occur by competitive or noncompetitive mechanisms. Competitive inhibition occurs when a drug or its metabolite competes with another drug for binding to the active site of an enzyme. Noncompetitive inhibition is the result of enzyme inactivation. The time to inhibition depends on the mechanism of inhibition and the half lives (short half lives-rapid onset of action; long half lives-delayed onset of interaction) of the respective drugs or their metabolites. For example, the onset of theophylline inhibition by erythromycin is delayed by several days, since it is a metabolite of erythromycin that is responsible for the competitive inhibition. Valproic acid is not an enzyme inducer, but rather is involved in competitive inhibition of substrates such as phenobarbital and lamotrigine [47].

Although most of these interactions involve the cytochrome P_{450} system, other enzyme systems or mechanisms may be responsible for drug-drug interactions. Allopurinol is a competitive inhibitor of xanthine oxidase which is responsible for oxidation of mercaptopurine to an inactive metabolite. When used concomitantly, patients may experience life threatening toxicity unless the dose of mercaptopurine is reduced. The same consideration should also be exercised when treating patients with azathioprine and allopurinol since azathioprine is metabolized to mercaptopurine. Another example of drug-drug interactions not involving the cytochrome P_{450} system is the effect of cimetidine or propranolol to reduce lidocaine clearance by decreasing hepatic blood flow.

In the ICU setting, it is paramount to consider the possibility of a drug-drug interaction whenever a patient is concomitantly receiving a drug capable of inducing or inhibiting drug metabolism and a drug with a narrow therapeutic index and the potential for serious adverse effects. If available, drug levels should be monitored closely.

Elimination

Most drug-drug interactions involving elimination from the body are the result of alterations in the renal processes of glomerular filtration rate (GFR), tubular secretion, or tubular reabsorption. NSAID's, which decrease GFR, may reduce the renal clearance of drugs such as digoxin and the aminoglycosides [63], or active metabolites (e.g. N-acetyl procainamide). Patients with preexisting renal impairment, hypertension, or congestive heart failure (CHF) appear to be at a greater risk for this interaction.

Competition for tubular secretion at the transport site for acidic or basic drugs or compounds may lead to decreased drug excretion. This mechanism has been used therapeutically in combining probenecid with β(beta)-lactam antibiotics. However, it may result in toxicity as well. For example, cimetidine decreases the tubular secretion of procainamide [64]. Tubular secretion may also be impaired via an interaction with renal tubular P-glycoprotein (PGP). This is the mechanism responsible for decreased renal excretion of digoxin by quinidine and amiodarone [65]. Therefore, both quinidine and amiodarone decrease digoxin's renal clearance as well as reducing its V_d by decreasing tissue binding.

Clinically significant drug interactions involving renal tubular reabsorption are rare. Lithium reabsorption is altered by drugs that affect proximal tubular sodium reabsorption. Renal clearance of lithium is reduced by loop and thiazide diuretics as well as NSAID's which increase proximal tubular sodium reabsorption [65]. More commonly, urinary pH is modified in the setting of acute poisoning to decrease reabsorption and enhance urinary excretion of a toxic compound (e.g. salicylates).

Pharmacodynamic Interactions

Pharmacodynamic drug interactions may result from summation of similar or opposing effects in patients receiving multiple drugs. Examples in the PICU setting of the former include CNS depression with benzodiazepines and opiates; neurotoxic effects from combined use of anticonvulsants with similar mechanism of action [48]; bleeding with any combination of warfarin, heparin, low molecular weight heparin, tissue plasminogen activator (TPA), and nonsteroidal anti-inflammatory drugs; hypotension with such agents as vasodilators, β(beta)-blockers, and propofol; hyperkalemia with potassium supplements, angiotensin-converting enzyme (ACE) inhibitors, or spironolactone; and hypokalemia with diuretics, amphotericin B, and β(beta) agonists. The risk of vancomycin associated nephrotoxicity is low when trough concentrations remain below 20. The risk increases three to fourfold, however, with concomitant use of aminoglycosides or other nephrotoxic agents [45]. Many drugs from a variety of classes have been implicated in the development of the serotonin syndrome [66–68]. These classes include amphetamines and derivatives (e.g. 3,4 methylenedioxymethamphetamine – ecstasy, cocaine, caffeine), MAO inhibitors, analgesics (e.g. cyclobenzaprine, meperidine, tramadol, fentanyl), antidepressants/mood stabilizers (e.g. buspirone, lithium, tricyclic antidepressants, SSRI's), antiemetics (metoclopramide, ondansitron), and miscellaneous agents such as detromethorphan, tryptophan, and linezolid. The latter possesses MAO inhibitor activity [68]. Most cases occur in patients on chronic therapy with an SSRI who receive or acutely ingest drugs that can increase serotonin levels at CNS receptors or heighten the response to serotonin at the receptors (e.g. lithium). However, other receptors such as NMDA, dopamine, and GABA may also be involved. The serotonin syndrome may also arise from a pharmacokinetic interaction. A 12 year old child taking sertraline chronically developed the syndrome when erythromycin (CYP3A4 inhibitor) was added [69]. Examples of summation of opposing effects would be the use of agonists and antagonists together such as albuterol and propranolol or the use of specific antagonists such as naloxone or flumazenil to reverse the effects of opiates or benzodiazepines, respectively. Pharmacodynamic interactions may also create a new pathophysiologic condition or exaggerate a condition only observed with one of the drugs. Examples of the former include psychiatric disturbances reported with combined valproic acid and leveteracetam [70]. Examples of the latter include precipitation of carbamazepine toxicity when leveteracetam is added to carbamazepine despite non toxic levels of the latter agent [47], and hyperammonemic encephalopathy with combined valproic acid and topiramate administration [71]. Anticonvulsant drugs, particularly phenytoin, carbamazepine, and Phenobarbital, may induce resistance to neuromuscular blocking agents. Although pharmacokinetic mechanisms (e.g. induction of metabolism, increased α(alpha)-1 glycoprotein resulting in increased protein binding) are mostly responsible, pharmacodynamic mechanisms may contribute as well by upregulation of acetylcholine receptors [72]. Pharmacodynamic drug interactions may also occur indirectly as previously mentioned under QT prolongation and torsades de pointes. Another example is diuretic induced hypokalemia may trigger digitalis toxicity. NSAID's, via sodium and water retention, may blunt the antihypertensive effects of ACE inhibitors, etc. or negate the benefits of diuretics in patients with CHF. Finally, pharmacodynamic interactions may be of benefit to the patient. For example, the addition of a low dose of lamotrigene to valproic acid can result in a profound synergistic effect to improve efficacy. However, tremors may also be exacerbated [47].

Herbal-Drug Interactions

These interactions may also occur on a pharmacokinetic or pharmacodynamic basis. Pharmacokinetic interactions, mediated by changes in the activity of drug metabolizing enzymes and/or the drug transporter, appear to be the most common types of interactions [73–75]. Reports of clinically significant interactions are limited and mostly involve St. John's wort with cyclosporine, anticoagulants, digoxin, antidepressants, and protease inhibitors [74–76]. St. John's wort induces cytochrome P_{450} activity, in the intestine and liver, and PGP in the intestine thus decreasing the plasma concentrations of the aforementioned drugs. The effect appears to be greater on intestinal compared to hepatic cytochrome P450 activity. With long term administration of St. John's wort, the area under the serum concentration time curve for orally administered midazolam is reduced by 50 % compared to a 20 % reduction observed following IV administration [75]. The INR may be decreased by 50 % when warfarin is administered to a patient receiving St. John's wort [77, 78] while organ rejection may occur due to subtherapeutic cyclosporine levels [79, 80].

Echinacea, a dietary supplement, appears to inhibit certain cytochrome P_{450} isoform (CYP2C9 and CYP1A2) while inducing CYP3A activity [75]. CYP2C9 and CYP1A2 are responsible for metabolism of such drugs as theophylline, phenytoin, and warfarin while the CYP3A isoform is responsible for the metabolism of such drugs as cyclosporine, midazolam, and tacrolimus. On the other hand, ginkgo and ginseng have been implicated in a number of reports without strong corroborating data [74]. There is a case report of imatinib hepatotoxicity because of a suspected interaction with Panex ginseng. Ginseng, by inhibiting CYP3A4 and intestinal PGP, may have increased the plasma concentration of imatinib and potentiated its toxicity [81].

Although there are a paucity of confirmed herbal-drug interactions in the literature, a variety of herbal therapies and foods including teas, cloves, garlic, ginger, and Allium satium to name a few, may have variable effects on cytochrome P_{450} isoforms. The potential for a significant interaction exists when patients receive drugs with a narrow therapeutic index after or while consuming these herbals or foods. Table 7.4 also summarizes known interactions between herbal and prescription medications involving cytochrome P_{450} isoforms.

As mentioned earlier, pharmacodynamic herb-drug interactions may also occur [74]. There are herbals with purported sedative, anticoagulant, antihypertensive, or antineoplastic effects to name a few. A similar potential exists for additive, synergistic, or antagonistic effects from herbal-drug interactions as may occur with combinations of drugs. For example, St. John's wort has been reported to trigger the serotonergic syndrome in patients receiving antidepressant medications [66]. Pharmacodynamic interactions may also arise with patients receiving anticoagulants [82]. Ginkgo, for example, has antiplatelet activity and has been implicated in cases of severe bleeding when used in combination with nonsteroidal anti-inflammatory agents. Of relevance in the PICU is the patient with prolonged or marked post operative bleeding. Javed et al. have recently reviewed the literature regarding herbal interactions with the coagulation system either alone or in combination with drugs. They identified 24 compounds with documented effects (most on platelet function) and 98 with theoretical risks [83].

Pharmaceutical Interactions

Pharmaceutical interactions result in drug inactivation when compounds are mixed together prior to administration in syringes, IV tubing or hyperalimentation fluid or during administration in the IV catheter. PICU's are frequently plagued with issues regarding IV compatibility because critically ill children often require multiple IV infusions through a limited number of vascular access sites. These children are commonly fluid overloaded and require concentrated medication infusions. To complicate matters further, compatibility information for the drug combination needed is often unavailable, poorly referenced, or does not include specific concentrations or diluents. Avoiding incompatibility/instability problems with concurrent medication infusions is important in order to optimize the therapeutic response and preserve vascular access.

Many factors influence drug compatibility such as temperature, drug concentration, ionic strength, pH, light exposure, and the length of time medications remain in contact. Physical incompatibilities are visible in the form of precipitation, turbidity, or a change in viscosity and may result in the loss of IV access (e.g. sodium bicarbonate and calcium). They are often due to inadequate solubility or acid-base reactions. On the other hand, chemical reactions are not always visible and are usually irreversible. Certain solutions may also contain preservatives such as benzyl alcohol and propylene glycol (e.g. pancuronium, lorazepam, heparin) to enhance stability that may result in serious adverse effects [84–86].

Proactive measures should be exercised to minimize drug incompatibilities. Be aware of factors that affect drug compatibility, do not co-administer incompatible drugs through the same line (e.g. epinephrine), take advantage of drug-delivery systems (e.g. Y-site administration), and always flush the catheter thoroughly between intermittent medication infusions. If compatibility is unknown, attempt to infuse the drugs/solutions through separate catheters. Closely monitor the patient's response to therapy if two medications of unknown compatibility must be infused together. If the patient is not obtaining the expected response from the medication, it may be that a chemical reaction has occurred. Creating compatibility charts with the medications and concentrations commonly used in your unit is extremely helpful to the PICU staff. Reviewing new compatibility information and upgrading the chart must be a continuous process. Appendix 3 lists common drug compatibilities and incompatibilities that we use as a guide in our PICU [87–91].

Drug-Food and Drug-Enteral Formula Interactions

Although there are many examples of drug-food interactions, very few are pertinent to the critical care setting. Table 7.5 includes the effects of foods on hepatic metabolism. Grapefruit juice interferes with CYP 3A3/A4 [75]. The predominant effect, however, is on intestinal rather than hepatic CYP 3A3/A4 activity. The consequence of this interaction is increased oral bioavailablity rather than decreased systemic clearance. Cruciferous vegetables such as cabbage, brussel sprouts, and cauliflower are potent inducers of CYP1A2. The most significant drug-food pharmacodynamic interaction is the blunted effect of warfarin when foods rich in Vitamin K are consumed. Enteral nutrition by tube feedings can decrease drug absorption and lead to therapeutic failures by binding the drug and/or competition for absorptive surface area in the intestine. There are a paucity of data evaluating drug-nutrient interactions for most drugs administered to ICU patients receiving continuous enteral nutrition. For most drugs studied, the rate but not extent of absorption is affected. There are a few exceptions most notably phenytoin, carbamazepine, warfarin, and ciprofloxacin [92–94]. There is no strategy that consistently obviates this interaction. We recommend flushing the tubing 1–2 h before drug administration and resuming feeds 1–2 h later. The bioavailability of some drugs may be reduced by adherence to the walls of the feeding tube (e.g. carbamazepine, diazepam solution) [93].

Drug-Disease Interactions

Disease states can alter the pharmacokinetics and pharmacodynamics of a drug, and conversely, a drug can interact with a disease to produce an adverse reaction. The most obvious example of these interactions is the effect of renal dysfunction on the pharmacokinetics of drugs cleared by the kidney. It is important to continuously evaluate the impact that a patient's changing renal function might have on a medica-

tion and adjust the dose or dosing interval accordingly. Renal replacement therapies will have varying effects on the clearance of drugs depending on the individual drug and type of replacement therapy [95]. However, these dosing recommendations may no longer be valid owing to new CRRT technology and methods augmenting drug removal [96]. Drugs metabolized by the liver are generally not affected until there is a significant degree of hepatic damage. However, dosing adjustments of hepatically cleared medications have to be made in the setting of overt liver failure. Other alterations in the pharmocologic properties of a drug are disease specific. For instance, the bioavailability of aspirin is significantly impaired during the acute phase of Kawaski disease, then increases dramatically when the patient becomes afebrile [97]. The pharmacokinetics of phenytoin are altered in the setting of severe head injury in children. The increased clearance of phenytoin in this patient population results in a requirement for higher than normal doses to achieve therapeutic serum concentrations [98, 99]. Protein binding is also altered due to decreased serum albumin levels and results in an elevated free fraction of phenytoin [99]. The Systemic Inflammatory Response Syndrome (SIRS) may interfere with hepatic drug metabolism. Pantoprazole clearance, mediated by CYP3A4 and CYP2C19, was reduced by 62 % in the presence of SIRS [100]. This supports the findings of Carcillo et al. [101]. Using antipyrene, a probe for CYP3A4, CYP1A2, CYP2C9, and other isoforms, they demonstrated a twofold reduction in clearance in septic children and a fourfold reduction in clearance in children with three or more organ failures. Antipyrene clearance was inversely related to interleukin-6 levels.

The pharmacodynamic action of a medication may also be altered by a patient's disease process. Critically ill children may require a higher area under the serum concentration time curve of pantoprezole to raise gastric pH [102]. Ketamine is an anesthetic agent that can be used for procedural sedation in the PICU. Although ketamine is a direct myocardial depressant, its administration generally results in increased blood pressure and heart rate caused by release of endogenous norepinephrine. In the setting of a patient with severe heart failure, however, ketamine's predominant effect may be myocardial depression resulting in adverse hemodynamic effects [103].

A drug may interact with a disease to produce a new pathophysiologic condition in a patient. Nonsteroidal anti-inflammatory drugs may precipitate acute renal failure in a patient with a low cardiac output state or septic shock. A drug may also exacerbate an underlying condition such as in an antihistamine lowering the seizure threshold in a patient with epilepsy. Table 7.6 lists some clinically important examples of interactions between drugs and diseases.

Table 7.6 Drug-disease interactions

Effect of disease on drug
Pharmacokinetic interactions
Renal failure
Increased free serum phenytoin concentration
Meperidine induced seizures due to accumulation of normeperidine metabolite
CHF
Decreased oral furosemide absorption
Decreased lidocaine clearance
Trauma
Increased phenytoin clearance and decreased protein binding
Viral infections and hepatic metabolism
Influenza and adenovirus inhibit theophylline, phenytoin, carbamazepine, and warfarin metabolism
SIRS and hepatic metabolism
Decreased cytochrome P_{450} enzyme activity
Pharmacodynamic interactions
Ketamine induced shock state in patients with severe heart failure
Sedatives precipitate encephalopathy in liver failure patients
Effect of drug on disease(adverse drug reactions)
New pathophysiologic condition
Reyes syndrome in patients receiving aspirin for juvenile rheumatoid arthritis
Acute renal failure in patients with low cardiac output or septic shock receiving NSAID's
Exacerbation of underlying disease
Decongestants and hypertension
β-blockers, NSAID's and asthma
β-agonists (e.g. albuterol), stimulants(e.g. methylphenidate) and supraventricular tachycardia
NSAID's and bleeding disorders
Steroids and diabetes
Phenothiazines, buproprion, antihistamines lower seizure threshold
β-blockers, calcium channel blockers and CHF
Sulfa, ceftriaxone and kernicterus in neonates with hyperbilirubinema

Drug Safety

An understanding of the principles discussed earlier is necessary to minimize the chance of producing adverse outcomes associated with drug therapy. However, knowledge of the science of pharmacology alone is inadequate to reduce adverse drug events (ADE's) to a minimum. Medication errors are a common cause of ADE's and have unfortunately been associated with fatalities in too many cases. Patients in the critical care unit are an especially vulnerable population due to the number of medications used and the complexity of their disease processes. The rate of ADE's in pediatric critical care units is 4.9 per 100 patient days, with a preventable rate of 2.1 per 100 patient days [104]. Errors can occur at any stage in the medication delivery process. One-third of serious medication errors occur during the ordering stage, one-third during medication administration and the remaining third are equally divided between the transcription and dispensing stages [105]. A single children's hospital study found a medication error rate of 5.7 errors per 100 medication orders, with most involving intravenous medications and occurring at the time the physician wrote the order [106]. The focus of error prevention is on the systems involved in medication prescription and delivery. It is well recognized that blaming an individual for making a human error, and strategies aimed at changing individual behaviors are not effective in preventing medication errors [107]. Systems which do not allow care providers to make an error are the most effective measures in dealing with preventable ADE's. Examples of simple error prevention solutions are oral medication syringes and enteral feeding tubing which will not allow connection to an intravenous catheter. Simple engineering changes such as these prevent the inadvertent, and often fatal, intravenous administration of products formulated for enteral use.

Technological strategies are being used more frequently in attempts to minimize medication errors. Computerized physician order entry (CPOE) has the potential to significantly decrease medication ordering errors in pediatric intensive care units [108]. However, the promise of this technology has not yet been shown to significantly decrease ADE's in PICU's [109] Implementation of CPOE requires a thoughtful approach and must be tailored to the workflow in an individual unit to avoid introducing new forms of errors/ adverse events [110]. CPOE is strengthened when paired with decision support software which helps guide clinicians in medication selection, dosing, prevention of medication interactions and avoidance of preventable allergic reactions [111]. Another promising technology is bar-coding. Bedside use of bar-coding technology, coupled with the use of an electronic medication administration record (eMAR) allows for identification of the patient receiving the medication, the drug being administered and matching of both with ordered medications. Bar-coding coupled with eMAR has been shown to significantly decrease medication administration errors in an adult hospital [112]. Infusion pumps with built in decision support software ("smart pumps") can be utilized to prevent dosing errors. Smart pumps can warn nurses when a medication dose is outside of an acceptable range and hard stops can be programmed which prevent the delivery of excessive medication [111]. Implementation of any technology often requires significant staff education and buy-in for the technology to be effective. The mere presence of CPOE, bar-coding and smart-pumps does not guarantee patient safety if the PICU staff is not well prepared and motivated to use the technology.

One well proven strategy to reduce drug errors in the PICU is the presence of a unit-based clinical pharmacist [113]. Combinations of various strategies aimed at eliminating medication errors in the PICU need to be investigated, and best practices in medication safety need to be shared among intensive care units world-wide.

References

1. Wilkinson GR. Pharmacokinetics - the dynamics of drug absorption, distribution, and elimination. In: Hardman JG, Limbard LE, Gilman AG, editors. Goodman & Gilman's the pharmacological basis of therapeutics. 10th ed. New York: McGraw-Hill; 2001. p. 3–29.
2. Ross EM, Kenakin TP. Pharmacodymanics - mechanism of drug action and the relationship between drug concentration and effect. In: Hardman JG, Limbard LE, Gilman AG, editors. Goodman & Gilman's the pharmacological basis of therapeutics. 10th ed. New York: McGraw-Hill; 2001. p. 31–43.
3. Spivey WH. Intraosseous infusions. J Pediatr. 1987;111:639–43.
4. Malinovsky JM, Lejus C, Servin F, et al. Plasma concentrations of midazolam after IV, nasal or rectal administration in children. Brit J Anaesth. 1993;70:617–20.
5. Kanto J. Midazolam: the first water-soluble benzodiazepine. Pharmacology, pharmacokinetics and efficacy in insomnia and anesthesia. Pharmacotherapy. 1985;5:138–55.
6. Taylor MB, Vine PR, Hatch DJ. Intramuscular midazolam premedication in young children. Anaesthesia. 1986;41:21–6.
7. Chiaretti A, Barone G, Rigante D, et al. Intranasal lidocaine and midazolam for procedural sedation in children. Arch Dis Child. 2011;96:160–3.
8. Holsti M, Dudley N, Schunk J, et al. Intranasal midazolam vs rectal diazepam for the home treatment of acute seizures in pediatric patients with epilepsy. Arch Pediatr Adolesc Med. 2010;164:747–53.
9. Bhattacharyya M, Kalra V, Gulati S. Intranasal midazolam vds rectal diazepam in acute childhood seizures. Pediatr Neurol. 2006;34:355–9.
10. Allegaert K, van den Anker JN, Naulaers G, et al. Determinants of drug metabolism in early neonatal life. Curr Clin Pharmacol. 2007;2:23–9.
11. Mouly S, Meune C, Bergmann J-F. Mini-series. Basic science. Uncertainty and inaccuracy of predicting CYP-mediated in vivo drug interactions in the ICU from in vitro models: focus on CYP3A4. Intensive Care Med. 2009;35:417–29.
12. Kearns GL, Abdel-Rahman SM, Alander SW, et al. Developmental pharmacology- drug disposition, action, and therapy in infants and children. N Engl J Med. 2003;349:1157–67.
13. Reed MD, Besunder JB. Developmental pharmacology: ontogenic basis of drug disposition. Pediatr Clin N Am. 1989;36:1053–74.
14. Besunder JB, Reed MD, Blumer JL. Principles of drug biodisposition in the neonate: a critical evaluation of the pharmacokinetic-pharmacodynamic interface. Clin Pharmacokinet. 1988;14:189–216, 261–86.
15. Agunod M, Yomaguchi N, Lopez R, et al. Correlative study of hydrochloric acid, pepsin, and intrinsic factor secretion in newborns and infants. Am J Dig Dis. 1969;14:400–14.
16. Friis-Hansen B. Water distribution in the foetus and newborn infant. Acta Paediatr. 1983;305(Suppl):7–11.
17. Radde IC. Drugs and protein binding. In: MacLeod SM, Radde IC, editors. Textbook of pediatric pharmacology. Littletown: PSG Publishing Co; 1985. p. 34.
18. Park MK, Ludden T, Arom KV, et al. Myocardial vs serum digoxin concentrations in infants and adults. Am J Dis Child. 1982;136:418–20.
19. Gorodischer R, Jusko WJ, Yaffe S. Tissue and erythrocyte distribution of digoxin in infants. Clin Pharmacol Ther. 1976;19:256–63.
20. Leeder JS, Kearns GL, Spielberg SP, et al. Understanding the relative roles of pharmacogenetics and ontogeny in pediatric drug development and regulatory science. J Clin Pharmacol. 2010;50:1377–87.
21. DeWildt SN, Kearns GL, Leeder JS, et al. Cytochrome P450 3A: ontogeny and drug disposition. Clin Pharmacokinet. 1999;37:485–505.
22. Anderson GD, Lynn AM. Optimizing pediatric dosing: a developmental pharmacologic approach. Pharmacotherapy. 2009;29:680–90.
23. Sumpter A, Anderson BJ. Pediatric pharmacology in the first year of life. Curr Opin Anaesthesiol. 2009;22:469–75.
24. Alam SN, Robert RJ, Fischer LJ. Age-related differences in salicylamide and acetaminophen conjugation in man. J Pediatr. 1977;90:130–5.
25. Miller RP, Roberts RJ, Fischer LJ. Acetaminophen elimination kinetics in neonates, children, and adults. Clin Pharmacol Ther. 1976;19:284–94.
26. Arant Jr BS. Developmental patterns of renal functional maturation compared in the human neonate. J Pediatr. 1978;92:705–12.
27. Leake RD, Trygstad CW. Gomerular filtration rate during the period of adaptation to extrauterine life. Pediatr Res. 1977;11:959–62.
28. West JR, Smith HW, Chasis H. Glomerular filtration rate, effective renal blood flow and maximal tubular excretory capacity in infancy. J Pediatr. 1948;32:10–8.
29. Leeder JS, Kearns GL. Pharmacogenetics in pediatrics. Pediatr Clin North Am. 1997;44:55–77.
30. Wang L, McLeod HL, Weinshilboum RM. Genomics and drug response. N Engl J Med. 2011;364:1144–53.
31. Wilkinson GR. Drug metabolism and variability among patients in drug response. New Engl J Med. 2005;352:2211–21.
32. Sindrup SH, Brosen K. The pharmacogentics of codeine hypoalgesia. Pharmacogenetics. 1995;5:335–46.
33. Ciszkowski C, Madadi P, Phillips MS, Lauwers AE, Koren G. Codeine, ultrarapid-metabolism genotype, and postoperative death. N Engl J Med. 2009;361:827–8.
34. Madadi M, Koren G, Cairns J, et al. Safety of codeine during breastfeeding. Fatal morphine poisoning in the breastfed neonate of a mother prescribed codeine. Can Fam Physician. 2007;53:33–5.
35. Brandolese R, Scordo MG, Spina E, et al. Severe phenytoin intoxication in a subject homozygous for CYP2C9*3. Clin Pharmacol Ther. 2001;70:391–4.
36. Epstein RS, Moyer TP, Aubert RE, O'Kane DJ, Xia F, Verbrugge RR, Gage BF, Teagarden JR. Warfarin genotyping reduces hospitalization rates. J Am Cool Cardiol. 2010;55:2804–12.
37. Kitzmiller JP, Groen DK, Phelps MA, Sadee W. Pharmacogenomic testing: relevance in medical practice why drugs work in some patients but not others. Cleve Clin J Med. 2011;78:243–57.
38. Tantisira KG, Lasky-Su J, Harada M, et al. Genomewide association between GLCCl1 and response to glucocorticoid therapy in asthma. N Engl J Med. 2011;365(13):1173–83.
39. Madadi P, Hildebrandt D, Gong IY, Schwartz UI, Ciszkowski C, Ross CJD, Sistonen J, Carelton BC, Hayden MR, Lauwers AE, Koren G. Fatal hydrocone overdose in a child: pharmacogenetics and drug interactions. Pediatrics. 2010;126:e986–9.
40. Gijsen V, Mital S, van Schaik RH, Soldin OP, van der Heiden IP, Nulman I, Koren G, de Wildt SN. Age and CYP3A5 genotype affect tacrolimus dosing requirements after transplant in pediatric heart recipients. J Heart Lung Transplant. 2011;30(12):1352–9.
41. Ishizaki T, Kubo M. Incidence of apparent Michaelis-Menten behavior of theophylline and its parameters (V_{max} and K_m) among asthmatic children and adults. Ther Drug Monit. 1987;9:11–20.
42. Carcillo JA, Fields AI, American College of Critical Care Medicine Task force Committee Members. Clinical practice parameters for hemodynamic support of pediatric and neonatal patients in septic shock. Crit Care Med. 2002;30:1365–78.
43. Reed MD, Blumer JL. Therapeutic drug monitoring in the pediatric intensive care unit. Pediatr Clin North Am. 1994;41:1227–43.

44. Kozer E, Parvez S, Minassian BA, et al. How high can we go with phenytoin? Ther Drug Monit. 2002;24:386–9.

45. Rybak M, Lomaestro B, Rotschafer JC, et al. Therapeutic monitoring of vancomycin in adult patients: a consensus review of the American Society of Health-System Pharmacists, the Infectious Diseases Society of America, and the Society of Infectious Diseases Pharmacists. Am J Health Syst Pharm. 2009;66:82–98.

46. Moura C, Prado N, Acurcio F. Potential drug-drug interactions associated with prolonged stays in the intensive care unit. Clin Drug Investig. 2011;31:309–16.

47. Johannessen Landmark C, Patsalos PN. Drug interactions involving the new second and third generation antiepileptic drugs. Expert Rev Neurother. 2010;10:119–40.

48. Perucca E. Clinically relevant drug interactions with antiepileptic drugs. Br J Clin Pharmacol. 2006;61:246–55.

49. Smithburger PL, Seybert AL, Armahizer MJ, et al. QT prolongation in the intensive care unit: commonly used medications and the impact of drug-drug interactions. Expert Opin Drug Saf. 2010;9:699–712.

50. Reuning RH, Geraets DR, Rocci ML, et al. Digoxin. In: Schentag JJ, Evans WE, Jusko WJ, editors. Applied pharmacokinetics: principles of therapeutic drug monitoring. 3rd ed. Vancouver: Applied Therapeutics Inc; 1992. p. 20–48.

51. Wadhwa NK, Schroeder TJ, O'Flaherty E, et al. The effect of oral metoclopramide on the absorption of cyclosporine. Transplant Proc. 1987;19:1730–3.

52. Hall TG, Cuddy PG, Glass CJ, et al. Effect of sucralfate on phenytoin bioavailability. Drug Intell Clin Pharm. 1986;20:607–11.

53. Nix DE, Watson WA, Handy L, et al. The effect of sucralfate pretreatment on the pharmacokinetics of ciprofloxacin. Pharmacotherapy. 1989;9:377–80.

54. Carter BL, Garnett WR, Pellock JM, et al. Effect of antacids on phenytoin bioavailability. Ther Drug Monit. 1981;3:333–40.

55. Sadowski DC. Drug interactions with antacids, mechanisms and clinical significance. Drug Saf. 1994;11:395–407.

56. Linday L, Dobkin JF, Wang TC, et al. Digoxin inactivation by the gut flora in infancy and childhood. Pediatrics. 1987;79:544–8.

57. Spriet I, Goyens J, Meersseman W, et al. Interaction between valproate and meropenam: a retrospective review. Ann Pharmacother. 2007;41:1130–6.

58. Mancl EE, Gidal BE. The effect of carbapenam antibiotics on plasma concentrations of valproic acid. Ann Pharmacother. 2009;43:2082–7.

59. Tsanaclis LM, Perucca AE, Routledge PA, Richens A. Effect of valproate on free plasma phenytoin concentrations. Br J Clin Pharmacol. 1984;18:17–20.

60. Davis RL, Berman W, Wernly JA, Kelly HW. Warfarin-nafcillin interaction. J Pediatr. 1991;118:300–3.

61. Nivoix Y, Ubeaud-Sequier G, Engel P, Leveque D, Herbrecht R. Drug-drug interactions of triazole antifungal agents in multimorbid patients and implications for patient care. Curr Drug Metab. 2009;10:395–409.

62. Janes J, Routledge PA. Recent developments in the management of paracetamol (acetaminophen) poisoning. Drug Saf. 1992;7:170–7.

63. Brouwers JRBJ, de Snet AGM. Pharmacokinetic-pharmacodynamic drug interactions with nonsteroidal anti-inflammatory drugs. Clin Pharmacokinet. 1994;27:462–85.

64. Kosoglou T, Valasses PH. Drug interactions involving renal transport mechanisms: an overview. Ann Pharmacother. 1989;23:116–22.

65. Nies AS. Principles of therapeutics. In: Hardman JG, Limbard LE, Gilman AG, editors. Goodman & Gilman's the pharmacological basis of therapeutics. 10th ed. New York: McGraw-Hill; 2001. p. 45–66.

66. Boyer EW, Shannon M. The serotonin syndrome. New Engl J Med. 2005;352:1112–20.

67. Ables AZ, Nagubilli R. Prevention diagnosis, and management of serotonin syndrome. Am Fam Physician. 2010;81:1139–42.

68. Steinberg M, Morin AK. Mild serotonin syndrome associated with concurrent linezolid and fluoxetine. Am J Health Syst Pharm. 2007;64:59–62.

69. Lee DO, Lee CD. Serotonin syndrome in a child associated with erythromycin and sertraline. Pharmacotherapy. 1999;19:894–6.

70. Siniscalchi A, Gallelli L, De Fazio S, et al. Psychic disturbances associated with sodium valproate plus levetiracetam. Ann Pharmacother. 2007;41:527–8. letter.

71. Wadzinski J, Franks R, Roane D, et al. Valproate-associated hyperammonemic encephalopathy. J Am Board Fam Med. 2007;20:499–502.

72. Soriano SG, Jeevendra Martyn JA. Antiepileptic-induced resistance to neuromuscular blockers: mechanisms and clinical significance. Clin Pharmacokinet. 2004;43:71–81.

73. Buck ML, Michel RS. Talking with families about herbal therapies. J Pediatr. 2000;136:673–8.

74. Williamson E. Drug interactions between herbal and prescription medicines. Drug Saf. 2003;26:1075–92.

75. Huang SM, Hall SD, Watkins P, Love LA, Serabjit-Singh C, Betz JM, et al. Drug interactions with herbal products and grapefruit juice: a conference report. Clin Pharmacol Ther. 2004;75:1–12.

76. Henderson L, Yue QY, Bergquist C, Gerden B, Arlett P. St. John's wort (Hypericum perforatum): drug interactions and clinical outcomes. Br J Clin Pharm. 2002;54:349–56.

77. Ernst E. Second thoughts about safety of SJW. Lancet. 1999;354:2014–6.

78. Yue QY, Bergquist C, Gerden B. Safety of St John's wort. Lancet. 2000;355:576–7.

79. Barone GW, Gurley BJ, Ketel BL, Lightfoot ML, Abul-Ezz SR. Drug interaction between St John's wort and cyclosporine. Ann Pharmacother. 2000;34:1013–6.

80. Mai I, Kruger H, Budde K, et al. Hazardous pharmacokinetic interaction of Saint John's wort (Hypericum perforatum) with the immunosuppressant cyclosporine. Int J Clin Pharmacol Ther. 2000;38:500–2.

81. Bilgi N, Bell K, Ananthakrischnan AN, Atallah E. Imatinib and panex ginseng: a potential interaction resulting in liver toxicity. Ann Pharmacother. 2010;44:926–8.

82. Gardner P, Phillips R, Shaughnessy AF. Herbal and dietary supplement-drug interactions in patients with chronic illnesses. Am Fam Physician. 2008;78:808.

83. Javed F, Golagani A, Sharp H. Potential effects of herbal medicines and nutritional supplements on coagulation in ENT practice. J Laryngol Otol. 2008;122:116–9.

84. Chicella M, Jansen P, Parthiban A, et al. Propylene glycol accumulation associated with continuous infusion of lorazepam in pediatric intensive care patients. Crit Care Med. 2002;30:2752–6.

85. Glasgow AM, Boeckx RL, Miller MK, MacDonald MG, August GP. Hyperosmolality in small infants due to propylene glycol. Pediatrics. 1983;72:353–5.

86. Committee on Fetus and Newborn. Benzyl alcohol: toxic agent in neonatal units. Pediatrics. 1983;72:356–8.

87. Trissel LA. Handbook on injectable drugs. 11th ed. Bethesda: American Society of Health-System Pharmacists, Inc.; 2001.

88. Trissel LA, Leissing NC. Trissel's tables. Chicago: Multimatrix, Inc.; 1996.

89. Wedekind CA, Fidler BD. Compatibility of commonly used intravenous infusions in a pediatric intensive care unit. Crit Care Nurse. 2001;214:45–51.

90. Farrington E, Adcock K. Y-site drug compatibility with TPN. Pharmacy Practice News. 1997 May:49–51.

91. Catania PN. Critical care admixtures wall chart. In: King JC, Catania PN, editors. King guide to parenteral admixtures. Napa, CA: King Guide Publications, Inc; 2002.

92. Williams NT. Medication administration through enteral feeding tubes. Am J Health Syst Pharm. 2008;65:2347–57.

93. Wohlt PD, Zheng L, Gunderson S, et al. Recommendations for the use of medications with continuous enteral nutrition. Am J Health Syst Pharm. 2009;66:1458–67.

94. Dickerson RN, Garmon WM, Kuhl DA, et al. Vitamin K- independent warfarin resistance after concurrent administration of warfarin and continuous enteral nutrition. Pharmacotherapy. 2008;28:308–13.

95. Veltri MA, Neu AM, Fivush BA, et al. Drug dosing. Pediatr Drugs. 2004;6:45–65.

96. Mueller BA, Smoyer WE. Challenges in developing evidence-based drug dosing guidelines for adults and children receiving renal replacement therapy. Clin Pharmacol Ther. 2009;86:479–82.

97. Koren G, Shaffer F, Silverman E, et al. Determinants of low serum concentrations of salicylates in patients with Kawasaki disease. J Pediatr. 1988;112:663–7.

98. O'Mara NB, Jones PR, Anglin DL, et al. Pharmacokinetics of phenytoin in children with acute neurotrauma. Crit Care Med. 1995;23:1418–24.

99. Stowe CD, Lee KR, Storgion SA, et al. Altered phenytoin pharmacokinetics in children with severe, acute traumatic brain injury. J Clin Pharmacol. 2000;40:1452–61.

100. Pettersen G, Mouksassi M-S, Theoret Y, et al. Population pharmacokinetics of intravenous pantoprazole in paediatric intensive care patients. Br J Clin Pharmacol. 2009;67:216–27.

101. Carcillo JA, Doughty L, Kofos D, et al. Cytochrome P450 mediated-drug metabolism is reduced in children with sepsis-induced multiple organ failure. Intensive Care Med. 2003;29:980–4.

102. Pettersen G, Faure C, Litalien C, et al. Therapeutic failure of a single intravenous dose of pantoprazole in young intensive care children. Crit Care Med. 2005;33:A170.

103. Christ G, Mundigler G, Merhaut C, et al. Adverse cardiovascular effects of ketamine infusion in patients with catecholamine-dependent heart failure. Anaesth Intensive Care. 1997;25:255–9.

104. Agarwal S, Classen D, Larsen D, et al. Prevelance of adverse events in pediatric intensive care units in the United States. Pediatr Crit Care Med. 2010;11:558–78.

105. Leape LL, Bates DW, Cullen DJ, et al. Incidence of adverse drug events: ADE prevention study group. JAMA. 1995;274:35–43.

106. Kaushal R, Bates DW, Landrigan C, et al. Medication errors and adverse drug events in pediatric inpatients. JAMA. 2001;285:2114–20.

107. Scanlon MC, Karsh B-T. Value of human factors to medication and patient safety in the intensive care unit. Crit Care Med. 2010;38:S90–6.

108. Potts AL, Barr FE, Gregory DF, Wright L, Patel NR. Computerized physician order entry and medication errors in a pediatric critical care unit. Pediatrics. 2004;113:59–63.

109. van Rosse F, Maat B, Rademaker CMA, van Vught AJ, Egberts ACG, Bollen CW. The effect of computerized physician order entry on medication prescription errors and clinical outcome in pediatric and intensive care: a systematic review. Pediatrics. 2009;123:1184–90.

110. Han YY, Carcillo JA, Venkataraman ST, Clark RSB, Watson S, Nguyen TC, Bayir H, Orr RA. Unexpected increase in mortality after implementation of a commercially sold computerized physician order system. Pediatrics. 2005;116:1506–12.

111. Hassan E, Badawi O, Weber RJ, Cohen H. Using technology to prevent adverse drug events in the intensive care unit. Crit Care Med. 2010;38:S97–105.

112. Poon EG, Keohane CA, Yoon CS. Effect of bar-code technology on the safety of medication administration. N Engl J Med. 2010;362:1698–707.

113. Krupicka MI, Bratton SL, Sonnethal K, et al. Impact of a pediatric clinical pharmacist in the pediatric intensive care unit. Crit Care Med. 2002;30:919–21.

114. Reed MD, Blumer JL. Drug-drug interactions. In: Haddad LM, Shannon MW, Winchester JF, editors. Clinical management of poisoning and drug overdose. 3rd ed. Philadelphia: WB Saunders Co; 1998.

115. Prescott L. Paracetamol, alcohol, and the liver. Br J Clin Pharmacol. 2000;49:291–301.

Telemedicine in the Pediatric Intensive Care Unit

James P. Marcin, Madan Dharmar, and Candace Sadorra

Abstract

Telemedicine technologies involve real-time, live interactive high-definition video and audio communication that allow pediatric critical care physicians to have a virtual presence at the bedside of any critically ill child. Telemedicine use has been increasing and is expected to become a common tool in remote emergency departments, inpatient wards, and Intensive Care Units for pediatric care. There is increasing data to support new care models that incorporate telemedicine technologies result in higher care quality, more efficient resource use with improved cost-effectiveness, and higher patient, parent and remote provider satisfaction. As more research is conducted, the best use of these technologies will be better defined, and result in increased access to pediatric critical care expertise to a larger population of children in need of Pediatric Intensive Care Unit (PICU) services.

Keywords

Telemedicine • Tele-ICU • eICU • Pediatric critical care • Healthcare disparities • Quality of care

Introduction

The annual number of patients admitted to Intensive Care Units (ICUs) in the United States (US) is approximately five million and is increasing each year. Patient acuity, reflected by comorbid medical conditions, technology dependence, and severity of illness, is also on the rise. The care provided in the ICU is increasingly complex and requires state-of-the-art facilities, the most modern technologies, and a comprehensive team of specially trained multidisciplinary providers and ancillary personnel. As a result, care of ICU patients has become more complicated, and patients are increasingly exposed to failures in the care delivery that result in mistakes, complications, and even death. In fact, it is estimated that on average, every patient admitted to an average US ICU experiences 1.7 potentially life threatening errors each day, and each year some 50,000 patients die from preventable deaths [1].

In the past two decades, two major health system factors have been identified that maximize the chances of high care quality and minimize risks of mistakes and complications in the ICU. The first factor is the regionalization of specialty ICU services. ICU regionalization is a means of concentrating medical expertise and increasing patient volumes at designated referral and tertiary care hospitals. Higher patient volumes often result in increased care efficiency and improved patient outcomes. Well known examples include the regionalization of trauma, specialty surgical procedures, adult critical care, as well as neonatal and pediatric intensive care [2–8]. The second factor shown to improve outcomes and quality of care in the ICU is to ensure that all patients are actively cared for by critical care physicians. In both adult and pediatric ICUs, research demonstrates that critically ill patients have a lower risk of death, shorter ICU and hospital length of stay, and receive higher care quality when critical care physicians are involved in their management [9–12].

J.P. Marcin, MD, MPH (✉) • M. Dharmar, MBBS, PhD
C. Sadorra, BS
Department of Pediatrics, UC Davis Children's Hospital,
2516 Stockton Boulevard, Sacramento, CA 95817, USA
e-mail: jpmarcin@ucdavis.edu; mdharmar@ucdavis.edu;
candace.sadorra@ucdmc.ucdavis.edu

D.S. Wheeler et al. (eds.), *Pediatric Critical Care Medicine*,
DOI 10.1007/978-1-4471-6362-6_8, © Springer-Verlag London 2014

In fact, researchers estimate that ICU mortality is reduced by some 10–25 % when critical care physicians direct patient care compared to ICUs where critical care physicians have little to no involvement in patient care [9, 10].

Unfortunately, not all critically ill patients are cared for in regionalized ICUs, nor are they uniformly treated by critical care physicians. While regionalization improves patient care, by its design, it also creates disparities in access. Acutely ill patients living in non-urban areas, are by necessity treated and cared for in hospitals that lack full PICU services and critical care expertise [13], resulting in risk of both delays in care and inappropriate care [14, 15]. Magnifying this problem is the continued shortages of critical care physicians, for both adult and PICUs, which is expected to worsen in future years [16, 17].

Telemedicine is defined as the provision of health care over a distance using telecommunications technologies. It can be used to supplement efforts to both maintain the regionalization of ICU services as well as help specially trained critical care physicians participate in the care of critically ill patients in other locations. Telemedicine technologies can be used to more efficiently increase access to specialty care services, including critical care physicians, to patients living in underserved and remote communities and in community hospitals where the full spectrum of ICU and critical care services is not available [18, 19]. By importing specialty expertise using telemedicine, emergency departments, inpatient wards and intensive care units are given the means to increase their capacity to provide higher quality of care to critically ill patients. Critical care physicians can also increase their efficiency with these technologies so that their expertise can be shared with more patients at more than one ICU or hospital at a time. In addition, telemedicine use can potentially reduce patient transfers of less severely ill and injured children to referral centers, thus reserving limited ICU beds to those most in need of care at a regionalized center [20, 21]. For these reasons, the use of telemedicine in critical care is increasing, and is expected to become a technology that most centers will use in their future practice.

Although telemedicine can be part of the solution to disparities in access to critical care physicians and specialized care, it is not meant to obviate the transfer of critically ill patients in need of services at a regional ICU, nor is it meant to replace an on-site critical care physician. Instead, as numerous clinical programs across the country have demonstrated, telemedicine and remote monitoring technologies can be used by critical care providers to immediately share their expertise in a variety of clinical scenarios. In this chapter, we review how telemedicine can be used by pediatric critical care physicians. Specifically, we review how telemedicine can be used in remote hospital emergency departments, during the transport of critically ill children, in hospital inpatient wards, and in remote ICUs where pediatric critical care specialists are not immediately available.

The Use of Telemedicine in Emergency Departments

Past studies demonstrate shortcomings in care quality for acutely ill and injured children treated in EDs without pediatric expertise [14, 22–24]. These EDs are, at times, inadequately equipped to care for pediatric emergencies [22, 23, 25–27]. Further, personnel working in rural EDs, including physicians, nurses, pharmacists and support staff are often less experienced in caring for critically ill children. The relative lack of equipment, infrastructure and personnel experienced in delivering specialty care to children may result in delayed or incorrect diagnoses, suboptimal therapies, and imperfect medical management [3, 11, 28, 29]. As a consequence, acutely ill or injured children receive lower quality of care than children presenting to EDs in regionalized children's hospitals [14, 30–33].

Telemedicine is a practical means of delivering expertise to remote EDs where specialists are not otherwise available [34–40]. The benefit of this technology is that it provides the consultant (i.e., the pediatric critical care physician) the ability to see what is happening in the remote ED as if they were physically present. The consultant has access to high-definition patient views, the treating providers, the family, as well as monitors and equipment. Several controlled trials have compared the diagnostic accuracy, planned treatment and disposition plans of patients seen and treated in the ED supported with telemedicine compared to conventional ED care. In general, studies demonstrate equivalent results, supporting the concept that telemedicine can be used by emergency and critical care physicians to provide expert advice to remote EDs [35, 36, 41]. Specifically, in some clinical scenarios, it has been shown that patients treated over telemedicine have similar outcomes, including the need for diagnostic studies, the need for medical interventions, the frequency of return ED visits, and overall patient satisfaction compared to patients treated by in-person physicians [35, 41].

Two current examples where telemedicine has been successfully implemented in clinical ED programs are adult stroke care and to support physician extenders working in remote EDs. In several studies, neurologists providing telemedicine consultations in the evaluation and treatment of stroke patients have similar outcomes to neurologists providing consultations in-person [42–44]. This care model allows hospitals without around-the-clock access to neurologists to have immediate expert care. While this is one of the fastest growing applications of telemedicine in the ED, other specialists can similarly provide consultations from remote sites to various patient groups that need specialty care.

Telemedicine is also effective when used by emergency medicine and critical care physicians to supervise the care of other non-physician clinicians working in remote EDs [45, 46]. Galli et al., reported their experience with a care model where physician assistants staff several rural EDs, with an emergency medicine physician available for consultation using telemedicine from a university hospital [45]. In this model, where tens of thousands of patients have been treated in the rural EDs by the on-site physician assistants, patient outcomes and provider satisfaction are similar to the care provided when emergency medicine physicians staffed each of the rural EDs. In addition, this model of ED care resulted in lower total healthcare costs [47, 48].

Telemedicine use to provide immediate specialty consultations to pediatric patients in the ED has also been shown to improve the quality of care and increase provider, patient, and parent-guardian satisfaction [46, 49]. Two studies describe how pediatric critical care physicians use telemedicine to provide consultations to critically ill children presenting to several rural EDs [46, 49]. Heath et al., at the University of Vermont concluded that use of telemedicine was associated with improved patient care and was superior to telephone consultations [46, 50]. In another study by Dharmar et al., the overall care quality, measured using a previously validated implicit-review instrument [51], was higher for patients receiving telemedicine consultations in remote EDs than for patients who received telephone consultations and for patients who received no consultations [49]. These researchers also found that referring ED physicians reported that consultations more frequently prompted a change in diagnosis or therapeutic interventions than when consultations were provided by telephone. Finally, parent-guardian satisfaction and perceived quality of care were significantly higher when telemedicine was used compared to telephone for consultations obtained by the referring ED [49].

The Use of Telemedicine During Transport of Critically Ill Children

There are currently only a handful of US programs using telemedicine technologies during the transport of critically ill patients. The transport program goals are to use telecommunications technologies to transmit data, including electrocardiac and laboratory data, as well as video of the patient during transport. Unfortunately, this model is typically limited by inadequate mobile telecommunication services to provide adequate bandwidth for continuous data and video transmission. Currently, there are two primary methods of providing continuous telecommunication services: the first uses combined cell-phone services and the second uses internet connectivity with city-wide Wi-Fi or satellite services [52, 53]. While a few programs document anecdotal success with their transport telemedicine programs, researchers have yet to produce data documenting improved clinical outcomes with this telemedicine application.

In a recent study, the outcomes of simulated adult trauma patients were compared among scenarios using telemedicine and scenarios using telephone communications during transport [54]. The researchers found that use of telemedicine resulted in improved clinical outcomes including fewer episodes of desaturation, hypotension, and less tachycardia compared to identical simulated patients without telemedicine use. In addition, the researchers found that recognition rates for key physiological signs and the need for critical interventions were higher in the transport simulations with access to telemedicine [54].

Such data support the feasibility of using telemedicine during patient transport and raises possibilities that telemedicine can improve this phase of care. However, until more reliable and affordable telecommunications are available to evaluate telemedicine in transport, the effectiveness and/or benefit remain undetermined.

The Use of Telemedicine for Children Hospitalized in Intensive Care Units

PICUs are more regionalized and fewer in number than adult ICUs because children require critical care services less frequently than adults. As a result, acutely ill and injured children living in non-urban communities frequently require a medically complicated, expensive, and sometimes lengthy and risky transport in order to access specialty services. Despite the risks and potential for complications, lengthy transports are most often in the patient's best interest, given the expertise of the regionalized PICU. However, under some circumstances, transporting a pediatric patient a long distance may not be necessary if there is a close by facility with intermediate capabilities, such as a Level II PICU or adult ICU with pediatric capabilities [55]. In addition, children hospitalized at regional hospitals experience longer length of stays, greater resource utilization, and higher costs than similar children cared for at non-Children's hospitals [56–58]. Therefore, it is logical that some "mildly" or "moderately" ill children (e.g., a child with asthma who requires continuous albuterol or a child with known diabetes and mild diabetic ketoacidosis) can be cared for in a Level II PICU or other non-Children's hospital's ICU under the care of nurses and physicians competent in the care of such children with supervision from a pediatric critical care physician or pediatric critical care team using telemedicine and remote monitoring.

Telemedicine can be used by pediatric critical care physicians in a variety of clinical scenarios and for a broad range of applications [59]. Consultations, remote monitoring, and nurse-physician oversight can range from a model of intermittent, need-based consultations (the consultative model), to a bundled continuous monitoring and active involvement model (the continuous oversight model). In a consultative model, a pediatric critical care physician can provide bedside telemedicine consultations to a patient in a remote inpatient ward or ICU. Such consultations could prompt a variety of clinical interventions, including recommendations on diagnostic studies, medications, and/or other therapies. The consultation may also recommend transport to the regional PICU. This type of model could result in a one-time consultation and recommendations or lead to multiple videoconferencing interactions during the day or hospital stay [60, 61].

In the continuous oversight model, telemedicine can be used in combination with comprehensive remote monitoring by a critical care physician and nurse(s). In such a model, a remote team of physician(s) and nurse(s) are able to monitor many patient beds in sometimes several different ICUs. This care model could be more pro-active in implementing evidence-based guidelines and intervening prior to worsening care status or development of complications. This ICU telemedicine model can be created by centralizing existing ICU monitoring technologies and electronic health records, or can be contracted out to a third party specializing in remote ICU monitoring services.

Consultative Model

A pediatric critical care telemedicine program based on the consultative model has been successfully used in caring for mildly to moderately ill children in remote ICUs in Northern California [60]. In one model, pediatric critical care physicians from a regional PICU connect to the telemedicine unit at the bedside for consultations to a referring neonatologist, general pediatrician, adult critical care physician, and/or surgeon caring for an infant, child or adolescent in a combined Pediatric-Adult ICU. The bedside nurses also can initiate a request for assistance from either the physician or pediatric critical care nurse at the regional PICU. While the remote ICU does not have pediatric critical care physicians on staff, it does have a neonatal ICU, a pediatric service, a pediatric inpatient ward, and the nurses are required to maintain training in pediatric critical care nursing [60].

In this program, telemedicine consultations from pediatric critical care physicians are available 24 h per day, 7 days per week. Consultations consist of a full history (with referring physician, nurse, and/or parent-guardian) and physical exam which may require the use of telemedicine peripheral devices (such as a stethoscope, otoscope, ophthalmoscope and/or general exam camera) or reported physical findings from the bedside nurse or physician. The history and physical also includes the review of pertinent radiographs, medical records, and laboratories. Follow-up consultations can be conducted at the discretion of the consulting critical care

physician or as requested by the referring physician or bedside nurse. At any time after the initial or follow-up consultation, the patient can be transported to the regional PICU based on the specialty needs of the patient, patient stability, and at the discretion of the referring or consulting physicians, with consideration to nurse and physician comfort and parental preference.

Published data from this telemedicine program demonstrate clinical outcomes, including mortality and length of stay, similar to severity adjusted benchmark data from a set of national PICUs [60, 61]. This program resulted in a high degree of satisfaction among remote providers and parents-guardians, and allowed patients to remain in their local community, lessening the stress among family members. Consultations using this model also provide clinical expertise for patients requiring evaluation from other specialty services, including cardiology and ethics [62, 63]. Data from this program also demonstrated an overall reduction in healthcare costs due to more appropriate transport utilization and decreased utilization of the more costly, regional PICU [64].

Continuous Oversight Model

When telemedicine and videoconferencing is bundled with a remote monitoring or "tele-presence" ICU system, a more proactive care model involving critical care physicians and nurses can be used. In this model of care, the specialist may act as a consultant responsible for continuous patient monitoring but may also actively participate in patient management, including addition and titration of therapies, championing compliance with critical care best practices, and active communication with health care team members. Using this model, the initial research studies comparing pre-intervention to post-intervention outcomes suggested a non-statistically significant reduction in severity-adjusted ICU mortality, severity adjusted-hospital mortality, the incidence of some ICU complications, and decreased ICU length of stay [65, 66]. However, the studies found no overall reduction in hospital length of stay.

There have been several subsequent studies evaluating the impact of the continuous oversight ICU model of care in a variety of adult ICU settings. In a large study conducted at six ICUs in a large US health care system, a similar pre-intervention versus post-intervention study found that implementation of an integrated telemedicine and remote monitoring program did not have a large impact on evaluated care [67]. This study reported no difference in ICU mortality, hospital mortality, ICU length of stay or hospital length of stay. However, the researchers found that among the subset of patients with higher involvement of remote telemedicine providers, outcomes including survival, were improved [67]. Using the data from this study, another group of investigators researched the costs and cost-effectiveness of the tele-ICU program [68]. They found that daily average ICU and hospital costs after the implementation of the program increased by 28 % and 34 %, respectively. The investigators concluded that the cost-effectiveness of the continuous oversight program was limited to the most severely ill patients [68].

However, two more recent studies in smaller hospital settings found conflicting results. In one study, investigators conducted a pre-intervention versus post-intervention study and found no reduction in ICU mortality, hospital mortality, ICU length of stay, or hospital length of stay when the same continuous oversight model was implemented in four ICUs in two community hospitals [69]. In the same year in a similarly designed study of a single academic community hospital, the continuous oversight telemedicine program was associated with a statistically significant reduction in mortality from 21.4 % at baseline to 14.7 %. The investigators also found a significant reduction in ICU length of stay from 4.06 days at baseline to 3.77 days, which remained significant even after adjustment for case-mix and severity of illness [70].

There has been one meta-analysis that combined published data evaluating ICU telemedicine impact on patient outcomes. These researchers found that among 13 eligible studies involving 35 ICUs, there was a significant reduction in ICU mortality (pooled odds ratio, 0.80), but found no impact on in-hospital mortality for patients admitted to the ICU [71]. They also found that remote ICU telemedicine coverage was associated with a reduction in ICU length of stay by 1.3 days, but found no statistically significant reduction in hospital length of stay [71]. All studies included in this meta-analysis were assessments that compared pre-telemedicine measures to post-telemedicine measures. This study design is not ideal and subject to many biases. In addition, the meta-analysis contained a heterogeneous group of studies conducted on heterogeneous populations resulting in wide confidence intervals [72, 73].

Subsequent to the publication of this meta-analysis, researchers evaluated seven adult ICUs on two campuses of a single academic medical center where a similar continuous oversight ICU telemedicine program were implemented. These researchers found that the telemedicine program was associated with significant improvements in several clinical outcomes [74]. The adherence to critical care best practices, including guidelines for prevention of deep vein thrombosis, stress ulcers, ventilator-associated pneumonia, catheter-related bloodstream infections, and guidelines for cardiovascular protection all significantly improved. In addition, there was a relative reduction in unadjusted and risk-adjusted ICU mortality by 13 % and 20 %, respectively. Further, both risk-adjusted hospital mortality ICU and hospital length of stay were significantly decreased [74, 75].

The reasons why some continuous oversight telemedicine programs have resulted in significantly improved outcomes while others have not is likely multifactorial and related to how the programs were implemented and supported. In studies that found improved clinical outcomes, the remote critical care teams seemed to work more proactively and were involved in care of a greater proportion of patients. The studies that found no improvements in clinical outcomes tended to use telemedicine and remote monitoring technologies in a more reactive manner where the primary physicians limited participation of the remote critical care physicians to fewer patients. In addition, the studies that did not find improved outcomes with telemedicine did not have an ongoing clinical improvement program. In other words, the degree of benefit seems to be related to the extent to which the telemedicine and remote monitoring is accepted by the medical staff and whether the program is actively used to create sustainable ICU care changes [74].

Telemedicine Technologies

Telemedicine ICU consultations involve real time, live interactive high-definition video and audio communication between the specialist at the regional PICU and health care provider at the remote hospital. Therefore, in developing a telemedicine program that originates from a PICU, there are many technical challenges to address, considering the goal is to provide 24 h per day immediate assistance to critically ill infants and children. It is a requirement to have on-call systems for both clinicians, as well as the technical personnel at both remote hospitals and regional PICUs.

Telecommunication lines need to be reliable and have adequate bandwidth to maintain quality of service. This may require use of dedicated telecommunication lines, such as complete or fractionated T1 lines, Integrated Services Digital Network (ISDN), or some other private networking telecommunication systems. If the internet is used, connection speeds can vary, and resulting audio-video quality can be unreliable. Further, modifications to allow encryption must be made so that the communications are compliant with the Health Insurance Portability and Accountability Act (HIPAA). A common solution to this is built-in videoconferencing unit encryption and/or establishing a virtual private network (VPN) tunnel.

Careful consideration of the telemedicine imaging equipment is also needed. Remotely controlled videoconferencing devices offer a range of quality and can be wall mounted, pole mounted, or even mounted on mobile robotic platforms. Peripheral devices, such as high-resolution exam cameras, stethoscopes, and oto-ophthalmoscopes are available;

however, it may be easier to have the remote physician or nurse describe physical findings, such as pupillary responses, than to have a remote operator use the camera. In the continuous oversight telemedicine models, the connections for live feeds of cardiorespiratory and pressure monitors are needed, with the option for live feeds of ventilators or other monitoring devices. In some cases where these monitoring systems are not used, as in the consultative model, a remotely controlled video camera can be directed for close-up real-time monitor visualization and other equipment with interpretations similar to physical bedside interpretations.

The Future of Telemedicine in the PICU

It is expected that telemedicine use in pediatric critical care will increase. These technologies allow subspecialists to extend their expertise more quickly and further than could be done in the past. The potential advantages are numerous. Pediatric critical care physicians will be able to provide better consultations to remote locations, resulting in higher quality of care. The transport of children to the regional PICU may become more efficient and appropriate. Referring hospitals and physicians will ideally be supported to care for less ill patients that previously were referred to urban tertiary care centers. All of these goals are to the advantage of the patient, the patient's family, the remote physician, the local hospital, regional health care systems as well as the payers.

Relationships between remote and regionalized PICUs may be enhanced, as subspecialists can provide the latest information to their remote peers, and these peers can educate their urban peers about the practice of medicine in a non-regionalized, non-children's Hospital. We expect that telemedicine technologies will become more integrated into our daily care, just as computerized physician order entry and the electronic health records are becoming. Different models of care using different technologies will be used depending upon the needs of the patients, the remote hospitals, and the regional PICUs. Data will continue to be evaluated and updated to better understand telemedicine's impact on efficiency, clinical outcomes, and cost-effectiveness, to better define where, when and for whom the technologies are most clinically and economically effective.

References

1. Donchin Y, Gopher D, Olin M, et al. A look into the nature and causes of human errors in the intensive care unit. Crit Care Med. 1995;23(2):294–300.
2. Birkmeyer JD, Finlayson EV, Birkmeyer CM. Volume standards for high-risk surgical procedures: potential benefits of the leapfrog initiative. Surgery. 2001;130(3):415–22.
3. Phibbs CS, Bronstein JM, Buxton E, Phibbs RH. The effects of patient volume and level of care at the hospital of birth on neonatal mortality. JAMA. 1996;276(13):1054–9.
4. Tilford JM, Simpson PM, Green JW, Lensing S, Fiser DH. Volume-outcome relationships in pediatric intensive care units. Pediatrics. 2000;106(2 Pt 1):289–94.
5. Marcin JP, Li Z, Kravitz RL, Dai JJ, Rocke DM, Romano PS. The CABG surgery volume-outcome relationship: temporal trends and selection effects in California, 1998–2004. Health Serv Res. 2008;43(1 Pt 1):174–92.
6. Marcin JP, Song J, Leigh JP. The impact of pediatric intensive care unit volume on mortality: a hierarchical instrumental variable analysis. Pediatr Crit Care Med. 2005;6(2):136–41.
7. Finks JF, Osborne NH, Birkmeyer JD. Trends in hospital volume and operative mortality for high-risk surgery. N Engl J Med. 2011;364(22):2128–37.
8. Lorch SA, Myers S, Carr B. The regionalization of pediatric health care. Pediatrics. 2010;126(6):1182–90.
9. Pronovost PJ, Angus DC, Dorman T, Robinson KA, Dremsizov TT, Young TL. Physician staffing patterns and clinical outcomes in critically ill patients: a systematic review. JAMA. 2002;288(17):2151–62.
10. Blunt MC, Burchett KR. Out-of-hours consultant cover and case-mix-adjusted mortality in intensive care. Lancet. 2000;356(9231):735–6.
11. Pollack MM, Alexander SR, Clarke N, Ruttimann UE, Tesselaar HM, Bachulis AC. Improved outcomes from tertiary center pediatric intensive care: a statewide comparison of tertiary and nontertiary care facilities. Crit Care Med. 1991;19(2):150–9.
12. Pollack MM, Cuerdon TT, Patel KM, Ruttimann UE, Getson PR, Levetown M. Impact of quality-of-care factors on pediatric intensive care unit mortality. JAMA. 1994;272(12):941–6.
13. Kanter RK. Regional variation in child mortality at hospitals lacking a pediatric intensive care unit. Crit Care Med. 2002;30(1):94–9.
14. Dharmar M, Marcin JP, Romano PS, et al. Quality of care of children in the emergency department: association with hospital setting and physician training. J Pediatr. 2008;153(6):783–9.
15. Marcin JP, Dharmar M, Cho M, et al. Medication errors among acutely ill and injured children treated in rural emergency departments. Ann Emerg Med. 2007;50(4):361–7. 367.e361–2.
16. Angus DC, Kelley MA, Schmitz RJ, White A, Popovich Jr J. Caring for the critically ill patient. Current and projected workforce requirements for care of the critically ill and patients with pulmonary disease: can we meet the requirements of an aging population? JAMA. 2000;284(21):2762–70.
17. Pediatrician workforce statement. Pediatrics. 2005;116(1):263–9.
18. Marcin J, Ellis J, Mawis R, Nagrampa E, Nesbitt T, Dimand R. Telemedicine and the medical home: providing pediatric subspecialty care to children with special health care needs in an underserved rural community. Pediatrics. 2004;113(1 Pt 1):1–6.
19. Marcin JP, Ellis J, Mawis R, Nagrampa E, Nesbitt TS, Dimand RJ. Using telemedicine to provide pediatric subspecialty care to children with special health care needs in an underserved rural community. Pediatrics. 2004;113(1 Pt 1):1–6.
20. Haskins PA, Ellis DG, Mayrose J. Predicted utilization of emergency medical services telemedicine in decreasing ambulance transports. Prehosp Emerg Care. 2002;6(4):445–8.
21. Tsai SH, Kraus J, Wu HR, et al. The effectiveness of video-telemedicine for screening of patients requesting Emergency Air Medical Transport (EAMT). J Trauma. 2007;62(2):504–11.
22. Athey J, Dean JM, Ball J, Wiebe R, Melese-d'Hospital I. Ability of hospitals to care for pediatric emergency patients. Pediatr Emerg Care. 2001;17(3):170–4.
23. McGillivray D, Nijssen-Jordan C, Kramer MS, Yang H, Platt R. Critical pediatric equipment availability in Canadian hospital emergency departments. Ann Emerg Med. 2001;37(4):371–6.
24. Bowman SM, Zimmerman FJ, Christakis DA, Sharar SR, Martin DP. Hospital characteristics associated with the management of pediatric splenic injuries. JAMA. 2005;294(20):2611–7.

25. Middleton KR, Burt CW. Availability of pediatric services and equipment in emergency departments: United States, 2002–03. Adv Data. 2006;367:1–16.

26. Gausche-Hill M, Schmitz C, Lewis RJ. Pediatric preparedness of US emergency departments: a 2003 survey. Pediatrics. 2007;120(6):1229–37.

27. Bourgeois FT, Shannon MW. Emergency care for children in pediatric and general emergency departments. Pediatr Emerg Care. 2007;23(2):94–102.

28. Tilford JM, Roberson PK, Lensing S, Fiser DH. Improvement in pediatric critical care outcomes. Crit Care Med. 2000;28(2):601–3.

29. Keeler EB, Rubenstein LV, Kahn KL, et al. Hospital characteristics and quality of care. JAMA. 1992;268(13):1709–14.

30. Seidel JS, Henderson DP, Ward P, Wayland BW, Ness B. Pediatric prehospital care in urban and rural areas. Pediatrics. 1991;88(4):681–90.

31. Seidel JS, Hornbein M, Yoshiyama K, Kuznets D, Finklestein JZ, Jr. St Geme JW. Emergency medical services and the pediatric patient: are the needs being met? Pediatrics. 1984;73(6):769–72.

32. Durch J, Lohr KN, Institute of Medicine (U.S.), Committee on Pediatric Emergency Medical Services. Emergency medical services for children. Washington, DC: National Academy Press; 1993.

33. Durch JS, Lohr KN. From the Institute of Medicine. JAMA. 1993;270(8):929.

34. Lambrecht CJ. Emergency physicians' roles in a clinical telemedicine network. Ann Emerg Med. 1997;30(5):670–4.

35. Brennan JA, Kealy JA, Gerardi LH, et al. Telemedicine in the emergency department: a randomized controlled trial. J Telemed Telecare. 1999;5(1):18–22.

36. Brennan JA, Kealy JA, Gerardi LH, et al. A randomized controlled trial of telemedicine in an emergency department. J Telemed Telecare. 1998;4 Suppl 1:18–20.

37. Stamford P, Bickford T, Hsiao H, Mattern W. The significance of telemedicine in a rural emergency department. IEEE Eng Med Biol Mag. 1999;18(4):45–52.

38. Rogers FB, Ricci M, Caputo M, et al. The use of telemedicine for real-time video consultation between trauma center and community hospital in a rural setting improves early trauma care: preliminary results. J Trauma. 2001;51(6):1037–41.

39. Latifi R, Hadeed GJ, Rhee P, et al. Initial experiences and outcomes of telepresence in the management of trauma and emergency surgical patients. Am J Surg. 2009;198(6):905–10.

40. Hicks LL, Boles KE, Hudson ST, et al. Using telemedicine to avoid transfer of rural emergency department patients. J Rural Health. 2001;17(3):220–8.

41. Kofos D, Pitetti R, Orr R, Thompson A. Telemedicine in pediatric transport: a feasibility study. Pediatrics. 1998;102(5):E58.

42. Emsley H, Blacker K, Davies P, O'Donnell M. Telestroke. When location, location, location doesn't matter. Health Serv J. 2010;120(6227):24–5.

43. Demaerschalk BM, Hwang HM, Leung G. Cost analysis review of stroke centers, telestroke, and rt-PA. Am J Manag Care. 2010;16(7):537–44.

44. Pervez MA, Silva G, Masrur S, et al. Remote supervision of IV-tPA for acute ischemic stroke by telemedicine or telephone before transfer to a regional stroke center is feasible and safe. Stroke. 2010;41(1):e18–24.

45. Galli R, Keith JC, McKenzie K, Hall GS, Henderson K. TelEmergency: a novel system for delivering emergency care to rural hospitals. Ann Emerg Med. 2008;51(3):275–84.

46. Heath B, Salerno R, Hopkins A, Hertzig J, Caputo M. Pediatric critical care telemedicine in rural underserved emergency departments. Pediatr Crit Care Med. 2009;10(5):588–91.

47. Henderson K. TelEmergency: distance emergency care in rural emergency departments using nurse practitioners. J Emerg Nurs. 2006;32(5):388–93.

48. Duchesne JC, Kyle A, Simmons J, et al. Impact of telemedicine upon rural trauma care. J Trauma. 2008;64(1):92–7; discussion 97–8.

49. Dharmar M, Romano PS, Kuppermann N, Nesbitt TS, Cole SL, Andrada ER, Vance C, Harvey DJ, Marcin JP. Impact of critical care telemedicine consultations on children in rural emergency departments. Crit Care Med. 2013;41(10):2388–95.

50. Dharmar M, Marcin JP. A picture is worth a thousand words: critical care consultations to emergency departments using telemedicine. Pediatr Crit Care Med. 2009;10(5):606–7.

51. Dharmar M, Marcin JP, Kuppermann N, et al. A new implicit review instrument for measuring quality of care delivered to pediatric patients in the emergency department. BMC Emerg Med. 2007;7:13.

52. Qureshi A, Shih E, Fan I, et al. Improving patient care by unshackling telemedicine: adaptively aggregating wireless networks to facilitate continuous collaboration. AMIA Proc Annu Symp. 2010;2010:662–6.

53. Hsieh JC, Lin BX, Wu FR, Chang PC, Tsuei YW, Yang CC. Ambulance 12-lead electrocardiography transmission via cell phone technology to cardiologists. Telemed J E Health. 2010;16(8):910–5.

54. Charash WE, Caputo MP, Clark H, et al. Telemedicine to a moving ambulance improves outcome after trauma in simulated patients. J Trauma. 2011;71(1):49–55.

55. Rosenberg DI, Moss MM. Guidelines and levels of care for pediatric intensive care units. Crit Care Med. 2004;32(10):2117–27.

56. Merenstein D, Egleston B, Diener-West M. Lengths of stay and costs associated with children's hospitals. Pediatrics. 2005;115(4):839–44.

57. Odetola FO, Gebremariam A, Freed GL. Patient and hospital correlates of clinical outcomes and resource utilization in severe pediatric sepsis. Pediatrics. 2007;119(3):487–94.

58. Gupta RS, Bewtra M, Prosser LA, Finkelstein JA. Predictors of hospital charges for children admitted with asthma. Ambul Pediatr. 2006;6(1):15–20.

59. Dharmar M, Smith AC, Armfield NR, Trujano J, Sadorra C, Marcin JP. Telemedicine for children in need of intensive care. Pediatr Ann. 2009;38(10):562–6.

60. Marcin JP, Nesbitt TS, Kallas HJ, Struve SN, Traugott CA, Dimand RJ. Use of telemedicine to provide pediatric critical care inpatient consultations to underserved rural Northern California. J Pediatr. 2004;144(3):375–80.

61. Marcin JP, Schepps DE, Page KA, Struve SN, Nagrampa E, Dimand RJ. The use of telemedicine to provide pediatric critical care consultations to pediatric trauma patients admitted to a remote trauma intensive care unit: a preliminary report. Pediatr Crit Care Med. 2004;5(3):251–6.

62. Huang T, Moon-Grady AJ, Traugott C, Marcin J. The availability of telecardiology consultations and transfer patterns from a remote neonatal intensive care unit. J Telemed Telecare. 2008;14(5):244–8.

63. Kon AA, Rich B, Sadorra C, Marcin JP. Complex bioethics consultation in rural hospitals: using telemedicine to bring academic bioethicists into outlying communities. J Telemed Telecare. 2009;15(5):264–7.

64. Marcin JP, Nesbitt TS, Struve S, Traugott C, Dimand RJ. Financial benefits of a pediatric intensive care unitbased telemedicine program to a rural adult intensive care unit: impact of keeping acutely ill and injured children in their local community. Telemed J E Health. 2004;10:1–5.

65. Rosenfeld BA, Dorman T, Breslow MJ, et al. Intensive care unit telemedicine: alternate paradigm for providing continuous intensivist care. Crit Care Med. 2000;28(12):3925–31.

66. Breslow MJ, Rosenfeld BA, Doerfler M, et al. Effect of a multiple-site intensive care unit telemedicine program on clinical and economic outcomes: an alternative paradigm for intensivist staffing. Crit Care Med. 2004;32(1):31–8.

67. Thomas EJ, Lucke JF, Wueste L, Weavind L, Patel B. Association of telemedicine for remote monitoring of intensive care patients with mortality, complications, and length of stay. JAMA. 2009;302(24):2671–8.

68. Franzini L, Sail KR, Thomas EJ, Wueste L. Costs and cost-effectiveness of a telemedicine intensive care unit program in 6 intensive care units in a large health care system. J Crit Care. 2011;26(3):329.e321–6.

69. Morrison JL, Cai Q, Davis N, et al. Clinical and economic outcomes of the electronic intensive care unit: results from two community hospitals. Crit Care Med. 2010;38(1):2–8.

70. McCambridge M, Jones K, Paxton H, Baker K, Sussman EJ, Etchason J. Association of health information technology and teleintensivist coverage with decreased mortality and ventilator use in critically ill patients. Arch Intern Med. 2010;170(7): 648–53.

71. Young LB, Chan PS, Lu X, Nallamothu BK, Sasson C, Cram PM. Impact of telemedicine intensive care unit coverage on patient outcomes: a systematic review and meta-analysis. Arch Intern Med. 2011;171(6):498–506.

72. Smith AC, Armfield NR. A systematic review and meta-analysis of ICU telemedicine reinforces the need for further controlled investigations to assess the impact of telemedicine on patient outcomes. Evid Based Nurs. 2011;14(4):102–3. Epub 2011 Aug 2.

73. Kahn JM. Intensive care unit telemedicine: promises and pitfalls. Arch Intern Med. 2011;171(6):495–6.

74. Lilly CM, Cody S, Zhao H, et al. Hospital mortality, length of stay, and preventable complications among critically ill patients before and after tele-ICU reengineering of critical care processes. JAMA. 2011;305(21):2175–83.

75. Kahn JM. The use and misuse of ICU telemedicine. JAMA. 2011;305(21):2227–8.

Quality Improvement Science in the PICU

9

Matthew F. Niedner

Abstract

This chapter describes important aspects of health-care quality, what it is, and how to engage clinical providers in improvement efforts. The case for improving healthcare quality is outlined, with an emphasis on the special considerations within the pediatric intensive care unit setting. Common terminology to facilitate an understanding of quality is reviewed – including near misses, preventable and non-preventable adverse events. Models for understanding system and process performance are discussed – including the system of profound knowledge, aims oriented change, Plan-Do-Study-Act applications of the scientific method, and features of high reliability organizations. Provided is a basic tool kit for implementing change through the use of error proofing, process control, lean engineering, standardization, checklists, and protocols. Additionally, an introductory review of statistical process control and understanding variation through control charts is provided.

Keywords

Quality Improvement • Patient Safety • Medical Errors • Reliability • Translational Research

What Is Health-Care Quality?

In *To Err Is Human*, the Institute of Medicine (IOM) defined *health-care quality* as "the degree to which health services increase the likelihood of desired outcomes" and *patient safety* as "freedom from accidental injury because of medical care or medical errors" [1]. These two concepts are fundamentally linked, of course, and many notable voices have explicitly cited safety as the key dimension of quality, including the IOM, the Leapfrog Group, the Institute for Healthcare Improvement (IHI), the National Quality Forum (NQF), and even Hippocrates – *primum non nocere*. Other chapters of this textbook will focus more explicitly on patient safety, unintended harm, and the prevention of

specific health-care associated complications. This chapter focuses on improvement models, general strategies, and practical concepts that can be applied in efforts to improve health-care quality.

The IOM outlined six dimensions of health-care quality [2]. The most fundamental attribute is that care should be safe. Care must also be effective and appropriately dispensed—that is, care must be provided to all who could benefit and not to those unlikely to benefit (avoiding underuse and overuse). Care should be patient-centered—respectful of and responsive to individual patient preferences, needs, and values, as opposed to provider or organizational motives. Quality care is timely—the right care to the right person at the right time—with waits and delays eliminated or minimized. Care should be efficient, actively seeking to identify and eliminate all forms of waste, be it time, equipment, supplies, or energy. The final dimension of care outlined by the IOM is equitability—the provision of care that does not vary in quality because of personal characteristics such as sex, ethnicity, geographic location, and socioeconomic status. It is a tall order, but ultimately attainable.

M.F. Niedner, MD
Pediatric Intensive Care Unit, Division of Critical Care Medicine, Department of Pediatrics, University of Michigan Medical Center, Mott Children's Hospital, F-6894 Mott #0243,
1500 East Medical Center Dr, Ann Arbor, MI 48109-0243, USA
e-mail: mniedner@med.umich.edu

D.S. Wheeler et al. (eds.), *Pediatric Critical Care Medicine*,
DOI 10.1007/978-1-4471-6362-6_9, © Springer-Verlag London 2014

The terms quality assurance (QA), quality control (QC), and quality improvement (QI) are often used interchangeably in colloquial parlance, however, each has a slightly different meaning. The primary objective of QA is to demonstrate that a service or product meets a set of pre-defined expectations or requirements. This is achieved by comparing actual processes and/or outcomes to those specified criteria. QC involves the systematic use of performance monitoring and corrective methods to ensure that a service or product conforms to a desired standard. QI refers to the betterment or enhancement of a product or service compared to current, historical, or benchmark states. The term continuous quality improvement (CQI) is used to describe ongoing or iterative QI efforts.

Engaging Healthcare Providers in Quality Improvement

In spite of the known risks to patients from deficits in health-care quality and safety countermeasures, most clinicians do not deliberately employ QI principles in their work, often believing that the responsibility for "systems issues" resides with the hospital administration [3–5]. Most clinicians focus on an understanding of pathophysiology and extrapolate treatment focusing on these principles. Figure 9.1 shows the translational research sequence of studies that transpire going from bench to bedside to practice guidelines. Research guided primarily by physiologic principles occurs in the early stages of translational research (e.g., T1 and T2). Late translational research (T3), such as implementation science, performance reliability, or improvement sustainability, is often confounded by local phenomena (e.g., staffing ratios, case mix), individualism (e.g., clinicians' experience base, leadership style), human factors (e.g., psychology, ergonomics), and nonmedical disciplines (e.g., business, economics, information technology, industrial engineering). These factors impact the generalizability of many quality and safety interventions. Tragically, the vast majority of discovery from T3 translational research is never published or disseminated—a lost opportunity in terms of the knowledge that *can* be extrapolated [3].

In 2001, the IOM report, *Crossing the Quality Chasm*, elaborated on strategic solutions to improve safety and quality in health-care, emphasizing the importance of systems-based analysis, correction of latent defects in complex systems, transparency, multi-professional and multi-institutional collaboration [2]. Perhaps most importantly was the emphasis on overcoming the culture of individual blame and reliance on imperfect humans to simply try harder or do better. The IOM argued that imperfections in human performance should be expected, and that systems should be designed to anticipate and mitigate their impact on patient outcomes. With the sentinel IOM reports, important health-care stakeholders have made significant commitments to address these issues [6]. In 1999, the Accreditation Council for Graduate Medical Education began requiring competence in systems-based practice for physicians in training. In 2005, the American Board of Medical Specialties outlined the kinds of patient-safety and quality-improvement content

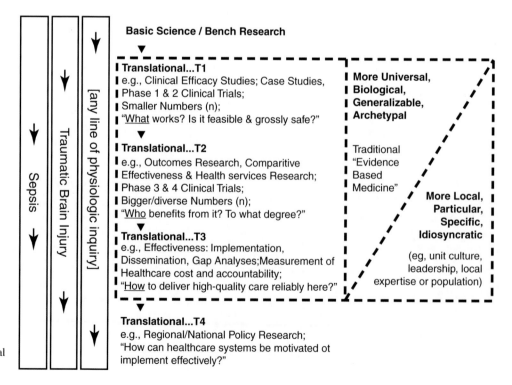

Fig. 9.1 A model of translational research stages

that should be included on board-examination questions in all medical specialties [7]. In 2007, on the heels of pay-for-performance approaches pioneered by some third-party payers, the Centers for Medicare & Medicaid Services declared that there would no longer be reimbursement for the additional costs associated with certain preventable medical complications – and many other insurers are now following suit [8, 9]. Most recently, in 2010, the Maintenance of Certification (MOC) program for physicians went beyond the traditional requirements—such as periodic examinations, continuing education, state credentialing—and required for the first time a practice performance assessment [10]. To maintain certification, physicians out of training must now demonstrate their ability to assess the quality of care they provide compared with peers or national benchmarks – and be able to apply the best evidence through follow-up assessments [11]. This latest element of MOC has only begun to play out, but it clearly represents a significant intent to encourage physicians to engage in clinical QI more substantively.

In the context of increasing public pressure for transparency, financial incentives for performance, as well as legal and regulatory drivers for improved patient safety and health-care quality, there is a rapidly flourishing academic dimension to QI. Some of the methodologies to analyze quality and safety in health-care with academic rigor are still in development, relatively young, and under adaptation from other industries and disciplines—and many are not familiar to practicing clinicians nor embedded in medical education [12]. Such analytic tools from human-factors engineering, psychology, industrial engineering and manufacturing are increasingly finding their way into the traditional stomping grounds of peer-reviewed medical literature [13]. Finally, calls for scholarly accounts of quality and safety endeavors—along with publication guidelines for proper peer review—have appeared in recent years [14, 15].

The Case for Health-Care Quality as a Priority for Pediatric Critical Care

The Pediatric Intensive Care Unit (PICU) is a place of converging threats to quality and safety—in essence, a canary in the coal mine. All the challenges that adult medicine has in defining, measuring, and improving health-care quality are amplified in pediatrics, where evidence for best practice is more limited, the data infrastructure less robust, and the potential loss of quality-adjusted life-years greater [16]. Furthermore, ICUs, emergency departments, and operating rooms are the locations where defects in care delivery are most prolific [1].

In the PICU, workflow is unpredictable, diverse, complex, technical, stressful, and invasive—often with little margin for error, as critically ill patients may succumb to insults that healthier patients might tolerate. Care must be multidisciplinary, with no one role—physician, nurse, respiratory therapist, pharmacist, or social worker—able to have mastery of all the information and skills necessary to treat the patient optimally. This makes the ICU critically dependent on teamwork and communication that must both function reliably in short time frames—and some of the most common and refractory sources of error are teamwork and communication failures [17]. There is a very high volume of "sharp end" activities—the point of care where all propagated defects emerging from the system actually reach the patient—a medicine injected, a catheter inserted, a chest shocked. Yet in spite of the pervasive risks in the PICU, adverse outcomes from errors are camouflaged. In general, more deaths occur in PICUs than in any other care units within a pediatric hospital, and adverse outcomes, although unwanted, are not unexpected. A death in a general-care unit stands out in bold relief and is scrutinized deeply for what went wrong—but how is it clearly discerned when morbidity or mortality in the PICU is from progressive refractory critical illness or from unrecognized (or unreported) medical errors slipping under the radar of awareness?

Pediatric critical-care medicine as a discipline has taken the initiative in asserting a voice at the national level regarding measures of performance quality and safety, instead of waiting for external entities to select or mandate such measures as targets for public reporting and pay-for-performance [18]. The density of error potential, the high level of vigilance, and the abundance of objective patient data make the ICU a locale that lends itself to measuring quality. Indeed, the NQF recently endorsed 48 quality measures, of which 23 are relevant to PICU care, and 7 are explicit measures of PICU performance. There are only 13 pediatric-specific measures, making PICU-specific measure representative of more than half of the NQF-endorsed measures for pediatric care (Fig. 9.2) [19]. Similarly, Medicare's recent announcement of numerous nonreimbursed "never events" included 8 metrics highly relevant to the PICU, although none that are PICU-specific (Fig. 9.2) [9].

The health-care industry has a fairly woeful track record of reliably delivering contemporary best practice. It is estimated that adults typically receive recommended, evidence-based care about 55 % of the time, with little variation among acute, chronic, and preventive care [20]. Although PICU-specific data on best-practice compliance are scarce, general pediatric data from a similar analysis suggest performance that is comparable to adult care on average, but a larger variability based on type of care [21]. Children receive an estimated 68 % of indicated care for acute medical problems, 53 % for chronic medical conditions, and 41 % for preventive care. What is more, data derived from such audits do not include many errors unrelated to widely accepted best

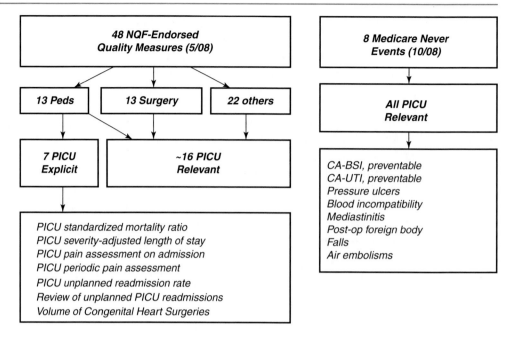

Fig. 9.2 Quality & safety measures endorsed by national entities. *CABSI* catheter-associated bloodstream infection, *CAUTI* catheter-associated urinary tract infection, *NQF* National Quality Forum

practices, nor those invisible to the audit methodology. In a survey of pediatric physicians and nurses, half filed incident reports on <50 % of their own errors, and a third did so <20 % of the time [22]. It is reasonable to conclude that most practitioners in the PICU are only aware of the tip of the iceberg when it comes to near-misses, preventable harm, and opportunities for improving healthcare quality.

Many quality and safety initiatives developed in the ICU find wide application in other medical environments and service lines. This not only makes the PICU fertile ground for the development of interventions relevant to pediatrics at large but also makes the PICU well positioned to further develop QI science itself [23]. If the PICU is to be the canary in the coal mine, then it can also be an incubator of improvement innovation.

Models for Understanding Quality

As experimental statistician George Box observed, "All models are wrong, but some are useful" [24]. Models, of course, provide an artificial structure for knowledge that reflects complex phenomena accurately enough to better enable understanding—ideally well enough to enable meaningful interpretation and constructive action. Clearly, healthcare quality is complex, but models can help us grasp what is essential. A few of the more common and useful models for improvement are touched on here.

A high-level perspective on managing quality is encapsulated by Deming's system of profound knowledge [25]. This model is comprised of these four domains:

1. *Appreciation of a system*: understanding the overall processes involving suppliers, producers, and customers (or

recipients) of goods and services; insight into the interdependence and dynamism of complex institutions; recognition of how the whole is greater than the sum of parts.

2. *Knowledge of variation*: understanding the range and causes of variation in quality (e.g., common versus special cause); ability or access to statistical sampling in measurements.

3. *Theory of knowledge (or epistemology)*: understanding the merits and limitations of what is knowable, how we come to understand through experimentation, and the roles of modeling, prediction, and justification.

4. *Knowledge of psychology*: understanding concepts of human nature, including inter-individual variation, communication styles, beliefs, assumptions, intrinsic/extrinsic motivation, and the will to change; insight into the collective impact of individual psychology toward the behavior of groups, morale, and teamwork.

Perhaps one of the simplest ways to think of QI is as a strategy to close the gap between actual practice and best known practice. The estimated time lag for scientific knowledge generated in randomized clinical trials to be routinely accepted into medical practice is 17 years, a rather shocking testimony to the size and persistence of the gap, and a provocative invitation to close it [2]. Figure 9.3 is one depiction of how QI fits in the context of actual, best, and idealized performance. If the graph is taken as a survival or time-to-adverse-event curve from some identified measure of quality or safety, one can assume that the ideal outcome is 100 % perfect over time. Much conventional research is focused on closing the gap between current best practice and such an idealized practice—that is, taking the best known mousetrap and incrementally making it better. In contrast, much QI is focused on closing the gap between actual practice and best

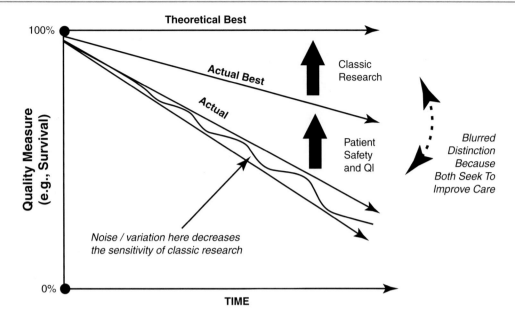

Fig. 9.3 A comparison of classic research versus quality improvement. Classic prospective interventional research and quality improvement (QI) both seek to move clinical care closer to an idealized theoretical best outcome. Classic research often focuses on novel means – such as more sensitive diagnostics or superior therapeutics. QI often focuses on closing the gap between common practice and established best practice—such as thru standardization, decision-support, and automation. Reducing errors and performance variation in operations through quality control can reduce the noise introduced into measures of research interest, thereby improving the sensitivity of research efforts. Thus, clinical research and clinical QI are synergistic

known practice—that is, taking the best designed mousetrap already known and ensuring that it deploys flawlessly every time it is indicated (and not when it isn't) in the specific local context of deployment. Complex systems and multi-step successes are often a basis for the gap between actual and best practice. If one is to start with valid, evidence-based health-care guidelines, many steps must be executed correctly for the best care to reach a patient. Staff must be aware of the evidence, accept it sufficiently, know how to apply it, work in a care environment that makes it feasible, remember to do it real-time, have agreement from the care team and consumer, and ensure that the care is actually performed in the right time, place, and manner. If each of these steps were to occur with 95 % fidelity, best care would be delivered only about 70 % of the time.

It is not uncommon for classic research and QI interventions to be confused, as they both are seeking to improve patient outcomes in data-driven ways, although typically through different mechanisms. Classic research and QI are often touted as serial, but in truth they are concurrent and synergistic. Classic research in early translational stages (T1/T2) certainly defines many of the best known practices that QI agents strive to implement in later translational work. Yet improvements in the consistency and reliability of baseline clinical performance can reduce noise, improving the sensitivity of analyses aimed at detecting small incremental improvements in best practice (Fig. 9.3). For example, if children are not dying or having prolonged hospitalizations due to nosocomial infections,

Hierarchy of Defects	Methods to Remediate
System Vulnerabilities *(Risk of Failure)* ⬇	*[MORE PROACTIVE]* ⇧ Failure Mode & Effects Analysis Reduce Steps (simplify / "lean")
Near Misses *(Failure, No Harm)* ⬇	Reliable Steps (process control) Root Cause Analysis (RCA)
Adverse Events *(Harm)*	⇩ *[MORE REACTIVE]*

Fig. 9.4 Hierarchy of defects and methods to remediate

medication errors, and surgical complications, then sensitivity will be increased when trying to detect the impact of a novel intervention on survivorship and length of stay.

Another useful QI model relates to the hierarchy of defects in a complex system. *Latent system risks, near-misses*, and *actual harm* are points along a continuum. Figure 9.4 demonstrates how this continuum matches up to methods commonly employed to remediate such defects. There is a long-standing debate between whether it is more advantageous to measure risk, errors, or harm—but in truth, each has advantages and disadvantages, and all are widely used. A brief consideration of each measurement follows.

Table 9.1 Types of waste in the lean model

Type of waste	Definition	Heath care examples
Correction	Rework because of defects, poor quality, mistakes	Revising incomplete or illegible forms
		Order entry error
Overproduction	Producing the wrong things or producing more/sooner/faster than required by downstream processes	Unused or too-frequent laboratory testing
		Too frequent clinic appointments
Motion/ movement	Unnecessary physical activity (motion) by people or relocation (movement) of people/materials	Walking to office supplies or exam room
		Searching for misplaced equipment or chart
		Multiple patient room transfers
Waiting	People, machine, and information idle time	Patient waiting in waiting room
		Providers waiting for lab results
Inventory	Information, material, or consumers in queue or stock	Stacks of medical notes to be dictated
		Excess stored supplies in stock room
Processing	Unnecessary or redundant handling or processing	Reentry of patient demographics
		Repeat collection of data
Underutilization	Tasking staff below their capacity or abilities	Nurse tending phones to refill prescriptions
		Surgeon operating on one patient per day

Detection and elimination of latent defects in a complex system provides the ideal solution to improving quality and safety, as it is the furthest point upstream from harming a patient. Failure Modes and Effects Analysis (FMEA) is one powerful strategy to identify ways in which a complex system can fail on the basis of known historical performance of constituent parts of a device or process. This allows potential defects to be designed out of the system (or planned countermeasures to be devised) before a design actually culminates in an actual product or active process. FMEA is widely used in manufacturing and engineering industries where device performance is fairly predictable (as with an intravenous pump or telemetry unit), but it is increasingly applied in the service industry—even though human factors and dynamic phenomena are more difficult to model [17]. Limitations of analyzing latent system vulnerabilities include: lack of good historical performance data upon which to base the model, the risk of unforeseen perturbations in complex and interdependent systems, unpredictable and dynamic changes in the system, lack of intuitive guidance to the sources of risk, and the theoretical nature of some assumptions and conclusions in the absence of measurable errors or harm.

Another top-tier tool in system improvement is process streamlining through the elimination of waste—be it time, energy, materials, or process complexity. As Albert Einstein said, "Make everything as simple as possible, but not simpler" [26]. If a desired outcome can be achieved in fewer steps without loss of fidelity or performance, it will likely be safer, because eliminating unnecessary steps removes some opportunities for errors to creep into a system and simultaneously reduces the number of variables when trying to understand ongoing failures. Furthermore, elimination of waste improves value from a cost–benefit perspective. This kind of streamlining to optimize value-added output is the basis for lean design, originally applied to production lines but increasingly applied to service lines. The contemporary paradigm of lean production and management is based on the Toyota Production System, and lean strategies have been successfully adapted to health care [27–29]. Specific examples of the kinds of waste identified and eliminated in the health-care setting are outlined in Table 9.1. A full description of lean methodology is beyond the scope of this chapter, but exhaustive resources are available for the interested student [30, 31].

Progressing along the ladder from latent defect to harm, the next step closer to patients is error. The most widely accepted criteria for medical error is failure of a planned action to be completed as intended (an error of execution) or the use of a wrong plan to achieve an aim (an error of planning), whether by commission or omission [32]. Thus the drug overdose due to a decimal error may be considered an error of execution by commission, whereas the treatment of mistaken septic shock instead of the actual adrenal crisis might be viewed as an error of planning where proper care was omitted. If the error results in no harm, it is commonly labeled a *near-miss*, whereas if harm occurs, it is considered a *preventable adverse event*. This should be considered distinct from *non-preventable adverse events* for which ways to avoid the known complication are not established—that is, harm occurring as a consequence of medical care but in the absence of an error (such as with the risk of cardiotoxicity from chemotherapy). Because errors resulting in near-misses are far more common than errors resulting in preventable harm, near-misses provide an attractive target for monitoring and measuring quality and safety on a continuous basis. Analysis of near-misses in an iterative manner can help generate hypotheses for root causes more rapidly than if only harmful events are considered. Focusing on errors and can be particularly helpful when related outcome measures are too rare or catastrophic to be acceptable guideposts (e.g., deaths).

Such error-based surveillance (e.g., compliance with a best practice) is particularly helpful when there is good evidence for key steps or processes firmly established in the medical literature. The ability to identify and monitor compliance with important process measures provides actionable data to an improvement team about how to reduce unnecessary variation and close the gap between actual performance and desired best practice (Fig. 9.3). This is the basis of process control—often associated with the Six Sigma management strategy employed widely in many sectors of industry, including health care.

Although there are advantages to error-based quality-performance analyses, there are notable limitations to acknowledge. Error and near-miss rates vary widely depending on the definitions used for error, surveillance methods, and even the safety culture of the reporting unit [33, 34]. Furthermore, measures of errors are most helpful if they can be expressed as rates (errors divided by opportunities for that error type), but often there is no denominator available [18]. Even the numerators can be circumspect because many errors go unreported, and there is an attention bias that favors identification of errors of commission (rather than omission) and errors resulting in harm (rather than near-misses) [22]. Thus, error-based quality assessment may be better applied as a local qualitative and semi-quantitative improvement strategy, rather than an as comparative performance tool [35.]

The measure of actual harm to patients is a final measure of quality and safety in the current hierarchy being discussed (Fig. 9.4). From a high-principled perspective, one can consider harm to the patient a failure to have detected and mitigated the latent system defects and combination of conspiring errors. Although risk and near-miss analyses are more proactive, harm analysis is a more reactive process—there is no putting the genie back in the bottle. From a pragmatic perspective, it is like adding insult to injury to witness harm and not try to learn from it. It is worth noting that all errors are not created equal . . . those resulting in harm may be distinct from those that do not, and harmful errors can implicate defects not necessarily apparent in near-misses [36]. Several organizations have proposed injury-based trigger tools that can be used to provide systematic surveillance measures of harm, such as the Agency for Healthcare Research and Quality's general and pediatric-specific Patient Safety Indicators, the IHI's Global Trigger Tool, and others [18, 37–39]. Some of these metrics and tools focus on types of harm that are assumed to be preventable or largely so, whereas other tools for measuring harm are inclusive of all readily identifiable harm. One key advantage to measuring all harm is that it provides an opportunity to question the boundary between preventable and unpreventable injuries. If the goal in health care is to eliminate or reduce all harm to patients, then including measures of harm considered unpreventable by traditional medical standards can direct our attention toward innovative care or research. Indeed, it is our medical legacy that types of harm formerly deemed to be "a cost of doing business in the ICU" are now considered imminently preventable, as has been the case with many hospital-acquired infections [23, 40, 41].

Harm-based performance metrics have their limitations too, of course—the most obvious being that the patient is injured in some manner. Because unpreventable adverse events and deaths are, to some extent, expected in the PICU, such occurrences do not necessarily raise the specter of preventable error. When they are recognized, attribution may not be accurate. Furthermore, the retrospective nature of harm evaluation provokes numerous kinds of bias toward which human perceptions are prone—such as hindsight and outcome bias [42].

If the analysis and attribution of risk, error, or harm is significantly biased, incorrect, or overly simplistic, then the conclusions not only are invalid but also can lead to unnecessary and possibly counterproductive attempts at remediation. Therefore, all risk, error, and harm analysis—as well as planned responses—must be undertaken with such limits and pitfalls in mind. Finally, because all monitoring and corrective strategies have limitations and none are perfectly suited for all applications, it makes sense to employ multiple simultaneous approaches for a more robust quality-monitoring and safety-monitoring system. Doing so also helps create cross-validation between sources of perceived risks, error patterns, and actual harm—helping to overcome the weaknesses of each individual approach.

The Science of Quality Improvement

When considering QI science, especially late translational research (e.g., T3), an understanding of the "realistic evaluation" model put forward by Pawson and Tilley [43] is helpful to get past some of the constraints inherent in orthodox experimentation [44] (Fig. 9.5). In a nutshell, realistic evaluation seeks to explain variation in outcomes by analyzing the context that may have differentially enabled or disabled an intervention from having the postulated impact. Classic research methods use strategies to wash out variation and isolate the effect of an intervention—such as with randomization, prospective analysis, large sample sizes, blinding, and controlling for known confounders. In the face of conflicted literature on the efficacy of an intervention, a conventional approach might be to perform a meta-analysis—to essentially "lump" the studies together to see what the "true" effect is when analyzed with greater power. However compellingly large the sample size may become, there are many limitations to this method of understanding variation between studies [45–47]. Another way to interpret conflicting studies is to consider the unknown, unmeasured, or unrecognized

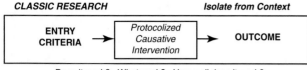

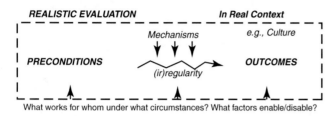

Fig. 9.5 Classic research versus realistic evaluation. Classic prospective interventional research often employs methods to "wash out" the influence of context and bias—such as through strict entry/exclusion criteria, large sample sizes, randomization, blinding, cluster analysis, etc. This largely obviates the need to explicitly understand, measure, or control for contextual variables that may be influencing outcomes—allowing the effects of the intervention to be isolated. This is an effective way to determine whether or not an intervention works and to what degree. In realistic evaluation, greater consideration is given to how uncontrolled preconditions are acted upon by a variety of mechanisms and/or interventions (which may not be carried out consistently) in a context of local idiosyncrasies (such as teamwork climate, staff experience, human factors). In a realistic evaluation of an intended intervention, differences it outcome might be interpreted based on what made the intervention perform as expected in some circumstances but not in others

contextual factors that altered the impact of an intervention (either positively or negatively) in different studies or sites. If influential contextual factors can be identified, implementing such enablers or eliminating disablers may allow an intervention to perform as intended. A good example of this is the impact of safety culture on certain unit outcomes, such as nosocomial infection rates, throughput delays, medication errors, and staff turnover [48–52]. Teamwork and safety climate have proven to be responsive to ICU-wide interventions, both positively and negatively, making interventional anthropology a growing domain of QI [49, 53].

Not only are the models for QI science often different from traditional biostatistical approaches, but the way measures are viewed and used also differ (Table 9.2) [54, 55]. Where classic research seeks to discover new knowledge in the scientific realm, improvement science seeks to operationalize it in real life. In research orthodoxy, unequivocal hard outcomes (e.g., death) are preferable to surrogate markers assumed to be correlated to them (e.g., multiple organ dysfunction scores). However, measures in improvement science are multidimensional, often with a hard outcome measure as an ultimate verification that improvement is occurring, but critically important process measures that serve as the tools to guide the specific improvement strategies employed. An important illustration of the difference

between QI process measures and traditional surrogate measures can be made with hand hygiene compliance. While the hard outcome measure of hospital-acquired infections (HAIs) can be measured, they are hopefully infrequent events and do not lend themselves to rapidly determining efficacy of interventions to reduce them. Hand hygiene compliance, however, can be measured frequently, and rapid-cycle improvement interventions can be built around such key processes contributing to HAIs without waiting for adverse events to occur.

Where classic research strives to have a rigorously consistent management protocol, improvement science constantly tweaks and refines management toward best practice. Whereas classic research seeks to eliminate or minimize biases, improvement scientists try to hold them sufficiently steady during testing to allow for causal inference. Classic research is typically powered a priori to definitively answer a primary question with statistical significance once all the data are gathered, and interim analyses are shunned to avoid spurious signals. Conversely, improvement science seeks to generate real-time and continuous data that can be interpreted and acted on simultaneously—sometimes using data trends to inform confidence in recent interventions and guide next steps from a probabilistic vantage point. For instance, if a QI intervention were inexpensive, safe, and minimally burdensome (e.g., a central line insertion checklist), then one might accept a different level of confidence in the statistical significance of local implementation than, say, if one were considering an intervention that is expensive, cumbersome, and accompanied by potential unintended consequences (e.g., a fast MRI scanner).

A large historical body of QI efforts is blighted in the eyes of many scientists as mere administrative window dressing—the rewriting of policies, the aesthetic revision of a patient portal Web site, the feel-good of patient-centered or family-centered niceties [56]. However, the modern patient-safety movement represents a sustained effort to use rigorous methods driven by data and testing. As the axiom goes, "In God we trust; all others bring data" [57]. At the core of science, be it classic research or QI, is the method. There are many ways to apply the scientific method, and the crucial challenge is to have sufficient knowledge of the tools and methods, to grasp their limitations, and to know which tool is right to apply to a particular problem at hand [5, 12, 55]. To this end, pioneers in the science of improvement have put forward an archetypal model for improvement that can serve as a fairly universal platform well suited for improvement work in health care [58, 59].

The model for improvement begins with a clear expression of aims in measurable and time-specific terms as it applies to a defined population. As the IHI's motto goes, "Soon is not a time . . . some is not a number." The model for improvement calls for clearly defining or developing new

Table 9.2 Comparison of measures in classic research versus quality improvement science

	Classic research	Improvement/safety science
Usual goals	Discovery of new knowledge; providing objective proof or basis; establishing best practice	Operationalize discoveries or best practice into routine care; ensure/monitor performance
Intervention or protocol	Single static protocol; first and last patient in protocol get same management; long timetables	Flexible/dynamic protocol or multiple serial tests; management adjusted freely based on learning; short and responsive timetables
Management of confounders	Identify, eliminate, exclude, and control for biases thru blinding, randomization, cross-over, etc	Identify and understand biases; stabilize biases during tests or interpret findings in bias context
Preferred measures	Hard and unequivocal outcomes; background data to ensure comparability	Blend of outcomes measures, relevant process measures, and possible balancing measures
Power and scale	Powered to definitively answer question and possibly explore post hoc analyses	Minimally sufficient data to meet confidence threshold for action or decision; successful tests scale up
Data interpretation	Data blinding; no interim peeking; data safety monitoring boards; classic biostatistics with significance thresholds	Real-time data; analyze & act on data simultaneously; statistical process control (control charts); data trends influence next steps

Based on data from Refs. [55, 57]

metrics to track progress toward the aim in quantitative ways—some combination of outcome, process, and balancing measures to know whether improvement is actually taking place independent of qualitative opinion. The crucial judgment step in this model is selecting the change to test. All improvement requires making changes, but not all changes result in improvement. Reliance on individuals with keen insight into the system complexities at hand as well as the operational realities is most helpful at this decision point, as an improvement team ideally selects from a host of possible changes the one(s) *most likely* to result in desirable change.

Once a candidate change is identified, the testing process can begin within the Plan → Do → Study → Act (PDSA) cycles. The PDSA structure is just a bare-bones expression of the scientific method as it is applied in the real work setting. PDSA is a decades-old construct offered by William Edwards Deming, PhD (Fig. 9.6), and is very analogous to the Six Sigma terminology for the scientific method as applied to process control—namely: Define, Measure, Analyze, Improve, Control [56]. The PDSA approach is not intended as a one-off pilot study, but instead a repetitive, rapid-cycle, action-oriented learning approach without necessarily waiting for complete stabilization of effect before another PDSA is undertaken. PDSA cycles that fail to meet hypotheses should be scrutinized for reasons, whereas PDSA cycles that suggest or result in clear improvement should be considered for refinement and scaling up. Therefore, all PDSA cycles should generate learning. In fact, failed PDSA cycles, if they are adequately analyzed, often teach improvement teams more about a system than successful PDSA cycles.

When interpreting measures for QI, one must understand the nuances to outcome, process, and balancing measures. Outcome measures indicate whether changes are actually leading to improvement and directly speak to the aim (e.g.,

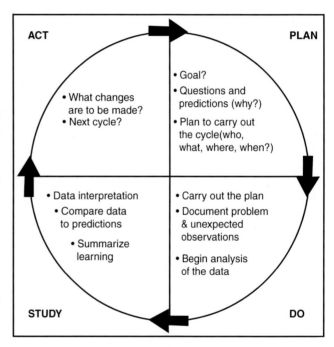

Fig. 9.6 The "Plan → Do → Study → Act" Cycle

central-line infection rates). Process measures relate to key activities or steps that are believed to drive the outcome measure (e.g., compliance with central-line insertion best practice). Balancing measures are sometimes selected to monitor whether changes intended to improve one part of a system are causing new problems in other parts of the system (e.g., procedure cart equipment costs). The key distinction is between "looking good" versus "doing well." Figure 9.7 depicts a model relating outcome measures and process measures. Predicated on the historical pressures of external audits to measure compliance with mandated processes (e.g., Joint Commission mandates), one might be tempted to believe that high compliance with process measures are preferable.

Fig. 9.7 Process measures versus outcome measures

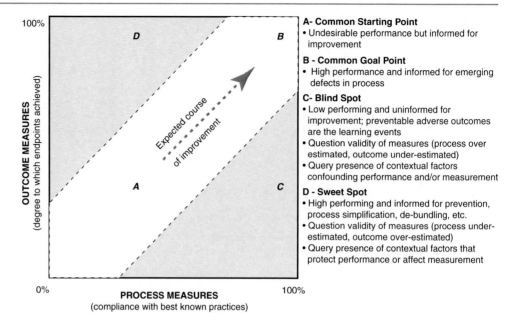

A- **Common Starting Point**
• Undesirable performance but informed for improvement

B - **Common Goal Point**
• High performance and informed for emerging defects in process

C- **Blind Spot**
• Low performing and uninformed for improvement; preventable adverse outcomes are the learning events
• Question validity of measures (process over estimated, outcome under-estimated)
• Query presence of contextual factors confounding performance and/or measurement

D - **Sweet Spot**
• High performing and informed for prevention, process simplification, de-bundling, etc.
• Question validity of measures (process under-estimated, outcome over-estimated)
• Query presence of contextual factors that protect performance or affect measurement

However, such a state can cripple an improvement team's ability to target interventions at defects in the real drivers of an outcome. If the outcome measure is perfect (e.g., zero central-line infections), then high compliance in a process measure may, in fact, reflect the etiology of the high performance (point B of Fig. 9.7). However, if the outcome measure is less than perfect, but the process measures (e.g., compliance with central-line insertion) show ideal practice, then either the wrong process measures have been selected or the measurement process is fallible – and the improvement team is blinded as to what to do next (point C of Fig. 9.7). When the process measures are less than perfect and the outcome measure is poor, the improvement team has insight into how to improve (point A of Fig. 9.7). Similarly, if the process measures are imperfect but performance is good for the outcome measure, an improvement team may be well poised to make improvements before additional adverse events occur (point D of Fig. 9.7). The outcome measure is the proof, whereas the process measures serves as informants that help an improvement team close the gap between actual and best practices. However, either can be miscalibrated, depending on surveillance techniques, staff members' perceptions of psychological safety, local response to error, safety culture, and so forth. In essence, an improvement team wants process measures that are "graded" as critically as possible to reveal all possible areas for improvement. Nonpunitive response to error (e.g., noncompliance) can help generate the honesty, accuracy, and transparency necessary to improve outcome measures.

One additional model worth discussing relates to high-reliability organizations (HRO). In industries with particularly complex and high-risk characteristics, some organizations have managed to contain errors and harm with remarkable effectiveness [60–62]. Examples include nuclear power plants, aircraft-carrier flight decks, and commercial aviation. Characteristic features of the context where development of an HRO is salient include: environments rich with the possibility for errors to occur, high-stakes error potential that can result in significant harm, high-pressure psychology with an unforgiving social or political milieu, opaque and delicate operations where learning through experimentation is difficult, and system complexity such that no one person can have mastery of the numerous and nuanced processes or technology involved. Although this may seem to describe health care in general (and pediatric critical care specifically), there are no known examples of health-care units achieving the kind of safety and reliability performance as HROs in other industries—but that does not mean that the health-care industry cannot learn from these examples. What, then, are the characteristic features of an HRO? They were outlined succinctly by Weick and Sutcliffe as follows [60]:

1. *Preoccupation with failure*: Small, seemingly inconsequential errors are regarded as a symptom that something serious is wrong. There is a commitment to finding and analyzing the "half-events" and to treating all failures as learning opportunities in a nonpunitive and transparent manner.

2. *Sensitivity to operations*: Attention is given to what is happening on the front line by all levels in the organization. Effective teamwork and a culture of safety are considered crucial. Data on processes and system performance are built into daily work and emerge visibly to promote situational awareness.

3. *Reluctance to simplify*: Excusing or explaining away errors is avoided. Diversity in experience, perspective, and opinion are encouraged. The questioning of assumptions is respected and supported, being viewed as a form of loyal dissent.

4. *Commitment to resilience*: There is an assumption that errors will occur, and there is a commitment to detect, contain, and recover from errors that do happen. The concept of fail-safe is not that a person or system will not fail but that something will inevitably fail and everyone will still be kept safe regardless.

5. *Deference to expertise*: Decision making and problem solving deeply engages people with the most related knowledge and expertise—typically the frontline workers, as opposed to top-down leadership.

Understanding Variation Through Statistical Process Control

As mentioned in Deming's system of profound knowledge, it is crucial for QI teams to understand variation in data to be able to avoid making errors in interpretation. However many QI teams do not, practically speaking, have sufficient biostatistical training to have confidence in real-time interpretation of continuous data streams generated by their efforts. This can stymie aims-oriented, data-driven, rapid-cycle PDSA improvement work. One accessible solution to this dilemma is for improvement teams to develop a working knowledge of statistical process control (SPC) [63–65]. The basic component of SPC is the control chart (also known as a Shewart chart) which serves as a graphical heuristic. It is not a hypothesis test but rather is constructed to generate insights into temporal signals in a complex system under a wide range of unknowable circumstances, both future and past.

To grasp the essence of a control chart, imagine a conventional bell-shaped curve turned 90°on its side to give a horizontal set of lines corresponding to the mean and standard deviations (Fig. 9.8). Time is represented on the x-axis, and the performance metric on the y-axis. Sigma is similar to standard deviation, but depends on the type of control chart being used and is generally more sensitive to detect outlying data as signals. The plus and minus three-sigma boundaries are called the upper and lower control limits, respectively. Accepting distributions of data within plus-or-minus three sigma of the mean (i.e., within a total range of six sigma) affords a rational way to minimize type I and type II errors. When data are outside this range, the system is considered *out of control*.

Unlike a bell-shaped curve where data are collapsed into one time bin, a control chart plots data over the additional axis of time (Fig. 9.8), providing insight into signals that emerge from the sequence of data being measured. The practical power of SPC is that people who are not statisticians can bring significant statistical rigor to their quantitative data in an intuitive format by understanding just a handful of simple rules to distinguish special-cause variation (i.e., signal) from common cause variation (i.e., noise) (Fig. 9.9) [20]. These rules are fairly intuitive for anyone with a basic grasp of probabilities. For instance, any single data point more than three sigma (roughly equivalent to three standard deviations) from the mean should stand out as a signal to which an attributable cause should be sought. So should a series of nine points on the same side of the mean line—tantamount to flipping nine consecutive heads with a coin.

SPC is rooted in venerated time series analysis and is an available function in most advanced biostatistical software packages. Yet such data can be readily maintained in simple spreadsheets, typically by entering numerators and denominators on whatever data-collection cycle is appropriate (e.g., weekly, monthly, quarterly). This allows QI teams to collect, interpret, and act on data in real time, without the bottleneck created by relying on a statistician to intermittently decipher

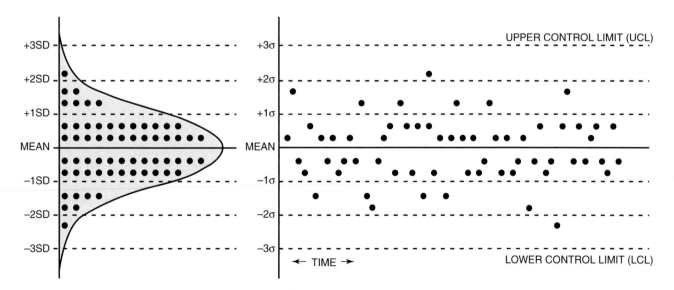

Fig. 9.8 Analogy of a bell-shaped distribution to control chart data

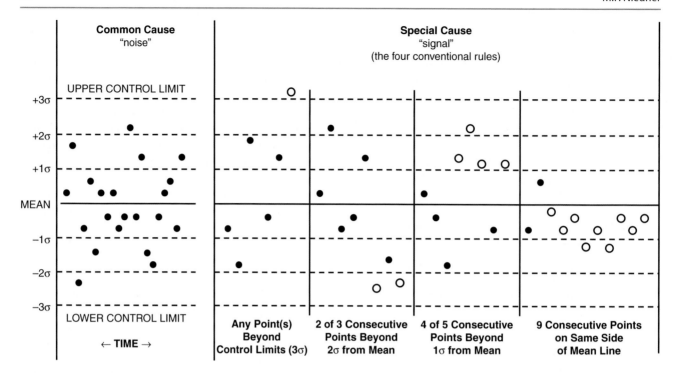

Fig. 9.9 Conventional rules for special cause variation in a control chart

signals and noise. Some expertise is required in selecting the correct type of control chart when getting started, because just as with traditional biostatistics, the nature of the measure (e.g., continuous, integer, categorical) determines the proper control chart to use—although one control chart visually appears much the same as the next one. Knowing when to reset mean lines also requires judgment, but generally speaking, break-points in the data are suggested by special cause variation in the data rather than by arbitrary cut points (e.g., fiscal year) or before-versus-after intervention timeframes (as is more common in classical time series analysis).

SPC can help "tell the story" of an improvement project, showing if a performance measure is in control, is exhibiting instability, is consistent over time, is showing improvement in response to interventions, or is showing decay in the context of neglect. SPC can help keep QI teams from mistaking noise for signal (i.e., false positive or type I error) and signal for noise (false negative or type II error). Figure 9.10 provides an example using catheter-associated bloodstream infection rates. Data point 'A' might seem high, but it does not meet the rules for special-cause variation; therefore reacting to this signal may represent energy wasted on random variation. Conversely, the mean line change at point 'B' represents a small but statistically significant change in the outcome measure that might have gone unrecognized without a control chart or periodic statistical testing.

Some traditionalists prefer P values or confidence intervals to describe variation; however, this often collapses time as a dimension (e.g., pre- versus post-intervention analyses)

and reduces rich graphic information into a few simple numbers. Confidence intervals and P values can still be derived from the primary data using classic biostatistical methods for additional verification, but determining the equivalent P values of a control chart "misses the point," according to Deming, who asserted that the intent and purpose of continuous QI is distinct from other forms of experimentation. Among other things, the P value of a control chart would depend on gross variability, the number of points plotted, and the number of rules used for special-cause variation (more than the conventional 4 can be used). However, a very rough estimation of the statistical rigor of a typical control chart can be made. If a control chart with normally distributed data were interpreted with the four conventional rules, the chances of either missing a real signal or seeing a false signal in 30 plotted points would be roughly 1 in 50–200 (or a P value of 0.02–0.005).

A Few Key Tools and Change Concepts for Quality Improvement

Many organizational change concepts, improvement tools, and safety strategies can be applied in an ICU—and it can certainly be helpful to have a wide variety of approaches at one's disposal, because some quality and safety problems lend themselves better to particular types of approaches. Although a description of the many possible tools and concepts is beyond the scope of this chapter, some approaches

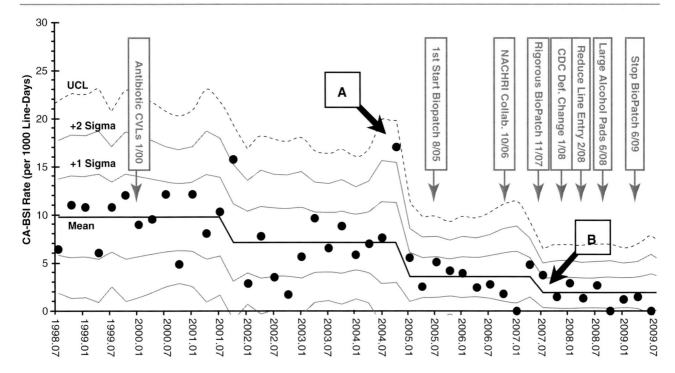

Fig. 9.10 Example of a control chart of catheter-associated blood-stream infections, annotated with key tests of change. *CABSI* catheter-associated bloodstream infection, *CDC* Centers for Disease Control and Prevention, *NACHRI* National Association of Children's Hospitals and Related Institutions

are more common and readily accessible than others. A few of the more practical ideas are reviewed in the following paragraphs.

One central strategy to improve quality and safety is error-proofing. Error-proofing methods have been categorized and ranked in a number of ways, including a binary codification. Level 1 error-proofing effectively achieves total prevention of an error, whereas level 2 simply makes errors less likely. Level 1 error-proofing is clearly preferable but unfortunately more difficult to identify or devise. An example of level 1 error-proofing is a forced function achieved by anesthesia-machine medical-gas connections, whereby a pin system allows only the oxygen hose to be connected to the oxygen source, air-to-air and vacuum-to-vacuum, thereby disallowing a misconnect that would be possible if hose connectors were universal. Level 2 error-proofing methods are much more prolific yet individually insufficient. Often multiple level 2 strategies will be deployed for an additive or synergistic effect. Examples of level 2 error-proofing include color coding, decision-support tools, and pop-up warnings in computer order-entry systems. In contrast to this binary classification, error-prevention strategies can also be considered along a continuum of general effectiveness (Table 9.3). Unfortunately, the easiest and most reflexive strategies often gain the least traction by themselves—even when they provide a necessary foundation for higher-order error-proofing strategies.

Gawande and Pronovost have championed the use of checklists to help overcome the incredible complexity of modern medicine [66–68]. When checklists were first used in aviation, it was with a growing understanding that even the most experienced and venerated pilots could be confounded by the huge number of variables and sequential steps in a complex procedure (e.g., taking off in a World War II bomber) and that failure to execute seemingly minor steps (e.g., releasing the lock on the flaps) could result in catastrophe (e.g., crashing at takeoff). Fundamentally, checklists identify a minimum set of high-value practices immediately before an action or in real time during a process. Checklists primarily help mitigate errors of ineptitude (i.e., the failure to apply knowledge) but can also combat errors of ignorance (i.e., the absence of knowledge). Pronovost, for instance, demonstrated that use of a central-line insertion checklist helped correct preprocedural hand washing by physicians dramatically – in spite of the fact that physicians know that hand hygiene is an important practice. Furthermore, the effectiveness of rounding checklists to address daily goals is enhanced with explicit verbal prompting by team members rather than by passive completion by one rounding team member – reinforcing the QI tenant that it is not merely *what* is implemented, but *how effectively* it is implemented [69].

Evidence-based protocols or pathways (commonly manifested as order sets) help to guide care toward best or preferred practices and can provide cues to remember easy-to-forget nuances and exceptions. Somewhat distinct from checklists, protocols are often more detailed and may not be necessarily by used in real time. Protocols primarily

Table 9.3 Error reduction hierarchy

More common, less effective	**Education & encouragement**: providing information to staff and cultivating intentions
↕	**Clear rules & policies**: setting explicit expectation consistent with best practice in concrete/written/available form
	Audits: creating data to detect defects in care that can promote situational awareness and/or be acted upon
	Simulation: creating opportunities for staff to practice and leadership to assess adherence to rules & policies
	Standardization: implementation of protocols/pathways to reduce unnecessary variation and improve predictability
	Checklists, double-checks, closed-loop communication: promotes attention and adherence to critical steps real-time
	Simplification, lean engineering: eliminates unnecessary steps or distractions where errors can be introduced
	Making the easy way the right way (or hard to do it wrong): capitalize on human factors/nature to do it the easiest way
	Automation & computerization: machines can perform more reliably than humans (if effectively designed/implemented)
Less common, more effective	**Forcing functions**: a physical constraint that makes a misuse nearly impossible without deliberate modification or override

help mitigate errors of ignorance, but like checklists, they can also reduce errors of ineptitude. Checklists and protocols both help reduce unnecessary variation, which can promote predictability and thereby reduce errors of communication and teamwork. Both checklists and protocols can also combat errors of supervision (i.e., the lack thereof) and have been touted to help focus the mind on important opportunities for customization of care by leaving unspecified modifiable factors outside the scope of the tool. Checklists and protocols, alongside more advanced electronic health record systems, can also function as decision-support tools that effectively improve the quality of care while simultaneously reducing costs [70–72].

There are, however, substantial challenges to the acceptance of standardized care, use of checklists, implementation of protocols, and effectiveness of automated decision support. Experienced by many physicians as "cookbook medicine," such tools admittedly do not always accommodate the wide range of practitioner experience nor facilitate innovation or creative problem solving. As the old NASA saying goes about astronauts, "There are two ways to die in space: (1) not following the procedure exactly as written and (2) following the procedure *exactly* as written." It is probably fair to say that one has to know the rules to know when to break them – but not knowing the rules is a recipe for failure.

Another common tool in the improvement-science arsenal is optimizing the visual workspace [73–75]. The Five-S mnemonic is often invoked, standing for (1) *sort/scrap* what is needed versus not needed; (2) *straighten* (or *set in order*) to make a workspace organized, labeled, ergonomic; (3) *scrub/shine/sweep* to eliminate messes that obscure the organization; (4) *standardize* to make it easy for everyone to

maintain and anticipate; and (5) *sustain order* with clear role responsibilities and discipline. Reducing unnecessary clutter and putting things in consistent order reduces search time for key materials and eliminates the wasteful warehousing of unnecessary items. Reported benefits have included improved efficiency, situational awareness, fewer lost items, streamlined supply chains, and improved staff and consumer satisfaction.

Root cause analysis (RCA) is, at its simplest level, a problem-solving methodology. Numerous formal RCA approaches have been well described in the literature, including fishbone diagrams and the "Five Whys" method of Toyota [76]. A robust RCA often illustrates the "Swiss cheese" model of error, where multiple latent defects (holes in the cheese), none of which alone are hugely problematic, all align to allow an error to propagate through the system and reach the patient. As already alluded to, an analysis of recognized errors or harm can provide constructive organizational learning. Such analysis is often undertaken in a fairly informal way, such as through qualitative discussion at morbidity and mortality reviews. However, formal RCA tools undertaken in an iterative manner can improve the likelihood of discovering latent defects in complex systems while simultaneously reducing some of the shortcomings of anecdotal analyses previously cited [42]. The overarching goal is to identify and eliminate causes of problems rather than to address immediately obvious "symptoms." RCAs can, but do not always, reveal system problems that will cause harm again if root causes are not recognized and addressed. Clearly, not all system problems are revealed by single events, so RCA is best undertaken as an iterative process, where recurrent themes are sought and contextualized. Often, categorical contributors are plotted on a Pareto chart (e.g., a histogram ordered from high to low prevalence) to visually depict where the preponderance of errors or harm seem to arise. This can provide an area of focus for consideration of risk from latent defects in such domains.

Summary

At no other time have health-care quality and patient safety recognition been of greater import than they are now. The modern patient-safety movement continues to grow at an unprecedented pace, both at pragmatic and academic levels. The PICU is an environment rich with the potential for risk, error, and harm. It is also full of dedicated, bright, vigilant people who have a wealth of clinical and operational information at their fingertips. This creates a very fertile environment to be able to engage in and pioneer quality-improvement science. PICUs across the United States have reduced historical rates of central-line infections, ventilator-associated pneumonias, harmful medication errors, unplanned extubations, and other adverse events [41, 53, 77, 78]. Sustainability of such improvements is patchy, and enhancements of positive dimensions of care more elusive [79, 80]. Often, the ingredients lacking for QI to flourish in a PICU are (1) local know-how, (2) leaders committed to a quality-improvement vision, and (3) the time and resources of frontline staff members to execute such a vision. Table 9.4 offers a few practical tips for local PICU leaders who want to run QI initiatives. The development of clinical leaders with a quality-improvement vision

Table 9.4 Tips for leading quality & safety initiatives from the trenches

Help set the proper scope/frequency of testing:
Usually smaller, more often, more variety of tests
Be a part of the testing:
Get first-hand experience, be wary of over-delegation
Distinguish bad ideas versus poor implementation:
Don't let good ideas fail because of poor execution
Allow operations to evolve:
Question habits/assomptions, prevent ruts/stagnation.
Engage higher order improvement strategies:
Think sustainability & reliability (not brute force)
Good leaders don't hoard information:
Create situational awareness for teams/frontline/staff
Be transparent, share data, network:
Never ask frontline for info that you don't feed back
Strive to have content and improvement expert in same body:
Use "quality coaches" to acquire skills, not substitute for them
Grow quality improvement leaders in your unit (instead of recruiting);
Support and educate frontline staff; identify who can actually "do" it
Don't wait until you're "ready":
Have teams meeting regularly to "do"; start before you're ready

and the procurement of resources to undertake "optional" initiatives remain real challenges for many PICUs, yet one can hope that the growing safety movement and national health-care reforms will continue to attack these voids with a constructive mixture of carrots and sticks [81].

References

1. Kohn LT, Corrigan J, Donaldson MS. To err is human: building a safer health system. Washington, DC: National Academy Press; 2000. p. xxi, 287.
2. Institute of Medicine (U.S.). Committee on Quality of Health Care in America. Crossing the quality chasm: a new health system for the 21st century. Washington, DC: National Academy Press; 2001. p. xx, 337.
3. Audet AM, Doty MM, Shamasdin J, Schoenbaum SC. Measure, learn, and improve: physicians' involvement in quality improvement. Health Aff (Millwood). 2005;24:843–53.
4. Milstein A, Adler NE. Out of sight, out of mind: why doesn't widespread clinical quality failure command our attention? Health Aff (Millwood). 2003;22:119–27.
5. Berwick DM, Nolan TW. Physicians as leaders in improving health care: a new series in Annals of Internal Medicine. Ann Intern Med. 1998;128:289–92.
6. Improvement IfH. The imperative for quality: a call for action to medical schools and teaching hospitals. Acad Med. 2003;78:1085–9.
7. Kachalia A, Johnson JK, Miller S, Brennan T. The incorporation of patient safety into board certification examinations. Acad Med. 2006;81:317–25.
8. Rowe JW. Pay-for-performance and accountability: related themes in improving health care. Ann Intern Med. 2006;145:695–9.
9. Epstein AM. Pay for performance at the tipping point. N Engl J Med. 2007;356:515–7.
10. Miller SH. American Board of Medical Specialties and repositioning for excellence in lifelong learning: maintenance of certification. J Contin Educ Health Prof. 2005;25:151–6.
11. American Board of Medical Specialties. About ABMS: maintenance of certification. www.abms.org/Maintenance_of_Certification. Accessed 11 Apr 2012.
12. Berwick DM. The science of improvement. JAMA. 2008;299:1182–4.
13. Reason JT. The human contribution: unsafe acts, accidents and heroic recoveries. Farnham/Burlington: Ashgate; 2008. p. x, 295.
14. Davidoff F, Batalden P, Stevens D, Ogrinc G, Mooney S. Publication guidelines for quality improvement in health care: evolution of the SQUIRE project. Qual Saf Health Care. 2008;17 Suppl 1:i3–9.
15. Speroff T, James BC, Nelson EC, Headrick LA, Brommels M. Guidelines for appraisal and publication of PDSA quality improvement. Qual Manag Health Care. 2004;13:33–9.
16. Shaller D. Implementing and using quality measures for children's health care: perspectives on the state of the practice. Pediatrics. 2004;113:217–27.
17. Donchin Y, Gopher D, Olin M, et al. A look into the nature and causes of human errors in the intensive care unit. Crit Care Med. 1995;23:294–300.
18. Scanlon MC, Mistry KP, Jeffries HE. Determining pediatric intensive care unit quality indicators for measuring pediatric intensive care unit safety. Pediatr Crit Care Med. 2007;8:S3–10.
19. National Quality Forum issue brief: strengthening pediatric quality measurement and reporting. J Healthc Qual. 2008;30:51–5.
20. McGlynn EA, Asch SM, Adams J, et al. The quality of health care delivered to adults in the United States. N Engl J Med. 2003;348:2635–45.

21. Mangione-Smith R, DeCristofaro AH, Setodji CM, et al. The quality of ambulatory care delivered to children in the United States. N Engl J Med. 2007;357:1515–23.

22. Taylor JA, Brownstein D, Christakis DA, et al. Use of incident reports by physicians and nurses to document medical errors in pediatric patients. Pediatrics. 2004;114:729–35.

23. Winters B, Dorman T. Patient-safety and quality initiatives in the intensive-care unit. Curr Opin Anaesthesiol. 2006;19:140–5.

24. Box G. Robustness in the strategy of scientific model building. In: Launer RL, Wilkinson WG, editors. Robustness in statistics. New York: Academic; 1979.

25. Carder B, Ragan P. Measurement matters: how effective assessment drives business and safety performance. Milwaukee: ASQ Quality Press; 2005. p. ix, 221.

26. Sessions R. How a 'difficult' composer gets that way. New York Times. New York, NY, 1950. p. 89.

27. Jimmerson C, Weber D, Sobek 2nd DK. Reducing waste and errors: piloting lean principles at Intermountain Healthcare. Jt Comm J Qual Patient Saf. 2005;31:249–57.

28. Kim CS, Spahlinger DA, Kin JM, Billi JE. Lean health care: what can hospitals learn from a world-class automaker? J Hosp Med. 2006;1:191–9.

29. Chalice R, American Society for Quality. Improving healthcare using Toyota lean production methods: 46 steps for improvement. Milwaukee: ASQ Quality Press; 2007. p. xiv, 302.

30. Liker JK. The Toyota way: 14 management principles from the world's greatest manufacturer. New York: McGraw-Hill; 2004. p. xxii, 330.

31. Liker JK, Meier D. The Toyota way fieldbook: a practical guide for implementing Toyota's 4Ps. New York: McGraw-Hill; 2006. p. xx, 475.

32. Reason JT. Human error. Cambridge/New York: Cambridge University Press; 1990. p. xv, 302.

33. Milch CE, Salem DN, Pauker SG, Lundquist TG, Kumar S, Chen J. Voluntary electronic reporting of medical errors and adverse events. An analysis of 92,547 reports from 26 acute care hospitals. J Gen Intern Med. 2006;21:165–70.

34. Wilmer A, Louie K, Dodek P, Wong H, Ayas N. Incidence of medication errors and adverse drug events in the ICU: a systematic review. Qual Saf Health Care. 2010;19(5):e7.

35. Savage I, Cornford T, Klecun E, Barber N, Clifford S, Franklin BD. Medication errors with electronic prescribing (eP): two views of the same picture. BMC Health Serv Res. 2010;10:135.

36. Resar RK, Rozich JD, Classen D. Methodology and rationale for the measurement of harm with trigger tools. Qual Saf Health Care. 2003;12 Suppl 2:ii39–45.

37. Agency for Healthcare Research and Quality Guide to Patient Safety Indicators, Version 3.0a (May 1, 2006). http://www.quality-indicators.ahrq.gov/Downloads/Modules/PSI/V30/psi_guide_v30a.pdf. Accessed 5 May 2011.

38. McDonald KM, Davies SM, Haberland CA, Geppert JJ, Ku A, Romano PS. Preliminary assessment of pediatric health care quality and patient safety in the United States using readily available administrative data. Pediatrics. 2008;122:e416–25.

39. Resar RK, Rozich JD, Simmonds T, Haraden CR. A trigger tool to identify adverse events in the intensive care unit. Jt Comm J Qual Patient Saf. 2006;32:585–90.

40. Sandora TJ. Prevention of healthcare-associated infections in children: new strategies and success stories. Curr Opin Infect Dis. 2010;23:300–5.

41. Miller MR, Griswold M, Harris 2nd JM, et al. Decreasing PICU catheter-associated bloodstream infections: NACHRI's quality transformation efforts. Pediatrics. 2010;125:206–13.

42. Cook RI. A brief look at the new look at complex system failure, error, safety, and resilience. Chicago: Cognitive Technologies Laboratory; 2005.

43. Pawson R, Tilley N. Realistic evaluation. London/Thousand Oaks: Sage; 1997. p. xvii, 235.

44. Godfrey MM, Melin CN, Muething SE, Batalden PB, Nelson EC. Clinical microsystems, Part 3. Transformation of two hospitals using microsystem, mesosystem, and macrosystem strategies. Jt Comm J Qual Patient Saf. 2008;34:591–603.

45. Shapiro S. Is meta-analysis a valid approach to the evaluation of small effects in observational studies? J Clin Epidemiol. 1997;50:223–9.

46. Feinstein AR. Meta-analysis: statistical alchemy for the 21st century. J Clin Epidemiol. 1995;48:71–9.

47. Bailar 3rd JC. The promise and problems of meta-analysis. N Engl J Med. 1997;337:559–61.

48. Huang DT, Clermont G, Kong L, et al. Intensive care unit safety culture and outcomes: a US multicenter study. Int J Qual Health Care. 2010;22:151–61.

49. Pronovost PJ, Berenholtz SM, Goeschel C, et al. Improving patient safety in intensive care units in Michigan. J Crit Care. 2008;23:207–21.

50. Pronovost P, Sexton B. Assessing safety culture: guidelines and recommendations. Qual Saf Health Care. 2005;14:231–3.

51. Mohr DC, Burgess Jr JF, Young GJ. The influence of teamwork culture on physician and nurse resignation rates in hospitals. Health Serv Manage Res. 2008;21:23–31.

52. Jain M, Miller L, Belt D, King D, Berwick DM. Decline in ICU adverse events, nosocomial infections and cost through a quality improvement initiative focusing on teamwork and culture change. Qual Saf Health Care. 2006;15:235–9.

53. Abstoss K, Shaw B, Owens T, Juno J, Commiskey E, Niedner M. Increasing medication error reporting rates while reducing harm through simultaneous cultural and system-level interventions in an intensive care unit. BMJ Qual Saf. 2011;20:914–22.

54. Davidoff F. Heterogeneity is not always noise: lessons from improvement. JAMA. 2009;302:2580–6.

55. Solberg LI, Mosser G, McDonald S. The three faces of performance measurement: improvement, accountability, and research. Jt Comm J Qual Improv. 1997;23:135–47.

56. Speroff T, O'Connor GT. Study designs for PDSA quality improvement research. Qual Manag Health Care. 2004;13:17–32.

57. Lloyd RC. In God we trust; all others bring data. Front Health Serv Manage. 2007;23:33–8; discussion 43–5.

58. Langley GJ. The improvement guide: a practical approach to enhancing organizational performance. San Francisco: Jossey-Bass; 2009. p. xxi, 490.

59. The Breakthrough Series: IHI's Collaborative Model for Achieving Breakthrough Improvement. IHI Innovation Series white paper. Institute for Healthcare Improvement. Cambridge, MA; 2003.

60. Weick KE, Sutcliffe KM. Managing the unexpected: resilient performance in an age of uncertainty. San Francisco: Jossey-Bass; 2007. p. xii, 194.

61. Nance JJ. Why hospitals should fly: the ultimate flight plan to patient safety and quality care. Bozeman: Second River Healthcare Press; 2008. p. ix, 225.

62. United States. Agency for Healthcare Research and Quality, Lewin Group. Becoming a high reliability organization: operational advice for hospital leaders. Rockville: Agency for Healthcare Research and Quality; 2008. p. 33.

63. Benneyan JC, Lloyd RC, Plsek PE. Statistical process control as a tool for research and healthcare improvement. Qual Saf Health Care. 2003;12:458–64.

64. Mohammed MA, Worthington P, Woodall WH. Plotting basic control charts: tutorial notes for healthcare practitioners. Qual Saf Health Care. 2008;17:137–45.

65. Thor J, Lundberg J, Ask J, et al. Application of statistical process control in healthcare improvement: systematic review. Qual Saf Health Care. 2007;16:387–99.

66. Gawande A. The checklist manifesto: how to get things right. New York: Metropolitan Books; 2009.

67. Gawande A. The checklist: if something so simple can transform intensive care, what else can it do? New Yorker. 2007. p. 86–101.

68. Pronovost P, Needham D, Berenholtz S, et al. An intervention to decrease catheter-related bloodstream infections in the ICU. N Engl J Med. 2006;355:2725–32.

69. Weiss C, Moazed F, McEvoy C, Singer B, Szleifer I. Prompting physicians to address a daily checklist and process of care and clinical outcomes. Am J Respir Crit Care Med. 2011;184:680–6.

70. Amarasingham R, Plantinga L, Diener-West M, Gaskin DJ, Powe NR. Clinical information technologies and inpatient outcomes: a multiple hospital study. Arch Intern Med. 2009;169:108–14.

71. Kawamoto K, Houlihan CA, Balas EA, Lobach DF. Improving clinical practice using clinical decision support systems: a systematic review of trials to identify features critical to success. BMJ. 2005;330:765.

72. Linder JA, Ma J, Bates DW, Middleton B, Stafford RS. Electronic health record use and the quality of ambulatory care in the United States. Arch Intern Med. 2007;167:1400–5.

73. 5S: A lean method to cut the clutter. OR Manager. 2007;23(3):15. Retrieved 11 Apr 2012, from ProQuest Nursing & Allied Health Source. (Document ID: 1244435041).

74. Hubbard R. Case study on the 5S program: the five pillars of the visual workplace. Hosp Mater Manage Q. 1999;20:24–8.

75. Waldhausen JH, Avansino JR, Libby A, Sawin RS. Application of lean methods improves surgical clinic experience. J Pediatr Surg. 2010;45:1420–5.

76. Gupta P, Varkey P. Developing a tool for assessing competency in root cause analysis. Jt Comm J Qual Patient Saf. 2009;35:36–42.

77. Brilli RJ, Sparling KW, Lake MR, et al. The business case for preventing ventilator-associated pneumonia in pediatric intensive care unit patients. Jt Comm J Qual Patient Saf. 2008;34:629–38.

78. Sadowski R, Dechert RE, Bandy KP, et al. Continuous quality improvement: reducing unplanned extubations in a pediatric intensive care unit. Pediatrics. 2004;114:628–32.

79. 5 Million Lives Campaign. How-to guide: sustainability and spread. Cambridge, MA: Institute for Healthcare Improvement; 2008. Available at www.ihi.org

80. NHS Modernisation Agency. Improvement leader's guide to sustainability and spread. Ipswich, England: Ancient House Printing Group; 2002.

81. Levy FH, Brilli RJ, First LR, et al. A new framework for quality partnerships in Children's Hospitals. Pediatrics. 2011;127:1147–56.

Matthew C. Scanlon

Abstract

Preventable harm is an unfortunate reality of care in the PICU. While this harm may result from infections, medication errors, diagnostic error, procedure complications among other causes, valid and reliable metrics are largely unavailable. Based on safety science, the problem of to harm to patients is a system problem of hazards and risks and not one of errors. Improvement, in turn, depends on thoughtful design and redesign of systems of care delivery.

Keywords

Patient Safety • Systems • PICU • Hazards

Introduction

The field of patient safety is one that is evolving – both in our understanding of the scope and nature of the problem, as well as solutions. In many ways, the problems associated with harm to patients during care are similar to issues that arise in caring for a patient with a significant illness in the Pediatric Intensive Care Unit (PICU). Both reflect a need to understand the role and interactions of complex systems along with the simultaneous requirement to promote recovery while treating underlying causes. Patient safety can be considered as the freedom from preventable injury [1]. This definition is notable for the purposeful exclusion of the concept of error. Despite the pervasive belief that harm to patients is a problem with human error, patient harm is instead the result of systems of which humans are an integral part. That said, this definition is also limited in focusing exclusively on harm without consideration for importance of hazards and risk to safety that exist within systems of care. This inclusion of risks may seem theoretical if not impractical.

M.C. Scanlon, MD
Department of Pediatric Critical Care,
Medical College of Wisconsin, Children's Hospital of Wisconsin,
9000 W. Wisconsin Ave MS 681, Milwaukee, WI 53226, USA
e-mail: mscanlon@mcw.edu

However, an appreciation of the systems nature of the patient safety problem will provide the basis for looking beyond harm.

The Challenge of Measurement of the Patient Safety Events

To characterize the failure to assure patient safety as simply an "event" is not far from characterizing the strife in Ireland as "the Troubles" or the engagement between the United States and North Vietnam as simply a "conflict". In each of these cases, the selected euphemism grossly underestimates the magnitude of the scope and significance. Depending on the data one includes, harm from healthcare ranges from the sixth to third leading cause of death in the United States [2, 3]. Hospital acquired infections alone have been linked to nearly 100,000 deaths annually [4]. Unfortunately, the nature and complexity of causes coupled with the lack of robust measures prevents accurate measurement of the exact scope of iatrogenic harm to patients. The lack of valid and reliable measures can be attributed to several things. First, many patient safety "measures" target the detection of errors. However, the different methods of detecting errors (voluntary reporting, chart review, and direct observation) [5] find different errors from different steps in the care delivery

D.S. Wheeler et al. (eds.), *Pediatric Critical Care Medicine*,
DOI 10.1007/978-1-4471-6362-6_10, © Springer-Verlag London 2014

process. As a result, the lack of an accurate count of the "number of errors" prevents identifying a numerator to establish a true rate. At best, one might be able to create a rate of "identified errors" over opportunities for error.

Even if there was a gold standard for error rates, the overwhelming majority of errors do not lead to harm. While the identification of errors may help identify opportunities for improving systems, a focus on errors also creates a reactive environment where one is chasing the last identified error rather than proactively improving systems of care. This reactive approach is aggravated by well-documented issues of hindsight bias, severity bias, and retrospective simplification of both processes of care and the decision making involved in performing in a complex system [6, 7]. As a result, there is an argument to focus on measuring harm instead of errors. From a PICU context, this approach works well for things like measuring central line-associated blood stream infections (CA-BSI) but less so for events like ventilator-associated pneumonia (VAP) in which there are not robust measures. Even an arguably well-defined CA-BSI purely describes an association and not a causal relationship. The same is true for catheter-associated urinary tract infections (CA-UTIs). The fact that not all harm events reflect failure in care delivery can be seen with other harm detection strategies. For instance, trigger tools, whether pediatric- or PICU-focused, have notoriously poor positive and negative predictive values [8–10]. As a result, a PICU team could waste valuable resources responding to "false positive" triggers. The same limitations exist with other screening tools including the Agency for Healthcare Research and Quality's Patient Safety Indicators and Pediatric Quality Indicators [11, 12]. A final limitation of harm-based metrics resides with the fact that one must wait for harm to occur to have a learning opportunity. As a result, both harm- and error-based metrics have limitations. Their role in identifying potential systems failure is significant but an exclusive focus on them results in a reactive game of "whack-a-mole."

Looking beyond the healthcare, other industries continue to learn from and attempt to prevent both errors and harm while focusing their efforts on identifying, understanding and eliminating hazards- those things that increase the risk of errors and harm. Whether providing safety equipment to workers building skyscrapers or designing technology to make it unlikely or even impossible to use incorrectly, these industries target hazards and risks, which, in turn, minimize the likelihood of human error leading to harm.

Though healthcare providers and leaders may not focus safety efforts on risk mitigation and elimination, healthcare hazards and risk are ubiquitous. One example is the use of multiple concentrations of a medication existing in a medication cabinet. For instance, if an ICU has both heparin concentrations of 10,000 units per milliliter and 10 units per milliliter in the cabinet with clear indications for use

associated with each medication, then a hazard exists. If a nurse inadvertently obtained the wrong concentration, an under- or over-dose would result and be viewed as a medication error. If the medication error reached the patient, then harm may occur. However, simply the presence of both concentrations of heparin is a hazard to patient safety. Regardless of whether or not either an error occurs and does or does not reach the patient, a significant source of risk of harm exists. How other industries reliably identify, analyze and reduce similar risks will be explored later in this chapter. Importantly, the answer depends on a solid understanding of systems and systems thinking.

What Harm and Risk Exists in PICUs

While early patient safety work identified the risk associated with PICUs, the lack of certainty about the true rate of harm from healthcare relates to the lack of gold standards for measurement as well as disagreements about causation and preventability [13–15]. Regardless of the lack of gold standard for measuring harm, PICUs are certainly high risk environments based on the complexity of care, the diversity of patients in age, diagnoses, acuity, and the range of tools and technologies that exist there. In the absence of robust data supporting true prevalence rates of errors and harm in the PICU setting, a consideration of the nature of known types of harm will be made.

To date, medication errors and adverse drug events (harm from medication errors) have been perceived as the most notorious of patient safety events. Medication errors have been the focus of measurement and a range of interventions and are relatively common, even though measurable harm from medication errors is detected less frequently. The reason for the relatively high known frequency of medication errors may rest with the sheer complexity of the medication process as well as the volume of medications used in the PICU and the added challenges of weight-based dosing in a broad range of patients. Unfortunately, there is also very little, if any, evidence that efforts at preventing medication errors in *any healthcare setting* has led to reduction in harm. This is despite technologies ranging from "smart" infusion pumps to computer physician order entry (CPOE) to bar coded medication administration. Potts' study in the PICU at Vanderbilt illustrates the seeming paradox nicely. Despite showing a significant reduction in the number of medication errors as a result of the introduction of CPOE, there was no evidence of reduction in adverse drug events (ADEs) [16]. The reason for this is twofold: most errors do not lead to harm, and most "safety technology" appears to be best at preventing the errors least likely to cause harm [17].

A second known cause of harm in the PICU is hospital-acquired infections (HAIs). CA-BSIs remain both a very real problem and a success story in PICUs. Leveraging the foundational work of Peter Pronovost and the central venous line (CVL) insertion bundle, a large group of PICUs worked with the National Association of Children's Hospitals and Related Institutions to decrease what was previously viewed as an unavoidable infection [18, 19]. In this study, 29 PICUs reduced the average CA-BSI rate by 43 %. Importantly, a key component of this initiative was the use of a CVL maintenance bundle. Unfortunately, VAP and CA-UTI have less clear of evidence bases to support improvement bundles [20, 21]. Additionally, viral infections and surgical site infections are known to be sources of other significant infections acquired during PICU hospitalization [22].

Other sources of harm in the PICU setting include direct injuries (decubitus ulcers, intravenous catheter infiltrates, falls, and catheter associated blood clots), miscommunication leading to misdiagnoses, delayed diagnoses, incorrect treatment or delayed treatment, and failure to rescue. Each of these represents harm that was not fundamentally associated with a patient's underlying condition and could potentially be prevented with a focus on redesigning systems of care in the PICU.

Systems, Systems Thinking and Patient Safety in PICUs

An 8-year-old child presents to an emergency room with septic shock. The adult emergency department provider orders an initial fluid bolus of 20 ml/kg, only to then instruct the nursing staff to stop the infusion because of the child's increased respiratory distress and falling oxygen saturations. This decision is made despite a heart rate of 175 beats per minute, hypotension, and poor perfusion. The provider elects to intubate the patient's trachea and use high positive end-expiratory pressure to treat the low saturations. Upon intubation, the child arrests and dies, despite attempts at resuscitation.

This vignette poses an all too common dilemma for pediatric intensivists: should one continue to treat the patient as a whole at the potential cost to aggravating a single organ system. The "organocentric" approach of stopping the fluids to protect the lungs resulted in insufficient volume resuscitation, arguably inadequate preload at the time of conversion to positive pressure ventilation, and a potentially preventable death. Pediatric intensivists understand that patients are not simply a group of unrelated and independent organ systems that should be addressed without respect for the interactions between these various systems. Similarly, intensivists realize that anything done to address one physiologic system has potential implications for all the other systems. While a patient can be viewed as a microsystem of the mitochondria existing (and interacting) with a larger microsystem of a cell which, in turn,

exists and interacts with a larger microsystems of organelles, organs and even regions of the body, the patient is more than the sum of these many systems. Ironically, few healthcare providers (or healthcare leaders) understand that healthcare organizations also represent a similar series of nested, interacting microsystems. A patient receiving extracorporeal life support (ECLS) in a room in the PICU represents the many systems comprising the patients as well as the systems of the ECLS pump, monitors, infusion pumps, catheters and numerous healthcare providers. This microsystem of the patient in a room exists in a larger system of the pod of the PICU, which is a subsystem of the PICU at large, the wing of the hospital, the hospital and the larger healthcare system. Like a collection of interactive matryoshka dolls, these many different levels of systems interact and a change to any one system influences all other systems [23].

Though understanding what constitutes a physiologic system may be second nature to intensivists, the use of the term "systems" in the context of patient safety can be achieved through considering models of system. One model that is readily applicable to patient safety scenarios is the SEIPS system model [24]. This model describes systems as having five major elements that interact: *people* who use *tools and technologies* to perform *tasks* within specific e*nvironments*, all with the broader context of an *organization*. Applying this model, safety is an emergent property of the system- something that is more than the sum of its parts. Consequently, seldom are patient safety problems (including human error and violations of safety rules) the fault of individuals working within the system. Instead, these problems result from the interactions of system elements. Safety (or the lack of safety) is produced by systems interactions. Therefore, to successfully improve safety, systems thinking requires the thoughtful redesign of systems.

An appreciation of both systems thinking and the concept of patient safety as an emergent property of a system leads to some important observations. First, people (be it nurses, physicians, pharmacists, managers or healthcare leaders) cannot assure safety by their actions alone. Even if a person performs flawlessly at all times, whether or not safe care occurs is the result of the interaction of the hypothetically perfect person with all other people involved, as well as the tools and technologies, tasks, environment and organization. Practically, this is important when dealing with individuals who resist efforts to improve safety because they have never, to their knowledge, caused harm to a patient. For instance, an intensivist refuses to participate in a process to limit variations in handoffs in a PICU based on the fact that they believe their handoffs are flawless. While they may consistently provide complete and succinct information when signing out to an on-call team, the ultimate success of the handoff communication depends on more than the actions of that one intensivist. Instead, the success of the handoff also depends on other elements of the system including the hearing, processing, memory and understanding of the recipient, any potential misunderstandings of jargon or abbreviations, the influence of distractions including background noise and competing demands such as other sick patients, tools to aid communication, and even the physical layout of the PICU. The intensivist in question may indeed perform perfectly every time. However, their perfection, in the context of a system, is inadequate to assure safety.

A second important observation of systems and systems thinking is that changes to any of the system components results in an impact on all the other systems components as well as whether care remains safe or unsafe. This concept was demonstrated in the case vignette when the emergency medicine provider intubated the hypovolemic patient, resulting in inadequate venous return and preload with a subsequent arrest. Acting on one of the patient's system elements by intubating the patient resulted in dramatic consequences for other systems elements including the heart. Switching to healthcare delivery as a system, an illustration of the implication of acting on systems might occur with hiring a new cardiothoracic surgeon. Regardless of how skilled the surgeon is at tasks including diagnosis, surgery and communication, safe outcomes depend on how the surgeon interacts with their patients, other members of the medical team, the new tools and technology they must use, the physical environment and the organization's rules, policies and culture. The role of systems is made even clearer if the new cardiothoracic surgeon, despite acclimation to the new system, is placed in a different environment the next time they were tasked with placing a patient safely on cardiopulmonary bypass. While one might ask, "So what if they did this in a different operating room?" outcomes would be far less certain if the operation was moved to the hospital's cafeteria or parking lot.

The emphasis on understanding systems and the need to redesign systems is paramount to improving safety in the PICU. This understanding helps explain why some "safety solutions" have led to dramatic improvement in the safety of patients while others have had little or even negative impact.

Improving Safety in the PICU: A Systems Approach

With an understanding of the systems nature of healthcare, pediatric critical care providers can learn from the safety model used in almost all other industries. First, these industries do learn from accidents (harm events). Both accidents and errors are studied extensively. However, the goal of this work is not to make humans "perform better." Instead, this information is used to redesign systems to reduce or eliminate the possibility of future events. Thus, the three central functions of a safety system become: (1) hazard/risk identification, (2) hazard/risk analysis, and (3) hazard/risk reduction. First, organizations (including PICUs) should proactively seek out hazards in their environment. Individuals can practice this behavior while working in the unit, e.g., looking for incorrectly dispensed medications or fall risks, while managers and leaders model risk identification at the level of patient care units and the hospital. The second step involves an analysis of this nature of the real or potential hazard. In the case of spilled water on the floor posing a fall risk, unit staff do not need to perform an elaborate analysis; instead they can move to step three and eliminate the hazard by cleaning up the spill. In the case of the heparin concentration mix up, the analysis begins by asking "could the event that happened at hospital x happen here?" The pharmacy and units would look to see whether both concentrations are currently stocked. If only one concentration is stocked on a unit, they might explore whether it would be possible for the incorrect concentration to be accidentally stocked. If either condition exists, then the third step is to remove the second heparin dose and redesign the heparin stocking process to assure a mix up could never occur.

More familiar examples of this approach likely exist in the reader's respective ICU. For instance, planned or existing CPOE implementations are intended to eliminate risks of error and harm associated with illegible handwriting, math errors, incomplete orders, medication allergies, or drug interactions. The components of the central venous catheter insertion bundle also are attempts to standardize the elimination of hazards to harm. In other words, failing to properly gown and glove or prepare and drape a patient will not necessarily result in a blood stream infection. However, either omission *increases the risk of an infection*. Thus, by systematically forcing providers to perform all known activities associated with risk reduction, the likelihood of a blood stream infection is dramatically reduced.

Importantly, not all steps to eliminate hazards and reduce risk are equal. The Occupational Safety and Health Administration publish a hierarchy for reducing harm to people (Fig. 10.1) [25]. The least effective approach is **training and education**. Note that this is the least effective approach, not an ineffective approach. Well-designed training can be effective. However, such training is difficult to develop and not typically seen in the setting of critical care. More effective is the use of **administrative controls**. These include policies and procedures, protocols, warnings and alerts. Examples might include a procedure for titrating heparin infusions or an alert in a computer order entry system. In each case, the goal of these interventions is to modify human behavior. However, these are often limited either the lack of applicability, fatigue, distractions, emergencies or a host of other real world factors.

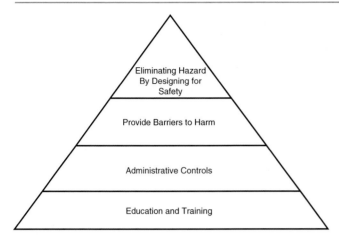

Fig. 10.1 Hierarchy to reduce harm

Even more effective is the **use of barriers** to reduce or mitigate hazards and harm. A well-known example from the anesthesia world is the creation of anesthetic gas connections that cannot be accidentally interchanged and misconnected. These specialized connections are in stark contrast to the interchangeable connections used in medication delivery. Another example from the ICU setting is the use of locked cabinets (including electronic automated dispensing cabinets) to limits access to medications. By locking medications away, the intent it to limit, though not eliminate the likelihood of a drug complication. Finally, the thoughtful and purposeful **use of design** to eliminate hazards is the most effective strategy to avoid drug complications. An example from the ICU setting includes the removal of any non-single concentrations of a medication from the care setting such as multiple concentrations of heparin or opioids in an ICU. By redesigning the medication delivery system to eliminate these hazards, it becomes impossible to have a drug complication attributable to the known cause.

Special Safety Topics

An exhaustive discussion of all possible safety topics in the PICU is impossible for a chapter. However, a few specific topics merit note. These include standardization, culture, and fatigue.

Standardization has become increasingly popular in healthcare settings as a purported safety solution. Without doubt, standardization is a good way to reduce cost; it is far less expensive to stock a single concentration of a medication than three. In the heparin example, standardization also is safer. However, it is arguable that no PICU provider would suggest a single standardized size of endotracheal tube for all patients. Nor would they standardize use of gentamicin to one dose regardless of a patient's age or renal function. Thus the

challenge for provider and leaders is to identify when standardization makes sense. Regardless of standardizing supplies, tools or even processes, one must consider the context that these things are used in and whether standardizing them still meets the needs of users all or nearly all of the time. Even then, any standardization must allow for exceptions when the now standardized tool or process doesn't fit. In contrast, if standardization will not meet the needs of the vast majority of those working in a system, then these efforts may create new problems including the need for users to break rules or work around processes to get work done. As a result, the patient safety should replace the call for standardization with what an HFE professional might describe as *thoughtful standardization when appropriate for a given context* [26].

Culture and a "culture of safety" are also hot topics in patient safety. It is well recognized that rigidly hierarchical culture of healthcare providers that discourages questioning plans is associated with intimidation and failure to communicate valid concerns. However, the result has been a misguided effort to "change culture" as if changing a light bulb or bandage. Culture can be viewed as the product of a person's experiences. In the context of the SEIPS model of systems, the role of culture appears in at least two of the system elements. First, the "people" involved in a given system each come with their own respective cultures and values which may influence their decisions, behaviors and interaction both with other people and the other four system elements. Further, depending on their role in the organization, any given person might also bring their professional culture to interactions. At the same time, the organization (be it clinic, hospital, health system or another type) has a culture that influences will influence decisions about the creation and enforcement of policies and rules, how people are treated by the organization, decision-making about tasks and tools/technology, as well as the design of the environment. The role of culture both at the level of an individual and the organization are consistent with and explain the perceived importance of culture to patient safety. In this context, culture is changed through creating new experiences such as not punishing people for honest mistakes and errors but instead learning from these errors and improving systems of care delivery.

Finally, **fatigue** has increasingly been an issue in the context of critical care medicine. Studies have revealed performance deficits and behavior changes in healthcare trainees, among others [27, 28]. However, the intervention of changing staffing models in PICUs and other settings to reduce fatigue has amplified the hazards associated with suboptimal handoff communication. Again, we see how a people focused solution (shorter shifts), which is well intended and arguably safer, has the unintended but predictable consequence of creating more handoffs and thus increased risk of communication breakdown. Thus while fatigue is clearly a detriment to performance and should be avoided among critical care providers of all roles, the best solution to lower fatigue while assuring safety remains unclear.

Patient Safety in the PICU

PICUs are high hazard and high-risk environments because of the heterogeneity of patients, their complexity and severity and the complexity of the work and tools required to care for these patients. The fact that more opportunities to prevent harm are not being identified in PICUs may reflect limited detection methods. However, time after time, safe care occurs because people compensate for suboptimal systems of care delivery. Thus any effort to further improve the safety of care in the PICU requires a thorough understanding of systems coupled with improvement efforts that consider the changes to all elements of a system.

References

1. Kohn LT, Corrigan JM, Donaldson MS. Why do errors happen? In: Kohn LT, Corrigan JM, Donaldson MS, editors. To err is human: building a safer health system. Washington, DC: National Academy Press; 1999.
2. Brennan TA, Leape LL, et al. Incidence of adverse events and negligence in hospitalized patients. N Engl J Med. 1991;324:370–6.
3. Office of the Inspector General. Adverse events in hospitals: national incidence among medicare beneficiaries. Available at http://oig.hhs.gov/oei/reports/oei-06-09-00090.pdf. Accessed 10 Apr 2012.
4. CDC. First state-specific healthcare-associated infections summary data report: January-June, 2009. Released 27 May 2010. Available at http://www.cdc.gov/hai/statesummary.html. Accessed 10 Apr 2012.
5. Flynn EA, Barker KN, Pepper GA, et al. Comparison of methods for detecting medication errors in 36 hospitals and skilled nursing facilities. Am J Health Syst Pharm. 2002;59(5):436–46.
6. Cook RI. A brief look at the new look in complex system failure, error, safety & resilience. 2005. Available at http://ctlab.org/publications.cfm. Accessed 10 April 2012.
7. Caplan RA, Posner KL, Cheney FW. Effect of outcome on physician judgments of appropriateness of care. JAMA. 1991;265(15):1957–60.
8. Sharek PJ, Horbar JD, et al. Adverse events in the neonatal intensive care unit: development, testing and findings of an NICU-focused trigger tool to identify harm in North American NICUs. Pediatrics. 2006;118:1332–40.
9. Takata GS, Mason W, et al. Development, testing and findings of a pediatric-focused trigger tool to identify medication-related harm in US children's hospitals. Pediatrics. 2008;121:e927–35.
10. Agarwal S, Classen D, Larsen G, et al. Prevalence of adverse events in pediatric intensive care units in the United States. Pediatr Crit Care Med. 2010;11(5):568–78.
11. Scanlon MC, Miller M, Harris JM, Schulz K, Sedman A. Targeted chart review of pediatric patient safety events identified by the AHRQ PSI methodology. J Patient Saf. 2006;2:191–7.
12. Scanlon M, Harris JM, Levy F, Sedman A. Evaluation of the Agency for Healthcare Research and Quality Pediatric Indicators. Pediatrics. 2008. doi:10.1542/peds.2007-3247.
13. Kaushal R, Bates DW, et al. Medication errors and adverse drug events in pediatric inpatients. JAMA. 2001;285:2114–20.
14. Folli HL, Poole RL, et al. Medication error prevention by clinical pharmacists in two children's hospitals. Pediatrics. 1987;79:718–22.
15. Raju TNK, Kecskes S, et al. Medication errors in neonatal and paediatric intensive-care units. Lancet. 1989;2:374–6.
16. Potts MJ, Phelan KW. Deficiencies in calculation and applied mathematics skills in pediatrics among primary care interns. Arch Pediatr Adolesc Med. 1996;150:748–52.
17. Wang, Herzog, Kaushal, et al. Prevention of pediatric medication errors by hospital pharmacists and the potential benefit of computerized physician order entry. Pediatrics. 2007;119:e77–85.
18. Pronovost P, Needham D, et al. An intervention to decrease catheter-related bloodstream infections in the ICU. N Engl J Med. 2006;355:2725–32.
19. Miller MR, Griswold M, Harris 2nd JM, et al. Decreasing PICU catheter-associated bloodstream infections: NACHRI's quality transformation efforts. Pediatrics. 2010;125:206–13.
20. Jarvis WR, Edwards JR, Culver DH, et al. Nosocomial infection rates in adult and pediatric intensive care units in the United States. National Nosocomial Infections Surveillance System. Am J Med. 1991;91:185s–91.
21. Elward AM, Warren DK, Fraser VJ. Ventilator-associated pneumonia in pediatric intensive care unit patients: risk factors and outcome. Pediatrics. 2002;109:758–64.
22. Raymond J, Aujard Y. Nosocomial infections in pediatric patients: a European, multicenter prospective study. Infect Control Hosp Epidemiol. 2000;21:260–3.
23. Karsh BT, Holden RJ, Alper SJ, et al. A human factors engineering paradigm for patient safety: designing to support the performance of the healthcare professional. Qual Saf Health Care. 2006;15:i59–65.
24. Carayon P, Hundt AS, Karsh BT, et al. Work system design for patient safety: the SEIPS model. Qual Saf Health Care. 2006;15:I50–8.
25. Occupational Safety and Health Administration. Hazard control. Available at http://www.osha.gov/SLTC/etools/safetyhealth/mod4_factsheets_hazctrl.html. Accessed 10 Apr 2012.
26. Scanlon MC, Karsh BT. The value of human factors to medication and patient safety in the ICU. Crit Care Med. 2010;38:S90–6.
27. Dinges DF, Pack F, Williams K, et al. Cumulative sleepiness, mood disturbance and psychomotor vigilance performance decrements during a week of sleep restricted to 4–5 hours per night. Sleep. 1997;20:267–77.
28. Landrigan CP, Rothschild JM, Cronin JW, et al. Effect of reducing interns work hours on serious medical errors in intensive car units. N Engl J Med. 2004;351:1838–48.

Folafoluwa Olutobi Odetola

Abstract

Pediatric critical care involves the delivery of care to children with severe illness or in need of close cardiopulmonary monitoring after a surgical procedure. In areas of the world where these critical care services are available and accessible, mortality has been on the decline over the past two decades. This gratifying result of intensive care and of biomedical advancement as a whole, has led to ever-increasing calls for measurement of the functional status and quality of life of survivors of critical illness. The ultimate goal of pediatric intensive care is to provide survival without impairment. Implicit in this assertion is the need to ensure that a child who survives intensive care is able to perform daily activities in a manner and range considered normal, meet basic needs, fulfill roles, and maintain health and well-being. The ensuing treatise will highlight the fact that majority of critically ill children survive hospitalization, however; they might be impaired or disabled thereafter. It is being increasingly recognized that while a child with disability resulting from critical illness, might adjust over time and be able to rate the quality of their life as good, normal, or acceptable; impairment (and resulting disability), is a poor outcome for pediatric intensive care. Focus on survival status alone will lead to omission of these vital patient-centered outcomes of functional status and quality of life. In the ensuing discourse, outcomes of critical care will be defined, along with methods to measure them. It will be evident that very few studies of functional status and health-related quality of life have been performed in pediatric intensive care, a pressing concern that needs to be addressed to enlighten important stakeholders, including patients and their caregivers, governmental and other regulatory agencies, and critical care providers about the value of pediatric intensive care that reaches far beyond survival status.

Keywords

Mortality • Child health outcomes • Health-related quality of life

Introduction

Pediatric intensive care is a rapidly growing field of child health care that focuses on the care of children with severe illness or who require intensive monitoring after complex surgery. Biomedical advances over the past several decades have led to reduced overall child mortality with which has come the realization that many children live with residual comorbid illnesses and impairment of function. Given this evolution of patient-centered outcomes over time among children with critical illness, it has become increasingly important to evaluate the immediate, short-term, and long-term outcomes of pediatric intensive care, elucidate opportunities to improve child health outcomes, and help inform

F.O. Odetola, MD, MPH (✉)
Pediatrics and Communicable Diseases,
University of Michigan Hospital and Health Systems,
300 North Ingalls Street, Room 6C07, Ann Arbor,
MI 48109-5456, USA
e-mail: fodetola@med.umich.edu

D.S. Wheeler et al. (eds.), *Pediatric Critical Care Medicine*,
DOI 10.1007/978-1-4471-6362-6_11, © Springer-Verlag London 2014

health care policy-making regarding the value of pediatric intensive care. The goal of intensive care is not only survival but survival with good quality of life and functional health status. The traditional measures of mortality and morbidity provide information about the lowest level of health, but reveal little about the other important aspects of an individual's level of health including dysfunction and disability associated with diseases and injuries. Health outcome assessors and the public have recently realized that, with advances in medicine leading to better treatment and cure of diseases, and delayed mortality; an important dimension was missing from the traditional health paradigm: the quality of a person's life. In essence, although biochemical measures and morbidity data may indicate the need for treatment, they do not always correlate with the way people feel [1, 2].

Thorough and objective assessment of the end-result of pediatric intensive care is a growing field of endeavor with major implications of importance to stakeholders including patients and their families, health care administrators, health care professionals in the intensive care unit and hospital, health care service and policy researchers, and insurance payers. In this vein, a germane question is increasingly being asked by stakeholders: "is mortality on the decline, and if so, how do survivors feel and function after an episode of critical illness, and at what cost to patients, health care givers, and society? Research into outcomes of pediatric intensive care aims to answer these important questions. In this chapter, information will be provided to allow readers adequately discriminate between the various terms used to describe child health outcomes, and understand the methods used to objectively and rigorously measure and report these outcomes, and their inherent limitations. The reader will hopefully become conversant with the *why* (rationale), *what* (definitions), and *how* (methods) of pediatric critical care outcomes research.

Rationale for Pediatric Critical Care Outcomes Research

Arrival to the pediatric intensive care unit (PICU) is often accompanied with uncertainty regarding the end-result of care which takes place in this intensely intimidating environment. Caregivers often are troubled with questions regarding their loved ones, including survival, management of symptoms while in the PICU, and functional capacity in the short-term and long-term time horizons after hospitalization. They also struggle with perceived helplessness regarding their inability to take control and "save" their loved ones from critical illness. Fortunately, most children will survive the PICU stay, however; there may be impairment in one or more domains of health status that might beg the question: "What is the quality of survival for those who

survive childhood critical illness" Given the expected longer life expectancy of children in comparison with adults, this question begets yet another: "after surviving critical illness, should the length (quantity) of life and the quality of life be regarded as separate constructs or not?" As a first step, a clear delineation of the terms used to describe child health outcomes is needed.

Definition of Outcome Measures

Careful determination of terms to describe outcomes for children who undergo intensive care is important, albeit not straightforward. They include survival status (survival versus death) in the short and long-term, functional health status, health-related quality of life (HRQOL), quality-adjusted life years, and societal outcomes, including resource utilization and economic burden.

Survival Status

Survival after critical illness is the main goal of pediatric intensive care. A "hard core" measure devoid of elaborate interpretation, survival status is the patient-centered outcome measure of utmost importance to patients, caregivers, and health care personnel. In the PICU, survival is often not guaranteed at the outset, a burgeoning concern the more severely ill the child is, and the longer the course in the PICU. Child mortality within PICUs across North America and Europe has fallen dramatically over the past 20 years, from above 20 % [3] to 3–8 % currently [4]. The timing of measurement of mortality is important, and most mortality prediction models are designed to predict mortality at the outset of intensive care, illustrating the role of the patient's premorbid illness state, and the impact of pre-ICU care, on outcomes, that might not be influenced by the care provided within the ICU. Also, the farther out from ICU discharge the measurement of the mortality end-point is, the more likely it is for non-ICU factors to influence mortality. Reports of declining all-cause mortality among critically ill children in developed countries, while heartwarming, raises the issue of ever-increasing difficulty in obtaining adequate sample size of subjects for studies in pediatric critical care that assign mortality as a primary or the sole study outcome measure [5].

Functional Health Status

Functional health status is a child's ability to perform daily activities that are essential to meet basic needs, fulfill roles, and maintain health and well-being. Surviving critical illness free of impairment of bodily function is the most sought after goal of critical care. Unfortunately, such picture-perfect outcome is not always achieved, given a host of factors broadly categorized into patient, social, and health care delivery factors, among a litany of factors that could potentially influence ultimate clinical patient outcomes. These factors include, but are not limited, to:

1. Patient factors: Diagnoses, patient illness severity, response/non-response to therapy.
2. Social factors: Access to care, demographic, geopolitical and social determinants of child health, including poverty, social-economic status, and family structure.
3. Health care delivery factors: These include quality-of-care factors such as timing, effectiveness, and availability, of appropriate health care resources.

Impairment of functional health status is referred to as *morbidity*, a term which encompasses a spectrum of limitation of age-appropriate activities. Morbidity refers to the impairment of a patient's functional health status encompassing cognitive and physical status (including organ-system dysfunction), and the ability to perform activities of daily living. Morbidity encompasses various terms that describe various (and progressive) degrees of limitation of age-appropriate activities including impairment, disability, and handicap. Impairment refers to any loss or abnormality of physiologic or anatomic structure. Disability, on the other hand, is any restriction or loss of ability (attributable to impairment) in performing an activity in a manner and range considered normal for a human being. Handicap is a disadvantage for a given individual, resulting from a disability or impairment, which limits or prevents the fulfillment of a role that is normal for that individual (depending on age, sex, social and cultural factors).

Assessment of organ dysfunction as a measure of morbidity has gained greater importance with the decline in PICU mortality, with the aim of determining the impact of physiologic insult to the patient and the presence or otherwise, of clinical response to treatment. The acquisition of multiple organ dysfunction might be a harbinger of death, or at the very least, a pointer to the low likelihood of immediate or short term return to a state of physiological well-being, if ever. In the PICU, the specific organ systems involved, the severity of the impairment of function and multiplicity of organ dysfunction are important determinants of survival [6–8]. Of note, acquisition of organ dysfunction among survivors of critical illness may be associated with impairment of functional status and HRQOL, imposing an extra burden on healthcare providers [9].

Several organ dysfunction scales are used in critical care research, including SOFA-Sequential Organ Dysfunction Assessment [10], MODS-Multiple Organ Dysfunction Score [11], and LOD-Logistic Organ Dysfunction Score for adult patients [12]; and the PELOD (PEdiatric Logistic Organ Dysfunction) score [13], and P-MODS (Pediatric Multiple Organ Dysfunction Score) [14], among critically ill children. These organ dysfunction scales permit measurement of patient baseline illness severity, progression of illness severity over time within the ICU, determination of delta scores (change in scores over time, relative to the baseline score), and cumulative scores during the ICU stay [15]. A recent measure of morbidity gaining popularity in critical care research is the concept of organ failure-free days, which encompasses mortality and morbidity. Essentially, these are the number of days over a fixed time interval, that the patient is alive and free of organ failure, as defined by the researchers [15].

Available tools to measure functional health status in children include the MARK-Multi-attribute health classification system for children 2 years and older [16], Wee Functional Independence (WeeFim) measure for children 6 months–8 years [17], Vineland Adaptive Behavioral Scales (VABS) for children from birth to 19 years [18], POPC – PCPC (Pediatric Overall Performance Category – Pediatric Cerebral Performance Category) [19], and most recently, the FSS (Functional Status Scale) [20]. Only the POPC-PCPC tools were developed specifically for PICU patients, while the MARK has been validated and used in a PICU population [21]. The FSS was developed using data from hospitalized children including PICU patients [20].

It is very important to carefully assign the aforementioned descriptors of functional status while assessing non-fatal outcomes for survivors of intensive care in children, particularly given the evolving stages of development and growth observed in many of these children for whom the functional limitation is a part of life. Szilagyi et al. have described child health as a multi-dimensional state, with difficulty in defining both health and disability since children are developing and changing rapidly, and normative values are "moving targets" [22]. They cautioned that there was a world of difference between the concept of health and normative functioning by age, due simply to developmental progression. Functional health status differs importantly from HRQOL, which introduces an additional domain of social well-being.

Health-Related Quality Of Life

HRQOL assesses the patient's total well-being encompassing physical, mental, and psychosocial determinants. Health, as defined by the World Health Organization is "a state of complete physical, mental, and social well-being and not merely the absence of disease, or infirmity" [23]. By extension, health in childhood refers to the ability to participate fully in developmentally appropriate physical, psychological (or mental), or social tasks. Measures of HRQOL incorporate these all-encompassing definitions of health because they, in addition to physical and mental status, attempt to assess important environmental and social-demographic factors, including poverty, which may play a very significant role in child growth, development, and health-related functional status. Unlike disease or death, HRQOL is a health concept that covers the full spectrum of health and is not inherently positive or negative in its orientation. It is more likely than other health outcomes to reflect broad consequences of disease or injury and is rapidly gaining acceptance as a measurable outcome. HRQOL measures are also increasingly considered valid indicators of service needs and intervention outcomes.

Domains measured in HRQOL include pain and impairment, functional status and mobility, social role, satisfaction and perceptions, and death. As similarly described earlier for a child's functional health status, several factors influence a child's HRQOL, many of which are operant after a child's discharge from the PICU [24]. They include social-demographic factors, family function, symptoms of disease, adherence to medication regimens, etc. Tools used to measure HRQOL need to be valid (measure what they intend to measure) and be reproducible (test-retest reliability) [25]. They can be disease-specific or generic, with the generic tools being subject to limitations of not being as responsive to changes in specific illnesses over time, as are the disease-specific tools. Among the existing pediatric HRQOL tools are the MARK [16], Child Health Questionnaire for children 2 months–15 years [26], Adolescent Child Health and Illness Profile for children 11–17 years [27], Functional Status Measure for children 0–16 years [28], and the Pediatric Quality of Life Inventory (PedsQL) for children 2–18 years [29]. By being brief and available as both a child report and an accompanying parent report, the PedsQL is believed to address the major limitations which have bedeviled pediatric HRQOL instruments, such as being time-consuming and dependent on potentially subjective parental report [24]. Specifically, the parents' cultural, social, and educational background [30, 31], mental health status [32], specific experience with the child, and their overall concerns or perception of health problems in the child [33], may influence their responses, and their perspective may differ from that of the child. Also, parental understanding and interpretations of questions might differ as to what is considered a functional disability, or there may be denial or undue concern, with resultant under- or over-reporting of problems.

Although health policy researchers have advocated for incorporation of assessments of children's HRQOL as the principal outcome for health service studies [34]; very few studies incorporate HRQOL assessment. For instance, only 1.7 % of literature in a methodological review of studies of adult critical care, included quality of life measures [35] despite a consensus statement that "future outcome evaluation of intensive care should incorporate quality of life" [36]. Of note, no data exist regarding the frequency of use of HRQOL measures in pediatric critical care research. It is

hoped that HRQOL measurement will progressively gain wider use in clinical trials and effectiveness research among critically ill children.

Studies of HRQOL and health status of survivors of pediatric intensive care with long-term follow up beyond 1 year after PICU discharge, have been done in the Netherlands, Australia, and Switzerland [3, 37–39], while studies performed in the U.S. have focused on functional outcome at PICU discharge [40, 41], hospital discharge [19], and 6 months after hospital discharge [41]. The studies reported varying follow up times and used different tools of measurement making comparison of the results difficult. However, mortality rates ranged from 5 to 20 % with rates being higher in the studies with longer follow up periods. There was functional impairment, of varying degrees, in 25–65 % of the survivors. Fortunately, most of these children with functional deficits at PICU discharge, improved over time. HRQOL has been reported as good in the majority of PICU survivors with poor assessment being associated with prolonged PICU stay, malignant neoplasm, and the presence of comorbid illness [37].

Severity of Illness as an Important Mediator of Outcomes

While there are various determinants of outcomes of ICU care, severity of illness is the exposure or mediating variable that appears to have the largest contributing impact to patient outcomes. Multiple tools have been used to measure illness severity within the adult ICU population, including the APACHE (Acute Physiology and Chronic Health Evaluation) [42], SAPS (Simplified Acute Physiology Score) [43, 44], and MPM (Mortality Prediction Model) [45]. In the PICU population, the most commonly used severity of illness assessment tools are the PRISM (Pediatric Risk of Mortality) [4] and the PIM (Pediatric Index of Mortality) [46]. Assessment of illness severity is important as a prognostic tool for groups of ICU patients but not individual patients. Also, assessment of patient illness severity is an integral portion of the benchmarking of ICU performance within and between hospitals. Given that the tools are used to predict survival outcomes among critically ill individuals, it is vitally important to re-calibrate them over time with advancement in diagnostic capability, and technology [47].

Methods of Outcome Assessment: Pathways to Studying Outcomes

Given the various measurable end-points that intensive care could conceivably result in, investigation into these outcomes could be conducted in various ways. However, as a rule, prior to performing research, the scientific investigator

Fig. 11.1 Structure-process-outcome model

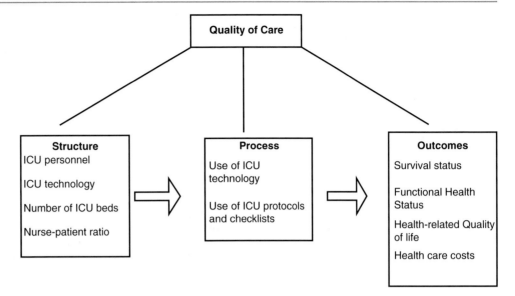

needs to always answer certain important questions in a consistent and stepwise manner:

1. Is the research question important and likely to inspire innovation?

   Rationale: Scientific inquiry requires thoughtful pondering and careful determination of the need to conduct the research, the outcome to measure, the study population of interest, and the potential implications of the study findings.

2. Can the research question generate hypotheses that can be tested?

   Rationale: Research aims and hypotheses are the foundation on which the study is built.

3. Is the study feasible and are the investigators capable of executing the study?

   Rationale: Careful selection of important outcome measures and potential exposure variables must be accompanied by appropriate expertise in research methods.

4. Which research methods should be employed to ensure that data can be collected, managed, and analyzed with scientific rigor?

   Rationale: Selection and application of appropriate research methods will permit reproducibility of the work, and enhance the validity of the study. For instance, outcome assessment instruments need to be validated within the study population [21].

5. Will the research findings be internally and externally valid?

   Rationale: It is important that the study findings answer the research question directly (internal validity), and be generalizable to the general population from which the study sample was obtained (external validity).

After careful consideration of the significance and goals of the research, researchers will often attempt to methodologically address research questions within a framework that places the research in context. This thematic approach, often invisible to the reader, might be the driving force behind the inquiry in the first place. On the other hand, the assessment of health outcomes might be driven by stakeholders, such as government agencies and pharmaceutical companies, who might directly or indirectly influence the scope of the assessment. To illustrate the thematic or paradigmatic approach to health outcome assessment, two conceptual approaches to the study of outcomes research in pediatric critical care will be discussed.

Structure-Process-Outcomes Model

Donabedian described quality of care as being highly related to the interplay of certain features inherent to the work place [48]. Interaction of these features, namely; structure, processes, and outcomes of care; could lead to good or bad quality of care (Fig. 11.1). Structure refers to the attributes of the care setting, which in the PICU setting, pertains to *material resources* (e.g. number of PICU beds, and availability of various PICU technology including mechanical ventilators, hemodialysis machines, and extracorporeal membrane oxygenation, among others), *human resources* (e.g. the number and qualifications of available personnel including intensivists, nurses, respiratory therapists, pharmacists, and other ancillary staff), and *organizational structure* (closed versus open units, presence/absence of step-down or intermediate care units, PICU admission and discharge policies, etc.). Process measures in the PICU address the actual treatments that are delivered to patients, and the manner in which intensive care is delivered. For instance, process of care assessment within the PICU might include the use of technology; including the timing of use, (since it is generally believed that the earlier ICU therapy is initiated the better the outcome), the competence of the user, and the ability to interpret data generated from use of the technology. Outcomes are the end-results of the care provided.

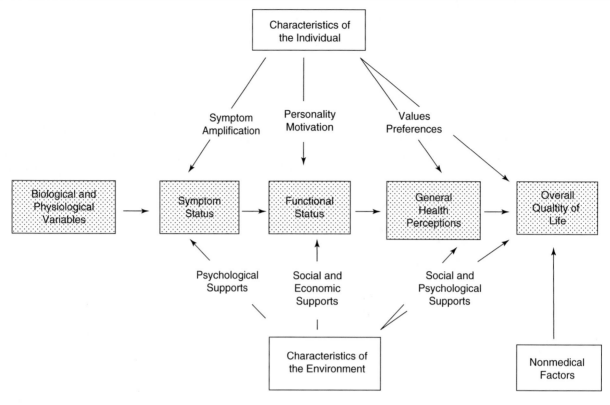

Fig. 11.2 Relationships among measures of patient outcome in a health-related quality of life conceptual model (Reprinted from Wilson and Cleary [57]. With permission from American Medical Association)

It is suggested that good processes and good structure should lead to good outcomes. Are structure and process linked to outcomes in intensive care? Structure – outcome relationships have been demonstrated for multiple structural attributes in the ICU; for instance, Pollack et al. have described improved odds of severity-adjusted survival for critically ill children treated at tertiary versus non-tertiary PICUs [49], and in PICUs with fellow trainees versus those without [50]. It has, however, been difficult to consistently demonstrate salutary effects of process measures on health outcomes. To illustrate, clinically significant differences have been associated with the application of specific processes with outcomes, such as, among the critically ill adult population, a survival benefit of restrictive red blood cell transfusion strategy versus a liberal transfusion strategy [51], and use of low tidal volume versus large tidal volume ventilation in acute respiratory distress syndrome [52]. On the other hand, some process interventions have not been associated with beneficial patient outcomes [53–55], with subsequent reduction in their use [56]. Importantly, some of the statistical models used to predict outcomes of adult [42, 45] and pediatric intensive care [46], incorporate process of care measures.

HRQOL Model

This conceptual model developed by Wilson and Cleary [57] emphasizes the inter-relationship that exists between various domains of non-fatal outcomes of care, with HRQOL as the centerpiece (Fig. 11.2). It also highlights the distinction between various measures of HRQOL.

- *Biological & physiological variables*: Diagnoses, laboratory values, measures of physiological function, and findings on clinical examination.
- *Symptom status*: Physical and psychosocial symptoms; such as pain, anxiety, fear, and depression, etc.
- *Functional status*: Ability to perform specified tasks, such as activities of daily living.
- *General health perceptions*: This domain assesses the patient's subjective global rating of health. It is an assessment often performed among older children, adolescents, and adults who are cognitively able to understand the constructs involved.
- *Overall quality of life*: Includes HRQOL and other measures of satisfaction with life.

As illustrated in Fig. 11.2, it is crucial to appreciate the potential confounding influence of various patient-level,

Table 11.1 Some important terms used in epidemiologic outcomes research

Type I (alpha) error: false-positive – the null hypothesis is rejected rather than accepted. Determines the p-value or threshold of statistical significance for hypothesis testing
Type II (beta) error: false-negative – the null hypothesis is accepted rather than rejected. Determines the power of a study (power = 1 minus beta). Most studies accept power of 0.80 or 0.90
Bias: systematic error that results in incorrect estimation of the association between exposure and outcomes. Bias should be mitigated by careful design and conduct of the study, and not by statistical analysis. Examples are selection bias and observer bias [58]
Confounding: the mixing of the effect of an exposure variable on the outcome, with the effect of a third variable. This extra variable must be associated with the exposure variable, and also with the outcome independent of the exposure variable. The observed relationship between the exposure variable and the outcome may be partly or wholly, due to the confounder. Confounding can be mitigated by the use of several epidemiological methods including randomization, stratification, matching, and multivariate analysis [59]

environmental and non-clinical factors on outcomes among survivors of critical illness. Assessment of outcomes in a prospective manner is therefore laden with some amount of uncertainty. Specifically, several environmental and non-clinical factors appear to increasingly influence long-term patient outcomes the more removed a patient is from the actual episode of critical illness and intensive care. Morrison et al. described this observation in their study of HRQOL among survivors of pediatric intensive care at their hospital in Australia [37]. They observed that the longer the time of outcome assessment from the episode of intensive care, the more likely it was for respondents to report better quality of life. They opined the finding could be the result of improvement in functional status over time or greater adjustment to disability over time [37].

Types of Outcome Research

Outcomes research studies could be broadly classified into randomized clinical trials and observational studies.

1. *Randomized Controlled clinical Trials (RCT)*: Are conducted to investigate the impact of interventions in the ICU, including the use of technology, new therapies, or various processes of care (e.g. ventilator strategy, red blood cell transfusion strategies). RCTs have the advantage of ameliorating study bias that could be introduced by imbalance of baseline patient characteristics; and also unequal distribution of confounders (Table 11.1), which could influence the relationship between the intervention and the outcome of interest. RCTs are, however, expensive to conduct, are often subject to concerns of generalizability that plague all human subjects' research, and seldom measure patient-centered outcomes.
2. *Observational Studies*: Devoid of randomization of study subjects, these studies might involve primary data collection (e.g. medical chart abstraction), or secondary data analysis, often conducted on large data sets collected for purposes other than research. Observational studies that assess outcomes include cohort, case-control, and cross-sectional studies. In cohort studies, subjects are followed over time until the outcome of interest occurs (prospective design), or conversely, could be studied after the outcome has occurred (retrospective design), with the study geared towards understanding of the factors that might be associated with the observed outcome. Case-control studies involve identification of patients who are either exposed (cases) or not exposed (controls) to a factor or disease, and subsequent ascertainment of outcomes attributable to this factor. Cross-sectional studies permit a broad snapshot of study variables of interest at a specific point in time, without any follow-up period. Cross-sectional studies therefore suffer from inability to evaluate the time-varying impact of different variables on outcomes of intensive care. It is very important to address the effects of bias and confounding on study findings in outcomes research (Table 11.1). Multiple methods exist to address confounding in observational studies including randomization, matching, stratification, and multivariate analysis [58, 59]. More recently, analytical methods such as propensity analysis and instrumental variable analysis have been incorporated from the social sciences and economics, as additional tools to ameliorate confounding, and to determine the causal relationships, respectively, in observational studies [60, 61].

RCTs are conducted in a controlled setting, and are largely, efficacy studies. Gaining prominence are comparative effectiveness research (CER) studies, which occur in the real world setting, and involve observations rather than experiments. CER studies evaluate how health care is delivered, how it could be improved and made more efficient and affordable, to positively impact population health outcomes. It is important to foster both RCTs and observational studies in pediatric critical care, utilizing methods applied in both fields of research.

In outcomes research, it is important to deploy appropriate methods to measure the outcome and ensure the study findings are valid. The effect size (statistically important difference between study arms) being targeted, the probabilities of type I error (alpha) and type II error (Table 11.1), and the proportion of the population with the disease under study (cohort or intervention studies), or exposed to the variable of interest (case-control studies) will influence the required sample size. The sample size will ultimately influence both the ability to arrive at the correct answer to the research question, and the external validity of the study.

Health Resource Utilization and Costs

Measures of clinical outcomes are closely linked to measures of health resource use such as duration of PICU and hospital stay, and costs of PICU and hospital care. Compared with critically ill adults, the expected life span of a child who survives critical illness is expected to be longer. Therefore, therapy is often administered to them with the belief that they will benefit society for a longer time if they survive. Notwithstanding, careful evaluation of therapeutic modalities in the research and real world settings is essential to ensure maximal benefit to the patient and to society. While this treatise is not focused on economic costs of pediatric intensive care, since very few clinical trial studies incorporate economic evaluation, readers are encouraged to review books that address evaluation of health care costs, taking the patient, hospital, or societal perspective [62]. ICU technology is expensive and not always beneficial; therefore economic evaluation of ICU technology is important and should be pursued routinely in outcomes research assigning survival status, functional status and HRQOL as outcome measures [63, 64]. It is imperative that measures of PICU efficiency which rely on resource use and costs, account for patient illness severity and case mix [65, 66].

The Future of Outcomes Research in Pediatric Intensive Care

In many areas of the world where PICU facilities are available, there is declining PICU mortality from disease and injuries. While it is unknown what the practice of intensive care will be in the decades to come, it is evident that overall child health outcomes can be enhanced by employing multifaceted approaches to improve disease and injury prevention, and by dissemination of proven, evidence-based intensive care, subjected to rigorous research; to geographic locales with minimal or no ICU services. While systems biology (genomics, proteomics, and metabolomics) aims to ultimately define and influence human composition and function at the genetic level, to usher in an era of personalized care [67]; it is also vitally important to keep the holistic

child-focused view in mind. It will be very important, therefore, to fund and espouse methodologically rigorous and germane research into biological, social, behavioral, and epidemiologic determinants of child health outcomes.

Research into the fatal and non-fatal outcomes of pediatric intensive care will require a concerted effort to improve the definitions and methods used to assess outcomes, develop inter-disciplinary collaborative linkages with professionals outside of intensive care, including rehabilitation clinicians, psychologists, neuro-developmental clinicians, traumatologists, health policy and health services researchers, amongst others; to conduct methodologically rigorous and relevant research. Only then will we optimize and sustain the gains made in increased survival status, improved ability to live and function independently, and optimal quality of life, for survivors of childhood critical illness.

References

1. Gill TM, Feinstein AR. A critical appraisal of the quality of quality-of-life measurements. JAMA. 1994;272:619–26.
2. NIH. Quality of life assessment: practice, problems and promise-proceedings of a workshop. Bethesda: NIH; 1993.
3. Butt W, Shann F, Tibballs J, Williams J, Cuddihy L, Blewett L, et al. Long-term outcome of children after intensive care. Crit Care Med. 1990;18:961–5.
4. Pollack MM, Patel KM, Ruttimann UE. PRISM III: an updated pediatric risk of mortality score. Crit Care Med. 1996;24:743–52.
5. Randolph AG, Lacroix J. Randomized clinical trials in pediatric critical care: rarely done but desperately needed. Pediatr Crit Care Med. 2002;3:102–6.
6. Johnston JA, Yi MS, Britto MT, Mrus JM. Importance of organ dysfunction in determining hospital outcomes in children. J Pediatr. 2004;144:595–601.
7. Wilkinson JD, Pollack MM, Ruttimann UE, Glass NL, Yeh TS. Outcome of pediatric patients with multiple organ system failure. Crit Care Med. 1986;14:271–4.
8. Typpo KV, Petersen NJ, Hallman DM, Markovitz BP, Mariscalco MM. Day 1 multiple organ dysfunction syndrome is associated with poor functional outcome and mortality in the pediatric intensive care unit. Pediatr Crit Care Med. 2009;10:562–70.
9. Buysse CM, Raat H, Hazelzet JA, Hop WC, Maliepaard M, Joosten KF. Surviving meningococcal septic shock: health consequences and quality of life in children and their parents up to 2 years after pediatric intensive care unit discharge. Crit Care Med. 2008;36: 596–602.
10. Vincent JL, Moreno R, Takala J, Willatts S, De Mendonça A, Bruining H, et al. The SOFA (Sepsis-related Organ Failure Assessment) score to describe organ dysfunction/failure. Intensive Care Med. 1996;22:707–10.
11. Marshall JC, Cook DJ, Christou NV, Bernard GR, Sprung CL, Sibbald WJ. Multiple organ dysfunction score: a reliable descriptor of a complex clinical outcome. Crit Care Med. 1995;23:1638–52.
12. Le Gall JR, Klar J, Lemeshow S, Saulnier F, Alberti C, Artigas A, et al. The Logistic Organ Dysfunction system. A new way to assess organ dysfunction in the intensive care unit. JAMA. 1996;276: 802–10.
13. Leteurtre S, Martinot A, Duhamel A, Proulx F, Grandbastien B, Cotting J, et al. Validation of the paediatric logistic organ dysfunction (PELOD) score: prospective, observational, multicentre study.

Lancet. 2003;19(362):192–7 [Erratum in: Lancet 2006;367:897; author reply 900–2. Lancet 2006;367:902].

14. Graciano AL, Balko JA, Rahn DS, Ahmad N, Giroir BP. The Pediatric Multiple Organ Dysfunction Score (P-MODS): development and validation of an objective scale to measure the severity of multiple organ dysfunction in critically ill children. Crit Care Med. 2005;33:1484–91.

15. Marshall JC. Measuring treatment outcomes in intensive care: mortality, morbidity, and organ dysfunction. In: Sibbald WJ, Bion JF, editors. Evaluating critical care: using health services research to improve quality: update in intensive care and emergency medicine; 35. Berlin/Heidelberg/New York: Springer; 2001. p. 69–85.

16. Torrance GW, Boyle MH, Horwood SP. Application of multi-attribute utility theory to measure social preferences for health states. Oper Res. 1982;30:1043–69.

17. Msall ME, DiGaudio K, Rogers BT, LaForest S, Catanzaro NL, Campbell J, et al. The Functional Independence Measure for Children (WeeFIM). Conceptual basis and pilot use in children with developmental disabilities. Clin Pediatr (Phila). 1994;33:421–30.

18. Sparrow S, Balla DA, Cicchetti DV. Vineland adaptive behavior scales. Interview Edition, Survey Form Manual. A revision of the Vineland Social Maturity Scale by E. A. Doll. Circle Pines: American Guidance Service; 1984.

19. Fiser DH. Assessing the outcome of pediatric intensive care. J Pediatr. 1992;121:68–74.

20. Pollack MM, Holubkov R, Glass P, Dean JM, Meert KL, Zimmerman J, Eunice Kennedy Shriver National Institute of Child Health and Human Development Collaborative Pediatric Critical Care Research Network, et al. Functional Status Scale: new pediatric outcome measure. Pediatrics. 2009;124:e18–28.

21. Gemke RJBJ, Bonsel GJ. Reliability and validity of a comprehensive health status measure in a heterogeneous population of children admitted to intensive care. J Clin Epidemiol. 1996;49: 327–33.

22. Szilagyi PG, Schor EL. The health of children. Health Serv Res. 1998;33:1001–39.

23. Preamble to the Constitution of the World Health Organization as adopted by the International Health Conference, New York, 19–22 June 1946; signed on 22 July 1946 by the representatives of 61 States (Official Records of the World Health Organization, no. 2, p. 100) and entered into force on 7 April 1948.

24. Knight TS, Burwinkle TM, Varni JW. Health-related quality of life. In: Sobo EJ, Kurtin PS, editors. Child health services research: applications, innovations, and insights. 1st ed. San Francisco: Jossey-Bass; 2003. p. 209–41.

25. Kutsogiannis DJ, Noseworthy T. Health-related quality of life: during and following critical care. In: Sibbald WJ, Bion JF, editors. Evaluating critical care: using health services research to improve quality: update in intensive care and emergency medicine; 35. Berlin/Heidelberg/New York: Springer; 2001. p. 86–103.

26. Landgraf JM, Maunsell E, Speechley KN, Bullinger M, Campbell S, Abetz L, et al. Canadian-French, German and UK versions of the Child Health Questionnaire: methodology and preliminary item scaling results. Qual Life Res. 1998;7:433–45.

27. Starfield B, Riley AW, Green BF, Ensminger ME, Ryan SA, Kelleher K, et al. The adolescent child health and illness profile. A population-based measure of health. Med Care. 1995;33:553–66.

28. Stein RE, Jessop DJ. Functional status II(R). A measure of child health status. Med Care. 1990;28:1041–55 [Erratum in: Med Care 1991;29:following 489].

29. Varni JW, Seid M, Rode CA. The PedsQL: measurement model for the pediatric quality of life inventory. Med Care. 1999;37:126–39.

30. Bruijnzeels MA, Van der Wouden JC, Foets M, Prins A, Van der Heuvel WJA. Validity and accuracy of interview and diary data on children's medical utilization in the Netherlands. J Epidemiol Community Health. 1998;52:65–9.

31. Bruijnzeels MA, Foets M, Van der Wouden JC, Prins A, Van der Heuvel WJA. Measuring morbidity of children in the community: a comparison of interview and diary data. Int J Epidemiol. 1998;27: 96–100.

32. Ferguson DM, Lynskey MT, Horwood LJ. The effect of maternal depression on maternal ratings of child behavior. J Abn Child Psychol. 1993;21:245–69.

33. Ireys HT, Silver EJ. Perception of the impact of a child's chronic illness: does it predict maternal mental health? J Dev Behav Pediatr. 1996;17:77–83.

34. Forrest CB, Simpson L, Clancy C. Child health services research. Challenges and opportunities. JAMA. 1997;277:1787–93.

35. Heyland DK, Guyatt G, Cook DJ, Meade M, Juniper E, Cronin L, Gafni A. Frequency and methodologic rigor of quality-of-life assessments in the critical care literature. Crit Care Med. 1998;26: 591–8.

36. Predicting outcome in ICU patients. 2nd European conference in intensive care medicine. Intensive Care Med. 1994;20:390–7.

37. Morrison AL, Gillis J, O'Connell AJ, Schell DN, Dossetor DR, Mellis C. Quality of life of survivors of pediatric intensive care. Pediatr Crit Care Med. 2002;3:1–5.

38. Gemke RJ, Bonsel GJ, Van Vught AJ. Long term survival and state of health after pediatric intensive care. Arch Dis Child. 1995;73: 196–201.

39. Ambuehl J, Karrer A, Meer A, Riedel T, Schibler A. Quality of life of survivors of paediatric intensive care. Swiss Med Wkly. 2007; 137:312–6.

40. Ruttimann UE, Pollack MM, Fiser DH. Prediction of three outcome states from pediatric intensive care. Crit Care Med. 1996;24:78–85.

41. Fiser DH, Long N, Roberson PK, et al. Relationship of pediatric overall performance category and pediatric cerebral performance category scores at pediatric intensive care unit discharge with outcome measures collected at hospital discharge and 1-and 6-month follow-up assessments. Crit Care Med. 2000;28:2616–20.

42. Zimmerman JE, Kramer AA, McNair DS, et al. Acute Physiology and Chronic Health Evaluation (APACHE) IV: hospital mortality assessment for today's critically ill patients. Crit Care Med. 2006;34:1297–310.

43. Metnitz PG, Moreno RP, Almeida E, Jordan B, Bauer P, Campos RA, SAPS 3 Investigators, et al. SAPS 3 – From evaluation of the patient to evaluation of the intensive care unit. Part 1: objectives, methods and cohort description. Intensive Care Med. 2005;31: 1336–44.

44. Moreno RP, Metnitz PG, Almeida E, Jordan B, Bauer P, Campos RA, SAPS 3 Investigators, et al. SAPS 3 – From evaluation of the patient to evaluation of the intensive care unit. Part 2: development of a prognostic model for hospital mortality at ICU admission. Intensive Care Med. 2005;31:1345–55 [Erratum in: Intensive Care Med 2006;32:796].

45. Lemeshow S, Teres D, Klar J, Avrunin JS, Gehlbach SH, Rapoport J. Mortality Probability Models (MPM II) based on an international cohort of intensive care unit patients. JAMA. 1993;270:2478–86.

46. Slater A, Shann F, Pearson G; Pediatric Index of Mortality (PIM) Study Group. PIM2: a revised version of the Pediatric Index of Mortality. Intensive Care Med. 2003;29:278–85.

47. Tilford JM, Roberson PK, Lensing S, Fiser DH. Differences in pediatric ICU mortality risk over time. Crit Care Med. 1998;26:1737–43.

48. Donabedian A. The quality of care. How can it be assessed? JAMA. 1988;260:1743–8.

49. Pollack MM, Alexander SR, Clarke N, Ruttimann UE, Tesselaar HM, Bachulis AC. Improved outcomes from tertiary center pediatric intensive care: a statewide comparison of tertiary and nontertiary care facilities. Crit Care Med. 1991;19:150–9.

50. Pollack MM, Patel KM, Ruttimann E. Pediatric critical care training programs have a positive effect on pediatric intensive care mortality. Crit Care Med. 1997;25:1637–42.

51. Hébert PC, Wells G, Blajchman MA, Marshall J, Martin C, Pagliarello G, et al. A multicenter, randomized, controlled clinical trial of transfusion requirements in critical care. Transfusion Requirements in Critical Care Investigators, Canadian Critical Care Trials Group. N Engl J Med. 1999;340:409–17.

52. National Heart, Lung, and Blood Institute ARDS Clinical Trials Network. Higher versus lower positive end-expiratory pressures in patients with the acute respiratory distress syndrome. N Engl J Med. 2004;351:327–36.

53. Clermont G, Kong L, Weissfeld LA, Lave JR, Rubenfeld GD, Roberts MS, NHLBI ARDS Clinical Trials Network, et al. The effect of pulmonary artery catheter use on costs and long-term outcomes of acute lung injury. PLoS One. 2011;6:e22512. Epub 2011 Jul 21.

54. Connors Jr AF, Speroff T, Dawson NV, Thomas C, Harrell Jr FE, Wagner D, SUPPORT Investigators, et al. The effectiveness of right heart catheterization in the initial care of critically ill patients. JAMA. 1996;276:889–97.

55. Heyland DK, Cook DJ, King D, Kernerman P, Brun-Buisson C. Maximizing oxygen delivery in critically ill patients: a methodologic appraisal of the evidence. Crit Care Med. 1996;24:517–24.

56. Wiener RS, Welch HG. Trends in the use of the pulmonary artery catheter in the United States, 1993–2004. JAMA. 2007;298:423–9.

57. Wilson IB, Cleary PD. Linking clinical variables with health-related quality of life. A conceptual model of patient outcomes. JAMA. 1995;273:59–65.

58. Hennekens CH, Buring JE. Analysis of epidemiologic studies: evaluating the role of bias. In: Mayrent SL, editor. Epidemiology in medicine. Boston/Toronto: Little, Brown and Company; 1987. p. 272–86.

59. Hennekens CH, Buring JE. Analysis of epidemiologic studies: evaluating the role of confounding. In: Mayrent SL, editor. Epidemiology in medicine. Boston/Toronto: Little, Brown and Company; 1987. p. 287–323.

60. McClellan M, McNeil BJ, Newhouse JP. Does more intensive treatment of acute myocardial infarction in the elderly reduce mortality? Analysis using instrumental variables. JAMA. 1994;272:859–66.

61. Odetola FO, Tilford JM, Davis MM. Variation in the use of intracranial-pressure monitoring and mortality in critically ill children with meningitis in the United States. Pediatrics. 2006;117:1893–900.

62. Folland S, Goodman AC, Stano M. The economics of health and health care. 6th ed. Upper Saddle River: Pearson Prentice Hall; 2010.

63. Roberts TE, The Extracorporeal Membrane Oxygenation Economics Working Group. Economic evaluation and randomised controlled trial of extracorporeal membrane oxygenation: UK collaborative trial. BMJ. 1998;317:911–5.

64. Peek GJ, Elbourne D, Mugford M, Tiruvoipati R, Wilson A, Allen E, et al. Randomised controlled trial and parallel economic evaluation of conventional ventilatory support versus extracorporeal membrane oxygenation for severe adult respiratory failure (CESAR). Health Technol Assess. 2010;14:1–46.

65. Chalom R, Raphaely RC, Costarino Jr AT. Hospital costs of pediatric intensive care. Crit Care Med. 1999;27:2079–85.

66. Sinzobahamvya N, Kopp T, Photiadis J, Arenz C, Schindler E, Haun C, et al. Surgical management of congenital heart disease: correlation between hospital costs and the Aristotle complexity score. Thorac Cardiovasc Surg. 2010;58:322–7.

67. Browman G, Hebert PC, Coutts J, Stanbrook MB, Flegel K, Macdonald N. Personalized medicine: a windfall for science, but what about patients? CMAJ. 2011;183:E1277.

Resident and Nurse Education in Pediatric Intensive Care Unit

Girish G. Deshpande, Gwen J. Lombard, and Adalberto Torres Jr.

Abstract

In the current age of exponential increase in medical knowledge, advances in technology, and electronic data gathering, education of resident physicians and nurses in Pediatric Intensive Care is imperative. Resident physicians are spending less time caring for critically ill patients due to restricted work hours, mandatory didactics attendance and continuity clinics. Attending physicians have less protected time dedicated to education due to administrative and research demands. Nurses working in Pediatric Intensive Care are required to possess extensive clinical skills that are increasingly complex. Educators need to explore new avenues of providing training to both resident physicians and nurses. Using different modalities of simulation appears to be the most appealing solution by providing necessary training in safe and effective environment. This chapter explores several different avenues of improving education in Pediatric Intensive Care.

Keywords

Resident Education • Nurse Education • Pediatric Intensive Care Unit • Web-based education • Simulation training • Factors impacting resident education

To study the phenomenon of disease without books is to sail an uncharted sea; while to study books without seeing patients is not to go sea at all. – Sir William Osler

Introduction

Learning is a lifelong process; and this is especially necessary in medicine, which continues to evolve each day. Dreyfus and Dreyfus [1] described the stages of learning that individuals go through during their professional lives. These five stages are novice, advanced beginner, competent, proficient, and expert. Brenner applied this model in a study of the nursing profession. Expertise develops when the clinician tests, and refines propositions, hypotheses, and principle-based expectations in actual practice situations [2]. Hands on experience is essential for the development of the physician or nurse. In professional education, learners grow into teachers and teachers continue to be learners. The medical student becomes the first year resident and also a teacher of other medical students. More senior residents are teaching their juniors. The ever-changing practice of medicine requires physicians and nurses to engage in continued learning. Newer Accreditation Council for Graduate Medical Education (ACGME) guidelines intended to

G.G. Deshpande, MD
Department of Pediatrics, Children's Hospital of Illinois,
530 NE Glen Oak Ave, Peoria, IL 61637, USA
e-mail: girish@uic.edu

G.J. Lombard, PhD, RN
Department of Neurosurgery, University of Florida,
100 S. Newell Drive, 100265,
Gainesville, FL 32610-0265, USA
e-mail: lombard@neurosurgery.ufl.edu

A. Torres Jr., MD, MS (✉)
Department of Pediatrics, Nemours Children's Hospital,
13535 Nemours Pkwy, Orlando, FL 32827, USA
e-mail: altorres@uic.edu

D.S. Wheeler et al. (eds.), *Pediatric Critical Care Medicine*,
DOI 10.1007/978-1-4471-6362-6_12, © Springer-Verlag London 2014

promote safe and effective patient care delivery, to improve quality and professionalism, and to promote resident well being, have created challenges in providing education to the trainees especially those in the Intensive Care Unit (ICU) environment [3, 4]. We as educators need to create new avenues and re-explore old ones to promote training in the ICU environment.

Uniqueness of Pediatric Intensive Care Units

Pediatric intensive care units (PICUs) are unique learning environments in several respects, including (1) the wide patient age range, (2) the patient illness severity, (3) the need for rapid treatment of unstable patients, (4) seasonal variations in workload and training opportunities, (5) continually changing technology and medications, and (6) the wide range of provider experience level. Patient age range varies from preterm neonates to adults. For example, adults undergoing repair for congenital heart disease may be admitted to a PICU if preferred by their cardiovascular surgeon. Many adults with life-long pediatric illnesses or conditions such as cystic fibrosis, cerebral palsy etc., may be admitted to the PICU because of their small size, familiarity with the PICU staff, or the referral preference of their primary physician.

Seasonal variations of certain diseases, especially infectious illnesses, cause large fluxes in both workload and learning opportunities for residents and new nurses. For example, the residents rotating through the PICU during respiratory syncytial virus season have a greater chance of performing tracheal intubations and learning respiratory pathophysiology than residents rotating through in the summer, which are more likely to see near-drowning or trauma.

Teaching PICUs are generally located in the regional referral institutions and therefore, they often attract more complex and severely ill patients from local community hospitals. Illnesses range from status asthmaticus to smoke inhalation, from diabetic ketoacidosis to adrenal crisis, from meningitis to head injury, and from sepsis to child abuse. Often a rapid deterioration in a patient's condition demands rapid interventions limiting time spent discussing therapeutic options with the resident or nurse.

The constantly evolving technology and endless introduction of new medications also make the PICU more challenging for learners who have to understand the basic principles while trying to conquer new information. Learners in the PICU face a daunting task of acquiring both new skills and knowledge while simultaneously caring for critically ill patients. They are also expected to develop self-directed and life-long learning skills [5]. At any time in the PICU there is a wide variety of professionals in training, which adds to the learning environment complexity. Although, to new residents and nurses, the PICU may appear alarmingly chaotic,

intimidating, unforgiving, and unnerving, it offers a unique learning experience where they can expand their knowledge base, sharpen their clinical skills, and learn the value of a good clinical team.

Resident Education Techniques

Residents receive training and education through different formats such as patient care rounds, morning reports, didactics (conferences, grand rounds), small group discussions, mock codes and organized focused courses such as Pediatric Advanced Life Support provider course. Didactics, the most widely used format, has been well documented to be unsuccessful in changing physician performance and patient outcomes [6, 7]. Hence, medical educators have moved on to more interactive formats such as problem based learning (PBL) and computer assisted learning (CAL). Problem-based learning is designed for small groups that work together and independently on information gathering and problem-solving. The instructor (facilitator) selects the clinical scenario to enhance learner's cognitive and problem-solving abilities. Studies have shown PBL has a little effect on self-directed learning [8–10]. David and Patel provide an excellent review of PBL in pediatrics [11].

Advances in computer technology and accessibility combined with Internet access for medical resource have pushed CAL to the forefront of medical education format. One of the most informative and useful Web sites of pediatric intensive care is PedsCCM (http://www.pedsccm.org). Besides providing clinical tools, evidence-based reviews of applicable literature, and clinical guidelines pertaining to care of critically ill children, it also gives links to other informative websites, e.g. eMedicine.Medscape (http://emedcine.medscape.com/pediatrics_cardiac), a free online reference for Pediatric Critical Care topics [12].

The Pediatric Resident Committee, a subcommittee of the Pediatric Section of the Society of Critical Care Medicine (SCCM), developed a PICU Course to form a core curriculum for medical students and residents in pediatric critical care medicine. The slide presentations, authored by members of the Resident Education Committee are available for download at a nominal fee to computer/server from a new SCCM website, LearnICU.org [13]. Originally, the presentations were designed to provide a template for attending led didactic sessions. The presentations have been modified for self-learning to provide residents flexibility to view as many presentations as possible during time that is convenient to them. This site also offers a pre and post-test to registered users, but composite scores of the residents are not available to respective program directors. Evaluation of this resource's impact on resident learning is lacking. Although there is insufficient evidence to assert that CAL is more effective than traditional methods, learners perform better when CAL supplements traditional methods [14]. Learners must possess basic computer literacy to take full advantage of this valuable and growing resource [15].

An active learning strategy that has been incorporated into medical school education for greater than 10 years [16] and is now being implemented into resident training is team-based learning (TBL). TBL fosters individual and group accountability as small group of learners work together to solve clinical problems. TBL employs three-phases: (1) advanced preparation by individuals, (2) readiness assurance via individual and group testing, and (3) problem-solving in small groups. Although there are no published reports of TBL being applied in pediatrics, there is evidence of TBL maintaining a learned clinical skill, i.e. patient alcohol screening and brief intervention, in family medicine residents [17].

Mock codes offer an opportunity to teach important critical thinking skills. Regular participation in mock codes prepares the resident to perform in crisis situations when there is little time to discuss therapeutic options and assistance with team building. Mock codes allow residents to participate not only in different roles but also in different settings. A successful mock code program has several benefits, one of which is working with nurses during a *crisis* when the consequences of mistakes are removed from patients [18].

Resident Education in Pediatric Critical Care

For more than 100 years, medical education has occurred in community settings. In the mid-nineteenth century, physicians were educated through preceptorships and apprenticeships. With the introduction of the full-time university post-Flexner model (1910), education shifted to the universities and their teaching hospitals, where most pediatric education was teacher centered [19]. In 1987, in a summary of a report by the American Board of Pediatrics regarding the future training of pediatricians, Cleveland and Brownlee [20] commented that the current training programs did not adequately prepare pediatric residents for practice and recommended emphasis on ambulatory or community-based training.

The *Final report of the FOPE (Future of Pediatric Education) II Pediatric Generalists of the Future Workgroup (2000)* describes the core attributes, skills, and competencies of the future generalist pediatrician and outlines implications of these requirements for residency training and continuing medical education [21]. The authors state that residents must be assured excellent training in the stabilization of critically ill or injured children to manage their problems appropriately in an acute care setting. This expectation requires sufficient experience in critical care medicine with older infants

and children to be able to provide leadership to a team stabilizing a critically ill patient. A working knowledge of pediatric advanced life support and advanced pediatric life support techniques and algorithms, in addition to the knowledge base to construct a differential diagnosis for further care, is essential [21].

The ACGME guidelines group the intensive care experience of both Neonatal ICU and PICU together to be a minimum of 5 and a maximum of 6 months, of which minimum 3 and maximum 4 block months in NICU (level II or III) and 2 block months in PICU. Any additional call hours in PICU are not included in calculation of intensive care time. Guidelines also state that the curricula in PICU must be structured to, (1) familiarize residents with the special multidisciplinary and multi-organ implications of fluid, electrolyte, and metabolic disorders; (2) trauma, nutrition, and cardiorespiratory management; (3) infection control; and (4) recognition and management of congenital anomalies in pediatric patients. It must also be designed to teach the following:

1. recognition and management of isolated and multi-organ system failure and assessment of reversibility;
2. understanding organ system dysfunction variation by patient age;
3. integration of clinical assessment and laboratory data to formulate management and therapeutic plans for critically ill patients;
4. invasive and noninvasive techniques for monitoring and supporting pulmonary, cardiovascular, cerebral, and metabolic functions;
5. participation in PICU admission, discharge, and patient transfer decision making;
6. resuscitation, stabilization, and transportation of ICU patients;
7. understanding appropriate physician roles for the pediatrician and intensivist in these settings;
8. participation in preoperative and postoperative management of surgical patients, including understanding appropriate physician roles for the pediatrician and the intensivist in this settings;
9. evaluation and management critically ill patients following traumatic injury [3].

Residents are expected to use the on-line log provided by the ACGME for documentation of all procedures. The program directors must be able to show the competence of each resident for each procedure using this document. In addition to PALS training, the residents must have sufficient training in the following skills: (1) basic and advanced life support; (2) endotracheal intubation; (3) placement of intraosseous lines (demonstration in a skills lab or PALS course is sufficient); (4) placement of intravenous lines; (5) arterial puncture; (6) venipuncture; (7) umbilical artery and vein catheterization; (8) lumbar puncture; (9) bladder

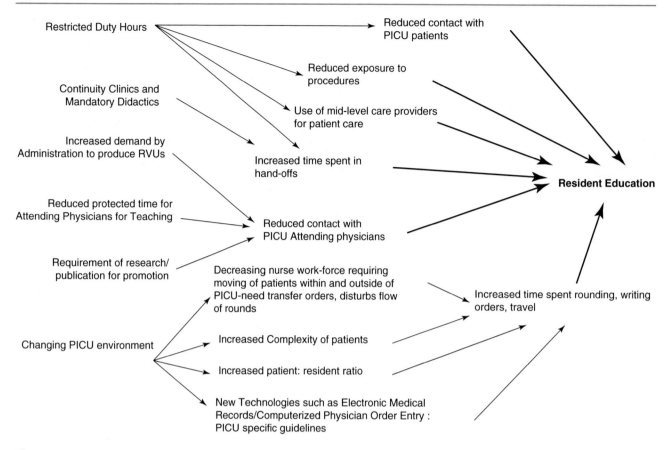

Fig. 12.1 Factors impacting resident education in pediatric critical care unit

catheterization; (10) wound care and suturing of lacerations; (11) procedural sedation and pain management; (12) chest tube placement and thoracentesis [3]. The remaining procedures listed in the ACGME document are more applicable outside of the PICU.

In July 2010, the ACGME implemented new standards for supervision and duty hours for residency programs. The 80-h work week averaged over 4-weeks is unchanged for all residents. The duty period of first year residents must not exceed 16 h in duration, while the intermediate and senior residents may be scheduled to a maximum of 24 h of continuous duty, with an additional 4 h permitted for handing off patients to another practitioner or, in unusual circumstances, remaining with an acutely ill patient. The new guidelines strongly suggest "strategic napping" especially after 16 h of continuous duty between 10 PM and 8 AM [22]. Resident education has been impacted by these changes overall but especially in intensive care units. The survey of program directors by Chudgar et al. showed resident availability, clinical workload, lack of faculty protected time for and lack of education funding as perceived education barriers. Resident delivered patient care, a core teaching method, has also suffered by reducing continuity of care, and increasing patient care transitions [4]. Figure 12.1 summarizes various factors that impact today's resident education in PICU; most have

negative effects on training. Introduction of new technologies such as electronic medical records, computerized order entry, and introduction of new guidelines may both improve care safety and consistency but may also demand more resident time [23]. The service needs for ICUs have been increasing over the past several decades, with advances in technology, improved monitoring, and the survival of more chronically ill and technology dependent children. Increasing complexity of care provides educational opportunities, but may increase the time spent in rounding [23].

An emphasis on ambulatory and community pediatric rotations has occurred over past decade, with pediatric residents spending less time caring for hospitalized patients. The new duty hours rule from the Residency Review Committee [22] limits residents to spend 80 h per week (averaged over a 4-week period) in clinical and academic activities. Residents' continuity clinics also significantly reduce (10–30 %) inpatient care time. In addition, housestaff are expected to attend morning reports, didactic conferences, and grand rounds all of which require them to be relieved of patient care responsibilities. Other responsibilities of residents in the PICU include admitting patients, managing care inclusive of some procedures, collecting patient or clinical data (laboratory, imaging, and other tests), clarifying pharmacy data, participating in nursing discussions/clarifications, and making

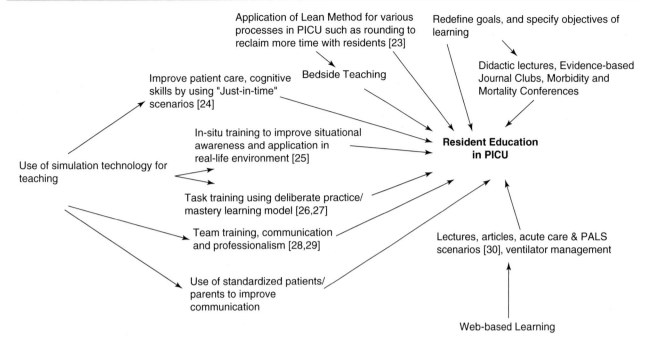

Fig. 12.2 Solutions proposed to enhance education in PICU

home care arrangements at the time of discharge of patients. Application of Lean Methodology geared towards resident education may be beneficial [23]. For example, having mid-level care providers to perform some repetitive responsibilities such as writing of total parenteral nutrition may free residents for other activities. Figure 12.2 offers some solutions implemented by educators in various fields to ameliorate current educational barriers [23–30]. One approach taken to meet PICU service needs has been to hire mid-level care providers or physician extenders such as advanced nurse practitioners and physician assistants. However, this alternative can be expensive, and has been reported to shift hospital support from resident education to service needs [31]. In addition, training these allied health professionals creates competition for learning opportunities between the house-staff and the physician extenders in smaller or slower PICUs.

Evaluation of Residents

Resident performance is assessed in six areas to the level expected of a new practitioner: patient care, medical knowledge, interpersonal skills and communication, practice-based learning and improvement, professionalism, and system-based practice. The ACGME website [32] also provides several tools to evaluate resident performance. The expectations for the residents in these six areas are as follows:

Patient care: Residents must be able to provide family-centered patient care that is culturally effective, developmentally and age appropriate, compassionate, and effective for the treatment of disease and the promotion of health.

Medical knowledge: Residents must demonstrate knowledge of established and evolving biomedical, clinical, epidemiologic, and social–behavioral sciences and application of this knowledge to patient care.

Practice-based learning and improvement: This involves the investigation and evaluation of care of patients, the appraisal and assimilation of scientific evidence, and improvements in inpatient care.

Interpersonal and communication skills: Residents must be able to demonstrate interpersonal and communication skills that result in effective information exchange and teaming with patients, their families, and professional associates.

Professionalism: Residents must demonstrate a commitment to carrying out professional responsibilities, adherence to ethical principles, and sensitivity to diversity.

System-based practice: This is manifested by actions that demonstrate an awareness of and responsiveness to the larger context and system of health care, as well as the ability to call effectively on other resources in the system to provide optimal health care.

Educating New Graduate Nurses

Nurses require ongoing education to face challenges related to increased care complexity including new medication education, electronic medical charting, in-servicing new technologies such as ventilators and monitoring devices, and learning new care guidelines. Nurses often must learn while carrying a full clinical workload. New graduate nurses in the PICU have to simultaneously learn hospital policies and procedures and the pathophysiologies of the wide array of pediatric illnesses, while acquiring practical bedside skills (e.g., invasive catheter care). Clinical demands during periods of high census, high acuity, and/or inadequate staffing can disrupt the preceptor–novice relationship and create stress on the novice nurse that can be potentially detrimental to both learning and patient safety [33].

Strategies used to facilitate critical care learning by nurses include formal orientation programs, PBL, concept mapping, nursing narratives, learning contracts, and reflective practices [34–37]. The major limiting factor for learning identified by PICU nurses was time constraints [38]. Students had a strong preference for courses in which theory and content were related to practice, making learning more relevant. A nurturing environment with knowledgeable preceptors, peer support, flexible work schedule, and multiformat educational approach (e.g., lectures, videos, case studies) has been successful in improving graduate nurse retention in the PICU [39, 40]. To meet regulatory standards, hospital orientation and annual competency validation, nurse educators often use a skills lab or fair to assess knowledge and psychomotor skills. This however does not address integration of clinical judgment. Simulation based education can offer opportunities to develop decision-making skills and integration of critical care procedures and concepts into the employee competency curriculum [41]. Computer-assisted learning resources are available for critical care nurses [42] and can even facilitate learning critical nursing skills [43]. Interested readers are referred to excellent references that deal with conceptual [44, 45] and practical [46–48] learning principles for critical care nurses.

Nursing care in the PICU requires meticulous attention to detail and good communication skills to provide the best care to the critically ill child. Patients are treated with a multitude of medications and infusions; a small error in calculation, composition, or administration could cause morbidity or mortality. The graduate nurse discovers early in their PICU education whether she or he possesses the ability to thrive in this highly challenging environment.

Use of Simulators in Medical Education

Experiential learning or learner-centered teaching has been accepted as a useful strategy for educators in the PICU to employ. According to Kolb [49], it is through repeated learning experiences that learners' thoughts are formed and reformed. Guided practice allows learners to assimilate key concepts, attitudes, and skills. Skills to be learned in the PICU are hands on, procedural, or problem solving. Problem-solving skills include making decisions when adequate information is not available or in the presence of conflicting information. Occasionally, clinical problems are encountered that come with little guidance from the literature or experience to help manage the case.

Medical education has been based on apprenticeship techniques since the era of Hippocrates. Medical simulation offers the potential for the evolution of new teaching paradigms for the new millennium [5]. The use of human patient simulators and reflective practice has recently come to the forefront of critical care education [5, 15, 50]. High-fidelity simulators are full-bodied mannequins that breathe, talk, blink, have a palpable pulse, make urine, and have audible bowel sounds similar to patients [50]. Simulators such as those made by METI (Medical Education Technology Inc., Sarasota, FL; www.meti.com) and Laerdal (Laerdal Medical Corp., Wappingers Falls, NY; www.laerdal.com) are becoming increasingly available in large academic medical centers. High-fidelity simulators provide ideal opportunities for experiential learning and hands-on practice with use of real instruments with real-time patient reactions to students' actions. The simulators provide a number of prescribed cases for students. In addition, real patient cases and data can be used to create scenarios that recreate what happened in the unit. Simulators can also be used to maintain skills that may be used rarely in the PICU, such as cardiopulmonary resuscitation [51]. Simulators can create adverse situations such as esophageal intubation or dislodged endotracheal tubes that in real life could be life threatening and hence cannot be deliberately created. It is mandatory that physicians recognize such situations immediately and manage them correctly and swiftly. Reducing error in high-risk situations (i.e., codes) can be addressed through strategies such as crisis resource management training using simulation [52].

Simulators are educational tools that allow students to learn new skills in a safe environment. Scenarios can be played out so that learners can see the results of their actions without having the attending or instructors having to step in and correct their actions or decisions. The use of videotape provides an objective, time-coded record of trainee communication and actions and creates a powerful stimulus for learning during facilitated debriefing. Because the activities in the simulator pose no risk to patients or to professional liability, trainees are allowed to witness the natural evolutions of mistakes without the need for intervention by senior faculty [53]. Simulators can also be used for learner assessment and evaluation [54, 55]. This is especially important for the competencies in residency education and being able to document a resident's ability to perform critical skills and procedures [56]. Thus, in a new era of exponentially increasing medical knowledge and ever-decreasing patient contact, simulation may offer an answer. According to Christine McGuire, Professor of Medical Education at the University of Illinois, simulation offers an opportunity to leverage the advantages of experiential learning and reflective practices through three defining characteristics: simulation imitates but does not duplicate reality, offers almost limitless opportunities to *go wrong*, and provides corrective feedback as a guide to future action [55]. Yager et al. has recently published an excellent review of simulation literature regarding its use in pediatric critical care and emergency medicine [57]. Andreatta et al., in their recent study showed progressive improvement in patient survival following pediatric cardiopulmonary arrest associated with an increase in number of mock codes over the 4-year study period [58]. This is the first study to link pediatric simulation based teaching to an important clinical outcome.

Conclusion

The PICU offers a unique learning environment. There are several models for adult learning, and success depends on the learner stage, methods used, and skill of the instructor/facilitator. Teaching residents all the knowledge base and procedural skills required by ACGME during their limited work hours is a challenge being faced by intensivists across the country. A combination of the many available educational approaches should be tailored to meet local educational needs while conforming to national standards. High-fidelity simulators appear to be a safe and effective way to teach and evaluate residents, fellows, and nurses inside or outside of the PICU environment.

References

1. Dreyfus HL, Dreyfus SE. Mind over machine: the power of human intuition and expertise in the era of the computer. New York: The Free Press; 1986.
2. Brenner P. From novice to expert: excellence and power in clinical nursing practice. Upper Saddle River: Prentice Hall Health; 2001.
3. ACGME Program Requirements for GME in Pediatrics July 1, 2007. www.acgme.org/acWebsite/downloads/RRC_ProgReq/320_pediatrics_07012007.pdf. Last accessed 28 Jan 2012.
4. Chudgar SM, Cox CE, Que LG, et al. Current teaching and evaluation methods in critical care medicine: has the Accreditation Council for Graduate Medical Education affected how we practice and teach in the intensive care unit? Crit Care Med. 2009;37:49–60.
5. Dunn W, editor. Simulators in critical care and beyond. Des Plaines: Society of Critical Care Medicine; 2004.
6. Davis D, Thomson MA, Oxman A, Andrew D, Haynes RB. Changing physician performance: a systematic review of the effect of continuing medical education strategies. JAMA. 1995;274:700–5.
7. Davis D, Thomson O'Brien MA, Freemantle N, et al. Impact of formal continuing medical education. Do conferences, workshops, rounds, and other traditional continuing education activities change physician behavior or health care outcomes? JAMA. 1999;282:867–74.
8. Colliver JA. Effectiveness of problem-based learning curricula: research and theory. Acad Med. 2000;75:259–66.
9. Colliver JA. Educational theory and medical education practice: a cautionary note for medical school faculty. Acad Med. 2002;77:1217–20.
10. Ozuah P, Curtis J, Stein R. Impact of problem based learning on residents' self-directed learning. Arch Pediatr Adolesc Med. 2001;155:669–72.
11. David TJ, Patel L. Adult learning theory, problem based learning, and paediatrics. Arch Dis Child. 1995;73:357–63.
12. Pediatrics: cardiac diseases and critical care medicine articles. http://emedicine.medscape.com/pediatric_cardiac. Last accessed 28 Jan 2012.
13. Resident ICU course. http://www.learnicu.org/Fundamentals/RICU/Pages/PICUModules.aspx. Last accessed 26 Jan 2012.
14. Tegtmeyer K, Ibsen L, Goldstein B. Computer-assisted learning in critical care: from ENIAC to HAL. Crit Care Med. 2001;29:N177–82.
15. Vozenilek J, Huff S, Reznek M, Gordon J. See one, do one, teach one: advanced technology in medical education. Acad Emerg Med. 2004;11:1149–54.
16. Parmalee D, Michaelsen LK. Team-based learning: it's here and it WORKS! (letter). Acad Med. 2010;85:1658.
17. Shellenberger S, Seale JP, Harris DL, et al. Applying team-based learning in primary care residency programs to increase patient alcohol screening and brief interventions. Acad Med. 2009;84:340–6.
18. Tegtmeyer K. Education in the age of the 80-hour work week. In: Tegtmeyer K, editor. Current concepts in pediatric critical care. Des Plaines: Society of Critical Care Medicine; 2005. p. 135–42.
19. American Academy of Pediatrics, Committee on Community Health Services. Community pediatrics: an annotated bibliography. Grove Village: American Academy of Pediatrics; 2002.
20. Cleveland W, Brownlee R. American Board of Pediatrics, future training of pediatricians: summary report of a series of conferences sponsored by the American Board of Pediatrics. Pediatrics. 1987;80:451–7.
21. Leslie L, Rappo P, Abelson H, Jenkins R, Sewall S. Final report of the FOPE II pediatric generalist of the future workgroup. Pediatrics. 2000;106:1199–223.
22. ACGME: common program requirements (effective July 1, 2010). http://www.acgme.org/acWebSite/home/Common_Program_Requirements_07012010.pdf. Last accessed 28 Jan2012.
23. Vats A, Goin KH, Fortenberry JD. Lean analysis of a pediatric intensive care unit physician group rounding process to identify inefficiencies and opportunities for improvement. Pediatr Crit Care Med. 2011;12:415–21.
24. Nishisaki A, Donoghue AJ, Colborn S, et al. Effect of just-in-time simulation training on tracheal intubation procedure safety in the pediatric intensive care unit. Anesthesiology. 2010;113:214–23.
25. Weinstock PH, Kappus LJ, Garden A, Burns JP. Simulation at the point of care, reduced cost, in situ training via a mobile cart. Pediatr Crit Care Med. 2009;10:176–82.
26. Wayne BD, Butter J, Siddall VJ, et al. Mastery learning of advanced cardiac life support skills by internal medicine residents using simulation technology and deliberate practice. J Gen Intern Med. 2006;21:251–6.
27. Barsuk JH, McGaghie WC, Cohen ER, O'Leary KJ, Wayne DB. Simulation-based mastery learning reduces complications during central venous catheter insertion in a medical intensive care unit. Crit Care Med. 2009;37:2697–701.
28. Nishisaki A, Nguyen J, Colborn S, et al. Evaluation of multidisciplinary simulation training on clinical performance and team behavior during tracheal intubation procedures in a pediatric intensive care unit. Pediatr Crit Care Med. 2011;12:406–14.
29. Frengley RW, Weller J, Torrie J, et al. The effect of a simulation-based training intervention on the performance of established critical care unit teams. Crit Care Med. 2011;12:1–7.
30. Ventre KM, Collingridge DS, DeCarlo D, Schwild HA. Performance of a consensus scoring algorithm for assessing pediatric advanced life support competency using a computer screen-based simulator. Pediatr Crit Care Med. 2009;10:623–35.

31. Carraccio C, Berman M. Intensive care: impact on resident education. Clin Pediatr. 1994;33:625–7.

32. Pediatric general competencies. http://www.acgme.org/acWebsite/RRC_320/320_gencomp.pdf. Last accessed 28 Jan 2012.

33. Endacott R, Scholes J, Freeman M, Cooper S. The reality of clinical learning in critical care settings: a practitioner: student gap? J Clin Nurs. 2003;12:778–85.

34. Dobbin K. Applying learning theories to develop teaching strategies for the critical care nurse. Don't limit yourself to the formal classroom lecture. Crit Care Nurs Clin North Am. 2001;13:1–11.

35. Prioux DM, Bourcier BJ. Graduate nurses in the intensive care unit. Crit Care Nurse. 2008;28:44–52.

36. Chunta KS, Katrancha ED. Using problem-based learning in staff development: strategies for teaching registered nurses and new graduate nurses. J Contin Educ Nurs. 2010;41:557–64.

37. Dix G, Hughes SJ. Strategies to help students learn effectively. Nurs Stand. 2004;18:39–42.

38. Hewitt-Taylor J, Gould D. Learning preferences of paediatric intensive care nurses. J Adv Nurs. 2002;38:288–95.

39. Janvrin S. Introducing new graduates into pediatric intensive care. A thorough on-the-job program turns anxious graduates into confident beginning practitioners. Nurs Manag 1990;21:967.

40. Race TK, Skees J. Changing tides: improving outcomes through mentorship on all levels of nursing. Crit Care Nurs Q. 2010;33:163–74.

41. Cato DL, Murray M. Use of simulation training in the intensive care unit. Crit Care Nurs Q. 2010;33:44–51.

42. Bove L. Computer-assisted education for critical care nurses. Crit Care Nurs Clin North Am. 2001;13:73–81.

43. DeAmicis P. Interactive videodisc instruction is an alternative method for learning and performing a critical nursing skill. Comput Nurs. 1997;15:155–8.

44. Kinney MR. Education for critical care nursing. Annu Rev Nurs Res. 1990;8:161–76.

45. Kuiper R, Pesut D. Promoting cognitive and metacognitive reflective reasoning skills in nursing practice: self-regulated learning theory. J Adv Nurs. 2004;45:381–91.

46. Dickerson P. 10 tips to help learning. J Nurses Staff Dev. 2003;19:240–6.

47. Hohler S. Creating an environment conductive to adult learning. AORN J. 2003;77:833–5.

48. Campbell J, Bell-Scott W. Unique solutions in pediatric critical care. Pediatr Nurs. 2001;27:483–91.

49. Kolb DA. Experiential learning: experience as the source of learning and development. Englewood Cliff: Prentice Hall; 1984.

50. Friedrich MJ. Practice makes perfect: risk free medical training with patient simulators. JAMA. 2002;288:2808–12.

51. Fiedor M. Pediatric simulation: a valuable tool for pediatric medical education. Crit Care Med. 2004;32(Suppl):S72–4.

52. Cheng A, Donoghue A, Gilfoyle E, Eppich W. Simulation-based crisis resource management training for pediatric critical care medicine: a review for instructors. Pediatr Crit Care Med. 2012;13: 197–203.

53. Halamek L, Kaegi DM, Gaba DM, et al. Time for a new paradigm in pediatric medical education: teaching neonatal resuscitation in a simulated delivery room environment. Pediatrics. 2000;106:e45.

54. Boulet JR, Murray D, Kras J, et al. Reliability and validity of a simulation-based acute care skills assessment for medical students and residents. Anesthesiology. 2003;99:1270–80.

55. Tekian A, McGuire CH, McGaghie WC. Innovative simulations for assessing professional competence: from paper and pencil to virtual reality. Chicago: University of Illinois at Chicago, Department of Medical Education; 1999.

56. Hugh DJ, Kurrek MM, Cohen MM, Cleave-Hogg D. The validity of performance assessments using simulation. Anesthesiology. 2001;95:36–42.

57. Yager PH, Lok J, Klig JE. Advances in simulation for pediatric critical care and emergency medicine. Curr Opin Pediatr. 2011;23:293–7.

58. Andreatta P, Saxton E, Thompson M, Annich G. Simulation-based mock codes significantly correlate with improved pediatric patient cardiopulmonary arrest survival rates. Pediatr Crit Care Med. 2011;12:33–8.

Epidemiology of Critical Illness

13

R. Scott Watson and Mary Elizabeth Hartman

Abstract

Knowledge of the incidence, prevalence, and natural history of disease informs the development of treatments to improve outcomes, the care delivered at the bedside, and the health policy that influences the systems of medical care for critically ill children. In this chapter, we discuss several issues related to clinical epidemiology in critical care and summarize some of the large-scale work that has been done examining the epidemiology of quintessential critical illnesses in children. There are a number of challenges in performing epidemiologic research in critical care, not the least of which is related to a core principle of epidemiology, which is the need to be able to reliably and validly identify diseases or conditions of interest In critical care, definitions of the syndromes that most consider quintessential critical care "diseases" lack gold standard tests by which to validate them. Despite these challenges, researchers have found mortality for many conditions is improving, and the use of ICU services is increasing. Critical care is provided to hundreds of thousands of children in the US annually, and the number and volume of pediatric ICUs has been increasing over the past two decades, to a greater extent than both the US pediatric population and hospital beds for children. Over 7,000 US children are treated for acute lung injury each year, and more than 100,000 infants and older children are mechanically ventilated. Severe sepsis occurs in over 42,000 US children annually, and is a leading cause of death. Rates of ICU care for asthma, the most common chronic disease in childhood, are increasing at the same time that hospitalization rates are decreasing. The thoughtful use of the tools of clinical epidemiology can facilitate advances in pediatric critical care, help us refine their application, and let us understand their ramifications.

Keywords

Epidemiology • Incidence • Critical care • Acute lung injury • Mechanical ventilation • Sepsis • Status asthmaticus • Intensive care units

R.S. Watson, MD, MPH (✉)
Department of Pediatric Critical Care Medicine,
Children's Hospital of Pittsburgh of UPMC,
4401 Penn Avenue, Pittsburgh, PA 15224, USA
e-mail: watsonrs@upmc.edu

M.E. Hartman, MD, MPH
Department of Pediatric Critical Care Medicine,
St. Louis Children's Hospital, Washington University in St. Louis,
8116, 8th Floor NWT, St. Louis, MO 63110, USA
e-mail: hartman_m@kids.wustl.edu

The clinical epidemiology of critical illness is vital to inform clinical care, meaningful patient-oriented research, and health policy. Knowledge of risk factors for disease aids in prevention of disease, timely intervention to treat it, and selection of study populations. Describing the natural history of disease informs the development of treatments to improve outcomes and the care delivered at the bedside. Understanding the burden of disease influences the prioritization of research efforts and the allocation of health care resources. However, there are a number of challenges in

D.S. Wheeler et al. (eds.), *Pediatric Critical Care Medicine*,
DOI 10.1007/978-1-4471-6362-6_13, © Springer-Verlag London 2014

performing epidemiologic research in critical care, not the least of which is related to a core principle of epidemiology. Delineating the epidemiology of a disease or condition starts with the ability to identify it, both reliably (different investigators classify a patient in the same way as each other and over time) and validly (the classification distinguishes people with the disease from those without it). In critical care, this may be conceptually straightforward but is operationally challenging. In this chapter, we discuss several issues related to clinical epidemiology in critical care and summarize some of the large-scale work that has been done examining the epidemiology of critical illnesses in children.

Challenges of Defining a Population in Critical Care

Critical illness is made up of a heterogeneous group of disorders that share a risk of organ dysfunction, long-term morbidity, and mortality. However, definitions of the syndromes that most consider quintessential critical care "diseases" (sepsis, acute respiratory distress syndrome (ARDS), and even organ failure) lack gold standard tests by which to validate them. By necessity, then, definitions have been developed by consensus and expert opinion. While these definitions represent a substantial improvement over the prior state of phenomenological disarray, they still suffer from limitations in reliability and validity [1–4]. Even the minimum degree of organ dysfunction, or risk thereof, that suggests that a patient is "critically" ill is often debated.

Another challenge to identifying patients with critical illness is that critical illness is often defined by where its care takes place (in the intensive care unit [ICU]) and the interventions used to treat it (e.g., mechanical ventilation (MV), infusions of medications to support hemodynamics, continuous renal replacement therapy). While convenient, these definitions are significantly limited. The definition of an illness cannot rely on the availability of an ICU bed or on the resources available to providers. Care that is provided in an ICU in one country or region may be provided on the ward in another (and even within a given hospital, the availability of ICU beds may change with hospital and ICU census). Critical illness nearly always begins prior to ICU admission and can last beyond ICU discharge. The timing and use of interventions vary markedly by provider, even when controlling for patient factors, such as severity of illness. It is therefore much more straightforward determining which patients received an intervention than which patients actually "needed" one [5–9]. Nonetheless, with the increasing availability of large scale databases and increasing numbers of large-scale epidemiologic studies using prospectively collected data, the size and scope of pediatric critical illness is beginning to be characterized.

Epidemiology of Children Receiving Critical Care Services

National estimates of the overall use of ICU services for children are limited. Extrapolating from a survey conducted in 2001 by Randolph and colleagues [10], in which pediatric ICU (PICU) directors were asked to report their annual number of PICU admissions, at least 230,000 children were admitted to PICUs that year. In preliminary work based on hospital discharge data from states representing a third of the US pediatric population, Hartman et al. estimated that 315,000 children 1 month to 19 years of age received intensive care services in the US in 2005 (in PICUs, neonatal ICUs, and adult ICUs admitting children) [11]. These patients represented 13.5 % of pediatric hospitalizations. The population-based incidence of ICU care in infants at least 1 month old was over three times that of older children. Hospital mortality was 2.3 % (or over 7,100 deaths nationally), was similar across age groups, and was consistent with that reported in Randolph and colleagues' survey (2.9 %) [10]. Mean hospital costs were $19,600 per patient, and total ICU costs were $6 billion nationally [11]. In Washington, DC, the rate of emergency ICU admissions of children less than 14 years old was 166 per 100,000, with higher rates for families with lower socioeconomic status [12]. In England and Wales, the rate of PICU admission was 98 per 100,000 children less than 16 years of age, representing 0.1 % of the pediatric population. Overall mortality was 4.9 %, and higher rates of admission and mortality were also found among those with lower socioeconomic status [13].

Angus et al. studied ICU services at the end of life for children and adults and found that one in five Americans who died in the US in 1999 did so after receiving ICU care [14]. Although many more adults died, children were more likely to receive ICU services at the end of life. Nearly half of infants and one third of older children who died in 1999 received ICU care. Subsequent preliminary analyses of a similar pediatric sample found that 76 % of deaths of hospitalized children 1 month to 19 years of age involved ICU care during the hospitalization [11].

Despite the limitations of using a geographic definition of critical illness, our understanding of the magnitude of critical illness among children is enhanced by information about the provision of pediatric critical care services [15]. Although only 9 % of counties in the US have PICUs and 99 % of PICU are located in urban counties [16], the relative importance of critical care for hospitalized children is on the rise. The number of US pediatric hospital beds overall has been decreasing since the 1980s, but the number of ICU beds for children has been increasing. In 1989, Pollack and others identified 276 pediatric-specific ICUs (PICUs) in the US, with an average of 528 admissions per year [17]. Pediatric intensivists were available in 73 % of the units, and reported mortality was 5.5 %. In 2001, Randolph and colleagues found that the number of PICUs increased to 349, with an average of 672 admissions per year, pediatric intensivists available in 94 %, and mortality of 2.9 % [10]. Between 1995 and 2001, the number of PICU beds increased by 24 % and outpaced population growth of children by 17.5 %. The number of beds per child varied substantially by region—from 1 per 15,250 children in Arkansas, Louisiana, and Texas to 1 per 27,440 in New England. Whether this variation reflects different regional pediatric critical care needs is unknown.

The reason for the increasing numbers of PICU beds is also unclear and likely multifactorial. It may reflect changes in referral patterns, with an increasing number of smaller hospitals providing care for patients previously transferred to larger units. Although this would be somewhat surprising in light of increasing evidence that higher volume units have better severity-adjusted outcomes than their smaller counterparts [18–23], healthcare financing affords incentives to provide intensive care services even at smaller hospitals. On the other hand, patients who remain at smaller hospitals may be less severely ill than those who are transferred to tertiary care and may merely require additional monitoring that is not available on the wards of many hospitals.

Perhaps the most important factor in the increasing demand for PICU services is an increasing number of children in the population living with chronic medical conditions. Success in the treatment of extremely low birth weight babies, genetic disorders, cancer, cystic fibrosis, and organ transplant recipients have lead to longer life expectancies and decreased mortality rates. These successes have also led to an increased number of children living at increased risk of critical illness [24–28]. In a population-based study at a tertiary PICU in New York, almost half (45 %) of all unscheduled admissions to the PICU were for patients with chronic health conditions, 32 % of whom received technology-assisted care (such as MV, oxygen, tracheostomies, and intravenous therapies) [29]. Children with chronic conditions were 3.3 times more likely than healthy children to have an unscheduled PICU admission, and those receiving technology-assisted care were 373 times more likely. The most common conditions were neurological, accounting for 15 % of all unscheduled admissions. Similarly, 23 % of all admissions (both scheduled and unscheduled) to a large, tertiary PICU had preexisting neurodevelopmental disorders [30]. Although hospital mortality was only 3 %, patients were discharged with significantly greater needs for ventilatory and nutritional technology support than they had on admission. In addition to increasing the number of PICU admissions, children with chronic illness may require lengthy PICU stays. Indeed, former premature babies admitted to the PICU consumed more healthcare resources than their non-premature counterparts, including longer lengths of stay and higher rates of MV [31].

Epidemiology of Mechanical Ventilation and ARDS/ALI

The provision of MV for acute respiratory failure was a major motivating factor in the development of intensive care units and is one of the hallmarks of critical care. National estimates of respiratory failure among infants and children have been derived from analyses of administrative records of patients receiving mechanical ventilation. Of course, some patients are ventilated in the ICU for reasons other than for respiratory failure (such as for extreme hemodynamic instability or after prolonged surgery). Therefore, the incidence of MV is higher than the incidence of respiratory failure. Rates of mechanical ventilation were higher in neonates than in any other age group (80,000 babies per year, or 1.8 % of US neonates) [32]. Although very low birth weight babies had extremely high rates of MV (52 %/year), one-third of ventilated neonates were of normal birth weight. Hospital mortality was 11.1 %, and total US hospital costs were $4.4 billion in 1994. Preliminary work examining older children found that 35,000 children aged 1–19 years were ventilated in the US in 1999 [33]. Duration of MV was 4 or more days in over a third of patients. Most were ventilated for medical (as opposed to surgical) reasons, and the most common associated condition was severe sepsis (in 35 %). Hospital mortality (13.8 %) was higher than that of neonates, and estimated national hospital costs were lower ($1 billion).

The epidemiology of ARDS and ALI is challenging to determine in multicenter studies, as it requires the collection of detailed physiologic data. Nonetheless, several good population-based estimates of children with these disorders, using the American-European Consensus Conference definitions [34], are now available. In Australia and New Zealand, a study of 13 ICUs (including eight of the nine PICUs in those countries) found 2.96 cases of ALI per 100,000 children less than 16 years of age per year. Most of these cases (88 %) met ARDS criteria. Mortality was 35 % for children with ALI and 44 % for children with ARDS [35]. In Germany, a prospective population-based study of ARDS in children 1 month to 18 years old found only seven new cases of ARDS in 3 months (Feb, June, April) at 94 ICUs. These cases represented 1.5 % of ventilated children and a population-based incidence of 3.1 per 100,000 per year [36]. The authors estimated that 500 children develop ARDS in Germany annually.

In the US, ALI/ARDS has been systematically assessed in a comprehensive study in King County, Washington. Among children 6 months to 15 years of age, 12.8 per 100,000 per year developed ALI, 74 % of whom met ARDS criteria. This projected to 7,700 cases of pediatric ALI in the US annually, 5,700 of whom had ARDS. The most common risk factor was severe sepsis, and the hospital mortality was 18 % [37]. The age-adjusted incidence in patients 15 years and older was 86.2/100,000/year (which projects to 190,600 cases per year nationally) in 1999–2000 [1]. Hospital mortality was 38.5 %, and both incidence and mortality increased with age.

Epidemiology of Sepsis

Not only is the treatment of sepsis an integral component of critical care, but sepsis also provides a good example of how defining a syndrome, even broadly, facilitates its study. In 1992, the American College of Chest Physicians/Society of Critical Care Medicine Consensus Conference met to standardize the definitions of sepsis and severe sepsis so that they might be more clearly applied in research and clinical practice [38]. The group defined *sepsis* as a systemic inflammatory response syndrome resulting from infection, *severe sepsis* as sepsis associated with organ dysfunction, hypoperfusion or hypotension, and *septic shock* as sepsis with arterial hypotension despite adequate fluid resuscitation [38]. These definitions now frequently serve as criteria for inclusion in randomized controlled trials for sepsis therapies [39–45] and are increasingly employed by medical practitioners around the world. One of the significant advantages for use of standard terminology is that it facilitated quantifying the magnitude of sepsis. Sepsis and severe sepsis are much more common than previously realized, and they are important causes of serious morbidity and mortality in both children and adults.

The US Centers for Disease Control (CDC) lists septicemia ("a systemic disease associated with organisms or their toxins in the blood") as the seventh leading cause of death for children age 1–4 years, and eighth for children 5–9 years [46]. Other investigators have examined severe sepsis specifically, applying consensus definitions to large administrative datasets containing records of US hospitalizations. In 1995, over 42,000 children younger than 20 years old were hospitalized with severe sepsis in the US, and 4,400 of them died (for a hospital mortality of 10.3 %) [47]. Compared to other conditions in the CDC's leading causes of death, severe sepsis deaths exceeded all but three among infants and all but one among older children. Almost half of children with severe sepsis (48 %) were less than 1 year old. Severe sepsis was more common among boys than girls and more common in children with underlying illness. Analyses of data from 2005 found that the population-based incidence of pediatric severe sepsis in the US increased by 59 %, the total number of cases per year rose to more than 75,000, and the case-fatality rate fell to 8.9 % [48]. The three most common pathogens for children with severe sepsis in the US were staphylococcus (all types), streptococcus (all types), and fungus, though viral etiologies were not examined [47].

In a single-center study in Montreal, Proulx et al. examined the incidence of sepsis and related conditions in a university pediatric intensive care unit [49]. This group examined 1,058 admissions to their PICU between 1991 and 1992, and identified 245 cases of sepsis (23 % of all PICU admissions), 46 cases of severe sepsis (4 %), and 25 cases of septic shock (2 %). Mortality among the children with sepsis was 6 % [49]. In this and multiple other studies, mortality after sepsis is higher among children with underlying disease, especially among children with cancer and those who have undergone bone marrow transplantation [47, 50, 51].

In addition to being at risk of in-hospital morbidity and mortality, children with severe sepsis are at risk for hospital readmission and post-discharge mortality. A study of children hospitalized with severe sepsis in Washington State over 15 years showed that 47 % of children surviving the hospitalization were readmitted to the hospital, with a median time to readmission of 3 months. Post-discharge mortality was 6.5 %, with a median time to death of approximately 13 months [52].

Multiple organ dysfunction (MOD) is often associated with severe sepsis. Details about its pathophysiology are poorly understood, and its effects on mortality are still being studied. Kutko et al. studied 96 cases of septic shock in 80 patients at a large academic PICU over 2 years to determine the impact of MOD on mortality in septic shock [53]. Over 70 % of sepsis cases occurred in patients with cancer (19 % of whom had undergone a bone marrow transplant), and half occurred in patients with neutropenia. Indwelling catheters were present in over 58 % of cases. MOD was present in almost 73 % of cases at some point in time during the PICU course, and mortality for this group was 36 %. In Proulx's sepsis cohort, discussed above, 29 % developed MOD, with a mortality of 32 % [49]. A finding common among these studies was that there were few or no deaths among previously healthy children and no deaths among patients without MOD.

Epidemiology of Status Asthmaticus

As the most common chronic disease among children, asthma's epidemiology has been extensively studied, and increasing numbers of investigators have examined the epidemiology of status asthmaticus. Asthma affects 5–7 % of US children. Its prevalence increased from 1980 to 1996 and leveled off between 1997 and 2000. It is one of the most common reasons for pediatric hospitalization in the US [54], and hospitalization rates increased between 1980 and the mid-1990s [55, 56]. In 2000, there were 152,000 pediatric hospital admissions for asthma, which generated a total US hospital charges of $835 million (2 % of US healthcare charges for children) [57].

Although status asthmaticus is a common reason for ICU admission, only an average of 8 % of children hospitalized with asthma at pediatric centers require PICU care [58]. Between 1992 and 2006, the population-based rate of hospital admission for status asthmaticus decreased by 50 %, while the rate of ICU admission more than tripled, and the use of MV was unchanged [59]. The use of invasive MV varies substantially by center (from 3 to 47 % of PICU patients [5–9]), by region of the US (from 6 to 27 % of PICU patients at pediatric centers [58]), and by year (from 8 to 18 % of ICU patients between 1992 and 2001 in a single state [60]). This variation persists even when controlling for severity of illness [5], and children with Medicaid insurance have higher rates of intubation and longer lengths of stay than patients with commercial insurance, even when controlling for severity of illness [61].

Mortality rates in children with asthma are increasing [55, 56, 62, 63], but death is still uncommon after patients are admitted to the hospital. Two recent, large studies found 0.3–0.4 % hospital mortality among patients admitted to tertiary PICUs [5, 58], and 2.8 % mortality among intubated patients [5]. Mortality is highest in adolescents (twice that of younger children), and children of African American decent are more than four times as likely to die from asthma as white children [55]. Risk factors for asthma-related death include previous life-threatening attacks, severe disease, recent hospital admission or emergency room visit, poor adherence to medical regimens [64, 65], and prior history of asthma-induced respiratory failure requiring mechanical ventilation [66]. Some patients with near-fatal asthma (requiring mechanical ventilation or resulting in unconsciousness) have been found to have decreased sensitivity to hypoxia and blunted perception of dyspnea [67].

Conclusion

Improving definitions of the syndromes that characterize critical illness, the development of efficient information technology, and the creation of extensive databases that include PICU patients have enabled large-scale epidemiologic research to be conducted in critical care. As evident from the above discussion, however, this work is incomplete. We need better estimates of basic critical care syndromes and interventions. We also need to examine further reasons for variation in care, the relationship between risk factors of disease, hospital course, and post-discharge outcome, and how public health and medical interventions affect the incidence and outcome of critical illness in children.

Recent and impending developments in the healthcare of children will affect the epidemiology of pediatric critical illness. Populations of children known to be at high risk for critical illness (e.g., premature babies, technology-dependent or immunosuppressed children) continue to grow. New vaccines may decrease the rate of severe sepsis in previously healthy children. Genetic and immunologic analysis will identify children at high or low risk of severe illness and sequelae. They will enhance our therapeutic effectiveness by allowing us to provide specific treatments to children based on more robust information regarding the likelihood of responsiveness [68]. The success of pediatric critical care study networks will increase our knowledge about the efficacy and effectiveness of interventions for critical illness and will enhance our understanding of the natural history of critical illness. The thoughtful use of the tools of clinical epidemiology can facilitate these advances, help us refine their application, and let us understand their ramifications.

References

1. Rubenfeld GD, Caldwell E, Peabody E, et al. Incidence and outcomes of acute lung injury. N Engl J Med. 2005;353:1685–93.
2. Goss CH, Brower RG, Hudson LD, Rubenfeld GD. Incidence of acute lung injury in the United States. Crit Care Med. 2003;31:1607–11.
3. Rubenfeld GD, Caldwell E, Granton J, Hudson LD, Matthay MA. Interobserver variability in applying a radiographic definition for ARDS. Chest. 1999;116:1347–53.
4. Rangel-Frausto MS, Pittet D, Costigan M, Hwang T, Davis CS, Wenzel RP. The natural history of the systemic inflammatory response syndrome (SIRS). A prospective study. JAMA. 1995;273:117–23.
5. Roberts JS, Bratton SL, Brogan TV. Acute severe asthma: differences in therapies and outcomes among pediatric intensive care units. Crit Care Med. 2002;30:581–5.
6. Bungard TJ, Ghali WA, Teo KK, McAlister FA, Tsuyuki RT. Why do patients with atrial fibrillation not receive warfarin? Arch Intern Med. 2000;160:41–6.
7. Bungard TJ, McAlister FA, Johnson JA, Tsuyuki RT. Underutilisation of ACE inhibitors in patients with congestive heart failure. Drugs. 2001;61:2021–33.
8. Sim I, Cummings SR. A new framework for describing and quantifying the gap between proof and practice. Med Care. 2003;41:874–81.
9. Bickell NA, McEvoy MD. Physicians' reasons for failing to deliver effective breast cancer care: a framework for underuse. Med Care. 2003;41:442–6.
10. Randolph AG, Gonzales CA, Cortellini L, Yeh TS. Growth of pediatric intensive care units in the United States from 1995 to 2001. J Pediatr. 2004;144:792–8.
11. Hartman ME, Watson RS, Millbrandt EB, Angus DC, Linde-Zwirble WT. The size and scope of pediatric critical care in the US. Critical Care Medicine 2008; 36(12S):A79.
12. Naclerio AL, Gardner JW, Pollack MM. Socioeconomic factors and emergency pediatric ICU admissions. Ann N Y Acad Sci. 1999;896:379–82.
13. Parslow RC, Tasker RC, Draper ES, et al. Epidemiology of critically ill children in England and Wales: incidence, mortality, deprivation and ethnicity. Arch Dis Child. 2009;94:210–5.
14. Angus DC, Barnato AE, Linde-Zwirble WT, et al. Use of intensive care at the end of life in the United States: an epidemiologic study. Crit Care Med. 2004;32:638–43.
15. Odetola FO, Clark SJ, Freed GL, Bratton SL, Davis MM. A national survey of pediatric critical care resources in the United States. Pediatrics. 2005;115:e382–6.
16. Odetola FO, Miller WC, Davis MM, Bratton SL. The relationship between the location of pediatric intensive care unit facilities and child death from trauma: a county-level ecologic study. J Pediatr. 2005;147:74–7.
17. Pollack MM, Cuerdon TC, Getson PR. Pediatric intensive care units: results of a national survey. Crit Care Med. 1993;21:607–14.
18. Tilford JM, Simpson PM, Green JW, Lensing S, Fiser DH. Volume-outcome relationships in pediatric intensive care units. Pediatrics. 2000;106:289–94.

19. Birkmeyer JD, Siewers AE, Finlayson EVA, et al. Hospital volume and surgical mortality in the United States. N Engl J Med. 2002;346:1128–37.

20. Dudley RA, Johansen KL, Brand R, Rennie DJ, Milstein A. Selective referral to high-volume hospitals: estimating potentially avoidable deaths. JAMA. 2000;283:1159–66.

21. Kahn JM, Goss CH, Heagerty PJ, Kramer AA, O'Brien CR, Rubenfeld GD. Hospital volume and the outcomes of mechanical ventilation. N Engl J Med. 2006;355:41–50.

22. Kahn JM, Linde-Zwirble WT, Wunsch H, et al. Potential value of regionalized intensive care for mechanically ventilated medical patients. Am J Respir Crit Care Med. 2008;177:285–91.

23. McLeod L, French B, Dai D, Localio R, Keren R. Patient volume and quality of care for young children hospitalized with acute gastroenteritis. Arch Pediatr Adolesc Med. 2011;165:857–63.

24. Newacheck PW, Taylor WR. Childhood chronic illness: prevalence, severity, and impact. Am J Public Health. 1992;82:364–71.

25. Reiss J, Gibson R. Health care transition: destinations unknown. Pediatrics. 2002;110:1307–14.

26. Feudtner C, Hays RM, Haynes G, Geyer JR, Neff JM, Koepsell TD. Deaths attributed to pediatric complex chronic conditions: national trends and implications for supportive care services. Pediatrics. 2001;107:E99.

27. Hack M. Consideration of the use of health status, functional outcome, and quality-of-life to monitor neonatal intensive care practice. Pediatrics. 1999;103:319–28.

28. Noble L. Developments in neonatal technology continue to improve infant outcomes. Pediatr Ann. 2003;32:595–603.

29. Dosa NP, Boeing NM, Ms N, Kanter RK. Excess risk of severe acute illness in children with chronic health conditions. Pediatrics. 2001;107:499–504.

30. Graham RJ, Dumas HM, O'Brien JE, Burns JP. Congenital neurodevelopmental diagnoses and an intensive care unit: defining a population. Pediatr Crit Care Med. 2004;5:321–8.

31. Slonim AD, Patel KM, Ruttimann UE, Pollack MM. The impact of prematurity: a perspective of pediatric intensive care units. Crit Care Med. 2000;28:848–53.

32. Angus DC, Linde-Zwirble WT, Griffin M, Clermont G, Clark RH. Epidemiology of neonatal respiratory failure in the US: projections from California and New York. Am J Respir Crit Care Med. 2001; 164:1154–60.

33. Watson RS, Linde-Zwirble WT, Hartman ME, Clermont G, Angus DC. Epidemiology of mechanical ventilation in non-infant US children. Crit Care Med. 2002;30(Suppl):A131.

34. Bernard GR, Artigas A, Brigham KL, et al. The American-European Consensus Conference on ARDS. Definitions, mechanisms, relevant outcomes, and clinical trial coordination. Am J Respir Crit Care Med. 1994;149:818–24.

35. Erickson S, Schibler A, Numa A, et al. Acute lung injury in pediatric intensive care in Australia and New Zealand: a prospective, multicenter, observational study. Pediatr Crit Care Med. 2007;8:317–23.

36. Bindl L, Dresbach K, Lentze MJ. Incidence of acute respiratory distress syndrome in German children and adolescents: a population-based study. Crit Care Med. 2005;33:209–12.

37. Zimmerman JJ, Akhtar SR, Caldwell E, Rubenfeld GD. Incidence and outcomes of pediatric acute lung injury. Pediatrics. 2009;124:87–95.

38. Definitions for sepsis and organ failure and guidelines for the use of innovative therapies in sepsis. American College of Chest Physicians/Society of Critical Care Medicine Consensus Conference. Crit Care Med. 1992;20:864–74.

39. Annane D, Sebille V, Charpentier C, et al. Effect of treatment with low doses of hydrocortisone and fludrocortisone on mortality in patients with septic shock. JAMA. 2002;288:862–71.

40. Rivers E, Nguyen B, Havstad S, et al. Early goal-directed therapy in the treatment of severe sepsis and septic shock. N Engl J Med. 2001;345:1368–77.

41. Briegel J, Forst H, Haller M, et al. Stress doses of hydrocortisone reverse hyperdynamic septic shock: a prospective, randomized, double-blind, single-center study. Crit Care Med. 1999;27:723–32.

42. Reinhart K, Meier-Hellmann A, Beale R, et al. Open randomized phase II trial of an extracorporeal endotoxin adsorber in suspected Gram-negative sepsis. Crit Care Med. 2004;32:1662–8.

43. Molnar Z, Mikor A, Leiner T, Szakmany T. Fluid resuscitation with colloids of different molecular weight in septic shock. Intensive Care Med. 2004;30:1356–60.

44. Bertolini G, Iapichino G, Radrizzani D, et al. Early enteral immunonutrition in patients with severe sepsis: results of an interim analysis of a randomized multicentre clinical trial. Intensive Care Med. 2003;29:834–40.

45. Busund R, Koukline V, Utrobin U, Nedashkovsky E. Plasmapheresis in severe sepsis and septic shock: a prospective, randomised, controlled trial. Intensive Care Med. 2002;28:1434–9.

46. Center for Disease Control. National Vital Statistics Report. 2002;50(16):1–36.

47. Watson RS, Carcillo JA, Linde-Zwirble WT, Clermont G, Lidicker J, Angus DC. The epidemiology of severe sepsis in children in the United States. Am J Respir Crit Care Med. 2003;167:695–701.

48. Hartman ME, Linde-Zwirble WT, Angus DC, Watson RS. Trends in the epidemiology of pediatric severe sepsis. Pediatric Critical Care Medicine. 2013;14(7):686–93.

49. Proulx F, Fayon M, Farrell CA, Lacroix J, Gauthier M. Epidemiology of sepsis and multiple organ dysfunction syndrome in children. Chest. 1996;109:1033–7.

50. Fiser RT, West NK, Bush AJ, Sillos EM, Schmidt JE, Tamburro RF. Outcome of severe sepsis in pediatric oncology patients. Pediatr Crit Care Med. 2005;6:531–6.

51. Proulx F, Joyal JS, Mariscalco MM, Leteurtre S, Leclerc F, Lacroix J. The pediatric multiple organ dysfunction syndrome. Pediatr Crit Care Med. 2009;10:12–22.

52. Czaja AS, Zimmerman JJ, Nathens AB. Readmission and late mortality after pediatric severe sepsis. Pediatrics. 2009;123:849–57.

53. Kutko MC, Calarco MP, Flaherty MB, et al. Mortality rates in pediatric septic shock with and without multiple organ system failure. Pediatr Crit Care Med. 2003;4:333–7.

54. McCormick MC, Kass B, Elixhauser A, Thompson J, Simpson L. Annual report on access to and utilization of health care for children and youth in the United States–1999. Pediatrics. 2000;105: 219–30.

55. Akinbami LJ, Schoendorf KC. Trends in childhood asthma: prevalence, health care utilization, and mortality. Pediatrics. 2002; 110:315–22.

56. Fulwood R, Parker S, Hurd SS. Asthma–United States, 1980–1987. MMWR Morb Mortal Wkly Rep. 1990;39:493–7.

57. Owens PL, Thompson J, Elixhauser A, Ryan K. Care of children and adolescents in U.S. Hospitals. Rockville: AHRQ; 2003. Report No. AHRQ Publication No. 04-0004.

58. Bratton SL, Odetola FO, McCollegan J, Cabana MD, Levy FH, Keenan HT. Regional variation in ICU care for pediatric patients with asthma. J Pediatr. 2005;147:355–61.

59. Hartman ME, Linde-Zwirble WT, Angus DC, Watson RS. Trends in admissions for pediatric status asthmaticus in New Jersey over a 15-year period. Pediatrics. 2010;126:e904–11.

60. Hartman ME, Linde-Zwirble WT, Watson RS, Angus DC. Changes in incidence, management, and care of pediatric status asthmaticus over the last decade. Crit Care Med. 2005;33(Suppl):A4.

61. Bratton SL, Roberts JS, Watson RS, Cabana M. Intensive care of pediatric asthma: differences in outcome and medicaid insurance. Pediatr Crit Care Med. 2002;3:234–8.

62. Centers for Disease Control and Prevention. Asthma mortality and hospitalization among children and young adults, United States, 1980–1993. MMWR CDC Surveill Summ. 1996;45:350–3.

63. Serafini U. Can fatal asthma be prevented? – a personal view. Clin Exp Allergy. 1992;22:576–88.

64. Greenberger PA, Patterson R. The diagnosis of potentially fatal asthma. N Engl Reg Allergy Proc. 1988;9:147–52.

65. Lowenthal M, Patterson R, Greenberger PA, Grammer LC. The application of an asthma severity index in patients with potentially fatal asthma. Chest. 1993;104:1329–31.

66. Rea HH, Scragg R, Jackson R, Beaglehole R, Fenwick J, Sutherland DC. A case-control study of deaths from asthma. Thorax. 1986;41: 833–9.

67. Kikuchi Y, Okabe S, Tamura G, et al. Chemosensitivity and perception of dyspnea in patients with a history of near-fatal asthma. N Engl J Med. 1994;330:1329–34.

68. Israel E, Chinchilli VM, Ford JG, et al. Use of regularly scheduled albuterol treatment in asthma: genotype-stratified, randomised, placebo-controlled cross-over trial. Lancet. 2004;364:1505–12.

Ethics in the Pediatric Intensive Care Unit: Controversies and Considerations

14

Rani Ganesan and K. Sarah Hoehn

Abstract

Pediatric intensivists face ethical challenges every day. In this chapter, we will highlight areas that are integral to the practice of pediatric critical care medicine, from informed consent to the provision of palliative care. We will describe situations where pediatric patients can make their independent decisions, as well as situations where parents are not the optimal decision maker. The doctrine of double effect will be described, along with other key elements to withdrawing and withholding technological support. We will review policy guidelines and consensus statements, and include resources for resolving difficult cases. Finally, we will address challenges for the caregiver, as not all difficult cases may be resolved. The goal is that this chapter will provide information to facilitate the practice of pediatric critical care medicine in challenging times.

Keywords

Ethics • Withdrawing life support • Withholding life support • Informed consent • Decision making • Palliative care

Introduction

Care to critically ill pediatric patients requires a unique balance of modern technology, conscientious care providers, and the involvement of patients and their families. Fortunately, the majority of children treated in the PICU recover to an acceptable level of independent function and overall health [1–3]. Occasionally, when caring for children with complex medical issues and unclear prognoses, clinicians may be challenged with moral distress, ethical dilemmas and doubt [4]. These feelings may stem from concerns about resource utilization, patient suffering, and undue burden for outcomes that

may be considered unacceptable [4]. Redirection of care away from curative treatments to symptomatic relief and palliative care can be difficult for families, patients and some health care providers [4]. Such decisions may be difficult because pediatric practice uses the 'best interest' standard, and some families and care provider cannot accept that palliative care is ever in a child's best interest.

As children get older, more weight is given to their ideas about their medical care. This may blur the lines of parental permission, informed consent and assent. These ambiguous pediatric care areas may lead to conflict amongst clinicians within the care team or between caregivers and the patient and/or family. At such times, careful ethical analysis combined with an understanding of state and Federal laws, respectful listening, and collegial communication is essential to resolve the issues.

This chapter will begin with a discussion of consent, age and development – appropriate autonomous decision-making, and the provision care guided by patient 'best interest'. We will further discuss the delivery of palliative care to pediatric patients, including medication use at the end of life. Using

R. Ganesan, MD
Department of Pediatrics, Rush University Medical Center,
1653 W Congress Pkwy Murdock 622, Chicago, IL 60612, USA
e-mail: sarah1220@comcast.net

K.S. Hoehn, MD, MBe (✉)
University of Kansas Medical Center,
3901 Rainbow Blvd, Kansas City, KS 66160, USA
e-mail: shoehn@kumc.edu

D.S. Wheeler et al. (eds.), *Pediatric Critical Care Medicine*,
DOI 10.1007/978-1-4471-6362-6_14, © Springer-Verlag London 2014

accepted definitions of cardiac and brain death, we will address challenges surrounding organ donation. These topics will be described in the broader context of policies and recommendations by the American Academy of Pediatrics (AAP). The chapter will conclude with a discussion and recognition of the impact of caring for critically ill children on caregivers.

Informed Consent/Parental Permission

> …parents are free to become martyrs themselves. However, it does not follow that they are free, in identical circumstances, to make martyrs of their children before they have reached the age of full and legal discretion when they can make that choice for themselves. –United States Supreme Court Prince v. Massachusetts 321 U.S. 158 (1944)

It was only in the twentieth century that children were legally recognized as subjects and not as objects or property [5]. The first statement describing consent in the pediatric population was released in 1976 [6]. The process of informed consent is a procedure to ensure patients understand all anticipated treatment or procedure risks and benefits. Only patients with appropriate decision-making capacity and legal empowerment can give informed consent. Therefore, informed consent has limited direct application in pediatrics. Although minor patients are not legally empowered to give informed consent, their willingness, or assent, to participate in research trials or certain treatments, should be considered [5–8]. For the majority of pediatric patients, permission to treat is obtained from the parent with the child's assent whenever appropriate.

Informed Consent

In order to obtain true informed consent, the necessary elements required for appropriate decision-making must be understood [6]. To ensure that decisions are being made in his/her own best interest, the patient must be capable of giving consent. The patient's diagnosis must be explained in simple terms that are easy to comprehend. Along with describing the risk and benefits of the offered treatments, alternatives and their respective risk and benefits must also be discussed (Table 14.1). The consequences of foregoing recommended therapies and interventions should be thoroughly explained, and the patient must demonstrate an understanding of the possible outcomes. If a language barrier exists, consent should be obtained through a trained medical interpreter. Informed consent can only be obtained when a capable patient demonstrates an understanding of his diagnosis and all treatments options with respective risks and benefits.

As described before, direct application of informed consent is limited in pediatric patients. Various state statutes

Table 14.1 Informed consent

Provision of information
Explanations, in understandable language, of the nature of the ailment or condition, the nature of proposed diagnostic steps and/ or treatment and the probability of their success, the existence and nature of the risks involved, and the existence, potential benefits and risks of recommended alternative treatment (including the choice of no treatment)
Assessment of the patient's understanding of the above information
Assessment, if only tacit, of the capacity of the patient or surrogate to make the necessary decision
Assurance, insofar as is possible, that the patient has the freedom to choose among the medical alternatives without coercion or manipulation
AAP policy statement, *Informed consent, parental permission, and assent in pediatric practice*

allow minor patients to seek care and provide informed consent for family planning, to treat sexually transmitted diseases, receive mental healthcare or substance-abuse rehabilitation [6, 7]. Although these statutes allow for informed consent by a minor, it does not guarantee privacy. The Family Planning Act [9] is the only federal law that requires confidentiality for minor patients. All providers should be knowledgeable of their respective state and Federal laws for informed consent and confidentiality related to care of minor patients [7].

Frequently, we face unique challenges when obtaining informed consent for patients in the PICU due to life-threatening circumstances and social circumstances that may surround necessary treatments and procedures. According to the AAP 2011 policy on consent for pediatric emergency medical services, "medical screening examination and any medical care necessary and likely to prevent imminent and significant harm to a pediatric patient with an emergency medical condition should not be withheld or delayed because of problems obtaining consent" [10].

Parental Permission

For most pediatric care, parental permission is obtained instead of informed consent [10]. Parents know their child well and their affection will lead them to make decisions in the child's best interest [6, 10]. However in some child abuse cases, the parent's ability to make decisions in the child's best interest comes into question [11]. Forgoing life-sustaining medical treatments may pose a conflict of interest with fear that the legal charges could change from assault to manslaughter or murder [11]. In these cases, the AAP and legal counsel advocate that a guardian ad litem be appointed by the court [11].

The unaccompanied minor is another circumstance where treatment of a minor may not require parental permission. According to current federal law under the Emergency

Medical Treatment and Active Labor Act (EMTALA), a medical screening examination is mandated for every patient seeking treatment in an Emergency Department of any hospital that participates in programs that receive federal funding, independent of consent or reimbursement status [12]. This law protects providers and unaccompanied minors when evaluating for and treating life and limb threatening conditions [12].

Assent

Our legal obligation to treat a pediatric patient according to the wishes of his legal guardian must not overshadow our ethical responsibility to respect the child's willingness, or assent, to participate in his/her care. Weithorn et al. demonstrated that patients as young as 9 years old can weigh important pieces of information when presented with medical scenarios [13]. Limited data suggests that adolescents, especially 14 years and older, may have the ability to make informed health care decisions similar to adults [13].

Emancipated Minor and Mature Minor Exceptions

The emancipated minor and mature minor are additional circumstances that legally preclude the requirement for parental permission in order to treat. The mature minor is a principle that deems the minor patient as mature and capable of making medical and welfare decisions in their own best interest. It is decided on a case by case basis, and states vary as to whether such status can be granted by a physician, or reserved for judge's to assign. The mature minor must demonstrate sufficient maturity and understand the risks and benefits of the decision he/she is making [6].

Emancipated minors have full legal authority to make their own medical decisions. The legal system recognizes independent living, marriage, pregnancy or parenthood, and military duty as causes for emancipation [6]. These also vary by state, so it is crucial to know one's local laws. In summary, children should participate in age and developmentally appropriate discussion and medical-decision making when feasible [5–8].

Communication in the Pediatric Intensive Care Unit

Communication is the skill or art of conveying meaningful information through words, visual cues, and body language. Whether discussing a new cancer diagnosis or the need to repeat a chest radiograph, patients' and parents' stress related to a hospitalization and the disease can be under-estimated [7]. Parents in a PICU have reported that they want communication that is *Honest, Inclusive, Compassionate, Clear and Comprehensive, and Coordinated* [14]. This can be remembered using the acronym HICCC [14]. In an effort to enable and foster family-centered care and patient involvement, parents and children are encouraged to participate in-patient rounds and discussions. Routine multidisciplinary conferences provide the opportunity to re-evaluate long-term goals of care [15–17].

Provision of End of Life Care in the Pediatric Intensive Care Unit

In the PICU, children can receive life saving interventions from intubation and ventilation, dialysis and even extracorporeal membrane oxygenation. The transition from heroic measures to setting limits on interventions can be difficult to navigate. Despite limitations of technological support, families should be assured that symptom management will be aggressively provided to keep their child comfortable. Often times, resuscitation status is addressed first to set the initial stage for any limitations of care.

Do-not-attempt-resuscitation (DNAR) is legally defined as withholding cardiopulmonary resuscitation (which may include intubation, defibrillation, and chest compressions) in the event of an acute cardiopulmonary arrest. DNAR does not address limitations of the treatments that may prevent an acute arrest (i.e., antibiotics, corticosteroids, pain medications, blood products, etc) [18]. Families and patients may think that DNAR is synonymous with do not treat or withdrawal of support. Sanders et al. described the term partial do-not-attempt-resuscitation order and how it may represent a fundamental misunderstanding of the patient's prognosis and/or is erroneously used interchangeably with advanced directives or other care limitations [19]. A recent study reported that supplemental steroids and pain medications were interventions most commonly added after DNAR orders are implemented suggesting that patient comfort was not prioritized until after limits were set [18]. Advance directives are a legal document where an individual specifies medical treatments to be provided or withheld, if he/she becomes unable to express decisions for himself. All patients with legal decision making capacity should be asked about advance directives to comply with federal regulations.

Use of Medication at the End of Life

After a decision has been made to withdraw technological support, the next hurdle is planning how to manage symptoms after removal of support therapies. Medication use at the end of life is an integral part of pediatric critical care medicine. Patients in the intensive care unit often develop tachyphylaxis to sedatives and analgesics, therefore dosages may need to be adjusted prior to the withdrawal of life sustaining therapy [20]. For patients that have received narcotics and sedatives as infusions, a reasonable starting dose is bolus administration of the patient's hourly doses which may be titrated to treat discomfort during end of life care [20]. It is crucial to understand the goals of treatment, which are to mitigate pain and suffering.

The moral doctrine of double effect guides our end of life care [21]. The doctrine of double effect maintains that an action is permissible even if it results in a bad outcome, provided that (a) the bad outcome, although a known risk, was not the intended consequence, (b) the action intended was a good outcome (i.e. comfort), (c) the bad outcome was not the means to the good outcome, and (d) the action was justified by the proportionality of risks and benefits [21]. Therefore an appropriate dose of medication to treat air hunger is acceptable, even if it may cause respiratory depression [22]. Medication should be titrated to effect with rational doses.

Given the doctrine of double effect, use of neuromuscular blocking agents (NMBA) cannot be justified as the intent is to prevent movement and ability to breath [23]. If a patient has received NMBAs, it is ideal to document return of neuromuscular function (either clinical movement or train of four). There are rare clinical situations where neuromuscular blockade is markedly prolonged due to impaired drub metabolism secondary to multi-organ system failure and prolonged infusion of NMBAs such that it may be unrealistic to wait for return of motor function [23]. In these situations, one must insure adequate administration of analgesics and sedatives. In general, routine train of four monitoring with titration of NMBA to 1–2 twitches or daily "drug holidays" where the NMBA infusion is stopped till the patient initiates a respiratory effort prevent profound overdose and prevent this situation [23].

Withholding Artificially Provided Fluids and Nutrition

Withholding and withdrawing artificially provided fluids and nutrition continue to be controversial and potentially difficult for both caregivers and families. Families may be concerned their loved ones experience hunger or thirst. Withholding or withdrawing non-oral nutritional and hydration support does not prevent patients from being safely fed when signs and symptoms related to thirst and/or hunger are present. The AAP "concludes that the withdrawal of medically administered fluids and nutrition for pediatric patients is ethically acceptable in limited circumstances" [24].

Unilateral Decision Making and Futility

Often times, difficult decisions at the end of life create concern and moral distress among caregivers, especially if the health care providers disagree with the family medical decisions. Sometimes in these cases, pediatric critical care practitioners will seek a unilateral DNAR order or attempt to withdraw support under a futility policy. Unilateral DNAR orders are not universally accepted in pediatrics, and pediatric futility policies have had mixed results [25, 26]. Consultation with medical administration, palliative care and the ethics service are strongly recommended.

A recent survey of pediatric intensivists reported that physicians did not support the concept of unilateral decision making [27]. For a hypothetical case of an infant with severe hypoxic ischemic encephalopathy and intestinal failure, the majority of physicians (83.7 %) would not enact a unilateral DNAR. In the case where a child met neurological criteria for death, 54.3 % of surveyed physicians said they would support unilateral DNAR in the event of a cardiac arrest, yet a third (33.1 %) would continue mechanical ventilation [27]. In most scenarios, intensivists cited consultation from the ethics committee (53.8–76.6 %) as the most appropriate way to resolve the conflict [27]. Qualitative data revealed intensivists prefer to honor a families' wishes and work to achieve consensus with support from a multidisciplinary team rather than unilateral DNAR to address these conflicts. Therefore, the authors recommended supporting families struggling with difficult decisions and supporting health care providers when they disagree with decisions that are made.

Conflict Resolution

When these difficult cases arise, pediatric critical care practitioners can utilize institutional ethics committees [28]. In cases of ongoing and persistent conflict between the health care team and family, care should be taken to be respectful of the parents' wishes and to support the medical team dealing with the challenging issues.

Pursuit or refusal of medical treatments can result in conflict between medical caregivers and families of critically ill children. Ultimately, medical decisions are made by the child's legal guardian with advice from healthcare providers [6]. If the medical team thinks that the parents or legal guardian are making decisions that are not in the best interest of the child and are likely to harm the patient, then consultation with the ethics committee is recommended. This provides a forum for all parties to discuss the issues, improve communication and hopefully achieve consensus [28].

Parents may deny their children potentially lifesaving therapies or continue unnecessarily burdensome treatments

Table 14.2 Key policy statements from the American Academy of Pediatrics

Committee on Bioethics, *Guidelines on Foregoing Life-sustaining Medical Treatment*. Pediatrics, 1994. 93(3): 532–536
Shaddy RE, Denne SC, and the Committee on Drugs and the Committee on Pediatric Research. *Guidelines for the ethical conduct of studies to evaluate drugs in pediatric populations*. Pediatrics, 2010. 125(4): 850–860
Committee on Bioethics, *Informed consent, parental permission, and assent in pediatric practice*. Pediatrics, 1995. 95(2): 314–317
Committee on Bioethics, *Ethics and the Care of Critically Ill Infants and Children*. Pediatrics, 1996. 98(1): 149–152
Committee on Bioethics, *Religious Objections to Medical Care*. Pediatrics, 1997. 99(2): 279–281
Nakagawa TA, Ashwa S, Mathur M, Mysore M. *Clinical report-guidelines for the determination of brain death in infants and children: an update of the 1987 task force recommendations*. Pediatrics, 2011. 128: e720–740
Committee on Bioethics and Committee on Hospital Care, *Palliative Care for Children*. Pediatrics, 2000. 106(2): 351–357
Committee on Pediatric Emergency Medicine and Committee on Bioethics, *Consent for Emergency Medical Services for Children and Adolescents*. Pediatrics, 2011. 128: 427
Committee on Child Abuse and Neglect and Committee on Bioethics, *Forgoing Life-Sustaining Medical Treatment in Abused Children*. Pediatrics, 2000. 106(5): 1151–1153
Committee on Bioethics, *Institutional Ethics Committees*. Pediatrics, 2001. 107(1): 205–209
Committee on Hospital Care and Section on Surgery, *Pediatric Organ Donation and Transplantation*. Pediatrics, 2002. 109(5): 982–984
Committee on Pediatric Emergency Medicine, *Consent for Emergency Medical Services for Children and Adolescents*. Pediatrics, 2003. 111(3): 703–706

because of religious or spiritual beliefs. In some cases, Federal and state legislative activity have exempted parents from claims of child abuse and neglect based on religious belief. "The AAP opposes such exemptions as harmful to children and advocates that children, regardless of parental religious beliefs, deserve effective medical treatments when such treatment is likely to prevent substantial harm or suffering or death" [29]. The Academy encourages practitioners to demonstrate sensitivity to religious beliefs; support legislation that holds parents who endanger their children by withholding medical care accountable and responsible; support the repeal of religious exemption laws; and advocate for religious and child advocacy organizations to collaboratively develop structured education programs that educate the public about parents' legal responsibility to obtain necessary medical care for their children [29]. Whenever possible, practitioners and parents should make decisions in the best interest of children while minimizing burden. Table 14.2 includes a list of AAP policy statements and consensus guidelines that may be useful to the pediatric critical care practitioner struggling with conflicts. In order to preserve the integrity and trust of the

parent-provider relationship, threatening or seeking state legal intervention should be the last resort in conflict resolution.

Declaring Death and Organ Donation

Declaration of Death

According to the Uniform Determination of Death Act, an individual is considered legally dead if they have irreversible cessation of circulatory and respiratory functions, or irreversible cessation of function of the entire brain including brain stem. Widjicks' review described criteria used to establish brain death, which is now widely accepted [30]. Timely diagnosis of death avoids prolonged and unnecessary life support, allows families to grieve, and may increase consent for organ donation with improved success in procurement and donation of organs [31].

The AAP recently endorsed updated brain death guidelines [32]. Notable changes compared to earlier (1987 report in Pediatrics) guidelines supported by the AAP included the recommended observation period. Twelve hours was recommended for all pediatric patients over 30 days of age. The new guidelines require the absence of confounding factors (i.e., use of high dose sedatives, NMBA, hypothermia, hemodynamic instability, profound metabolic derangement), two clinical examination showing no neurological function, and two apnea tests that document no respiratory effort. The new guidelines did not recommend ancillary confirmatory studies unless the clinical examination or apnea test could not be fully performed (due to medication or patient instability) [32]. In addition, these guidelines recommend the clinical examinations be performed by two different attending physicians, and that a 24 h waiting period be utilized prior to starting the process of declaration of brain death after cardiopulmonary resuscitation or other hypoxemic injury [32].

Organ Donation

Prior to and during the 1960s, organs were retrieved after irreversible cessation of circulatory and respiratory functions, or cardiac death, was declared. In 1968, a definition of death based on neurologic criteria was issued [33]. From that point, organs were used primarily after death caused by irreversible cessation of brain function because of superior graft function compared to organ procured after cardiac death. However, the increasing gap between candidates for transplantation and potential dead organ donors with increasing deaths on the waiting list revived interest in donation after circulatory death, also known as DCD. The United Network for Organ Sharing and the Organ Procurement and Transplant

Network finalized and issued rules for donation after cardiac death in 2007. The process begins when a potential donor is identified after the decision has been made to withdraw life sustaining therapies and death is expected to occur rapidly, usually in an hour or less.

The Centers for Medicare and Medicaid mandate that all cases of imminent death be reported to the local Organ Procurement Organization (OPO). Early communication with the critical care team allows time to assess if the child is eligible to donate and enables the OPO to be readily available after the family and critical care team have agreement that withdrawal of care is in the patient's best interest. As the AAP statement outlines: the OPO should approach discussions with parents of the potential donor regarding organ donation [34]. This is important to both avoid perceptions of conflict of interest and trained requestors have been proven to be more effective in obtaining consent for donation than physicians [33]. After the family makes the decision withdraw life-sustaining medical treatments and consents to donate organs, life-sustaining therapies are withdrawn under controlled conditions. This may happen in the PICU, in the operating room, or in the perioperative area.

Despite the location, the pediatric critical care medicine provider continues to be responsible for the patient, including titration of medications and declaration of death. One study reported an average of 4 mcg/kg fentanyl and 0.1 mg/kg lorazepam titrated by the pediatric intensivist [35]. It is imperative that the physician who is responsible for withdrawal of technological support and declaration of death is not directly involved with the procurement process. After cardiorespiratory function ceases, there is a mandatory waiting period before organ recovery begins. This waiting period varies from 75 s to 10 min [35, 36]. The recommended period from the Institute of Medicine is 5 min, but times as short as 75 s have been used to cardiac donation after cardiac death. The Society for Critical Care Medicine recommendation is for a 2 min waiting period after cessation of circulatory function. If the patient does not die within 60–90 min after withdrawal of support, their organs are no longer routinely acceptable for donation. The family should be aware of that possibility, and further care will be directed by the pediatric intensive care team.

Ethical Issues Related to Donation After Cardiac Death

Although organ donation after cardiac death was the primary criteria used to declare death prior to donation before 1968, the practice poses interesting ethical concerns today, including cause of death, definition of cardiac death, and support of the family throughout the process. Patients are protected under the "dead donor rule" which states that organ donation

should not hasten death. To avoid claims of coercion or conflict of interest, conversations regarding potential organ donation should not be initiated until the family has decided to withdraw life-sustaining therapies, or the family has independently approached the team about possible organ donation.

Research in the Pediatric Intensive Care Unit

Currently, many therapeutic interventions used for pediatric patients have been extrapolated from adult research and practice. With the Pediatric Research Equity Act and the US FDA Modernization Act there is more motivation for pharmaceutical companies to conduct drug research studies in children [37]. The AAP supports this, "The AAP believes it is unethical to deny children appropriate access to existing and new therapeutic agents. It is the combined responsibility of the pediatric community, pharmaceutical industry and regulatory agencies to design, approve and conduct high quality studies in children" [37].

According to the US Code of Federal Regulation, research involving children should: (1) involve no greater than minimal risk (2) greater than minimal risk but presenting the prospect of direct benefit to clinical subjects or (3) involving no greater than minimal risk and no prospect of direct benefit to individual subjects but likely to yield generalizable knowledge about the subjects' disorder or condition [38]. There is a fourth condition, which is for research that is not otherwise approvable but presents opportunities to understand, prevent or alleviated a serious problem that affects the health or welfare of children. This category must be approved by the FDA and/or US Department of Health and Human Services [38]. With research integrity and safety as top priorities, the pediatric population will remain protected as we conduct research to improve provision of care.

Caring for the Caregiver

> When health is absent; Wisdom cannot reveal itself; Art cannot manifest; Strength cannot fight; Wealth becomes useless, and intelligence cannot be applied –Herophilus, Greek physician and pioneer of human anatomy

Choosing a career that involves caring for critically ill children is as taxing as it is noble. Despite the known incidence of psychiatric ailments, burnout and substance abuse in healthcare providers, the medical community continues to be slow in providing structured programs geared to alleviate the impact of these job-related injuries. People of certain personality types may be drawn to a career in medicine. Gabbard et al. described the compulsive triad (doubt, feelings of guilt, and an over exaggerated sense of responsibility) as central personality characteristics of many normal physicians [39]. Indicators of burnout are present as early as medical school. Dyrbye et al. described higher overall psychological distress among US and Canadian medical students relative to both the general population and age-matched peers [40]. Woluschuk et al. claimed that some students experience a deterioration of optimism and empathy and development of cynicism [41]. Good psychological health has been related to improved performance in healthcare. Hojat et al. showed that psychosocial characteristics and health predicted clinical competency better than admission test scores [42]. Dyrbye et al. demonstrated that stability in mental and physical health equipped physicians with the emotional and physical demands to care for patients [40].

While staying on par with the ACGME's attempts to improve housestaff quality of life and patient care with restriction of work hours, provision and access to other support systems are equally important. Honest discussions, bereavement debriefing sessions and use of readily available crisis counselors should be advocated as healthy coping strategies [43]. Meaningful lifestyle choices should be modeled by senior mentors to younger physicians. In addition to individual successes, teamwork and collegiality should be encouraged as paths to medical achievements.

As we care for children in the PICU, we often face decisions and dilemmas that challenge our job performance, work-life balance, and moral compass. We should utilize resources available to us, including national policies, colleagues and institutional ethics committees if needed. Ultimately, the way we navigate through these difficulties defines us as clinicians and as people.

References

1. Morrison W. Mortality, morbidity and pediatric critical care. Pediatr Crit Care Med. 2010;11(5):630–1.
2. Morrison AL, Gillis J, O'Connell A, Schell D, Dossetor D, Mellis C. Quality of life of survivors of pediatric intensive care. Pediatr Crit Care Med. 2002;3(1):1–5.
3. Taylor A, Butt W, Ciardulli M. The functional outcome and quality of life of children after admission to an intensive care unit. Intensive Care Med. 2003;29:795–800.
4. Knapp C, Thompson L. Factors associated with perceived barriers to pediatric palliative care: a survey of pediatricians in Florida and California. Palliat Med. 2012;26(3):268–74.
5. Streuli J, Michel M, Vayena E. Child's rights in pediatrics. Eur J Pediatr. 2011;170:9–14.
6. Committee on Bioethics. Informed consent, parental permission, and assent in pediatric practice. Pediatrics. 1995;95(2):314–7.
7. Levetown M, Committee of Bioethics. Technical report – communicating with children and families: from everyday interactions to sill in conveying distressing information. Pediatrics. 2008;121(5):e1441–60.
8. Committee on Bioethics and Committee on Hospital Care. Palliative care for children. Pediatrics. 2000;106(2):351–7.
9. Family Planning Act. US Department of Health & Human Services. http://www.hhs.gov/opa/familyplanning/index.html. Accessed 20 Apr 2012.
10. Committee on Pediatric Emergency Medicine and Committee on Bioethics. Policy statement – consent for emergency medical services for children and adolescents. Pediatrics. 2011;128(2):427–33.
11. Committee on Child Abuse and Neglect and Committee on Bioethics. Forgoing life-sustaining medical treatment in abused children. Pediatrics. 2000;106:1151–3.
12. Emergency Medical Treatment and Active Labor Act (EMTALA). Centers for Medicare & Medicaid Services. https://www.cms.gov/emtala. Accessed 20 Apr 2012.
13. Weithorn LA, Campbell SB. The competency of children and adolescents to make informed decisions. Child Dev. 1982;53(6): 1589–98.
14. DeLemos D, Chen M, Romer A, Brydon K, Kastner K, Anthony B, Hoehn KS. Building trust through communication in the intensive care unit: HICCC. Pediatr Crit Care Med. 2010;11(3):378–84.
15. Davidson JE, Powers K, Hedayat KM, Tieszen M, Kon AA, Shepard E, Spuhler V, Todres ID, Levy M, Barr J, Ghandi R, Hirsch G, Armstrong D. Clinical practice guidelines for support of the family in the patient-centered intensive care unit: American College of Critical Care Medicine Task Force 2004–2005. Crit Care Med. 2007;35(2):605–22.
16. Aronson PL, Yau J, Helfaer MA, Morrison W. Impact of family presence during pediatric intensive care unit rounds on the family and medical team. Pediatrics. 2009;124(4):1119–25.
17. Phipps L, Bartke C, Spear D, Jones L, Foerster C, Killian M, Hughes J, Hess J, Johnson D, Thomas N. Assessment of parental presence during bedside pediatric intensive care unit rounds: effect on duration, teaching, and privacy. Pediatr Crit Care Med. 2007;8(3):220–4.
18. Baker J, Kane J, Rai S, Howard S, PCS Research Working Group, Hinds P. Changes in medical care at a pediatric oncology referral center after placement of a do-not-resuscitate order. J Palliat Med. 2010;13(11):1349–52.
19. Sanders A, Schepp M, Baird M. Partial do-not-resuscitate orders: a hazard to patient safety and clinical outcomes? Crit Care Med. 2011;39(1):14–8.
20. Partridge JC, Wall SN. Analgesia for dying infants whose life support is withdrawn or withheld. Pediatrics. 1997;99(1):76–9.
21. Sulmasy DP, Pellegrino ED. The rule of double effect: clearing up the double talk. Arch Intern Med. 1999;159(6):545–50.
22. Luce JM, Alpers A. End-of-life care: what do the American courts say? Crit Care Med. 2001;29(2 Suppl):N40–5.
23. Truog RD, et al. Pharmacologic paralysis and withdrawal of mechanical ventilation at the end of life. N Engl J Med. 2000; 342(7):508–11.
24. Diekema DS, Botkin JR. Forgoing medically provided nutrition and hydration in children. Pediatrics. 2009;124(2):813–22.
25. Fine RL. Point: The Texas Advance Directives Act effectively and ethically resolves disputes about medical futility. Chest. 2009; 136(4):963–7.
26. Truog RD. Counterpoint: The Texas Advance Directives Act is ethically flawed. Chest. 2009;136(4):968–73.
27. Morparia K, Dickerman M, Hoehn KS. Futility: unilateral decision making is not the default for pediatric intensivists. Pediatric Critical Care Medicine. 2012;13(5):e311–5.
28. Committee on Bioethics. Institutional ethics committees. Pediatrics. 2001;107(1):205–9.
29. Committee on Bioethics. Religious objections to medical care. Pediatrics. 1997;99(2):279–81.
30. Widjicks E. The diagnosis of brain death. N Engl J Med. 2001; 344:1215–21.
31. Steinbrook R. Organ donation after cardiac death. N Engl J Med. 2007;357(3):209–12.

32. Nakagawa TA, Ashwa S, Mathur M, Mysore M. Clinical report-guidelines for the determination of brain death in infants and children: an update of the 1987 task force recommendations. Pediatrics. 2011;128:e720–40.

33. A definition of irreversible coma: report of the Ad Hoc Committee of the Harvard Medical School to Examine the Definition of Brain Death. JAMA. 1968;205:337–40.

34. Committee on Hospital Care, Section on Surgery and Section of Critical Care. Pediatric organ donation and transplantation. Pediatrics. 2011;125(4):823–8.

35. Boucek MM, Mashburn C, Dunn SM, Frizell R, Edwards L, Pietra B, Campbell D. Pediatric heart transplantation after declaration of cardiocirulatory death. N Engl J Med. 2008;359(7):709–14.

36. Bernat JL, D'Alessandro AM, Port FK, Bleck TP, Heard SO, Medina J, Rosenbaum SH, Devita MA, Gaston RS, Merion RM, Barr ML, Marks WH, Nathan H, O'Connor K, Rudow DL, Leichtman AB, Schwab P, Ascher NL, Metzger RA, McBride V, Graham W, Wagner D, Warren J, Delmonico FL. Report of a national conference on donation after cardiac death. Am J Transplant. 2006;6:281–91.

37. Shaddy RE, Denne SC, Committee on Drugs and the Committee on Pediatric Research. Guidelines for the ethical conduct of studies to evaluate drugs in pediatric populations. Pediatrics. 2010;125(4):850–60.

38. Code of Federal Regulations. Title 45-Public welfare. Part 46-Protection of Human Subjects. Subpart D: Additional protections for children involved as subjects in research. Rockville: Department of Health and Human Services; 2005. Available at: www.hhs.gov/ohrp/humansubjects/guidance/45cfr46.htm#subpartd.

39. Gabbard GO. The role of compulsiveness in normal the physician. JAMA. 1985;254(20):2926–9.

40. Dyrbye L, Thomas M, Shanafelt T. Systemic review of depression, anxiety, and other indicators of psychological distress among US and Canadian medical students. Acad Med. 2006;81:354–73.

41. Woloschuk W, Harasym PH, Temple W. Attitude change during medical school: a cohort study. Med Educ. 2004;38:522–34.

42. Hojat M, Robeson M, Damjanov I, Veloski JJ, Glaser K, Gonnella JS. Students' psychosocial characteristics as predictors of academic performance in medical school. Acad Med. 1993;68:635–7.

43. Keene E, Hutton N, Hall B, Rushton C. Bereavement debriefing sessions: an intervention to support health care professionals in managing their grief after the death of a patient. Pediatr Nurs. 2010;36(4):185–9.

Kelly Nicole Michelson and Linda B. Siegel

Abstract

Pediatric palliative care seeks to treat suffering and achieve the best possible quality of life for patients facing serious or potentially life-limiting illnesses. The goals and values of the child and family should direct decision making and guide care. Curative care may be continued with increased attention to symptom management and the psychosocial needs of the family. Palliative care focuses on six domains: (1) support of the family unit; (2) communication about treatment goals with the child and family; (3) ethics and shared decision making; (4) pain and other symptom relief; (5) care continuity; and 6) grief and bereavement support. After providing a comprehensive palliative care definition and discussion of pediatric intensive care unit (PICU) patients who might benefit from palliative care, this chapter reviews: the integration of palliative care into the PICU, focusing on the six defined domains; the importance of attending to the emotional needs of healthcare professionals; and practical considerations during the peri-death and bereavement periods. This review is intended to aid pediatric intensivists as they treat and guide patients confronted with serious or potentially life-limiting illnesses and their families. By adhering to the principles of palliative care, intensivists assume a privileged role and can positively impact patients, families, and health care professionals during challenging times.

Keywords

Palliative care • Quality-of-life • Decision making • Dying • Bereavement

Introduction

Clinicians in the pediatric intensive care unit (PICU) often save lives of critically ill children who decades ago died despite medical care. But even now not all children survive. When curative therapies do not exist or therapies impose excessive, unacceptable burden, the intensive nature of care continues even as goals change. Care of patients with serious or potentially life-limiting illnesses and their families shapes not only the life and death of the patients, but also the experience of everyone around them, including healthcare professionals. Pediatric intensivists have the unique opportunity and responsibility to help patients and their families navigate the challenges faced by serious or potentially life-limiting illnesses, and through their interactions can mitigate suffering for all involved.

K.N. Michelson, MD, MPH (✉)
Division of Pediatric Critical Care Medicine, Department of Pediatrics, Ann and Robert H. Lurie Children's Hospital of Chicago, 225 E. Chicago Avenue, 73 Chicago, IL 60611-2605, USA
e-mail: kmichelson@luriechildrens.org

L.B. Siegel, MD, FAAP
Divisions of Pediatric Critical Care Medicine and Pediatric Palliative CareCohen, Children's Medical Center, 2690-01 76th Avenue, New Hyde Park, NY 11040, USA
e-mail: lsiegs64@gmail.com

The Definition of Palliative Care

Many individuals mistakenly regard palliative care as care focused solely on the dying patient. However, palliative care is not the same as hospice care, a Medicare benefit for

D.S. Wheeler et al. (eds.), *Pediatric Critical Care Medicine*,
DOI 10.1007/978-1-4471-6362-6_15, © Springer-Verlag London 2014

patients who have forsaken curative care and are predicted to survive less than 6 months. The World Health Organization (WHO) defines palliative care as "an approach that improves the quality of life of patients and their families facing the problem associated with life-threatening illness, through the prevention and relief of suffering by means of early identification and impeccable assessment and treatment of pain and other problems, physical, psychosocial and spiritual" [1]. The WHO goes on to define palliative care for children as "the active total care of the child's body, mind and spirit, and also involves giving support to the family. It begins when illness is diagnosed, and continues regardless of whether or not a child receives treatment directed at the disease" [1].

Palliative care focuses on treating suffering and improving quality of life in all phases of life [2]. In part, palliative care mirrors all care delivered in the PICU. The distinguishing features of pediatric palliative care include a comprehensive focus addressing patients' and families' emotional and spiritual needs; symptom management; and the unique needs of children with serious or potentially life-limiting illnesses and their families [3]. To meet these unique needs the Initiative for Pediatric Palliative Care identified six domains of care: (1) support of the family unit; (2) communication with the child and family about treatment goals; (3) ethics and shared decision making; (4) relief of pain and other symptoms; (5) continuity of care; and (6) grief and bereavement support [4]. Through individualized patient- and family-centered care, palliative care seeks to address these six domains.

Epidemiology of Palliative Care Patients in the PICU

Of the 55,000 annual pediatric deaths in the United States [5–7], more than 56 % occur in the hospital [5]. Within hospitals, studies show that 50–82 % of all pediatric deaths occur in the PICU [6, 8–10]. PICU deaths account for 3–8 % of PICU admissions [8, 11–14], and occur in children with a wide range of medical problems, from chronic conditions such as neurodegenerative disorders or congenital heart disease to acute conditions such as trauma or sudden infant death syndrome (SIDS) [11, 12, 15]. The median PICU length of stay prior to death ranges from 2 to 13 days [11–13]. Forty to 65 % of PICU deaths follow a decision to withdraw or limit life-sustaining treatments [11–13, 16–19]. Approximately 15–23 % of patients experience brain death and a little over 10 % die without any limitation of life-sustaining therapies or advance directive [19, 20].

In considering PICU patients who would benefit from palliative care, one must include more than those who are imminently dying. The majority of palliative care patients have complex, chronic conditions and typically greater than one major diagnosis [21, 22]. Such patients often require multiple PICU admissions during their lives. In a study of palliative care patients at multiple centers in the United States and Canada, 58 % of patients had their initial palliative care consult encounter as an inpatient, and just under a fifth of these consultations occurred while the patient remained in an intensive care unit (ICU) [22]. Among consults initiated in an ICU setting, 65 % of patients were still alive 30 days later. This illustrates the expanded focus of palliative care to include patients with serious or potentially life-limiting conditions and not limit the benefits of palliative care to those actively dying.

Integration of Palliative Care in the Critical Care Setting

As noted in the WHO definition, palliative care ideally begins when a serious or potentially life-limiting illness is diagnosed. The American Academy of Pediatrics (AAP) also recommends that "At diagnosis of a life-threatening or terminal condition, it is important to offer an integrated model of palliative care that continues throughout the course of illness, regardless of the outcome" [23]. One challenge to integrating palliative care into the ICU setting is concomitantly offering and implementing life-extending and/or potentially curative therapies while discussing and addressing the needs of those with a high likelihood of death. Although the goals are not mutually exclusive, the focus of the medical and palliative care teams must evolve to reflect changes in the patient's illness and disease trajectory. Figure 15.1 shows how both curative and palliative care can complement each other through the course of a patient's illness.

The Interdisciplinary Palliative Care Team

Just as patients in the PICU have complicated diseases requiring input from multiple subspecialists, so too do palliative care patients require care from people in multiple disciplines. Typically palliative care teams include a physician and/or a nurse practitioner and/or other medically trained professional, a social worker, a chaplain, and a child-life specialist. Additional involvement from music, art, physical, and occupational therapists is desirable. Ideally, a team of specialists follows an individual patient throughout the course of his/her illness to minimize the introduction of new care providers during times of stress, such as admission to the PICU. The ability to achieve such continuity depends on the organizational structure of each institution.

Fig. 15.1 Integration of palliative and curative care. The focus of palliative care shifts and adjusts to the individual needs of a patient and his/her family throughout the continuum of illness during life and after death (Adapted from Liben et al. [66] and Lanken et al. [67])

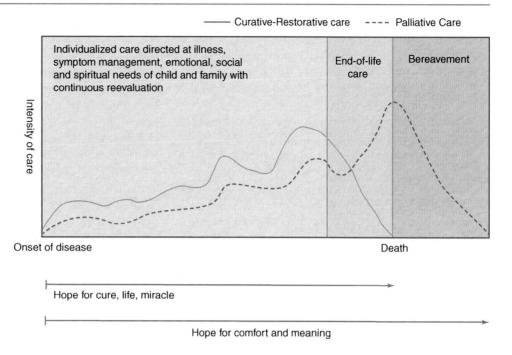

Fig. 15.2 Lines of communication in the PICU. Care of PICU patients involves multiple people resulting in complicated networks of communication among those involved

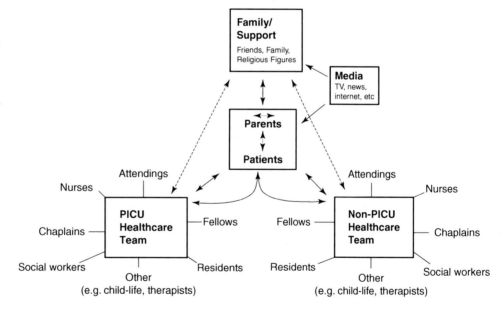

Family-Centered Communication

Palliative care seeks to provide patient- and family-centered care through individualizing goals and therapies ideally reflecting the needs and values of those involved. Family-centered, goal-directed care relies on good communication within the health care team and between health care providers. To quote a prominent expert, "Let us communicate with each other clearly, compassionately, and collaboratively, as we strive to improve the quality of life for children including, when necessary, that part of life that is dying" [24]. Clinicians must provide families with information and

options, but must also understand each family's perspective, ideals, and goals.

Lines of communication in the PICU are multiple and complex (Fig. 15.2). Communication occurs in different settings: daily rounds; impromptu conversations at the bedside during times of relative calm (e.g. with a stable patient) and acute stress (e.g. during an active resuscitation); formal family meetings; and sometimes spontaneous encounters outside the PICU (e.g. in the hallway). Regardless of the setting, clinicians should use evidence-based strategies shown to improve communication. These include: explore and focus on family values and preferences [25]; allow families ample opportunity to speak [25, 26]; acknowledge emotions expressed by family members; provide assurance that all efforts will be made to limit patient suffering [27]; include expressions of non-abandonment [27, 28]; and support the family's decision regarding continuation or withdrawal of life-sustaining therapies [27].

Communication about palliative care patients must also address communication among health care professionals both inside and out of the PICU. Multiple studies demonstrate challenges related to and negative impact from lack of adequate care coordination among different services [29–31]. Palliative care teams can help convey the family's values, preferences, and goals to the other medical care teams involved. Efforts should also be made to ensure detailed communication among medical team members regarding the child's physiological status and key psychosocial information. Good communication among healthcare professionals can minimize the amount of conflicting information families receive and build trust between families and healthcare professionals.

Goals of Care and Decision Making

Defining care goals provides a framework for clinicians and parents to direct medical decision making. Goals may change over time from cure to limiting suffering, staying out of the hospital, or may remain focused on prolonging life [2]. Realistic goal setting relies on honest communication about diagnosis, prognosis, and the burdens and benefits of each treatment option. Defining goals also requires that clinicians accept realistic prognostic assessments. The Institute for Medicine Report, "When Children Die" states "If physicians cannot fully face a child's poor prognosis and then appropriately communicate their assessment to families, timely reexamination of the goals of care and corresponding adjustments in care plans may be delayed."

Medical decisions in pediatrics are generally made by parents who give informed permission for procedures and treatment. Informed consent is designed to protect the ethical value of personal autonomy for patients [32], but requires a competent patient to make decisions. Children under the age of 18 are not considered legally competent except in rare situations. Each state has unique statutes regarding mature and emancipated minors. Parents have legal decision making authority for their minor children because our society assumes that parents act in their child's best interest.

Situations involving older children and adolescents require additional consideration. According to the AAP, decision making involving older children and adolescents should include, as much as possible, the child's assent [32]. According to the AAP committee on bioethics the key steps to obtaining assent from a child or adolescent include:

explaining the child's condition in a developmentally appropriate way; explaining the tests and treatments and what to expect; assessing the child's understanding of the information; asking if the child is willing to accept the proposed care (unless the child will not be allowed to dissent) [33]. Including the child in discussions becomes more critical when considering decisions about palliative care, such as: symptom management; limiting or discontinuing disease specific treatment; determining do not attempt resuscitate (DNAR) status; or considering withdrawal of life-sustaining therapy. Reports suggest that children living with chronic diseases may have better understanding of death than other similar aged children and are capable of engaging in conversations about these topics [2, 34–36].

Advanced care planning is becoming the norm in adults, offering competent adults an opportunity to express how they want to spend the end of their life and limit, or not, medical interventions if they become incapacitated. Minors can also complete advanced care planning documents. Though not legally binding, such documents give the child an opportunity to express his/her thoughts and feelings and can help parents and caregivers make decisions in keeping with the child's wishes [37]. Completing an advanced directive can also help to begin a conversation with the child about the potentially life-limiting nature of his/her disease. "My wishes" is one example of an advanced care document designed for children [38]. Palliative care teams can also create their own forms to include language appropriate for different ages and situations.

Adolescents should certainly be included in conversations about medical care goals and decisions. Many people believe that older adolescents should be allowed to make their own decisions pertaining to end of life care [33], although no research validates this as better or worse for the teen or family. Ideally, the palliative care team, primary team, and families can agree about how to include the child or adolescent in decision making. If consensus cannot be reached ethics consultation may be helpful; however, it is preferable to avoid legal intervention when making end of life decisions [33].

Symptom Management

Children living with serious or life-threatening conditions may suffer from many difficult to control symptoms, both physical and emotional. Pain, fatigue, nausea, depression and anorexia are just a few common symptoms confronted by palliative care teams. Because a complete review of symptom management is outside the scope of this chapter, we focus our discussion on basic concepts related to pain management and refer the reader to other sources for a more detailed review of symptom management for pediatric palliative care patients [2, 39–42].

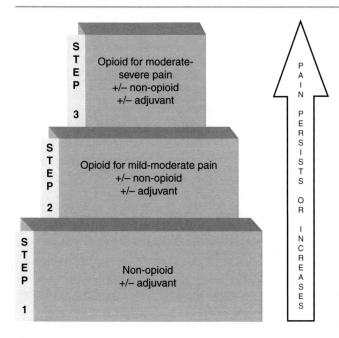

Fig. 15.3 World Health Organization three step ladder approach to pain management (Adapted from Pain Relief Ladder. http://www.who.int/cancer/palliative/painladder/en/. Accessed November 8th, 2011. With permission from World Health Organization)

Initial pain management should start with the WHO concepts: drugs should be dosed around the clock to achieve steady state; the least invasive form of therapy possible should be used; and the WHO analgesic ladder should be used to increase the potency of medications as needed [39] (Fig. 15.3). Myths that lead to inadequate pain relief include fear that prolonged opioid use will cause addiction or that use of opioids will hasten death [43]. Children with chronic pain often develop tolerance to opioids and may require extremely high doses, but, with proper use, psychological addiction rarely occurs in children [43]. Regarding concerns about hastening death, studies show that increasing opioid doses at the end of life do not result in shorter time to death [44, 45].

Narcotics are the mainstay therapy for pain management in the PICU. When choosing a narcotic, intensivists should consider, among other things: route of administration, drug half-life, and side effect profiles. Side effects, such as sedation, nausea, and constipation should be anticipated and treated prophylactically when possible. Patients and families should be appropriately counseled about the side effects of narcotics and the potential for developing tolerance. Constipation is almost universal among those treated with narcotics, so a bowel regimen should be used to mitigate this unpleasant problem [39].

Children followed by palliative care teams often suffer from different types of pain. Neuropathic pain, pain from injury to the central or peripheral nervous system, can be harder to control than nociceptive pain, pain from injury to

the body. N-methyl-D-aspartate receptor antagonists such as ketamine, methadone, gabapentin or pregabalin can be useful for neuropathic pain when traditional opioids are not successful [39, 46]. Adjuvant pain treatments should also be considered, including antidepressants which may also aid sleep and anticonvulsants. Surgery, radiation, or other interventions to treat the underlying disease can offer palliation even if aggressive disease modifying treatments have been discontinued. Select patients may require tunneled epidurals or nerve blocks [42, 47].

Studies describe an increased use of complementary and alternative medicine (CAM) in pediatrics [48]. In oncology, the use of CAM has been reported in 29 % of children during the palliative phase of the disease in one study [49] and 82 % after failure of frontline therapy in another study [50]. CAM therapies include biochemical treatments (herbs, dietary supplements), lifestyle changes (nutrition, exercise, biofeedback, hypnosis), biomechanical therapies (massage, chiropractor) and bioenergetic therapies (acupuncture, acupressure, Reiki) [48]. Despite the sparse data on the risks and benefits of specific CAM therapies, a willingness to consider non-traditional therapies shows respect for families' beliefs and can strengthen the relationship between the team and the family. An assessment of potential harm versus benefit is necessary before approving any individual therapy [48].

Rarely, when a child is imminently dying, he/she may have symptoms that are unresponsive to the usual medications. When these symptoms are intolerable, the child may benefit from palliative sedation [48]. Palliative sedation involves the administration of sedatives until the patient is comfortable and able to tolerate burdensome symptoms. This may or may not result in unconsciousness [48]. The goals of the patient and family should be explored prior to initiating palliative sedation, as some children may prefer to be conscious despite pain or other symptoms. Because palliative sedation seeks to achieve patient comfort, and not death, as its primary goal, it differs clinically, ethically and legally from euthanasia and physician assisted suicide [51].

Spiritual Distress

In order to provide comprehensive care to the child and family, attention must be paid to spiritual distress [2, 52]. Spirituality is defined by experts as "...the aspect of humanity that refers to the way individuals seek and express meaning and purpose and the way they experience their connectedness in the moment, to self, to others, to nature, and to the significant or sacred" [53]. Religion may or may not be part of one's spirituality. Children with serious or life-threatening diseases and their families may suffer from existential concerns and benefit from exploring these issues. Attention to spiritual issues allows children and their families the opportunity to find meaning in the face of disease and potential death. All members of the healthcare team should be comfortable assessing for spiritual distress and referring to the chaplain for management.

Attention to Siblings

During the terminal phase of a child's disease, health care professionals tend to focus primarily on the child and his/her parents. But we must also prioritize siblings. Data shows that approximately 73 % of children followed by a palliative care team have siblings [22]. For many families, the tendency is to protect and shield siblings from death and the dying process. However, research demonstrates that excluding siblings may hinder sibling bereavement [54, 55]. Experts encourage healthcare professionals to involve siblings through information sharing and when appropriate, interactions with the patient in the hospital and even during the dying period [56–58]. Parents often need guidance in communicating with the siblings about the child's illness [59]. Such guidance should be individualized to the sibling's developmental stage, background, and temperament. Guidance is ideally, but not necessarily, provided by a child-life specialist.

Practical Considerations During the Peri-death Period in the PICU

Whether by preference or circumstance, many families experience their child's death in the PICU. Attention to simple but important practical considerations that modify the PICU environment as a child is dying can help support the family and meet their needs (Table 15.1). When it becomes clear that the child is imminently dying, systems should be in place to implement modifications to the environment that allow families time and space to create memories and be with their child.

Table 15.1 Considerations during the dying period in the PICU

Evaluate all treatments and medications and discontinue those not contributing to quality of life with the agreement of the family
Offer opportunities for memory making
Hand/foot prints or molds
Taking photographs
Preserving a lock of hair
Offer the opportunity to hold bedside ceremonies
Consider relaxing visiting hours
Provide a private space for families
Allow families to hold and/or lay with their child
Allow families to bathe and/or dress their child
Prepare families for what happens after the child dies: shrouding and transfer to the morgue, autopsy, funeral home
Allow families as much time as they need with the child after death

When a child is actively dying in the hospital, healthcare professionals may spend less time with the patient and family, perhaps because of personal discomfort with death, not knowing what to say, or feeling that one has nothing to offer. However, such avoidance may lead families to feel abandoned. Regular visits from the healthcare team lets families know they are supported. Often, just listening is enough. Families will remember these acts of kindness [60, 61].

Bereavement

Addressing family bereavement starts in the PICU. Memory making activities should be offered (Table 15.1) as they may significantly impact a family's bereavement process [62–64]. Prior to leaving the hospital, families should receive written materials and contact information for bereavement support services. There should be a plan for someone from the healthcare team to follow-up with the family a few weeks (or sooner if necessary) after the child's death. Such contact provides families an opportunity to ask questions, discuss their child's illness, or express their need for support. If an autopsy was performed, a meeting should be planned, preferably in person, to discuss the autopsy results and give the family an opportunity to ask questions. Many bereavement teams call or send a card on the child's birthday and anniversary of the child's death to let the family know the child has not been forgotten.

Caring for Healthcare Professionals

Healthcare professionals may encounter difficult emotional challenges when caring for children with serious or life-limiting conditions and their families. For some, providing such care can engender a sense of suffering and burden. Even providers who find this work meaningful are at risk for burnout or compassion fatigue, a disorder similar to post-traumatic stress but which affects those witnessing the suffering or trauma of others [65]. Systems should be in place to address the emotional needs of healthcare professionals. Helpful approaches after a patient death include: giving professionals time before taking on a new patient; having group debriefing sessions following a death or difficult experience; allowing staff time off to attend the funeral or wake; arranging a memorial service in the hospital for staff; and providing individual counseling as needed. Even a moment of silence after the death of a patient or a verbal acknowledgement that a life was lost can be helpful.

Conclusion

The cure-directed, technology-dependent, emotionally charged PICU environment may appear to be a challenging place to incorporate palliative care. However, delivering quality whole person, family-centered care that focuses on goals, symptom management, psychosocial and spiritual needs for children with serious or potentially life-limiting illnesses is necessary, feasible and enriching. It is with duty and privilege that intensivists have the opportunity to guide others as they face the challenges associated with serious illness or death.

References

1. WHO. Definition of palliative care. http://www.who.int/cancer/palliative/definition/en/. Accessed 4 Oct 2011.
2. Klick JC, Hauer J. Pediatric palliative care. Curr Probl Pediatr Adolesc Health Care. 2010;40(6):120–51.
3. Lenton S, Goldman A, Eaton N, Southall D. Development and epidemiology. In: Golman A, Hain R, Liben S, editors. Oxford textbook of palliative care for children. Oxford: Oxford University Press; 2007. p. 3–13.
4. Truog RD, Meyer EC, Burns JP. Toward interventions to improve end-of-life care in the pediatric intensive care unit. Crit Care Med. 2006;34(11 Suppl):S373–9.
5. Committee on Palliative and End-of-Life Care for Children and Their Families Board on Health Sciences Policy, Institute of Medicine. Field MJ, Behrman RE (eds). When Children Die: Improving Palliative and End-of-life Care for Children and Their Families. Washington, DC: The National Academies Press; 2003.
6. Feudtner C, Connor SR. Epidemiology and health services research. In: Carter BS, Levetown M, editors. Palliative care for infants, children, and adolescents: a practical handbook. Baltimore: The Johns Hopkins University Press; 2004. p. 3–22.
7. Kochanek KD, Murphy SL, Anderson RN, Scott C. Deaths: final data for 2002. Natl Vital Stat Rep. 2004;53(5):1–115.
8. Lantos JD, Berger AC, Zucker AR. Do-not-resuscitate orders in a children's hospital. Crit Care Med. 1993;21(1):52–5.
9. McCallum DE, Byrne P, Bruera E. How children die in hospital. J Pain Symptom Manag. 2000;20(6):417–23.
10. Carter BS, Howenstein M, Gilmer MJ, Throop P, France D, Whitlock JA. Circumstances surrounding the deaths of hospitalized children: opportunities for pediatric palliative care. Pediatrics. 2004;114(3):e361–6.
11. Vernon DD, Dean JM, Timmons OD, Banner Jr W, Allen-Webb EM. Modes of death in the pediatric intensive care unit: withdrawal and limitation of supportive care. Crit Care Med. 1993;21(11):1798–802.
12. Garros D, Rosychuk RJ, Cox PN. Circumstances surrounding end of life in a pediatric intensive care unit. Pediatrics. 2003; 112(5):e371.
13. Burns JP, Mitchell C, Outwater KM, et al. End-of-life care in the pediatric intensive care unit after the forgoing of life-sustaining treatment. Crit Care Med. 2000;28(8):3060–6.
14. Randolph AG, Gonzales CA, Cortellini L, Yeh TS. Growth of pediatric intensive care units in the United States from 1995 to 2001. J Pediatr. 2004;144(6):792–8.
15. Sands R, Manning JC, Vyas H, Rashid A. Characteristics of deaths in paediatric intensive care: a 10-year study. Nurs Crit Care. 2009;14(5):235–40.
16. Ryan CA, Byrne P, Kuhn S, Tyebkhan J. No resuscitation and withdrawal of therapy in a neonatal and a pediatric intensive care unit in Canada. J Pediatr. 1993;123(4):534–8.
17. Mink RB, Pollack MM. Resuscitation and withdrawal of therapy in pediatric intensive care. Pediatrics. 1992;89(5):961–3.
18. Levetown M, Pollack MM, Cuerdon TT, Ruttimann UE, Glover JJ. Limitations and withdrawals of medical intervention in pediatric critical care. JAMA. 1994;272(16):1271–5.
19. Lee KJ, Tieves K, Scanlon MC. Alterations in end-of-life support in the pediatric intensive care unit. Pediatrics. 2010;126(4):e859–64.
20. Pleacher KM, Roach ES, Van der Werf W, Antommaria AH, Bratton SL. Impact of a pediatric donation after cardiac death program. Pediatr Crit Care Med. 2009;10(2):166–70.
21. Feudtner C, Hays RM, Haynes G, Geyer JR, Neff JM, Koepsell TD. Deaths attributed to pediatric complex chronic conditions: national trends and implications for supportive care services. Pediatrics. 2001;107(6):E99.
22. Feudtner C, Kang TI, Hexem KR, et al. Pediatric palliative care patients: a prospective multicenter cohort study. Pediatrics. 2011;127(6):1094–101.
23. American Academy of Pediatrics. Committee on Bioethics and Committee on Hospital Care. Palliative care for children. Pediatrics. 2000;106(2 Pt 1):351–7.
24. Feudtner C. Collaborative communication in pediatric palliative care: a foundation for problem-solving and decision-making. Pediatr Clin N Am. 2007;54(5):583–607, ix.
25. Curtis JR, Engelberg RA, Wenrich MD, Shannon SE, Treece PD, Rubenfeld GD. Missed opportunities during family conferences about end-of-life care in the intensive care unit. Am J Respir Crit Care Med. 2005;171(8):844–9.
26. McDonagh JR, Elliott TB, Engelberg RA, et al. Family satisfaction with family conferences about end-of-life care in the intensive care unit: increased proportion of family speech is associated with increased satisfaction. Crit Care Med. 2004;32(7):1484–8.
27. Stapleton RD, Engelberg RA, Wenrich MD, Goss CH, Curtis JR. Clinician statements and family satisfaction with family conferences in the intensive care unit. Crit Care Med. 2006;34(6):1679–85.
28. West HF, Engelberg RA, Wenrich MD, Curtis JR. Expressions of nonabandonment during the intensive care unit family conference. J Palliat Med. 2005;8(4):797–807.
29. Meert KL, Eggly S, Pollack M, et al. Parents' perspectives on physician-parent communication near the time of a child's death in the pediatric intensive care unit. Pediatr Crit Care Med. 2008;9(1):2–7.
30. Meyer EC, Ritholz MD, Burns JP, Truog RD. Improving the quality of end-of-life care in the pediatric intensive care unit: parents' priorities and recommendations. Pediatrics. 2006;117(3):649–57.
31. Michelson K, Emanuel L, Brinkman P, Carter A, Clayman M, Frader J. Pediatric intensive care unit family conferences: one mode of communication for discussing end-of-life care decisions. Pediatr Crit Care Med. 2011;12(6):e336–e343.
32. Freyer DR. Care of the dying adolescent: special considerations. Pediatrics. 2004;113(2):381–8.
33. Informed consent, parental permission, and assent in pediatric practice. Committee on Bioethics, American Academy of Pediatrics. Pediatrics. 1995;95(2):314–7.
34. Hinds PS, Drew D, Oakes LL, et al. End-of-life care preferences of pediatric patients with cancer. J Clin Oncol. 2005;23(36):9146–54.
35. Levetown M. Communicating with children and families: from everyday interactions to skill in conveying distressing information. Pediatrics. 2008;121(5):e1441–60.
36. Weir RF, Peters C. Affirming the decisions adolescents make about life and death. Hastings Cent Rep. 1997;27(6):29–40.
37. Zinner SE. The use of pediatric advance directives: a tool for palliative care physicians. Am J Hosp Palliat Care. 2008 Dec-2009 Jan;25(6):427–30.
38. Dignity Aw. My wishes. http://www.agingwithdignity.org/. Accessed 7 Oct 2011.
39. Friedrichsdorf SJ, Kang TI. The management of pain in children with life-limiting illnesses. Pediatr Clin N Am. 2007;54(5):645–72, x.

40. Ullrich CK, Mayer OH. Assessment and management of fatigue and dyspnea in pediatric palliative care. Pediatr Clin N Am. 2007;54(5):735–56, xi.

41. Symptom care. In: Goldman A, Hain R, Liben S, editors. Oxford textbook of palliative care for childrens. Great Clarendon Street: Oxford University Press; 2006. p. 231–509.

42. Wolfe J, Hinds PS, Sourkes B. Textbook of interdisciplinary pediatric palliative care. Philadelphia: Elsevier/Saunders; 2011.

43. Friedrichsdorf SJ. Pain management in children with advanced cancer and during end-of-life care. Pediatr Hematol Oncol. 2010;27(4): 257–61.

44. Thorns A, Sykes N. Opioid use in last week of life and implications for end-of-life decision-making. Lancet. 2000;356(9227):398–9.

45. Sykes N, Thorns A. The use of opioids and sedatives at the end of life. Lancet Oncol. 2003;4(5):312–8.

46. Sang CN. NMDA-receptor antagonists in neuropathic pain: experimental methods to clinical trials. J Pain Symptom Manag. 2000;19(1 Suppl):S21–5.

47. Anghelescu DL, Faughnan LG, Baker JN, Yang J, Kane JR. Use of epidural and peripheral nerve blocks at the end of life in children and young adults with cancer: the collaboration between a pain service and a palliative care service. Paediatr Anaesth. 2010;20(12):1070–7.

48. Kemper KJ, Vohra S, Walls R. American Academy of Pediatrics. The use of complementary and alternative medicine in pediatrics. Pediatrics. 2008;122(6):1374–86.

49. Tomlinson D, Hesser T, Ethier MC, Sung L. Complementary and alternative medicine use in pediatric cancer reported during palliative phase of disease. Support Care Cancer. 2011;19(11):1857–63.

50. Paisley MA, Kang TI, Insogna IG, Rheingold SR. Complementary and alternative therapy use in pediatric oncology patients with failure of frontline chemotherapy. Pediatr Blood Cancer. 2011;56(7):1088–91.

51. Kirk TW, Mahon MM. National Hospice and Palliative Care Organization (NHPCO) position statement and commentary on the use of palliative sedation in imminently dying terminally ill patients. J Pain Symptom Manag. 2010;39(5):914–23.

52. McSherry M, Kehoe K, Carroll JM, Kang TI, Rourke MT. Psychosocial and spiritual needs of children living with a life-limiting illness. Pediatr Clin North Am. 2007;54(5):609–29, ix–x.

53. Puchalski C, Ferrell B, Virani R, et al. Improving the quality of spiritual care as a dimension of palliative care: the report of the Consensus Conference. J Palliat Med. 2009;12(10):885–904.

54. Giovanola J. Sibling involvement at the end of life. J Pediatr Oncol Nurs. 2005;22(4):222–6.

55. Lauer ME, Mulhern RK, Bohne JB, Camitta BM. Children's perceptions of their sibling's death at home or hospital: the precursors of differential adjustment. Cancer Nurs. 1985;8(1):21–7.

56. Hilden JM, Watterson J, Chrastek J. Tell the children. J Clin Oncol. 2003;21(9 Suppl):37s–9s.

57. Duncan J, Joselow M, Hilden JM. Program interventions for children at the end of life and their siblings. Child Adolesc Psychiatr Clin N Am. 2006;15(3):739–58.

58. Nolbris M, Hellstrom AL. Siblings' needs and issues when a brother or sister dies of cancer. J Pediatr Oncol Nurs. 2005;22(4): 227–33.

59. Williams J, Koocher G. Medical crisis counseling on a pediatric intensive care unit: case examples and clinical utility. J Clin Psychol Med Settings. 1999;6(3):249–58.

60. Kars M, Grypdonck M, Beishuizen A, Meijer-van den Bergh E, van Delden J. Factors influencing parental readiness to let their child with cancer die. Pediatr Blood Cancer. 2010;54(7): 1000–8.

61. Knapp C, Contro N. Family support services in pediatric palliative care. Am J Hosp Palliat Care. 2009 Dec-2010 Jan 2009;26(6): 476–82.

62. Alexander KV. The one thing you can never take away. MCN Am J Matern Child Nurs. 2001;26(3):123–7.

63. Riches G, Dawson P. Lost children, living memories: the role of photographs in processes of grief and adjustment among bereaved parent. Death Stud. 1998;22(2):121–40.

64. Lundqvist A, Nilstun T, Dykes AK. Experiencing neonatal death: an ambivalent transition into motherhood. Pediatr Nurs. 2002;28(6):621–5, 610.

65. Kearney MK, Weininger RB, Vachon ML, Harrison RL, Mount BM. Self-care of physicians caring for patients at the end of life: "Being connected… a key to my survival". JAMA. 2009;301(11):1155–64, E1151.

66. Liben S, Papadatou D, Wolfe J. Paediatric palliative care: challenges and emerging ideas. Lancet. 2008;371(9615):852–64.

67. Lanken PN, Terry PB, Delisser HM, et al. An official American Thoracic Society clinical policy statement: palliative care for patients with respiratory diseases and critical illnesses. Am J Respir Crit Care Med. 2008;177(8):912–27.

Evidence-based Pediatric Critical Care Medicine

Donald L. Boyer and Adrienne G. Randolph

Abstract

Evidence-based medicine (EBM) strives to find the optimal course of action for a given clinical question by merging the best available scientific evidence with expert clinical judgment that incorporates a patient's values and preferences. Although learning how to apply the concepts and principles of EBM is not intuitive, most clinicians become facile with modest effort. This chapter will describe the evolution of EBM from clinical and epidemiologic principles and research. We review the process of EBM in detail, including EBM core concepts related to articles on diagnosis, therapy, harm, and prognosis. We conclude by discussing the role of EBM in the PICU, emphasizing challenges and future directions.

Keywords

Evidence-based clinical practice (EBCP) • Evidence-based medicine (EBM) • Critical appraisal, critical care

A Clinical Scenario Raises Important Clinical Questions

Evidence-based medicine (EBM) is the "conscientious, explicit and judicious use of current evidence in making decisions about the care of individual patients" [1]. Despite increasing acceptance of the role of EBM in clinical practice over the last two decades, many clinicians are unaware of EBM's history and do not understand the rigorous systematic approach that the practice of EBM requires. To improve this understanding, we will review the origins of clinical research leading up to the era of EBM to explain why EBM came about. We start this chapter with a clinical scenario to which we will repeatedly refer. We then briefly describe the stepwise approach to some of the EBM core topics as applied to this and other patient encounters. Ways to keep up with the evidence and efficiently find evidence will be reviewed and we will also address challenges to practicing EBM in the pediatric intensive care unit (PICU).

Clinical Scenario

A 7 year-old male is admitted to the PICU after being involved in a motor vehicle accident. At the scene he was hypertensive and bradycardic with asymmetric pupils, an irregular respiratory pattern and a Glasgow Coma Score (GCS) of 6. He was intubated in the field and Emergency Medical Services (EMS) personnel attempted to hyperventilate for suspected elevated intracranial pressure (ICP). Upon arrival to the PICU, he underwent central line placement and was started on an infusion of hypertonic saline and narcotic and benzodiazepine drips for pain and sedation. A few hours after PICU admission, his blood pressure and heart rate normalized.

D.L. Boyer, MD
Department of Anesthesiology and Critical Care Medicine, The Children's Hospital of Philadelphia and the Perelman School of Medicine at the University of Pennsylvania, Philadelphia, PA, USA

A.G. Randolph, MD, MSc (✉)
Division of Critical Care Medicine, Department of Anesthesia, Perioperative and Pain Medicine, Children's Hospital Boston, 300 Longwood Avenue, Boston, MA 02115, USA
e-mail: Adrienne.Randolph@childrens.harvard.edu

D.S. Wheeler et al. (eds.), *Pediatric Critical Care Medicine*,
DOI 10.1007/978-1-4471-6362-6_16, © Springer-Verlag London 2014

This patient's presentation raises numerous types of questions:

- **Etiology**: By what mechanism does traumatic brain injury cause elevated ICP? Why do patients with elevated ICP demonstrate hypertension, bradycardia and abnormal respirations and how often do these findings present as a constellation?
- **Diagnosis**: How likely is the constellation of findings (hypertension, bradycardia and abnormal respirations) indicative of elevated ICP? What is the gold standard for diagnosis of diffuse axonal injury following traumatic brain injury?
- **Treatment**: What is the role of hypertonic saline as an osmotic agent following traumatic brain injury? How does this compare to other osmotic agents like mannitol? Would induced hypothermia be beneficial for this patient?
- **Harm**: Is hypotension after traumatic brain injury causing hypoperfusion associated with worse neurologic outcomes? Is hyperglycemia harmful?
- **Prognosis**: What predictions can be made about survivability following such an injury? What expectations can be given to the family regarding cognitive outcomes if the child survives?

Questions related to etiology or the "background" of the clinical problem are foundational, focusing on the core of our medical knowledge. Questions related to diagnosis, treatment, harm and prognosis are considered 'foreground' questions and are at the core of EBM. Clinicians often rely on expertise – their own or those of consultants – to answer the above questions. One problem with reliance on clinical expertise alone is that it can lead to variable and sometimes contradictory guidance, leaving the clinician unclear about the optimal approach. EBM – also known as evidence-based clinical practice or EBCP – aims to answer "foreground" questions by integrating the best available evidence with clinician expertise taking into account individual patient preferences and values [2].

The Need for EBM

Led by Dr. David Sackett in the early 1980s, a group of clinical epidemiologists at McMaster University published a series of articles in the *Canadian Medical Association Journal* designed to help clinicians interpret clinical research. They coined the term "critical appraisal" to emphasize the need to thoughtfully examine and assess the reliability of research studies and applicability to specific patients [3]. At the time of David Sackett's initial introduction of critical appraisal, the biomedical literature was expanding at a rate of 6–7 % per year, thereby increasing tenfold every 35–50 years [4]. Clinicians were overwhelmed at the exponential expansion of clinical literature yet altering clinical practice with solid

evidence occurred very slowly, impeding the probability that the evidence could improve patient's lives.

Many of the illustrative historical clinical research examples given below are excerpted from a book entitled *Clinical Trials* by Pocock [5] and the James Lind Library, "created to help people understand fair tests of treatments in health care" (www.jameslindlibrary.org). Starting in 1753, one of the first published clinical studies was by Lind entitled *The Treatise of the Scurvy* [6]. Below is a modified excerpt of this study:

> I took 12 patients with the scurvy on board the Salisbury at sea. The cases were as similar as I could have them…they lay together in one place…and had one diet common to all. Two of these were ordered one quart of cider a day. Two others took 25 gutts of elixir vitriol…Two others took two spoonfuls of oranges and one lemon given to them each day…Two others took the bigness of a nutmeg. The most sudden and visible good effects were perceived from the use of oranges and lemons, one of those who had taken them being at the end of 6 days fit for duty…The other…was appointed to nurse the sick.

This study is important for two reasons. One is that it was the first strong "evidence" that vitamin C could be used to treat and prevent scurvy. The other is that Lind understood some basic features of good study design. He controlled for differences between patients by identifying those at the same level of illness. He controlled for other influences on outcome by giving patients the same diet, except for the interventions, and the same amount of sunlight and other environmental exposures. He also had two patients in each treatment arm because, although one patient could improve just by chance, the likelihood of two patients improving by chance alone was lower. Interestingly, despite this evidence, it was over five decades before lemon juice became standard fare on British naval ships. Delays in the application of evidence are still a major problem more than two and a half centuries later.

Another early clinical researcher was Louis who established clinical trials and epidemiology on a scientific footing [5]. In the 1800s, bleeding was the standard treatment for numerous serious and minor ailments across the U.S. and Europe. In 1835, Louis urged the need for the exact observation of patient outcome, knowledge of the natural progression of untreated controls, precise disease definition prior to treatment, and careful observation of deviations from intended treatment [7]. Louis' careful comparisons, showed no differences in the outcomes of patients with a variety of disorders who were bled and not bled. His findings led to the slow but eventual decline of bleeding as a standard treatment [5] – although it took over a century before bleeding was completely out of vogue.

In the early days of much of clinical medicine, especially for surgery, anesthesia, and critical care, early procedures and therapies led to dramatic improvements. With such profoundly clear benefits, the need for large numbers and control groups went by the wayside. Lister in 1870 [8] reported a before-after study of antiseptics for amputation operations, reporting a 43 % rate of mortality in 35 cases before antiseptic use versus a 15 % mortality rate in 40 cases afterwards. Although he focused on the small sample size and erroneously claimed the difference was not statistically significant, a more important problem with before-after studies such as this one is that many other things could have changed in the interim to explain the effect. Newer anesthetic methods, newer surgical techniques, and better basic hygiene could underlie the difference in mortality rates rather than antiseptic use.

The first randomized controlled trial was published in 1948 [9], when streptomycin plus bedrest was compared to bedrest alone to treat pulmonary tuberculosis [10]. The novel features of this trial, besides the randomized assignment to groups, were that outcome assessors were blinded to the treatment allocation and that multiple clinicians assessed outcome and had to come to consensus. This introduces a factor that clinical trials are designed to control for which is called "bias". Bias is a systematic difference between the research question and the actual question answered by the study that may cause the study to give a wrong answer [11]. Carefully designed studies minimize bias. Bias can come from patient variables (e.g., patients in one group being more ill at baseline), predictor variables (e.g., patients in one group are treated differently, besides the intervention), outcome variables (e.g., outcome assessors know patient treatment arm assignment and this influences their assessment), or from the placebo effect. EBM focuses on assessment of study design to ensure that steps were taken to minimize bias to optimize the trial's chances for the real answer to the question to emerge.

In the late 1950s through the 1960s, there was a rapid growth of clinical studies and especially of randomized controlled trials. For some therapies such as penicillin, the impact on disease was so great that observational studies of small numbers of patients showing dramatic recovery [12, 13] led to widespread use at the end of World War II saving thousands of soldier's lives. It is also true, however, that dramatic appearing results from clinician observation can be refuted by subsequent randomized trials, and that randomized trials can reveal larger treatment effects that were dampened by non-randomized studies. An example of the first is the rise and fall of "gastric freeze" for duodenal ulcer [14]. This intervention rose to be the standard of care in the 1960s based upon the clinical experience of major opinion leaders and published statements such as "Since April 1961, no patients with duodenal ulcer disease have been operated upon on the senior author's surgical service. This circumstance in itself bespeaks the confidence in the method by patients as well as surgeons" [15]. Thousands of gastric freezing machines were subsequently sold. A proper randomized trial finally led to the abolishment of gastric freeze for duodenal

ulcers because there was no difference in rates of subsequent surgery for ulcer disease, gastrointestinal hemorrhage, or hospitalization for intractable pain in patients randomized to the sham treatment versus the gastric freeze [16].

An example of how a randomized trial can lead to more rapid implementation of a promising intervention due to stronger results is from the Salk Polio vaccine trial [5, 17, 18]. In 1954, the annual incidence of polio was 1 in 2,000 people. Polio was epidemic but hit some geographic areas harder than others. Because of this, studies of preventive interventions with control groups within the same geographic regions were needed. Two studies were planned. Some health care regional authorities opted for an observed control approach where second graders were vaccinated while first and third graders served as unvaccinated controls. One million children participated in this study. Health authorities in other regions were concerned that bias could be introduced if the physician diagnosing polio, a diagnosis not always made with certainty, could guess whether or not the child received the vaccine. These practitioners opted for a blinded randomized controlled trial in which 800,000 children participated. The results were clear: in the randomized study the polio vaccine was highly effective with a 70 % reduction in polio and all four deaths occurred in the control group. The observed control study also showed better outcomes in the vaccinated group, however, children in both groups who declined participation in the study had better outcomes, making the results difficult to interpret. The data from the randomized, controlled trial eliminated much of the confusion from this observational control study and therefore provided the impetus for vaccination mandates.

The 1960s through 1980s were years of rapid growth of the clinical literature with the publication of many thousands of clinical trials. Advances in computerization facilitated management of large datasets, the growth of statistical methods, and searching for medical information. Medical practice was still based, however, on the expertise of the individual practitioner and there was no systematic method for practitioners to assess and incorporate published findings into their practice.

The EBM Process and Approaching the EBM Core Topics

McMaster University in Ontario, Canada served as the birthplace of EBM. *Clinical Epidemiology: a Basic Science for Clinical Medicine* was authored by Drs. Sackett, Haynes, and Tugwell and published in 1985 [19]. Dr. Gordon Guyatt later coined the term "evidence-based medicine" and with his colleagues published the principles of EBM in a series of articles in *JAMA* starting in 1993 entitled "Users' Guides to the Medical Literature" [20]. Each guide has the same

Table 16.1 Primary validity criteria for articles addressing therapy or prevention, diagnosis, prognosis and risk or harm

Type of study	Validity criteria
Therapy or prevention [21, 22]	Was the assignment of patients to treatments randomized?
	Were all of the patients who entered the trial properly accounted for and attributed at its conclusion?
	Was follow-up complete?
	Were patients analyzed in the groups to which they were randomized?
Diagnosis [23, 24]	Was there an independent, blind comparison with a reference standard?
	Did the patient sample include an appropriate spectrum of the sort of patients to whom the diagnostic test will be applied in clinical practice?
Prognosis [25]	Was there a representative and well-defined sample of patients at a similar point in the course of disease?
	Was follow-up sufficiently long and complete?
Harm [26]	Were there clearly identified comparison groups that were similar with respect to important determinants of outcome, other than the one of interest?
	Were the outcomes and exposures measured in the same way in the groups being compared?
	Was follow-up sufficiently long and complete?

structure: I. Are the results valid? (Using different validity criteria for different types of questions.); II. What are the results? (Including the effect size and its precision.); and III. Are these results applicable to my patient?

Assessing the validity of a study as the initial step can save the reader time. Fancy statistics will not fix a weak study design. If the study is not valid, there is no reason to read further. If the study design is of high quality and the study reports a statistically significant result, the next step is to ensure that the confidence interval around the treatment effect increases our confidence that the treatment is beneficial. If the study reports no effect, it is important to ensure that the study had sufficient power to test the hypothesis. Even if the study is valid, the sample size was large enough, and the confidence interval appropriately narrow, the study may not be applicable to your specific patient's situation based upon differences in their demographic or clinical status as well as their individual preferences and values.

Table 16.1 shows the Users' Guide primary validity criteria for questions about therapy or prevention [21, 22], diagnosis [23, 24], prognosis [25], and risk or harm [26] showing how criteria differ for each question type. To practice EBM, it is important to focus the clinical question and to choose and apply the correct Users' Guide criteria. There are over 25 Users' Guides currently available for different topics. Many are included in a series of articles edited by Dr. Deborah Cook that were published in *Critical Care Medicine* using critical care examples [27]. The *JAMA* Users' Guide series has also been incorporated into a book and pocket guide entitled Users' Guides to the Medical Literature [28].

To practice EBM is more than accessing and understanding the Users' Guides. EBM is defined as the conscientious, explicit and judicious application of current best evidence to the care of individual patients [29]. The practice of EBM requires the integration of clinical expertise and critical appraisal to determine the applicability and quality of available evidence. Practitioners of EBM make a commitment to use a systematic approach to search for, critically appraise,

synthesize, and apply evidence in their clinical practice [29]. To do this requires a five-step approach called the Evidence Cycle [28] often referred to as 'The 5 As':

1. **Assess** the patient and the problem to determine the pertinent issues (e.g., differential diagnosis, treatment, prognosis, risk of harm).
2. **Ask** a clear answerable clinical question that guides your search for the best available evidence.
3. **Acquire** the best evidence through efficient searching and from appropriate sources.
4. **Appraise** the evidence you have retrieved using a systematic method to evaluate it for validity, importance, and usefulness.
5. **Apply** the evidence to a particular patient and to their unique values and preferences.

Step 1: Assessing the Patient

The method of EBCP relies first on clinical expertise to assess the patient and incorporate all of the relevant clinical data. Clinical expertise is essential. With a comprehensive understanding of pathophysiology and by taking a thorough history and performing a rational clinical examination, the clinical problem(s) will be identified. The problem could involve a differential diagnosis, a treatment decision, a determination of prognosis, or a weighing of risk and benefit. Using clinical skills forms the basis for moving forward to the next steps in the Evidence Cycle.

Step 2: Asking Effective Clinical Questions

A critical step is to identify one or two key issues arising from the assessment to develop a focused and answerable clinical question. Doig and Simpson [30] put forth the mnemonic 'PICO' to detail the critical aspects of a well-formulated clinical question. The question should clearly entail the *P*atient/*P*opulation of interest, the *I*ntervention (or exposure) and its *C*omparison/*C*ontrol in evaluating an *O*utcome of interest. (Some have advocated expanding this to 'PICOT' to stress the importance of considering what *T*ype of study is most desirable, considering the

Fig. 16.1 Hierarchy of evidence. The "5S" evolution of information services for evidence-based healthcare decisions is a hierarchy of evidence designed to demonstrate the progression from original scientific articles all the way to the individual patient whereby escalating levels of evidence synthesis results in patient-specific decision support based upon best-existing evidence (Based on data from Haynes [49])

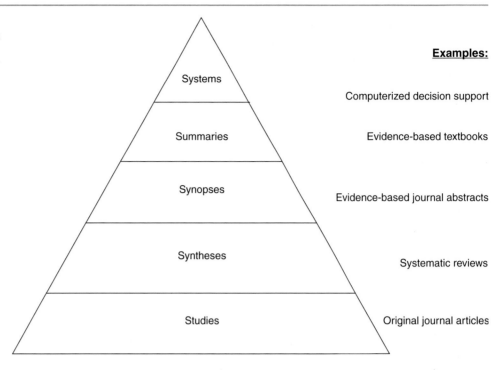

Systems

Summaries

Synopses

Syntheses

Studies

Examples:

Computerized decision support

Evidence-based textbooks

Evidence-based journal abstracts

Systematic reviews

Original journal articles

hierarchy of evidence shown in Fig. 16.1. Asking the most specific question for a given patient scenario allows for the most efficient acquisition of available literature.

Step 3: Acquire (Finding and Keeping Up with the Evidence) High-quality systematic evidence reviews, when available, save an enormous amount of time [4]. Although reviews that do not take an evidence-based systematic approach can be helpful in describing the physiology and pathology of a problem, they often present data in ways that are slanted to support the opinion of the expert author. Using a systematic approach to search for, critically appraise, synthesize, and present the results minimizes the potential for bias. The Cochrane Collaboration publishes an updated database of systematic reviews – all referenced in PubMed – that uses a rigorous and standardized review methodology developed and refined by expert methodologists (www.cochrane.org).

Efficiently finding evidence in online medical search engines such as PubMed, a National Library of Medicine platform for searching MEDLINE, requires using the right terminology such as Medical Subject Headings (MeSH). There are search criteria developed by Dr. Brian Haynes for using PubMed to identify relevant articles that will yield a higher sensitivity (retrieving all relevant articles) and specificity (not retrieving irrelevant articles) [31–34]. PubMed has a special search feature found under Clinical Tools on the home page called "Clinical Queries" This search tool is based upon the work of Dr. Haynes and colleagues that automatically filters searches based on the type of clinical study and searches specifically for systematic reviews allowing the clinician to set the search criteria broadly or narrowly.

Information overload is a constant problem plaguing clinicians. Given that research relevant to the pediatric intensive care setting may be found in the areas of internal medicine, neurology, surgery, trauma, infectious disease as well as hospital epidemiology, neonatology, pediatrics, radiology, oncology, and many other specialties, it can seem impossible to keep up with the literature [35]. Journal clubs that critically appraise relevant studies can save time. The PedsCCM Evidence-Based Journal Club (http:// PedsCCM.org) identifies articles across a range of medical journals, reviews them using the Users' Guide approach, and now publishes a select number in *Pediatric Critical Care Medicine*.

Additionally, a recent scoping review by Duffett et al. is an excellent consolidation of the available RCTs in pediatric critical care. The authors have made these accessible to clinicians and researchers at epicc.mcmaster.ca and have underscored the need for more high-quality evidence in order to support clinical decision-making in our patient population [36].

Returning to the patient presentation at the beginning of this chapter, suppose that the question we seek to answer is the role of hyperosmolar therapy in the management of pediatric TBI. Following the hierarchy of evidence, individual studies provide the foundation by which stronger evidence is based. Optimally, the practitioner would find a systems-level body of evidence in the form of practice guidelines, clinical pathways, or evidence-based textbook summaries that are frequently updated as new evidence arises. Turning to the question of hyperosmolar therapy and its role in the treatment of pediatric TBI for example, a clinician may stop after a literature search that reveals one of several individual articles pertaining to the use of hyperosmolar agents in severe TBI. However, more optimal evidence exists in the form of a set of guidelines published in 2012 which address the role of multiple treatments and management approaches and would be discovered upon a more exhaustive literature search [37, 38]. Updated from the 2003 set of guidelines, this revised clinical guide incorporates the GRADE approach to rate topics [39], providing a starting point for our clinical question. Chapter 8 of the pediatric TBI guidelines [38] specifically addresses the question of hyperosmolar agents in severe pediatric TBI and provides a summary of relevant articles. This allows a clinician to review the strength of the recommendation based upon the available evidence up to the time of the publication of the guideline. Because there is a 2 month to 1 year gap between development of a guideline and the timing of publication, it would be important to review further articles published after 2011 and determine if they would influence the recommendations in the guideline.

Step 4: Critical Appraisal

Appraisal of the acquired literature is unarguably the most important step in the application of evidence to clinical practice. Poorly designed studies, publications wrought with bias or unaccounted-for confounders and studies with improper statistical analysis or unfounded conclusions can lead clinicians to the wrong conclusion. As shown in Table 16.1, each type of study – therapy, diagnosis, prognosis, harm, etc. – should be appraised for validity using the validity criteria relevant for the type of study in question.

Returning to the hyperosmolar therapy question in severe pediatric TBI, we will review the EBM criteria (Table 16.1) for a therapy article. The first aspect of appraisal involves the validity of results and incorporates several key components to strengthen the findings. One must ask if patients in the intervention and control groups started with the same prognosis. While there may be confounders that are difficult to control for or even unknown to the investigating team, all attempts should be made to ensure prognostic equality between the groups in order to ensure that any difference is truly due to the intervention studied. Patient randomization is the optimal method for ensuring equal distribution of known factors that can influence patient outcome between the groups. Randomization can be done in multiple ways and to be most effective, should be a concealed process by which allocation into study arms cannot be affected by clinician bias. Following initial prognostic balancing at time of enrollment, the reader should consider whether enrollees maintained prognostic balance throughout the duration of the study. This is accomplished through blinding at as many levels as possible (i.e., study participant, investigator, data collector, and statistician). Finally,

prognostic balance can be assessed at the conclusion of the study by evaluation of how complete follow-up was, whether patients were analyzed in the groups in which they were randomized (intention-to-treat analysis) and whether or not the trial was stopped early.

Once you are convinced the results are likely to be valid, it is now worth your time to review them identifying the point estimate and the confidence interval around it. A point estimate is simply the observed treatment effect from the study with the knowledge that the "true" treatment effect is likely different from that observed, secondary to a multitude of factors (i.e., confounders). To address this discrepancy between the point estimate and what may be a different "true" effect, a confidence interval is calculated. The confidence interval is simply a range of values within which the reader can be confident that the true effect lies. It is standard to use the 95 % confidence interval which defines the range that includes the true effect 95 % of the time, provided that the study was well-designed and executed with minimal bias [40].

Step 5: Apply the Evidence

The final aspect of a critical appraisal for a therapy article addresses the applicability of the results to patient care [41]. This can perhaps become one of the more challenging aspects of EBM since many well-developed studies work to minimize confounders by studying a relatively homogenous group, thereby limiting generalizability to a broader patient base. In assessing the applicability to patient care for a therapy article, there are three key questions to address:

1. Were those patients being studied similar to my patients?
2. Were all of the patient-important outcomes considered?
3. Are the likely treatment benefits worth the potential harms and costs?

The subspecialty of pediatric critical care in the specialty of pediatrics is a small and relatively new field. Although the amount and quality of evidence are improving, practicing evidence-based pediatric critical care medicine can be challenging, often requiring assessment of evidence collected in critically ill adult populations or non-critically ill children, and then determining if it is applicable to your critically ill pediatric patient. For the patient presentation at the beginning of this chapter, some questions have an evidence-base in critically ill children while for other questions, extrapolation from best-available literature must suffice until more studies specific to pediatric critical care are conducted.

Even in valid studies reporting therapeutic efficacy, incorporation of a patient and family's preferences and values is essential to the practice of EBM. How to elicit preferences of critically ill patients and their families and how to incorporate them into clinical encounters is a chal-

Table 16.2 Ten steps to changing behavior to implement evidence in practice

Start with a manageable problem and specify an achievable goal
Key ingredients: teamwork and leadership
Do an environmental scan
Develop a formal proposal
Understand the current behavior
Create a data collection system
Decide how to report results to your target audience
Select and introduce behavior change strategies
Reevaluate performance and modify behavior as necessary
Conclusion and the final step (or "move on to the next project!")

Reprinted from Cook et al. [48]. With permission from McGraw Hill

lenging frontier for pediatric critical care EBM meriting much further study [42].

Evidence-Based Clinical Practice in Pediatric Critical Care: Challenges and Next Steps

There are numerous challenges to practicing EBM in the PICU. As we have shown, learning the principles of EBM is a time-consuming but clearly surmountable task. Although evidence focused on critically ill children is still sparse, the amount of high quality evidence is growing. Most clinical interventions have a modest effect yielding a 25 % or lower relative risk reduction. This means that clinical trials powered to identify a reduction in mortality requires enrollment of over 700 patients per group or 1,400 patients for two groups even if baseline mortality is as high as 25 % (assuming alpha 0.05, 80 % power, 25 % risk reduction). Finding 1,400 children with severe sepsis or acute respiratory distress syndrome is a challenge even if 50 or more pediatric centers are enrolling subjects [43, 44]. Fortunately, research networks such as The Pediatric Acute Lung Injury and Sepsis Investigator's (PALISI) Network (http://palisi.org) [45, 46] are facilitating performance of trials across large numbers of PICUs.

One aspect of practicing evidence-based pediatric critical care medicine involves the assessment of whether we are actually doing so. The gap between the availability of strong evidence and the application of evidence in practice is huge. It is likely that as few as 20 % of effective interventions actually reach patients [47]. Changing clinician behavior is one of the most challenging aspects of implementing EBM. Cook and colleagues have developed a pragmatic approach and in Table 16.2 we list their ten steps for changing clinician behavior and implement evidence into clinical practice [48].

EBM is a paradigm shift away from the practice of medicine based on clinical expertise alone. Uninformed colleagues sometimes misinterpret EBM and accuse it of being "cookbook medicine" and potentially harmful to the patient. This is an uninformed opinion. Prior to widespread acceptance of EBM, developers of guidelines and protocols rarely graded the level of evidence underlying each recommendation. Knowing how strong the evidence is behind clinical recommendations allows clinicians to make informed decisions prior to application. It also helps to reassure colleagues that although clinical expertise is hard to define, one cannot effectively practice EBM without sound clinical judgment that comes from a wealth of patient experience.

Although our introduction to EBM has been brief, we attempted to highlight the foundational principles as well as the challenges to practicing evidence-based pediatric critical care medicine. One website developed to help clinicians practice EBM in the PICU and other specialties is JAMA Evidence (http://www.jamaevidence.com). This website includes learning tools, calculators, podcasts and education guides and contains links to other options such as applications for smartphones and PDAs. We hope that this brief introduction to EBM has supplied high quality sources for learning more about EBM.

References

1. Sackett DL, Rosenberg WM, Gray JA, Haynes RB, Richardson WS. Evidence based medicine: what it is and what it isn't. BMJ. 1996;312(7023):71–2.
2. Evidence-Based Medicine Working Group. Evidence-based medicine. A new approach to teaching the practice of medicine. JAMA. 1992;268(17):2420–5.
3. Sackett DL, Parkes J. Teaching critical appraisal: no quick fixes. CMAJ. 1998;158(2):203–4.
4. Oxman AD, Guyatt GH. Guidelines for reading literature reviews. CMAJ. 1988;138(8):697–703.
5. Pocock SJ. Clinical trials: a practical approach. Chichester: Wiley; 1983.
6. Lind J. A treatise of the scurvy. In three parts. Containing an inquiry into the nature, causes and cure, of that disease. Together with a critical and chronological view of what has been published on the subject. Edinburgh: A Kincaid and A Donaldson; 1753.
7. Louis PCA. Recherches sur les effets de la saignée dans quelques maladies inflammatoires et sur l'action de l'émétique et des vésicatoires dans la pneumonie. Paris: Librairie de l'Académie royale de médecine; 1835.
8. Lister J. Effects of the antiseptic system of treatment upon the salubrity of a surgical hospital. Lancet. 1870;1:40–2.
9. Doll R. Controlled trials: the 1948 watershed. BMJ. 1998; 317(7167):1217–20.
10. Medical Research Council Streptomycin in Tuberculosis Trials Committee. Streptomycin treatment for pulmonary tuberculosis. BMJ. 1948;ii:769–82.
11. Newman TB, Browner WS, Hulley SB. Enhancing causal inference in observational studies. In: Hulley SB, Cummings SR, editors. Designing clinical research. Philadelphia: Williams and Wilkins; 2005. p. 98–109.
12. Mahoney JF, Arnold RC, Sterner BL, Harris A, Zwally MR. Landmark article Sept 9, 1944: penicillin treatment of early syphilis: II. By J.F. Mahoney, R.C. Arnold, B.L. Sterner, A. Harris and M.R. Zwally. JAMA. 1984;251(15):2005–10.
13. Rosenberg DH, Arling PA. Landmark article Aug 12, 1944: penicillin in the treatment of meningitis. By D.H.Rosenberg and P.A.Arling. JAMA. 1984;251(14):1870–6.

14. Maio LL. Gastric freezing: an example of the evaluation and medicine therapy by randomized clinical trials. In: Bunker JP, Barnes BA, Mosteller F, editors. Costs, risks & benefits of surgery. New York: Oxford; 1977. p. 198–211.

15. Wangensteen OH, Peter ET, Nicoloff DM, Walder AI, Sosin H, Bernstein EF. Achieving "physiological gastrectomy" by gastric freezing. A preliminary report of an experimental and clinical study. JAMA. 1962;180:439–44.

16. Ruffin JM, Grizzle JE, Hightower NC, McHardy G, Shull H, Kirsner JB. A co-operative double-blind evaluation of gastric "freezing" in the treatment of duodenal ulcer. N Engl J Med. 1969;281(1):16–9.

17. Francis T, Korns RF, Voight RB, Boisen M, Hemphill FM, Napier JA, et al. An evaluation of the 1954 poliomyelitis vaccine trials. Am J Public Health. 1955;45(5, Part 2):1–63.

18. Meier P. The biggest public health experiment ever: the 1954 field trial of the Salk poliomyelitis vaccine. In: Tanur JM, editor. Statistics: a guide to the unknown. San Francisco: Holden-Day; 1972. p. 2–13.

19. Sackett DL, Haynes RB, Tugwell P. Clinical epidemiology: a basic science for clinical medicine. Toronto: Little Brown & Company; 1985.

20. Oxman AD, Sackett DL, Guyatt GH. Users' guides to the medical literature I. How to get started. The Evidence-Based Medicine Working Group. JAMA. 1993;270(17):2093–5.

21. Guyatt GH, Sackett DL, Cook DJ. Users' guides to the medical literature. II. How to use an article about therapy or prevention. A. Are the results of the study valid? Evidence-Based Medicine Working Group. JAMA. 1993;270(21):2598–601.

22. Guyatt GH, Sackett DL, Cook DJ. Users' guides to the medical literature. II. How to use an article about therapy or prevention. B. What were the results and will they help me in caring for my patients? Evidence-Based Medicine Working Group. JAMA. 1994;271(1):59–63.

23. Jaeschke R, Guyatt GH, Sackett DL. Users' guides to the medical literature. III. How to use an article about a diagnostic test. B. What are the results and will they help me in caring for my patients? The Evidence-Based Medicine Working Group. JAMA. 1994;271(9):703–7.

24. Jaeschke R, Guyatt G, Sackett DL. Users' guides to the medical literature. III. How to use an article about a diagnostic test. A. Are the results of the study valid? Evidence-Based Medicine Working Group. JAMA. 1994;271(5):389–91.

25. Laupacis A, Wells G, Richardson WS, Tugwell P. Users' guides to the medical literature V. How to use an article about prognosis. Evidence-Based Medicine Working Group. JAMA. 1994;272(3):234–7.

26. Levine M, Walter S, Lee H, Haines T, Holbrook A, Moyer V. Users' guides to the medical literature IV. How to use an article about harm. Evidence-Based Medicine Working Group. JAMA. 1994;271(20):1615–9.

27. Cook DJ, Sibbald WJ, Vincent JL, Cerra FB. Evidence based critical care medicine; what is it and what can it do for us? Evidence Based Medicine in Critical Care Group. Crit Care Med. 1996;24(2):334–7.

28. Guyatt G, Rennie D, Meade MO, Cook DJ. Users' Guides to the Medical Literature: a manual for evidence-based clinical practice. 2nd ed. New York: McGraw Hill; 2008.

29. Sackett DL. Evidence-based medicine. Semin Perinatol. 1997;21(1):3–5.

30. Doig GS, Simpson F. Efficient literature searching: a core skill for the practice of evidence-based medicine. Intensive Care Med. 2003;29(12):2119–27.

31. Haynes RB, McKibbon KA, Walker CJ, Mousseau J, Baker LM, Fitzgerald D, et al. Computer searching of the medical literature. An evaluation of MEDLINE searching systems. Ann Intern Med. 1985;103(5):812–6.

32. Haynes RB, Wilczynski N, McKIBBON KA, Walker CJ, Sinclair JC. Developing optimal search strategies for detecting clinically sound studies in MEDLINE. J Am Med Inform Assoc. 1994;1(6):447–58.

33. Haynes RB, McKibbon KA, Wilczynski NL, Walter SD, Werre SR. Optimal search strategies for retrieving scientifically strong studies of treatment from Medline: analytical survey. BMJ. 2005;330(7501):1179.

34. Haynes RB, Wilczynski N. Finding the gold in MEDLINE: clinical queries. ACP J Club. 2005;142(1):A8–9.

35. Cook DJ, Meade MO, Fink MP. How to keep up with the critical care literature and avoid being buried alive. Crit Care Med. 1996;24(10):1757–68.

36. Duffett M, Choong K, Hartling L, Menon K, Thabane L, Cook DJ. Randomized controlled trials in pediatric critical care: a scoping review. Critical Care. 2013;17:R256.

37. Kochanek PM, Carney N, Adelson PD, Ashwal S, Bell MJ, Bratton S, et al. Guidelines for the acute medical management of severe traumatic brain injury in infants, children, and adolescents – Second Edition. Pediatr Crit Care Med. 2012;13(Suppl):S1–82.

38. Kochanek PM, Carney N, Adelson PD, Ashwal S, Bell MJ, Bratton S, et al. Guidelines for the acute medical management of severe traumatic brain injury in infants, children, and adolescents– Second Edition. Chapter 8. Hyperosmolar therapy. Pediatr Crit Care Med. 2012;13(Suppl):S36–41.

39. Atkins D, Briss PA, Eccles M, Flottorp S, Guyatt GH, Harbour RT, et al. Systems for grading the quality of evidence and the strength of recommendations II: pilot study of a new system. BMC Health Serv Res. 2005;5(1):25.

40. Guyatt G, Jaeschke R, Heddle N, Cook D, Shannon H, Walter S. Basic statistics for clinicians: 2. Interpreting study results: confidence intervals. CMAJ. 1995;152(2):169–73.

41. Dans AL, Dans LF, Guyatt GH, Richardson S. Users' guides to the medical literature: XIV How to decide on the applicability of clinical trial results to your patient. Evidence-Based Medicine Working Group. JAMA. 1998;279(7):545–9.

42. Guyatt GH, Haynes RB, Jaeschke RZ, Cook DJ, Green L, Naylor CD, et al. Users' Guides to the Medical Literature: XXV Evidence-based medicine: principles for applying the Users' Guides to patient care. Evidence-Based Medicine Working Group. JAMA. 2000;284(10):1290–6.

43. Randolph AG, Meert KL, O'Neil ME, Hanson JH, Luckett PM, Arnold JH, et al. The feasibility of conducting clinical trials in infants and children with acute respiratory failure. Am J Respir Crit Care Med. 2003;167(10):1334–40.

44. Santschi M, Jouvet P, Leclerc F, Gauvin F, Newth CJ, Carroll CL, et al. Acute lung injury in children: therapeutic practice and feasibility of international clinical trials. Pediatr Crit Care Med. 2010;11(6):681–9.

45. Randolph AG, Wypij D, Venkataraman ST, Hanson JH, Gedeit RG, Meert KL, et al. Effect of mechanical ventilator weaning protocols on respiratory outcomes in infants and children: a randomized controlled trial. JAMA. 2002;288(20):2561–8.

46. Willson DF, Thomas NJ, Markovitz BP, Bauman LA, DiCarlo JV, Pon S, et al. Effect of exogenous surfactant (calfactant) in pediatric acute lung injury: a randomized controlled trial. JAMA. 2005;293(4):470–6.

47. Glasziou P, Haynes B. The paths from research to improved health outcomes. ACP J Club. 2005;142(2):A8–10.

48. Cook DJ, Wall RJ, Foy R, Akl EA, Guyatt G, Schunemann H, et al. Changing behavior to apply best evidence in practice. In: Guyatt G, Rennie D, Meade MO, Cook DJ, editors. Users' Guides to the medical literature: a manual for evidence-based clinical practice. 2nd ed. New York: McGraw Hill; 2008. p. 721–42.

49. Haynes RB. Of studies, syntheses, synopses, summaries, and systems: the "5S" evolution of information services for evidence-based healthcare decisions. Evid Based Med. 2006;11(6):162–4.

Catherine K. Allan, Ravi R. Thiagarajan, and Peter H. Weinstock

Abstract

As attention to patient safety and the contribution of human factors to medical errors has increased, the use of simulation has rapidly become an important tool to train clinicians at the individual and team level in a structured environment without risk to patients. Drawing on work done in other high risk industries, most notably the aviation industry, pioneers in medical simulation in the 1980s developed immersive simulation environments in which practitioners could interact with the patient simulator and the clinical environment, allowing trainees to engage in real-time clinical problem solving. Simulation has since been broadly applied in critical care medicine, with applications including multidisciplinary team training focusing on principles of effective teamwork, skills-based training, competency assessment and systems testing to identify latent safety threats. Simulation-based training programs are maximally effective when they are developed and delivered using rigorous, structured processes that adhere to principles of adult learning theory. Important components of this process include formal needs assessment, development of scenarios appropriately targeted to the level of the learner, and structured debriefing to aid learners in processing the simulation event. Recent innovations in simulation technology, such as development of high fidelity infant and pediatric-specific task trainers, are expanding the role of simulation in pediatric critical care medicine.

Keywords

Simulation • Patient safety • Medical education • Critical care • Skills training • Teamwork

Adverse Events and Medical Error in the Intensive Care Unit: Rationale for a Robust Training Model

The landmark IOM report "To Err is Human: building a safer health system" brought patient safety and error prevention to the forefront of modern healthcare [1]. Since that time, a mounting literature has broadened our understanding of the pervasive nature and causes of medical errors across acute care sub-specialties. The intensive care unit (ICU) environment - comprised of a multitude of technologies, large interdisciplinary provider teams, critically ill patients, high emotionality, and fatiguing work schedules – represents a particularly high stakes environment for human error and systems failures [2, 3]. This is compounded by the need for

C.K. Allan, MD (✉)
Division of Cardiac Intensive, Department of Cardiology,
Boston Children's Hospital, 300 Longwood Ave.,
Boston, MA 02115, USA
e-mail: catherine.allan@cardio.chboston.org

R.R. Thiagarajan, MBBS, MPH
Department of Cardiology, Boston Children's Hospital,
300 Longwood Ave., Boston, MA 02115, USA
e-mail: ravi.thiagarajan@cardio.chboston.org

P.H. Weinstock, MD, PhD
Division of Critical Care, Department of Anesthesia, Perioperative and Pain Medicine, Boston Children's Hospital, Boston, MA USA
e-mail: peter.wienstock@childrens.harvard.edu

ICU providers to rapidly and accurately integrate large volumes of complex data to make critical decisions. Such decision-making may be hampered by the increased cognitive load related to high levels of sensory input in the loud and chaotic environment of the ICU, potentially leading to human error and patient harm.

Studies of human errors and adverse events in the ICU highlight the danger inherent in this environment. Utilizing 24 h patient observations, Donchin et al. reported an average of 1.7 errors per patient per day, 30 % of which were rated as potentially leading to significant deterioration in patient status or death if not identified and managed promptly [4]. A multicenter chart review of 15 pediatric ICUs (PICUs) documented 1488 adverse events in 734 patients, with at least one adverse event identified for 62 % of subjects. Importantly, 45 % of these adverse events were classified as preventable [5]. Furthermore, analysis of errors and adverse events in the ICU has demonstrated that nearly half of factors contributing to critical incidents are related to non-technical skills such as teamwork and communication [6, 7]. Similarly, studies of teams involved in both actual and simulated resuscitations [8–10] have demonstrated the positive impact of effective leadership; teams lead by individuals who are able to organize a team, avoid task fixation, and voice a mental model for the event had improved performance measured by indicators such as hands on time when providing chest compressions and time to defibrillation following recognition of ventricular fibrillation. These performance indicators are clinically important given that early defibrillation and increased CPR fraction have both been associated with improved survival following cardiac arrest [11–13]. The importance of specific teamwork skills has been acknowledged in recent resuscitation guidelines from the American Heart Association, including Pediatric Advanced Life Support Guidelines [14]. Thus, incorporating multidisciplinary teamwork training into ICU teaching curriculum may help decrease preventable non-technical errors and may improve ICU patient outcomes.

Heritage of Medical Simulation as a Tool to Mitigate Human Error

High stakes industries outside of medicine, including aviation and nuclear power, have long appreciated that human factors, including gaps in teamwork, contribute substantially to accidents and catastrophic failures. As a result, these industries have responded by investing heavily in simulation-based training. In commercial and military aviation, simulation-based teamwork training is a mandatory aspect of maintenance of certification. Given the growing appreciation of the role of human factors in patient safety, it is perhaps not surprising that the lessons of the aviation industry have been transferred to medical training. Indeed, since the introduction of immersive simulation in the late 1980s [15], simulation has been applied broadly among both acute and non-acute care areas of medicine [16–18] – covering the gamut of applications – including clinical skills, competency assessment, teamwork training, as well as rapid cycle improvement via identification of latent system safety threats at the point of clinical care delivery.

Simulation has particular appeal in pediatrics, a field in which high risk crisis events, such as cardiopulmonary arrests, are relatively infrequent [19]. Low event rates, though an overall positive marker of child health, create a "pediatric training paradox [20]," leading to an unfavorable "volume-outcome relationship" and hence high rates of ill-prepared providers when it comes to pediatric resuscitation [21–23]. In addition, current pressures in health care education, including work-hour restrictions [24] and low thresholds for senior physician involvement have placed limitations on trainee experience as well as opportunities for feedback, that may potentially delay the acquisition of clinical proficiency prior to completion of clinical training. Simulation can overcome these limitations by providing on-demand, structured experiences across the gamut of training, practice, immediate feedback and assessment all at the 'simulated bedside'.

Early forays into medical simulation were predominantly directed at using human patient simulators to teach technical skills. The earliest computer-controlled physiology simulator, Sim One, was designed to teach intubation skills to anesthesia residents [15]. Also developed in the late 1960s, the Harvey Cardiology Patient Simulator was a part task trainer designed to teach skills in examination of the cardiovascular system [25]. It wasn't until the 1980s that one of the early precursors of today's high fidelity physiology-based patient manikin simulators was created by David Gaba and colleagues at Stanford. Gaba created a simulation environment, CASE (Comprehensive Anesthesia Simulation Environment) that utilized a commercially available intubation head and thorax as well as a series of computer simulators that interfaced with real operating room equipment (patient monitors, anesthesia machine, etc.) to realistically recreate patient physiology. Gaba's innovative environment was the first that allowed participants to interact in a realistic manner with the simulated patient, including providing medications, interpreting findings from clinical monitors, and using real anesthetic equipment, thus allowing participants to most fully engage in real time clinical problem solving [26]. In addition, Gaba recognized early on the value of the simulated environment for specific training around human factors. Gaba and his colleagues went on to adapt principles from the aviation industry to develop "Anesthesia Crisis Resource Management" (ACRM), a training program that focused on teaching effective coordination and utilization of resources to optimize outcomes from anesthesia crises [27].

Table 17.1 Fundamental principles of crisis resource management training

CRM principle	Key components
Communication	Use of names
	Closed loop
	Explicit
	Channeled through event manager
Role clarity	Clear event manager
	Explicit task assignments
	Frequent task updates
Personnel support	Identify and mobilize appropriate supporting personnel
Resource utilization	Identify and mobilize material resources
	Utilize hospital emergency protocols and procedures
Global assessment	Maintain situational awareness
	Avoid fixation
	Frequent team updates by event manager

This work was the foundation for teamwork training as we know it today.

Simulation-Based Teamwork Training in Pediatric Critical Care

Curriculum

In aviation, teamwork and communication skills are taught through a simulation-based program called Crew Resource Management [28–30], which is required at initial licensure and with every license renewal cycle for every commercial pilot [31]. Organizational psychology research in high risk industries has identified essential characteristics of effective teamwork which form the foundation of this training. These characteristics are defined by five broad concepts described by Eduardo Salas as the "Big 5" of team work, including team leadership, mutual performance monitoring, back-up behavior, adaptability, and team orientation [32]. These behaviors are supported by coordinating mechanisms such as closed-loop communication and the development of shared mental models. These principles have been widely adopted and, for the purposes of training, both the "Big 5" and coordinating processes have been translated into specific and measurable behaviors in high acuity medical fields, first by David Gaba in anesthesia, under the moniker "Crisis Resource Management" (CRM) Training [33], later incorporated into training programs in critical care [34, 35], emergency medicine [36], and surgery [37]. The principles of CRM include [33] (Table 17.1):

1. *Effective communication* – including the use of explicit, closed loop communication directed at specific individuals;

2. *Role clarity* – encompassing both leadership and followership [38]. Key leadership priorities include organization of the team through explicit task assignments, avoiding task fixation, and generating a shared mental model for the management of the crisis event through frequent updates of global assessment. Followership includes taking on explicit task assignments, providing updates on progression of task completion and offering assistance or information to the event manager including against an authority gradient;

3. *Personnel support* – including identification, mobilization, and appropriate utilization of personnel resources, including expert consultants.

4. *Resource utilization* – referring to a working knowledge and ability to apply hospital emergency procedures and protocols and to mobilize material resources necessary for successful event navigation;

5. *Global assessment* – traditionally a central goal and purpose of the event manager, global assessment, or *situational awareness*, is encouraged in all team members. Strategies include frequent reassessment of patient status, etiology of event, and treatment plans.

Delivery Modes

Early CRM training had been traditionally delivered at stand-alone dedicated centers. More recent iterations include on-site/hospital-based centers, along with an increasing number of "in-situ" applications, delivering the technology directly to the point of clinical care. Table 17.2 reviews the pros and cons of these different delivery modes. While both stand-alone and on-site Simulation Centers hold the advantage of dedicated space, and reductions in interruptions, "in-situ" simulation can enhance accessibility to full native teams. Additionally, in-situ simulation activities can efficiently capture nuances of the clinical environment and in so doing also allow for potentially valuable identifications of latent safety threats [20, 39]. Given the heterogeneity of the PICU, inclusion of CRM training in situ allows the opportunity to incorporate many scenarios that cover the spectrum of emergencies potentially encountered in the PICU and incorporate management strategies into the technical aspects of emergency event management beyond those provided by Pediatric Advanced Life Support Guidelines [34].

Outcomes of CRM Training

CRM training has become widespread in acute care areas of medicine such as the PICU. Several levels of evidence suggest that CRM training is effective in improving team function. In a meta-analysis of studies evaluating the effect of

Table 17.2 Pros and cons of various simulation delivery modes

	Off-site center	On-site center	In-situ simulation
Benefits	No interruptions	Accessibility	Convenient to full team
	Dedicated space	Convenient to full team	Lower cost
		Integration into clinical day	Accessibility
			Integration into clinical day
			Useful for systems probing
Limitations	Cost	Cost	Higher risk cancellations
	Travel	Space constraints	"Mixing" of clinical and simulation equipment
	Challenging to train full team remote from clinical area	Potential for interruptions	Exposure to patients and families
	Generic "clinical" space	Generic "clinical" space	

CRM training on team function [40], Salas et al. identified 4 levels of outcomes of teamwork training – cognitive (self-assessment of knowledge gains following training), affective (perceived effectiveness of team coordination and communication), behavioral processes (measures of communication, self-correction, etc.), and performance outcomes – and concluded that team training is effective in each. However, in this meta-analysis medical teams were relatively underrepresented, and studies reviewed were quite heterogeneous. Multiple studies cite increased self-efficacy/preparedness and comfort among participants of CRM training [34, 36, 41]. Behavioral processes are measured in simulator-based studies and have demonstrated improved performance of both teamwork-related skills and clinical skills following participation in CRM training. Thomas et al. demonstrated that interns who participated in a modified Neonatal Resuscitation Program (NRP) training with additional teamwork training exhibited greater teamwork behavior, including information sharing, assertion of patient's clinical status, and inquiry of other team members, compared to those who underwent standard NRP training alone [35]. Measurement of performance outcomes of CRM training, and in particular translation to improved outcomes at the patient bedside, have proven more challenging. Challenges include random/unpredictable nature of emergency events that makes debriefing of the events in a timely fashion difficult. Thus the opportunity to identify deficiencies in teamwork and its impact on patient outcome may be lost. Furthermore, issues related to patient privacy may limit retrospective access to patient information that can help in understanding the impact of team performance on patient outcomes during an event. Similarly, primary outcomes such as patient morbidity and mortality are susceptible to multiple confounding variables. Despite these barriers, a growing literature lends support to the notion that CRM training improves team function and improves delivery of care during critical events. For example, Morey et al. demonstrated a significant improvement in observed performance among emergency department (ED) teams from multiple sites who had undergone formal training as compared to those who did not. In addition, this group documented a significant decrease in observed clinical error rates in EDs in which the training was implemented compared to no change in error rate in EDs without training over the same time period [42].

Implementation of a compulsory team training program to a subset of operating room teams in the U.S. Department of Veterans Affairs (VA) system was associated with an 18 % reduction in annual mortality rate compared with 7 % in those centers that did not undergo team training and a similar decrease in morbidity [43, 44]. Likewise, a growing body of literature around obstetrical team training also supports the notion that effective utilization of teamwork principles correlates to improved delivery of care, and that simulation-based training can improve outcomes. Timely performance of critical medical interventions, specifically time between onset of seizures and administration of intravenous magnesium sulfate for eclampsia, correlated with effective utilization of teamwork principles [45]. Particular teamwork factors associated with improved clinical efficiency in this critical intervention included verbal declaration of the presence and nature of the crisis, use of closed-loop communication, and fewer exits from the labor room during the emergency, a surrogate for effective resource utilization [46]. Furthermore, clinical knowledge of management of obstetric emergencies, skills in the simulator setting, or attitudes towards teamwork and patient safety did not correlate with timely administration of magnesium sulfate [47], suggesting that these factors alone are not sufficient for effective team performance. The effectiveness of obstetrical teamwork training on performance in the clinical realm is demonstrated by a significant decrease in the interval between diagnosis of cord prolapse and emergency cesarean delivery from 25 to 14.5 min (p < 0.001) in the pre versus post-training era in a large maternity center in the United Kingdom which instituted service-wide obstetrical team training [48].

Simulation as a Teaching Tool: Principles of Practice

Simulation-Based Curricula Founded on Principles of Adult Learning Theory

Much of the appeal of simulation comes from its ability to afford individuals and teams opportunities for deliberative practice [49] of knowledge, skills, and attitudes, all within a safe and structured environment far from patient harm. Effective simulation-based teaching requires a rigorous approach to both curriculum design and implementation with each based firmly on principles of adult learning theory, formal needs assessments, and use of structured debriefing by skilled facilitators. Well-designed simulation-based curricula are designed to successfully capture/engage the largest audience of learners. David Kolb described four types of adult learners [50] based on two axes of learning preferences related to (1) knowledge acquisition (via *concrete experience* vs. more *abstract conceptualization*) and (2) knowledge processing (via *reflection* vs. *active experimentation*). Consequently, effective curricula engage each type of learner within a single setting by creating a so-called "cycle of learning" touching on each quadrant [51]. For example, an emotionally engaging simulation experience is followed by a structured debriefing focused on self-reflection followed by conceptualization and generalization of newly identified principles followed by application and experimentation with new learned concepts through subsequent simulation experiences. In this way, medical simulation is uniquely suited to "step through" the so-called Kolb Learning Cycle – from experiencing to analyzing to applying to experimenting and back to new experiences.

Simulation Scenario Design

Adult learning theory also dictates that curricula must be highly relevant to the learner, thus curriculum development should begin with a formal needs assessment of the participant pool and key stakeholders to assess prior knowledge and identify key training objectives. For multidisciplinary courses, such as team training, needs assessments should include representation from all disciplines that represent the native team. Simulation scenarios and didactics can then be built which specifically address objectives, or competencies, identified by this needs assessment. A structured approach to scenario design which provides explicit opportunities to observe performance related to these core competencies or objectives strengthens a simulation-based curriculum [52]. In addition, complexity of the scenarios should be matched to the level of expertise of the learners and to the complexity of the learning objective. For example, the degree of technical realism required may vary based on learner expertise. Activities focused primarily on clinical or procedural skills – "high signal" courses – may use simple skills trainers in a simulation lab to meet the learning objectives of a novice student learning a new procedural skill. A more experienced clinician who has already acquired basic knowledge of a procedure and some degree of automaticity may benefit from having the procedural skill presented in an immersive environment that closely replicates real life practice, complete with background noise and cognitive distractors which requires the clinician to simultaneously perform the procedure and attend to clinical decision making. Not only is such a "high noise" scenario unnecessary for novices, it may actually impair procedural learning at a stage when novices need to focus on mastering individual steps of a procedure. Similarly, higher "noise" scenarios are appropriate to target CRM principles for multidisciplinary teams of experienced practitioners. The ratio of "signal to noise" in a simulation scenario occurs along a spectrum from the novice to experienced practitioner.

During the design and implementation phase of a scenario attention must be given to the realism of the scenario. Realism has been divided into three separate spheres – technical, conceptual, and emotional – each important in the process of engagement of learners during simulation [53]. Technical realism, which refers to the degree to which manikins, trainers, and other equipment, replicate real life, may suffer from intrinsic limitations of technology. However, attention to simple technical details, such as utilization of equipment identical to that found in the clinical environment, may significantly enhance engagement even when some limitations of technical reality cannot be overcome. Just as the balance of "signal to noise" requirements varies for novice through expert practitioners, the degree of technical realism required for optimal learner engagement varies with level of expertise [54], and this should help guide utilization of costly resources for simulation.

Equally important to engagement, particularly for experienced practitioners, is the idea of conceptual realism [53, 55], which encompasses features of simulation related to theoretical frameworks under which clinicians practice or make decisions. Simplified, does the context of this clinical case make sense? Are the clinical events of this simulation unfolding in a way that is similar to what practitioners would experience during a real life event? A high degree of attention to conceptual reality may help maintain learner engagement when there are limitations to technical reality [55]. This attention to conceptual realism may be particularly important for expert practitioners. Finally, *emotional* reality refers to the way that learners engage or feel within the simulation environment, and is particularly relevant in more complex simulations that examine relationships, such as in team training programs [53].

Debriefing

Simulation encounters have been described as "the raw data out of which learning is created [56]." Simulation-based learning affords opportunity for practice without risk of patient harm, however, practice alone is not sufficient for performance improvement, but must be linked with opportunities for immediate feedback or debriefing either during or following an encounter with the simulator. Studies from both clinical skills and teamwork focused simulations have suggested that performance may not improve in the absence of structured debriefing or feedback [57, 58]. In a survey of European Simulation Centers, simulation participants regarded debriefing as the most important element of the experience, and indicated that a poorly conducted debriefing could be seen as harmful [59]. Similarly, a systematic review of studies of simulation-based education identified feedback as the most important curricular element [60]. Debriefing, as a core component of the total simulation-based learning experience, is evidenced by the development of multiple 'train-the-trainer' courses internationally as well as the requirement of faculty training for simulator program credentialing among several accrediting societies and organizations [61]. Additionally, tools for rating debriefing effectiveness, such as the Debriefing Assessment for Simulation in Healthcare (DASH) [62], have been developed with work currently under way to validate these tools [63].

Multiple debriefing methodologies have been described, [64–66], and despite subtle differences, each contains common elements (Fig. 17.1) [56]:

1. *Set and maintain an environment of psychological safety* [67] to encourage active self-reflection on the part of learners as the basis for practice change. Fundamental to this is the idea that the facilitator must present a supportive and respectful environment for reflection. Strategies to accomplish this include explicit outlining of the debriefing process, including learning objectives, the structure of the debriefing, and clear ground rules for debriefing such as respect and confidentiality around both the simulation and the debriefing [68].
2. *Assist learners in processing a simulation experience in the context of their prior knowledge and experience* [56].
3. *Help learners identify performance gaps and strategies to close these gaps* [64, 65]. Ideally, identification of strategies to close performance gaps will not be a fully prescriptive process, but will involve participants strategizing as individuals or as a team ways to change performance. Efforts are made to move the debriefing from aspects of individual performance in the simulation to more general-

izable principles of practice that are relevant and applicable to all learners [56].

4. *Provide facilitator and course designers with critical information about whether the curriculum, including but not limited to the simulation and debriefing, addresses the intended learning objectives of the course.* In essence, the debriefing provides important feedback for ongoing course development.

Optimal debriefing methodology varies based on learning objectives, degree of expertise of learners, composition of the group of learners, and time available for debriefing. Most debriefing strategies are built on a framework that leads participants through (1) a description of the event, (2) analysis of the experience, and (3) application of new learning to the real work environment. However, the way in which facilitators achieve this will differ greatly depending on the factors outlined above. Dismukes and colleagues [69] described three levels of facilitation that dictate the degree and manner to which the facilitator participates in the debriefing:

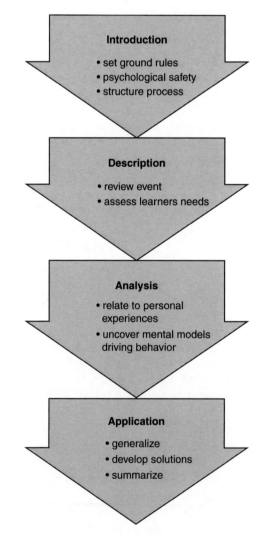

Fig. 17.1 Framework for debriefing in simulation-based teaching

1. *High impact debriefing* requires lower facilitator involvement, with the facilitator motivating the discussion with open ended questions and use of silence/pauses to allow for reflection, adding to discussion only when necessary. This type of debriefing is most often applied to human factor team training and is most useful when participants have both a high level of technical expertise as well as ability to be self-reflective, and when the group as a whole can reflect on the experience, analyze, and generate ideas for change. Facilitator techniques in this type of debriefing include use of open-ended questions and carefully timed pauses to facilitate reflection.

2. *Intermediate impact debriefing*, encourages participants to engage in independent discussion, but requires increased facilitator input to promote deeper analysis and understanding of the experience. Techniques here might include rewording or rephrasing questions in different ways to draw answers from the group or asking the same question of several different participants to uncover different interpretations or meanings and to facilitate discussion.

3. *Low impact debriefing* requires continuous facilitator involvement and is useful with novice participants engaged in focused "high signal" curricula (e.g. procedural skills, algorithms). Techniques here include pausing the scenario or activity followed by serial questions to lead participants through a step-wise analysis, recapping, and direct answering of questions for participants. The extreme of this approach might be considered frank *instruction*, in which direct side-by-side mentoring is used during a simulation when teaching novice learners procedural skills (e.g. IV placement) with minute to minute corrective feedback.

Applications of Simulation-Based Skills Training in Critical Care Training

Simulation-based skills training has a significant history grounded largely in surgical fields, with a significant body of evidence supporting the use of surgical skills trainers such as laparoscopic surgery trainers to support skill acquisition through deliberate practice incorporating rigorous assessment and feedback [70, 71]. As a result of recent work hour restrictions, as well as increasing oversight (both at the residency and fellowship level), pediatric trainees, particularly in high acuity environments, often experience limited opportunities for practice of procedures at the bedside. In this context, simulation-based skills training overcomes many of these obstacles and provides an important supplement to the traditional apprenticeship model [72]. While simulation-based skills training has utility and applicability in the pediatric critical care environment, broad applicability of this educational modality will be greatly enhanced by the continued development of pediatric-specific skills trainers that accurately replicate important nuances of neonatal or infant anatomy.

Resuscitation Training

Simulation-based studies have documented deficiencies in several crucial resuscitations skills among pediatric residents who have undergone traditional BLS and PALS training, including timely and correct performance of basic resuscitative measures such as bag mask ventilation, intubation, defibrillation, and provision of CPR [73–76]. Skills-based training has gained broad acceptance in pediatric critical care medicine, with many pediatric critical care medicine training programs offering a simulation-based skills and teamwork training program ("bootcamp") for fellows such as that described by Nishisaki et al [77].

Procedural Training

The efficacy of simulation-based skills training programs have been demonstrated in multiple studies relevant to critical care medicine. Simulation-based central venous catheter placement training curricula have been demonstrated to contribute to decreased CVL infection rates and increased proficiency in CVL placement by resident physicians [78, 79]. Sekiguchi et al demonstrated a reduction in complications from 32.9 % to 22.9 % in the 6 months pre-training compared to 6 month post-training period following implementation of mandatory simulation-based CVL training for all resident housestaff [80]. Placement failure rates also decreased from 22.8 % to 16.0 %, p<.01. Predictably, the greatest improvement was seen from the pre-training to post-training period among the least experienced providers. Previously, the direct application of similar training programs in the pediatric intensive care unit has been limited by the lack of commercially available pediatric and infant-specific vascular access skills trainers. However, recent efforts to overcome the limitations of commercially-available skills trainers in infant and pediatric populations have led to the development of specialized high-fidelity integrated trainers that address nuances of vascular access and anatomy in infants and children. For example, Allan et al. described a curriculum for teaching emergent infant ECMO cannulation skills to cardiac surgery residents and fellows using a novel integrated cannulation skills trainer in a highly contextualized environment with ongoing cardiopulmonary resuscitation. The study demonstrated significant outcomes in the simulator environment, including decreased cannulation time and improvement in a novel composite ECMO cannulation score technical medical aspects of cannulation management that were sustained at 3 months [81].

Airway Management

Simulation is frequently used as a tool to teach airway management skills [82], and some clinical programs require ongoing simulation-based training as an indicator of competency in airway management [83]. While multiple studies have demonstrated improved airway management skills in the simulator setting following simulation-based teaching and practice [84, 85], translation to improved patient care is less clear. Hall et al demonstrated equivalent performance on orotracheal intubation of patients in the operating room for paramedic students trained for 10 h using high fidelity simulation compared to those who performed 15 human intubations in the operating room [86]. However, Nishisaki et al. demonstrated no improvement in either first intubation or overall intubation success rates for pediatric residents who participated in a "just in time, just in place" airway management training module compared to those who didn't [87]. One salient difference between the two training programs that could account for translation of skills to the clinical environment by Hall et al. but not by Nishisaki et al is the substantially longer spent in simulator-based training in the study by Hall et. al. (10 h vs 20 min initial training plus 10 min skill refreshers prior to each call). No studies have systematically investigated the relationship between duration and frequency of training in the simulator and acquisition and retention of skills applicable to the clinical environment.

Other Applications of Simulation to the Pediatric Critical Care Environment

While the most common applications of simulation-based training are in the realms of team and procedural skills training, additional simulation-based curricula have been reported that may be highly applicable in the pediatric critical care environment. These include:

1. *Actor-based relational and communication training* (e.g. delivery of bad news and discussions of end of life care) to increase caregiver comfort and skill in family-centered care. A need for additional training around effective techniques for delivering bad news has been identified among resident trainees and more experienced clinicians [88–90], and residents cite less preparation and greater discomfort around delivering bad news in a pediatric versus adult setting [89]. The use of "standardized parents" with observation and feedback is a feasible means of teaching communication skills [91], and studies suggest greater efficacy than more traditional role-play based programs [92].

2. *Latent safety threat analysis* via high fidelity simulation delivered to the point of clinical care, both to identify latent safety threats in a clinical environment and to identify common practice deficiencies during critical events or procedures. Additionally, in situ simulation has been used to identify safety threats around implementation of new and high risk procedures in the operating room [93], prior to opening of new clinical care areas [94], and for low frequency, high-risk events such as cannulation for Extracorporeal Membrane Oxygenator (ECMO) therapy [95]. Studies of team and individual performance in the simulator have diagnosed pervasive deficiencies in key resuscitation skills such as initiation of airway management, defibrillation, and CPR performance as well as types and frequency of medication errors during resuscitation events [96]. Knowledge gained through these studies can be used to inform development of curricula and training programs to address deficiencies in knowledge and skills and to modify the clinical environment and care processes to enhance safety.

Conclusion

Medical simulation, via on-demand experiences well tailored to the adult learner within safe/structured yet authentic environments, offers new paradigms in the training and practice of pediatric critical care. The pedagogy provides unique opportunity for ICU providers to maintain skills and proficiency for managing infrequent but life threatening events and thereby has tremendous implications on patient safety. Simulation has been used effectively in a growing number of pediatric critical care domains, including teamwork, clinical/procedural skills and competency, as well as a robust quality improvement tool to identify deficiencies of practice and latent safety threats. Maximum effectiveness of simulation requires process-driven curricular planning and implementation that optimally leverages adult learning principles, taught by skilled facilitators. Future research should continue to work to uncover the impact on the quality, consistency and safety of care delivered to the patient bedside as simulation-based training continues to define itself as a new frontier in continuing medical education.

References

1. Kohn LT, Corrigan J, Donaldson MS. To err is human: building a safer health system. Washington, DC: National Academy Press; 2000.
2. Donchin Y, Seagull FJ. The hostile environment of the intensive care unit. Curr Opin Crit Care. 2002;8(4):316–20.
3. St. Pierre M, Hofinger G, Buerschaper C. Crisis management in acute care settings. Berlin: Springer; 2008. p. 234.
4. Donchin Y, et al. A look into the nature and causes of human errors in the intensive care unit. Crit Care Med. 1995;23(2):294–300.

5. Agarwal S, et al. Prevalence of adverse events in pediatric intensive care units in the United States. Pediatr Crit Care Med. 2010;11(5):568–78.
6. Reader T, et al. Non-technical skills in the intensive care unit. Br J Anaesth. 2006;96(5):551–9.
7. Reader TW, Flin R, Cuthbertson BH. Communication skills and error in the intensive care unit. Curr Opin Crit Care. 2007;13(6):732–6.
8. Cooper S, Wakelam A. Leadership of resuscitation teams: 'Lighthouse Leadership'. Resuscitation. 1999;42(1):27–45.
9. Hunziker S, et al. Hands-on time during cardiopulmonary resuscitation is affected by the process of teambuilding: a prospective randomised simulator-based trial. BMC Emerg Med. 2009;9:3.
10. Marsch SC, et al. Human factors affect the quality of cardiopulmonary resuscitation in simulated cardiac arrests. Resuscitation. 2004;60(1):51–6.
11. Christenson J, et al. Chest compression fraction determines survival in patients with out-of-hospital ventricular fibrillation. Circulation. 2009;120(13):1241–7.
12. Chan PS, et al. Delayed time to defibrillation after in-hospital cardiac arrest. N Engl J Med. 2008;358(1):9–17.
13. Ali B, Zafari AM. Narrative review: cardiopulmonary resuscitation and emergency cardiovascular care: review of the current guidelines. Ann Intern Med. 2007;147(3):171–9.
14. Kleinman ME, et al. Part 14: pediatric advanced life support: 2010 American Heart Association Guidelines for Cardiopulmonary Resuscitation and Emergency Cardiovascular Care. Circulation. 2010;122(18 Suppl 3):S876–908.
15. Cooper JB, Taqueti VR. A brief history of the development of mannequin simulators for clinical education and training. Postgrad Med J. 2008;84(997):563–70.
16. Eppich WJ, Adler MD, McGaghie WC. Emergency and critical care pediatrics: use of medical simulation for training in acute pediatric emergencies. Curr Opin Pediatr. 2006;18(3):266–71.
17. Yager PH, Lok J, Klig JE. Advances in simulation for pediatric critical care and emergency medicine. Curr Opin Pediatr. 2011;23(3):293–7.
18. Dull KE, Bachur RG. Simulation in the pediatric emergency department. Clin Pediatr. 2012;51(8):711–7.
19. de Mos N, et al. Pediatric in-intensive-care-unit cardiac arrest: incidence, survival, and predictive factors. Crit Care Med. 2006;34(4):1209–15.
20. Weinstock PH, et al. Toward a new paradigm in hospital-based pediatric education: the development of an onsite simulator program. Pediatr Crit Care Med. 2005;6(6):635–41.
21. Hannan EL, et al. Relationship between provider volume and mortality for carotid endarterectomies in New York State. Stroke J Cereb Circ. 1998;29(11):2292–7.
22. Hannan EL, et al. Pediatric cardiac surgery: the effect of hospital and surgeon volume on in-hospital mortality. Pediatrics. 1998;101(6):963–9.
23. Marx WH, et al. The relationship between annual hospital volume of trauma patients and in-hospital mortality in New York State. J Trauma. 2011;71(2):339–46.
24. ACGME. Approved Standards. 2011. Available from: http://www. acgme-2010standards.org/approved-standards.html. Accessed 22 Mar 2013.
25. Gordon MS, et al. "Harvey," the cardiology patient simulator: pilot studies on teaching effectiveness. Am J Cardiol. 1980;45(4):791–6.
26. Gaba DM, DeAnda A. A comprehensive anesthesia simulation environment: re-creating the operating room for research and training. Anesthesiology. 1988;69(3):387–94.
27. Howard S, et al. Anesthesia crisis resource management training: teaching anesthesiologists to handle critical incidents. Aviat Space Environ Med. 1992;63(9):763–70.
28. Helmreich RL, et al. How effective is cockpit resource management training? Exploring issues in evaluating the impact of programs to enhance crew coordination. Flight saf dig. 1990;9(5):1–17.
29. Helmreich RL, et al. Cockpit resource management: exploring the attitude-performance linkage. Aviat Space Environ Med. 1986;57(12 Pt 1):1198–200.
30. Helmreich RL, et al. Preliminary results from the evaluation of cockpit resource management training: performance ratings of flightcrews. Aviat Space Environ Med. 1990;61(6):576–9.
31. Federal Aviation Administration; Advanced Qualifications Program; Frequency of Training and Evaluation. [cited 2012 12/05/2012]; Available from: http://www.faa.gov/training_testing/ training/aqp/more/frequency/. Accessed 22Mar 2013.
32. Salas E, Sims DE, Burke CS. Is there a "big five" in teamwork? Small Group Res. 2005;36:555–99.
33. Gaba D, Fish K, Howard SK. Crisis management in anesthesiology. New York: Churchill Linvigstone; 1994.
34. Allan CK, et al. Simulation-based training delivered directly to the pediatric cardiac intensive care unit engenders preparedness, comfort, and decreased anxiety among multidisciplinary resuscitation teams. J Thorac Cardiovasc Surg. 2010;140(3):646–52.
35. Thomas EJ, et al. Teaching teamwork during the Neonatal Resuscitation Program: a randomized trial. J Perinatol. 2007;27(7):409–14.
36. Reznek M, et al. Emergency Medicine Crisis Resource Management (EMCRM): pilot study of a simulation-based crisis management course for emergency medicine. Acad Emerg Med. 2003;10(4):386–9.
37. Volk MS, et al. Using medical simulation to teach crisis resource management and decision-making skills to otolaryngology housestaff. Otolaryngol Head Neck Surg. 2011;145(1):35–42.
38. Cheng A, et al. Simulation-based crisis resource management training for pediatric critical care medicine: a review for instructors. Pediatr Crit Care Med. 2012;13(2):197–203.
39. Weinstock PH, et al. Simulation at the point of care: reduced-cost, in situ training via a mobile cart. Pediatr Crit Care Med. 2009;10(2):176–81.
40. Salas E, et al. Does team training improve team performance? A meta-analysis. Hum Factors. 2008;50(6):903–33.
41. Lighthall GK, et al. Use of a fully simulated intensive care unit environment for critical event management training for internal medicine residents. Crit Care Med. 2003;31(10):2437–43.
42. Morey JC, et al. Error reduction and performance improvement in the emergency department through formal teamwork training: evaluation results of the MedTeams project. Health Serv Res. 2002;37(6):1553–81.
43. Neily J, et al. Association between implementation of a medical team training program and surgical mortality. JAMA. 2010;304(15):1693–700.
44. Young-Xu Y, et al. Association between implementation of a medical team training program and surgical morbidity. Arch Surg. 2011;146(12):1368–73.
45. Siassakos D, et al. The management of a simulated emergency: better teamwork, better performance. Resuscitation. 2011;82(2):203–6.
46. Siassakos D, et al. Clinical efficiency in a simulated emergency and relationship to team behaviours: a multisite cross-sectional study. BJOG. 2011;118(5):596–607.
47. Siassakos D, et al. More to teamwork than knowledge, skill and attitude. BJOG. 2010;117(10):1262–9.
48. Siassakos D, et al. Retrospective cohort study of diagnosis-delivery interval with umbilical cord prolapse: the effect of team training. BJOG. 2009;116(8):1089–96.
49. Ericsson KA. Deliberate practice and acquisition of expert performance: a general overview. Acad Emerg Med. 2008;15(11):988–94.
50. Kolb DA. Experience as the source of learning and development. Englewood Cliffs: Prentice Hall; 1984.
51. Armstrong E, Parsa-Parsi R. How can physicians' learning styles drive educational planning? Acad Med. 2005;80(7):680–4.
52. Rosen MA, et al. Promoting teamwork: an event-based approach to simulation-based teamwork training for emergency medicine residents. Pediatr Crit Care Med. 2008;15(11):1190–8.

53. Rudolph JW, Simon R, Raemer DB. Which reality matters? Questions on the path to high engagement in healthcare simulation. Simul Healthc. 2007;2(3):161–3.

54. Curtis MT, Diazgranados D, Feldman M. Judicious use of simulation technology in continuing medical education. J Contin Educ Health Prof. 2012;32(4):255–60.

55. Dieckmann P, Gaba D, Rall M. Deepening the theoretical foundations of patient simulation as social practice. Simul Healthc. 2007;2(3):183–93.

56. Lederman LC. Debriefing: toward a systematic assessment of theory and practice. Simul Gaming. 1992;23(2):145–60.

57. Mahmood T, Darzi A. The learning curve for a colonoscopy simulator in the absence of any feedback: no feedback, no learning. Surg Endosc. 2004;18(8):1224–30.

58. Savoldelli GL, et al. Value of debriefing during simulated crisis management: oral versus video-assisted oral feedback. Anesthesiology. 2006;105(2):279–85.

59. Rall M, Manser T, Howard S. Key elements of debriefing for simulator training. Eur J Anaesthesiol. 2000;17:516–7.

60. Issenberg SB, et al. Features and uses of high-fidelity medical simulations that lead to effective learning: a BEME systematic review. Med Teach. 2005;27(1):10–28.

61. SSH Society for Simulation in Healthcare. Certified Healthcare Simulation Educator Information. Available from: http://www.ssih. org/certification. Accessed on 22 Mar 2013.

62. Center for Medical Simulation. Debriefing Assessment for Simulation in Healthcare © (DASH)©. http://www.harvardmedsim.org/dash.html. Accessed 22 Mar 2013.

63. Brett-Fleegler M, et al. Debriefing assessment for simulation in healthcare: development and psychometric properties. Simul Healthc. 2012;7(5):288–94.

64. Rudolph JW, et al. There's no such thing as "nonjudgmental" debriefing: a theory and method for debriefing with good judgment. Simul Healthc. 2006;1(1):49–55.

65. Rudolph JW, et al. Debriefing with good judgment: combining rigorous feedback with genuine inquiry. Anesthesiol Clin. 2007;25(2):361–76.

66. Zigmont JJ, Kappus LJ, Sudikoff SN. The 3D model of debriefing: defusing, discovering, and deepening. Semin Perinatol. 2011;35(2):52–8.

67. Edmondson A. Psychological safety and learning behavior in work teams. Adm Sci Q. 1999;44:350–83.

68. Fanning RM, Gaba DM. The role of debriefing in simulation-based learning. Simul Healthc. 2007;2(2):115–25.

69. McDonnell LK, Jobe KK, Dismukes RK. Facilitating LOS debriefings: synopsis of a training manual. In: Dismukes RK, Smith GM, editors. Facilitation and debriefing in aviation training operations. Aldershot: Ashgate; 2000. p. 26–49.

70. Larsen CR, et al. The efficacy of virtual reality simulation training in laparoscopy: a systematic review of randomized trials. Acta Obstet Gynecol Scand. 2012;91(9):1015–28.

71. Vassiliou MC, et al. FLS and FES: comprehensive models of training and assessment. Surg Clin N Am. 2010;90(3):535–58.

72. Rodriguez-Paz JM, et al. Beyond "see one, do one, teach one": toward a different training paradigm. Qual Saf Health Care. 2009;18(1):63–8.

73. Hunt EA, et al. Simulation of in-hospital pediatric medical emergencies and cardiopulmonary arrests: highlighting the importance of the first 5 minutes. Pediatrics. 2008;121(1):e34–43.

74. Hunt EA, et al. Delays and errors in cardiopulmonary resuscitation and defibrillation by pediatric residents during simulated cardiopulmonary arrests. Resuscitation. 2009;80(7):819–25.

75. Shilkofski NA, Nelson KL, Hunt EA. Recognition and treatment of unstable supraventricular tachycardia by pediatric residents in a simulation scenario. Simul Healthc. 2008;3(1):4–9.

76. Sutton RM, et al. Quantitative analysis of chest compression interruptions during in-hospital resuscitation of older children and adolescents. Resuscitation. 2009;80(11):1259–63.

77. Nishisaki A, et al. A multi-institutional high-fidelity simulation "boot camp" orientation and training program for first year pediatric critical care fellows. Pediatr Crit Care Med. 2009;10(2):157–62.

78. Khouli H, et al. Performance of medical residents in sterile techniques during central vein catheterization: randomized trial of efficacy of simulation-based training. Chest. 2011;139(1):80–7.

79. Barsuk JH, et al. Simulation-based mastery learning reduces complications during central venous catheter insertion in a medical intensive care unit. Crit Care Med. 2009;37(10):2697–701.

80. Sekiguchi H, et al. A pre-rotational simulation-based workshop improves the safety of central venous catheter insertion: results of a successful internal medicine house staff training program. Chest. 2011;140(3):652–8.

81. Allan CK, et al. An ECMO cannulation curriculum featuring a novel integrated skills trainer leads to improved performance among Pediatric Cardiac Surgery Trainees. Simulation Healthc. 2013;8(4):221–8.

82. Silverman E, et al. Nonsurgical airway management training for surgeons. J Surg Educ. 2008;65(2):101–8.

83. Losek JD, et al. Tracheal intubation practice and maintaining skill competency: survey of pediatric emergency department medical directors. Pediatr Emerg Care. 2008;24(5):294–9.

84. Binstadt E, et al. Simulator training improves fiber-optic intubation proficiency among emergency medicine residents. Acad Emerg Med. 2008;15(11):1211–4.

85. Goldmann K, Steinfeldt T. Acquisition of basic fiberoptic intubation skills with a virtual reality airway simulator. J Clin Anesth. 2006;18(3):173–8.

86. Hall RW. Simulation of electronic and geometric degrees of freedom using a kink-based path integral formulation: application to molecular systems. J Chem Phys. 2005;122(16):164112.

87. Nishisaki A, et al. Effect of just-in-time simulation training on tracheal intubation procedure safety in the pediatric intensive care unit. Anesthesiology. 2010;113(1):214–23.

88. Birkeland AL, et al. Breaking bad news: an interview study of paediatric cardiologists. Cardiol Young. 2011;21(3):286–91.

89. Dube CE, et al. Self-assessment of communication skills preparedness: adult versus pediatric skills. Ambul Pediatr. 2003;3(3):137–41.

90. Fallowfield L, Jenkins V. Communicating sad, bad, and difficult news in medicine. Lancet. 2004;363(9405):312–9.

91. Gough JK, et al. Simulated parents: developing paediatric trainees' skills in giving bad news. J Paediatr Child Health. 2009;45(3):133–8.

92. Bosse HM, et al. Peer role-play and standardised patients in communication training: a comparative study on the student perspective on acceptability, realism, and perceived effect. BMC Med Educ. 2010;10:27.

93. Rodriguez-Paz JM, et al. A novel process for introducing a new intraoperative program: a multidisciplinary paradigm for mitigating hazards and improving patient safety. Anesth Analg. 2009;108(1):202–10.

94. Geis GL, et al. Simulation to assess the safety of new healthcare teams and new facilities. Simul Healthc. 2011;6(3):125–33.

95. Burton KS, et al. Impact of simulation-based extracorporeal membrane oxygenation training in the simulation laboratory and clinical environment. Simul Healthc. 2011;6(5):284–91.

96. Kozer E, et al. Prospective observational study on the incidence of medication errors during simulated resuscitation in a paediatric emergency department. BMJ. 2004;329(7478):1321.

M. Michele Mariscalco

Abstract

While the clinical disciplines who practice in the pediatric critical care unit are increasing, this chapter focuses primarily on physician career development, because research for the other medical disciplines is currently limited… Nonetheless, many of the career opportunities discussed in this chapter are also available to nurse practitioners and physician assistants. It is important to consider a career in "epochs", recognizing that career expertise develops over time, and focus may change. Never before have had so many opportunities existed in critical care. It is the skills sets we use as intensivists, which help us develop, not only as clinicians, but as educators, basic scientists, administrators, trialists, implementation scientists, patient safety and quality improvement specialists, and medical informatics officers.

Keywords

Clinical skill • Career development • Work force • Team science • Quality improvement

Introduction

To develop a "career" in pediatric critical care medicine requires a base framework from which to begin. Practitioners of pediatric critical care come from very different starting points as pediatricians, anesthesiologists, surgeons, nurses, physician assistants. For physicians as of 2013, there is no way to become an experienced practitioner in our field, without entering through a general specialty. Throughout this chapter I will highlight areas which I believe are areas open for career growth. While there are an increasing number of nurse practitioners and physician assistants working in pediatric intensive care units (PICUs), the literature primarily focuses on training, and manpower, and little on career development [1–6]. We will need increasing numbers of nurse practitioners and physician assistants to help staff our PICUs, but we know little of how to attract them, help them grow as clinicians, and retain them in our field (i.e. support their career development).

Developing "Mastery" in Clinical Pediatric Critical Care Medicine

A successful career in pediatric critical care requires that you become a "life-long learner". Many individuals equate this with opportunities to "teach to keep up their skills." While many outstanding teachers are life-long learners, there are those who teach who are not. A framework for skills acquisition that describes development stages, based on the Dreyfus and Dreyfus model, has been proposed. This has been particularly helpful to describe development into a skilled clinician [7]. See Table 18.1. Careful review of the table demonstrates that caregivers in the PICU begin their careers at different levels of skill acquisition. While it is possible that a physician assistant or nurse practitioner may begin at the beginner or advanced beginner stage (see Table 18.1), most

M.M. Mariscalco, MD
Department of Pediatrics,
University of Illinois College of Medicine at Urbana Champaign,
506 S. Mathews Ave, Urbana, IL 81801, USA
e-mail: mmariscalco@kumc.edu

D.S. Wheeler et al. (eds.), *Pediatric Critical Care Medicine*,
DOI 10.1007/978-1-4471-6362-6_18, © Springer-Verlag London 2014

Table 18.1 Principles of the Dreyfus and Dreyfus Model of Skill Development applied to the development of physician competence

Level	Characteristics
Novice	Rules driven, extensively uses 'analytic reasoning'; cannot easily prioritize information, synthesis is problematic, big picture is often missing
Advanced beginner	Quickly sorts through rules and information to identify relevant information based on past experience; uses analytical reasoning and pattern recognition; can move from concrete information to more general aspects
Competent	Is emotionally engaged and feels appropriate level of responsibility; experiences permit use of pattern recognition of common problems; uses analytic reasoning for complex or uncommon problems;
Proficient	Intuitive problem solving as past experience permits pattern recognition; ambiguity is acceptable; decision making is easier and deviations from "normal pattern" is more common; less experience in management than illness recognition, thereby using analytic reasoning for problem solving
Expert	Open to recognize the unexpected; perceptive to recognize when features do not fit the pattern; intuitive problem solving as well as problem recognition; clever
Master	Exercises practical wisdom; deeply committed to work; emotionally engaged at the highest level and is greatly concerned for right and wrong decisions; pursues ongoing learning and improvement; sees beyond the big picture to the bigger picture of culture and context

Adapted from Carraccio et al. [7]. With permission from Wolter Kluwers Health

pediatric critical care physicians should be "competent" at the completion of fellowship.

The Dreyfuss Model proposes that clinical reasoning is dependent on two processes: (1) the analytic method, and (2) the non-analytic method, or pattern-based recognition [7]. The analytic method refers to the hypothetico-deductive approach characteristic of the scientific method. The pattern recognition approach relies on the learner's ability to recognize relationships between past clinical experiences and what is currently occurring. These patterns are referred to as "illness scripts". Learners at all levels use both forms of reasoning in clinical practice. As one progresses through the Dreyfuss Model of Skill Development, use of the hypothetico-deductive lessens, and more pattern recognition increases. Intensivists become "proficient" in their skill development somewhere between 5 and 8 years out of fellowship. This is dependent on their clinical time in the PICU, case complexity, and learning styles. A career clinical intensivist should expect herself/himself to become a "master" somewhere a decade or so after completion of her/his training (Table 18.1). Experts align thoughts, feelings, and actions into intuitive problem recognition and situational responses and management. They are open to the unexpected, are clever, and very perceptive in discriminating features that do not "fit" the illness script [7].

As highlighted by Carraccio and colleagues, it is possible to become an "experienced non-expert." In this case, the ease of responding to the majority of clinical encounters leads to clinician complacency, emotional involvement diminishes with each encounter. The "experienced non expert" is at high risk of burn out. The expert (or expert transitioning to master) takes the mental resources "saved" in applying pattern recognition, and reinvests them in tackling the next level of problem. The progressive problem solving pushes one beyond a prior zone of comfort and is the hallmark of a master [7]. A master has a deep knowledge and much practical wisdom to impart. They recognize the much bigger picture of context and culture, with an intense level of commitment to the work that triggers an automatic and ongoing concern for right and wrong answers. Emotional engagement occurs at every level for the master. As one is developing a career, it is important to partner with a group of individuals who are at least proficient in their care of critically ill children. It is easier to become an expert or master, if one can "model" from colleagues. However, sometimes one must look outside your immediate critical care colleagues, if you do not find an expert or master. While masters of critical care are usually outstanding bedside leaders, they may or may not be division directors or departmental chairs as different skill sets are required for those leadership roles.

Workforce and Career Development

There are currently almost 1,900 individuals who are American Board of Pediatrics-certified subspecialists in Critical Care Medicine [8]. Their average age is 49.2 years with a decrease in the number of clinicians who are older than 60 years of age. In contrast, there are over 5,000 neonatologists, their average age is 55.6 years, with many neonatologists working well into their 70s. This may be as a result of the relative "youth" of critical care medicine as a subspecialty (established in the 1980s) compared to neonatology (which was established in the 1960s). The majority of certified pediatric critical care medicine physicians practice in academic health centers (71 %), while only 49 % of neonatologists do so [9]. Of pediatric subspecialists, only hematology-oncology physicians have a higher percentage of academicians (77 %). The Future of Pediatric Education II survey was sponsored by the American Academy of Pediatrics and American Board of Pediatrics in the early 2000s. Of those pediatricians who responded, 805 were pediatric critical care medicine physicians [10]. These individuals spent more than 50 % of their time in direct patient care, and the remainder of their time in teaching (15 %), administration (12–20 %), and research (7–14 %). For most critical care physicians, the majority of their time will be spent on clinical service, primarily in the intensive care unit, and it is likely that the majority of physicians will remain in academic health science centers in the near future [10]. Tracking critical care medicine practitioners and their career paths is important, but expensive, and has not been done well enough to adequately inform education/training leaders.

Surveys from 2001 to 2004 demonstrate that most PICUs have 24 h physician coverage (>70 %) with most having intensivist coverage, the larger units ≥ (greater than or equal to) 19 beds had the larger proportion of intensivist coverage [11]. A 2001 practices survey demonstrated that up to 42 % of all large PICUs had in house intensive coverage 24 h a day [12]. Outcomes improve with 24 h intensive care coverage, and increased mortality associated with night and weekend admissions appears to be mitigated when pediatric intensivists are present 24 h a day, though more recent data may not be as supportive of that conclusion [13–15]. PICUs will likely be staffed 24 h a day with physicians, and the majority will increasingly be intensivists. The ideal number of intensivists is not known, but the number of children to pediatric critical care physician is twice that of children to neonatologist (43,981 vs 19, 262) [8]. Telemedicine has been used to enhance care under critical care physician oversight in nonpediatric units, though results are mixed [16]. Telemedicine has also been shown to be feasible in PICU's, but there is no evidence of its equivalency to in-house care [17]. Thus at a time when critical care physicians remain limited in number, there is an expectation that physicians will continue to have much clinical responsibility, with overnight and in-house responsibilities. However many are also expected to actively contribute to the missions of academic and non-academic health centers: clinical care, education, and research.

Maintenance of Workforce

Critical care fellowship training has a drop-out rate of about 30 %, which has remained fairly constant for almost two decades [8]. Physician stress and burnout are particularly problematic in intensive care medicine. In a study by Fields and colleagues from 1995, 400 pediatric intensivists were surveyed. Up to 50 % were "burned out" or "at risk" of burnout [18]. There was no association between burnout status and the following: having fellows, having protected time for research and publications, frequency of being called at home, frequency of returning to the hospital when called at home, or the call schedule [18]. Those who were "burned out" or "at risk" reported that their work was not valued by others,

they felt less successful, felt their peers viewed them as less successful, they were less satisfied with their professional life, and they were less likely to routinely exercise or have outside interests. Burnout or burnout risk is also present in large number of adult ICU physicians [19, 20]. While working conditions increase the burnout potential, individual doctors' attitudes toward work are also affected by personality and learning style [21]. In a study of 18–20 year olds in Great Britain, followed longitudinally for 12 years after applying for medical school, researchers found that study habits and learning styles during school were associated with perception of work-related stress, burnout and satisfaction. Stress, burnout and satisfaction also correlated with personality trait [21]. This provocative article suggests working conditions may have less of an effect for an individual physician on burnout risk, than their own personality traits and learning style. As burnout risk is so great for critical care physicians, further work in this area is particularly important for our subspecialty, and will require engagement of educational specialists and psychologists in addition to clinicians.

Leadership and Team Science in Pediatric Critical Care

Evidence is accruing that critical care teams that include physicians, nurses, pharmacists, respiratory and physical therapists have better outcomes [22, 23]. The business world recognizes and values leadership and management skills, but medicine has been slow to embrace leadership training. The American College of Graduate Medical Education now requires critical care medicine fellowships to have curricula on administration, management, and resource utilization. Despite that, few of us feel prepared to handle the many PICU managerial issues. Most report feeling underprepared to manage team conflict, conflict with other groups, and effective stress management [24, 25]. Stockwell and colleagues examined attending leadership in one PICU, and scored these skills against achievement of patient goals. The older and more experienced clinicians had higher leadership scores. Those with the highest leadership scores also achieved the most patient goals [26]. The study highlights that leadership skills can be learned, trainees easily recognize good leaders, and good leadership skills impact patient outcome. Whether you will ever have a "managerial position" at your institution is actually not the point. All intensive care physicians should understand and apply leadership techniques because they are expected to lead the daily activities of the team [22].

The overarching principle of ICU management is building a culture in which all team members feel respected and empowered to participate. There is a list of well-described leadership styles, many of which are "situation- appropriate" [27].

For example an autocratic style (i.e. "top down") is appropriate when leading a resuscitation team, but not when trying to redesign a patient flow initiative, when a consensus-driven or "democratic" style is required. "Transformational" leaders do not simply direct individuals to complete tasks (as occurs with "transactional" leaders); rather they seek to empower team mates. This reinforces the team shared mission. Providing psychological safety leads to team member engagement and a willingness to "speak up" when there is a failure. The team leaders must be willing to hear, address/solve problems and then broadcast the results. This creates positive reinforcement for team members to continue to provide feedback. Transactive memory involves the division and coordination of responsibilities among team members, and appreciation of what each member brings to the team. Mutual accountability is the reciprocity of responsibility, i.e. tasks or obligations are not identical for each team member, but each member expects others to remain accountable to the team. Will a nurse "speak up" if s/he sees an attending physician not complying with an agreed upon process? The application of team science is ubiquitous across high accountability organization. Yet it remains inadequately explored in the PICU. Three areas that deserve further examination and implementation are: (1) formal education about teams (2) mindfully building strong teams; (3) collection and dissemination of data on high functioning critical care teams [22].

Job Activity and Career Development in Pediatric Critical Care

As outlined earlier in the chapter, the majority of pediatric critical care physicians practice in an academic health center [9]. This means that in addition to caring for patients, physicians will likely spend their time in other missions of academic health centers including teaching, research, and administration. There are misconceptions that physicians who work in "private practice" cannot/do not work at academic health centers or those who work in community health centers do not engage in any of the "traditional" missions of academic health centers. While there is a perception that academicians make substantially less than private practitioners, this again is a misconception, and depends on location, and institution. There should be an expectation that programs/institutions measure physician performance individually, and as a group. "Productivity" can and should be tied to "compensation", as in any business. At the Hospital for Sick Children (HSC) in Toronto, there has been a practice plan in place for most of the last 15 years to provide compensation and career development for all three missions in the Department of Pediatrics known as the Career Development and Compensation Plan (CDCP) [28]. HSC has developed six job activity profiles under the titles of "Clinician -Specialist, -Administrator, -Investigator, -Scientist, -Educator, -Teacher", with varying amounts of time dedicated to education, research, administration, and advancing clinical excellence [28]. With annual Departmental reviews (which determines annual financial bonus), and tri-annual peer review (which determines changes in guaranteed base salary), departmental members are compared "using the same stick" to themselves and other members of the department. HSC has now evaluated this pay for performance three times. There have been program modifications over the years, but it continues to have wide department support [29–31].

Intensivist as Educator

You cannot be an expert critical care practitioner without excellent communication skills. We often hone our "education" skills as we learn to improve our "communication skills." If you are in critical care medicine, you will be educating throughout your whole career, either formally or informally. Through residency and fellowship, there is an opportunity to increase teaching skills, with different level trainees. In addition generally there are "teaching" courses that are offered during fellowship. Almost every academic health center/medical school has an education group responsible for providing educational training opportunities, so these will likely be available to you even after fellowship training. As outlined in the previous section, you should receive compensation for the education you provide to trainees [28]. If your career path is as a clinician-teacher or clinician-educator, you will be expected to expend significant time to the education of trainees and others. For individuals who wish a major commitment to education administration and educational development or research in education, you should consider formal courses that lead to a Masters in Medical Education. There are workshops sponsored by the American Academy of Pediatrics, Accreditation Council for Graduate Medical Education, Association of American Medical Colleges, and the Pediatric Academic societies at their national meetings. Most departments will require an "educational portfolio" for promotion or evidence of productivity. So, early in your career, seek out what information that should be included in the portfolio, and add to the portfolio regularly. Keep a record of all learner evaluations in the portfolio, as invariably promotion or productivity quotas require you to have evidence that you have incorporated feedback into your educational activities. Many critical care physicians are the directors and associate directors of pediatric house staff education. If you wish to move your career along this path, visit the Association of Pediatric Program Directors web site and explore professional educational opportunities [32]. As residency clinical hours continue to decrease and as we look to build new teams of individuals (and train in those teams) there are significant opportunities to explore/study new models of care, training and evaluation [33–36].

RESEARCH…research…Translational Research and Implementation Science… and Mentoring

As pediatric subspecialists, we should improve the care of children. There have never been so many opportunities to do so, than at present. There has been a seismic shift in the definition of "research" over the last 15–20 years. While discoveries still begin "at the bench" with basic investigations at the molecular and cellular level, there is a new (renewed?) focus on translating the finding to the bedside (bench to bedside) which then "re-informs" studies at the bench. This is referred to often as "translational" research (or T1). T1 research requires input from specialists in molecular biology, genetics, and other basic sciences. However T1 research cannot occur in isolation. It also requires input from expert clinicians and individuals with "trial expertise" (or trialist) to ensure that new discoveries are brought to the patients. This has been the focus of the National Institutes of Health, with the development of the Clinical Translational Research Awards [37]. T1 Research has traditionally been the focus of training for many pediatricians, and the NIH is the leading (but not only) source of funding. If you choose to focus your career in this area you will require the following: (1) Time. This path requires substantial amounts of time and effort to successfully transition to a clinician/scientist. (2) Commitment. Commitment is needed by you, but also entails the commitment of your departmental chairperson, your division leader, your partners at work and your life-partner and family. These individuals are your support team. Pragmatically if your support team is not "behind you"…it is not going to happen. (3) Mentorship. Senior scientists are needed to help guide you initially. As you mature in your science, mentors are often replaced by "co-investigators", or "peer mentors". (4) Educational opportunities. You should search out courses that will help develop research skills. Many institutions have clinical scientist training programs (or a similar program with a different name). These programs provide training to clinicians who wish to become clinical scientists, often they are a master's level program. (5) Money. Your department should fund you initially. Nonetheless you should expect to obtain internal funding (from your school/health science center) or external funding fairly early in your career. There are specific funding mechanisms for junior investigators available from the NIH and professional organizations (American Academy of Pediatrics/Section on Critical Care, for example).

Another area of translation research seeks to close the gap and improve quality by "translating results from clinical studies (T1) into every day clinical practice. It is referred to as T2 research, and it occurs in the community and ambulatory care settings as well as in the hospital [37]. Skill sets required for T2 research are quite different than T1 and include skills in implementation science, clinical epidemiology, behavioral science, and informatics. The transition of paper records to an the electronic health record, and the incorporation of wireless technology [38, 39] provides exciting opportunities for research in evidence based care [40]. Funding opportunities are often sponsored by the Agency for Healthcare Research and Quality and non-governmental organizations. Work in this arena overlaps and in some areas parallels that of quality improvement and patient safety, often confusing clinicians, human subject committees and hospital administrators. Improving quality cannot occur without generating new knowledge. However comparative effectiveness research will not improve outcomes, unless they can rapidly be incorporated into practice. This requires a focus on health delivery research, a science that takes a systems view to improve health outcomes [41]. The Institute of Medicine called for a new "rapid learning healthcare system", to accelerate the generation of new evidence, apply and evaluate it. This shifts the paradigm from a "top down" approach, and instead incorporates all the stakeholders in the process: researchers, providers and patients [40]. The Patient Protection and Affordable Care Act created the Patient – Centered Outcomes Research Institute (PCORI). PCORI focuses on comparative effectiveness research which informs patients, clinicians, and purchasers in making health decisions [42]. While comparative effectiveness research is not new, PCORI emphasizes a "patient centeredness" approach.

What is clear is that there a plethora of opportunities for pediatric critical care clinicians to impact the care of critically ill children in robust, far ranging ways. However, this will require additional educational opportunities and new partnerships between hospitals and clinicians [43]. Opportunities to learn quality improvement abound, are offered by specific societies, large academic institutions (Mayo, Harvard, Columbia) and online courses such as from the Institute for Healthcare Improvement Open School [44]. As with T1 research, T2 work also requires time and mentoring. However mentors in this arena will more likely be industrial engineers, research psychologists with training in human factors, and individuals with expertise in informatics.

Mentorship is critical throughout one's work life, but particularly so during the early post fellowship years. There are several outstanding articles regarding the mentor/mentee dyad [45–48]. However, mentoring is not solely "senior clinician/scientist-younger clinician/scientist", it includes "peer mentoring" and a constellation of other relationships [49]. Healthy, helpful mentoring relationships are respectful of each other's times, and are focused, realistic and reflective. Mentoring relationships should benefit all involved. Mentors can be found in many corners of your health system and academic institutions. Mentors often are not physicians.

Career Development...beyond Pediatric Critical Care Medicine

As discussed above, burn-out is particularly problematic for intensive care physicians. As we are a "younger" subspecialty than neonatology and cardiology, it is not surprising that we have fewer practitioners who are practicing into their 60s and beyond [8]. What is unclear is to what extent the 'aging intensivist' is providing clinical care. Anecdotally, critical care practitioners are now counted amongst the leaders of academic and non-academic health centers, including chief executive officers, chancellors, and deans of colleges of medicine. In addition, we lead quality improvement, informatics and patient safety initiatives in health systems, and research centers in both large and small academic centers. It is unlikely that many of us began our career with these goals in mind. Nonetheless, as our clinical care naturally aligns our careers with those engaged in systemic and systematic change, and research to improve the care of some of the sickest it is unsurprising that many of us have followed these paths. However, we are just as likely to be authors and artists, and leaders for ethics committees and palliative care teams. Pediatric critical care as a subspecialty is a very big tent, and there are many opportunities to develop careers both aligned with pediatrics and critical care, and in many arenas that are tangential to our primary clinical focus.

References

1. Freed GL, Dunham KM, Loveland-Cherry C, Martyn KK, Moote MJ. Nurse practitioners and physician assistants employed by general and subspecialty pediatricians. Pediatrics. 2011;128(4):665–72.
2. Freed GL, Dunham KM, Loveland-Cherry CJ, Martyn KK. Pediatric nurse practitioners in the United States: current distribution and recent trends in training. J Pediatr. 2010;157(4):589–93, 593.e581.
3. Freed GL, Dunham KM, Moote MJ, Lamarand KE. Pediatric physician assistants: distribution and scope of practice. Pediatrics. 2010;126(5):851–5.
4. DeNicola L, Kleid D, Brink L, et al. Use of pediatric physician extenders in pediatric and neonatal intensive care units. Crit Care Med. 1994;22(11):1856–64.
5. Mathur M, Rampersad A, Howard K, Goldman GM. Physician assistants as physician extenders in the pediatric intensive care unit setting-A 5-year experience. Pediatr Crit Care Med. 2005;6(1):14–9.
6. Sorce L, Simone S, Madden M. Educational preparation and postgraduate training curriculum for pediatric critical care nurse practitioners. Pediatr Crit Care Med. 2010;11(2):205–12.
7. Carraccio CL, Benson BJ, Nixon LJ, Derstine PL. From the educational bench to the clinical bedside: translating the Dreyfus developmental model to the learning of clinical skills. Acad Med. 2008;83(8):761–7.
8. American Board of Pediatrics Workforce Data 2010–2011. https://www.abp.org/abpwebsite/stats/wrkfrc/workforcebook.pdf. Accessed 22 Jan 2013.
9. Freed GL, Dunham KM, Loveland-Cherry C, Martyn KK, Moote MJ. Private practice rates among pediatric subspecialists. Pediatrics. 2011;128(4):673–6.
10. Anderson MR, Jewett EA, Cull WL, Jardine DS, Outwater KM, Mulvey HJ. Practice of pediatric critical care medicine: results of the Future of Pediatric Education II survey of sections project. Pediatr Crit Care Med. 2003;4(4):412–7.
11. Odetola FO, Clark SJ, Freed GL, Bratton SL, Davis MM. A national survey of pediatric critical care resources in the United States. Pediatrics. 2005;115(4):e382–6.
12. Randolph AG, Gonzales CA, Cortellini L, Yeh TS. Growth of pediatric intensive care units in the United States from 1995 to 2001. J Pediatr. 2004;144(6):792–8.
13. Arias Y, Taylor DS, Marcin JP. Association between evening admissions and higher mortality rates in the pediatric intensive care unit. Pediatrics. 2004;113(6):e530–4.
14. Hixson ED, Davis S, Morris S, Harrison AM. Do weekends or evenings matter in a pediatric intensive care unit? Pediatr Crit Care Med. 2005;6(5):523–30.
15. Peeters B, Jansen NJ, Bollen CW, van Vught AJ, van der Heide D, Albers MJ. Off-hours admission and mortality in two pediatric intensive care units without 24-h in-house senior staff attendance. Intensive Care Med. 2010;36(11):1923–7.
16. Wilcox ME, Adhikari NK. The effect of telemedicine in critically ill patients: systematic review and meta-analysis. Crit Care. 2012;16(4):R127.
17. Yager PH, Cummings BM, Whalen MJ, Noviski N. Nighttime telecommunication between remote staff intensivists and bedside personnel in a pediatric intensive care unit: a retrospective study. Crit Care Med. 2012;40(9):2700–3.
18. Fields AI, Cuerdon TT, Brasseux CO, et al. Physician burnout in pediatric critical care medicine. Crit Care Med. 1995;23(8):1425–9.
19. Lederer W, Kinzl JF, Traweger C, Dosch J, Sumann G. Fully developed burnout and burnout risk in intensive care personnel at a university hospital. Anaesth Intensive Care. 2008;36(2):208–13.
20. Rama-Maceiras P, Parente S, Kranke P. Job satisfaction, stress and burnout in anaesthesia: relevant topics for anaesthesiologists and healthcare managers? Eur J Anaesthesiol. 2012;29(7):311–9.
21. McManus IC, Keeling A, Paice E. Stress, burnout and doctors' attitudes to work are determined by personality and learning style: a twelve year longitudinal study of UK medical graduates. BMC Med. 2004;2:29.
22. Manthous CA, Hollingshead AB. Team science and critical care. Am J Respir Crit Care Med. 2011;184(1):17–25.
23. Krupicka MI, Bratton SL, Sonnenthal K, Goldstein B. Impact of a pediatric clinical pharmacist in the pediatric intensive care unit. Crit Care Med. 2002;30(4):919–21.
24. Gasperino J, Brilli R, Kvetan V. Teaching intensive care unit administration during critical care medicine training programs. J Crit Care. 2008;23(2):251–2.
25. Stockwell DC, Pollack MM, Turenne WM, Slonim AD. Leadership and management training of pediatric intensivists: how do we gain our skills? Pediatr Crit Care Med. 2005;6(6):665–70.
26. Stockwell DC, Slonim AD, Pollack MM. Physician team management affects goal achievement in the intensive care unit. Pediatr Crit Care Med. 2007;8(6):540–5.
27. Bass BM. Bass and Stogdill's handbook of leadership: theory, research and managerial application. New York: Free Press; 1990.
28. O'Brodovich H. Career development and compensation: strategies for physicians in academic health science centers. A perspective from a Canadian academic health science center. J Pediatr. 2001;139(2):171–2.

29. O'Brodovich H, Pleinys R, Laxer R, Tallett S, Rosenblum N, Sass-Kortsak C. Evaluation of a peer-reviewed career development and compensation program for physicians at an academic health science center. Pediatrics. 2003;111(1):e26–31.

30. O'Brodovich H, Beyene J, Tallett S, MacGregor D, Rosenblum ND. Performance of a career development and compensation program at an academic health science center. Pediatrics. 2007;119(4):e791–7.

31. Daneman D, Kennedy J, Coyte PC. Evaluation of the Career Development and Compensation Program in the Department of Paediatrics at The Hospital for Sick Children. Healthc Q. 2010; 13(3):64–71.

32. Association of Pediatric Program Directors. www.appd.org. Accessed 22 Jan 2013.

33. Cutrer WB, Castro D, Roy KM, Turner TL. Use of an expert concept map as an advance organizer to improve understanding of respiratory failure. Med Teach. 2011;33(12):1018–26.

34. Roy KM, Miller MP, Schmidt K, Sagy M. Pediatric residents experience a significant decline in their response capabilities to simulated life-threatening events as their training frequency in cardiopulmonary resuscitation decreases. Pediatr Crit Care Med. 2011;12(3):e141–4.

35. Thammasitboon S, Mariscalco MM, Yudkowsky R, Hetland MD, Noronha PA, Mrtek RG. Exploring individual opinions of potential evaluators in a 360-degree assessment: four distinct viewpoints of a competent resident. Teach Learn Med. 2008;20(4):314–22.

36. Emlet LL, Al-Khafaji A, Kim YH, Venkataraman R, Rogers PL, Angus DC. Trial of shift scheduling with standardized sign-out to improve continuity of care in intensive care units. Crit Care Med. 2012;40(12):3129–34.

37. Woolf SH. The meaning of translational research and why it matters. JAMA. 2008;299(2):211–3.

38. Asch DA, Muller RW, Volpp KG. Automated hovering in health care – watching over the 5,000 hours. N Engl J Med. 2012;367(1):1–3.

39. Mandl KD, Kohane IS. Escaping the EHR trap – the future of health IT. N Engl J Med. 2012;366(24):2240–2.

40. Bloomrosen M, Detmer DE. Informatics, evidence-based care, and research; implications for national policy: a report of an American Medical Informatics Association health policy conference. J Am Med Inform Assoc. 2010;17(2):115–23.

41. Pronovost PJ, Goeschel CA. Time to take health delivery research seriously. JAMA. 2011;306(3):310–1.

42. Selby JV, Beal AC, Frank L. The Patient-Centered Outcomes Research Institute (PCORI) national priorities for research and initial research agenda. JAMA. 2012;307(15):1583–4.

43. Levy FH, Brilli RJ, First LR, et al. A new framework for quality partnerships in Children's Hospitals. Pediatrics. 2011;127(6):1147–56.

44. Improvement IfH. Institute for Healthcare Improvement Open School. Webpage for Institute for Healthcare Improvement Open School. Available at: http://www.ihi.org/offerings/IHIOpenSchool/Pages/default.aspx. Accessed 22 Jan 2013.

45. Detsky AS, Baerlocher MO. Academic mentoring – how to give it and how to get it. JAMA. 2007;297(19).

46. Lister G. Mentorship: lessons I wish I learned the first time. Curr Opin Pediatr. 2004;16(5):579–84.

47. Lane R. Mentoring and the development of the physician-scientist. J Pediatr. 2008;152(2):296–7.

48. Ramani S, Gruppen L, Kachur EK. Twelve tips for developing effective mentors. Med Teach. 2006;28(5):404–8.

49. Balmer D, D'Alessandro D, Risko W, Gusic ME. How mentoring relationships evolve: a longitudinal study of academic pediatricians in a physician educator faculty development program. J Contin Educ Health Prof. 2011;31(2):81–6.

Genetic Polymorphisms in Critical Illness and Injury

Mary K. Dahmer and Michael W. Quasney

Abstract

Most genes are variable in their nucleotide sequence. How this variability might influence the host's response to critical illness and injury and contribute to the overall outcome is largely unknown. Yet this genetic variability may help identify critically ill children who are at greatest risk for poor outcomes and modify our monitoring strategies currently used in the pediatric intensive care unit. In addition, this variability may yield insight into certain disease processes observed in this vulnerable population, and may identify novel therapeutic interventions that may improve outcomes. The technologies used in examining genetic variability in populations are rapidly changing and able to examine a large number of variations simultaneously. Future studies using well defined disease phenotypes and large numbers of children will be needed to better take advantage of the potential of genetic studies.

Keywords

Gene polymorphisms • Genomics • Proteomics

Introduction

Critical illness and injury illicit a highly complex, yet highly integrated response that is influenced by a number of factors. While some of these factors are specific to the inciting stimulus, other factors are specific to the host. One of these factors is the genetic make-up of the host. It is becoming increasingly evident that while there are many similarities in the pathways that are either up-regulated or down-regulated in response to a noxious stimulus, some variability exists and that this variability contributes to the overall response and outcome.

The vast majority of nuclear DNA is identical from one person to the next; however, there is a small fraction of DNA sequence (~0.1 %) that varies between individuals. These variations in DNA sequence contribute to the diversity of our physical characteristics, our physiology, and to some degree, our personality traits. Genetic variability also appears to be involved with susceptibility to some common diseases and response to environmental stimuli, as well as therapeutic responses to treatment. Genetic variations may also affect the severity of some common illnesses, thereby influencing the severity of illness. In this chapter, we will describe the types of genetic variations that exist, as well as some examples of genetic variations that appear to influence the severity of critical illness that we encounter as pediatric intensivists. We will discuss how genetic variations may influence susceptibility to, severity of, and outcome from critical illness and injury. We will also describe how these genetic variations may help to identify risk factors for complications in patients in the intensive care unit (ICU).

Genetic Polymorphisms

Most genes in the human genome are polymorphic; that is, there are small differences in DNA sequence. The sites within genes where variation occurs relatively commonly

M.K. Dahmer, PhD • M.W. Quasney, MD, PhD (✉)
Department of Pediatrics, Critical Care Medicine,
The University of Michigan, 1500 E. Medical Center Drive,
F6790/5243, Ann Arbor, MI 48109, USA
e-mail: mkdahmer@med.umich.edu; mquasney@med.umich.edu

D.S. Wheeler et al. (eds.), *Pediatric Critical Care Medicine*,
DOI 10.1007/978-1-4471-6362-6_19, © Springer-Verlag London 2014

(allele frequency between 1 and 50 %) are referred to as polymorphic sites. Single nucleotide polymorphisms (SNP) are single nucleotide substitutions for another nucleotide and are the most common type of human genetic variation. They can be common within a population, and by definition, a SNP is a variant nucleotide present at a frequency >1 % in the population. This is in contrast to mutations which are genetic variations found at a frequency of less than 1 % in the population and, are thereby, rarer. Other types of genetic variations include insertions or deletions of various numbers of nucleotides or the presence of a variable number of tandem repeats (VNTR) of short, repetitive DNA sequences.

Polymorphic sites may exist in coding and/or noncoding regions of the gene. When the polymorphic site exists in a noncoding region of the gene, such as the promoter region, it may affect the binding of transcription factors, altering the transcription of the gene and resulting in altered levels of the gene product. Polymorphic sites may also exist at the intron-exon junction, or splice junction, and alter the degree of splicing of the mRNA transcript. Polymorphic sites in the coding sequences of the gene may or may not change the amino acid of the gene product. SNPs that change the amino acid of the gene product are referred to as non-synonymous SNPs. Genetic variations may have no effect on the function of the gene product, or they may influence the activity and/or level of the resulting protein and dramatically affect biochemical pathways and processes.

Techniques Involved in Genotyping of Polymorphic Sites

Early examples of the extent of polymorphisms in the human genome were demonstrated using restriction enzymes that recognize and cut DNA at specific nucleotide sequences. Analyses of the size of the DNA fragments generated by these enzymes on human DNA demonstrated that the size of the cleavage products differed between individuals. These restriction fragment length polymorphisms (RFLPs) are generally due to a difference in a single nucleotide within the recognition site of the restriction enzyme.

There are a number of methods that can be used to determine the genotype of individuals at a polymorphic site of interest and whether the individuals are homozygous or heterozygous. Almost all these methods require amplification of the fragment of DNA containing the site of interest by the polymerase chain reaction (PCR) technique. PCR allows for the amplification of a specific region of the genome (in this case a region containing the polymorphic site) using small fragments of DNA that flank the

polymorphic site as primers for the PCR. More recently, with the increased interest in SNPs as tools for mapping genes and for candidate gene association studies, techniques for high throughput SNP genotyping have been developed. The underlying strategies for the newer high throughput techniques and the older more labor intensive techniques are both based first, on a reaction which discriminates which nucleotide is present at the polymorphic site, and then a technique that allows the identification of the product of the reaction. The chapter in the previous edition of this textbook discussed the older technologies of genotyping; however, we will briefly discuss here the basis for the high throughput techniques.

The first step in using SNP DNA microarrays is the fragmentation, denaturation of the genomic DNA into individual strands, and attachment of a fluorescent label. In Fig. 19.1, the two double-stranded copies of the gene (a_1b_1 and a_2b_2) have a polymorphic site at position -308, in which one allele is a guanine (G, on a_1) and the other allele is an adenine (A, on a_2); thus, at this particular allele in this gene, the individual is heterozygous. The microarray itself, commonly a glass plate, has many strands of very specific oligonucleotides (o_1, o_2, and o_3) covalently attached to the plate (upper right hand corner of Fig. 19.1). The specific oligonucleotides not only are designed to hybridize to the genomic DNA but specifically are designed to target the regions around the polymorphic site; hybridization occurs most optimally when there is complete hybridization. In this example, o_1 hybridizes to the a_1 strand while o_3 hybridizes to its complementary strand a_2. The oligonucleotide o_2 is designed to hybridize to another polymorphic gene not shown. In addition, the position on the microarray plate is precisely known for each oligonucleotide. The genomic DNA is then hybridized to the microarray. Those portions of the microarray plate where the oligonucleotides hybridize to the labeled genomic DNA fragments with the greatest efficiency fluoresce with the greater intensity. In this fashion, one can identify which alleles are present. High throughput SNP genotyping can also be performed using bead arrays and single base extension (Fig. 19.2).

In the last several years these newer high throughput techniques have been used for whole genome SNP analysis and are beginning to be used more commonly in studies of critically ill patients. These genome wide association studies (GWAS) are capable of genotyping over a million SNPs in a single assay. The bioinformatics and statistical testing required for such large amounts of data is challenging, but the potential rewards can be great. Recent studies have begun to use these techniques in critically ill patients [1–4], including adult trauma patients, in order to identify associations of SNPs with the development of acute lung injury (ALI) [3].

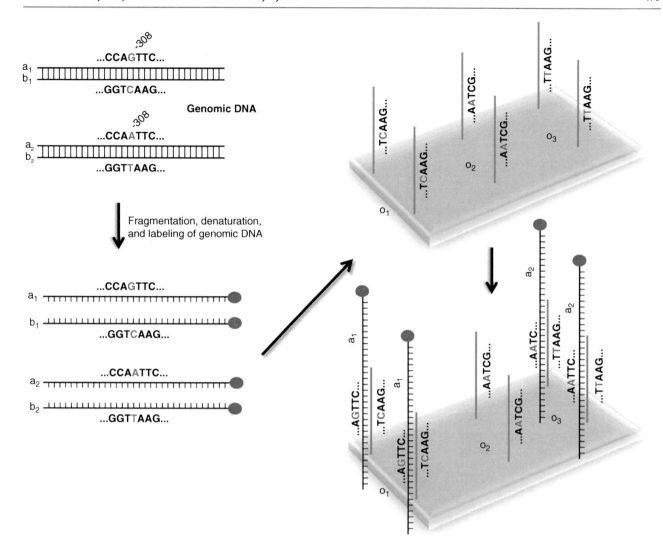

Fig. 19.1 Genotyping of polymorphic sites using DNA microarrays. Example of genotyping using microarray technology. The DNA containing a polymorphic site at position −308 (either a guanine (*G*) or adenine (*A*) is present on strands a_1 and a_2 respectively with either a cytosine (*C*) or thymine (*T*) on the complementary strands b_1 and b_2) is used as a template in a PCR reaction that incorporates a label indicated by the *oval*. Shown at the *top right* of the figure is the microarray with three different oligonucleotides, o_1–o_3, at three different positions on the microarray (though the arrays are usually made with >1,000,000 oliginucleotides) that are designed to anneal to labeled PCR products near polymorphic sites. The precise location on the array and the sequence of each of these oliginucleotides is known. The labeled PCR product made from genomic DNA is allowed to anneal to complementary oliginucleotides on the array as shown in the *lower right* of the figure. In this example, o_1 specifically targets one of two possible alleles at the polymorphic site on strand a_1 while o_3 targets the other allele at the same polymorphic site on strand a_2. Since both exist in the indicated sample, both regions of the array have fluorescence indicating that the patient is heterozygous at this polymorphic site. Alternatively, if the region of the array with o_3 does not fluoresce but the o_1 region does, the patient would be homozygous for a G at this site. The region of the array with the o_2 oligonucleotides did not fluoresce, and, hence, whatever gene and polymorphic site it was designed to detect was not present in the sample. By knowing the exact sequence of the oliginucleotides and their location on the array, >1,000,000 SNPs can be genotyped in this fashion on a single array

Influence of Genetic Polymorphisms in Sepsis

High inter-individual variability has been observed in the human response to pathogens. Most patients will recover and do well, while a small but significant portion will develop severe sepsis, and may develop multiple organ system failure, refractory hypotension, and die. This variability in the susceptibility to and outcome from sepsis, which is considered to be the most common cause of death in children in the world, has been attributed to a number of factors. These include the virulence of the etiologic agent and the length of time between onset of symptoms and initiation of treatment. However, the

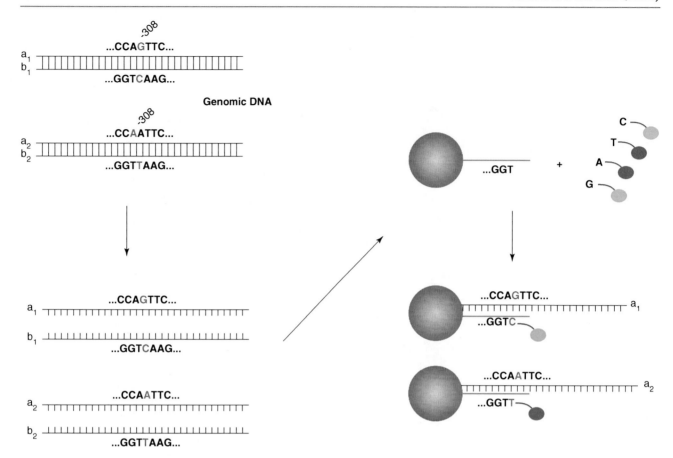

Fig. 19.2 Genotyping of polymorphic sites using bead and single base extension. Example of genotyping using probes attached to beads and single base extension. The genomic DNA contains a polymorphic site at position −308 (with either a guanine (*G*) or adenine (*A*) present on strand a_1 and a_2, respectively; and complementary strands b_1 or b_2 with either a cytosine (*C*) or thymine (*T*)). The beads each have an oligonucleotide probe covalently attached to them that is complementary to a region of genomic DNA with the specific polymorphic site of interest. In the example, the oligonucleotide ends in GGT and is one nucleotide short of the −308 polymorphic site. Denatured genomic DNA is allowed to anneal to complementary oligonucleotide probes on the bead array and the addition of a single base extension is performed using fluorescently labeled nucleotides. This allows for specific fluorescence to be detected on specific beads with probes for specific polymorphic sites. In the example shown the individual is a heterozygous (has one copy of each allele, A and G). Strand a_1 with the G allele incorporates a C with *green* fluorescence. Strand a_2 with the A allele incorporates a T with *red* fluorescence. A detector determines whether either green (homozygous G), or red (homozygous A) or both green and red are present (heterozygous)

genetic makeup of the host also appears to play an important role. For example, familial studies in which there were deaths due to severe infections demonstrated a strong genetic influence [5]. In this section we will discuss the evidence that genetic variability in specific genes plays a role in development of sepsis and its outcome (for reviews, see [6, 7]).

Genetic Variation in Genes Involved in the Recognition of Pathogens

The innate immune system plays a key role in the host response to pathogens and involves the early recognition of highly conserved pathogen-associated molecular patterns

(PAMPs) by receptors [8–10] and binding proteins. Both the recognition and subsequent response require many cellular proteins, most of which are polymorphic. Genetic variation within these polymorphic genes or their regulatory regions may influence the overall response to the stimulus by altering the number of functional receptors, their ability to recognize PAMPs, or their ability to transduce a signal through the cell membrane. Many of the genes coding for the proteins involved in these processes have been the target of candidate gene association studies.

Recognition of the stimulus, be it PAMP or other noxious stimuli, is the first step in the process. For pathogens causing sepsis, these receptors and binding proteins include molecules such as toll-like receptors, CD-14, lipopolysaccharide binding protein (LBP), mannose-binding lectin (MBL), and the Fcγ receptor (FcγR) genes (Table 19.1). We will discuss two examples of genes coding for proteins involved in the recognition of pathogens, the leukocyte Fcγ receptors and mannose binding lectin, in which genetic variations alter the ability to recognize a pathogenic stimulus and influence the severity of disease.

Table 19.1 Genetic polymorphisms in sepsis

Gene	Polymorphism[a]	Consequence of polymorphism	References
ACE	Insertion/deletion (I/D)	DD associated with increased serum and tissue levels; associated with more severe meningococcal disease DD associated with decreased risk of sepsis	[11, 12]
BPI	+545 G/C rs4358188 (+645 A/G, Lys216Glu)	Increased risk of gram – sepsis and mortality	[13]
CD14	−1145 G/A rs7524551 (−159 C/T)	Association with CD14 expression, MODS and sepsis Association with CD14 levels, MODS, sepsis, mortality, and gram – infections	[14–19]
FCγRIIa	rs1801274 (H131R)	Associated with decreased affinity to IgG_2 and opsonization; associated with increased risk of meningococcal and septic shock	[20–24]
HSPA1L	rs2227956 (−2437 C/T)	Associated with increased cytokine levels and liver failure but not sepsis-related morbidity	[25–27]
HSPA1B	(−1538 G/A)	Associated with increased cytokine levels and liver failure but not sepsis-related morbidity	[25–27]
HSP70-2	rs1061581 (+1267 G/A)	A allele associated with septic shock in adults with CAP	[28]
IL-1β and IL-1$_{RA}$	rs16944 (−511 T/C) Variable 86-bp repeat −1470 G/C rs1143627 (−31 C/T)	−511 allele associated with increased survival of meningococcemia; combination of IL-1β and IL-1$_{RA}$ alleles associated with decreased survival	[29–32]
IL-6	rs4800795 (−174 G/C) rs1800796 (−572 G/C)	Associated with increased IL-6 levels and risk of sepsis and severity of sepsis	[33]
IL-10	rs1800896 (−1082 G/A) rs1800871 (−819 C/T) rs1800872 (−592 C/A)	GCC haplotype associated with increased levels; associated with sepsis and some variations associated with mortality	[34–37]
LBP	rs1780616 (−1978 C/T) rs5741812 (−921 A/T) rs2232571 (−836 C/T) rs1780617 (−763 A/G) rs2232618 (26877 T/C Phe436Leu)	Severe sepsis for 4 SNP haplotype CATA; serum LBP increased and mortality for -836 C/T; Phe436Leu associated with sepsis in trauma cohort	[38–40]
TNF-β and LT-α	rs1800629 (−308 G/A) rs361525 (−238 G/A) Many others rs909253 (LT-α + 252 G/A)	Associated with increased TNF-α levels; associated with increased mortality in sepsis and bacteremia	[41–68]
MBL	rs11003125 (−550 G/C) rs7096206 (−221 G/C) rs5030737 (Arg$_{52}$Cys C/T) rs1800450 (Gly$_{54}$Asp G/A) rs1800451 (Gly$_{57}$Glu G/A)	−221 associated with MBL levels, sepsis, but not to mortality; structural variants associated with decreased levels and activity and increased risk of infection and severity of disease	[18, 69–74]
ND1	rs1599988 (m4216 T/C)	Associated with decreased NADH dehydrogenase 1 activity	[75, 76]
PAI-1	4G/5G	4G associated with increased levels; associated with septic shock and DIC in meningococcal disease	[77–82]
Protein C	rs1799808 (−1654 C/T) rs1799809 (−1641 G/A) rs2069912 (673 T/C)	CA haplotype (−1654 and −1641) and C allele associated with increased mortality in Asian populations; CG haplotype associated with more severe meningococcal disease in Caucasians	[83–85]
TIMP-1	rs4898 (372 T/C)	Associated with higher levels of TIMP-1 and higher 30-day mortality	[86]
TLR1	rs5743551 (−7202 A/G)	Associated with greater immune response, higher mortality and worse organ function	[87, 88]

(continued)

Table 19.1 (continued)

Gene	Polymorphism[a]	Consequence of polymorphism	References
TLR2	−16933 A/T	Associated with gram + sepsis but not survival	[18, 64, 89–94]
	rs1895830 (−15607 A/G)	Associated with cytokine expression	
	rs3804099 (597 C/T)	Associated with cytokine expression, MODS, and morbidity	
	2029 C/T (Arg677Trp)	Associated with mycobacterial infections	
	rs5743708 (2257 A/G, Arg753Gln)	Associated with increased severe bacterial infections, increased sepsis in African Americans	
TLR4	−2242 T/C	Associated with increased cytokine expression, sepsis-related morbidity, and MODS; gram − bacteremia; associated with increased risk of sepsis and mortality	[17, 94–96]
	rs4986790 (Asp299Gly)		
	Thr399Ile		
VEGF	rs3025039 (936 C/T)	Associated with development of AKI in patients with severe sepsis	[97]

ACE angiotensin converting enzyme, *BPI* bactericidal permeability increasing protein, *MODS* multi-organ dysfunction syndrome, *Ig* immunoglobulin, *HSP* heat shock protein, *CAP* community acquired pneumonia, *IL-1_{RA}* interleukin 1 receptor antagonist (GCC haplotype of the IL-10 promoter is defined by 3 single-site polymorphisms at −1082, −819, and −592), *LBP* lipopolysaccharide binding protein, *TNF* tumor necrosis factor, *LT* lymphotoxin, *MBL* mannose-binding lectin, *PAI* plasminogen activator inhibitor, *DIC* disseminated intravascular coagulation, *TIMP* tissue inhibitor of matrix metalloproteinase, *TLR* Toll-like receptor, *VEGF* vascular endothelial growth factor

[a]Terminology used for the various polymorphisms are the ones most commonly used in the literature and may refer to the nucleotide position, amino acid position, or name of the allele. This table is representative of polymorphisms examined in sepsis but does not include all such polymorphisms

Leukocyte Fcγ receptors bind to the constant region of IgG and are primarily responsible for the phagocytosis of IgG coated bacteria and subsequent induction of the inflammatory response [20, 98, 99]. The human Fcγ receptors are grouped into three classes which vary in their affinity for the various IgG subclasses. The FcγRI class consists of the FcγRIa receptor, the FcγRII class consists of FcγRIIa, FcγRIIb, FcγRIIc, and the FcγRIII class consists of FcγRIIIa and FcγRIIIb. Genetic polymorphisms affecting function have been described in some of the Fcγ receptors [20]. The FcγRIIIa has a polymorphism resulting in a change in amino acid 158 from a valine to a phenylalanine, which in turn affects its affinity for IgG_1, IgG_3 and IgG_4 [100, 101]. The gene coding for FcγRIIIb has a polymorphism that results in a four amino acid substitution (allotypes FcγRIIIb-NA1 or -NA2) resulting in differences in glycosylation [102]. This substitution alters the opsonization efficiency required for phagocytosis of IgG_1 and IgG_3-opsonized particles [103, 104]. Individuals homozygous for the FcγRIIIb-NA1 allotype appear to have more efficient phagocytosis. The FcγRIIa gene has a polymorphic site resulting in a variation of the amino acid at position 131; either a histidine (FcγRIIa-H131) or an arginine (FcγRIIa-R131) is present [105, 106]. This amino acid is in the extracellular domain of the receptor, and the FcγRIIa-R131 allotype binds the Fc portion of IgG_2 with lower affinity than the more common FcγRIIa-H131 allotype [106]. In vitro studies have demonstrated reduced phagocytosis of IgG_2 opsonized particles in cells from individuals homozygous for FcγRIIa-R131 compared to cells from individuals homozygous for FcγRIIa-H131 [107, 108]. IgG_2 is the main antibody subtype directed against encapsulated bacteria such as

Streptococcus pneumoniae, Haemophilus influenzae type b, and *Neisseria meningitides* and plays an important role in their phagocytosis [106, 109, 110]. Most gene association studies have demonstrated higher frequencies of the FcγRIIa-R131/R131 or FcγRIIIb-NA2/NA2 genotypes in patients with meningococcal disease [21–24, 111, 112] particularly in patients with severe meningococcal disease [23, 24] or fulminant meningococcal septic shock [21, 22] when compared with a healthy control population, though this finding is not entirely consistent [113, 114]. Associations between the FcγRIIa polymorphism and infection with other encapsulated bacteria or in patients with pneumonia have also been reported, though the associations are not always with the same allele [115–118]. Thus, genetic variations in the genes coding for at least two of the Fcγ receptors appear to influence the susceptibility to and outcome from certain infections.

Mannose binding lectin binds to surface oligosaccharides N-acetyl glucosamine and mannose on a number of different bacteria activating complement and acting as an opsonin that enhances phagocytosis. The heterotrimeric MBL protein contains a carbohydrate binding domain and a helical tail domain that is important in polymerization of the three peptides [119]. Polymerization of the heterotrimer is crucial for the stability of MBL. Three genetic variants have been described in the first exon of MBL that alter amino acids at positions 52, 54 and 57 and result in a diminished ability of the helical tails to polymerize. This results in an increased degradation of MBL [120–122] and reduced serum levels of MBL [122, 123]. Variants also exist in the promoter region that influence serum levels of MBL. Studies have demonstrated associations between these variants and increased susceptibility to infections in a number of cohorts, including children [69, 70, 124–128]. A recent systematic review demonstrated that genetic polymorphisms in the gene coding for MBL increase the susceptibility to pneumococcal and meningococcal diseases [29]. High risk alleles also appear to be independently associated with in-hospital and 90-day mortality and development of septic shock [71]. Thus, genetic variations in genes coding for receptors and binding proteins for pathogens appear to influence not only the susceptibility to infection but also the severity of and outcome from infection.

Genetic Variation in Genes Involved in the Response to Pathogens and Other Stimuli

TNF-α plays a key role in the biology and pathobiology of the innate immune response. As a pro-inflammatory cytokine, it contributes to further activation of the inflammatory response, and yet it also contributes to the development of the harmful effects of the response such as capillary leak, hypotension, acute respiratory distress syndrome (ARDS), and multiple organ system failure [129–133]. The pro-inflammatory effects of TNF-α are balanced by anti-inflammatory cytokines such as IL-10 [134–138]. An imbalance in these responses favoring a more exaggerated pro-inflammatory response contributes to the clinical manifestation of severe sepsis and septic shock. The mechanism by which this imbalance occurs leading to an exaggerated response may involve a high inoculum of pathogen, an ability of the pathogen to evade host defenses, or a delay in therapy. However, host genetic variability within genes coding for the pro-inflammatory and anti-inflammatory cytokines also affect this balance and could potentially influence the overall susceptibility to and outcome from the sepsis.

The genetic variants within the regulatory regions of the gene coding for TNF-α are perhaps the most extensively studied of all cytokines. Several single nucleotide polymorphisms located in the regulatory region of the gene coding for TNF-α have been identified that affect TNF-α production [41, 42, 139–144]. The most studied are the G to A transitions 308 and 238 base pairs upstream from the transcriptional start site for the TNF-α gene. In vitro studies have demonstrated that the rarer TNF-α−308A allele is associated with increased transcription [142] and increased secretion of TNF-α from LPS-stimulated macrophages [144] compared with the more common TNF-α−308G allele. In contrast, the more common TNF-α−238G allele is associated with higher TNF-α production in vitro compared with the rarer TNF-α−238A allele [145]. These polymorphisms lie near putative DNA binding sites for several transcription factors, and allele-specific binding of transcription factors has been

demonstrated [146–148]. Another polymorphism associated with higher levels of TNF-α is approximately 252 base pairs downstream from the transcriptional start site for the gene coding for lymphotoxin alpha (LT-α, also known as TNF-β) and approximately 3.2 kilobases upstream from the TNF-α gene [42, 140, 141]. This region either acts as an enhancer for the TNF-α gene or it is linked to a regulatory region further downstream. Thus, genetic variations in the regulatory regions of the gene coding for TNF-α influence the amount of TNF-α produced most likely through transcriptional regulatory mechanisms.

Many genetic association studies have examined the impact of TNF-α polymorphisms on the clinical presentation and/or outcome in sepsis [41–65, 141, 149]. A higher frequency of the TNF-α−308A allele has been demonstrated in adults who died from septic shock [44] and in children who died from meningococcal disease [149]. Even those children who are heterozygous at this position (TNF-α−308 G/A) appear to be at increased risk for more fulminant meningococcal disease and death compared with those children who were homozygous for the wild-type genotype (TNF-α−308 G/G) [149]. However, a recent meta-analysis reviewing 25 studies consisting of nearly 3,000 patients suggested that while those individuals with the A allele at the TNF-α−308 site were at higher risk for sepsis, there was not a statistically significant association with higher mortality [66]. The inconsistent findings of genetic association studies in critically ill populations have been noted by others [150] and one should be mindful of the limitations of such studies (see below).

Genetic variations in other genes coding for proteins not directly involved in the immune response but still believed to play a role in the pathobiology of sepsis have also been examined in critically ill patients (Table 19.1). In addition to an imbalance in the inflammatory response that may contribute to sepsis-induced systemic multi-organ system failure (MOSF), other molecular mechanisms may contribute to MOSF. One possible mechanism is an inhibition of the mitochondrial respiratory chain and a decrease of oxygen utilization. Consequently, genetic variations that impact mitochondrial genes involved in energy production might also impact outcomes from sepsis. The mitochondrial genome which codes for proteins involved in the electron transport chain as well as mitochondrial transfer and ribosomal RNAs has recently attracted interest in sepsis research. Due to the increased energy requirements in patients with sepsis, genetic variations that impact mitochondrial function might also impact outcomes in sepsis. One genetic variation is the T to C transition at 4216 (mT4216C) in the gene coding for NADH dehydrogenase I (*ND1*) which is thought to reduce the efficiency of complex I and impair the production of adenosine triphosphate (ATP) [151]. The C allele is associated with sepsis-related organ dysfunction or septic shock in burn patients [75] and organ dysfunction and mortality in other non-thermal trauma patients [76]. In both studies, the impact of this genetic variation was only observed in male adult Caucasians.

Other mechanisms involved in sepsis-induced MOSF are believed to involve endothelial dysfunction and intravascular fibrin deposition [152]. Widespread microthromboses are evident histologically [153]. Diminished activity of anticoagulants, or elevated levels of inhibitors of fibrinolysis, can lead to fibrin deposition, and serum levels of protein C, protein S and anti-thrombin III are decreased [154]. Plasminogen activator inhibitor 1 (PAI-1) is an inhibitor of fibrinolysis due to its ability to inhibit the potent fibrinolytic, plasminogen activator. Elevated plasma concentrations of PAI-1 have been observed in sepsis [155] and severe meningococcal disease [156] and high concentrations are correlated with mortality [157–159]. A single nucleotide insertion/deletion polymorphism exists within the promoter region of the gene coding for PAI-1 675 basepairs upstream from the transcriptional start site. This polymorphism influences the amount of PAI-1 produced with individuals homozygous for the 4G/4G genotype producing more PAI-1 than either individuals heterozygous (4G/5G) or homozygous for 5 guanines (5G/5G) [160, 161]. Children with the 4G/4G genotype who have meningococcal disease have higher plasma levels of PAI-1 [158] and an increased risk of death from sepsis compared with children with either the 4G/5G or 5G/5G genotypes [77, 78, 158, 162]. In addition, the 4G allele is associated with disseminated intravascular coagulation (DIC) in this population [79]. In adults, this polymorphism is not only associated with poor outcome from septic shock from multiple etiologies [80, 81, 163, 164] but also appears to be a marker for poor outcome after severe trauma [165]. However, not all studies demonstrate similar findings [166]. Nevertheless, there appears to be a strong association between the 4G/4G genotype in the PAI-1 gene, high plasma concentrations of PAI-1, and worse outcome in critical illness.

The influence of genetic variations in the gene coding for angiotensin I converting enzyme (ACE) in patients with sepsis has also been extensively studied. ACE is present in all tissues, particularly the pulmonary endothelium, and is primarily responsible for converting angiotensin I to angiotensin II. It is also involved in the metabolism of chemotactic peptides suggesting that it may play a role in the inflammatory response. Individuals have been shown to have variable plasma and tissue levels of ACE, and evidence suggests that these variable levels are due in part to genetic factors [167]. Specifically, an insertion (I)/deletion (D) of a 287 base repair repeat sequence in the noncoding intron 16 of the gene coding for ACE [168, 169] is associated with variable plasma levels; individuals with the DD genotype have higher plasma and tissue levels of ACE compared with individuals who are heterozygous or are homozygous for the insertion sequence [170, 171]. Association studies have suggested that the D/D genotype is associated with more severe meningococcal disease in children as measured by a higher predicted risk of mortality, greater prevalence of inotropic support and mechanical ventilation, and longer intensive care unit stay [11]. Several other studies have also examined the influence of the I/D polymorphism in sepsis with variable results [12, 166, 172–176]. A recent meta-analysis concluded that the D/D genotype was protective against the risk of sepsis but does not influence the severity of disease [177].

In summary, there are a number of genetic variants within the coding or regulatory regions of genes involved in the recognition and response to bacterial pathogens as well as other genes involved in the pathobiology of sepsis that appear to be associated with the development of, and/or outcome from sepsis (Table 19.1). While not all studies are in agreement, there does appear to be a growing body of evidence that genetic variations influence outcomes in critically ill patients. These findings may lead to the stratification of patients based on genetic risk factors and may also lead to genetic-based specific targeting of therapies.

Influence of Genetic Polymorphisms in Respiratory Failure and Lung Injury

Acute lung injury (ALI)/ARDS accounts for a significant proportion of all pediatric ICU admissions. For every 1,000 children admitted to pediatric ICUs, 9–16 meet the criteria for either ALI or ARDS. Several pediatric studies have used the American European Consensus Conference (AECC) criteria [178] for ARDS to determine the incidence rates to be from 1.4 cases/100,000/year to 9.5 cases/100,000/year [179–184]. The causes of ALI in children are numerous, and as in adults, community-acquired pneumonia (CAP) is the primary etiology. While the mortality in children with ARDS is high, upwards of 90 % in some high-risk cohorts, it has been steadily decreasing over the past several years. Although most children with CAP have minimal lung injury, a small but significant number develop respiratory failure and severe lung injury. This variability in the severity of lung injury in children with CAP raises the possibility that genetic variation influences the susceptibility to and severity of lung injury in this population. Table 19.2 lists many genes in which genetic variations have been reported to be associated with more severe lung disease, though most of these studies have been done in adult cohorts. We will discuss a few examples of genes that play a role in normal respiratory physiology for which data suggests that genetic variations may influence the degree of lung injury in children.

Table 19.2 Genetic polymorphisms associated with ALI

Gene	Polymorphism[a]	Consequence of polymorphism	References
ACE	Insertion/deletion	D/D associated with increased serum and tissue levels; associated with development of ALI	[185–187]
ANGPT2	rs2959811 rs2515475 rs1868554	Associated with variable plasma levels of angiopoietin-2 and development of ALI in adults with trauma	[188, 189]
CFTR	$(TG)_m T_n$	More TG's or fewer T's associated with more skipping of exon 9 and, therefore, less CFTR; associated with more severe lung injury in African American children with CAP	[190]
F5	rs6025 (Arg506Gln)	Associated with decreased mortality in Caucasian adults with ARDS	[191]
FAS	rs17447140 (−11341 A/T) rs2147420 (9325 G/A) rs2234978 (21541 C/T) rs1051070 (22484 A/T)	Haplotype associated with increased FAS mRNA in response to LPS and risk of ALI but not mortality	[192]
FTL	rs905238 rs918546 rs2230267	Frequency of SNPs higher in adult cohort with ARDS	[193]
HMOX2	rs1362626 rs2404579 rs2270366 rs1051308 rs7702	Frequency of specific genotypes and haplotypes lower in adults with ARDS	[193]
IL-1$_{RA}$	rs4251961 variable 86-bp repeat	Associated with variable levels of IL-1$_{RA}$ and VNTR associated with risk of severe lung injury in children	[194, 195]
IL-6	rs4800795 (−174 G/C) Several others	Associated with variable levels of IL-6 and haplotype associated with increased susceptibility to ARDS in adults	[196–199]
IRAK3	rs10506481	Associated with increased risk of ARDS in adults with sepsis	[200]
MBL2	rs1800451	Associated with lower levels of MBL and more severe sepsis and sepsis-induced ARDS	[201–203]
MIF	rs2070767 rs755622	Haplotypes associated with sepsis and ALI and both European-descent and African-descent populations	[204]
MYLK	rs9840993 rs4678047 rs28497577	Individual SNPs as well as haplotypes associated with increased risk of ALI especially in African American population	[205, 206]
NFE2L2 (Nrf2)	rs1754059 (−617 C/A)	A allele reduces activity of gene promoter and was associated with ALI in trauma patients	[207]
NFKBIA	rs3138053 (−881 A/G) rs2233406 (−826 C/T) rs2233409 (−297 C/T)	GTC haplotype is associated with ARDS	[208]
NQO1	rs689455 (−1221 A/C)	C allele associated with decreased transcription and lower incidence of ALI in trauma patients	[209]
PAI-1	4G/5G	4G associated with increased levels; associated with increased mortality in ALI	[82]
PBEF1	rs41496055	Associated with decreased transcription of PBEF and higher risk of ALI in adults with sepsis	[210]
PLAU	rs1916341 rs2227562 rs2227564 rs2227566 rs2227571 rs4065	CGCCCC haplotype associated with 60-day mortality and ventilator-free days but not risk for developing ALI in adults with sepsis	[211]
PPFIA1	rs471931	Associated with ALI in adults using GWAS	[3]
SFTPB	rs1130866 (+1580 C/A)	Associated with development of ALI and worse lung injury; allele may impact glycosylation and processing of protein	[212]

(continued)

Table 19.2 (continued)

Gene	Polymorphism[a]	Consequence of polymorphism	References
SOD3	rs1007991 rs8192291 rs2695232 rs2855262	GCCT haplotype associated with decreased ALI in adults with sepsis and lower mortality	[213]
TLR1	rs5743551 (−7202 A/G)	Associated with sepsis-induced ALI and mortality in adults	[87]
TNF-α	rs1800629 (−308 G/A)	A allele is associated with increased level of production and with mortality in patients with ARDS	[214]
VEGF	rs833061 (−460 C/T) rs2010963 (+405 C/G) rs3025039 (+936 C/T)	Specific genotypes and haplotypes associated with lower levels of VEGF and higher mortality in ARDS	[215, 216]

ACE angiotensin converting enzyme, *ANGPT2* angiopoietin-2, *CFTR* cystic fibrosis transmembrane conductance regulator, *F5* factor V Leiden, *FTL* ferritin light chain, *HMOX2* heme oxygenase 2, *IL-1_{RA}* interleukin 1 receptor antagonist, *IL-6* interleukin 6, *IRAK3* interleukin-1 receptor-associated kinase 3, *MBL* mannose-binding lectin, *MIF* macrophage migration inhibitory factor, *MYLK* myosin light chain kinase, *NFE2L2* nuclear factor (erythroid-derived)-like 2, *NFKBIA* nuclear factor kappa B inhibitor alpha, *NQO1* NADPH quinone oxidoreductase 1, *PAI-1* plasminogen activator inhibitor 1, *PBEF1* pre-B cell colony-enhancing factor 1, *PLAU* plasminogen activator urokinase, *PPFIA 1* Protein Tyrosine Phosphatase Receptor Type F Polypeptide-Interacting Protein Alpha-1, *SFTPB* surfactant protein B, *SOD* superoxide dismutase, *TLR1* Toll-like receptor 1, *TNF* tumor necrosis factor, *VEGF* vascular endothelial growth factor

[a]Terminology used for the various polymorphisms are the ones most commonly used in the literature and may refer to the nucleotide position, amino acid position, or name of the allele. This table is representative of polymorphisms examined in ALI but may not include all such polymorphisms

Several key components have been recognized in the pathophysiology of ALI (for review, see [217, 218]). These include inflammation, coagulation with alveolar fibrin deposition, vascular permeability, surfactant dysfunction, oxidative stress, and apoptosis. Many investigators have used the candidate gene approach to identify genetic variations in genes involved in these processes to determine if the frequency of the variations is different in a cohort with ALI compared with a cohort without ALI. For example, we and others have examined the frequency of a common genetic variation in the gene coding for surfactant protein B [212, 219]. This variation results in an amino acid change in exon 4 located in a region of the amino terminal pro-peptide which is thought to play a role in targeting of surfactant protein B to lamellar bodies. This amino acid change alters a glycosylation site in the pro-peptide of surfactant protein B and may disrupt trafficking of the protein. Several adult studies and our pediatric study provide evidence that individuals with this variation are more likely to have more severe lung injury as defined by the development of meeting ALI criteria or the need for mechanical ventilation.

As previously discussed, genetic association studies have progressed beyond examining the influence of a single genetic variation within a gene. Studies now examine a number of known variations in the gene in order to create haplotypes consisting of all the various combinations of SNPs within a gene. For example, for surfactant protein B, we examined seven genetic variations in a cohort of African American children with CAP and found two haplotypes which were associated with lung injury [212]. In addition, other recent studies have evaluated genetic variation in a group of genes involved in a specific biological pathway with the idea that variations within components of the pathway may influence the overall functionality of the pathway. One study using this approach examined variants in toll-like receptor signaling pathways, which identified a variant in the gene coding for toll interacting protein that is associated with protection from sepsis [220].

The final example involves the CFTR gene (*CFTR*), the gene coding for the cystic fibrosis transmembrane conductance regulator. We selected this gene for SNP analysis because influx of fluid into the alveoli due to increased permeability of the alveolar-capillary barrier is one of the hallmarks of ALI [221], and the ability to clear fluid rapidly is associated with improved outcome [222]. The clearance of alveolar fluid occurs through active ion transport [223], and CFTR has been shown to have a role in both cyclic adenosine monophosphate-stimulated fluid absorption and modulation of the epithelial sodium channel [224–226]. CFTR is an ATP-binding cassette transporter chloride channel expressed on epithelial cells in bronchi, bronchioles, and alveoli [224, 225, 227, 228]. *CFTR* contains 27 exons that are spliced together to give mature CFTR mRNA. Alternatively spliced transcripts are relatively common and levels vary between individuals [229]. Mutations in the *CFTR* gene cause cystic fibrosis (CF), a disease characterized by progressive injury to the lungs [230]. In vitro and ex vivo studies suggest that CFTR deficiency results in a dysregulated inflammatory response [231–236] and promotes LPS-induced lung injury in mice [234, 237].

The most studied mutation in *CFTR* results in the deletion of phenylalanine 508 (p.508del) in exon 10, part of the first nucleotide-binding domain; inheriting two p.508del mutations causes CF [230]. This mutation disrupts the processing and functioning of CFTR by causing mis-folding and retention in the endoplasmic reticulum [238, 239]. Individuals with CF have <5 % of normal CFTR activity [230]. Only two relatively common polymorphisms have been reported to affect the function of CFTR. One such polymorphism is the $(TG)_mT_n$ variable repeat region located in intron 8. Both in vitro and in vivo studies demonstrate association of either a higher number of TG repeats and/or a lower number of Ts with an increased proportion of mRNA transcripts missing exon 9 [240–244]. Mechanistic studies also indicate that different alleles at the $(TG)_mT_n$ site likely affect exon 9 skipping due to differences between alleles in affinity of the binding of splicing regulatory proteins [245, 246]. Exon 9 is essential for CFTR function as it, together with exons 10–12, encodes for the first nucleotide-binding domain, and mRNA transcripts without exon 9 do not produce functional CFTR [238, 247, 248]. In healthy individuals, 5–90 % of the CFTR transcripts are missing exon 9 [249], suggesting that CFTR activity present in healthy individuals varies over a broad range. Although the reduction of CFTR activity to <5 % of normal is observed in patients with CF, it is possible that other variants that reduce the level of functional CFTR to a lesser degree may still impact the risk of other lung disease [230]. We examined the $(TG)_mT_n$ alleles in a cohort of children with CAP. African American children with CAP who have the $(TG)_mT_n$ alleles that are associated with increased skipping of exon 9 were found to be more likely to require mechanical ventilation and develop ALI [190]. This suggests that less functional CFTR might contribute to more severe lung injury and that the genetic make-up of the host may contribute to this reduced functional CFTR.

As mentioned above, GWAS has begun to be used in the study of critically ill patients. One recent study used GWAS to examine genetic variations in an adult cohort to identify polymorphisms that might be associated with the development of ARDS [3]. This study is particular important in that it not only validated the association of previously identified SNPs with the development of ALI, but also identified a novel association of a variant in the gene coding for the protein liprin-α (*PPFIA1*) [250] suggesting the involvement of liprin-α in the pathogenesis of ALI. Liprin-α may affect localization of β1-integrins [251] that are involved in the pathogenesis of ALI through interactions with the extracellular matrix by altering cell adhesion and lung vascular permeability [252, 253]. Thus, GWAS may not only help identify new proteins associated with ALI leading to a better understanding of the pathophysiology but also may help identify new potential therapeutic targets.

Influence of Genetic Polymorphisms in Cardiopulmonary Bypass

Children with congenital heart lesions represent a significant number of patients in pediatric ICUs, and many of these children are in the immediate post-operative period after undergoing cardiopulmonary bypass (CPB). The use of CPB in both adults and children initiates an acute systemic inflammatory response that contributes to the development of post-operative complications, including multi-organ system dysfunction and failure [254–267]. The initiation of this inflammatory response is due to the surgical trauma itself, endotoxemia [268], ischemia and reperfusion [269], complement activation [270, 271], and the contact of blood with the non-physiological surfaces of the cardiopulmonary bypass circuitry. However, as in the response to pathogens, wide variability in the intensity of this inflammatory response has been observed. Whether genetic polymorphisms contribute to this variability in response and are associated with complications in the post-operative period is certainly of interest; if genetic variations do in fact impact the post-operative course, pre-operative genotyping of patients might identify those that are at greater risk prior to the stimulus and lead to interventions that might ameliorate the response.

As discussed above, genetic variations influence the levels of many of the pro-inflammatory and anti-inflammatory cytokines as well as other mediators. It is plausible, therefore, that the complications after exposure to cardiopulmonary bypass may be, in part, influenced by genetic variation. The IL-6 −572 C allele, IL-10 −592 C allele, IL-10 −1082 G allele, and TNF-α−308 A allele as well as another TNF-α promoter polymorphism at position −863 [272], have been shown to be associated with elevated levels of their respective cytokines and/or various post-operative complications in adults after CPB [263, 266, 273–283]. The pro-inflammatory cytokine IL-18, known to play an important role in promoting the production of Th2 cytokines and the pathogenesis of inflammatory diseases, has several regulatory polymorphisms. The −607 C allele is associated with the development of ALI in adults after CPB [284]. GWAS has been performed in adults who have undergone CPB and has identified three loci that are associated with post-operative ventricular dysfunction [285].

Association between genetic polymorphisms and complications in children who have undergone cardiac surgery is less well studied but two examples will be discussed. An association has been demonstrated between the ACE deletion polymorphism (D allele) and junctional ectopic tachycardia (JET), the most prevalent arrhythmia in the post-operative period in children undergoing CPB [286]. Elevated ACE and angiotensin II levels associated with the D allele have been well established and may contribute to a pro-arrhythmic state. Consistent with this idea are the observations demonstrating associations between the D allele and atrial fibrillation [287], reperfusion-induced ventricular arrhythmias [288], and prolonged atrioventricular nodal conductance [289].

A second example involves pulmonary artery hypertension, another complication in the post-operative period in children undergoing CPB for some congenital heart lesions.

Nitric oxide is known to mediate vascular smooth muscle relaxation and is produced from the catalysis of L-arginine to L-citrulline by endothelial nitric oxide synthase (eNOS). Two well-studied polymorphisms in the gene coding for eNOS, a 27 base pair variable nucleotide tandem repeat (VNTR) polymorphism in intron 4 and a G to T substitution at nucleotide position 894 in exon 7 that leads to a substitution of a glutamic acid at amino acid position 298 with aspartic acid (Glu298Asp), are associated with variable plasma NO levels [290]. Children undergoing CPB who have the Glu298Asp polymorphism are more likely to develop acute pulmonary hypertension in the post-operative period [291]. Thus, while the studies are limited, there are examples in children who undergo CPB in which genetic variations may influence the post-operative complications.

The discussions above suggest that an imbalanced inflammatory response may contribute to some of the post-operative complications and that genetic variations may contribute to the imbalance of the inflammatory mediators. These observations are important in that they point out that clinicians may be able to pre-operatively identify those children at risk for developing certain complications and develop therapeutic interventions that may attenuate the response. Recently, in a small trial, prophylactic peritoneal dialysis after CPB in children demonstrated a decrease in IL-8 and IL-6 levels at 24 h and improvement in several clinical outcome variables [267]. It would be interesting to determine if host genetics partially influenced the cytokine levels and whether peritoneal dialysis could be reserved for those patients more likely to develop higher cytokine levels and worse outcomes based on their genetic makeup.

Influence of Genetic Polymorphisms and Risk of Thrombosis

Thromboses are a significant problem in children in pediatric ICUs as they are exposed to a number of risk factors for thrombus formation [292–302]. Venous thromboembolism (VTE) have been reported in up to 50 % of critically ill children with central venous catheters though this prevalence is lower in more recent years [299, 302–306]. A number of well-described genetic variants in both pro-coagulant, anti-coagulant, and fibrinolytic pathways have been shown to increase the risk of thrombosis (Table 19.3); however, most of these have not been specifically studied in pediatric cohorts. Several of these variations alter the quantity or function of proteins in these pathways as well as platelet function and have been shown to be significant risk factors for thrombosis [307–313]. These include variations in genes coding for Factor V [314], prothrombin [315–318], antithrombin [319–323], protein C [324–327], protein S [328–333], methylentetrahydrofolate reductase [334],

endothelial nitric oxide synthase [335–337], α-fibrinogen [338–341], Factor XIII [338, 342–347] and PAI-1 [348–351].

The impact of genetic variants in VTE in otherwise healthy children has begun to be recognized [352]. The Arg506Gln polymorphism in the factor V gene (Factor V Leiden) has been reported to be present in 13–45 % of children with thromboembolism [353–356], and heterozygosity for this variant is associated with a sevenfold increase in risk for stroke and transient ischemic attacks in children [357]. However, very little data on the risk of these genetic variants in the development of thrombosis in critically ill children has been reported. In a cohort of neonates, no association was observed between several of these variants and umbilical catheter thrombosis [358]. However, the risk of thrombosis and bleeding with the use of anti-coagulants are both significant adverse events in the pediatric ICU, knowledge of a child's genetic polymorphisms in the genes coding for components of the coagulation system might identify children who are at greatest risk for these complications.

Pharmacogenomics: The Study of the Genomics of Drug Response and Adverse Effects

Genetic variations have long been known to influence the response to drug therapy as well as adverse drug reactions (for review, see [359–364]). They do so by affecting absorption, transport, binding to receptors, activation or inhibition of signal transduction pathways, metabolism, and elimination. Furthermore, these genetic variations may not only help explain why some patients have the expected response to drug therapies while others experience toxicities or therapeutic failures, but also provide a mechanism to help clinicians predict how an individual patient might respond. Table 19.4 lists some examples of genes in which variations have been shown to influence the action of drugs commonly used in pediatric intensive care units.

The best described examples of genetic polymorphisms that influence drug response are those that are found in genes coding for enzymes involved in drug metabolism (Table 19.4). Two examples will be briefly described here in order to demonstrate the clinical relevance of such genetic variations. Thiopurine S-methyltransferase (TPMT) is an enzyme primarily responsible for inactivation of the thiopurines, mercaptopurine and azathioprine, used as immunosuppressants and chemotherapeutic drugs. Genetic polymorphisms in the gene coding for TPMT result in a nonfunctioning enzyme; thus, patients receiving mercaptopurine or azathioprine who inherit the loss of function allele accumulate high concentrations of the active metabolites and are

Table 19.3 Genetic polymorphisms examined for associations with risk of thrombosis

Gene	Polymorphism[a]	Consequence of polymorphism
Factor V	rs6205 (G1691A) (Factor V Leiden)	Resists activated Protein C; increased risk of VTE in Caucasians but not African Americans
Prothrombin	rs1799963 (G20210A)	Increased levels; associated with risk of VTE in Caucasians
Antithrombin	Multiple sites	Decreased levels and activity
Protein C	Multiple sites in promoter	Decreased levels; associated with risk of venous thrombosis
Protein S	Multiple sites	Decreased levels; associated with increased thrombosis
PAI-1	4G/5G	Increased PAI-1 levels, increased risk of thrombosis
α-Fibrinogen	rs6050 (Thr312Ala)	Affects structure/function and FXIII cross-linking; associated with pulmonary embolism
Methylentetrahydrofolate reductase	**rs**1801133 (C677T)	Decreased enzymatic activity; increased levels of homocysteine; minimal association with VTE in Caucasians but significant association with VTE in Asians
Endothelial nitric oxide synthase	rs1799983 (G894T; Glu298Asp)	Less stable enzyme; associated with restenosis of stents; associated with myocardial infarcts
Factor XIII A	rs5985 (Val34Leu)	Increased cleavage and activation; associated with DVT

VTE venous thromboembolism, *DVT* deep thromboembolism, *UTR* untranslated region

[a]Terminology used for the various polymorphisms are the ones most commonly used in the literature and may refer to the nucleotide position, amino acid position, or name of the allele. This table is representative of polymorphisms examined in thrombosis but does not include all such polymorphisms

Table 19.4 Genes in which polymorphisms alter drug effects

Gene	Examples of specific drugs or drug class	Consequence of polymorphism
G6PD[a]	Rasburicase, dapsone	Deficiency associated with risk of severe hemolysis
β₂-adrenergic receptor	Albuterol, terbutaline	Decreased bronchodilation
β₁-adrenergic receptor	β₁-agonists	Decreased cardiovascular response
G$_s$ protein α	β-blockers	Decreased antihypertensive effect
Thiopurine methyltransferase	azathioprine, thioguanine, mercaptopurine	Variation associated with increased risk of myelotoxicity
Urea cycle disorder deficiency	Valproic acid	Hyperammonemic encephalopathy
Vitamin K reductase	Warfarin	Altered drug exposure
ALOX5[b]	Leukotriene receptor antagonists	Decreased effect on FEV₁
Protein C	Warfarin	Deficiency associated with tissue necrosis
Serotonin transporter	Antidepressants, antipsychotics	Decreased antidepressant and clozapine response
N-acetyltransferase 2	Rifampin, hydralazine	Increased hepatotoxicity with slow acetylation genotypes
[c]CYP2C9	Warfarin, phenytoin, losartan celecoxib	Alters drug exposure; increased anticoagulant effects of warfarin
CYP2D6	Risperidone, tramadol, codeine, clozapine, metoprolol, propranolol, propafenone, aspirin, caffeine, acetaminophen	Alters drug exposure; decreased codeine analgesia; increased antidepressant toxicity
CYP3A4/3A5/3A7	Midazolam, steroids, calcium channel blockers	Alters drug exposure; altered clearance of midazolam and steroids
CYP2C19	Omeprazole, voriconazole, pantoprazole, diazepam;	Alters drug exposure
	Clopidogrel	Poor metabolizers have diminished response

[a]*G6PD* Glucose-6-phophate dehydrogenase

[b]*ALOX5* arachidonate 5-lipooxygenase

[c]*CYP* cytochrome p-450; this table is representative of genes in which polymorphisms have been shown to alter drug effects but does not include all such genes and their polymorphisms

at risk for developing life-threatening haematopoietic toxicities [365–367]. Clinical diagnostic tests are available for detecting the SNPs in the TPMT gene that result in TPMT deficiency thereby allowing for the identification of patients at high risk for thiopurine toxicities. Patients receiving mercaptopurine or azathioprine who are genetically predisposed to be TPMT-deficient have been treated successfully for their oncologic diseases using approximately 5–10 % of the conventional dose of the thiopurines [365, 366] without the toxicities. This represents a good example of modifying drug therapy based on an individual's genetic makeup.

A second example of a genetic variation that influences drug response involves the gene coding for cytochrome P-450 2C19 (*CYP2C19*) which is involved in the metabolism of several drugs. Anti-platelet therapies such as clopidogrel are becoming increasingly used in the pediatric population particularly in children with complex congenital heart disease and stroke [368]. Clopidogrel is a potent inhibitor of the platelet $P2Y_{12}$ adenosine diphosphate (ADP) receptor, but large inter-individual variation in effectiveness has been observed and common genetic variations appear to account for much of this variability. Once absorbed in the gastrointestinal tract, 85 % of clopidogrel is hydrolyzed in the liver to create inactive metabolites while 15 % is metabolized to the active metabolite by CYP450 enzymes, particularly CYP2C19 [369, 370]. The active metabolite inhibits platelet function by irreversibly inhibiting the $P2Y_{12}$ ADP receptor located on the surface of platelets and prevents the binding of ADP. This prevents the G_i subunit from inhibiting adenylate cyclase resulting in an increase in cyclic adenosine monophosphate (cAMP) production which prevents activation of phosphoinositide 3-kinase (PI3K). This results in decreased expression of glycoprotein IIb/IIIa which mediates fibrinogen binding and subsequent platelet aggregation, endothelial adherence, and thrombus formation [371]. Thus, clopidogrel inhibits platelet aggregation by blocking the initial step in this pathway, but only after conversion to the active metabolite by CYP2C19.

Common loss of function alleles have been described in the gene coding for CYP2C19 with allelic frequencies of about 15 % in Caucasian and African American populations and about 30 % in Asian populations. Studies have suggested an association between the presence of CYP2C19 polymorphisms, less clopidogrel active metabolite generation, and decreased clopidogrel responsiveness, as measured by platelet function and adverse clinical outcomes [372–374]. These are just two examples of many that exist in which genetic variations in genes involved in the mechanism of action of drugs used in the PICU can influence the therapeutic response as well as adverse drug reactions. However, keep in mind that most of these studies have been performed in adult populations and developmental differences in the expression in many of these genes exist that will also impact the overall therapeutic response.

Limitations and Study Design Issues in Genetic Association Studies

Investigators have used the candidate gene approach, pathway based analysis, and GWAS in examining the influence of genetic variations in critically ill populations (and, indeed other populations with complex phenotypes). Each approach has advantages and disadvantages, and some of the limitations have been reviewed previously [375]. In addition, several study design issues need to be considered regardless of the approach to be used. First, it is important that the correct control population is used for comparison. For example, in some sepsis studies the frequency of a polymorphism in the group of patients with septic shock is compared with the frequency of the polymorphism in a healthy control population. However, healthy individuals may not be the appropriate control population as they may not have been exposed to the same pathogens to which the patients with septic shock were exposed. A more appropriate control group for comparison might be a group of patients with a similar infection who did not develop septic shock. Population stratification is a second issue that needs to be considered. The frequency of many of the SNPs varies between racial and ethnic groups and so comparisons should only be made within similar groups and correction for population stratification even within these groups should be considered. Power estimates and sample size are significant issues both for candidate gene approaches and GWAS; GWAS frequently examine several hundred to over a thousand subjects making the costs to use this approach high and the feasibility daunting for some diseases found in the PICU. For any gene association study, replication in independent data sets is crucial given the often spurious results, although replication cohorts are often difficult to obtain in pediatric studies. In addition, other variables can influence the outcome of patients and must be tested in appropriate statistical modeling for the degree of their effect. For example, age, co-morbid conditions, nutritional status, variability in treatment strategies, and even socioeconomic status may be independent predictors of mortality [376, 377]. There should be a thoughtful evaluation of the technical aspects of the genotyping with mention of genotyping success and error rates. Finally, the functionality of the genetic variants should be discussed; many of the SNPs that are examined are not functional but may rather be linked to the causative variation.

Conclusion

In summary there is little doubt that host genetic variation is responsible for some of the variable disease presentation, response to therapy and final outcome observed in critically ill children, but the *degree* of the influence of genetic variations remains to be determined. Identification of genetic polymorphisms that will ultimately be useful in identifying critically ill children who are at increased risk for more severe disease or are more likely to benefit from a specific therapy will allow for a more individualized approach to treatment. Carefully controlled studies examining gene variants alone and in combination with other clinically important characteristics will be required to determine whether patient treatment can be tailored more specifically to an individual child's genetic make-up.

References

1. Freeman BD, Buchman TG, McGrath S, Tabrizi AR, Zehnbauer BA. Template-directed dye-terminator incorporation with fluorescence polarization detection for analysis of single nucleotide polymorphisms implicated in sepsis. J Mol Diagn. 2002;4(4):209–15.
2. Freeman BD, Buchman TG, Zehnbauer BA. Template-directed dye-terminator incorporation with fluorescence polarization detection for analysis of single nucleotide polymorphisms associated with cardiovascular and thromboembolic disease. Thromb Res. 2003;111(6):373–9.
3. Christie JD, Wurfel MM, Feng R, O'Keefe GE, Bradfield J, Ware LB, Christiani DC, Calfee CS, Cohen MJ, Matthay M, et al. Genome wide association identifies PPFIA1 as a candidate gene for acute lung injury risk following major trauma. PLoS One. 2012; 7(1):e28268.
4. Mikacenic C, Reiner AP, Holden TD, Nickerson DA, Wurfel MM. Variation in the TLR10/TLR1/TLR6 locus is the major genetic determinant of interindividual difference in TLR1/2-mediated responses. Genes Immun. 2013;14(1):52–7.
5. Sorensen TI, Nielsen GG, Andersen PK, Teasdale TW. Genetic and environmental influences on premature death in adult adoptees. N Engl J Med. 1988;318(12):727–32.
6. Dahmer MK, Randolph A, Vitali S, Quasney MW. Genetic polymorphisms in sepsis. Pediatr Crit Care Med. 2005;6(3 Suppl):S61–73.
7. Wong HR. Genetics and genomics in pediatric septic shock. Crit Care Med. 2012;40(5):1618–26.
8. Akira S, Takeda K, Kaisho T. Toll-like receptors: critical proteins linking innate and acquired immunity. Nat Immunol. 2001;2(8):675–80.
9. Akira S, Takeda K. Toll-like receptor signalling. Nat Rev Immunol. 2004;4(7):499–511.
10. Akira S, Uematsu S, Takeuchi O. Pathogen recognition and innate immunity. Cell. 2006;124(4):783–801.
11. Harding D, Baines PB, Brull D, Vassiliou V, Ellis I, Hart A, Thomson AP, Humphries SE, Montgomery HE. Severity of meningococcal disease in children and the angiotensin-converting enzyme insertion/deletion polymorphism. Am J Respir Crit Care Med. 2002;165(8):1103–6.
12. Cogulu O, Onay H, Uzunkaya D, Gunduz C, Pehlivan S, Vardar F, Atlihan F, Ozkinay C, Ozkinay F. Role of angiotensin-converting enzyme gene polymorphisms in children with sepsis and septic shock. Pediatr Int. 2008;50(4):477–80.
13. Michalek J, Svetlikova P, Fedora M, Klimovic M, Klapacova L, Bartosova D, Elbl L, Hrstkova H, Hubacek JA. Bactericidal permeability increasing protein gene variants in children with sepsis. Intensive Care Med. 2007;33(12):2158–64.
14. Gu W, Dong H, Jiang DP, Zhou J, Du DY, Gao JM, Yao YZ, Zhang LY, Wen AQ, Liu Q, et al. Functional significance of CD14 promoter polymorphisms and their clinical relevance in a Chinese Han population. Crit Care Med. 2008;36(8):2274–80.
15. Baldini M, Lohman IC, Halonen M, Erickson RP, Holt PG, Martinez FD. A Polymorphism* in the 5′ flanking region of the CD14 gene is associated with circulating soluble CD14 levels and with total serum immunoglobulin E. Am J Respir Cell Mol Biol. 1999;20(5):976–83.
16. Gibot S, Cariou A, Drouet L, Rossignol M, Ripoll L. Association between a genomic polymorphism within the CD14 locus and septic shock susceptibility and mortality rate. Crit Care Med. 2002;30(5):969–73.
17. Barber RC, Chang LY, Arnoldo BD, Purdue GF, Hunt JL, Horton JW, Aragaki CC. Innate immunity SNPs are associated with risk for severe sepsis after burn injury. Clin Med Res. 2006;4(4): 250–5.
18. Sutherland AM, Walley KR, Russell JA. Polymorphisms in CD14, mannose-binding lectin, and toll-like receptor-2 are associated with increased prevalence of infection in critically ill adults. Crit Care Med. 2005;33(3):638–44.
19. Barber RC, Aragaki CC, Chang LY, Purdue GF, Hunt JL, Arnoldo BD, Horton JW. CD14-159 C allele is associated with increased risk of mortality after burn injury. Shock. 2007;27(3):232–7.
20. van Sorge NM, van der Pol WL, van de Winkel JG. FcgammaR polymorphisms: implications for function, disease susceptibility and immunotherapy. Tissue Antigens. 2003;61(3):189–202.
21. Bredius RG, Derkx BH, Fijen CA, de Wit TP, de Haas M, Weening RS, van de Winkel JG, Out TA. Fc gamma receptor IIa (CD32) polymorphism in fulminant meningococcal septic shock in children. J Infect Dis. 1994;170(4):848–53.
22. Domingo P, Muniz-Diaz E, Baraldes MA, Arilla M, Barquet N, Pericas R, Juarez C, Madoz P, Vazquez G. Associations between Fc gamma receptor IIA polymorphisms and the risk and prognosis of meningococcal disease. Am J Med. 2002;112(1):19–25.
23. Platonov AE, Kuijper EJ, Vershinina IV, Shipulin GA, Westerdaal N, Fijen CA, van de Winkel JG. Meningococcal disease and polymorphism of FcgammaRIIa (CD32) in late complement component-deficient individuals. Clin Exp Immunol. 1998;111(1):97–101.
24. Platonov AE, Shipulin GA, Vershinina IV, Dankert J, van de Winkel JG, Kuijper EJ. Association of human Fc gamma RIIa (CD32) polymorphism with susceptibility to and severity of meningococcal disease. Clin Infect Dis. 1998;27(4):746–50.
25. Schroder O, Schulte KM, Ostermann P, Roher HD, Ekkernkamp A, Laun RA. Heat shock protein 70 genotypes HSPA1B and HSPA1L influence cytokine concentrations and interfere with outcome after major injury. Crit Care Med. 2003;31(1):73–9.
26. Schroeder S, Reck M, Hoeft A, Stuber F. Analysis of two human leukocyte antigen-linked polymorphic heat shock protein 70 genes in patients with severe sepsis. Crit Care Med. 1999;27(7):1265–70.
27. Bowers DJ, Calvano JE, Alvarez SM, Coyle SM, Macor MA, Kumar A, Calvano SE, Lowry SF. Polymorphisms of heat shock protein-70 (HSPA1B and HSPA1L loci) do not influence infection or outcome risk in critically ill surgical patients. Shock. 2006;25(2):117–22.
28. Waterer GW, ElBahlawan L, Quasney MW, Zhang Q, Kessler LA, Wunderink RG. Heat shock protein 70-2+1267 AA homozygotes have an increased risk of septic shock in adults with community-acquired pneumonia. Crit Care Med. 2003;31(5):1367–72.
29. Brouwer MC, de Gans J, Heckenberg SG, Zwinderman AH, van der Poll T, van de Beek D. Host genetic susceptibility to pneumococcal and meningococcal disease: a systematic review and meta-analysis. Lancet Infect Dis. 2009;9(1):31–44.
30. Read RC, Cannings C, Naylor SC, Timms JM, Maheswaran R, Borrow R, Kaczmarski EB, Duff GW. Variation within genes encoding interleukin-1 and the interleukin-1 receptor antagonist influence the severity of meningococcal disease. Ann Intern Med. 2003;138(7):534–41.
31. Endler G, Marculescu R, Starkl P, Binder A, Geishofer G, Muller M, Zohrer B, Resch B, Zenz W, Mannhalter C. Polymorphisms in the interleukin-1 gene cluster in children and young adults with systemic meningococcemia. Clin Chem. 2006;52(3):511–4.

32. Wen AQ, Gu W, Wang J, Feng K, Qin L, Ying C, Zhu PF, Wang ZG, Jiang JX. Clinical relevance of IL-1beta promoter polymorphisms (-1470, -511, and -31) in patients with major trauma. Shock. 2010;33(6):576–82.

33. Michalek J, Svetlikova P, Fedora M, Klimovic M, Klapacova L, Bartosova D, Hrstkova H, Hubacek JA. Interleukin-6 gene variants and the risk of sepsis development in children. Hum Immunol. 2007;68(9):756–60.

34. Zeng L, Gu W, Chen K, Jiang D, Zhang L, Du D, Hu P, Liu Q, Huang S, Jiang J. Clinical relevance of the interleukin 10 promoter polymorphisms in Chinese Han patients with major trauma: genetic association studies. Crit Care. 2009;13(6):R188.

35. Stanilova SA, Miteva LD, Karakolev ZT, Stefanov CS. Interleukin-10-1082 promoter polymorphism in association with cytokine production and sepsis susceptibility. Intensive Care Med. 2006;32(2):260–6.

36. Wattanathum A, Manocha S, Groshaus H, Russell JA, Walley KR. Interleukin-10 haplotype associated with increased mortality in critically ill patients with sepsis from pneumonia but not in patients with extrapulmonary sepsis. Chest. 2005;128(3):1690–8.

37. Accardo Palumbo A, Forte GI, Pileri D, Vaccarino L, Conte F, D'Amelio L, Palmeri M, Triolo A, D'Arpa N, Scola L, et al. Analysis of IL-6, IL-10 and IL-17 genetic polymorphisms as risk factors for sepsis development in burned patients. Burns. 2012;38(2):208–13.

38. Flores C, Perez-Mendez L, Maca-Meyer N, Muriel A, Espinosa E, Blanco J, Sanguesa R, Muros M, Garcia JG, Villar J. A common haplotype of the LBP gene predisposes to severe sepsis. Crit Care Med. 2009;37(10):2759–66.

39. Chien JW, Boeckh MJ, Hansen JA, Clark JG. Lipopolysaccharide binding protein promoter variants influence the risk for Gram-negative bacteremia and mortality after allogeneic hematopoietic cell transplantation. Blood. 2008;111(4):2462–9.

40. Zeng L, Gu W, Zhang AQ, Zhang M, Zhang LY, Du DY, Huang SN, Jiang JX. A functional variant of lipopolysaccharide binding protein predisposes to sepsis and organ dysfunction in patients with major trauma. Ann Surg. 2012;255(1):147–57.

41. Appoloni O, Dupont E, Vandercruys M, Andriens M, Duchateau J, Vincent JL. Association of tumor necrosis factor-2 allele with plasma tumor necrosis factor-alpha levels and mortality from septic shock. Am J Med. 2001;110(6):486–8.

42. McArthur JA, Zhang Q, Quasney MW. Association between the A/A genotype at the lymphotoxin-alpha+250 site and increased mortality in children with positive blood cultures. Pediatr Crit Care Med. 2002;3(4):341–4.

43. Dumon K, Rossbach C, Harms B, Gorelov V, Gross-Weege W, Schneider EM, Goretzki PE, Roher HD. Tumor necrosis factor-alpha (TNF-alpha) gene polymorphism in surgical intensive care patients with SIRS. Langenbecks Arch Chir Suppl Kongressbd. 1998;115(Suppl I):387–90.

44. Mira JP, Cariou A, Grall F, Delclaux C, Losser MR, Heshmati F, Cheval C, Monchi M, Teboul JL, Riche F, et al. Association of TNF2, a TNF-alpha promoter polymorphism, with septic shock susceptibility and mortality: a multicenter study. JAMA. 1999;282(6):561–8.

45. Nuntayanuwat S, Dharakul T, Chaowagul W, Songsivilai S. Polymorphism in the promoter region of tumor necrosis factor-alpha gene is associated with severe meliodosis. Hum Immunol. 1999;60(10):979–83.

46. Tang GJ, Huang SL, Yien HW, Chen WS, Chi CW, Wu CW, Lui WY, Chiu JH, Lee TY. Tumor necrosis factor gene polymorphism and septic shock in surgical infection. Crit Care Med. 2000;28(8):2733–6.

47. Waterer GW, Quasney MW, Cantor RM, Wunderink RG. Septic shock and respiratory failure in community-acquired pneumonia have different TNF polymorphism associations. Am J Respir Crit Care Med. 2001;163(7):1599–604.

48. Majetschak M, Obertacke U, Schade FU, Bardenheuer M, Voggenreiter G, Bloemeke B, Heesen M. Tumor necrosis factor gene polymorphisms, leukocyte function, and sepsis susceptibility in blunt trauma patients. Clin Diagn Lab Immunol. 2002;9(6):1205–11.

49. O'Keefe GE, Hybki DL, Munford RS. The G-->A single nucleotide polymorphism at the -308 position in the tumor necrosis factor-alpha promoter increases the risk for severe sepsis after trauma. J Trauma. 2002;52(5):817–25; discussion 825–6.

50. Calvano JE, Um JY, Agnese DM, Hahm SJ, Kumar A, Coyle SM, Calvano SE, Lowry SF. Influence of the TNF-alpha and TNF-beta polymorphisms upon infectious risk and outcome in surgical intensive care patients. Surg Infect (Larchmt). 2003;4(2):163–9.

51. Gallagher PM, Lowe G, Fitzgerald T, Bella A, Greene CM, McElvaney NG, O'Neill SJ. Association of IL-10 polymorphism with severity of illness in community acquired pneumonia. Thorax. 2003;58(2):154–6.

52. Schaaf BM, Boehmke F, Esnaashari H, Seitzer U, Kothe H, Maass M, Zabel P, Dalhoff K. Pneumococcal septic shock is associated with the interleukin-10-1082 gene promoter polymorphism. Am J Respir Crit Care Med. 2003;168(4):476–80.

53. Treszl A, Kocsis I, Szathmari M, Schuler A, Heninger E, Tulassay T, Vasarhelyi B. Genetic variants of TNF-[FC12]a, IL-1beta, IL-4 receptor [FC12]a-chain, IL-6 and IL-10 genes are not risk factors for sepsis in low-birth-weight infants. Biol Neonate. 2003;83(4):241–5.

54. Zhang D, Li J, Jiang ZW, Yu B, Tang X. Association of two polymorphisms of tumor necrosis factor gene with acute severe pancreatitis. J Surg Res. 2003;112(2):138–43.

55. Zhang DL, Li JS, Jiang ZW, Yu BJ, Tang XM, Zheng HM. Association of two polymorphisms of tumor necrosis factor gene with acute biliary pancreatitis. World J Gastroenterol. 2003;9(4):824–8.

56. Barber RC, Aragaki CC, Rivera-Chavez FA, Purdue GF, Hunt JL, Horton JW. TLR4 and TNF-alpha polymorphisms are associated with an increased risk for severe sepsis following burn injury. J Med Genet. 2004;41(11):808–13.

57. Gordon AC, Lagan AL, Aganna E, Cheung L, Peters CJ, McDermott MF, Millo JL, Welsh KI, Holloway P, Hitman GA, et al. TNF and TNFR polymorphisms in severe sepsis and septic shock: a prospective multicentre study. Genes Immun. 2004;5(8):631–40.

58. Jaber BL, Rao M, Guo D, Balakrishnan VS, Perianayagam MC, Freeman RB, Pereira BJ. Cytokine gene promoter polymorphisms and mortality in acute renal failure. Cytokine. 2004;25(5):212–9.

59. Nakada TA, Hirasawa H, Oda S, Shiga H, Matsuda K, Nakamura M, Watanabe E, Abe R, Hatano M, Tokuhisa T. Influence of toll-like receptor 4, CD14, tumor necrosis factor, and interleukine-10 gene polymorphisms on clinical outcome in Japanese critically ill patients. J Surg Res. 2005;129(2):322–8.

60. Watanabe E, Hirasawa H, Oda S, Shiga H, Matsuda K, Nakamura M, Abe R, Nakada T. Cytokine-related genotypic differences in peak interleukin-6 blood levels of patients with SIRS and septic complications. J Trauma. 2005;59(5):1181–9; discussion 1189–90.

61. Garnacho-Montero J, Aldabo-Pallas T, Garnacho-Montero C, Cayuela A, Jimenez R, Barroso S, Ortiz-Leyba C. Timing of adequate antibiotic therapy is a greater determinant of outcome than are TNF and IL-10 polymorphisms in patients with sepsis. Crit Care. 2006;10(4):R111.

62. Sipahi T, Pocan H, Akar N. Effect of various genetic polymorphisms on the incidence and outcome of severe sepsis. Clin Appl Thromb Hemost. 2006;12(1):47–54.

63. Jessen KM, Lindboe SB, Petersen AL, Eugen-Olsen J, Benfield T. Common TNF-alpha, IL-1 beta, PAI-1, uPA, CD14 and TLR4 polymorphisms are not associated with disease severity or outcome from Gram negative sepsis. BMC Infect Dis. 2007;7:108.

64. McDaniel DO, Hamilton J, Brock M, May W, Calcote L, Tee LY, Vick L, Newman DB, Vick K, Harrison S, et al. Molecular analysis

of inflammatory markers in trauma patients at risk of postinjury complications. J Trauma. 2007;63(1):147–57; discussion 157–8.

65. Menges T, Konig IR, Hossain H, Little S, Tchatalbachev S, Thierer F, Hackstein H, Franjkovic I, Colaris T, Martens F, et al. Sepsis syndrome and death in trauma patients are associated with variation in the gene encoding tumor necrosis factor. Crit Care Med. 2008;36(5):1456–62, e1451–6.

66. Teuffel O, Ethier MC, Beyene J, Sung L. Association between tumor necrosis factor-alpha promoter -308 A/G polymorphism and susceptibility to sepsis and sepsis mortality: a systematic review and meta-analysis. Crit Care Med. 2010;38(1):276–82.

67. Stuber F, Udalova IA, Book M, Drutskaya LN, Kuprash DV, Turetskaya RL, Schade FU, Nedospasov SA. 308 tumor necrosis factor (TNF) polymorphism is not associated with survival in severe sepsis and is unrelated to lipopolysaccharide inducibility of the human TNF promoter. J Inflamm. 1995;46(1):42–50.

68. Song Z, Song Y, Yin J, Shen Y, Yao C, Sun Z, Jiang J, Zhu D, Zhang Y, Shen Q, et al. Genetic variation in the TNF gene is associated with susceptibility to severe sepsis, but not with mortality. PLoS One. 2013;7(9):e46113.

69. Koch A, Melbye M, Sorensen P, Homoe P, Madsen HO, Molbak K, Hansen CH, Andersen LH, Hahn GW, Garred P. Acute respiratory tract infections and mannose-binding lectin insufficiency during early childhood. JAMA. 2001;285(10):1316–21.

70. Hibberd ML, Sumiya M, Summerfield JA, Booy R, Levin M. Association of variants of the gene for mannose-binding lectin with susceptibility to meningococcal disease. Meningococcal Research Group. Lancet. 1999;353(9158):1049–53.

71. Garnacho-Montero J, Garcia-Cabrera E, Jimenez-Alvarez R, Diaz-Martin A, Revuelto-Rey J, Aznar-Martin J, Garnacho-Montero C. Genetic variants of the MBL2 gene are associated with mortality in pneumococcal sepsis. Diagn Microbiol Infect Dis. 2012;73(1):39–44.

72. Arcaroli J, Fessler MB, Abraham E. Genetic polymorphisms and sepsis. Shock. 2005;24(4):300–12.

73. Huh JW, Song K, Yum JS, Hong SB, Lim CM, Koh Y. Association of mannose-binding lectin-2 genotype and serum levels with prognosis of sepsis. Crit Care. 2009;13(6):R176.

74. Ozkan H, Koksal N, Cetinkaya M, Kilic S, Celebi S, Oral B, Budak F. Serum mannose-binding lectin (MBL) gene polymorphism and low MBL levels are associated with neonatal sepsis and pneumonia. J Perinatol. 2012;32(3):210–7.

75. Huebinger RM, Gomez R, McGee D, Chang LY, Bender JE, O'Keeffe T, Burris AM, Friese SM, Purdue GF, Hunt JL, et al. Association of mitochondrial allele 4216C with increased risk for sepsis-related organ dysfunction and shock after burn injury. Shock. 2010;33(1):19–23.

76. Gomez R, O'Keeffe T, Chang LY, Huebinger RM, Minei JP, Barber RC. Association of mitochondrial allele 4216C with increased risk for complicated sepsis and death after traumatic injury. J Trauma. 2009;66(3):850–7; discussion 857–8.

77. Haralambous E, Hibberd ML, Hermans PW, Ninis N, Nadel S, Levin M. Role of functional plasminogen-activator-inhibitor-1 4G/5G promoter polymorphism in susceptibility, severity, and outcome of meningococcal disease in Caucasian children. Crit Care Med. 2003;31(12):2788–93.

78. Geishofer G, Binder A, Muller M, Zohrer B, Resch B, Muller W, Faber J, Finn A, Endler G, Mannhalter C, et al. 4G/5G promoter polymorphism in the plasminogen-activator-inhibitor-1 gene in children with systemic meningococcaemia. Eur J Pediatr. 2005;164(8):486–90.

79. Binder A, Endler G, Muller M, Mannhalter C, Zenz W. 4G4G genotype of the plasminogen activator inhibitor-1 promoter polymorphism associates with disseminated intravascular coagulation in children with systemic meningococcemia. J Thromb Haemost. 2007;5(10):2049–54.

80. Garcia-Segarra G, Espinosa G, Tassies D, Oriola J, Aibar J, Bove A, Castro P, Reverter JC, Nicolas JM. Increased mortality

in septic shock with the 4G/4G genotype of plasminogen activator inhibitor 1 in patients of white descent. Intensive Care Med. 2007;33(8):1354–62.

81. Madach K, Aladzsity I, Szilagyi A, Fust G, Gal J, Penzes I, Prohaszka Z. 4G/5G polymorphism of PAI-1 gene is associated with multiple organ dysfunction and septic shock in pneumonia induced severe sepsis: prospective, observational, genetic study. Crit Care. 2010;14(2):R79.

82. Sapru A, Hansen H, Ajayi T, Brown R, Garcia O, Zhuo H, Wiemels J, Matthay MA, Wiener-Kronish J. 4G/5G polymorphism of plasminogen activator inhibitor-1 gene is associated with mortality in intensive care unit patients with severe pneumonia. Anesthesiology. 2009;110(5):1086–91.

83. Binder A, Endler G, Rieger S, Geishofer G, Resch B, Mannhalter C, Zenz W. Protein C promoter polymorphisms associate with sepsis in children with systemic meningococcemia. Hum Genet. 2007;122(2):183–90.

84. Russell JA, Wellman H, Walley KR. Protein C rs2069912 C allele is associated with increased mortality from severe sepsis in North Americans of East Asian ancestry. Hum Genet. 2008;123(6):661–3.

85. Chen QX, Wu SJ, Wang HH, Lv C, Cheng BL, Xie GH, Fang XM. Protein C -1641A/-1654C haplotype is associated with organ dysfunction and the fatal outcome of severe sepsis in Chinese Han population. Hum Genet. 2008;123(3):281–7.

86. Lorente L, Martin MM, Plasencia F, Sole-Violan J, Blanquer J, Labarta L, Diaz C, Borreguero-Leon JM, Jimenez A, Paramo JA, et al. The 372 T/C genetic polymorphism of TIMP-1 is associated with serum levels of TIMP-1 and survival in patients with severe sepsis. Crit Care. 2013;17(3):R94.

87. Wurfel MM, Gordon AC, Holden TD, Radella F, Strout J, Kajikawa O, Ruzinski JT, Rona G, Black RA, Stratton S, et al. Toll-like receptor 1 polymorphisms affect innate immune responses and outcomes in sepsis. Am J Respir Crit Care Med. 2008;178(7):710–20.

88. Thompson CM, Holden TD, Rona G, Laxmanan B, Black RA, O'Keefe GE, Wurfel MM. Toll-like receptor 1 polymorphisms and associated outcomes in sepsis after traumatic injury: a candidate gene association study. Ann Surg. 2013.

89. Chen KH, Gu W, Zeng L, Jiang DP, Zhang LY, Zhou J, Du DY, Hu P, Liu Q, Huang SN, et al. Identification of haplotype tag SNPs within the entire TLR2 gene and their clinical relevance in patients with major trauma. Shock. 2011;35(1):35–41.

90. Kang TJ, Chae GT. Detection of toll-like receptor 2 (TLR2) mutation in the lepromatous leprosy patients. FEMS Immunol Med Microbiol. 2001;31(1):53–8.

91. Thuong NT, Hawn TR, Thwaites GE, Chau TT, Lan NT, Quy HT, Hieu NT, Aderem A, Hien TT, Farrar JJ, et al. A polymorphism in human TLR2 is associated with increased susceptibility to tuberculous meningitis. Genes Immun. 2007;8(5):422–8.

92. Lorenz E, Mira JP, Cornish KL, Arbour NC, Schwartz DA. A novel polymorphism in the toll-like receptor 2 gene and its potential association with staphylococcal infection. Infect Immun. 2000;68(11):6398–401.

93. Moore CE, Segal S, Berendt AR, Hill AV, Day NP. Lack of association between toll-like receptor 2 polymorphisms and susceptibility to severe disease caused by Staphylococcus aureus. Clin Diagn Lab Immunol. 2004;11(6):1194–7.

94. Chen K, Wang YT, Gu W, Zeng L, Jiang DP, Du DY, Hu P, Duan ZX, Liu Q, Huang SN, et al. Functional significance of the toll-like receptor 4 promoter gene polymorphisms in the Chinese Han population. Crit Care Med. 2010;38(5):1292–9.

95. Lorenz E, Mira JP, Frees KL, Schwartz DA. Relevance of mutations in the TLR4 receptor in patients with gram-negative septic shock. Arch Intern Med. 2002;162(9):1028–32.

96. Shalhub S, Junker CE, Imahara SD, Mindrinos MN, Dissanaike S, O'Keefe GE. Variation in the TLR4 gene influences the risk of organ failure and shock posttrauma: a cohort study. J Trauma. 2009;66(1):115–22; discussion 122–3.

97. Cardinal-Fernandez P, Ferruelo A, El-Assar M, Santiago C, Gomez-Gallego F, Martin-Pellicer A, Frutos-Vivar F, Penuelas O, Nin N, Esteban A, et al. Genetic predisposition to acute kidney injury induced by severe sepsis. J Crit Care. 2013;28(4):365–70.

98. van der Pol W, van de Winkel JG. IgG receptor polymorphisms: risk factors for disease. Immunogenetics. 1998;48(3):222–32.

99. Shashidharamurthy R, Zhang F, Amano A, Kamat A, Panchanathan R, Ezekwudo D, Zhu C, Selvaraj P. Dynamics of the interaction of human IgG subtype immune complexes with cells expressing R and H allelic forms of a low-affinity Fc gamma receptor CD32A. J Immunol. 2009;183(12):8216–24.

100. Koene HR, Kleijer M, Algra J, Roos D, von dem Borne AE, de Haas M. Fc gammaRIIIa-158V/F polymorphism influences the binding of IgG by natural killer cell Fc gammaRIIIa, independently of the Fc gammaRIIIa-48L/R/H phenotype. Blood. 1997;90(3):1109–14.

101. Wu J, Edberg JC, Redecha PB, Bansal V, Guyre PM, Coleman K, Salmon JE, Kimberly RP. A novel polymorphism of FcgammaRIIIa (CD16) alters receptor function and predisposes to autoimmune disease. J Clin Invest. 1997;100(5):1059–70.

102. Huizinga TW, Kleijer M, Tetteroo PA, Roos D, von dem Borne AE. Biallelic neutrophil Na-antigen system is associated with a polymorphism on the phospho-inositol-linked Fc gamma receptor III (CD16). Blood. 1990;75(1):213–7.

103. Salmon JE, Edberg JC, Kimberly RP. Fc gamma receptor III on human neutrophils: allelic variants have functionally distinct capacities. J Clin Invest. 1990;85:1287–95.

104. Salmon JE, Millard SS, Brogle NL, Kimberly RP. Fc gamma receptor IIIb enhances Fc gamma receptor IIa function in an oxidant-dependent and allele-sensitive manner. J Clin Invest. 1995;95(6):2877–85.

105. Warmerdam PA, van de Winkel JG, Gosselin EJ, Capel PJ. Molecular basis for a polymorphism of human Fc gamma receptor II (CD32). J Exp Med. 1990;172(1):19–25.

106. Warmerdam PA, van de Winkel JG, Vlug A, Westerdaal NA, Capel PJ. A single amino acid in the second Ig-like domain of the human Fc gamma receptor II is critical for human IgG2 binding. J Immunol. 1991;147(4):1338–43.

107. Salmon JE, Edberg JC, Brogle NL, Kimberly RP. Allelic polymorphisms of human Fc gamma receptor IIA and Fc gamma receptor IIIB. Independent mechanisms for differences in human phagocyte function. J Clin Invest. 1992;89(4):1274–81.

108. Sanders LA, Feldman RG, Voorhorst-Ogink MM, de Haas M, Rijkers GT, Capel PJ, Zegers BJ, van de Winkel JG. Human immunoglobulin G (IgG) Fc receptor IIA (CD32) polymorphism and IgG2-mediated bacterial phagocytosis by neutrophils. Infect Immun. 1995;63(1):73–81.

109. Siber GR, Schur PH, Aisenberg AC, Weitzman SA, Schiffman G. Correlation between serum IgG-2 concentrations and the antibody response to bacterial polysaccharide antigens. N Engl J Med. 1980;303(4):178–82.

110. Herrmann DJ, Hamilton RG, Barington T, Frasch CE, Arakere G, Makela O, Mitchell LA, Nagel J, Rijkers GT, Zegers B, et al. Quantitation of human IgG subclass antibodies to Haemophilus influenzae type b capsular polysaccharide. Results of an international collaborative study using enzyme immunoassay methodology. J Immunol Methods. 1992;148(1–2):101–14.

111. van der Pol WL, Huizinga TW, Vidarsson G, van der Linden MW, Jansen MD, Keijsers V, de Straat FG, Westerdaal NA, de Winkel JG, Westendorp RG. Relevance of Fcgamma receptor and interleukin-10 polymorphisms for meningococcal disease. J Infect Dis. 2001;184(12):1548–55.

112. Fijen CA, Bredius RG, Kuijper EJ. Polymorphism of IgG Fc receptors in meningococcal disease. Ann Intern Med. 1993;119(7 Pt 1):636.

113. Tezcan I, Berkel AI, Ersoy F, Sanal O, Kanra G. Fc gamma receptor allotypes in children with bacterial meningitis. A preliminary study. Turk J Pediatr. 1998;40(4):533–8.

114. Smith I, Vedeler C, Halstensen A. FcgammaRIIa and FcgammaRIIIb polymorphisms were not associated with meningococcal disease in Western Norway. Epidemiol Infect. 2003;130(2):193–9.

115. Lieke A, Sanders M, vdW JGJ. Fcgamma receptor IIa (CD32) heterogeneity in patients with recurrent bacterial respiratory tract infections. J Infect Dis. 1994;170:854–61.

116. Yee AM, Phan HM, Zuniga R, Salmon JE, Musher DM. Association between FcgammaRIIa-R131 allotype and bacteremic pneumococcal pneumonia. Clin Infect Dis. 2000;30(1):25–8.

117. Endeman H, Cornips MC, Grutters JC, van den Bosch JM, Ruven HJ, van Velzen-Blad H, Rijkers GT, Biesma DH. The Fcgamma receptor IIA-R/R131 genotype is associated with severe sepsis in community-acquired pneumonia. Clin Vaccine Immunol. 2009;16(7):1087–90.

118. Sole-Violan J, Garcia-Laorden MI, Marcos-Ramos JA, de Castro FR, Rajas O, Borderias L, Briones ML, Herrera-Ramos E, Blanquer J, Aspa J, et al. The Fcgamma receptor IIA-H/H131 genotype is associated with bacteremia in pneumococcal community-acquired pneumonia. Crit Care Med. 2011;39(6):1388–93.

119. Sastry K, Herman GA, Day L, Deignan E, Bruns G, Morton CC, Ezekowitz RA. The human mannose-binding protein gene. Exon structure reveals its evolutionary relationship to a human pulmonary surfactant gene and localization to chromosome 10. J Exp Med. 1989;170(4):1175–89.

120. Turner MW. Mannose-binding lectin (MBL) in health and disease. Immunobiology. 1998;199(2):327–39.

121. Lipscombe RJ, Sumiya M, Hill AV, Lau YL, Levinsky RJ, Summerfield JA, Turner MW. High frequencies in African and non-African populations of independent mutations in the mannose binding protein gene. Hum Mol Genet. 1992;1(9):709–15.

122. Sumiya M, Super M, Tabona P, Levinsky RJ, Arai T, Turner MW, Summerfield JA. Molecular basis of opsonic defect in immunodeficient children. Lancet. 1991;337(8757):1569–70.

123. Madsen HO, Garred P, Thiel S, Kurtzhals JA, Lamm LU, Ryder LP, Svejgaard A. Interplay between promoter and structural gene variants control basal serum level of mannan-binding protein. J Immunol. 1995;155(6):3013–20.

124. Summerfield JA, Ryder S, Sumiya M, Thursz M, Gorchein A, Monteil MA, Turner MW. Mannose binding protein gene mutations associated with unusual and severe infections in adults. Lancet. 1995;345(8954):886–9.

125. Summerfield JA, Sumiya M, Levin M, Turner MW. Association of mutations in mannose binding protein gene with childhood infection in consecutive hospital series. BMJ. 1997;314(7089):1229–32.

126. Garred P, Madsen HO, Halberg P, Petersen J, Kronborg G, Svejgaard A, Andersen V, Jacobsen S. Mannose-binding lectin polymorphisms and susceptibility to infection in systemic lupus erythematosus. Arthritis Rheum. 1999;42(10):2145–52.

127. Gomi K, Tokue Y, Kobayashi T, Takahashi H, Watanabe A, Fujita T, Nukiwa T. Mannose-binding lectin gene polymorphism is a modulating factor in repeated respiratory infections. Chest. 2004;126(1):95–9.

128. Roy S, Knox K, Segal S, Griffiths D, Moore CE, Welsh KI, Smarason A, Day NP, McPheat WL, Crook DW, et al. MBL genotype and risk of invasive pneumococcal disease: a case-control study. Lancet. 2002;359(9317):1569–73.

129. Tracey KJ, Beutler B, Lowry SF, Merryweather J, Wolpe S, Milsark IW, Hariri RJ, Fahey 3rd TJ, Zentella A, Albert JD, et al. Shock and tissue injury induced by recombinant human cachectin. Science. 1986;234(4775):470–4.

130. van Hinsbergh VW, Bauer KA, Kooistra T, Kluft C, Dooijewaard G, Sherman ML, Nieuwenhuizen W. Progress of fibrinolysis during tumor necrosis factor infusions in humans. Concomitant increase in tissue-type plasminogen activator, plasminogen activator inhibitor type-1, and fibrin(ogen) degradation products. Blood. 1990;76(11):2284–9.

131. Wheeler AP, Jesmok G, Brigham KL. Tumor necrosis factor's effects on lung mechanics, gas exchange, and airway reactivity in sheep. J Appl Physiol. 1990;68(6):2542–9.

132. Furman WL, Strother D, McClain K, Bell B, Leventhal B, Pratt CB. Phase I clinical trial of recombinant human tumor necrosis factor in children with refractory solid tumors: a Pediatric Oncology Group study. J Clin Oncol. 1993;11(11):2205–10.

133. Selleri C, Sato T, Anderson S, Young NS, Maciejewski JP. Interferon-gamma and tumor necrosis factor-alpha suppress both early and late stages of hematopoiesis and induce programmed cell death. J Cell Physiol. 1995;165(3):538–46.

134. Nathan C. Points of control in inflammation. Nature. 2002;420(6917):846–52.

135. Cohen J. The immunopathogenesis of sepsis. Nature. 2002; 420(6917):885–91.

136. Palsson-McDermott EM, O'Neill LA. Signal transduction by the lipopolysaccharide receptor, toll-like receptor-4. Immunology. 2004;113(2):153–62.

137. Calvano SE, Xiao W, Richards DR, Felciano RM, Baker HV, Cho RJ, Chen RO, Brownstein BH, Cobb JP, Tschoeke SK, et al. A network-based analysis of systemic inflammation in humans. Nature. 2005;437(7061):1032–7.

138. Seeley EJ, Matthay MA, Wolters PJ. Inflection points in sepsis biology: from local defense to systemic organ injury. Am J Physiol Lung Cell Mol Physiol. 2012;303(5):L355–63.

139. Wilson AG, di Giovine FS, Blakemore AI, Duff GW. Single base polymorphism in the human tumour necrosis factor alpha (TNF alpha) gene detectable by NcoI restriction of PCR product. Hum Mol Genet. 1992;1(5):353.

140. Pociot F, Briant L, Jongeneel CV, Molvig J, Worsaae H, Abbal M, Thomsen M, Nerup J, Cambon-Thomsen A. Association of tumor necrosis factor (TNF) and class II major histocompatibility complex alleles with the secretion of TNF-alpha and TNF-beta by human mononuclear cells: a possible link to insulin-dependent diabetes mellitus. Eur J Immunol. 1993;23(1):224–31.

141. Stuber F, Petersen M, Bokelmann F, Schade U. A genomic polymorphism within the tumor necrosis factor locus influences plasma tumor necrosis factor-alpha concentrations and outcome of patients with severe sepsis. Crit Care Med. 1996;24(3):381–4.

142. Wilson AG, Symons JA, McDowell TL, McDevitt HO, Duff GW. Effects of a polymorphism in the human tumor necrosis factor alpha promoter on transcriptional activation. Proc Natl Acad Sci U S A. 1997;94(7):3195–9.

143. Higuchi T, Seki N, Kamizono S, Yamada A, Kimura A, Kato H, Itoh K. Polymorphism of the 5'-flanking region of the human tumor necrosis factor (TNF)-alpha gene in Japanese. Tissue Antigens. 1998;51(6):605–12.

144. Louis E, Franchimont D, Piron A, Gevaert Y, Schaaf-Lafontaine N, Roland S, Mahieu P, Malaise M, De Groote D, Louis R, et al. Tumour necrosis factor (TNF) gene polymorphism influences TNF-alpha production in lipopolysaccharide (LPS)-stimulated whole blood cell culture in healthy humans. Clin Exp Immunol. 1998;113(3):401–6.

145. Huizinga TW, Westendorp RG, Bollen EL, Keijsers V, Brinkman BM, Langermans JA, Breedveld FC, Verweij CL, van de Gaer L, Dams L, et al. TNF-alpha promoter polymorphisms, production and susceptibility to multiple sclerosis in different groups of patients. J Neuroimmunol. 1997;72(2):149–53.

146. Kroeger KM, Carville KS, Abraham LJ. The -308 tumor necrosis factor-alpha promoter polymorphism effects transcription. Mol Immunol. 1997;34(5):391–9.

147. Baseggio L, Bartholin L, Chantome A, Charlot C, Rimokh R, Salles G. Allele-specific binding to the -308 single nucleotide polymorphism site in the tumour necrosis factor-alpha promoter. Eur J Immunogenet. 2004;31(1):15–9.

148. Suriano AR, Sanford AN, Kim N, Oh M, Kennedy S, Henderson MJ, Dietzmann K, Sullivan KE. GCF2/LRRFIP1 represses tumor

149. Nadel S, Newport MJ, Booy R, Levin M. Variation in the tumor necrosis factor-alpha gene promoter region may be associated with death from meningococcal disease. J Infect Dis. 1996;174(4):878–80.

150. Clark MF, Baudouin SV. A systematic review of the quality of genetic association studies in human sepsis. Intensive Care Med. 2006;32(11):1706–12.

151. Ross OA, McCormack R, Maxwell LD, Duguid RA, Quinn DJ, Barnett YA, Rea IM, El-Agnaf OM, Gibson JM, Wallace A, et al. mt4216C variant in linkage with the mtDNA TJ cluster may confer a susceptibility to mitochondrial dysfunction resulting in an increased risk of Parkinson's disease in the Irish. Exp Gerontol. 2003;38(4):397–405.

152. Aird WC. Vascular bed-specific hemostasis: role of endothelium in sepsis pathogenesis. Crit Care Med. 2001;29(7 Suppl):S28–34; discussion S34–25.

153. Faust SN, Levin M, Harrison OB, Goldin RD, Lockhart MS, Kondaveeti S, Laszik Z, Esmon CT, Heyderman RS. Dysfunction of endothelial protein C activation in severe meningococcal sepsis. N Engl J Med. 2001;345(6):408–16.

154. Fourrier F, Lestavel P, Chopin C, Marey A, Goudemand J, Rime A, Mangalaboyi J. Meningococcemia and purpura fulminans in adults: acute deficiencies of proteins C and S and early treatment with antithrombin III concentrates. Intensive Care Med. 1990;16(2):121–4.

155. Paramo JA, Perez JL, Serrano M, Rocha E. Types 1 and 2 plasminogen activator inhibitor and tumor necrosis factor alpha in patients with sepsis. Thromb Haemost. 1990;64(1):3–6.

156. Brandtzaeg P, Joo GB, Brusletto B, Kierulf P. Plasminogen activator inhibitor 1 and 2, alpha-2-antiplasmin, plasminogen, and endotoxin levels in systemic meningococcal disease. Thromb Res. 1990;57(2):271–8.

157. Kornelisse RF, Hazelzet JA, Savelkoul HF, Hop WC, Suur MH, Borsboom AN, Risseeuw-Appel IM, van der Voort E, de Groot R. The relationship between plasminogen activator inhibitor-1 and proinflammatory and counterinflammatory mediators in children with meningococcal septic shock. J Infect Dis. 1996;173(5):1148–56.

158. Hermans PW, Hibberd ML, Booy R, Daramola O, Hazelzet JA, de Groot R, Levin M. 4G/5G promoter polymorphism in the plasminogen-activator-inhibitor-1 gene and outcome of meningococcal disease. Meningococcal Research Group. Lancet. 1999;354(9178):556–60.

159. Zenz W, Muntean W, Gallistl S, Zobel G, Grubbauer HM. Recombinant tissue plasminogen activator treatment in two infants with fulminant meningococcemia. Pediatrics. 1995;96(1 Pt 1):144–8.

160. Dawson SJ, Wiman B, Hamsten A, Green F, Humphries S, Henney AM. The two allele sequences of a common polymorphism in the promoter of the plasminogen activator inhibitor-1 (PAI-1) gene respond differently to interleukin-1 in HepG2 cells. J Biol Chem. 1993;268(15):10739–45.

161. Eriksson P, Kallin B, van 't Hooft FM, Bavenholm P, Hamsten A. Allele-specific increase in basal transcription of the plasminogen-activator inhibitor 1 gene is associated with myocardial infarction. Proc Natl Acad Sci U S A. 1995;92(6):1851–5.

162. Westendorp RG, Hottenga JJ, Slagboom PE. Variation in plasminogen-activator-inhibitor-1 gene and risk of meningococcal septic shock. Lancet. 1999;354(9178):561–3.

163. Wingeyer SP, de Larranaga G, Cunto E, Fontana L, Nogueras C, San Juan J. Role of 4G/5G promoter polymorphism of Plasminogen Activator Inhibitor-1 (PAI-1) gene in outcome of sepsis. Thromb Res. 2010;125(4):367–9.

164. Huq MA, Takeyama N, Harada M, Miki Y, Takeuchi A, Inoue S, Nakagawa T, Kanou H, Hirakawa A, Noguchi H. 4G/5G

necrosis factor alpha expression. Mol Cell Biol. 2005;25(20): 9073–81.

Polymorphism of the plasminogen activator inhibitor-1 gene is associated with multiple organ dysfunction in critically ill patients. Acta Haematol. 2012;127(2):72–80.

165. Menges T, Hermans PW, Little SG, Langefeld T, Boning O, Engel J, Sluijter M, de Groot R, Hempelmann G. Plasminogen-activator-inhibitor-1 4G/5G promoter polymorphism and prognosis of severely injured patients. Lancet. 2001;357(9262):1096–7.

166. Tsantes A, Tsangaris I, Kopterides P, Nikolopoulos G, Kalamara E, Antonakos G, Kapsimali V, Gialeraki A, Dimopoulou I, Orfanos S, et al. Angiotensin converting enzyme (ACE) insertion/deletion (I/D) polymorphism and circulating ACE levels are not associated with outcome in critically ill septic patients. Clin Chem Lab Med. 2012;50(2):293–9.

167. Cambien F, Alhenc-Gelas F, Herbeth B, Andre JL, Rakotovao R, Gonzales MF, Allegrini J, Bloch C. Familial resemblance of plasma angiotensin-converting enzyme level: the Nancy Study. Am J Hum Genet. 1988;43(5):774–80.

168. Rigat B, Hubert C, Alhenc-Gelas F, Cambien F, Corvol P, Soubrier F. An insertion/deletion polymorphism in the angiotensin I-converting enzyme gene accounting for half the variance of serum enzyme levels. J Clin Invest. 1990;86(4):1343–6.

169. Rigat B, Hubert C, Corvol P, Soubrier F. PCR detection of the insertion/deletion polymorphism of the human angiotensin converting enzyme gene (DCP1) (dipeptidyl carboxypeptidase 1). Nucleic Acids Res. 1992;20(6):1433.

170. Costerousse O, Allegrini J, Lopez M, Alhenc-Gelas F. Angiotensin I-converting enzyme in human circulating mononuclear cells: genetic polymorphism of expression in T-lymphocytes. Biochem J. 1993;290(Pt 1):33–40.

171. Tiret L, Rigat B, Visvikis S, Breda C, Corvol P, Cambien F, Soubrier F. Evidence, from combined segregation and linkage analysis, that a variant of the angiotensin I-converting enzyme (ACE) gene controls plasma ACE levels. Am J Hum Genet. 1992;51(1):197–205.

172. John Baier R, Loggins J, Yanamandra K. Angiotensin converting enzyme insertion/deletion polymorphism does not alter sepsis outcome in ventilated very low birth weight infants. J Perinatol. 2005;25(3):205–9.

173. Bunker-Wiersma HE, Koopmans RP, Kuipers TW, Knoester H, Bos AP. Single nucleotide polymorphisms in genes of circulatory homeostasis in surviving pediatric intensive care patients with meningococcal infection. Pediatr Crit Care Med. 2008;9(5):517–23.

174. Villar J, Flores C, Perez-Mendez L, Maca-Meyer N, Espinosa E, Blanco J, Sanguesa R, Muriel A, Tejera P, Muros M, et al. Angiotensin-converting enzyme insertion/deletion polymorphism is not associated with susceptibility and outcome in sepsis and acute respiratory distress syndrome. Intensive Care Med. 2008;34(3):488–95.

175. Davis SM, Clark EA, Nelson LT, Silver RM. The association of innate immune response gene polymorphisms and puerperal group A streptococcal sepsis. Am J Obstet Gynecol. 2010;202(3):308.e301. 8.

176. Spiegler J, Gilhaus A, Konig IR, Kattner E, Vochem M, Kuster H, Moller J, Muller D, Kribs A, Segerer H, et al. Polymorphisms in the Renin-Angiotensin system and outcome of very-low-birthweight infants. Neonatology. 2010;97(1):10–4.

177. Hou X, Zhang P, Nie W, Tang S, Wang J, Zhang Q, Wan Z, Zhang B, Song B. Association between angiotensin-converting enzyme I/D polymorphism and sepsis: a meta-analysis. J Renin Angiotensin Aldosterone Syst. 2013 [Epub ahead of print].

178. Bernard GR, Artigas A, Brigham KL, Carlet J, Falke K, Hudson L, Lamy M, Legall JR, Morris A, Spragg R. The American-European Consensus Conference on ARDS. Definitions, mechanisms, relevant outcomes, and clinical trial coordination. Am J Respir Crit Care Med. 1994;149(3 Pt 1):818–24.

179. Zimmerman JJ, Akhtar SR, Caldwell E, Rubenfeld GD. Incidence and outcomes of pediatric acute lung injury. Pediatrics. 2009;124(1):87–95.

180. Bindl L, Dresbach K, Lentze MJ. Incidence of acute respiratory distress syndrome in German children and adolescents: a population-based study. Crit Care Med. 2005;33(1):209–312.

181. Kneyber MC, Brouwers AG, Caris JA, Chedamni S, Plotz FB. Acute respiratory distress syndrome: is it underrecognized in the pediatric intensive care unit? Intensive Care Med. 2008;34(4):751–4.

182. Erickson S, Schibler A, Numa A, Nuthall G, Yung M, Pascoe E, Wilkins B. Acute lung injury in pediatric intensive care in Australia and New Zealand: a prospective, multicenter, observational study. Pediatr Crit Care Med. 2007;8(4):317–23.

183. Hu X, Qian S, Xu F, Huang B, Zhou D, Wang Y, Li C, Fan X, Lu Z, Sun B. Incidence, management and mortality of acute hypoxemic respiratory failure and acute respiratory distress syndrome from a prospective study of Chinese paediatric intensive care network. Acta Paediatr. 2010;99(5):715–21.

184. Lopez-Fernandez Y, Azagra AM, de la Oliva P, Modesto V, Sanchez JI, Parrilla J, Arroyo MJ, Reyes SB, Pons-Odena M, Lopez-Herce J, et al. Pediatric Acute Lung Injury Epidemiology and Natural History study: incidence and outcome of the acute respiratory distress syndrome in children. Crit Care Med. 2012;40(12):3238–45.

185. Adamzik M, Frey U, Sixt S, Knemeyer L, Beiderlinden M, Peters J, Siffert W. ACE I/D but not AGT (-6)A/G polymorphism is a risk factor for mortality in ARDS. Eur Respir J. 2007;29(3):482–8.

186. Marshall RP, Webb S, Bellingan GJ, Montgomery HE, Chaudhari B, McAnulty RJ, Humphries SE, Hill MR, Laurent GJ. Angiotensin converting enzyme insertion/deletion polymorphism is associated with susceptibility and outcome in acute respiratory distress syndrome. Am J Respir Crit Care Med. 2002;166(5):646–50.

187. Jerng JS, Yu CJ, Wang HC, Chen KY, Cheng SL, Yang PC. Polymorphism of the angiotensin-converting enzyme gene affects the outcome of acute respiratory distress syndrome. Crit Care Med. 2006;34(4):1001–6.

188. Su L, Zhai R, Sheu CC, Gallagher DC, Gong MN, Tejera P, Thompson BT, Christiani DC. Genetic variants in the angiopoietin-2 gene are associated with increased risk of ARDS. Intensive Care Med. 2009;35(6):1024–30.

189. Meyer NJ, Li M, Feng R, Bradfield J, Gallop R, Bellamy S, Fuchs BD, Lanken PN, Albelda SM, Rushefski M, et al. ANGPT2 genetic variant is associated with trauma-associated acute lung injury and altered plasma angiopoietin-2 isoform ratio. Am J Respir Crit Care Med. 2011;183(10):1344–53.

190. Baughn JM, Quasney MW, Simpson P, Merchant D, Li SH, Levy H, Dahmer MK. Association of cystic fibrosis transmembrane conductance regulator gene variants with acute lung injury in African American children with pneumonia*. Crit Care Med. 2012;40(11):3042–9.

191. Adamzik M, Frey UH, Riemann K, Sixt S, Lehmann N, Siffert W, Peters J. Factor V Leiden mutation is associated with improved 30-day survival in patients with acute respiratory distress syndrome. Crit Care Med. 2008;36(6):1776–9.

192. Glavan BJ, Holden TD, Goss CH, Black RA, Neff MJ, Nathens AB, Martin TR, Wurfel MM. Genetic variation in the FAS gene and associations with acute lung injury. Am J Respir Crit Care Med. 2011;183(3):356–63.

193. Lagan AL, Quinlan GJ, Mumby S, Melley DD, Goldstraw P, Bellingan GJ, Hill MR, Briggs D, Pantelidis P, du Bois RM, et al. Variation in iron homeostasis genes between patients with ARDS and healthy control subjects. Chest. 2008;133(6):1302–11.

194. Reiner AP, Wurfel MM, Lange LA, Carlson CS, Nord AS, Carty CL, Rieder MJ, Desmarais C, Jenny NS, Iribarren C, et al. Polymorphisms of the IL1-receptor antagonist gene (IL1RN) are

associated with multiple markers of systemic inflammation. Arterioscler Thromb Vasc Biol. 2008;28(7):1407–12.

195. Patwari PP, O'Cain P, Goodman DM, Smith M, Krushkal J, Liu C, Somes G, Quasney MW, Dahmer MK. Interleukin-1 receptor antagonist intron 2 VNTR polymorphism and respiratory failure in children with community acquired pneumonia. Pediatr Crit Care Med. 2008;9:553–9.

196. Marshall RP, Webb S, Hill MR, Humphries SE, Laurent GJ. Genetic polymorphisms associated with susceptibility and outcome in ARDS. Chest. 2002;121(3 Suppl):68S–9.

197. Sutherland AM, Walley KR, Manocha S, Russell JA. The association of interleukin 6 haplotype clades with mortality in critically ill adults. Arch Intern Med. 2005;165(1):75–82.

198. Nonas SA, Finigan JH, Gao L, Garcia JG. Functional genomic insights into acute lung injury: role of ventilators and mechanical stress. Proc Am Thorac Soc. 2005;2(3):188–94.

199. Flores C, Ma SF, Maresso K, Wade MS, Villar J, Garcia JG. IL6 gene-wide haplotype is associated with susceptibility to acute lung injury. Transl Res. 2008;152(1):11–7.

200. Pino-Yanes M, Ma SF, Sun X, Tejera P, Corrales A, Blanco J, Perez-Mendez L, Espinosa E, Muriel A, Blanch L, et al. Interleukin-1 receptor-associated kinase 3 gene associates with susceptibility to acute lung injury. Am J Respir Cell Mol Biol. 2010;45(4):740–5.

201. Gong MN, Zhou W, Williams PL, Thompson BT, Pothier L, Christiani DC. Polymorphisms in the mannose binding lectin-2 gene and acute respiratory distress syndrome. Crit Care Med. 2007;35(1):48–56.

202. Ip WK, Chan KH, Law HK, Tso GH, Kong EK, Wong WH, To YF, Yung RW, Chow EY, Au KL, et al. Mannose-binding lectin in severe acute respiratory syndrome coronavirus infection. J Infect Dis. 2005;191(10):1697–704.

203. Garcia-Laorden MI, Sole-Violan J, Rodriguez de Castro F, Aspa J, Briones ML, Garcia-Saavedra A, Rajas O, Blanquer J, Caballero-Hidalgo A, Marcos-Ramos JA, et al. Mannose-binding lectin and mannose-binding lectin-associated serine protease 2 in susceptibility, severity, and outcome of pneumonia in adults. J Allergy Clin Immunol. 2008;122(2):368–74. 374.e361–2.

204. Gao L, Flores C, Fan-Ma S, Miller EJ, Moitra J, Moreno L, Wadgaonkar R, Simon B, Brower R, Sevransky J, et al. Macrophage migration inhibitory factor in acute lung injury: expression, biomarker, and associations. Transl Res. 2007;150(1):18–29.

205. Gao L, Grant A, Halder I, Brower R, Sevransky J, Maloney JP, Moss M, Shanholtz C, Yates CR, Meduri GU, et al. Novel polymorphisms in the myosin light chain kinase gene confer risk for acute lung injury. Am J Respir Cell Mol Biol. 2006;34(4):487–95.

206. Christie JD, Ma SF, Aplenc R, Li M, Lanken PN, Shah CV, Fuchs B, Albelda SM, Flores C, Garcia JG. Variation in the myosin light chain kinase gene is associated with development of acute lung injury after major trauma. Crit Care Med. 2008;36(10):2794–800.

207. Marzec JM, Christie JD, Reddy SP, Jedlicka AE, Vuong H, Lanken PN, Aplenc R, Yamamoto T, Yamamoto M, Cho HY, et al. Functional polymorphisms in the transcription factor NRF2 in humans increase the risk of acute lung injury. FASEB J. 2007;21(9):2237–46.

208. Zhai R, Zhou W, Gong MN, Thompson BT, Su L, Yu C, Kraft P, Christiani DC. Inhibitor kappaB-alpha haplotype GTC is associated with susceptibility to acute respiratory distress syndrome in Caucasians. Crit Care Med. 2007;35(3):893–8.

209. Reddy AJ, Christie JD, Aplenc R, Fuchs B, Lanken PN, Kleeberger SR. Association of human NAD(P)H:quinone oxidoreductase 1 (NQO1) polymorphism with development of acute lung injury. J Cell Mol Med. 2009;13(8B):1784–91.

210. Ye SQ, Simon BA, Maloney JP, Zambelli-Weiner A, Gao L, Grant A, Easley RB, McVerry BJ, Tuder RM, Standiford T,

et al. Pre-B-cell colony-enhancing factor as a potential novel biomarker in acute lung injury. Am J Respir Crit Care Med. 2005;171(4):361–70.

211. Arcaroli J, Sankoff J, Liu N, Allison DB, Maloney J, Abraham E. Association between urokinase haplotypes and outcome from infection-associated acute lung injury. Intensive Care Med. 2008;34(2):300–7.

212. Dahmer MK, O'Cain P, Patwari PP, Simpson P, Li SH, Halligan N, Quasney MW. The influence of genetic variation in surfactant protein B on severe lung injury in black children. Crit Care Med. 2011;39(5):1138–44.

213. Arcaroli JJ, Hokanson JE, Abraham E, Geraci M, Murphy JR, Bowler RP, Dinarello CA, Silveira L, Sankoff J, Heyland D, et al. Extracellular superoxide dismutase haplotypes are associated with acute lung injury and mortality. Am J Respir Crit Care Med. 2009;179(2):105–12.

214. Gong MN, Zhou W, Williams PL, Thompson BT, Pothier L, Boyce P, Christiani DC. 308GA and TNFB polymorphisms in acute respiratory distress syndrome. Eur Respir J. 2005;26(3):382–9.

215. Zhai R, Gong MN, Zhou W, Thompson TB, Kraft P, Su L, Christiani DC. Genotypes and haplotypes of the VEGF gene are associated with higher mortality and lower VEGF plasma levels in patients with ARDS. Thorax. 2007;62(8):718–22.

216. Medford AR, Keen LJ, Bidwell JL, Millar AB. Vascular endothelial growth factor gene polymorphism and acute respiratory distress syndrome. Thorax. 2005;60(3):244–8.

217. Ware LB. Pathophysiology of acute lung injury and the acute respiratory distress syndrome. Semin Respir Crit Care Med. 2006;27(4):337–49.

218. Matthay MA, Zemans RL. The acute respiratory distress syndrome: pathogenesis and treatment. Annu Rev Pathol. 2011;6:147–63.

219. Quasney MW, Waterer GW, Dahmer MK, Kron GK, Zhang Q, Kessler LA, Wunderink RG. Association between surfactant protein B + 1580 polymorphism and the risk of respiratory failure in adults with community-acquired pneumonia. Crit Care Med. 2004;32(5):1115–9.

220. Song Z, Yin J, Yao C, Sun Z, Shao M, Zhang Y, Tao Z, Huang P, Tong C. Variants in the toll-interacting protein gene are associated with susceptibility to sepsis in the Chinese Han population. Crit Care. 2011;15(1):R12.

221. Ware LB, Matthay MA. The acute respiratory distress syndrome. N Engl J Med. 2000;342(18):1334–49.

222. Matthay MA. Alveolar fluid clearance in patients with ARDS: does it make a difference? Chest. 2002;122(6 Suppl):340S–3.

223. Matthay MA, Robriquet L, Fang X. Alveolar epithelium: role in lung fluid balance and acute lung injury. Proc Am Thorac Soc. 2005;2(3):206–13.

224. Fang X, Fukuda N, Barbry P, Sartori C, Verkman AS, Matthay MA. Novel role for CFTR in fluid absorption from the distal airspaces of the lung. J Gen Physiol. 2002;119(2):199–207.

225. Fang X, Song Y, Hirsch J, Galietta LJ, Pedemonte N, Zemans RL, Dolganov G, Verkman AS, Matthay MA. Contribution of CFTR to apical-basolateral fluid transport in cultured human alveolar epithelial type II cells. Am J Physiol Lung Cell Mol Physiol. 2006;290(2):L242–9.

226. Regnier A, Dannhoffer L, Blouquit-Laye S, Bakari M, Naline E, Chinet T. Expression of cystic fibrosis transmembrane conductance regulator in the human distal lung. Hum Pathol. 2008;39(3):368–76.

227. Nagel G, Szellas T, Riordan JR, Friedrich T, Hartung K. Non-specific activation of the epithelial sodium channel by the CFTR chloride channel. EMBO Rep. 2001;2(3):249–54.

228. Reddy MM, Light MJ, Quinton PM. Activation of the epithelial Na+ channel (ENaC) requires CFTR Cl- channel function. Nature. 1999;402(6759):301–4.

229. Bremer S, Hoof T, Wilke M, Busche R, Scholte B, Riordan JR, Maass G, Tummler B. Quantitative expression patterns of multidrug-resistance P-glycoprotein (MDR1) and differentially spliced cystic-fibrosis transmembrane-conductance regulator mRNA transcripts in human epithelia. Eur J Biochem. 1992;206(1):137–49.

230. Davis PB. Cystic fibrosis since 1938. Am J Respir Crit Care Med. 2006;173(5):475–82.

231. Hunter MJ, Treharne KJ, Winter AK, Cassidy DM, Land S, Mehta A. Expression of wild-type CFTR suppresses NF-kappaB-driven inflammatory signalling. PLoS One. 2010;5(7):e11598.

232. Tirouvanziam R, de Bentzmann S, Hubeau C, Hinnrasky J, Jacquot J, Peault B, Puchelle E. Inflammation and infection in naive human cystic fibrosis airway grafts. Am J Respir Cell Mol Biol. 2000;23(2):121–7.

233. Vandivier RW, Richens TR, Horstmann SA, deCathelineau AM, Ghosh M, Reynolds SD, Xiao YQ, Riches DW, Plumb J, Vachon E, et al. Dysfunctional cystic fibrosis transmembrane conductance regulator inhibits phagocytosis of apoptotic cells with proinflammatory consequences. Am J Physiol Lung Cell Mol Physiol. 2009;297(4):L677–86.

234. Vij N, Mazur S, Zeitlin PL. CFTR is a negative regulator of NFkappaB mediated innate immune response. PLoS One. 2009;4(2):e4664.

235. Weber AJ, Soong G, Bryan R, Saba S, Prince A. Activation of NF-kappaB in airway epithelial cells is dependent on CFTR trafficking and Cl- channel function. Am J Physiol Lung Cell Mol Physiol. 2001;281(1):L71–8.

236. Mueller C, Braag SA, Keeler A, Hodges C, Drumm M, Flotte TR. Lack of cystic fibrosis transmembrane conductance regulator in CD3+ lymphocytes leads to aberrant cytokine secretion and hyperinflammatory adaptive immune responses. Am J Respir Cell Mol Biol. 2011;44(6):922–9.

237. Su X, Looney MR, Su HE, Lee JW, Song Y, Matthay MA. Role of CFTR expressed by neutrophils in modulating acute lung inflammation and injury in mice. Inflamm Res. 2011;60(7):619–32.

238. Strong TV, Wilkinson DJ, Mansoura MK, Devor DC, Henze K, Yang Y, Wilson JM, Cohn JA, Dawson DC, Frizzell RA, et al. Expression of an abundant alternatively spliced form of the cystic fibrosis transmembrane conductance regulator (CFTR) gene is not associated with a cAMP-activated chloride conductance. Hum Mol Genet. 1993;2(3):225–30.

239. Pissarra LS, Farinha CM, Xu Z, Schmidt A, Thibodeau PH, Cai Z, Thomas PJ, Sheppard DN, Amaral MD. Solubilizing mutations used to crystallize one CFTR domain attenuate the trafficking and channel defects caused by the major cystic fibrosis mutation. Chem Biol. 2008;15(1):62–9.

240. Chu CS, Trapnell BC, Curristin S, Cutting GR, Crystal RG. Genetic basis of variable exon 9 skipping in cystic fibrosis transmembrane conductance regulator mRNA. Nat Genet. 1993;3(2):151–6.

241. Chu CS, Trapnell BC, Murtagh Jr JJ, Moss J, Dalemans W, Jallat S, Mercenier A, Pavirani A, Lecocq JP, Cutting GR, et al. Variable deletion of exon 9 coding sequences in cystic fibrosis transmembrane conductance regulator gene mRNA transcripts in normal bronchial epithelium. EMBO J. 1991;10(6):1355–63.

242. Cuppens H, Lin W, Jaspers M, Costes B, Teng H, Vankeerberghen A, Jorissen M, Droogmans G, Reynaert I, Goossens M, et al. Polyvariant mutant cystic fibrosis transmembrane conductance regulator genes. The polymorphic (Tg)m locus explains the partial penetrance of the T5 polymorphism as a disease mutation. J Clin Invest. 1998;101(2):487–96.

243. Pagani F, Buratti E, Stuani C, Baralle FE. Missense, nonsense, and neutral mutations define juxtaposed regulatory elements of splicing in cystic fibrosis transmembrane regulator exon 9. J Biol Chem. 2003;278(29):26580–8.

244. Niksic M, Romano M, Buratti E, Pagani F, Baralle FE. Functional analysis of cis-acting elements regulating the alternative splicing of human CFTR exon 9. Hum Mol Genet. 1999;8(13):2339–49.

245. Buratti E, Baralle FE. Characterization and functional implications of the RNA binding properties of nuclear factor TDP-43, a novel splicing regulator of CFTR exon 9. J Biol Chem. 2001;276(39):36337–43.

246. Dujardin G, Buratti E, Charlet-Berguerand N, Martins de Araujo M, Mbopda A, Le Jossic-Corcos C, Pagani F, Ferec C, Corcos L. CELF proteins regulate CFTR pre-mRNA splicing: essential role of the divergent domain of ETR-3. Nucleic Acids Res. 2010;38(20):7273–85.

247. Delaney SJ, Rich DP, Thomson SA, Hargrave MR, Lovelock PK, Welsh MJ, Wainwright BJ. Cystic fibrosis transmembrane conductance regulator splice variants are not conserved and fail to produce chloride channels. Nat Genet. 1993;4(4):426–31.

248. Gregory RJ, Rich DP, Cheng SH, Souza DW, Paul S, Manavalan P, Anderson MP, Welsh MJ, Smith AE. Maturation and function of cystic fibrosis transmembrane conductance regulator variants bearing mutations in putative nucleotide-binding domains 1 and 2. Mol Cell Biol. 1991;11(8):3886–93.

249. Chu CS, Trapnell BC, Curristin SM, Cutting GR, Crystal RG. Extensive posttranscriptional deletion of the coding sequences for part of nucleotide-binding fold 1 in respiratory epithelial mRNA transcripts of the cystic fibrosis transmembrane conductance regulator gene is not associated with the clinical manifestations of cystic fibrosis. J Clin Invest. 1992;90(3):785–90.

250. Serra-Pages C, Medley QG, Tang M, Hart A, Streuli M. Liprins, a family of LAR transmembrane protein-tyrosine phosphatase-interacting proteins. J Biol Chem. 1998;273(25):15611–20.

251. Asperti C, Pettinato E, de Curtis I. Liprin-alpha1 affects the distribution of low-affinity beta1 integrins and stabilizes their permanence at the cell surface. Exp Cell Res. 2010;316(6):915–26.

252. Reutershan J, Ley K. Bench-to-bedside review: acute respiratory distress syndrome - how neutrophils migrate into the lung. Crit Care. 2004;8(6):453–61.

253. Crosby LM, Waters CM. Epithelial repair mechanisms in the lung. Am J Physiol Lung Cell Mol Physiol. 2010;298(6):L715–31.

254. Butler J, Rocker GM, Westaby S. Inflammatory response to cardiopulmonary bypass. Ann Thorac Surg. 1993;55(2):552–9.

255. te Velthuis H, Jansen PG, Oudemans-van Straaten HM, Sturk A, Eijsman L, Wildevuur CR. Myocardial performance in elderly patients after cardiopulmonary bypass is suppressed by tumor necrosis factor. J Thorac Cardiovasc Surg. 1995;110(6):1663–9.

256. Cremer J, Martin M, Redl H, Bahrami S, Abraham C, Graeter T, Haverich A, Schlag G, Borst HG. Systemic inflammatory response syndrome after cardiac operations. Ann Thorac Surg. 1996;61(6):1714–20.

257. Khabar KS, elBarbary MA, Khouqeer F, Devol E, al-Gain S, al-Halees Z. Circulating endotoxin and cytokines after cardiopulmonary bypass: differential correlation with duration of bypass and systemic inflammatory response/multiple organ dysfunction syndromes. Clin Immunol Immunopathol. 1997;85(1):97–103.

258. Wan S, LeClerc JL, Vincent JL. Inflammatory response to cardiopulmonary bypass: mechanisms involved and possible therapeutic strategies. Chest. 1997;112(3):676–92.

259. Gilliland HE, Armstrong MA, McMurray TJ. Tumour necrosis factor as predictor for pulmonary dysfunction after cardiac surgery. Lancet. 1998;352(9136):1281–2.

260. Paparella D, Yau TM, Young E. Cardiopulmonary bypass induced inflammation: pathophysiology and treatment. An update. Eur J Cardiothorac Surg. 2002;21(2):232–44.

261. Schmartz D, Tabardel Y, Preiser JC, Barvais L, d'Hollander A, Duchateau J, Vincent JL. Does aprotinin influence the inflammatory response to cardiopulmonary bypass in patients? J Thorac Cardiovasc Surg. 2003;125(1):184–90.

262. Clark SC. Lung injury after cardiopulmonary bypass. Perfusion. 2006;21(4):225–8.

263. Allen ML, Hoschtitzky JA, Peters MJ, Elliott M, Goldman A, James I, Klein NJ. Interleukin-10 and its role in clinical immunoparalysis following pediatric cardiac surgery. Crit Care Med. 2006;34(10):2658–65.

264. Warren OJ, Smith AJ, Alexiou C, Rogers PL, Jawad N, Vincent C, Darzi AW, Athanasiou T. The inflammatory response to cardiopulmonary bypass: part 1 – mechanisms of pathogenesis. J Cardiothorac Vasc Anesth. 2009;23(2):223–31.

265. Warren OJ, Watret al, de Wit KL, Alexiou C, Vincent C, Darzi AW, Athanasiou T. The inflammatory response to cardiopulmonary bypass: part 2 – anti-inflammatory therapeutic strategies. J Cardiothorac Vasc Anesth. 2009;23(3):384–93.

266. Jouan J, Golmard L, Benhamouda N, Durrleman N, Golmard JL, Ceccaldi R, Trinquart L, Fabiani JN, Tartour E, Jeunemaitre X, et al. Gene polymorphisms and cytokine plasma levels as predictive factors of complications after cardiopulmonary bypass. J Thorac Cardiovasc Surg. 2012;144(2):467–73. 473 e461–462.

267. Sasser WC, Dabal RJ, Askenazi DJ, Borasino S, Moellinger AB, Kirklin JK, Alten JA. Prophylactic peritoneal dialysis following cardiopulmonary bypass in children is associated with decreased inflammation and improved clinical outcomes. Congenit Heart Dis. 2013 [Epub ahead of print].

268. Jansen NJ, van Oeveren W, Gu YJ, van Vliet MH, Eijsman L, Wildevuur CR. Endotoxin release and tumor necrosis factor formation during cardiopulmonary bypass. Ann Thorac Surg. 1992;54(4):744–7; discussion 747–8.

269. Lindal S, Gunnes S, Lund I, Straume BK, Jorgensen L, Sorlie D. Myocardial and microvascular injury following coronary surgery and its attenuation by mode of reperfusion. Eur J Cardiothorac Surg. 1995;9(2):83–9.

270. Chenoweth DE, Cooper SW, Hugli TE, Stewart RW, Blackstone EH, Kirklin JW. Complement activation during cardiopulmonary bypass: evidence for generation of C3a and C5a anaphylatoxins. N Engl J Med. 1981;304(9):497–503.

271. Kirklin JK, Westaby S, Blackstone EH, Kirklin JW, Chenoweth DE, Pacifico AD. Complement and the damaging effects of cardiopulmonary bypass. J Thorac Cardiovasc Surg. 1983;86(6):845–57.

272. Boehm J, Hauner K, Grammer J, Dietrich W, Wagenpfeil S, Braun S, Lange R, Bauernschmitt R. Tumor necrosis factor-alpha -863 C/A promoter polymorphism affects the inflammatory response after cardiac surgery. Eur J Cardiothorac Surg. 2011;40(1):e50–4.

273. Gaudino M, Andreotti F, Zamparelli R, Di Castelnuovo A, Nasso G, Burzotta F, Iacoviello L, Donati MB, Schiavello R, Maseri A, et al. The -174G/C interleukin-6 polymorphism influences postoperative interleukin-6 levels and postoperative atrial fibrillation. Is atrial fibrillation an inflammatory complication? Circulation. 2003;108 Suppl 1:II195–9.

274. Galley HF, Lowe PR, Carmichael RL, Webster NR. Genotype and interleukin-10 responses after cardiopulmonary bypass. Br J Anaesth. 2003;91(3):424–6.

275. Schroeder S, Borger N, Wrigge H, Welz A, Putensen C, Hoeft A, Stuber F. A tumor necrosis factor gene polymorphism influences the inflammatory response after cardiac operation. Ann Thorac Surg. 2003;75(2):534–7.

276. Tomasdottir H, Hjartarson H, Ricksten A, Wasslavik C, Bengtsson A, Ricksten SE. Tumor necrosis factor gene polymorphism is associated with enhanced systemic inflammatory response and increased cardiopulmonary morbidity after cardiac surgery. Anesth Analg. 2003;97(4):944–9.

277. Yende S, Quasney MW, Tolley E, Zhang Q, Wunderink RG. Association of tumor necrosis factor gene polymorphisms and prolonged mechanical ventilation after coronary artery bypass surgery. Crit Care Med. 2003;31(1):133–40.

278. Grunenfelder J, Umbehr M, Plass A, Bestmann L, Maly FE, Zund G, Turina M. Genetic polymorphisms of apolipoprotein E4 and tumor necrosis factor beta as predisposing factors for increased inflammatory cytokines after cardiopulmonary bypass. J Thorac Cardiovasc Surg. 2004;128(1):92–7.

279. Podgoreanu MV, White WD, Morris RW, Mathew JP, Stafford-Smith M, Welsby IJ, Grocott HP, Milano CA, Newman MF, Schwinn DA. Inflammatory gene polymorphisms and risk of postoperative myocardial infarction after cardiac surgery. Circulation. 2006;114(1 Suppl):I275–81.

280. Bittar MN, Carey JA, Barnard JB, Pravica V, Deiraniya AK, Yonan N, Hutchinson IV. Tumor necrosis factor alpha influences the inflammatory response after coronary surgery. Ann Thorac Surg. 2006;81(1):132–7.

281. Yoon SZ, Jang IJ, Choi YJ, Kang MH, Lim HJ, Lim YJ, Lee HW, Chang SH, Yoon SM. Association between tumor necrosis factor alpha 308G/A polymorphism and increased proinflammatory cytokine release after cardiac surgery with cardiopulmonary bypass in the Korean population. J Cardiothorac Vasc Anesth. 2009;23(5):646–50.

282. Wang JF, Bian JJ, Wan XJ, Zhu KM, Sun ZZ, Lu AD. Association between inflammatory genetic polymorphism and acute lung injury after cardiac surgery with cardiopulmonary bypass. Med Sci Monit. 2010;16(5):CR260–5.

283. Jia X, Tian Y, Wang Y, Deng X, Dong Z, Scafa N, Zhang X. Association between the interleukin-6 gene -572G/C and -597G/A polymorphisms and coronary heart disease in the Han Chinese. Med Sci Monit. 2010;16(3):CR103–8.

284. Chen S, Xu L, Tang J. Association of interleukin 18 gene polymorphism with susceptibility to the development of acute lung injury after cardiopulmonary bypass surgery. Tissue Antigens. 2010;76(3):245–9.

285. Fox AA, Pretorius M, Liu KY, Collard CD, Perry TE, Shernan SK, De Jager PL, Hafler DA, Herman DS, DePalma SR, et al. Genome-wide assessment for genetic variants associated with ventricular dysfunction after primary coronary artery bypass graft surgery. PLoS One. 2011;6(9):e24593.

286. Borgman KY, Smith AH, Owen JP, Fish FA, Kannankeril PJ. A genetic contribution to risk for postoperative junctional ectopic tachycardia in children undergoing surgery for congenital heart disease. Heart Rhythm. 2013;8(12):1900–4.

287. Fatini C, Sticchi E, Gensini F, Gori AM, Marcucci R, Lenti M, Michelucci A, Genuardi M, Abbate R, Gensini GF. Lone and secondary nonvalvular atrial fibrillation: role of a genetic susceptibility. Int J Cardiol. 2007;120(1):59–65.

288. Hamdi HK, Castellon R. A genetic variant of ACE increases cell survival: a new paradigm for biology and disease. Biochem Biophys Res Commun. 2004;318(1):187–91.

289. Watanabe H, Kaiser DW, Makino S, MacRae CA, Ellinor PT, Wasserman BS, Kannankeril PJ, Donahue BS, Roden DM, Darbar D. ACE I/D polymorphism associated with abnormal atrial and atrioventricular conduction in lone atrial fibrillation and structural heart disease: implications for electrical remodeling. Heart Rhythm. 2009;6(9):1327–32.

290. Tsukada T, Yokoyama K, Arai T, Takemoto F, Hara S, Yamada A, Kawaguchi Y, Hosoya T, Igari J. Evidence of association of the ecNOS gene polymorphism with plasma NO metabolite levels in humans. Biochem Biophys Res Commun. 1998;245(1):190–3.

291. Loukanov T, Hoss K, Tonchev P, Klimpel H, Arnold R, Sebening C, Karck M, Gorenflo M. Endothelial nitric oxide synthase gene polymorphism (Glu298Asp) and acute pulmonary hypertension post cardiopulmonary bypass in children with congenital cardiac diseases. Cardiol Young. 2011;21(2):161–9.

292. Derish M, Smith D, Frankel L. Venous catheter thrombus formation and pulmonary embolism in children. Pediatr Pulmonol. 1995;20:349–54.

293. DeAngelis GA, McIlhenny J, Willson DF, Vittone S, Dwyer 3rd SJ, Gibson JC, Alford BA. Prevalence of deep venous thrombosis in the lower extremities of children in the intensive care unit. Pediatr Radiol. 1996;26(11):821–4.

294. Beck C, Dubois J, Grignon A, Lacroix J, David M. Incidence and risk factors of catheter-related deep vein thrombosis in a pediatric intensive care unit: a prospective study. J Pediatr. 1998;133(2):237–41.

295. Massicotte MP, Dix D, Monagle P, Adams M, Andrew M. Central venous catheter related thrombosis in children: analysis of the Canadian Registry of Venous Thromboembolic Complications. J Pediatr. 1998;133(6):770–6.

296. Donnelly KM. Venous thromboembolic disease in the pediatric intensive care unit. Curr Opin Pediatr. 1999;11(3):213–7.

297. Casado-Flores J, Barja J, Martino R, Serrano A, Valdivielso A. Complications of central venous catheterization in critically ill children. Pediatr Crit Care Med. 2001;2(1):57–62.

298. Gutierrez JA, Bagatell R, Samson MP, Theodorou AA, Berg RA. Femoral central venous catheter-associated deep venous thrombosis in children with diabetic ketoacidosis. Crit Care Med. 2003;31(1):80–3.

299. Hanson SJ, Punzalan RC, Greenup RA, Liu H, Sato TT, Havens PL. Incidence and risk factors for venous thromboembolism in critically ill children after trauma. J Trauma. 2010;68(1):52–6.

300. Faustino EV, Lawson KA, Northrup V, Higgerson RA. Mortality-adjusted duration of mechanical ventilation in critically ill children with symptomatic central venous line-related deep venous thrombosis. Crit Care Med. 2011;39(5):1151–6.

301. Higgerson RA, Lawson KA, Christie LM, Brown AM, McArthur JA, Totapally BR, Hanson SJ. Incidence and risk factors associated with venous thrombotic events in pediatric intensive care unit patients. Pediatr Crit Care Med. 2011;12(6):628–34.

302. Hanson SJ, Punzalan RC, Christensen MA, Ghanayem NS, Kuhn EM, Havens PL. Incidence and risk factors for venous thromboembolism in critically ill children with cardiac disease. Pediatr Cardiol. 2012;33(1):103–8.

303. David M, Andrew M. Venous thromboembolic complications in children. J Pediatr. 1993;123(3):337–46.

304. Krafte-Jacobs B, Sivit CJ, Mejia R, Pollack MM. Catheter-related thrombosis in critically ill children: comparison of catheters with and without heparin bonding. J Pediatr. 1995;126(1):50–4.

305. Talbott GA, Winters WD, Bratton SL, O'Rourke PP. A prospective study of femoral catheter-related thrombosis in children. Arch Pediatr Adolesc Med. 1995;149(3):288–91.

306. van Ommen CH, Heijboer H, Buller HR, Hirasing RA, Heijmans HS, Peters M. Venous thromboembolism in childhood: a prospective two-year registry in The Netherlands. J Pediatr. 2001;139(5):676–81.

307. Miletich JP, Prescott SM, White R, Majerus PW, Bovill EG. Inherited predisposition to thrombosis. Cell. 1993;72(4):477–80.

308. De Stefano V, Finazzi G, Mannucci PM. Inherited thrombophilia: pathogenesis, clinical syndromes, and management. Blood. 1996;87(9):3531–44.

309. Spek CA, Reitsma PH. Genetic risk factors for venous thrombosis. Mol Genet Metab. 2000;71(1–2):51–61.

310. Voetsch B, Loscalzo J. Genetics of thrombophilia: impact on atherogenesis. Curr Opin Lipidol. 2004;15(2):129–43.

311. Gohil R, Peck G, Sharma P. The genetics of venous thromboembolism. A meta-analysis involving approximately 120,000 cases and 180,000 controls. Thromb Haemost. 2009;102(2):360–70.

312. Kunicki TJ, Williams SA, Nugent DJ. Genetic variants that affect platelet function. Curr Opin Hematol. 2012;19(5):371–9.

313. Anderson JA, Lim W, Weitz JI. Genetics of coagulation: what the cardiologist needs to know. Can J Cardiol. 2013;29(1):75–88.

314. Bertina RM, Koeleman BP, Koster T, Rosendaal FR, Dirven RJ, de Ronde H, van der Velden PA, Reitsma PH. Mutation in blood coagulation factor V associated with resistance to activated protein C. Nature. 1994;369(6475):64–7.

315. Poort SR, Rosendaal FR, Reitsma PH, Bertina RM. A common genetic variation in the 3′-untranslated region of the prothrombin gene is associated with elevated plasma prothrombin levels and an increase in venous thrombosis. Blood. 1996;88(10):3698–703.

316. Bertina RM. The prothrombin 20210 G to A variation and thrombosis. Curr Opin Hematol. 1998;5(5):339–42.

317. Ceelie H, Bertina RM, van Hylckama Vlieg A, Rosendaal FR, Vos HL. Polymorphisms in the prothrombin gene and their association with plasma prothrombin levels. Thromb Haemost. 2001;85(6):1066–70.

318. Perez-Ceballos E, Corral J, Alberca I, Vaya A, Llamas P, Montes R, Gonzalez-Conejero R, Vicente V. Prothrombin A19911G and G20210A polymorphisms' role in thrombosis. Br J Haematol. 2002;118(2):610–4.

319. Erdjument H, Lane DA, Ireland H, Di Marzo V, Panico M, Morris HR, Tripodi A, Mannucci PM. Antithrombin Milano, single amino acid substitution at the reactive site, Arg393 to Cys. Thromb Haemost. 1988;60(3):471–5.

320. Lane DA, Erdjument H, Thompson E, Panico M, Di Marzo V, Morris HR, Leone G, De Stefano V, Thein SL. A novel amino acid substitution in the reactive site of a congenital variant antithrombin. Antithrombin pescara, ARG393 to pro, caused by a CGT to CCT mutation. J Biol Chem. 1989;264(17):10200–4.

321. Caso R, Lane DA, Thompson EA, Olds RJ, Thein SL, Panico M, Blench I, Morris HR, Freyssinet JM, Aiach M, et al. Antithrombin Vicenza, Ala 384 to Pro (GCA to CCA) mutation, transforming the inhibitor into a substrate. Br J Haematol. 1991;77(1):87–92.

322. Lane DA, Olds RJ, Boisclair M, Chowdhury V, Thein SL, Cooper DN, Blajchman M, Perry D, Emmerich J, Aiach M. Antithrombin III mutation database: first update. For the Thrombin and its Inhibitors Subcommittee of the Scientific and Standardization Committee of the International Society on Thrombosis and Haemostasis. Thromb Haemost. 1993;70(2):361–9.

323. Lane DA, Olds RJ, Thein SL. Antithrombin III: summary of first database update. Nucleic Acids Res. 1994;22(17):3556–9.

324. Reitsma PH, Bernardi F, Doig RG, Gandrille S, Greengard JS, Ireland H, Krawczak M, Lind B, Long GL, Poort SR, et al. Protein C deficiency: a database of mutations, 1995 update. On behalf of the Subcommittee on Plasma Coagulation Inhibitors of the Scientific and Standardization Committee of the ISTH. Thromb Haemost. 1995;73(5):876–89.

325. Spek CA, Greengard JS, Griffin JH, Bertina RM, Reitsma PH. Two mutations in the promoter region of the human protein C gene both cause type I protein C deficiency by disruption of two HNF-3 binding sites. J Biol Chem. 1995;270(41):24216–21.

326. Spek CA, Koster T, Rosendaal FR, Bertina RM, Reitsma PH. Genotypic variation in the promoter region of the protein C gene is associated with plasma protein C levels and thrombotic risk. Arterioscler Thromb Vasc Biol. 1995;15(2):214–8.

327. Aiach M, Nicaud V, Alhenc-Gelas M, Gandrille S, Arnaud E, Amiral J, Guize L, Fiessinger JN, Emmerich J. Complex association of protein C gene promoter polymorphism with circulating protein C levels and thrombotic risk. Arterioscler Thromb Vasc Biol. 1999;19(6):1573–6.

328. Reitsma PH, Ploos van Amstel HK, Bertina RM. Three novel mutations in five unrelated subjects with hereditary protein S deficiency type I. J Clin Invest. 1994;93(2):486–92.

329. Duchemin J, Gandrille S, Borgel D, Feurgard P, Alhenc-Gelas M, Matheron C, Dreyfus M, Dupuy E, Juhan-Vague I, Aiach M. The Ser 460 to Pro substitution of the protein S alpha (PROS1) gene is a frequent mutation associated with free protein S (type IIa) deficiency. Blood. 1995;86(9):3436–43.

330. Gandrille S, Borgel D, Eschwege-Gufflet V, Aillaud M, Dreyfus M, Matheron C, Gaussem P, Abgrall JF, Jude B, Sie P, et al.

Identification of 15 different candidate causal point mutations and three polymorphisms in 19 patients with protein S deficiency using a scanning method for the analysis of the protein S active gene. Blood. 1995;85(1):130–8.

331. Gomez E, Poort SR, Bertina RM, Reitsma PH. Identification of eight point mutations in protein S deficiency type I – analysis of 15 pedigrees. Thromb Haemost. 1995;73(5):750–5.

332. Koenen RR, Tans G, van Oerle R, Hamulyak K, Rosing J, Hackeng TM. The APC-independent anticoagulant activity of protein S in plasma is decreased by elevated prothrombin levels due to the prothrombin G20210A mutation. Blood. 2003;102(5):1686–92.

333. Koenen RR, Gomes L, Tans G, Rosing J, Hackeng TM. The Ser460Pro mutation in recombinant protein S Heerlen does not affect its APC-cofactor and APC-independent anticoagulant activities. Thromb Haemost. 2004;91(6):1105–14.

334. Fukasawa M, Matsushita K, Kamiyama M, Mikami Y, Araki I, Yamagata Z, Takeda M. The methylentetrahydrofolate reductase C677T point mutation is a risk factor for vascular access thrombosis in hemodialysis patients. Am J Kidney Dis. 2003;41(3):637–42.

335. Shimasaki Y, Yasue H, Yoshimura M, Nakayama M, Kugiyama K, Ogawa H, Harada E, Masuda T, Koyama W, Saito Y, et al. Association of the missense Glu298Asp variant of the endothelial nitric oxide synthase gene with myocardial infarction. J Am Coll Cardiol. 1998;31(7):1506–10.

336. Gorchakova O, Koch W, von Beckerath N, Mehilli J, Schomig A, Kastrati A. Association of a genetic variant of endothelial nitric oxide synthase with the 1 year clinical outcome after coronary stent placement. Eur Heart J. 2003;24(9):820–7.

337. Heil SG, Den Heijer M, Van Der Rijt-Pisa BJ, Kluijtmans LA, Blom HJ. The 894 G > T variant of endothelial nitric oxide synthase (eNOS) increases the risk of recurrent venous thrombosis through interaction with elevated homocysteine levels. J Thromb Haemost. 2004;2(5):750–3.

338. Carter AM, Catto AJ, Kohler HP, Ariens RA, Stickland MH, Grant PJ. alpha-fibrinogen Thr312Ala polymorphism and venous thromboembolism. Blood. 2000;96(3):1177–9.

339. Standeven KF, Grant PJ, Carter AM, Scheiner T, Weisel JW, Ariens RA. Functional analysis of the fibrinogen Aalpha Thr312Ala polymorphism: effects on fibrin structure and function. Circulation. 2003;107(18):2326–30.

340. Ozbek N, Atac FB, Yildirim SV, Verdi H, Yazici C, Yilmaz BT, Tokel NK. Analysis of prothrombotic mutations and polymorphisms in children who developed thrombosis in the perioperative period of congenital cardiac surgery. Cardiol Young. 2005;15(1):19–25.

341. Standeven KF, Ariens RA, Grant PJ. The molecular physiology and pathology of fibrin structure/function. Blood Rev. 2005;19(5):275–88.

342. Alhenc-Gelas M, Reny JL, Aubry ML, Aiach M, Emmerich J. The FXIII Val 34 Leu mutation and the risk of venous thrombosis. Thromb Haemost. 2000;84(6):1117–8.

343. Ariens RA, Philippou H, Nagaswami C, Weisel JW, Lane DA, Grant PJ. The factor XIII V34L polymorphism accelerates thrombin activation of factor XIII and affects cross-linked fibrin structure. Blood. 2000;96(3):988–95.

344. Balogh I, Szoke G, Karpati L, Wartiovaara U, Katona E, Komaromi I, Haramura G, Pfliegler G, Mikkola H, Muszbek L. Val34Leu polymorphism of plasma factor XIII: biochemistry and epidemiology in familial thrombophilia. Blood. 2000;96(7):2479–86.

345. Margaglione M, Bossone A, Brancaccio V, Ciampa A, Di Minno G. Factor XIII Val34Leu polymorphism and risk of deep vein thrombosis. Thromb Haemost. 2000;84(6):1118–9.

346. Wartiovaara U, Mikkola H, Szoke G, Haramura G, Karpati L, Balogh I, Lassila R, Muszbek L, Palotie A. Effect of Val34Leu polymorphism on the activation of the coagulation factor XIII-A. Thromb Haemost. 2000;84(4):595–600.

347. Van Hylckama VA, Komanasin N, Ariens RA, Poort SR, Grant PJ, Bertina RM, Rosendaal FR. Factor XIII Val34Leu polymorphism, factor XIII antigen levels and activity and the risk of deep venous thrombosis. Br J Haematol. 2002;119(1):169–75.

348. Sartori MT, Wiman B, Vettore S, Dazzi F, Girolami A, Patrassi GM. 4G/5G polymorphism of PAI-1 gene promoter and fibrinolytic capacity in patients with deep vein thrombosis. Thromb Haemost. 1998;80(6):956–60.

349. Segui R, Estelles A, Mira Y, Espana F, Villa P, Falco C, Vaya A, Grancha S, Ferrando F, Aznar J. PAI-1 promoter 4G/5G genotype as an additional risk factor for venous thrombosis in subjects with genetic thrombophilic defects. Br J Haematol. 2000;111(1):122–8.

350. Sartori MT, Danesin C, Saggiorato G, Tormene D, Simioni P, Spiezia L, Patrassi GM, Girolami A. The PAI-1 gene 4G/5G polymorphism and deep vein thrombosis in patients with inherited thrombophilia. Clin Appl Thromb Hemost. 2003;9(4):299–307.

351. Akhter MS, Biswas A, Ranjan R, Meena A, Yadav BK, Sharma A, Saxena R. Plasminogen activator inhibitor-1 (PAI-1) gene 4G/5G promoter polymorphism is seen in higher frequency in the Indian patients with deep vein thrombosis. Clin Appl Thromb Hemost. 2010;16(2):184–8.

352. Ohga S, Ishiguro A, Takahashi Y, Shima M, Taki M, Kaneko M, Fukushima K, Kang D, Hara T. Protein C deficiency as the major cause of thrombophilias in childhood. Pediatr Int. 2012;55(3):267–71.

353. Nowak-Gottl U, Koch HG, Aschka I, Kohlhase B, Vielhaber H, Kurlemann G, Oleszcuk-Raschke K, Kehl HG, Jurgens H, Schneppenheim R. Resistance to activated protein C (APCR) in children with venous or arterial thromboembolism. Br J Haematol. 1996;92(4):992–8.

354. Manco-Johnson MJ. Disorders of hemostasis in childhood: risk factors for venous thromboembolism. Thromb Haemost. 1997;78(1):710–4.

355. Uttenreuther-Fischer MM, Vetter B, Hellmann C, Otting U, Ziemer S, Hausdorf G, Gaedicke G, Kulozik AE. Paediatric thrombo-embolism: the influence of non-genetic factors and the role of activated protein C resistance and protein C deficiency. Eur J Pediatr. 1997;156(4):277–81.

356. Hagstrom JN, Walter J, Bluebond-Langner R, Amatniek JC, Manno CS, High KA. Prevalence of the factor V leiden mutation in children and neonates with thromboembolic disease. J Pediatr. 1998;133(6):777–81.

357. Herak DC, Antolic MR, Krleza JL, Pavic M, Dodig S, Duranovic V, Brkic AB, Zadro R. Inherited prothrombotic risk factors in children with stroke, transient ischemic attack, or migraine. Pediatrics. 2009;123(4):e653–60.

358. Turebylu R, Salis R, Erbe R, Martin D, Lakshminrusimha S, Ryan RM. Genetic prothrombotic mutations are common in neonates but are not associated with umbilical catheter-associated thrombosis. J Perinatol. 2007;27(8):490–5.

359. Vesell ES. Pharmacogenetic perspectives gained from twin and family studies. Pharmacol Ther. 1989;41(3):535–52.

360. Meyer UA, Zanger UM. Molecular mechanisms of genetic polymorphisms of drug metabolism. Annu Rev Pharmacol Toxicol. 1997;37:269–96.

361. Guengerich FP, Hosea NA, Parikh A, Bell-Parikh LC, Johnson WW, Gillam EM, Shimada T. Twenty years of biochemistry of human P450s: purification, expression, mechanism, and relevance to drugs. Drug Metab Dispos. 1998;26(12):1175–8.

362. Evans WE, Relling MV. Pharmacogenomics: translating functional genomics into rational therapeutics. Science. 1999;286(5439):487–91.

363. Meyer UA. Pharmacogenetics – five decades of therapeutic lessons from genetic diversity. Nat Rev Genet. 2004;5(9):669–76.

364. Empey PE. Genetic predisposition to adverse drug reactions in the intensive care unit. Crit Care Med. 2010;38(6 Suppl):S106–16.

365. Evans WE, Horner M, Chu YQ, Kalwinsky D, Roberts WM. Altered mercaptopurine metabolism, toxic effects, and dosage requirement in a thiopurine methyltransferase-deficient child with acute lymphocytic leukemia. J Pediatr. 1991;119(6):985–9.

366. Evans WE, Hon YY, Bomgaars L, Coutre S, Holdsworth M, Janco R, Kalwinsky D, Keller F, Khatib Z, Margolin J, et al. Preponderance of thiopurine S-methyltransferase deficiency and heterozygosity among patients intolerant to mercaptopurine or azathioprine. J Clin Oncol. 2001;19(8):2293–301.

367. Weinshilboum R. Inheritance and drug response. N Engl J Med. 2003;348(6):529–37.

368. Gentilomo C, Huang YS, Raffini L. Significant increase in clopidogrel use across U.S. children's hospitals. Pediatr Cardiol. 2011;32(2):167–75.

369. Ancrenaz V, Daali Y, Fontana P, Besson M, Samer C, Dayer P, Desmeules J. Impact of genetic polymorphisms and drug-drug interactions on clopidogrel and prasugrel response variability. Curr Drug Metab. 2010;11(8):667–77.

370. Scott SA, Sangkuhl K, Gardner EE, Stein CM, Hulot JS, Johnson JA, Roden DM, Klein TE, Shuldiner AR. Clinical pharmacogenetics implementation consortium guidelines for cytochrome P450-2C19 (CYP2C19) genotype and clopidogrel therapy. Clin Pharmacol Ther. 2013;90(2):328–32.

371. Cattaneo M. The platelet P2Y(1)(2) receptor for adenosine diphosphate: congenital and drug-induced defects. Blood. 2011;117(7):2102–12.

372. Mega JL, Close SL, Wiviott SD, Shen L, Hockett RD, Brandt JT, Walker JR, Antman EM, Macias W, Braunwald E, et al. Cytochrome p-450 polymorphisms and response to clopidogrel. N Engl J Med. 2009;360(4):354–62.

373. Simon T, Verstuyft C, Mary-Krause M, Quteineh L, Drouet E, Meneveau N, Steg PG, Ferrieres J, Danchin N, Becquemont L. Genetic determinants of response to clopidogrel and cardiovascular events. N Engl J Med. 2009;360(4):363–75.

374. Mega JL, Close SL, Wiviott SD, Shen L, Walker JR, Simon T, Antman EM, Braunwald E, Sabatine MS. Genetic variants in ABCB1 and CYP2C19 and cardiovascular outcomes after treatment with clopidogrel and prasugrel in the TRITON-TIMI 38 trial: a pharmacogenetic analysis. Lancet. 2010;376(9749):1312–9.

375. Vitali SH, Randolph AG. Assessing the quality of case-control association studies on the genetic basis of sepsis. Pediatr Crit Care Med. 2005;6(3 Suppl):S74–7.

376. Garau J, Aguilar L, Rodriguez-Creixems M, Dal-re R, Perez-Trallero E, Rodriguez M, Bouza E. Influence of comorbidity and severity on the clinical outcome of bacteremic pneumococcal pneumonia treated with beta-lactam monotherapy. J Chemother. 1999;11(4):266–72.

377. Garnacho-Montero J, Garcia-Cabrera E, Diaz-Martin A, Lepe-Jimenez JA, Iraurgi-Arcarazo P, Jimenez-Alvarez R, Revuelto-Rey J, Aznar-Martin J. Determinants of outcome in patients with bacteraemic pneumococcal pneumonia: importance of early adequate treatment. Scand J Infect Dis. 2010;42(3):185–92.

Genomics in Critical Illness

20

Hector R. Wong

Abstract

The term "genomics" has morphed into an umbrella term to describe broadly the large-scale study of genes, gene products, gene variants, and their impact on health and disease. This chapter reviews the impact of genomics on critical illness and injury. The chapter will also review other "omics" such as proteomics, pharmacogenomics, epigenetics, lipidomics, and metabolomics. Gene association studies attempt to link gene variants with susceptibility to and outcomes from various forms of critical illness. Genome wide expression studies have been leveraged to elucidate novel therapeutic pathways and targets, gene expression-based subclasses of critical illness, and the discovery of candidate diagnostic and stratification biomarkers. Other "omics" disciplines are also leading to novel insights regarding the pathobiology of critical illness. For example, the discovery of neutrophil gelatinase-associated lipocalin as an early biomarker of acute kidney injury is based on trancriptomic and proteomic studies involving animals models. Comparative genomics has led to the discovery of important signaling mechanisms relevant to critical illness. For example, the discovery of Toll-like receptor 4 as the primary receptor for lipopolysaccharide is the product of comparative genomics. Finally, epigenetics is beginning to provide clues as to why recovery from critical illness may be associated for prolonged risk for subsequent critical illness. Overall, genomics-centered studies continue to evolve in the field of critical care medicine and hold the promise of substantially advancing our understanding and approach to various forms of critical illness.

Keywords

Gene expression • Proteomics • Biomarkers • Pathways • Genetics • Metabolomics • Polymorphisms • Sepsis • Acute lung injury • Genes • Transcriptomics • Microarray

Introduction

The origin of the term "genomics" is credited to T.H. Roderick of the Jackson Laboratory, Bar Harbor, Maine, during the launching of a new journal, *Genomics*, which sought to serve

H.R. Wong, MD
Division of Critical Care Medicine,
Cincinnati Children's Hospital Medical Center,
University of Cincinnati College of Medicine,
3333 Burnet Avenue, Cincinnati, OH 45229, USA
e-mail: hector.wong@cchmc.org

a "new discipline born from a marriage of molecular and cell biology with classical genetics and fostered by computational science" [1]. Since that time, for many individuals, the term "genomics" has morphed into more of an umbrella term to broadly describe the large scale study of genes, gene products, gene variants, and their impact on health and disease. This chapter will use this broader conceptual framework for reviewing the impact of genomics on critical illness and injury. The chapter will also review other "omics" such as pharmacogenomics, epigenomics, lipidomics, and metabolomics.

Gene Association Studies

It is highly plausible that much of the pathology and heterogeneity (e.g. sepsis and acute lung injury) that we encounter in the intensive care unit is substantially influenced by genetic variability. Indeed, almost 25 years ago Sorenson et al. convincingly demonstrated that premature death from infection has a stronger (although undefined) component than premature death from cardiovascular disease or cancer [2]. Despite these compelling data, however, unambiguous and well validated evidence linking specific genetic variations with critical illness have remained relatively elusive.

Most investigations attempting to link genetic variation with critical illness have focused on gene polymorphisms, defined as the regular occurrence (>1 %), in a population, of two or more alleles at a particular chromosome location. The most frequent type of polymorphism is called a single nucleotide polymorphism (SNP): a substitution, deletion, or insertion of a single nucleotide that occurs in approximately 1 per every 1,000 base pairs of human DNA. SNPs can result in an altered protein, a change in the level of normal protein expression, or no discernable change in protein function.

When SNPs cause a change in an amino acid they are said to be non-synonymous or missense SNPs (Fig. 20.1), and these are typically the type of SNPs that can lead to a change in protein function. SNPs in the promoter region of a gene or in the 3′ un-translated region can lead to changes in protein expression. Most SNPs occur in either non-coding regions or they are synonymous SNPs (i.e. variants that code for the same amino acid; Fig. 20.1) and therefore have no known direct effect on phenotype. These types of SNPs, however, may be worthy of study because although they are not causal variants they may be co-inherited along with the causal variant by a process known as linkage disequilibrium (LD), which refers to the non-random association of alleles at two or more chromosome locations, as measured by formal statistical methods. Related to the concept of LD is that of haplotype, which refers to a set of SNPs on a single chromosome that are statistically associated and typically co-inherited. These haplotype "blocks" consist of multiple linked polymorphisms and can be identified by haplotype tag SNPs. The International HapMap project is developing a haplotype map of the entire human genome as means to more effectively enable genetic association studies [3].

A classic approach to assess the impact of genetic variants on disease involves linkage analysis, which follows family members (pedigrees) for co-segregation of the disease of interest and genetic variants. This type of approach is appropriate and feasible for monogenic diseases with relatively distinct phenotypes (e.g. cystic fibrosis), but is generally not applicable to common ICU conditions such as sepsis and acute lung injury, as it is not often feasible to obtain

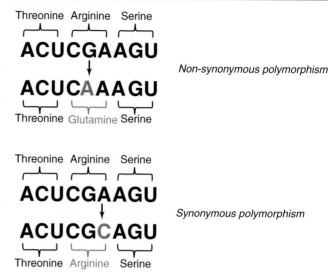

Fig. 20.1 Examples of non-synonymous and synonymous substitution polymorphisms. In the *top panel*, a change in the second amino acid for the arginine codon, from a "G" to an "A", leads to a change in the amino acid to glutamine (non-synonymous). In the *bottom panel*, a change in the third amino acid for the arginine codon, from an "A" to a "C" does not change the amino acid (synonymous)

unambiguous histories of critical illness in family members and it is not biologically plausible that sepsis or acute lung injury are monogenic syndromes. Consequently, the most common study design in the setting of critical illness is an association study, of which there are two types: case-control and cohort studies [4].

Apart from study design, another important factor in conducting genetics research in critical illness involves choosing the method for assessing genetic variation. The two primary choices are genome-wide association studies (GWAS) and candidate gene association studies. GWAS involves the simultaneous interrogation of thousands of polymorphisms. This approach is comprehensive, discovery-oriented, and relatively bias free in that the investigator makes no a priori assumptions regarding associations between any particular polymorphism and the disease of interest. This approach is relatively expensive, but cost is progressively becoming less of an issue with rapid advances in sequencing and chip technology. The main challenge that comes with GWAS is the need for a large number of patients and the application of appropriate and complex statistical methods to reduce the rate of false discovery.

Candidate gene association studies are more focused and more rooted in the traditional scientific method (i.e. hypothesis testing). In this approach the investigator focuses on a specific polymorphism, or a discrete set of polymorphisms, based on known biology, that potentially links a candidate gene to the disease of interest. This approach is less daunting from an analysis standpoint, but can be limited by investigator bias and has high potential for missing causal polymorphisms. Whichever of the two approaches one chooses, there

Table 20.1 Characteristics of an ideal genetic association study

The study should have an a priori hypothesis
Large sample size and small p values
The association between the gene and the disease of interest should have biological plausibility
The allele should affect the gene product in a physiologically meaningful way
There should be an initial study and an independent replication (validation)
The gene association should be observed in the context of both family- and population-based control cohorts
Cases should be clearly defined and should represent a spectrum of disease severity
Cases and controls should be well matched for environmental risk factors
Cases and controls should be well matched for ethnicity
Potential confounders should be presented and statistically analyzed
Allele equilibrium should be reported (Hardy-Weinberg equilibrium)
Power calculations should be targeted toward detection of a positive association

are a number of factors that impact the quality (or lack thereof) of an "ideal" gene association study. These qualities have been reviewed elsewhere [5–7] and are summarized in Table 20.1.

A large number of gene association studies have been published in the critical care literature and the reader is directed toward some recent reviews on the topic [8–12]. Table 20.2 provides a selected group of studies focused on sepsis [13–30]. Gene association studies should be conducted in the critically ill population. The heterogeneous clinical responses and presentations that we observe daily at the bedside provide the necessary general rationale that genetic polymorphisms have an important impact on our patients, in terms of disease susceptibility and disease outcome. While conducting these studies in the context of critical illness is particularly challenging, we must nonetheless seek to conduct these studies with as much rigor as that of our colleagues in other fields. One potential solution to meeting

Table 20.2 Selected gene association studies related to sepsis

Reference	Gene/polymorphism	Main findings
Lorenz et al. [22]	Toll-like receptor 4 (TLR4) polymorphisms that reduce responsiveness to endotoxin (Asp299Gly and Thr39Ile)	The TLR4 Asp299Gly allele was found exclusively in adult patients with septic shock. Patients with the TLR4 Asp299Gly/Thr399Ile alleles had a higher prevalence of gram negative infections
Agnese et al. [13]	TLR4 polymorphisms: Asp299Gly and Thr39Ile	Adult patients with these alleles had a higher incidence of gram negative infections
Multiple	TLR4 polymorphisms: Asp299Gly and Thr39Ile	Children with the Asp299Gly allele have increased risk of urinary tract infection [20], but this allele does not appear to influence susceptibility to or severity of meningococcal septic shock in children [14, 28]
Kutukculer et al. [21]	TLR2 polymorphism that reduces responsiveness to cell wall components of gram positive bacteria (Arg753Gln)	Children with recurrent infections were more frequently heterozygous for the Arg753Gln allele
Tabel et al. [29]	TLR2 polymorphism: Arg753Gln	Children with the Arg753Gln had a higher incidence of urinary tract infections
Mira et al. [25]	Tumor necrosis factor-α (TNFα) promoter polymorphism: TNF1 (guanine at -308A and TNF2 (adenosine at -308A). TNF2 allele associated with increased production of TNFα	TNF2 associated with susceptibility to septic shock and death due to septic shock
Nadel et al. [26]	TNF1 and TNF2 alleles	More deaths and increased illness severity in children with the TNF2 allele and meningococcal sepsis
McArthur et al. [23]	Lymphotoxin-α: +250A and +250G. +250A allele associated with increased TNFα production	Bacteremic children with the AA genotype had a higher mortality rate from sepsis
Read et al. [27]	Polymorphisms of interleukin-1 (IL1B (−511)) and IL-1 receptor antagonist (IL1RN(+2018))	Patients with the IL1B(−511) allele were more likely to survive meningococcal sepsis. The combination of the IL1B(−511) and the rare IL1RN(+2018) allele decreased the likelihood of surviving meningococcal sepsis
Endler et al. [16]	Multiple polymorphisms for the IL-1 locus	The IL1RA(+2018) polymorphism was associated with risk of meningococcal disease and with its outcome
Michalek et al. [24]	IL-6 polymorphisms (G-174>C and G-572>C)	Both polymorphisms could be predictors of risk of development and/or predictors of sepsis severity in children
Balding et al. [15]	Polymorphisms for IL-6, IL-1, TNFα, IL-10, and IL-1Ra	The IL-6(−174) G/G and the IL-10(−1082) A/A genotypes were more frequent among nonsurvivors of meningococcal sepsis
Multiple [17–19, 30]	Deletion/insertion (4G/5G) polymorphism of the plasminogen-activator inhibitor type-1 (PAI-1) promoter region. The 4G allele is associated with higher PAI-1 plasma levels	The 4G allele increases susceptibility to and severity of septic shock, and increased risk of mortality in children with meningococcal sepsis

this challenge is the development of multi-institutional and multi-national research consortia specifically dedicated to gene association studies.

Genome-Wide Expression Profiling

Genome-wide expression profiling (a.k.a. transcriptomics) refers to the simultaneous and efficient measurement of steady-state mRNA abundance of thousands of transcripts from a given tissue source. The general approach involves variations of microarray technology [31–33], and there is a new, potentially more powerful technique referred to as RNA Sequencing (RNA Seq) [34]. While gene expression profiling has important limitations, this discovery-oriented approach has nonetheless provided an unprecedented opportunity to gain a broader, genome-level "picture" of complex and heterogeneous clinical syndromes encountered in critical care medicine. In addition, this genome-level approach has the potential to reduce investigator bias, and thus increase discovery capability, in as much as all genes are potentially interrogated, rather than a specific set of genes chosen by the investigator based on a priori and potentially biased assumptions. Genome-wide expression profiling in sepsis will be discussed below as an example of how this approach can be applied to critically ill patients. All of the studies discussed below have used the blood compartment as the RNA source.

Several fundamental physiologic and biologic principles of the sepsis paradigms are derived from experiments involving human volunteers subjected to intravenous endotoxin challenge [35–38]. More recently, the genome-level response during experimental human endotoxemia has been studied using microarray technology [39–41]. For example, Talwar et al. compared eight volunteers challenged with intravenous endotoxin to four controls challenged with saline [39]. Mononuclear cell-specific RNA was obtained at four different time points after endotoxin challenge and analyzed via microarray. As expected, a large number of transcripts related to inflammation and innate immunity were substantially up regulated in response to endotoxin challenge. Interestingly, the peak transcriptomic response to the single endotoxin challenge occurred within six hours and mRNA levels generally returned to control levels within 24 h. The investigators also reported endotoxin-mediated differential regulation of over 100 genes not typically associated with acute inflammation.

Genome-wide expression has also been conducted in critically ill patients with sepsis and septic shock. These studies present considerable experimental challenges due to the inherent heterogeneity of clinical sepsis and septic shock. Nonetheless, several studies have provided novel insight into the overall genome-level response to sepsis [42–53]. A common theme across many of these studies is the massive up

regulation of inflammation- and innate immunity-related genes in patients with sepsis and septic shock. These observations are not intrinsically novel, but they are consistent with the long-standing sepsis paradigms centered on a hyper-active inflammatory response, and thus provide a component of biological plausibility with regard to overall microarray data output in the context of clinical sepsis.

Another common paradigm in the sepsis field involves a two-phase model consisting of an initial hyper-inflammatory phase, followed by a compensatory anti-inflammatory phase, but this has been recently challenged, in large part due to the multiple failures of interventional clinical trials founded on this paradigm [54–56]. Recently, Tang et al. conducted a formal systematic review of a carefully selected group of microarray-based human sepsis studies [33]. The major conclusion of this systematic review is that, in aggregate, the transcriptome-level data does not consistently separate sepsis into distinct pro- and anti-inflammatory phases. This conclusion has been questioned [57], but is supported by several recent cytokine- and inflammatory mediator-based studies in clinical and experimental sepsis [58–60].

Another prevailing paradigm in the sepsis field involves the concept of immune-paralysis, or immune-suppression, which frames sepsis as an adaptive immune problem and the inability to adequately clear infection [61, 62]. Recently, this paradigm was elegantly corroborated in mice subjected to sepsis and rescued by administration of interleukin-7, an anti-apoptotic cytokine essential for lymphocyte survival and expansion [63, 64]. In studies focused on mononuclear cell-specific expression profiles, Tang et al. have reported early repression of adaptive immunity genes in patients with sepsis [48, 50]. Finally, multiple studies in children with septic shock have reported, and validated, early and persistent repression of adaptive immunity-related gene programs: *T cell activation, T cell receptor signaling, and antigen presentation* [42, 47, 51–53, 65–67]. Thus, the concept of adaptive immune dysfunction as an early and prominent feature of clinical sepsis and septic shock seems to be well supported by the available genome-wide expression data.

Developmental age is thought to be a major contributor to sepsis heterogeneity. Recently, a microarray-based study in children with septic shock corroborated this concept at the genomic level [68]. Four developmental age groups of children were compared based on whole-blood derived gene expression profiles. Children in the "neonate" group (<28 days of age) demonstrated a unique expression profile relative to older children. For example, children in the neonate group demonstrated widespread repression of genes corresponding to the triggering receptor expressed on myeloid cells 1 (TREM-1) pathway. TREM-1 is critical for amplification of the inflammatory response to microbial products and there has been recent interest in blockade of the TREM-1 signaling pathway in septic shock [69]. The observation that

TREM-1 signaling may not be relevant in neonates with septic shock, illustrates how some candidate therapeutic strategies for septic shock may not have biological plausibility in certain developmental age groups.

Apart from providing a broad, genome-level view of sepsis biology, as described above, genome-wide expression profiling also provides an opportunity to discover previously unrecognized, or unconsidered, targets and pathways relevant to sepsis biology. For example, using a combination of clinical expression profiling and in vitro approaches, Pathan et al. have identified interleukin-6 as a major contributor to myocardial depression in patients with meningococcal sepsis [70]. In another example, Pachot et al. identified a set of genes differentially regulated between adult survivors and non-survivors with septic shock. The gene most highly expressed in survivors, relative to non-survivors, was that of the chemokine receptor, CX3CR1 (fractalkine receptor) [44]. In a subsequent validation study, these same investigators provided further evidence supporting the novel concept that dysregulation of CX3CR1 in monocytes contributes to immune-paralysis in human sepsis [71].

A number of studies in children with septic shock have documented early and persistent repression of gene programs directly related to zinc homeostasis, in combination with low serum zinc concentrations [42, 47, 51, 53, 65]. Since normal zinc homeostasis is absolutely critical for normal immune function [72], these observations have raised the possibility of zinc supplementation as a potentially safe and low cost therapeutic strategy in clinical septic shock and other forms of critical illness [73–75]. Importantly, Knoell et al. have independently corroborated that zinc deficiency is detrimental, and that zinc supplementation is highly beneficial, in experimental sepsis [76, 77]. Additional studies by Knoell et al. have corroborated decreased plasma zinc concentrations in patients with sepsis, and that low plasma zinc concentrations correlate with higher illness severity [78]. Furthermore, plasma zinc concentrations correlate inversely with monocyte expression of the zinc transporter gene SLC39A8 (a.k.a. ZIP8) [78, 79]. Interestingly, microarray-based studies in children with septic shock have reported high level SLC39A8 expression in non-survivors, relative to survivors [53]. Despite the intriguing convergence of these data from independent laboratories, the safety and efficacy of zinc supplementation in clinical sepsis remains to be directly demonstrated and is a current area of active investigation.

In the aforementioned studies involving children with septic shock, metalloproteinase-8 (MMP-8) has consistently been the highest expressed gene in patients with septic shock, relative to normal controls [42, 47, 51–53, 65, 68]. In addition, MMP-8 is more highly expressed in patients with septic shock, compared to patients with sepsis, and in septic shock non-survivors, compared to septic shock survivors [80]. MMP-8 is also known as neutrophil collagenase because it is a neutrophil-derived protease that cleaves collagen in the extracellular matrix (ECM), but MMP-8 is also known to have other cellular sources and non-ECM substrates, including chemokines and cytokines [81]. The consistently high level expression of MMP-8 in clinical septic shock recently stimulated the formal study of MMP-8 in experimental sepsis. These studies demonstrated that either genetic ablation of MMP-8, or pharmacologic inhibition of MMP-8 activity, confers a significant survival advantage in a murine model of sepsis [80]. While these studies require further development and validation, the findings are intriguing given that there exist a number of drugs to effectively inhibit MMP-8 activity in the clinical setting [82].

Another potential application of genome-wide expression profiling is the discovery of candidate biomarkers [83]. A daily conundrum in the intensive care unit is the ability to distinguish which patients that meet criteria for systemic inflammatory response syndrome (SIRS) are infected, and which patients with SIRS are not infected. Accordingly, there are ongoing microarray-based efforts to discover diagnostic biomarkers for sepsis. Several investigators have reported genome-level signatures that can distinguish patients with SIRS (not infected) from patients with sepsis [43, 46, 50, 84]. A substantial amount of work, including validation, remains to be done in order to leverage these datasets into clinically applicable diagnostic biomarkers, but the datasets nonetheless provide a foundation for the derivation and development of diagnostic biomarkers for sepsis.

Investigators have also applied microarray technology to address other important diagnostic clinical challenges directly related to infection. Cobb et al. have reported an expression signature (the "ribonucleogram") having the potential to predict ventilator-associated pneumonia in critically ill blunt trauma patients up to 4 days before traditional clinical recognition [85, 86]. Similarly, Ramilo et al. have reported expression signatures that can distinguish Influenza A infection from bacterial infection, and E. coli infection from S. aureus infection, in hospitalized febrile children [87].

Another aspect of biomarker development in sepsis surrounds stratification (outcome) biomarkers. In theory, any gene that is consistently differentially regulated between survivors and non-survivors in a microarray dataset may warrant further investigation and validation as a potential stratification biomarker. As mentioned previously, Pachot et al., using a microarray data set, have identified CX3CR1 as a potential stratification biomarker in sepsis [44, 71]. Similarly, Nowak et al. have leveraged microarray data to identify chemokine (C-C motif) ligand 4 (CCL4) as a stratification biomarker in children with septic shock [88]. Both candidate stratification biomarkers, however, require further validation.

Interleukin-8 (IL-8) has emerged as a robust stratification biomarker in children with septic shock [89], and the rationale for pursuing IL-8 stemmed directly from

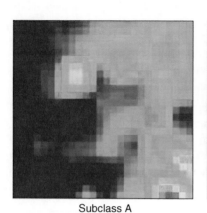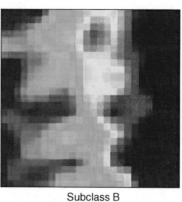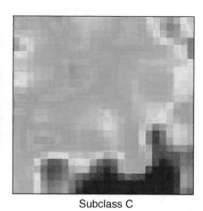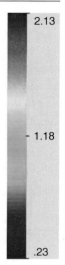

| Subclass A | Subclass B | Subclass C |

Fig. 20.2 Examples of gene expression mosaics for individual patients in septic shock subclasses A, B, and C, respectively [66, 67]. The expression mosaics represent the expression patterns of same 100-class defining genes corresponding to adaptive immunity, glucocorticoid receptor signaling, and the peroxisome proliferator-activated receptor-α

signaling pathway. The *color bar* on the right depicts the relative intensity of gene expression. Patients in subclass A have a higher level of illness severity as measured by mortality, degree of organ failure, and illness severity score

microarray-based studies that identified IL-8 as one of the more highly expressed genes in pediatric non-survivors of septic shock, compared to survivors [53]. Subsequent studies in a derivation cohort of patients demonstrated that serum IL-8 protein levels, measured within 24 h of presentation to the intensive care unit with septic shock, could predict survival in pediatric septic shock with a probability of 95 % [89]. The robustness of IL-8 as a stratification biomarker was subsequently validated in a completely independent cohort of children with septic shock. Consequently, it has been proposed that IL-8 could be used in future pediatric septic shock interventional trials as a means to *exclude* patients having a high likelihood of survival with standard care, as a means of improving the risk to benefit ratio of a given intervention. This type of stratification strategy would be particularly applicable for an intervention that carries more than minimal risk. Interestingly, it appears that IL-8-based stratification may not perform in a similarly robust manner in adults with septic shock [90], thus providing another example of how developmental age contributes to septic shock heterogeneity.

Currently, there is an ongoing effort to derive and validate a multi-biomarker sepsis outcome risk model in pediatric septic shock. The foundation of this effort is the relatively unbiased selection of a panel of candidate outcome biomarkers using microarray data from a large cohort of children with septic shock [83, 91].

Viewing septic shock as a highly heterogeneous syndrome implies the existence of "disease subclasses", in an analogous manner to that encountered in the oncology field [56]. Recently, there has been an attempt to identify septic shock subclasses in children based exclusively on genome-wide expression profiling [65]. Complete microarray data

from a large cohort of children with septic shock, representing the first 24 h of admission, were used to identify septic shock subclasses based exclusively on unsupervised hierarchical gene clustering. Patients with statistically similar gene expression patterns were grouped into one of three subclasses (subclasses "A", "B", or "C") and subsequently the clinical database was mined to determine if there were any phenotypic differences between the three subclasses. Patients in subclass A had a significantly higher level of illness severity as measured by mortality, organ failure, and illness severity score. In addition, the gene expression patterns that distinguished the subclasses were distilled to a 100 gene expression signature corresponding to adaptive immunity, glucocorticoid receptor signaling, and the peroxisome proliferator-activated receptor-α signaling pathway. Of note, the genes corresponding to these functional annotations were generally repressed in the subclass of patients with the higher level of illness severity (i.e. subclass A patients).

In a subsequent study, the expression patterns of the 100 subclass-defining genes were depicted using visually intuitive gene expression mosaics and shown to a panel of clinicians with no formal bioinformatic training and blinded to the actual patient subclasses (Fig. 20.2). The clinicians were able to allocate patients into the respective subclasses with a high degree of sensitivity and specificity [67]. The ability to identify a subclass of children with a higher illness severity was further corroborated when the gene expression-based subclassification strategy was applied to a separate validation cohort of children with septic shock [66]. Collectively, these studies demonstrate the feasibility of subclassifying patients with septic shock, in a clinically relevant manner, based on the expression patterns of a discrete set of genes having relevance to sepsis biology. These features are consistent with the concept of "theranostics" in which molecular based diagnostic tools also have the potential to direct therapy [92]. The availability of clinical microfluidics [93] and digital mRNA measurement technology [94] may allow for clinical feasibility of measuring the 100 class-defining genes in a timely manner that is suitable to direct patient care or stratification for clinical trials.

Proteomics

It is well known that the degree of mRNA expression does not necessarily correlate with the degree of protein expression, and that protein function is frequently dependent on post-translational modifications. Accordingly, an important limitation of the gene expression profiling approach described above, which is focused on mRNA expression, is that it provides no direct information regarding gene end products, proteins, which ultimately carry out gene function. Accordingly, the discipline of "proteomics" has evolved to address this limitation and proteomic approaches are being increasingly applied to critical illness [93, 95–98].

As the name implies, proteomics involves the large scale analysis, including structure and function, of proteins from biological fluids and tissues. The technological armamentarium for proteomic research includes two-dimensional gel electrophoresis, matrix-assisted laser desorption/ionization time-of-flight mass spectrometry (MALDI-TOF MS), liquid chromatography coupled to electrospray ionization-tandem MS (LC-ESI MS), surface-enhanced laser desorption/ionization coupled to TOF MS (SELDI-TOF MS), capillary electrophoresis coupled to MS, and protein microarrays [95, 96]. The broad concept of proteomics is analogous to that of transcriptomics: large scale analysis of the proteomic response during health and disease as a means of unbiased discovery.

One major application of proteomics is the discovery of candidate biomarkers [83, 99]. Human blood, a primary target for biomarker discovery and development, has been described as a highly comprehensive and readily accessible proteome potentially providing a representation of all body tissues during health and disease. However other tissues and body fluids (a.k.a. "proximal" fluids), as well as animal models, can be used for proteomics-based biomarker discovery. The discovery of neutrophil gelatinase-associated lipocalin (NGAL) as biomarker for acute kidney injury (AKI) well illustrates the discovery potential of proteomics, as well as the use of proximal fluids and animal models in the biomarker discovery phase.

NGAL is now recognized as a robust biomarker for AKI in certain populations of critically ill patients, including children [100–102]. NGAL was initially identified as a candidate AKI biomarker in rodent models of kidney ischemia [103, 104]. Analyses of the kidney parenchymal transcriptome and the urine proteome demonstrated that NGAL was one of the most abundant genes expressed in rodents subjected to experimental renal ischemia. The use of kidney tissue and urine as the biological materials was a key component of the discovery phase in that they directly represent, or are in close proximity to, the tissue of interest (i.e. the kidney), are therefore likely to be enriched for kidney-specific candidate biomarkers, and the urine proteome is several orders of magnitude less complex than the blood proteome. Thus, an unbiased approach based on biological samples from an experimental animal model enabled the discovery of a candidate diagnostic biomarker (i.e. NGAL) that may have not been readily evident using more traditional approaches.

Comparative Genomics

The ability to reliably and efficiently sequence entire genomes from a broad variety of species, including humans, has enabled the field of comparative genomics. At its most fundamental level, comparative genomics involves the analysis and comparison of genomes from different species as a means to better understand how species have evolved. Another application of comparative genomics, more directly relevant to critical care medicine, is to understand the function of human genes by examining their respective homologues in less complex organisms such as worms, flies, and mice. The identification of Toll-like receptor 4 (TLR4) as the pattern recognition receptor for lipopolysaccharide (LPS; endotoxin), and the programmed cell death process known as "apoptosis", are two relevant examples of how comparative genomics has impacted the field of critical care medicine.

TLR4 is now well known as the cellular receptor that allows cells to recognize and respond to LPS from gram negative bacteria, and several other TLRs are now known to be receptors for other classes of pathogens [105]. In addition, there is considerable interest in targeting TLR4 as a therapeutic strategy in clinical sepsis [106, 107]. The discovery of TLR4 as the LPS receptor has been comprehensively reviewed by Beutler and Poltorak [108]. Briefly, although it was known for some time that LPS was responsible for the clinical manifestations of gram negative sepsis, the cellular receptor for LPS remained unknown until data from *Drosophila* and mutant mice converged to identify TLR4 as the receptor for LPS. The Toll gene was recognized a key component of *Drosophila* immunity, and was subsequently found to have homology with the human interleukin-1 receptor. Relatively in parallel, mutant mice were discovered that were resistant to LPS, but highly susceptible to gram negative infections. Through a complex series of gene mapping experiments, the mutant locus conferring this abnormal response to LPS in mice was identified as TLR4, which was

Fig. 20.3 Schematic example of epigenetic regulation of gene expression. The *upper panel* illustrates the basic packaging of DNA into nucleosomes by winding around histone cores. The *middle panel* illustrates that the addition of three methyl groups to lysine 27 of histone subunit H3 leads to a DNA confirmation that does not allow for transcription factor binding to the gene promoter region, thus repressing gene expression. The *bottom panel* illustrates that the addition of three methyl groups to lysine 4 of histone subunit H3 leads to a DNA confirmation that allows transcription factor binding to the gene promoter region, thus facilitating gene expression

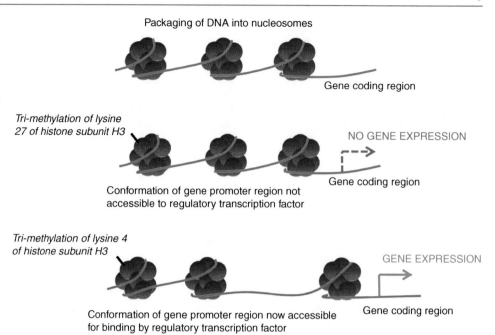

Packaging of DNA into nucleosomes

Gene coding region

Tri-methylation of lysine 27 of histone subunit H3

NO GENE EXPRESSION

Gene coding region

Conformation of gene promoter region not accessible to regulatory transcription factor

Tri-methylation of lysine 4 of histone subunit H3

GENE EXPRESSION

Conformation of gene promoter region now accessible for binding by regulatory transcription factor

Gene coding region

found to share components with the IL-1 signaling cascade. Thereafter, with the aid of comparative genomics, the human homologue of TLR4 was identified.

The process of programmed cell death, or apoptosis, has become a focus of critical care medicine research in several areas including traumatic brain injury [109], sepsis [110], and acute lung injury [111]. The history of our understanding of apoptosis and its mechanisms has been comprehensively reviewed by several authors [112, 113]. What we know today about apoptotic mechanisms began with observations in the roundworm, *C. elegans*, which produces 1,090 somatic cells during its development, but 131 of these cells are not present in the adult due to programmed cell death. The genes responsible for this process of programmed cell death in *C. elegans* were eventually identified, and subsequently human homologues were discovered through comparative genomics.

Epigenetics

Epigenetics refers to heritable changes in gene expression patterns that are not related to direct changes to the DNA sequence of a given gene [114]. The epigenetic mechanisms that regulate gene expression include chemical modifications of DNA (typically methylation), post-translational modifications of histones (typically acetylation, methylation, and/or phosphorylation), and micro-RNAs that regulate gene expression by binding specific mRNA molecules and targeting them for degradation. A key concept of epigenetic-mediated gene regulation is that the epigenetic modifications can be "inherited" (i.e. passed on to daughter cells) and can therefore lead to long lasting effects on gene expression.

A simplified example of epigenetic regulation of gene expression is provided in Fig. 20.3. Nucleosomes are the basic unit of DNA packaging into chromatin and chromosomes. A nucleosome consists of DNA segments wound around an octamer of histone proteins (two copies each of histones H2A, H2B, H3, and H4). The histone proteins can be modified by the addition (or removal) of methyl or acetyl groups to specific amino acids. These histone modifications can, in turn, alter DNA conformation and consequently alter the ability of transcription factors to bind DNA promoter regions. In the example provided in Fig. 20.3, the addition of three methyl groups to lysine 27 of histone subunit H3 leads to a DNA confirmation that does not allow transcription factor binding to the gene promoter, thus rendering the gene as being "off". Alternatively, the addition of three methyl groups to lysine 4 of histone subunit H3 leads to a DNA confirmation that allows transcription factor binding to the gene promoter, thus rendering the gene as being "on".

Of direct relevance to critical care medicine is the evolving concept that immunity- and inflammation-related genes are subject to epigenetic regulation [115]. For example, the phenomenon of endotoxin tolerance, whereby repeated exposure to endotoxin blunts subsequent cellular inflammatory responses, is mediated, in part by epigenetic mechanisms involving histone, chromatin, and DNA modifications [116–119]. In addition, production of some cytokines and chemokines by immune cells challenged with endotoxin appears to be partially dependent on epigenetic mechanisms [120, 121]. From a potential therapeutic standpoint, a recent study demonstrated that the administration of a compound that mimics acetylated histones disrupts chromatin complexes related to inflammatory responses in macrophages and confers protection in rodent models of sepsis [122].

As discussed in previous sections, an evolving paradigm in the sepsis field surrounds the concept of altered adaptive immunity and immune-suppression. Additionally, it is now well established that patients that recover from various forms of critical illness, sepsis in particular, are at increased risk of death for several years after discharge from the intensive care unit [123–125]. Evolving experimental data indicates that sepsis induces epigenetic changes in dendritic cells and lymphocytes that render the host immune deficient for a remarkably long period of time after the initial sepsis challenge [126–128]. Of note, one of the aforementioned genome-wide expression studies in children with septic shock reported the differential expression of a group of genes corresponding to gene networks involved in transcriptional repression and epigenetic regulation, in parallel with suppression of adaptive immunity genes [52]. Thus, it possible that our future approach to the recovering critically ill patient will need to take into consideration the epigenetic impact of critical illness.

Pharmacogenomics

The discipline of pharmacogenomics encompasses a blend of pharmacology, genomic data, and genomic technology [129]. There are two broad goals or applications of pharmacogenomics: understanding variations in drug metabolism and efficacy, and discovery of new pharmacologic targets.

Variability in patient responses to drugs is a very well-known clinical phenomenon in the intensive care unit, and much of this variability is based on genetic variation in key enzymes involved in drug metabolism [130]. The cytochrome P450 (CYP) system is responsible for liver metabolism of many drugs relevant to critical care medicine, and the isoenzymes that make up the P450 system are highly polymorphic. For example, a specific SNP of CYP3A can significantly reduce the metabolism of midazolam and tacrolimus [131, 132]. Another source of variability in patient responses to drugs is based on genetic variation of drug receptors. For example, the genes encoding for adrenoreceptors (α and β) have well described polymorphisms that alter response to various cardiovascular drugs used in the intensive care unit and can also impact survival in patients with heart failure [133]. Of particular relevance to pediatric critical care medicine, polymorphisms of the β2 adrenergic receptor are linked to altered responses to bronchodilators in patients with asthma [134].

The concept of "personalized medicine" is, in large part, centered on the knowledge obtained from the discipline of pharmacogenomics. However, while the goal of personalized medicine in the field of critical care is laudable, it has yet to be realized at the bedside of critically ill patients. One practical barrier is that a great deal of pharmacogenomic data potentially relevant to the critically ill patient is generated from healthy volunteers, rather than in the critical care setting and all of the attendant confounding factors such as shock, end organ failure, and poly-pharmacy. Nonetheless, technological advances have made it feasible to obtain pharmacogenomic data in critically ill patients in a clinically relevant time frame, thus bringing the concept of personalized medicine closer to the intensive care unit. The challenge going forward will be to conduct pharmacogenomics-based research in the critical care setting, with an emphasis on drugs with narrow therapeutic and toxic ranges, and that are substantially affected by genetic variation.

Other Branches of "Omics"

The widespread enthusiasm surrounding genomic medicine, coupled with rapidly advancing technologies, have fostered the development of other forms of "omic" disciplines centered on discovery via high throughput generation of large data sets. Metabolomics involves the large scale analysis of endogenous metabolites (e.g. amino acids, carbohydrates, lactate, acetate, etc.) in blood, urine, and other biological specimens. This approach is potentially highly complementary to transcriptomics and proteomics in that it provides information about the end products of gene function, and is now beginning to generate interest in the field of critical care medicine [135]. Lipidomics is conceptually related to metabolomics, but as the name implies, it is focused on large scale analysis of lipid metabolism within a biological system [136]. Degradomics focuses on large scale analysis and discovery of protease substrates [137]. The Human Microbiome Project was launched in 2008 to develop a comprehensive catalogue of the entire community of microorganisms that reside in five anatomical locations: oral, skin, vagina, gut, and respiratory tract. The project includes genome sequencing of the identified organisms, and has the ultimate goal of elucidating how the human microbiome contributes to health and disease. Finally, there is the demanding concept of the "interactome" which seeks to combine and integrate knowledge from the various "omics" fields under the umbrella of systems biology [138, 139].

Conclusion

Despite the widespread optimism surrounding the completion of the human genome project, the promise of genomic medicine has yet to be realized at the bedside of critically ill patients. The emerging data nonetheless provide hope that ongoing advances in genomic science will eventually lead to meaningful advances in our collective approach to critical illness. Realizing this goal will require substantial resources, thoughtful prioritization, multi-center collaborations, and interactions between diverse disciplines including genetics, complex statistics, computer science, molecular biology, physics, engineering, industry, and of course, the clinicians who provide critical care.

References

1. McKusick VA, Ruddle FH. Editorial: a new discipline, a new name, and new journal. Genomics. 1987;1:1–2.

2. Sorensen TI, Nielsen GG, Andersen PK, Teasdale TW. Genetic and environmental influences on premature death in adult adoptees. N Engl J Med. 1988;318(12):727–32.

3. Manolio TA, Collins FS. The HapMap and genome-wide association studies in diagnosis and therapy. Annu Rev Med. 2009;60:443–56.

4. Yende S, Kammerer CM, Angus DC. Genetics and proteomics: deciphering gene association studies in critical illness. Crit Care. 2006;10(4):227.

5. Hobson MJ, Wong HR. Genetic association research: understanding its challenges and limitations. Pediatr Crit Care Med. 2010;11(6):762–3.

6. Stalets E, Wong HR. Critically associating. Crit Care Med. 2009;37(4):1492–3.

7. Freely associating. Nat Genet. 1999;22:1–2.

8. Cornell TT, Wynn J, Shanley TP, Wheeler DS, Wong HR. Mechanisms and regulation of the gene-expression response to sepsis. Pediatrics. 2010;125(6):1248–58.

9. Flores C, Pino-Yanes MM, Casula M, Villar J. Genetics of acute lung injury: past, present and future. Minerva Anestesiol. 2010;76(10):860–4.

10. Gao L, Barnes KC. Recent advances in genetic predisposition to clinical acute lung injury. Am J Physiol Lung Cell Mol Physiol. 2009;296(5):L713–25.

11. Namath A, Patterson AJ. Genetic polymorphisms in sepsis. Crit Care Clin. 2009;25(4):835–56, x.

12. Sutherland AM, Walley KR. Bench-to-bedside review: association of genetic variation with sepsis. Crit Care. 2009;13(2):210.

13. Agnese DM, Calvano JE, Hahm SJ, Coyle SM, Corbett SA, Calvano SE, et al. Human toll-like receptor 4 mutations but not CD14 polymorphisms are associated with an increased risk of gram-negative infections. J Infect Dis. 2002;186(10):1522–5.

14. Allen A, Obaro S, Bojang K, Awomoyi AA, Greenwood BM, Whittle H, et al. Variation in toll-like receptor 4 and susceptibility to group A meningococcal meningitis in Gambian children. Pediatr Infect Dis J. 2003;22(11):1018–9.

15. Balding J, Healy CM, Livingstone WJ, White B, Mynett-Johnson L, Cafferkey M, et al. Genomic polymorphic profiles in an Irish population with meningococcaemia: is it possible to predict severity and outcome of disease? Genes Immunol. 2003;4(8):533–40.

16. Endler G, Marculescu R, Starkl P, Binder A, Geishofer G, Muller M, et al. Polymorphisms in the interleukin-1 gene cluster in children and young adults with systemic meningococcemia. Clin Chem. 2006;52(3):511–4.

17. Geishofer G, Binder A, Muller M, Zohrer B, Resch B, Muller W, et al. 4G/5G promoter polymorphism in the plasminogen-activator-inhibitor-1 gene in children with systemic meningococcaemia. Eur J Pediatr. 2005;164(8):486–90.

18. Haralambous E, Hibberd ML, Hermans PW, Ninis N, Nadel S, Levin M. Role of functional plasminogen-activator-inhibitor-1 4G/5G promoter polymorphism in susceptibility, severity, and outcome of meningococcal disease in Caucasian children. Crit Care Med. 2003;31(12):2788–93.

19. Hermans PW, Hibberd ML, Booy R, Daramola O, Hazelzet JA, de Groot R, et al. 4G/5G promoter polymorphism in the plasminogen-activator-inhibitor-1 gene and outcome of meningococcal disease. Meningococcal Research Group. Lancet. 1999;354(9178):556–60.

20. Karoly E, Fekete A, Banki NF, Szebeni B, Vannay A, Szabo AJ, et al. Heat shock protein 72 (HSPA1B) gene polymorphism and toll-like receptor (TLR) 4 mutation are associated with increased risk of urinary tract infection in children. Pediatr Res. 2007;61(3):371–4.

21. Kutukculer N, Yeniay BS, Aksu G, Berdeli A. Arg753Gln polymorphism of the human toll-like receptor-2 gene in children with recurrent febrile infections. Biochem Genet. 2007;45(7–8):507–14.

22. Lorenz E, Mira JP, Frees KL, Schwartz DA. Relevance of mutations in the TLR4 receptor in patients with gram-negative septic shock. Arch Intern Med. 2002;162(9):1028–32.

23. McArthur JA, Zhang Q, Quasney MW. Association between the A/A genotype at the lymphotoxin-alpha +250 site and increased mortality in children with positive blood cultures. Pediatr Crit Care Med. 2002;3(4):341–4.

24. Michalek J, Svetlikova P, Fedora M, Klimovic M, Klapacova L, Bartosova D, et al. Interleukin-6 gene variants and the risk of sepsis development in children. Hum Immunol. 2007;68(9):756–60.

25. Mira JP, Cariou A, Grall F, Delclaux C, Losser MR, Heshmati F, et al. Association of TNF2, a TNF-alpha promoter polymorphism, with septic shock susceptibility and mortality: a multicenter study. JAMA. 1999;282(6):561–8.

26. Nadel S, Newport MJ, Booy R, Levin M. Variation in the tumor necrosis factor-alpha gene promoter region may be associated with death from meningococcal disease. J Infect Dis. 1996;174(4):878–80.

27. Read RC, Cannings C, Naylor SC, Timms JM, Maheswaran R, Borrow R, et al. Variation within genes encoding interleukin-1 and the interleukin-1 receptor antagonist influence the severity of meningococcal disease. Ann Intern Med. 2003;138(7):534–41.

28. Read RC, Pullin J, Gregory S, Borrow R, Kaczmarski EB, di Giovine FS, et al. A functional polymorphism of toll-like receptor 4 is not associated with likelihood or severity of meningococcal disease. J Infect Dis. 2001;184(5):640–2.

29. Tabel Y, Berdeli A, Mir S. Association of TLR2 gene Arg753Gln polymorphism with urinary tract infection in children. Int J Immunogenet. 2007;34(6):399–405.

30. Westendorp RG, Hottenga JJ, Slagboom PE. Variation in plasminogen-activator-inhibitor-1 gene and risk of meningococcal septic shock. Lancet. 1999;354(9178):561–3.

31. Christie JD. Microarrays. Crit Care Med. 2005;33(12 Suppl): S449–52.

32. Gershon D. Microarray technology: an array of opportunities. Nature. 2002;416(6883):885–91.

33. Tang BM, Huang SJ, McLean AS. Genome-wide transcription profiling of human sepsis: a systematic review. Crit Care. 2010;14(6):R237.

34. Ozsolak F, Milos PM. RNA sequencing: advances, challenges and opportunities. Nat Rev Genet. 2011;12(2):87–98.

35. Boujoukos AJ, Martich GD, Supinski E, Suffredini AF. Compartmentalization of the acute cytokine response in humans after intravenous endotoxin administration. J Appl Physiol. 1993;74(6):3027–33.

36. DeLa Cadena RA, Suffredini AF, Page JD, Pixley RA, Kaufman N, Parrillo JE, et al. Activation of the kallikrein-kinin system after endotoxin administration to normal human volunteers. Blood. 1993;81(12):3313–7.

37. Suffredini AF, Fromm RE, Parker MM, Brenner M, Kovacs JA, Wesley RA, et al. The cardiovascular response of normal humans to the administration of endotoxin. N Engl J Med. 1989;321(5):280–7.

38. Suffredini AF, Harpel PC, Parrillo JE. Promotion and subsequent inhibition of plasminogen activation after administration of intravenous endotoxin to normal subjects. N Engl J Med. 1989;320(18):1165–72.

39. Talwar S, Munson PJ, Barb J, Fiuza C, Cintron AP, Logun C, et al. Gene expression profiles of peripheral blood leukocytes after endotoxin challenge in humans. Physiol Genomics. 2006;25(2):203–15.

40. Prabhakar U, Conway TM, Murdock P, Mooney JL, Clark S, Hedge P, et al. Correlation of protein and gene expression profiles of inflammatory proteins after endotoxin challenge in human subjects. DNA Cell Biol. 2005;24(7):410–31.

41. Calvano SE, Xiao W, Richards DR, Felciano RM, Baker HV, Cho RJ, et al. A network-based analysis of systemic inflammation in humans. Nature. 2005;437(7061):1032–7.

42. Cvijanovich N, Shanley TP, Lin R, Allen GL, Thomas NJ, Checchia P, et al. Validating the genomic signature of pediatric septic shock. Physiol Genomics. 2008;34(1):127–34.

43. Johnson SB, Lissauer M, Bochicchio GV, Moore R, Cross AS, Scalea TM. Gene expression profiles differentiate between sterile SIRS and early sepsis. Ann Surg. 2007;245(4):611–21.

44. Pachot A, Lepape A, Vey S, Bienvenu J, Mougin B, Monneret G. Systemic transcriptional analysis in survivor and non-survivor septic shock patients: a preliminary study. Immunol Lett. 2006;106(1):63–71.

45. Payen D, Lukaszewicz AC, Belikova I, Faivre V, Gelin C, Russwurm S, et al. Gene profiling in human blood leucocytes during recovery from septic shock. Intensive Care Med. 2008;34(8):1371–6.

46. Prucha M, Ruryk A, Boriss H, Moller E, Zazula R, Herold I, et al. Expression profiling: toward an application in sepsis diagnostics. Shock. 2004;22(1):29–33.

47. Shanley TP, Cvijanovich N, Lin R, Allen GL, Thomas NJ, Doctor A, et al. Genome-level longitudinal expression of signaling pathways and gene networks in pediatric septic shock. Mol Med. 2007;13(9–10):495–508.

48. Tang BM, McLean AS, Dawes IW, Huang SJ, Cowley MJ, Lin RC. Gene-expression profiling of gram-positive and gram-negative sepsis in critically ill patients. Crit Care Med. 2008;36(4):1125–8.

49. Tang BM, McLean AS, Dawes IW, Huang SJ, Lin RC. The use of gene-expression profiling to identify candidate genes in human sepsis. Am J Respir Crit Care Med. 2007;176(7):676–84.

50. Tang BM, McLean AS, Dawes IW, Huang SJ, Lin RC. Gene-expression profiling of peripheral blood mononuclear cells in sepsis. Crit Care Med. 2009;37(3):882–8.

51. Wong HR, Cvijanovich N, Allen GL, Lin R, Anas N, Meyer K, et al. Genomic expression profiling across the pediatric systemic inflammatory response syndrome, sepsis, and septic shock spectrum. Crit Care Med. 2009;37(5):1558–66.

52. Wong HR, Freishtat RJ, Monaco M, Odoms K, Shanley TP. Leukocyte subset-derived genomewide expression profiles in pediatric septic shock. Pediatr Crit Care Med. 2010;11(3):349–55.

53. Wong HR, Shanley TP, Sakthivel B, Cvijanovich N, Lin R, Allen GL, et al. Genome-level expression profiles in pediatric septic shock indicate a role for altered zinc homeostasis in poor outcome. Physiol Genomics. 2007;30(2):146–55.

54. Carlet J, Cohen J, Calandra T, Opal SM, Masur H. Sepsis: time to reconsider the concept. Crit Care Med. 2008;36(3):964–6.

55. Marshall JC. Such stuff as dreams are made on: mediator-directed therapy in sepsis. Nat Rev Drug Discov. 2003;2(5):391–405.

56. Marshall JC, Vincent JL, Fink MP, Cook DJ, Rubenfeld G, Foster D, et al. Measures, markers, and mediators: toward a staging system for clinical sepsis. A report of the Fifth Toronto Sepsis Roundtable, Toronto, Ontario, Canada, October 25–26, 2000. Crit Care Med. 2003;31(5):1560–7.

57. Russell JA. Gene expression in human sepsis: what have we learned? Crit Care. 2011;15(1):121.

58. Gogos CA, Drosou E, Bassaris HP, Skoutelis A. Pro- versus anti-inflammatory cytokine profile in patients with severe sepsis: a marker for prognosis and future therapeutic options. J Infect Dis. 2000;181(1):176–80.

59. Osuchowski MF, Welch K, Siddiqui J, Remick DG. Circulating cytokine/inhibitor profiles reshape the understanding of the SIRS/CARS continuum in sepsis and predict mortality. J Immunol. 2006;177(3):1967–74.

60. Osuchowski MF, Welch K, Yang H, Siddiqui J, Remick DG. Chronic sepsis mortality characterized by an individualized inflammatory response. J Immunol. 2007;179(1):623–30.

61. Hotchkiss RS, Karl IE. The pathophysiology and treatment of sepsis. N Engl J Med. 2003;348(2):138–50.

62. Hotchkiss RS, Opal S. Immunotherapy for sepsis – a new approach against an ancient foe. N Engl J Med. 2010;363(1):87–9.

63. Unsinger J, McGlynn M, Kasten KR, Hoekzema AS, Watanabe E, Muenzer JT, et al. IL-7 promotes T cell viability, trafficking, and functionality and improves survival in sepsis. J Immunol. 2010;184(7):3768–79.

64. Kasten KR, Prakash PS, Unsinger J, Goetzman HS, England LG, Cave CM, et al. Interleukin-7 (IL-7) treatment accelerates neutrophil recruitment through gamma delta T-cell IL-17 production in a murine model of sepsis. Infect Immun. 2010;78(11):4714–22.

65. Wong HR, Cvijanovich N, Lin R, Allen GL, Thomas NJ, Willson DF, et al. Identification of pediatric septic shock subclasses based on genome-wide expression profiling. BMC Med. 2009;7:34.

66. Wong HR, Cvijanovich NZ, Allen GL, Thomas NJ, Freishtat RJ, Anas N, et al. Validation of a gene expression-based subclassification strategy for pediatric septic shock. Crit Care Med. 2011;39:2511–7.

67. Wong HR, Wheeler DS, Tegtmeyer K, Poynter SE, Kaplan JM, Chima RS, et al. Toward a clinically feasible gene expression-based subclassification strategy for septic shock: proof of concept. Crit Care Med. 2010;38(10):1955–61.

68. Wynn JL, Cvijanovich NZ, Allen GL, Thomas NJ, Freishtat RJ, Anas N, et al. The influence of developmental age on the early transcriptomic response of children with septic shock. Mol Med. 2011;17(11–12):1146–56.

69. Bouchon A, Facchetti F, Weigand MA, Colonna M. TREM-1 amplifies inflammation and is a crucial mediator of septic shock. Nature. 2001;410(6832):1103–7.

70. Pathan N, Hemingway CA, Alizadeh AA, Stephens AC, Boldrick JC, Oragui EE, et al. Role of interleukin 6 in myocardial dysfunction of meningococcal septic shock. Lancet. 2004;363(9404):203–9.

71. Pachot A, Cazalis MA, Venet F, Turrel F, Faudot C, Voirin N, et al. Decreased expression of the fractalkine receptor CX3CR1 on circulating monocytes as new feature of sepsis-induced immunosuppression. J Immunol. 2008;180(9):6421–9.

72. Rink L, Haase H. Zinc homeostasis and immunity. Trends Immunol. 2007;28(1):1–4.

73. Cvijanovich NZ, King JC, Flori HR, Gildengorin G, Wong HR. Zinc homeostasis in pediatric critical illness. Pediatr Crit Care Med. 2009;10(1):29–34.

74. Heyland DK, Jones N, Cvijanovich NZ, Wong H. Zinc supplementation in critically ill patients: a key pharmaconutrient? JPEN J Parenter Enter Nutr. 2008;32(5):509–19.

75. Weitzel LR, Mayles WJ, Sandoval PA, Wischmeyer PE. Effects of pharmaconutrients on cellular dysfunction and the microcirculation in critical illness. Curr Opin Anaesthesiol. 2009;22(2):177–83.

76. Bao S, Liu MJ, Lee B, Besecker B, Lai JP, Guttridge DC, et al. Zinc modulates the innate immune response in vivo to polymicrobial sepsis through regulation of NF-kappaB. Am J Physiol Lung Cell Mol Physiol. 2010;298(6):L744–54.

77. Knoell DL, Julian MW, Bao S, Besecker B, Macre JE, Leikauf GD, et al. Zinc deficiency increases organ damage and mortality in a murine model of polymicrobial sepsis. Crit Care Med. 2009;37(4):1380–4.

78. Besecker BY, Exline MC, Hollyfield J, Phillips G, Disilvestro RA, Wewers MD, et al. A comparison of zinc metabolism, inflammation, and disease severity in critically ill infected and noninfected adults early after intensive care unit admission. Am J Clin Nutr. 2011;93(6):1356–64.

79. Knoell DL, Liu MJ. Impact of zinc metabolism on innate immune function in the setting of sepsis. Int J Vitam Nutr Res. 2010;80(4–5):271–7.

80. Solan PD, Dunsmore KE, Denenberg AG, Odom K, Zingarelli B, Wong HR. A novel role for matrix metalloproteinase-8 in sepsis. Crit Care Med. 2012;40:379–87.

81. Van Lint P, Libert C. Matrix metalloproteinase-8: cleavage can be decisive. Cytokine Growth Factor Rev. 2006;17(4):217–23.

82. Vanlaere I, Libert C. Matrix metalloproteinases as drug targets in infections caused by gram-negative bacteria and in septic shock. Clin Microbiol Rev. 2009;22(2):224–39, Table of Contents.

83. Kaplan JM, Wong HR. Biomarker discovery and development in pediatric critical care medicine. Pediatr Crit Care Med. 2011;12(2):165–73.

84. Lissauer ME, Johnson SB, Bochicchio GV, Feild CJ, Cross AS, Hasday JD, et al. Differential expression of toll-like receptor genes: sepsis compared with sterile inflammation 1 day before sepsis diagnosis. Shock. 2009;31(3):238–44.

85. Cobb JP, Moore EE, Hayden DL, Minei JP, Cuschieri J, Yang J, et al. Validation of the riboleukogram to detect ventilator-associated pneumonia after severe injury. Ann Surg. 2009;250(4):531–9.

86. McDunn JE, Husain KD, Polpitiya AD, Burykin A, Ruan J, Li Q, et al. Plasticity of the systemic inflammatory response to acute infection during critical illness: development of the riboleukogram. PLoS One. 2008;3(2):e1564.

87. Ramilo O, Allman W, Chung W, Mejias A, Ardura M, Glaser C, et al. Gene expression patterns in blood leukocytes discriminate patients with acute infections. Blood. 2007;109(5):2066–77.

88. Nowak JE, Wheeler DS, Harmon KK, Wong HR. Admission chemokine (C-C motif) ligand 4 levels predict survival in pediatric septic shock. Pediatr Crit Care Med. 2010;11(2):213–6.

89. Wong HR, Cvijanovich N, Wheeler DS, Bigham MT, Monaco M, Odoms K, et al. Interleukin-8 as a stratification tool for interventional trials involving pediatric septic shock. Am J Respir Crit Care Med. 2008;178(3):276–82.

90. Calfee CS, Thompson BT, Parsons PE, Ware LB, Matthay MA, Wong HR. Plasma interleukin-8 is not an effective risk stratification tool for adults with vasopressor-dependent septic shock. Crit Care Med. 2010;38(6):1436–41.

91. Standage SW, Wong HR. Biomarkers for pediatric sepsis and septic shock. Expert Rev Anti Infect Ther. 2011;9(1):71–9.

92. Pene F, Courtine E, Cariou A, Mira JP. Toward theragnostics. Crit Care Med. 2009;37(1 Suppl):S50–8.

93. Kotz KT, Xiao W, Miller-Graziano C, Qian WJ, Russom A, Warner EA, et al. Clinical microfluidics for neutrophil genomics and proteomics. Nat Med. 2010;16(9):1042–7.

94. Geiss GK, Bumgarner RE, Birditt B, Dahl T, Dowidar N, Dunaway DL, et al. Direct multiplexed measurement of gene expression with color-coded probe pairs. Nat Biotechnol. 2008;26(3):317–25.

95. Karvunidis T, Mares J, Thongboonkerd V, Matejovic M. Recent progress of proteomics in critical illness. Shock. 2009;31(6):545–52.

96. Nguyen A, Yaffe MB. Proteomics and systems biology approaches to signal transduction in sepsis. Crit Care Med. 2003;31(1 Suppl):S1–6.

97. Qian WJ, Petritis BO, Kaushal A, Finnerty CC, Jeschke MG, Monroe ME, et al. Plasma proteome response to severe burn injury revealed by 18O-labeled "universal" reference-based quantitative proteomics. J Proteome Res. 2010;9(9):4779–89.

98. Liu T, Qian WJ, Gritsenko MA, Xiao W, Moldawer LL, Kaushal A, et al. High dynamic range characterization of the trauma patient plasma proteome. Mol Cell Proteomics. 2006;5(10):1899–913.

99. Rifai N, Gillette MA, Carr SA. Protein biomarker discovery and validation: the long and uncertain path to clinical utility. Nat Biotechnol. 2006;24(8):971–83.

100. Haase M, Bellomo R, Devarajan P, Schlattmann P, Haase-Fielitz A. Accuracy of neutrophil gelatinase-associated lipocalin (NGAL) in diagnosis and prognosis in acute kidney injury: a systematic review and meta-analysis. Am J Kidney Dis. 2009;54(6):1012–24.

101. Devarajan P. Neutrophil gelatinase-associated lipocalin (NGAL): a new marker of kidney disease. Scand J Clin Lab Invest Suppl. 2008;241:89–94.

102. Mishra J, Dent C, Tarabishi R, Mitsnefes MM, Ma Q, Kelly C, et al. Neutrophil gelatinase-associated lipocalin (NGAL) as a biomarker for acute renal injury after cardiac surgery. Lancet. 2005;365(9466):1231–8.

103. Mishra J, Ma Q, Prada A, Mitsnefes M, Zahedi K, Yang J, et al. Identification of neutrophil gelatinase-associated lipocalin as a novel early urinary biomarker for ischemic renal injury. J Am Soc Nephrol. 2003;14(10):2534–43.

104. Devarajan P. Proteomics for biomarker discovery in acute kidney injury. Semin Nephrol. 2007;27(6):637–51.

105. Casanova JL, Abel L, Quintana-Murci L. Human TLRs and IL-1Rs in host defense: natural insights from evolutionary, epidemiological, and clinical genetics. Annu Rev Immunol. 2011; 29:447–91.

106. Kalil AC, Larosa SP, Gogate J, Lynn M, Opal SM. Influence of severity of illness on the effects of eritoran tetrasodium (E5564) and on other therapies for severe sepsis. Shock. 2011;36(4):327–31.

107. Tidswell M, LaRosa SP. Toll-like receptor-4 antagonist eritoran tetrasodium for severe sepsis. Expert Rev Anti Infect Ther. 2011;9(5):507–20.

108. Beutler B, Poltorak A. The sole gateway to endotoxin response: how LPS was identified as Tlr4, and its role in innate immunity. Drug Metab Dispos. 2001;29(4 Pt 2):474–8.

109. Zhang X, Chen Y, Jenkins LW, Kochanek PM, Clark RS. Bench-to-bedside review: apoptosis/programmed cell death triggered by traumatic brain injury. Crit Care. 2005;9(1):66–75.

110. Hotchkiss RS, Coopersmith CM, Karl IE. Prevention of lymphocyte apoptosis – a potential treatment of sepsis? Clin Infect Dis. 2005;41 Suppl 7:S465–9.

111. Tang PS, Mura M, Seth R, Liu M. Acute lung injury and cell death: how many ways can cells die? Am J Physiol Lung Cell Mol Physiol. 2008;294(4):L632–41.

112. Zakeri Z, Lockshin RA. Cell death: history and future. Adv Exp Med Biol. 2008;615:1–11.

113. Elmore S. Apoptosis: a review of programmed cell death. Toxicol Pathol. 2007;35(4):495–516.

114. Delcuve GP, Rastegar M, Davie JR. Epigenetic control. J Cell Physiol. 2009;219(2):243–50.

115. Carson WF, Cavassani KA, Dou Y, Kunkel SL. Epigenetic regulation of immune cell functions during post-septic immunosuppression. Epigenetics. 2011;6(3):273–83.

116. Chan C, Li L, McCall CE, Yoza BK. Endotoxin tolerance disrupts chromatin remodeling and NF-kappaB transactivation at the IL-1beta promoter. J Immunol. 2005;175(1):461–8.

117. El Gazzar M, Yoza BK, Chen X, Garcia BA, Young NL, McCall CE. Chromatin-specific remodeling by HMGB1 and linker histone H1 silences proinflammatory genes during endotoxin tolerance. Mol Cell Biol. 2009;29(7):1959–71.

118. El Gazzar M, Yoza BK, Chen X, Hu J, Hawkins GA, McCall CE. G9a and HP1 couple histone and DNA methylation to TNFalpha transcription silencing during endotoxin tolerance. J Biol Chem. 2008;283(47):32198–208.

119. Foster SL, Hargreaves DC, Medzhitov R. Gene-specific control of inflammation by TLR-induced chromatin modifications. Nature. 2007;447(7147):972–8.

120. Brogdon JL, Xu Y, Szabo SJ, An S, Buxton F, Cohen D, et al. Histone deacetylase activities are required for innate immune cell control of Th1 but not Th2 effector cell function. Blood. 2007;109(3):1123–30.

121. Tsaprouni LG, Ito K, Adcock IM, Punchard N. Suppression of lipopolysaccharide- and tumour necrosis factor-alpha-induced interleukin (IL)-8 expression by glucocorticoids involves changes in IL-8 promoter acetylation. Clin Exp Immunol. 2007;150(1):151–7.

122. Nicodeme E, Jeffrey KL, Schaefer U, Beinke S, Dewell S, Chung CW, et al. Suppression of inflammation by a synthetic histone mimic. Nature. 2010;468(7327):1119–23.

123. Czaja AS, Zimmerman JJ, Nathens AB. Readmission and late mortality after pediatric severe sepsis. Pediatrics. 2009;123(3): 849–57.

124. Quartin AA, Schein RM, Kett DH, Peduzzi PN. Magnitude and duration of the effect of sepsis on survival. Department of Veterans Affairs Systemic Sepsis Cooperative Studies Group. JAMA. 1997;277(13):1058–63.

125. Winters BD, Eberlein M, Leung J, Needham DM, Pronovost PJ, Sevransky JE. Long-term mortality and quality of life in sepsis: a systematic review. Crit Care Med. 2010;38(5):1276–83.

126. Ishii M, Wen H, Corsa CA, Liu T, Coelho AL, Allen RM, et al. Epigenetic regulation of the alternatively activated macrophage phenotype. Blood. 2009;114(15):3244–54.

127. Wen H, Dou Y, Hogaboam CM, Kunkel SL. Epigenetic regulation of dendritic cell-derived interleukin-12 facilitates immunosuppression after a severe innate immune response. Blood. 2008;111(4):1797–804.

128. Wen H, Schaller MA, Dou Y, Hogaboam CM, Kunkel SL. Dendritic cells at the interface of innate and acquired immunity: the role for epigenetic changes. J Leukoc Biol. 2008; 83(3):439–46.

129. Ma Q, Lu AY. Pharmacogenetics, pharmacogenomics, and individualized medicine. Pharmacol Rev. 2011;63(2):437–59.

130. Empey PE. Genetic predisposition to adverse drug reactions in the intensive care unit. Crit Care Med. 2010;38(6 Suppl):S106–16.

131. Relling MV, Hoffman JM. Should pharmacogenomic studies be required for new drug approval? Clin Pharmacol Ther. 2007;81(3):425–8.

132. Yu KS, Cho JY, Jang IJ, Hong KS, Chung JY, Kim JR, et al. Effect of the CYP3A5 genotype on the pharmacokinetics of intravenous midazolam during inhibited and induced metabolic states. Clin Pharmacol Ther. 2004;76(2):104–12.

133. Johnson JA, Liggett SB. Cardiovascular pharmacogenomics of adrenergic receptor signaling: clinical implications and future directions. Clin Pharmacol Ther. 2011;89(3):366–78.

134. Chung LP, Waterer G, Thompson PJ. Pharmacogenetics of beta2 adrenergic receptor gene polymorphisms, long-acting beta-agonists and asthma. Clin Exp Allergy. 2011;41(3):312–26.

135. Serkova NJ, Standiford TJ, Stringer KA. The emerging field of quantitative blood metabolomics for biomarker discovery in critical illnesses. Am J Respir Crit Care Med. 2011;184(6):647–55.

136. Wolf C, Quinn PJ. Lipidomics: practical aspects and applications. Prog Lipid Res. 2008;47(1):15–36.

137. Overall CM, Dean RA. Degradomics: systems biology of the protease web. Pleiotropic roles of MMPs in cancer. Cancer Metastasis Rev. 2006;25(1):69–75.

138. Namas R, Zamora R, An G, Doyle J, Dick TE, Jacono FJ, et al. Sepsis: something old, something new, and a systems view. J Crit Care. 2011;27(3):314.e1–11.

139. Vodovotz Y, Constantine G, Faeder J, Mi Q, Rubin J, Bartels J, et al. Translational systems approaches to the biology of inflammation and healing. Immunopharmacol Immunotoxicol. 2010;32(2):181–95.

Signal Transduction Pathways in Critical Illness and Injury

21

Timothy T. Cornell, Waseem Ostwani, Lei Sun,
Steven L. Kunkel, and Thomas P. Shanley

Abstract

Cells respond to environmental stimuli using an elaborate process to propagate and amplify a signal from the cell surface to the nucleus leading to initiation of gene induction in a process termed "signal transduction". The NFκB and MAPK pathways are two important pathways in the cellular responses during critical illness. Both pathways are composed of a series of kinases that utilize phosphorylation to activate downstream kinases. Once activated these pathways must be deactivated in order to reestablish homeostasis usually by a phosphatase. Additionally, intracellular inhibitors and epigenetic processes are important in regulating the activation of signal pathways.

Keywords

Signal transduction • NFκB • MAP kinase pathways • Phosphatases • Epigenetics • MicroRNA • Regulators of signal transduction • Histone modifications

T.T. Cornell, MD (✉)
Department of Pediatrics and Communicable Diseases,
C.S. Mott Children's Hospital University of Michigan,
1500 East Medical Center Drive, Mott F-6882/Box 5243,
Ann Arbor, MI 48104, USA
e-mail: ttcornel@med.umich.edu

W. Ostwani, MD
Department of Pediatric Critical Care Medicine, C.S. Mott
Children's Hospital, 1500 E. Medical Center Dr., Neuroscience
Hospital F6790/SPC 5243, Ann Arbor, MI 481095243, USA
e-mail: waseem@med.umich.edu

L. Sun, PhD
Department of Pediatrics and Communicable Diseases,
University of Michigan, C.S. Mott Children's Hospital,
Von Voigtlander Women's Hospital,
109 Zina Pitcher Place, BSRB 4478, Ann Arbor, MI 48103, USA
e-mail: leisun@med.umich.edu

S.L. Kunkel, MS, PhD
Department of Pathology, University of Michigan,
4107 Medical Science Building 1, 1301 Catherine Street,
Ann Arbor, MI 48105, USA
e-mail: slkunkel@umich.edu

T.P. Shanley, MD
Michigan Institute for Clinical and Health Research,
University of Michigan Medical School, 2800 Plymouth Road,
Building 400, Ann Arbor, MI 48109, USA
e-mail: tshanley@med.umich.edu

Introduction

One of the most important biologic functions that cells perform is to sense and respond to an external stimulus. Changes that occur in the extracellular environment must be *sensed* at the cell surface creating a signal that is propagated through the cytoplasm to the nucleus often resulting in the activation of the machinery responsible for transcription of genes and translation to proteins. Cells utilize highly conserved mechanistic principles and have adapted a broad array of specific pathways to accomplish this biologic task. The synonymous terms *signal transduction*, *cell signaling*, and *transmembrane signaling* have been used to define this conserved, fundamental cellular process. This field now comprises its own scientific entity [1] and a comprehensive review of all pertinent pathways is beyond the scope of this chapter. For this purpose, the reader is referred to recent, excellent, comprehensive text [1, 2]. The intent of the current chapter is to review some fundamental biologic processes involved in signal transduction and gene expression, introduce some of the key pathways currently focused on by investigators in critical care medicine, and emphasize the biologic relevance of these pathways to critical illness.

D.S. Wheeler et al. (eds.), *Pediatric Critical Care Medicine*,
DOI 10.1007/978-1-4471-6362-6_21, © Springer-Verlag London 2014

Historical Perspective of Signal Transduction

The science of signal transduction owes its origin to the field of endocrinology and hormonal biology. The concept of intracellular communication or *messaging* originated from Claude Bernard's work in the 1850s, when he described how *internal secretions* of the thyroid and adrenal glands were released into the circulation and had distant effects on various organs. Later, this concept was refined by Bayliss and Starling [3] who described *secretin* as a member of a large group of chemical messengers that ultimately came to be called *hormones*. This work was the initial summary of the biologic function by which a secreted product could affect a specific response in distal cells of a target organ. With the subsequent explosion of biochemical and molecular research tools, recent decades have witnessed extraordinary advances in our understanding of signal transduction pathways. At every level of this biologic principle—cell surface receptors that sense a stimulus, second messengers that propagate the signal, and numerous nuclear factors that regulate gene expression—advances have helped us better understand the pathophysiology of critical illnesses and provided hope of identifying novel targets that increase our therapeutic armamentarium.

Basic Overview of Signal Transduction

Signal transduction incorporates a series of mechanisms schematically arranged in a pathway that function to transmit a signal (generally from the cell surface) to the nuclear compartment where the machinery capable of mounting an adaptive cellular response, usually by affecting gene expression, exists (Fig. 21.1). Thus, the initial step involves engagement of a receptor by a stimulus followed by the generation of a signal that is then amplified and/or

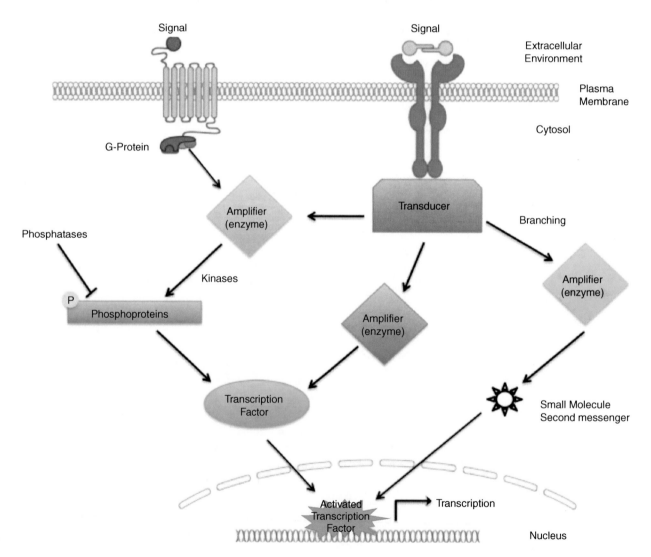

Fig. 21.1 Overview of signal transduction mechanisms

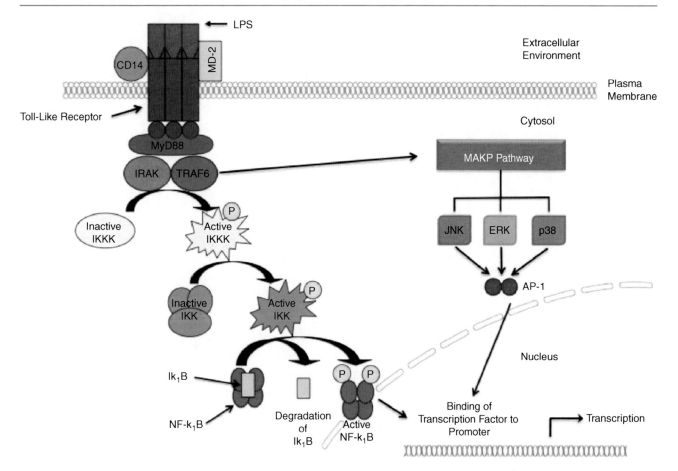

Fig. 21.2 Key signaling pathways in critical illness: nuclear factor-k B pathway and the mitogen-activated protein kinase pathways. *MyD88* myeloid differentiation adapter protein, *TRAF* TNF receptor-associated factor, *IRAK* Interleukin-1 receptor-associated kinase, *IKK* IκB kinase, *IκB* inhibitor of κB, *NF-κB* Nuclear factor-kappaB, *JNK* c-Jun N-terminal kinases, *ERK* Extracellular signal-regulated kinases, *AP-1* activator protein 1

propagated to the nuclear transcriptional and gene regulatory machinery allowing for de novo gene expression. To accomplish this with both specificity and fidelity, a number of strategies are used, including reversible phosphorylation of proteins, mobilization of calcium and other ions, activation of lipid-derived mediators, accumulation and/or degradation of cyclic nucleotides, and stimulation of G-coupled proteins. Finally, in the nuclear compartment, transcription activating factors facilitate the process of transcribing DNA to mRNA which in turn can be subjected to post-transcriptional modifications (e.g. destabilization or degradation) that influence the amount of mRNA translated to protein [4]. In light of the vast numbers of proteins playing a role in signaling (receptors, adaptor proteins, kinases, phosphatases, and so forth), complete understanding of the complexity of even a single pathway can be daunting. In this chapter, we highlight those pathways that have specific relevance to the biology of critical illness, specifically the Nuclear Factor-kappa B Pathway and the Mitogen-Activated Protein Kinase Pathways (Fig. 21.2).

Stimuli Triggering Signal Transduction

Signal transduction is initiated by any number of stimuli that influence cellular responses and activities. Among those stimuli relevant to critical care are circulating mediators (hormones, cytokines, and growth factors), osmolar changes, mechanical stress (such as shear, stretch) and pathogens; Table 21.1). Of particular importance to the pediatric critical care practitioner are those responses observed in the setting of an invading pathogen that are commonly responsible for the pathophysiologic consequence of severe sepsis.

Basic science investigators have identified an increasing number of molecular patterns expressed by pathogens; so-called *pathogen- (or microbial-) associated molecular patterns* or *PAMPS (or MAMPS)* that distinguish microbe from the human host. To sense these PAMPS, the innate immune system has adapted a series of germ-line encoded pattern-recognition receptors (PRRs). PRRs have specific affinity for conserved regions of PAMPS making these receptors key component in the interaction between host and pathogen.

Table 21.1 Factors initiating signal transduction events

Classes of factors	Examples
Circulating mediators	
Hormones	Cortisol, thyroid hormones catecholamines
Cytokines/chemokines	TNF-α, IL-1, IL-6, CXCL-8/IL-8, CCLT/MCP-1, IL-10
Growth factors	Insulin growth factor, GM-CSF
Pathogens	
Gram-negative bacteria	Lipopolysaccharide, CPG DNA
Gram-positive bacteria	Lipotechoic acid
Viruses	Capsid proteins, viral DNA/RNA
Fungi	Mannose
Biologic stresses (biotrauma)	
Mechanical stress	Mechanical ventilation, vascular resistance, trauma
Shear stress	Vasculopathies, hypercoagulation, hypertension
Osmotic stress	Hyper-, hyponatremia, osmolar therapies
In vivo, endogenous ligands	
Extracellular matrix proteins	Heparin sulfate
Cell-to-cell interactions	Leukocyte/platelet-endothelial cell interactions

GM-CSF granulocyte-macrophage colony-stimulating factor, *IL* interleukin, *TNF* tumor necrosis factor

The first and most well characterized PRRs are the Toll-like receptors (TLRs) [5]. TLRs are a key component in the innate immune response and mediate most of the inflammatory response encountered in critical care. As a prime example of receptors capable of initiating a signaling response, many but not all TLRs are cell membrane bound and possess an extracellular ligand-binding domain and usually an intracellular signaling domain or adapter protein that serves to transmit the signal across the cell membrane [6]. A numbers of receptor-based or cell membrane-based systems possess the capacity to undergo ligand binding and/or conformational changes that result in the initiation of the signal that then requires propagation through the cytosolic compartment. Crosstalk among the various receptors and the signal pathways they activate allow for the predictable response to the various PAMPs [5].

General Strategies for Signal Propagation

Upon initiation of the signal, a number of serial and/or parallel pathways that are comprised of transducing proteins or amplifiers regulate the amplification and/or propagation of the signal. One of the most common mechanisms employed by mammalian cells to propagate a signal is reversible phosphorylation of serine, threonine, and/or tyrosine residues on target proteins [7, 8]. To accomplish this, protein kinases,

one of the largest gene families known, facilitate the catalytic transfer of a γ-phosphate group from $Mg^{2+}ATP$ to these amino acid residues. An example of kinases that modulate inflammatory responses associated with sepsis and acute lung injury are the mitogen-activated protein (MAP) kinases, which includes the ERK, JNK, and p38 pathways, reviewed below [9, 10].

The activity of a kinase is generally measured in one of two ways—by determining the presence of phosphorylation of the target substrate using Western blot analysis or by directly measuring kinase activity using an in vitro kinase assay. In the latter case, the kinase of interest is specifically immunoprecipitated and then combined with a substrate for the kinase and a labeled source of phosphate (^{32}P-ATP or a fluorescent dye) so that phosphorylation of the substrate can be determined by subsequent radiography or fluorescence. It is imperative to note that, at any point in time, the phosphorylation state of a protein is maintained by a balance between the actions of kinases and possible dephosphorylation by enzymes called *protein phosphatases*. The phosphatases are proteins that hydrolyze the phosphoester bonds of phosphorylated serine, threonine, and tyrosine residues and thus provide the counter regulatory arm of reversible protein phosphorylation. Two large protein phosphatase families exist: serine (Ser)/threonine (Thr) and tyrosine (Tyr) phosphatases, which are reviewed later.

Several other mechanisms for signal propagation exist, including calcium mobilization, activation of lipid-derived mediators (e.g. ceramide pathway), changes in cyclic nucleotides (e.g. cAMP) and stimulation of G-coupled proteins, all of which have some relevance to critical care. For example, depolarization of the muscle cell opens membrane calcium channels that subsequently signal release of additional calcium stores in the sarcoplasmic reticulum to mediate optimal contraction of the myocyte. A principle proinflammatory mediator, platelet activating factor, increases the expression of the cell membrane, sphingolipid product, ceramide resulting in activation of inflammatory signaling pathways resulting in pulmonary edema formation [11]. Endothelin-1 mediates potent vasoconstriction through a G-protein coupled, endothelin (ETA) receptor [12]. Thus, numerous examples of these general signaling principles exist throughout diseases faced in the critical care unit.

Specific Pathways

As greater insight into disease states has been achieved, our understanding of the role of signal transduction pathways and the regulation, or dysregulation, of the signal transduction pathways in these pathologic states has substantially increased. Some of these pathways have been studied in both preclinical models and clinical states pertaining to critical illness, such as sepsis and acute lung injury. Increasingly, the importance of understanding the activation of certain pathways and the regulation of these pathways as a means to truly understand the clinical pathophysiologic states has become evident in recent years. Some of the notable examples of key pathways important in critical care are described in the following sections.

Nuclear Factor-k B Pathway

For signaling pathways to initiate a cellular change on the basis of *de novo* protein synthesis, transcription (DNA serving as the genetic template for mRNA production) must be initiated. Proteins that serve this function are called *transcriptional activation factors*. Among the important transcription factors examined in the context of critical care is Nuclear Factor-kappa B (NFκB) because of the large number of inflammatory genes induced by its activation (Table 21.2). Nuclear Factor-kappa B really refers to a series of proteins categorized as the so-called Rel family of transcription activation factors [13, 14], but the canonical NFκB is a heterodimer composed of two subunits, p50 and p65. This heterodimer, under most steady-state conditions, is anchored in the cytoplasm by an inhibitory subunit called *inhibitor of kappa B* (IκB), commonly the α-form, which is a member of a larger family of IκB-related proteins [15–17]. The NFκB pathway is activated in response to a variety of pathologic stimuli (e.g., lipopolysaccharide, biotrauma, and other PAMPs). One of the best-studied examples with relevance to critical care is activation by lipopolysaccharide. Binding of lipopolysaccharide to its receptor complex (TLR4/CD14/MD2), facilitated by lipopolysaccharide binding protein, results in the recruitment of the myeloid differentiation adapter protein, MyD88, to this receptor complex (Fig. 21.2). This process results in the recruitment of the interleukin-1 (IL-1) receptor associated kinase (IRAK), which undergoes auto-phosphorylation and recruits the additional adapter protein, TNF receptor associated factor-6 (TRAF-6) [18]. TRAF-6 then phosphorylates and activates an upstream, heterotrimeric member of the NFκB pathway, the IκB protein kinase complex (IκK-α, -β and -γ [also called NEMO]), resulting in IκB-α phosphorylation [19]. Once phosphorylated, IκB-α is targeted for polyubiquitination, a process that targets proteins for proteasomic degradation via the 26S proteasome. Upon degradation of IκB-α, the nuclear localization sequence of the p50 subunit is unmasked, and nuclear translocation of NFκB occurs (Fig. 21.2) [20]. NFκB then binds to a DNA sequence (a so-called *consensus sequence*) on those portions of chromatin in the promoter regions that are specifically recognized by NFκB to initiate transcription of a number of key inflammatory-related genes (see Table 21.2) [21]. Numerous clinical studies have associated

Table 21.2 Various genes regulated by nuclear factor-κB involved in critical illness

Cytokines and chemokines
Tumor necrosis factor-α
Interleukins-1, -2, -3, -6, and -12
CXCL8/interleukin 8
CXCL1/Gro-α
CXCL2/Gro-β
CCL3/Macrophage inflammatory protein (MIP)-1α
CCL2/Monocyte chemotactic protein (MCP)-1
CCL5/RANTES
CCL11/eotaxin
Growth factors
Granulocyte-macrophage colony stimulating factor (GM-CSF)
Macrophage colony-stimulating factor (M-CSF)
Macrophage colony-stimulating factor (M-CSF)
Adhesion molecules
Intracellular adhesion molecule (ICAM)-1
E-selectin
Vascular cell adhesion molecule (VCAM)-1
Miscellaneous
Inducible nitric oxide synthase (iNOS)
C-reactive protein
5-Lipoxygenase
Cyclooxygenase (COX)-2

certain disease states (e.g., sepsis, acute respiratory distress syndrome) with evidence of increased NFκB activation. For example, bronchoalveolar lavage–retrieved alveolar macrophages from patients with acute respiratory distress syndrome showed significantly greater activation of NFκB than did those of control patients [22]. In studies of septic shock in adults, increased binding activity of NFκB in circulating leukocytes positively correlated with severity of illness and also differentiated survivors from nonsurvivors [23–25]. Thus, these observations provide increasing support for the concept that the NFκB pathway may be a valid therapeutic target in these disease states. This description of the classic pathway of NFκB activation is probably simplistic as we continue to gain insight into the multiple levels of regulation of NFκB-driven gene activation. For example, the subunits of NFκB are subject to various post-translational modifications (e.g., phosphorylation and acetylation), with important consequences on subcellular localization, subunit composition, and interaction with co-activator and/or co-repressor proteins [26]. In addition, alternative pathways from the IκK/IκB-α pathway have been shown to activate NFκB [27]. As one example, the tyrosine phosphatase inhibitor pervanadate activated NFκB, but via tyrosine phosphorylation of IκB-α rather than serine phosphorylation and did not involve degradation of IκB-α [28].

An equally important task of the cell is to turn off activated pathways, and a well-described mechanism for deactivating NFκB involves its own inhibitor, IκB. Because the promoter region of the IκB-α gene contains NFκB consensus binding sites, NFκB activation induces de novo expression of its own inhibitor, IκB-α [29]. As a result, the newly synthesized IκBα can move to the cytosol and block ongoing NFκB activation by reforming the heterotrimeric complex with p50 and p65. In has also been shown that induced IκBα can bind activated NFκB in the nucleus and chaperone it to the cytoplasm to terminate NFκB-dependent transcription [30]. Recent investigations into the deactivation and regulation of NFκB suggest epigenetics mechanisms, specifically microRNA and histone acetylation, plan an important role (see Epigenetics section below) [31].

Mitogen-Activated Protein Kinase Pathways

Another transcription activating factor that mediates expression of a number of inflammation-related genes is activating protein-1 (AP-1). The AP-1 family consists of various homodimers and heterodimers of the Jun (e.g., c-Jun), Fos (e.g., c-fos), or activating transcription factor (e.g., ATF2) proteins (reviewed in [32]). Various combinations of these proteins have been described, although the most commonly described AP-1 *complex* is the heterodimer formed by c-jun and c-fos proteins. Activating protein-1 regulates a diverse set of cellular functions, including cell proliferation and growth, apoptosis, inflammation, and tissue morphogenesis. Activation of AP-1 occurs in response to propagation of the upstream signal by an interwoven cascade of pathways known

as the mitogen-activated protein kinase (MAPK) pathways (Fig. 21.2, reviewed in [33–36]). Three MAPK pathways exist: the c-Jun NH2-terminal kinase (JNK) pathway (also called the *stress-activated MAPK* [SAPK] pathway); the extracellular-regulated protein kinase (ERK) pathway; and the p38 mitogen-activated kinase (p38 MAPK). All members of these MAPK families undergo activation via phosphorylation of threonine and tyrosine residues by upstream MAPK kinases (MKKs or MEKs), which are in turn activated via phosphorylation by upstream MKK kinase (MKKKs or MEKKs) (Fig. 21.3) [36]. Diverse sets of stimuli activate these pathways can broadly influence a variety of cellular functions relevant to inflammation and critical illness.

p38 Mitogen-Activated Protein Kinase Pathway

The p38 family of MAPK is composed of various isoforms (two α isoforms and β1, β2, γ, and δ) whose expressions are dictated in large part by cellular and tissue localization. For example, leukocytes express predominantly p38α and p38δ isoforms. Similar to the NFκB pathway, a number of stimuli activate this pathway, notably lipopolysaccharide, TNF, IL-8, and platelet activating factor, which in turn mediates gene expression changes of several downstream targets described to play a critical role in numerous disease states (see Fig. 21.3) [34]. One of the key occurrences in acute lung injury is the infiltration of leukocytes from the vascular space

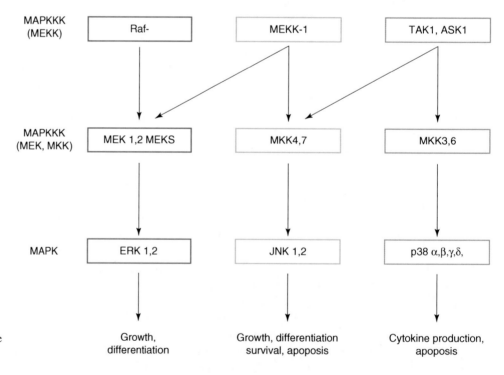

Fig. 21.3 Mitogen-activated protein kinase (*MAPK*) signal transduction pathways. MAPK (MEK, MKK), MAPK kinase; MAPKK (MEKK), MAPK kinase kinase

into the lung, which is mediated by a coordinated effort of cytokines, chemokines, integrins, and adhesion molecules. As a result of the genes regulated by p38, this pathway likely plays a central role in this pathogenesis. For example, lipopolysaccharide-induced expression of TNF-α from both neutrophils [37] and macrophages [38] is augmented by p38 activation via a process of mRNA stabilization. Similarly, TNF-α-mediated upregulation of E-selectin, which initiates the *rolling* phase of the leukocyte–endothelial cell adhesion cascade, is regulated in part through p38 activation of the transcription factor ATF2 [39]. The migration of adherent neutrophils from the vascular endothelium to the alveolus in acute lung injury is mediated by chemokines, such as CXCL8/IL-8, often induced by lipopolysaccharide or TNF-α, which is also dependent on p38 activation. Finally, the lung injury associated with infiltration of neutrophils into the airspace is at least in part caused by release of toxic oxygen radical species. Production of reactive oxygen species is catalyzed by NADPH oxidase of which a necessary subunit is the p47^{phox} protein. Phosphorylation and subsequent activation of p47^{phox} by the p38 pathway appears necessary to the assembly of this complex [40]. One of the important endogenous counterregulators of the p38 pathway is the dual-specific phosphatase MKP-1, which deactivates p38 via dephosphorylation as described below. Thus, given its ubiquitous role in mediating several events in leukocyte-mediated injury, the p38 MAPK pathway may be a valid target for inhibition in the hopes of attenuating inflammatory responses.

JNK Mitogen-Activated Protein Kinase Pathway

Three principal JNK protein kinases have been identified—JNK-1 and JNK-2, which are ubiquitously expressed, and JNK-3, which appears restricted to the brain. JNK protein kinases are also phosphorylated on threonine and tyrosine residues by upstream kinases (MKK4/SEK1 and MKK7) (see Fig. 21.3) [33, 35]. MKK4 is promiscuous in being capable of activating both the JNK and p38 MAPK pathways, while MKK7, which is primarily activated by proinflammatory cytokines, is generally restricted to JNK activation [41, 42]. Upstream from MKK4/MKK7, the MKKK MEKK-1 appears to be responsible for downstream activation of the JNK pathway [43, 44].

Using TNF-α as a stimulus, studies have elucidated the mechanisms by which initiation of the signal at the cell surface is transduced through MEKK-1, resulting in JNK activation. TNF-α binding to the adaptor protein TRAF-2 caused receptor oligomerization with consequent binding to and activation of MEKK-1 [45]. Endotoxin stimulation of monocytes also results in JNK activation with the observed downstream consequence of AP-1 complex formation and transcriptional activation of IL-1β expression [46, 47]. Similar to the observed counter-relationship between p38 and MKP-1, lipopolysaccharide induced JNK activation is negatively modulated by the endogenous serine-threonine phosphatase PP2A [47]. A physical association between JNK and the regulatory subunit PP2A-A/α, in addition to other reports of signal transduction complexes composed of MAP kinases and regulatory phosphatases in association with scaffolding proteins, suggests that these *signalosomes* may be critical regulatory components of inflammatory cell signal transduction pathways [48]. As on-going studies continue to unravel the mechanisms by which signals are transduced through these complex pathways, the precise roles of the JNK pathway in disease states such as sepsis and acute lung injury will be better understood to determine the validity of therapeutic measures aimed at its attenuation.

ERK Mitogen-Activated Protein Kinase Pathway

Although it was the first identified member of the MAPK pathways, less has been reported with regards to the potential role of the ERK pathway in inflammatory diseases such as sepsis and acute lung injury. Two ERK isoforms exist, denoted as ERK1 and ERK2. The principal MAPKKK that activates the ERK1/2 is Raf, which in turn activates the MAPKKs MEK1 and MEK2 (see Fig. 21.3) [49, 50]. Raf activation is initiated by the G-coupled protein Ras, that can be stimulated by a number of growth factors, including epidermal growth factor, platelet-derived growth factor, and transforming growth factor-β [51]. As a result, it is intuitive that ERK activation plays a primary role in cell growth and differentiation that may be vitally important to the repair process following tissue injury. The role for ERK does not appear restricted to this function, as investigators have reported additional functional consequences of ERK activation. For example, ERK activation was described following respiratory syncytial virus infection of lung epithelial cells, and production of CXCL8/IL-8 from these cells was attenuated by ERK inhibition, suggesting a role for ERK in viral induced chemokine production [52]. ERK has also been shown to be important in the regulation of the MAPK pathways through an interaction with the dual specific phosphatases [53]. Thus, while data implicating the ERK MAPK pathway in critical illnesses remain limited, this pathway may ultimately play an important role in pathogen-mediated (e.g., viral) cell activation (Table 21.3).

Table 21.3 Partial list of genes regulated by activating protein-1/mitogen-activated protein kinase pathways

Inflammatory mediators
  Tumor necrosis factor-α
  Interleukins-1, -2, -4, and -18
  Inducible nitric oxide synthase (iNOS)
  Arginine transporter
Transcriptional activators
  c-fos/c-jun (self-activating mechanism)
  Nuclear factor AT4
Adhesion molecules
  Intracellular adhesion molecule (ICAM)-1
  E-selectin
  P-selectin glycoprotein ligand (PSGL)-1
  Integrins (α, β₂ integrins)
Others
  P47^{phox} (component of NADPH oxidase complex)
  Fas ligand
  Tau (microtubule-associated protein)
  Cyclooxygenase (COX)-2

Table 21.4 Classes of phosphatases related to critical illness

Serine/threonine phosphatases	Tyrosine phosphatases
Protein phosphatase (PP) family	Cytosolic protein tyrosine phosphatases
PP1	SHP-1
PP2A	SHP-2
PP2B	PTP-1B
PPM Family	Receptor-like protein tyrosine phosphatases (RPTPs)
PP2C	CD45
	RPTPα
	Low-molecular weight protein tyrosine phosphatases
	T-cell protein tyrosine phosphatases
Novel members	Dual-specific phosphatases (DUSPs)
PP4/PPX	MKP-1 (DUSP-1)
PP6/PPV	MKP-2 (DUSP-4)
	MKP-3 (DUSP-6)
	MKP-5 (DUSP-10) CDC25

Regulation of Signal Transduction Pathway

Signal transduction activation is necessary for cell survival and subsequent response to environmental stimuli but equally as important as activation is the deactivation or resetting of the pathways once the stimuli are no longer present as a means of reestablishing cellular homeostasis. In fact, recent gene profiling in pediatric patients with septic shock suggests sepsis may result from down-regulation of several key immune function-related signal transduction pathways resulting in differential gene expression [54]. Although several regulatory mechanisms exist, the chapter highlights three that appear important in regulating cellular responses in critical illnesses: phosphatase activation, inducible protein regulators and epigenetic mechanisms.

Phosphatases as Regulators

As mentioned above, the phosphorylated state of a protein reflects a balance between phosphorylation mediated by protein kinases and dephosphorylation mediated by phosphatases. Protein phosphatases (PP) are categorized into three classes: those targeting serine and/or threonine residues (Ser/Thr phosphatases); those targeting tyrosine phosphorylated residues (Tyr phosphatases); and dual-specific phosphatases that can target either tyrosine or threonine residues (Table 21.4) [55]. Based on biochemical parameters, substrate specificity, and sensitivity to pharmacologic inhibitors, Ser/Thr protein phosphatases are further divided into two major classes. Type I phosphatases (e.g., PP1) can be inhibited by two heat-stable proteins known as Inhibitor-1 (I-1)

and Inhibitor-2 (I-2) and preferentially dephosphorylate the β-subunit of phosphorylase kinase. In contrast, type II PPs are insensitive to heat-stable inhibitors and preferentially dephosphorylate the α-subunit of phosphorylase kinase. Type II phosphatases are subdivided into spontaneously active (PP2A), Ca^{2+}-dependent (PP2B), and Mg^{2+}-dependent (PP2C) classes. Subtle but important structural differences in and around the catalytic site provide one component of substrate specificity. Also, additional regulatory proteins that bind to the catalytic subunits and in some instances comprise larger phosphatase complexes or holoenzymes afford additional substrate specificity [56]. Detailed structural and enzymatic biochemistries of the various phosphatases have been elucidated, but this discussion is beyond the objective of this chapter. Instead, for additional information on the formal biochemistry of these enzymes the reader is referred to other excellent reviews [57, 58].

Given the importance of reversible protein phosphorylation to a myriad of cellular functions, it is likely that the various phosphatases regulate several important physiologic processes regulated by signal transduction pathways. For example, PP1 participates in glycogen metabolism, muscle contraction, protein synthesis, intracellular protein transport, and cell cycle [59]. Despite its ubiquitous role in these homeostatic cellular functions, whether PP1 plays a role in signaling pathways relevant to critical illness remains to be more completely defined. In contrast, much data suggest that PP2A plays a key role in the endogenous regulation of inflammation-related signaling pathways.

For example, cell stimulation by either TNF-α or IFN-γ has been shown to activate sphingomyelinase, leading to the formation of ceramide. Ceramide is capable of mimicking the cytotoxicity of TNF-α and Fas by activating caspases that lead to apoptosis [60]. Of note, ceramide formation has also been described to activate what was previously termed *ceramide-activated protein phosphatase*, which has been identified as the trimeric form of PP2A [61]. As reviewed above, the AP-1 transcriptional activation pathway regulates expression of a number of inflammatory mediators. The upstream kinases in the MAPK pathways are activated via phosphorylation principally of serine and threonine residues and as such are logical targets of Ser/Thr phosphatases [62]. Inhibition of PP2A by the small-t antigen [63], I-2 [64], or okadaic acid [47, 65] has been shown to result in hyperphosphorylation and augmented activity of JNK. This increase in JNK activity was associated with increased AP-1–driven transcriptional activity and gene expression as evidenced by increased IL-1β expression [47] as well as IL-8 [65]. The data with regards to PP2A regulation of the NF-κB pathway are less clear. Addition of phosphatase inhibitors to human T cells caused an increased activation of NFκB that correlated with hyperphosphorylation of IκB-α, and only recombinant PP2A, but not PP1 or PP2C, could dephosphorylate IκB-α [66].

In another biologic model, it was shown that respiratory syncytial virus infection of epithelial cells caused a persistent activation of NFκB that was mediated by expression of the viral phosphoprotein P, which was shown to sequester and inhibit PP2A [67]. Together, these data suggest that PP2A may be a crucial negative modulator of the NFκB pathway. In contrast, Kray et al. [68] demonstrated that, in binding to the IκK-γ subunit, PP2A was necessary to fully achieve phosphorylation of IκK and activation of NFκB. Thus, although it appears certain that PP2A is a crucial modifier of important signal transduction cascades, what precise effects it has appears to depend on the stimulus, cell type, and pathway examined such that further investigation into the role of this Ser/Thr phosphatase is warranted.

One of the other families of phosphatases that are clearly important to regulation of inflammation-related signaling pathways is the dual-specificity phosphatases (DUSPs), which have been shown to be key modulators of the MAPK pathways, thus they are referred to as *MAPK phosphatases* (MKPs) [69]. Eleven MKPs have now been cloned all of which share a conserved catalytic domain and an amino-terminal non-catalytic domain. Several notable characteristics distinguish the MKPs from previously reviewed phosphates. First, some of the MKPs (e.g., MKP-1) are transcriptionally induced by the same stimuli that activate the MAPKs, such as lipopolysaccharide [53, 70]. Second, many of the MKPs show tremendous substrate specificity as exemplified by MKP-3 (Pyst1), which demonstrates nearly 100-fold more activity toward ERK2 than p38 [71]. Third, expression of some of the MKPs can be transient as shown for MKP-1, which can be targeted for ubiquitin mediated proteasomal degradation similar to IκB-α [72].

Finally, MAPK inactivation may be governed by specific protein–protein interactions with MKPs as demonstrated for MKP-3 whose binding of its noncatalytic domain to ERK2 results in substantial enhancement of MKP-3 phosphatase activity [73]. Thus, by modulation of the MAPK pathways the MKPs are key regulators of the inflammation.

Intracellular Protein Modulators

Three inducible intracellular proteins, IRAK-M, suppressors of cytokine signaling (SOCS) proteins and A20, are important in the regulation of key pathways activated by TLR stimulation. IRAK-M, a member of the IRAK family, is predominantly expressed in monocytes and macrophages [74–76] and regulates the production of IL-12, IL-6 and TNF-α in response to LPS stimulation [74]. Unlike other members of the IRAK family, IRAK-M has no kinase activity and the exact mechanism by which IRAK-M regulates TLR signaling has not been fully delineated.

A second inducible inhibitor of TLR signaling is the family of SOCS proteins. Eight SOCS proteins have been identified, each being induced by a variety of cytokines as well as PAMPS (e.g. LPS) [77]. SOCS regulates TLR signaling as an E3 ubiquitin ligase promoting the degradation of proteins involved in the signaling pathways activated by TLR stimulation [77]. An example of the importance of SOCS in regulating the pathways involved in cellular response in critical illness is the results from investigations regarding SOCS 1, whereby SOCS 1$^{-/-}$ mice were demonstrated to be hyper-responsive to LPS challenge resulting in increased serum levels of TNF-α as well as increased mortality [78, 79].

A20 is a third inducible enzyme that provides a negative feedback loop during NFκB activation [80]. Once activated NF-κB induces the expression of A20 [81], which in turn decreases NFκB activity via a ubiquitin-editing function in which A20 has both peptidase and ligase activity [82].

Epigenetic Mechanisms as Regulators

Epigenetics describes the processes involved in heritable changes in genomic function that are not passed on through changes in DNA sequences [83] and has only recently become a focus of intense investigation in the regulation of cellular responses to environmental stimuli. Three epigenetic mechanisms of regulation have been described: DNA methylation, histone post-translational modifications and non-coding RNA silencing. Of these three mechanisms, post-translational histone modifications and the specific non-coding RNA, microRNA, have been most extensively studied as being involved in critical illness.

Histone Modifications

Epigenetic modifications of chromatin structure play a crucial role in controlling gene expression by creating two conformations of chromatin: heterochromatin or euchromatin. Heterochromatin is tightly packed chromatin that limits access to the promotor regions of DNA thereby limiting gene induction and constitutes what is described as a "gene off" state. Euchromatin is a more loosely packed chromatin state that readily allows for access to the promoter regions constituting a so-called "gene on" state. Eukaryotic DNA is wound around an octomer of histone proteins (H2A, H2B, H3, H4), forming a nucleosome. Chromatin remodeling complexes (CRCs) are recruited to promoter sites by bound transcription factors and can modify histones resulting in either confirmation of the chromatin [84]. Possible histone modifications include methylation, phosphyloration and acetylation and have been linked to the regulation of the host inflammatory response [84]. Evidence suggesting a role of epigenetics in the regulation of cellular response to stimuli in critical illness includes the evidence that inhibition of histone deacetylase enzymes results in the reduced production of TNF-α and nitric oxide [85] as well as IL-10 [86] production in response to cellular stimulation. Histone deacetlyase inhibitors have also been shown to decrease the activation of macrophages and dendritic cells resulting in an imbalanced between Th1 and Th2 cells [87]. In addition to the immediate impact of histone modifications, Wen et al. showed that histone modifications regulate the dendritic cell production of IL-12 resulting in long-term immunosuppression [88]. Thus several lines of evidence suggest a regulatory role for histone modifications in response to the inflammatory response to pathogens.

microRNA

MicroRNAs are small 18–22 nucleotide strands of RNA that post-transcriptionally regulate cellular processes. They are transcribed non-coding regions of the genome into primary-miRNA complexes, which are cleaved into pre-miRNA, shorter stem-loop complexes, by the RNase Drosha [89]. Pre-miRNA is transported from the nucleus to the cytoplasm by the Exportin 5 complex. The pre-miRNA are then processed by the Dicer enzyme complex into mature-miRNA [90], which are loaded into the RNA-induced silencing complex (RISC) [89] where they combine with 3′-UTR region of the target mRNA resulting to the degradation or repression of the target mRNA [89].

Expression profiling of human monocytes following LPS stimulation revealed increases in miR-146a/b, miR-132 and miR-155 [91]. MiR-146 was subsequently shown to down regulate IRAK-1 and TRAF-6 [91]. IL-1β signaling is also negatively regulated by miR-146 regulating the production of both IL-8 and RANTES in lung alveolar epithelial cells [92]. Recently mir-146 has also been shown to interfere with the NFκB pathway by promoting the binding of the inhibitor RelB to NFκB binding sites in promoters [93]. Additionally, miR-155 was also found to be induced by TLR 2, 3, 4 and 9 ligands as well as TNF-α suggesting a broad acting role for miR-155 in the innate inflammatory host response [94]. In a mouse model of sepsis, miR-155 and mir-125b were both induced in response to LPS [95]; while studies in transgenic mice lacking functional miR-155 suggest a negative regulatory role for miR-155 in response to LPS [95]. Thus, while the extent to which microRNAs regulate the host inflammatory response is not fully defined, several lines of evidence are establishing their importance as a potential negative regulating mechanism.

Conclusion

Signal transduction provides the cellular basis for sensing extracellular changes or pathologic stresses and transmitting this signal to the transcriptional machinery capable of mounting a response on the basis of gene expression. The vast complexity, remarkable inter-connectedness, and substantial redundancy of the myriad of signal transduction pathways create an enormous challenge to deciphering their precise roles in biology, particularly in disease states as complex as those faced in the pediatric intensive care unit. In addition to this complexity, many of the scientific findings reported are often cell type-, stimulus-, and model-specific limiting the extrapolation of the data to other conditions. Thus, the goal remains to more fully understand the molecular processes at play using both a reductionist (i.e., single pathway) and a more comprehensive (i.e., genomics, proteomics, clinical studies) approach to identify potential therapeutic targets within a relevant pathway. Surely as our methodologic approaches advance, our understanding of the molecular and biochemical regulation of signaling pathways will continue to grow at an extraordinary rate. The key will be translating this improved understanding into more effective therapeutic approaches directed toward improving the outcomes of critically ill children. Signal transduction is the language of the cells; to achieve this lofty goal, we too must become fluent in this sophisticated molecular language.

References

1. Bradshaw RA, Dennis EA. Handbook of cell signaling. Amsterdam/San Diego: Academic Press; 2004.
2. Gomperts BD, Tatham PER, Kramer IM. Signal transduction. 2nd ed. Burlington/London: Elsevier/Academic; 2009.

3. Bayliss WM, Starling EH. The mechanism of pancreatic secretion. J Physiol. 1902;28(5):325–53.

4. Wong HR. Translation. Crit Care Med. 2005;33(12 Suppl):S404–6.

5. Kawai T, Akira S. Toll-like receptors and their crosstalk with other innate receptors in infection and immunity. Immunity. 2011; 34(5):637–50.

6. Dunne A, O'Neill LA. The interleukin-1 receptor/Toll-like receptor superfamily: signal transduction during inflammation and host defense. Sci STKE. 2003;25(171):re3.

7. Hunter T. Protein modification: phosphorylation on tyrosine residues. Curr Opin Cell Biol. 1989;1(6):1168–81.

8. Hunter T. Protein kinases and phosphatases: the yin and yang of protein phosphorylation and signaling. Cell. 1995;80(2):225–36.

9. Chang L, Karin M. Mammalian MAP kinase signalling cascades. Nature. 2001;410(6824):37–40.

10. Johnson GL, Lapadat R. Mitogen-activated protein kinase pathways mediated by ERK, JNK, and p38 protein kinases. Science. 2002;298(5600):1911–2.

11. Goggel R, Winoto-Morbach S, Vielhaber G, Imai Y, Lindner K, Brade L, Brade H, Ehlers S, Slutsky AS, Schutze S, Gulbins E, Uhlig S. PAF-mediated pulmonary edema: a new role for acid sphingomyelinase and ceramide. Nat Med. 2004;10(2):155–60.

12. Galie N, Manes A, Branzi A. The endothelin system in pulmonary arterial hypertension. Cardiovasc Res. 2004;61(2):227–37.

13. Bonizzi G, Karin M. The two NF-kappaB activation pathways and their role in innate and adaptive immunity. Trends Immunol. 2004;25(6):280–8.

14. Karin M. The NF-kappa B activation pathway: its regulation and role in inflammation and cell survival. Cancer J Sci Am. 1998;4 Suppl 1:S92–9.

15. Delhase M, Hayakawa M, Chen Y, Karin M. Positive and negative regulation of IkappaB kinase activity through IKKbeta subunit phosphorylation. Science. 1999;284(5412):309–13.

16. Delhase M, Karin M. The I kappa B kinase: a master regulator of NF-kappa B, innate immunity, and epidermal differentiation. Cold Spring Harb Symp Quant Biol. 1999;64:491–503.

17. Senftleben U, Karin M. The IKK/NF-kappa B pathway. Crit Care Med. 2002;30(1 Suppl):S18–26.

18. Qian Y, Commane M, Ninomiya-Tsuji J, Matsumoto K, Li X. IRAK-mediated translocation of TRAF6 and TAB2 in the interleukin-1-induced activation of NFkappa B. J Biol Chem. 2001;276(45):41661–7.

19. Baud V, Karin M. Signal transduction by tumor necrosis factor and its relatives. Trends Cell Biol. 2001;11(9):372–7.

20. Karin M, Ben-Neriah Y. Phosphorylation meets ubiquitination: the control of NF-[kappa]B activity. Annu Rev Immunol. 2000;18:621–63.

21. Wong HR, Shanley TP. Signal transduction pathways in acute lung injury: NF-kB and AP-1. In: Wong HRaS TP, editor. Molecular biology of acute lung injury. Norwell: Kluwer Academic Publishers; 2001. p. 1–16.

22. Jarrar D, Kuebler JF, Rue 3rd LW, Matalon S, Wang P, Bland KI, Chaudry IH. Alveolar macrophage activation after trauma-hemorrhage and sepsis is dependent on NF-kappaB and MAPK/ERK mechanisms. Am J Physiol Lung Cell Mol Physiol. 2002;283(4):L799–805.

23. Arnalich F, Garcia-Palomero E, Lopez J, Jimenez M, Madero R, Renart J, Vazquez JJ, Montiel C. Predictive value of nuclear factor kappaB activity and plasma cytokine levels in patients with sepsis. Infect Immun. 2000;68(4):1942–5.

24. Bohrer H, Qiu F, Zimmermann T, Zhang Y, Jllmer T, Mannel D, Bottiger BW, Stern DM, Waldherr R, Saeger HD, Ziegler R, Bierhaus A, Martin E, Nawroth PP. Role of NFkappaB in the mortality of sepsis. J Clin Invest. 1997;100(5):972–85.

25. Paterson RL, Galley HF, Dhillon JK, Webster NR. Increased nuclear factor kappa B activation in critically ill patients who die. Crit Care Med. 2000;28(4):1047–51.

26. Hoberg JE, Popko AE, Ramsey CS, Mayo MW. IkappaB kinase alpha-mediated derepression of SMRT potentiates acetylation of RelA/p65 by p300. Mol Cell Biol. 2006;26(2):457–71.

27. Lawrence T. The nuclear factor NF-kappaB pathway in inflammation. Cold Spring Harb Perspect Biol. 2009;1(6):a001651.

28. Imbert V, Rupec RA, Livolsi A, Pahl HL, Traenckner EB, Mueller-Dieckmann C, Farahifar D, Rossi B, Auberger P, Baeuerle PA, Peyron JF. Tyrosine phosphorylation of I kappa B-alpha activates NF-kappa B without proteolytic degradation of I kappa B-alpha. Cell. 1996;86(5):787–98.

29. Ito CY, Kazantsev AG, Baldwin Jr AS. Three NF-kappa B sites in the I kappa B-alpha promoter are required for induction of gene expression by TNF alpha. Nucleic Acids Res. 1994;22(18): 3787–92.

30. Arenzana-Seisdedos F, Thompson J, Rodriguez MS, Bachelerie F, Thomas D, Hay RT. Inducible nuclear expression of newly synthesized I kappa B alpha negatively regulates DNA-binding and transcriptional activities of NF-kappa B. Mol Cell Biol. 1995;15(5):2689–96.

31. McCall CE, El Gazzar M, Liu T, Vachharajani V, Yoza B. Epigenetics, bioenergetics, and microRNA coordinate gene-specific reprogramming during acute systemic inflammation. J Leukoc Biol. 2011;90(3):439–46.

32. Karin M, Liu Z, Zandi E. AP-1 function and regulation. Curr Opin Cell Biol. 1997;9(2):240–6.

33. Davis RJ. Signal transduction by the JNK group of MAP kinases. Cell. 2000;103(2):239–52.

34. Herlaar E, Brown Z. p38 MAPK signalling cascades in inflammatory disease. Mol Med Today. 1999;5(10):439–47.

35. Ip YT, Davis RJ. Signal transduction by the c-Jun N-terminal kinase (JNK) – from inflammation to development. Curr Opin Cell Biol. 1998;10(2):205–19.

36. Krishna M, Narang H. The complexity of mitogen-activated protein kinases (MAPKs) made simple. Cell Mol Life Sci. 2008;65(22):3525–44.

37. Nick JA, Avdi NJ, Young SK, Lehman LA, McDonald PP, Frasch SC, Billstrom MA, Henson PM, Johnson GL, Worthen GS. Selective activation and functional significance of p38alpha mitogen-activated protein kinase in lipopolysaccharide-stimulated neutrophils. J Clin Invest. 1999;103(6):851–8.

38. Mahtani KR, Brook M, Dean JL, Sully G, Saklatvala J, Clark AR. Mitogen-activated protein kinase p38 controls the expression and posttranslational modification of tristetraprolin, a regulator of tumor necrosis factor alpha mRNA stability. Mol Cell Biol. 2001;21(19):6461–9.

39. Read MA, Whitley MZ, Gupta S, Pierce JW, Best J, Davis RJ, Collins T. Tumor necrosis factor alpha-induced E-selectin expression is activated by the nuclear factor-kappaB and c-JUN N-terminal kinase/p38 mitogen-activated protein kinase pathways. J Biol Chem. 1997;272(5):2753–61.

40. Brown GE, Stewart MQ, Bissonnette SA, Elia AE, Wilker E, Yaffe MB. Distinct ligand-dependent roles for p38 MAPK in priming and activation of the neutrophil NADPH oxidase. J Biol Chem. 2004;279(26):27059–68.

41. Tournier C, Whitmarsh AJ, Cavanagh J, Barrett T, Davis RJ. Mitogen-activated protein kinase kinase 7 is an activator of the c-Jun NH2-terminal kinase. Proc Natl Acad Sci U S A. 1997; 94(14):7337–42.

42. Tournier C, Dong C, Turner TK, Jones SN, Flavell RA, Davis RJ. MKK7 is an essential component of the JNK signal transduction pathway activated by proinflammatory cytokines. Genes Dev. 2001;15(11):1419–26.

43. Xia Y, Makris C, Su B, Li E, Yang J, Nemerow GR, Karin M. MEK kinase 1 is critically required for c-Jun N-terminal kinase activation by proinflammatory stimuli and growth factor-induced cell migration. Proc Natl Acad Sci U S A. 2000;97(10):5243–8.

44. Yujiri T, Sather S, Fanger GR, Johnson GL. Role of MEKK1 in cell survival and activation of JNK and ERK pathways defined by targeted gene disruption. Science. 1998;282(5395):1911–4.

45. Baud V, Liu ZG, Bennett B, Suzuki N, Xia Y, Karin M. Signaling by proinflammatory cytokines: oligomerization of TRAF2 and TRAF6 is sufficient for JNK and IKK activation and target gene induction via an amino-terminal effector domain. Genes Dev. 1999;13(10):1297–308.

46. Hambleton J, Weinstein SL, Lem L, DeFranco AL. Activation of c-Jun N-terminal kinase in bacterial lipopolysaccharide-stimulated macrophages. Proc Natl Acad Sci U S A. 1996;93(7):2774–8.

47. Shanley TP, Vasi N, Denenberg A, Wong HR. The serine/threonine phosphatase, PP2A: endogenous regulator of inflammatory cell signaling. J Immunol. 2001;166(2):966–72.

48. Burack WR, Shaw AS. Signal transduction: hanging on a scaffold. Curr Opin Cell Biol. 2000;12(2):211–6.

49. Kolch W. Coordinating ERK/MAPK signalling through scaffolds and inhibitors. Nat Rev Mol Cell Biol. 2005;6(11):827–37.

50. Kolch W, Calder M, Gilbert D. When kinases meet mathematics: the systems biology of MAPK signalling. FEBS Lett. 2005;579(8):1891–5.

51. Thompson N, Lyons J. Recent progress in targeting the Raf/MEK/ERK pathway with inhibitors in cancer drug discovery. Curr Opin Pharmacol. 2005;5(4):350–6.

52. Chen W, Monick MM, Carter AB, Hunninghake GW. Activation of ERK2 by respiratory syncytial virus in A549 cells is linked to the production of interleukin 8. Exp Lung Res. 2000;26(1):13–26.

53. Cornell TT, Rodenhouse P, Cai Q, Sun L, Shanley TP. Mitogen-activated protein kinase phosphatase 2 regulates the inflammatory response in sepsis. Infect Immun. 2010;78(6):2868–76.

54. Shanley TP, Cvijanovich N, Lin R, Allen GL, Thomas NJ, Doctor A, Kalyanaraman M, Tofil NM, Penfil S, Monaco M, Odoms K, Barnes M, Sakthivel B, Aronow BJ, Wong HR. Genome-level longitudinal expression of signaling pathways and gene networks in pediatric septic shock. Mol Med. 2007;13(9–10):495–508.

55. Shanley TP. Phosphatases: counterregulatory role in inflammatory cell signaling. Crit Care Med. 2002;30(1 Suppl):S80–8.

56. Schillace RV, Scott JD. Organization of kinases, phosphatases, and receptor signaling complexes. J Clin Invest. 1999;103(6):761–5.

57. Mumby MC, Walter G. Protein serine/threonine phosphatases: structure, regulation, and functions in cell growth. Physiol Rev. 1993;73(4):673–99.

58. Barford D, Das AK, Egloff MP. The structure and mechanism of protein phosphatases: insights into catalysis and regulation. Annu Rev Biophys Biomol Struct. 1998;27:133–64.

59. Ceulemans H, Bollen M. Functional diversity of protein phosphatase-1, a cellular economizer and reset button. Physiol Rev. 2004;84(1):1–39.

60. Kolesnick R, Golde DW. The sphingomyelin pathway in tumor necrosis factor and interleukin-1 signaling. Cell. 1994;77(3):325–8.

61. Galadari S, Kishikawa K, Kamibayashi C, Mumby MC, Hannun YA. Purification and characterization of ceramide-activated protein phosphatases. Biochemistry. 1998;37(32):11232–8.

62. Chung H, Brautigan DL. Protein phosphatase 2A suppresses MAP kinase signalling and ectopic protein expression. Cell Signal. 1999;11(8):575–80.

63. Sontag E, Sontag JM, Garcia A. Protein phosphatase 2A is a critical regulator of protein kinase C zeta signaling targeted by SV40 small t to promote cell growth and NF-kappaB activation. EMBO J. 1997;16(18):5662–71.

64. Al-Murrani SW, Woodgett JR, Damuni Z. Expression of I2PP2A, an inhibitor of protein phosphatase 2A, induces c-Jun and AP-1 activity. Biochem J. 1999;341(Pt 2):293–8.

65. Cornell TT, Hinkovska-Galcheva V, Zlatarov N, Van way S, Shanley TP. Role of PP2A and ceramide in regulating TNF-alpha induced CXCL-8/IL-8 production in respiratory epithelium. Crit Care Med. 2007;35:A1.

66. Sun SC, Maggirwar SB, Harhaj E. Activation of NF-kappa B by phosphatase inhibitors involves the phosphorylation of I kappa B alpha at phosphatase 2A-sensitive sites. J Biol Chem. 1995;270(31):18347–51.

67. Bitko V, Barik S. Persistent activation of RelA by respiratory syncytial virus involves protein kinase C, underphosphorylated IkappaBbeta, and sequestration of protein phosphatase 2A by the viral phosphoprotein. J Virol. 1998;72(7):5610–8.

68. Kray AE, Carter RS, Pennington KN, Gomez RJ, Sanders LE, Llanes JM, Khan WN, Ballard DW, Wadzinski BE. Positive regulation of IkappaB kinase signaling by protein serine/threonine phosphatase 2A. J Biol Chem. 2005;280(43):35974–82.

69. Liu Y, Shepherd EG, Nelin LD. MAPK phosphatases–regulating the immune response. Nat Rev Immunol. 2007;7(3):202–12.

70. Nimah M, Zhao B, Denenberg AG, Bueno O, Molkentin J, Wong HR, Shanley TP. Contribution of MKP-1 regulation of p38 to endotoxin tolerance. Shock. 2005;23(1):80–7.

71. Groom LA, Sneddon AA, Alessi DR, Dowd S, Keyse SM. Differential regulation of the MAP, SAP and RK/p38 kinases by Pyst1, a novel cytosolic dual-specificity phosphatase. EMBO J. 1996;15(14):3621–32.

72. Brondello JM, Pouyssegur J, McKenzie FR. Reduced MAP kinase phosphatase-1 degradation after p42/p44MAPK-dependent phosphorylation. Science. 1999;286(5449):2514–7.

73. Camps M, Nichols A, Gillieron C, Antonsson B, Muda M, Chabert C, Boschert U, Arkinstall S. Catalytic activation of the phosphatase MKP-3 by ERK2 mitogen-activated protein kinase. Science. 1998;280(5367):1262–5.

74. Kobayashi K, Hernandez LD, Galan JE, Janeway Jr CA, Medzhitov R, Flavell RA. IRAK-M is a negative regulator of Toll-like receptor signaling. Cell. 2002;110(2):191–202.

75. Rosati O, Martin MU. Identification and characterization of murine IRAK-M. Biochem Biophys Res Commun. 2002;293(5):1472–7.

76. Wesche H, Gao X, Li X, Kirschning CJ, Stark GR, Cao Z. IRAK-M is a novel member of the Pelle/interleukin-1 receptor-associated kinase (IRAK) family. J Biol Chem. 1999;274(27):19403–10.

77. Yoshimura A, Naka T, Kubo M. SOCS proteins, cytokine signalling and immune regulation. Nat Rev Immunol. 2007;7(6):454–65.

78. Kinjyo I, Hanada T, Inagaki-Ohara K, Mori H, Aki D, Ohishi M, Yoshida H, Kubo M, Yoshimura A. SOCS1/JAB is a negative regulator of LPS-induced macrophage activation. Immunity. 2002;17(5):583–91.

79. Nakagawa R, Naka T, Tsutsui H, Fujimoto M, Kimura A, Abe T, Seki E, Sato S, Takeuchi O, Takeda K, Akira S, Yamanishi K, Kawase I, Nakanishi K, Kishimoto T. SOCS-1 participates in negative regulation of LPS responses. Immunity. 2002;17(5):677–87.

80. Coornaert B, Carpentier I, Beyaert R. A20: central gatekeeper in inflammation and immunity. J Biol Chem. 2009;284(13):8217–21.

81. Krikos A, Laherty CD, Dixit VM. Transcriptional activation of the tumor necrosis factor alpha-inducible zinc finger protein, A20, is mediated by kappa B elements. J Biol Chem. 1992;267(25):17971–6.

82. Wertz IE, O'Rourke KM, Zhou H, Eby M, Aravind L, Seshagiri S, Wu P, Wiesmann C, Baker R, Boone DL, Ma A, Koonin EV, Dixit VM. De-ubiquitination and ubiquitin ligase domains of A20 downregulate NF-kappaB signalling. Nature. 2004;430(7000):694–9.

83. Probst AV, Dunleavy E, Almouzni G. Epigenetic inheritance during the cell cycle. Nat Rev Mol Cell Biol. 2009;10(3):192–206.

84. Foster SL, Medzhitov R. Gene-specific control of the TLR-induced inflammatory response. Clin Immunol. 2009;130(1):7–15.

85. Choi Y, Park SK, Kim HM, Kang JS, Yoon YD, Han SB, Han JW, Yang JS, Han G. Histone deacetylase inhibitor KBH-A42 inhibits cytokine production in RAW 264.7 macrophage cells and in vivo endotoxemia model. Exp Mol Med. 2008;40(5):574–81.

86. Villagra A, Cheng F, Wang HW, Suarez I, Glozak M, Maurin M, Nguyen D, Wright KL, Atadja PW, Bhalla K, Pinilla-Ibarz J, Seto E, Sotomayor EM. The histone deacetylase HDAC11 regulates the

expression of interleukin 10 and immune tolerance. Nat Immunol. 2009;10(1):92–100.

87. Brogdon JL, Xu Y, Szabo SJ, An S, Buxton F, Cohen D, Huang Q. Histone deacetylase activities are required for innate immune cell control of Th1 but not Th2 effector cell function. Blood. 2007;109(3):1123–30.

88. Wen H, Dou Y, Hogaboam CM, Kunkel SL. Epigenetic regulation of dendritic cell-derived interleukin-12 facilitates immunosuppression after a severe innate immune response. Blood. 2008; 111(4):1797–804.

89. Carthew RW, Sontheimer EJ. Origins and mechanisms of miRNAs and siRNAs. Cell. 2009;136(4):642–55.

90. Lau PW, Macrae IJ. The molecular machines that mediate microRNA maturation. J Cell Mol Med. 2009;13(1):54–60.

91. Taganov KD, Boldin MP, Chang KJ, Baltimore D. NF-kappaB-dependent induction of microRNA miR-146, an inhibitor targeted to signaling proteins of innate immune responses. Proc Natl Acad Sci U S A. 2006;103(33):12481–6.

92. Perry MM, Moschos SA, Williams AE, Shepherd NJ, Larner-Svensson HM, Lindsay MA. Rapid changes in microRNA-146a expression negatively regulate the IL-1beta-induced inflammatory response in human lung alveolar epithelial cells. J Immunol. 2008; 180(8):5689–98.

93. El Gazzar M, Church A, Liu T, McCall CE. MicroRNA-146a regulates both transcription silencing and translation disruption of TNF-{alpha} during TLR4-induced gene reprogramming. J Leukoc Biol. 2011;90:509–19.

94. O'Connell RM, Taganov KD, Boldin MP, Cheng G, Baltimore D. MicroRNA-155 is induced during the macrophage inflammatory response. Proc Natl Acad Sci U S A. 2007;104(5):1604–9.

95. Tili E, Michaille JJ, Cimino A, Costinean S, Dumitru CD, Adair B, Fabbri M, Alder H, Liu CG, Calin GA, Croce CM. Modulation of miR-155 and miR-125b levels following lipopolysaccharide/TNF-alpha stimulation and their possible roles in regulating the response to endotoxin shock. J Immunol. 2007;179(8):5082–9.

Pro-inflammatory and Anti-inflammatory Mediators in Critical Illness and Injury

Jennifer A. Muszynski, W. Joshua Frazier, and Mark W. Hall

Abstract

Many forms of critical illness are characterized, at their onset, by a pro-inflammatory insult. Counter-regulatory, anti-inflammatory processes also exist in order to promote immunologic homeostasis. These processes are driven by, and modulate, the innate and adaptive arms of the immune system and are, in part, mediated by cytokines and chemokines. While surges in these pro-inflammatory mediators clearly produce many of the signs and symptoms of critical illness, the resultant anti-inflammatory surge has associated consequences as well. Systemic cytokine levels and leukocyte mRNA expression patterns suggest significant dysregulation of the inflammatory response in critical illness, though immune function testing is likely to be important as well. Severe reductions in innate and adaptive immune function following the onset of critical illness have been reported with increased risks for nosocomial infection and death across a wide array of adult and pediatric forms of critical illness. Immune monitoring and modulation trials are badly needed in the ICU, as growing evidence suggests that severe critical illness-induced immune suppression, or immunoparalysis, is reversible with potentially beneficial effects on outcomes. In addition, it appears that many of the therapies that are routinely used in critically ill children, including medications and transfusions, are likely to be inadvertently immunomodulatory. The role of these therapies, as well as the role of host genetics, on immunologic function and immunologic balance is poorly understood.

Keywords

Immune • Pro-inflammatory • Anti-inflammatory • Cytokine • Immunoparalysis

J.A. Muszynski, MD
Division of Critical Care Medicine,
The Ohio State University College of Medicine,
Nationwide Children's Hospital,
700 Children's Drive, Columbus, OH 43205, USA
e-mail: jennifer.muszynski@nationwidechildrens.org

W.J. Frazier, MD • M.W. Hall, MD (✉)
Division of Critical Care Medicine,
Nationwide Children's Hospital,
700 Children's Drive, Columbus, OH 43205, USA
e-mail: warrenjfrazier@nationwidechildrens.org;
mark.hall@nationwidechildrens.org

Introduction

Many of the processes that contribute to the development of critical illness (e.g. sepsis, trauma, cardiopulmonary bypass, major surgery) are characterized by an initial pro-inflammatory insult. Indeed, the classic signs and symptoms of sepsis including fever, capillary leak, and abnormal vascular tone can be replicated by the infusion of pro-inflammatory mediators into a healthy host [1]. In fact, it is often the exaggerated host response that is responsible for organ dysfunction in the setting of critical illness, rather than exogenous factors. For the vast majority of biological processes, however, counter-regulatory mechanisms exist to promote restoration of homeostasis. The inflammatory

D.S. Wheeler et al. (eds.), *Pediatric Critical Care Medicine*,
DOI 10.1007/978-1-4471-6362-6_22, © Springer-Verlag London 2014

response is no different, with multiple anti-inflammatory mediators playing this crucial role in restoring balance to the immune response in the setting of serious illness or injury. Unfortunately the scales can tip too far in the direction of these anti-inflammatory mediators, resulting in a form of acquired immunodeficiency that has, itself, been associated with adverse outcomes from critical illness in adults and children.

The regulation and function of the immune system in the setting of an inflammatory insult is exceedingly complex. Central themes, however, emerge and form the focus of this chapter which will provide a framework for understanding the importance of immunologic balance between pro- and anti-inflammatory forces in the critically ill patient. This will begin with a review of cellular elements and circulating mediators that comprise the inflammatory response in humans. Evidence for the role of both the pro- and anti-inflammatory responses in the pathogenesis of critical illness will then be reviewed. Finally the potential roles for immune monitoring and modulation in the critically ill or injured child will be discussed. While not an exhaustive review, this chapter provides a solid foundation for understanding the inflammatory response in the pediatric intensive care unit (PICU).

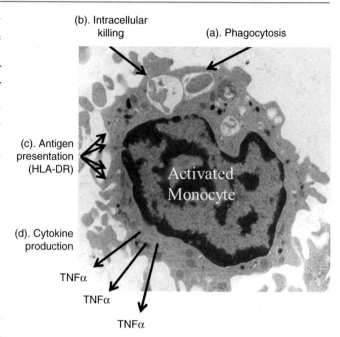

Fig. 22.1 Functions of an activated monocyte. This figure shows an electron micrograph of an activated monocyte (20,000X) that is engaged in phagocytosis of a pathogen (**a**) and intracellular killing (**b**). Other functions of activated innate immune cells include the presentation of processed antigen on cell-surface molecules such as HLA-DR (**c**) and the production of pro-inflammatory cytokines such as TNFα (alpha) (**d**)

Cellular Elements

Innate Immunity

The cellular elements of the immune system can be divided roughly into two groups: innate and adaptive immune cells. Innate immune cells include neutrophils, monocytes, macrophages, and dendritic cells. Most innate immune cells are of myeloid origin and respond to pathogens through ligation of receptors that recognize pathogen-associated molecular patterns (PAMPs). These PAMPs include broad classes of molecules which are not present on mammalian cells and include lipopolysaccharide (LPS), peptidoglycan (PG), lipoteichoic acid (LTA) and mannose. Examples of innate immune cell PAMP receptors include the toll-like receptors (TLR), NOD-like receptors (NLR), and mannose receptors (reviewed in [2, 3]). Interestingly, some innate immune cells can also be activated by damage- or danger-associated molecular patterns (DAMPs) including ATP, uric acid, heat shock proteins, and DNA (reviewed in [4]). In addition, innate immune cells can be activated, or their function further modulated, by the action of circulating cytokines.

Innate immune cells, once activated, should respond robustly from their first exposure to a PAMP. In contrast to adaptive immune cells, which typically require antigen presentation and a period of clonal expansion to achieve maximal responsiveness, an innate immune cell should produce a maximal response quickly. Accordingly, innate immune

cells are thought to drive the early inflammatory response to critical illness. The monocyte, by virtue of its broad array of functions and its accessibility in whole blood for study, is often viewed as a window into the innate immune system in critical illness. A normal, activated monocyte carries out all of the functions of the innate immune system, namely surveillance for and phagocytosis of pathogens, intracellular killing of pathogens, presentation of antigenic peptides on cell surface molecules such as human leukocyte antigen (HLA)-DR, and the production of pro-inflammatory cytokines which make the local environment more favorable for clearance of infection (Fig. 22.1).

Adaptive Immunity

Lymphocytes comprise the cellular elements of the adaptive immune system. They differ from innate immune cells in their lymphoid bone marrow origins, their typical requirement for antigen presentation in order to become activated, and the time course required for maximal response. Most lymphocyte responses, due to the time necessary for antigen presentation and clonal expansion, peak in the days following an insult, though this process is accelerated in the setting of repeated exposure to a given antigen (i.e. the memory response). Lastly, lymphocyte responses are notable for their extreme antigen specificity, with a given lymphocyte being capable of activation only by a highly distinct peptide sequence that is determined through gene rearrangement in the course of lymphocyte development.

Lymphocytes can be further classified into B cells and T cells. B cells, once activated, become plasma cells which are responsible for antibody production. T cells, by contrast, produce cytokines and modulate the local environment to perpetuate or resolve the inflammatory response. The naïve T cell can differentiate into one of a number of different subtypes depending on the cytokine milieu in which it becomes activated. Though the number of subtypes currently known exceeds the scope of this chapter, it is reasonable to mention a few. T-helper (T_H)-1 cells are CD4+ cells that produce pro-inflammatory cytokines, while T_H-2 cells typically produce anti-inflammatory cytokines. T_H17 cells are potently pro-inflammatory through their production of the cytokine interleukin (IL)-17 [5]. Conversely, regulatory T cells (T_{reg}) are potently anti-inflammatory through production of IL-10 and transforming growth factor (TGF)-β (beta), and through direct cell contact-mediated inhibition. T_{reg} can be identified by cell surface markers (CD4+, CD25+, CD127^{lo}) and by their expression of the transcription factor FOXP3 [6]. Lastly CD8+ cytotoxic T cells and natural killer (NK) cells serve as main lines of defense against virally infected and malignantly transformed cells.

Cytokines and Chemokines

Many of the clinical effects of systemic inflammation such as fever, capillary leak, and organ dysfunction are the results of actions of soluble mediators of the inflammatory response known as cytokines and chemokines. A limited list of these mediators, along with their cells of origin and actions, are listed in Table 22.1. These proteins are produced by innate and adaptive immune cells, as well as by vascular endothelium and other parenchymal cells. Pro-inflammatory cytokines act on immune and other cells in order to make the local environment more favorable to fighting infection or healing injured tissues. Chemokines serve as chemoattractants along whose concentration gradients immune cells migrate to the site of infection or injury. All of these things have the potential to be beneficial to the host in the setting of a localized infection. For example, elevated temperature, vasodilation, and increased capillary permeability (to allow immune cells and antimicrobial peptides access to the infected region) would improve the host's ability to contain and fight a localized infection. When these mediators spill over into the systemic circulation, however, they exert their effects in a widespread manner which results in the systemic inflammatory response syndrome (SIRS) and can lead to organ failure and death.

Table 22.1 Cytokines and chemokines

Mediator	Source		Effects
	Innate	Adaptive	
IL-1β (beta)	●		Innate immune cell and T-cell activation, fever, vasodilation
TNFα (alpha)	●	●	Innate immune cell and endothelial activation, fever, vasodilation, apoptosis
IFNγ (gamma)		●	Pro-inflammatory lymphocyte activation
IL-2		●	Pro-inflammatory lymphocyte activation
IL-17-1α (alpha)		●	Pro-inflammatory lymphocyte activation, innate immune cell activation, endothelial activation
GM-CSF	●	●	Innate immune cell growth and activation
MIF		●	Macrophage activation and inhibition of migration
IL-8	●		Neutrophil migration and activation
MIP	●	●	Innate immune cell migration and activation
MCP-1	●		Innate and adaptive cell migration
IP-10	●		Innate immune and T-cell migration
RANTES		●	Innate immune cell migration and activation
IL-6	●	●	Acute phase response, promotion of anti-inflammatory T-cell response
IL-10	●	●	Promotion of anti-inflammatory innate and adaptive immune cell phenotype
TGF-β (beta)	●	●	Promotion of anti-inflammatory innate and adaptive immune cell phenotype
sTNFr	●	●	Binding and inactivation of plasma TNFα (alpha)
IL-1ra	●		Blockade of IL-1β (beta) receptor action

White boxes represent pro-inflammatory cytokines, grey boxes represent chemokines, diagonally hatched box represents a mixed-function cytokine, vertically hatched boxes represent anti-inflammatory cytokines

IL interleukin, *TNF* tumor necrosis factor, *IFN* interferon, *GM-CSF* granulocyte macrophage colony-stimulating factor, *MIF* macrophage migration inhibitory factor, *MIP* macrophage inflammatory protein, *MCP* macrophage chemoattractant protein, *IP* interferon gamma-induced protein, *RANTES* chemokine regulated on activation of normal T-cells expressed and secreted, *TGF* transforming growth factor, *sTNFr* soluble TNF receptor, *IL-1ra* IL-1 receptor antagonist

Accordingly, counter-regulatory mechanisms exist which halt this pro-inflammatory cascade. Anti-inflammatory cytokines are produced in response to pro-inflammatory signals and serve to down-regulate the responsiveness of innate and/or adaptive immune cells (IL-10, TGFβ) or to inactivate pro-inflammatory mediators themselves (sTNFr, IL-1ra). Also, lymphocyte apoptosis is, as discussed below, a prominent sequela of critical illness, thereby further negatively regulating the inflammatory response [7]. Collectively, this process is known as the compensatory anti-inflammatory response syndrome (CARS). If this system works well, the host experiences a transient pro-inflammatory response which is limited to the area of local infection or injury and is promptly turned off by the anti-inflammatory response before systemic inflammation can result. In the setting of critical illness, however, a massive pro-inflammatory response often begets a pathologic anti-inflammatory response, both of which can have major consequences for the patient.

The Inflammatory Response in Critical Illness

Circulating Cytokine Levels

It has long been understood that an excess of pro-inflammatory mediators is harmful in the setting of critical illness. The timing of cytokine production is an important factor in understanding the inflammatory response in the ICU (Fig. 22.2). Cytokines such as TNFα and IL-1β tend to peak very early following a pro-inflammatory insult, and may be declining in the plasma by the time the patient reaches the ICU. Biomarkers such as IL-6 and IL-8 are produced by a wider variety of tissues in response to pro-inflammatory cytokines (as well as PAMP and DAMP signals) and elevations in their plasma levels are more sustained following the onset of illness. Accordingly, elevations in plasma levels of IL-6 [8–10] and/or IL-8 [11, 12] have been most consistently associated with adverse outcomes from critical illness and injury in adults and children. It should be noted that IL-6 is a pleiotropic cytokine, in that it induces the hepatic acute phase response and is, as such, pro-inflammatory, but is also is known to have anti-inflammatory properties [13]. It should also be understood that therapies targeting individual pro-inflammatory cytokines have been attempted without success in multiple clinical trials in the setting of sepsis in adults [14–16].

Not long after the TNFα and IL-1β signals begin to fade, plasma levels of anti-inflammatory cytokines such as IL-10 and IL1-ra begin to rise [17]. Again, because there is frequently a delay of hours or more between the time of illness onset and presentation to the ICU, many patients already have high plasma levels of anti-inflammatory mediators at the time of blood sampling. Perhaps paradoxically, systemic elevations of IL-10 have been associated with adverse outcomes from pediatric critical illness alongside elevations

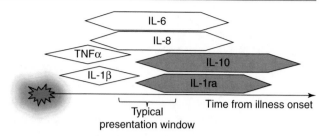

Fig. 22.2 Timeline of cytokine production following a pro-inflammatory insult. Pro-inflammatory innate immune cytokines including TNFα (alpha) and IL-1β (beta) are elaborated and fade quickly following illness onset. Plasma levels of these mediators may already be in decline by the time a critically ill patient presents to the ICU. This is followed by more sustained production of IL-6 and IL-8, often by non-immune cells, in response to the earlier TNFα (alpha) and IL-1β (beta) peaks. Compensatory upregulation of anti-inflammatory mediators such as IL-10 and IL-1ra follows

in markers of the pro-inflammatory response such as IL-6 [18–21]. This scenario of simultaneous activation of pro- and anti-inflammatory responses, sometimes referred to as the mixed cytokine response or "cytokine storm", can be explained in part by the overlapping time courses of cytokine elaboration and the ongoing production of pro-inflammatory mediators by injured parenchymal cells. Circulating plasma cytokine levels, however, are unlikely to be sufficient to fully characterize the immune response to critical illness.

Gene Expression Profiling

Several investigators have recently evaluated gene expression in circulating white blood cells in the setting of critical illness. Tang et al. [22, 23] and Wong et al. [24, 25] in adults and children respectively, have evaluated leukocyte mRNA expression levels in samples from septic patients and have found evidence for both activation and suppression of inflammation-related genes. The pediatric data speak most strongly to down-regulation of genes important for adaptive immune activation, with concomitant activation of genes important for signaling in innate immune cells [26–28]. Transcriptome analysis has also been carried out longitudinally in adults following critical traumatic injury. Xiao et al. similarly demonstrated upregulation in expression of innate immune signaling pathway elements with down-regulation of adaptive pathway members [29]. Together, these findings have resulted in competing models of the inflammatory response in critical illness and injury (Fig. 22.3). In the sequential model (a), an inflammatory stimulus results first in the SIRS response, followed temporally by the CARS response. In the simultaneous model (b), pro- and anti-inflammatory pathways are affected at the same time, with the severity and duration of activation being related to outcomes. In order to reconcile these models, it is necessary to evaluate *functional* aspects of the immune response in the critically ill patient.

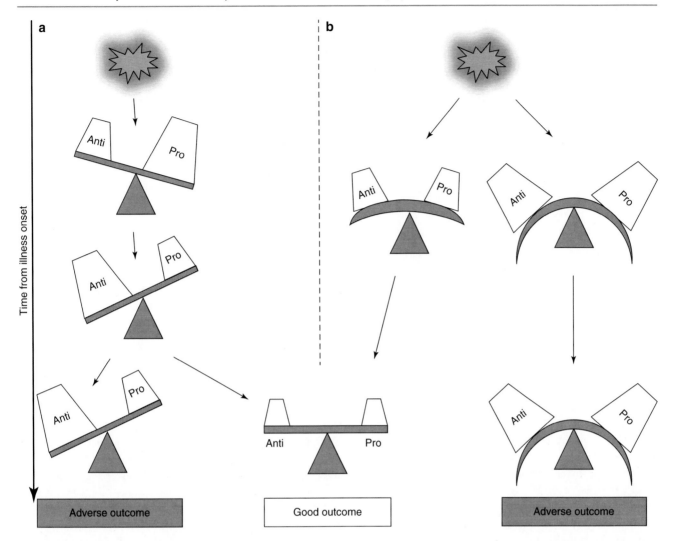

Fig. 22.3 Models of the immune response to critical illness. (**a**) *Sequential model*: An inflammatory stimulus results in a surge of pro-inflammatory mediators (SIRS) followed temporally by an anti-inflammatory phenotype (CARS) which, if persistent, is associated with increased risks for new infection and death. (**b**) *Simultaneous* *model*: In this model, pro- and anti-inflammatory systems are activated simultaneously, with the magnitude and duration of activation being predictive of adverse outcomes. In both models, restoration of immunologic balance is associated with favorable outcomes

Immunoparalysis

Innate Immunity

In the 1980s and 1990s, several investigators reported adverse outcomes associated with impaired innate immune function in the setting of adult trauma [30–32], surgery [33, 34], and sepsis [35]. These studies initially focused on reductions in monocyte HLA-DR expression as measured by flow cytometry, with levels <30 % being associated with increased risks for secondary infection and death. This severe reduction in antigen presenting capacity was termed "immunoparalysis" and is thought to be mediated by internalization of HLA-DR molecules from the monocyte cell surface in response to anti-inflammatory mediators such as IL-10 [36]. These findings have since

been confirmed in adults with transplantation [37], pancreatitis [38], burns [39], and septic shock [40]. In addition, marked reduction in monocyte HLA-DR expression has been associated with increased secondary infection and mortality risks in children with multiple organ dysfunction syndrome (MODS) [41] and following cardiopulmonary bypass [42].

The phenomenon of immunoparalysis extends beyond antigen presentation, however. As noted earlier, another important function of the monocyte is to produce pro-inflammatory mediators in response to a new challenge. This can be tested ex vivo by stimulation of whole blood with a standardized LPS-stimulation solution. Blood from normal subjects (adult or pediatric) produces robust amounts of TNFα (alpha) upon ex vivo LPS stimulation. Blood samples from subjects with innate immune

Table 22.2 Summary of clinical studies of innate immune function in critically ill children

Population	N	Findings	Reference
MODS	30	Reduced ex vivo LPS-induced TNFα (alpha) production capacity was associated with mortality. This was also associated with increased plasma IL-10 levels and monocyte mRNA levels of *IL10*	[45]
Sepsis-induced MODS	24	Reduced ex vivo LPS-induced TNFα (alpha) production capacity was associated with failure to recover neuroendocrine function and with mortality	[46]
MODS	70, 14	Reduced ex vivo LPS-induced TNFα (alpha) production capacity and monocyte HLA-DR expression were associated with increased risks for secondary infection and mortality. In a small, associated randomized controlled trial, GM-CSF was effective in reversing immunoparalysis with an associated reduction in secondary infection risk	[41]
CPB	82	Post-operative reduction in monocyte HLA-DR expression was associated with increased risk for development of sepsis/SIRS	[42]
CPB	36	Post-operative reduction in ex vivo LPS-induced TNFα (alpha) production capacity and elevation in plasma IL-10 levels were associated increased risk of post-operative complications	[20]
CPB	92	Post-operative reduction in ex vivo LPS-induced TNFα (alpha) production capacity and elevation in plasma IL-10 levels were associated with increased risk for development of secondary infection. Epigenetic modification of the *IL10* promoter region is implicated	[19]
Influenza	52	First multi-center study of innate immune function in critically ill children demonstrated a strong association between early reduction in ex vivo LPS-induced TNFα (alpha) production capacity and mortality from influenza. This association was strongest in children co-infected with *S. aureus*	[18]
RSV	80	Reduced ex vivo LPS-induced TNFα (alpha) production capacity was associated with increased disease severity and longer ICU stay	[47]

MODS multiple organ dysfunction syndrome, *CPB* cardiopulmonary bypass, *RSV* respiratory syncytial virus

suppression make *reduced* amounts of TNFα upon ex vivo stimulation. Depending on the stimulation protocol being used, specific thresholds of ex vivo LPS-induced TNFα production capacity can be identified that can identify the immunoparalyzed patient. Severe reductions in TNFα response have been associated with adverse outcomes in adults with trauma [43], and sepsis [44] as well as in children with MODS [41, 45, 46], respiratory syncytial virus (RSV) infection [47], influenza infection [18], and children following cardiopulmonary bypass [19, 20]. A summary of innate immune function studies in critically ill children to date is presented in Table 22.2. In sum, despite transcriptome-level and plasma cytokine level data suggesting activation of the innate immune response, functional data suggest a net *suppression* of antigen presenting capacity and cytokine production capacity in many children and adults who experience morbidity and mortality from critical illness.

Adaptive Immunity

Lymphocytes also appear to be affected by the wave of immune suppression that often follows the onset of critical illness. Hotchkiss et al. have repeatedly demonstrated marked lymphocyte apoptosis in adult sepsis non-survivors [48, 49]. Further, they have demonstrated impaired lymphocyte cytokine production capacity and upregulation of the pro-apoptotic/inhibitory PD-1 receptor on the remaining lymphocytes in their septic patients [49].

A strong relationship between severe lymphopenia (absolute lymphocyte count <1,000 cells/mm^3) and secondary infection and mortality risks has also been reported in children with MODS [50]. Lastly, it appears that highly anti-inflammatory regulatory T cells are resistant to the pro-apoptotic environment in critical illness. Venet and Monneret have demonstrated increased relative [51] and absolute numbers [52] of immunosuppressive T_{reg} in adults with septic shock.

Reversal of Immunoparalysis

A growing body of evidence suggests that immunoparalysis is reversible, potentially with beneficial effects on outcomes. Interferon-γ has been used to improve monocyte function ex vivo [53], and in vivo [44] in critically ill adults. Granulocyte macrophage colony-stimulating factor (GM-CSF) has also been used in the ICU to restore innate immune function in adults in vivo [54–56]. To date there has been a single small pediatric randomized controlled trial which also suggested that ex vivo LPS-induced TNFα production capacity could be restored in immunoparalyzed children with MODS using GM-CSF therapy, with an accompanying reduction in risk for the development of secondary infection [41]. It is noteworthy that in these adult and pediatric studies, restoration of innate immune function was *not* associated with an increase in systemic inflammation as measured by plasma cytokine levels. Treatment of critical illness-induced adaptive immune suppression in adults has also been proposed using agents such as IL-7 and anti-PD-1 therapy [57].

Tipping the Scales

In addition to overt immunomodulation with drugs like GM-CSF, along with intentional immunosuppression with agents like myeloablative chemotherapy, glucocorticoids, and transplant rejection prophylaxis, it is essential to acknowledge the inadvertent ways in which ICU therapies affect immune function. Many of the agents that make up the ICU pharmacopeia have immunomodulatory properties that are distinct from their intended uses. For example, opiates [58, 59], benzodiazepines [60], and insulin [61] have anti-inflammatory properties. Catecholamines can be both pro- and anti-inflammatory [62]. Red blood cell transfusion may well be immunosuppressive as well, particularly as a function of increasing storage age [63–65].

Conclusion

The restoration of balance between pro- and anti-inflammatory mediators is crucial to recovery from critical illness while maintaining host defense against new infection and promoting organ recovery. The natural compensatory mechanisms for restoring homeostasis are often themselves dysfunctional in the highly artificial environment of the ICU, in which patients are often shepherded through massive inflammatory insults only to suffer complications related to secondary, acquired immunosuppression. Specific etiologies of immunoparalysis, particularly genetic determinants, remain elusive, but evidence is mounting that the achievement of normal innate and adaptive immune function is both possible and important for uncomplicated recovery. It remains unknown whether innate or adaptive immune function (or both) represents the most appropriate target for therapy in the immunoparalyzed individual. Additional research is needed to understand the immunomodulatory effects of our ICU therapies, to identify optimal immune monitoring regimens, and to design immunostimulatory therapies to promote immunologic balance in the critically ill child.

References

1. van Eijk LT, Dorresteijn MJ, Smits P, van der Hoeven JG, Netea MG, Pickkers P. Gender differences in the innate immune response and vascular reactivity following the administration of endotoxin to human volunteers*. Crit Care Med. 2007;35(6):1464–9.
2. Uematsu S, Akira S. Toll-like receptors (TLRs) and their ligands. Handb Exp Pharmacol. 2008;183:1–20.
3. Martinon F, Tschopp J. NLRs join TLRs as innate sensors of pathogens. Trends Immunol. 2005;26(8):447–54.
4. Kuipers MT, van der Poll T, Schultz MJ, Wieland CW. Bench-to-bedside review: damage-associated molecular patterns in the onset of ventilator-induced lung injury. Crit Care (Lond). 2011;15(6):235.
5. Romagnani S. Human Th17 cells. Arthritis Res Ther. 2008; 10(2):206.
6. Tang Q, Bluestone JA. The Foxp3+ regulatory T cell: a jack of all trades, master of regulation. Nat Immunol. 2008;9(3):239–44.
7. Hotchkiss RS, Tinsley KW, Karl IE. Role of apoptotic cell death in sepsis. Scand J Infect Dis. 2003;35(9):585–92.
8. Kellum JA, Kong L, Fink MP, et al. Understanding the inflammatory cytokine response in pneumonia and sepsis: results of the Genetic and Inflammatory Markers of Sepsis (GenIMS) Study. Arch Intern Med. 2007;167(15):1655–63.
9. Fioretto JR, Martin JG, Kurokawa CS, et al. Interleukin-6 and procalcitonin in children with sepsis and septic shock. Cytokine. 2008;43(2):160–4.
10. Doughty LA, Kaplan SS, Carcillo JA. Inflammatory cytokine and nitric oxide responses in pediatric sepsis and organ failure. Crit Care Med. 1996;24(7):1137–43.
11. Wong HR, Cvijanovich N, Wheeler DS, et al. Interleukin-8 as a stratification tool for interventional trials involving pediatric septic shock. Am J Respir Crit Care Med. 2008;178(3):276–82.
12. Ozturk H, Yagmur Y, Ozturk H. The prognostic importance of serum IL-1beta, IL-6, IL-8 and TNF-alpha levels compared to trauma scoring systems for early mortality in children with blunt trauma. Pediatr Surg Int. 2008;24(2):235–9.
13. Steensberg A, Fischer CP, Keller C, Moller K, Pedersen BK. IL-6 enhances plasma IL-1ra, IL-10, and cortisol in humans. Am J Physiol Endocrinol Metab. 2003;285(2):E433–7.
14. Abraham E, Anzueto A, Gutierrez G, et al. Double-blind randomised controlled trial of monoclonal antibody to human tumour necrosis factor in treatment of septic shock. NORASEPT II Study Group. Lancet. 1998;351(9107):929–33.
15. Opal SM, Fisher Jr CJ, Dhainaut JF, et al. Confirmatory interleukin-1 receptor antagonist trial in severe sepsis: a phase III, randomized, double-blind, placebo-controlled, multicenter trial. The Interleukin-1 Receptor Antagonist Sepsis Investigator Group. Crit Care Med. 1997;25(7):1115–24.
16. Fisher Jr CJ, Dhainaut JF, Opal SM, et al. Recombinant human interleukin 1 receptor antagonist in the treatment of patients with sepsis syndrome. Results from a randomized, double-blind, placebo-controlled trial. Phase III rhIL-1ra Sepsis Syndrome Study Group. JAMA. 1994;271(23):1836–43.
17. Andreasen AS, Krabbe KS, Krogh-Madsen R, Taudorf S, Pedersen BK, Moller K. Human endotoxemia as a model of systemic inflammation. Curr Med Chem. 2008;15(17):1697–705.
18. Hall MW, Geyer SM, Guo CY, et al. Innate immune function and mortality in critically ill children with influenza: a multicenter study. Crit Care Med. 2013;41(1):224–36.
19. Cornell TT, Sun L, Hall MW, et al. Clinical implications and molecular mechanisms of immunoparalysis after cardiopulmonary bypass. J Thorac Cardiovasc Surg. 2012;143(5):1160–6.e1.
20. Allen ML, Hoschtitzky JA, Peters MJ, et al. Interleukin-10 and its role in clinical immunoparalysis following pediatric cardiac surgery. Crit Care Med. 2006;34(10):2658–65.
21. Doughty L, Carcillo JA, Kaplan S, Janosky J. The compensatory anti-inflammatory cytokine interleukin 10 response in pediatric sepsis-induced multiple organ failure. Chest. 1998;113(6):1625–31.
22. Tang BM, McLean AS, Dawes IW, Huang SJ, Lin RC. The use of gene-expression profiling to identify candidate genes in human sepsis. Am J Respir Crit Care Med. 2007;176(7):676–84.
23. Tang BM, Huang SJ, McLean AS. Genome-wide transcription profiling of human sepsis: a systematic review. Critical Care (Lond). 2010;14(6):R237.
24. Wong HR, Cvijanovich N, Allen GL, et al. Genomic expression profiling across the pediatric systemic inflammatory response syndrome, sepsis, and septic shock spectrum. Crit Care Med. 2009; 37(5):1558–66.

25. Wong HR. Genetics and genomics in pediatric septic shock. Crit Care Med. 2012;40(5):1618–26.

26. Shanley TP, Cvijanovich N, Lin R, et al. Genome-level longitudinal expression of signaling pathways and gene networks in pediatric septic shock. Mol Med (Camb). 2007;13(9–10):495–508.

27. Wong HR, Freishtat RJ, Monaco M, Odoms K, Shanley TP. Leukocyte subset-derived genomewide expression profiles in pediatric septic shock. Pediatr Crit Care Med. 2010;11(3):349–55.

28. Wong HR, Shanley TP, Sakthivel B, et al. Genome-level expression profiles in pediatric septic shock indicate a role for altered zinc homeostasis in poor outcome. Physiol Genomics. 2007;30(2):146–55.

29. Xiao W, Mindrinos MN, Seok J, et al. A genomic storm in critically injured humans. J Exp Med. 2011;208(13):2581–90.

30. Livingston DH, Appel SH, Wellhausen SR, Sonnenfeld G, Polk Jr HC. Depressed interferon gamma production and monocyte HLA-DR expression after severe injury. Arch Surg. 1988;123(11):1309–12.

31. Ditschkowski M, Kreuzfelder E, Rebmann V, et al. HLA-DR expression and soluble HLA-DR levels in septic patients after trauma. Ann Surg. 1999;229(2):246–54.

32. Giannoudis PV, Smith RM, Windsor AC, Bellamy MC, Guillou PJ. Monocyte human leukocyte antigen-DR expression correlates with intrapulmonary shunting after major trauma. Am J Surg. 1999;177(6):454–9.

33. Asadullah K, Woiciechowsky C, Docke WD, et al. Very low monocytic HLA-DR expression indicates high risk of infection–immunomonitoring for patients after neurosurgery and patients during high dose steroid therapy. Eur J Emerg Med. 1995;2(4):184–90.

34. Cheadle WG, Mercer-Jones M, Heinzelmann M, Polk Jr HC. Sepsis and septic complications in the surgical patient: who is at risk? Shock (Augusta Ga). 1996;6 Suppl 1:S6–9.

35. Volk HD, Reinke P, Krausch D, et al. Monocyte deactivation–rationale for a new therapeutic strategy in sepsis. Intensive Care Med. 1996;22 Suppl 4:S474–81.

36. Fumeaux T, Pugin J. Role of interleukin-10 in the intracellular sequestration of human leukocyte antigen-DR in monocytes during septic shock. Am J Respir Crit Care Med. 2002;166(11):1475–82.

37. Reinke P, Volk HD. Diagnostic and predictive value of an immune monitoring program for complications after kidney transplantation. Urol Int. 1992;49(2):69–75.

38. Ho YP, Sheen IS, Chiu CT, Wu CS, Lin CY. A strong association between down-regulation of HLA-DR expression and the late mortality in patients with severe acute pancreatitis. Am J Gastroenterol. 2006;101(5):1117–24.

39. Venet F, Tissot S, Debard AL, et al. Decreased monocyte human leukocyte antigen-DR expression after severe burn injury: correlation with severity and secondary septic shock. Crit Care Med. 2007;35(8):1910–7.

40. Monneret G, Lepape A, Voirin N, et al. Persisting low monocyte human leukocyte antigen-DR expression predicts mortality in septic shock. Intensive Care Med. 2006;32(8):1175–83.

41. Hall MW, Knatz NL, Vetterly C, et al. Immunoparalysis and nosocomial infection in children with multiple organ dysfunction syndrome. Intensive Care Med. 2011;37(3):525–32.

42. Allen ML, Peters MJ, Goldman A, et al. Early postoperative monocyte deactivation predicts systemic inflammation and prolonged stay in pediatric cardiac intensive care. Crit Care Med. 2002;30(5):1140–5.

43. Flach R, Majetschak M, Heukamp T, et al. Relation of ex vivo stimulated blood cytokine synthesis to post-traumatic sepsis. Cytokine. 1999;11(2):173–8.

44. Docke WD, Randow F, Syrbe U, et al. Monocyte deactivation in septic patients: restoration by IFN-gamma treatment. Nat Med. 1997;3(6):678–81.

45. Hall MW, Gavrilin MA, Knatz NL, Duncan MD, Fernandez SA, Wewers MD. Monocyte mRNA phenotype and adverse outcomes from pediatric multiple organ dysfunction syndrome. Pediatr Res. 2007;62(5):597–603.

46. Marquardt DJ, Knatz NL, Wetterau LA, Wewers MD, Hall MW. Failure to recover somatotropic axis function is associated with mortality from pediatric sepsis-induced multiple organ dysfunction syndrome. Pediatr Crit Care Med. 2010;11(1):18–25.

47. Mella C, Suarez-Arrabal MC, Lopez S, et al. Innate immune dysfunction is associated with enhanced disease severity in infants with severe respiratory syncytial virus bronchiolitis. J Infect Dis. 2013;207(4):564–73.

48. Hotchkiss RS, Tinsley KW, Swanson PE, et al. Sepsis-induced apoptosis causes progressive profound depletion of B and CD4+ T lymphocytes in humans. J Immunol. 2001;166(11):6952–63.

49. Boomer JS, To K, Chang KC, et al. Immunosuppression in patients who die of sepsis and multiple organ failure. JAMA. 2011;306(23):2594–605.

50. Felmet KA, Hall MW, Clark RS, Jaffe R, Carcillo JA. Prolonged lymphopenia, lymphoid depletion, and hypoprolactinemia in children with nosocomial sepsis and multiple organ failure. J Immunol. 2005;174(6):3765–72.

51. Monneret G, Debard AL, Venet F, et al. Marked elevation of human circulating CD4 + CD25+ regulatory T cells in sepsis-induced immunoparalysis. Crit Care Med. 2003;31(7):2068–71.

52. Venet F, Pachot A, Debard AL, et al. Increased percentage of CD4 + CD25+ regulatory T cells during septic shock is due to the decrease of CD4 + CD25- lymphocytes. Crit Care Med. 2004;32(11):2329–31.

53. Hershman MJ, Appel SH, Wellhausen SR, Sonnenfeld G, Polk Jr HC. Interferon-gamma treatment increases HLA-DR expression on monocytes in severely injured patients. Clin Exp Immunol. 1989;77(1):67–70.

54. Nierhaus A, Montag B, Timmler N, et al. Reversal of immunoparalysis by recombinant human granulocyte-macrophage colony-stimulating factor in patients with severe sepsis. Intensive Care Med. 2003;29(4):646–51.

55. Rosenbloom AJ, Linden PK, Dorrance A, Penkosky N, Cohen-Melamed MH, Pinsky MR. Effect of granulocyte-monocyte colony-stimulating factor therapy on leukocyte function and clearance of serious infection in nonneutropenic patients. Chest. 2005;127(6):2139–50.

56. Meisel C, Schefold JC, Pschowski R, et al. GM-CSF to reverse sepsis-associated immunosuppression: a double-blind randomized placebo-controlled multicenter trial. Am J Respir Crit Care Med. 2009;180(7):640–8.

57. Hotchkiss RS, Opal S. Immunotherapy for sepsis–a new approach against an ancient foe. N Engl J Med. 2010;363(1):87–9.

58. Nair MP, Schwartz SA, Polasani R, Hou J, Sweet A, Chadha KC. Immunoregulatory effects of morphine on human lymphocytes. Clin Diag Lab Immunol. 1997;4(2):127–32.

59. Singhal PC, Kapasi AA, Franki N, Reddy K. Morphine-induced macrophage apoptosis: the role of transforming growth factor-beta. Immunology. 2000;100(1):57–62.

60. Zavala F. Benzodiazepines, anxiety and immunity. Pharmacol Ther. 1997;75(3):199–216.

61. Marik PE, Raghavan M. Stress-hyperglycemia, insulin and immunomodulation in sepsis. Intensive Care Med. 2004;30(5):748–56.

62. Bergmann M, Sautner T. Immunomodulatory effects of vasoactive catecholamines. Wien Klin Wochenschr. 2002;114(17–18):752–61.

63. Muszynski J, Nateri J, Nicol K, Greathouse K, Hanson L, Hall M. Immunosuppressive effects of red blood cells on monocytes are related to both storage time and storage solution. Transfusion. 2012;52(4):794–802.

64. Baumgartner JM, Silliman CC, Moore EE, Banerjee A, McCarter MD. Stored red blood cell transfusion induces regulatory T cells. J Am Coll Surg. 2009;208(1):110–9.

65. Offner PJ, Moore EE, Biffl WL, Johnson JL, Silliman CC. Increased rate of infection associated with transfusion of old blood after severe injury. Arch Surg. 2002;137(6):711–6; discussion 716–7.

Katherine Mason

Abstract

The study of mediators and pathways of oxidative stress and nitrosative stress have been underway for decades, but the role of free radicals in the pathogenesis and treatment of disease remains incompletely understood. Recent years have seen a rapid escalation in research concerning the links between cellular mechanisms of disease and the clinical management of injury and illness. Reactive oxygen species and reactive nitrogen species are now understood to play a significant role in disordered cellular processes as well as having key regulatory roles in normal cellular physiology and healing. This chapter is focused on oxidative and nitrosative stress as it translates to the practice of pediatric critical care. The first part of this chapter reviews some fundamental concepts of oxidative and nitrosative regulation and stress. The roles of reactive oxygen and nitrogen species in select aspects of normal cellular homeostasis and physiologic function including endothelial function, immune system regulation and mitochondrial respiration are presented in the second part. The final section of this chapter discusses the role of these free radicals in select disease states chosen for their particular relevance to pediatric critical care.

Keywords

Reactive Oxygen Species • Reactive Nitrogen Species • Redox Homeostasis • Oxidative Stress • Nitrosative Stress • Antioxidants • Nitric Oxide • Superoxide

Introduction

Reactive Oxygen Species and Reactive Nitrogen Species

Reactive Oxygen Species (ROS) are oxygen-containing molecules that react avidly with proteins, nucleic acids, and lipids. The bioactivity of macromolecules can be changed by ROS via oxidation, cross-linking, denaturation and altered tertiary and quaternary structure of proteins, DNA breakage and mispairing, and the peroxidation of lipids and aldehyde generation. While some ROS such as hydrogen peroxide (H_2O_2) contain paired electrons, they are most frequently free radicals, containing a highly reactive unpaired electron. The primary ROS is superoxide (O_2^{-}) which is produced by the reaction of an electron with one of the two unpaired electrons in the outer shell of molecular oxygen. Superoxide can be produced by electron shift in heme proteins, arachidonic acid metabolism, and direct radiant injury to molecular oxygen, as well as by enzymes of the cytochrome P450 and nitric oxide synthase (NOS) families, xanthine oxidase, nitric oxide synthase, and aldehyde oxidase [1–7]. However, physiologically relevant superoxide is predominantly produced by the reaction of electrons leaked from complexes I and III in the mitochondrial electron transport chain with molecular oxygen [8–10]. It is suggested that approximately 1–3 % of the O_2 reduced in mitochondria becomes O_2^{-} by means of this electron leak [11–15].

K. Mason, MD
Department of Pediatrics, Rainbow Babies Children's Hospital,
11100 Euclid Avenue, Cleveland, OH 44106, USA
e-mail: katherine.mason@uhhospitals.org

D.S. Wheeler et al. (eds.), *Pediatric Critical Care Medicine*,
DOI 10.1007/978-1-4471-6362-6_23, © Springer-Verlag London 2014

O_2^- itself is a relatively weak oxidizing substance and exerts most of its biologic effects through its derivatives: hydrogen peroxide (H_2O_2), hydroxyl radical ($OH\cdot$), hydroperoxyl radical ($HOO\cdot$) and others. O_2^- can react with nitric oxide ($NO\cdot$) to form the very potent oxidant peroxynitrite. Superoxide dismutase (SOD) converts two O_2^- into hydrogen peroxide (H_2O_2). Unlike other ROS, H_2O_2 can diffuse away from the site of its production, undergo subsequent metabolism and exert effects at targets some distance from the original site of generation.

In the presence of reduced transition metals such as Fe(II), hydrogen peroxide can be converted to the hydroxyl radical ($OH\cdot$) in a process known as the Fenton reaction. The hydroxyl radical is an extremely potent oxidant capable of abstracting an electron from nearly any biomolecule. The reaction of H_2O_2 with transition metals also results in oxidizing intermediates that are intrinsically capable of significant oxidative damage. Although the biochemical availability of transition metals such as iron are tightly regulated in normal physiologic conditions, the potential for interaction with ROS is readily apparent under common conditions such as the release of free hemoglobin through traumatic membrane disruption. Overexpression of enzymes capable of binding these transition metals and thus preventing reactions with ROS and RNS has been shown to be protective against oxidative stress in sepsis, further indicating the role of transition metals and ROS in the evolution of pathologic conditions such as sepsis [16].

While ROS were initially described in the 1950s, it wasn't until 1980 that Furchgott and Zawadski began publishing research on an endothelial-derived relaxation factor that subsequently came to be identified as nitric oxide [17]. $NO\cdot$ was found in diverse cell types and determined to be an important signaling molecule for a vast array of additional physiologic functions including immune regulation, neurotransmission, cellular adhesion, and others [3]. Nitric oxide synthase (NOS) is the enzyme responsible for the generation of nitric oxide ($NO\cdot$) through the oxidation of L-arginine. There are three subtypes of NOS, two that are constitutively expressed, calcium dependent forms and one rapidly inducible, calcium independent form. Research on the various roles of $NO\cdot$ expanded rapidly, and in 1998 the Nobel Prize in Physiology and Medicine was awarded to Drs. Furchgott, Ignarro, and Murad for their extensive study of the role of nitric oxide in physiology and disease. Research on $NO\cdot$ led to the identification of bioactive nitrogen oxide derivatives now referred to as reactive nitrogen species (RNS). Nitric oxide itself has multiple known physiologic effects, some of which are discussed below. The reaction of superoxide ($O_2\cdot$) with nitric oxide ($NO\cdot$) yields peroxynitrite ($ONOO^-$). Nitric oxide and peroxynitrite are examples of reactive nitrogen species (RNS).

Antioxidants

Under physiologic conditions the continuous low level production of ROS is counterbalanced by their clearance. Nonenzymatic compounds such as proteins, amino acids, glutathione, ascorbate (vitamin C), and alpha-tocopherol (vitamin E) are important ROS scavengers, serving as substrates for oxidation by ROS and RNS and consuming them in the process. Serum proteins are low affinity substrates for ROS/RNS but they are present in such large quantities that they function as a major mechanism for clearance. Oxidation of proteins interferes with tertiary and quaternary structure. Unfolding and partial degradation of proteins exposes more sites susceptible to oxidation and nitrosylation, thereby rendering them higher affinity substrates and further accelerating their reaction with ROS/RNS. Proteolytic degradation is thus accelerated, facilitating the consumption and breakdown of ROS/RNS from the cell.

Scavenging of basal levels of ROS/RNS by proteins and other anti-oxidant compounds is quite effective in physiologic conditions and is an important part of maintaining redox regulation and the homeostasis of oxidative metabolism. However, it has been demonstrated that high levels of ROS/RNS can directly inhibit proteosomal activity resulting in the intracellular accumulation of dysfunctional oxidized and nitrosylated proteins and further loss of oxidative homeostasis [18–20].

In addition to proteins and other antioxidants with low specific activity toward ROS/RNS there are a number of enzymes that facilitate the conversion of potentially toxic ROS/RNS into molecular oxygen and water, or into intermediates that are ultimately metabolized into nontoxic products. Superoxide dismutase (SOD), glutathione peroxidase, thioredoxins, and catalase are enzymatic antioxidants that regulate the clearance of ROS and RNS. These antioxidants exert their protective effects through (a) acting as an essential cofactor for detoxifying enzymes, (b) directly scavenging singlet oxygen and the hydroxyl radical and (c) participating in the regeneration of other anti-oxidant compounds [21–24].

The balance between ROS/RNS production and antioxidant activity is termed redox regulation and the normal physiologic balance referred to as redox homeostasis. Under normal physiologic conditions, ROS/RNS have several important regulatory and signaling roles that will be considered in the section below. Oxidative stress and nitrosative stress are the terms given to the condition in which the production of ROS/RNS overwhelms the counter-regulatory antioxidant systems, promoting the transition from the important tightly regulated physiologic functions of ROS/RNS to pathophysiologic states.

Redox Homeostasis and Physiologic Function

ROS and RNS are key regulators of a myriad of important physiologic functions. A few chosen for their particular relevance to the practice of pediatric critical care are herein reviewed.

Endothelial Relaxation and Adherence Properties

NO· is critical to the regulation of smooth muscle relaxation and vascular tone. Endogenous nitric oxide is produced by three nitric oxide synthase (NOS) subtypes. Neuronal nitric oxide synthase (nNOS) and endothelial nitric oxide synthase (eNOS) are the two calcium-sensitive constitutive types while the activity of the inducible nitric oxide synthase (iNOS) type is dependent upon increased transcription of the iNOS gene [25, 26]. Exogenous nitric oxide is now used widely in pediatric ICUs to treat common conditions characterized by endothelial pathology including respiratory failure, pulmonary hypertension and respiratory distress associated with prematurity [27–32].

Nitric Oxide (NO·) inhibits platelet and neutrophil adhesion to endothelium [33–37]. NO· activates guanylyl cyclase, inhibits phosphoinositide 3-kinase, inhibits cyclooxygenase-1 and reduces platelet adhesion through a cGMP-dependent reduction in intracellular calcium [38, 39]. Conversely, reactive oxygen species promote leukocyte and platelet adhesion and aggregation [35, 40–43].

Immune Responses

Superoxide radicals, H_2O_2, and hypochloric acid (HOCL) are produced through the activity of NAD(P)H oxidase, superoxide dismutase (SOD), and myeloperoxidase, respectively. These reactive oxygen species are an important part of the oxidative burst in activated neutrophils, a critical response to pathogens [44, 45]. Although each of these reactive oxygen species is part of the normal host response to pathogens, deficiencies of the enzymes responsible for their formation do not manifest uniformly. Most clinicians will be familiar with X-linked Chronic Granulomatous Disease (CGD) as a serious disorder of immunity characterized by abnormal killing of bacteria and fungi despite normal or near normal neutrophil recruitment and phagocytosis. In this condition neutrophil NAD(P)H oxidase activity is absent or deficient. The neutrophils of affected individuals are unable to generate superoxide (O_2^-). Although a relatively weak oxidant,

(O_2^-) is the precursor to other ROS having direct cytotoxic effects on pathogens. Before the condition was well characterized and medical treatment widely utilized CGD was uniformly fatal in early life. Despite treatment with effective antibiotics, immunomodulatory therapies and recently bone marrow transplant the disease still carries a significant burden of morbidity and mortality due to severely impaired (O_2^-) production. A recent study published by Kuhn et.al demonstrated a clear association between residual (O_2^-) production and survival in patients with CGD, highlighting the critical role of phagocyte derived NAD(P)H oxidase activity in normal host immunity [46].

Non-phagocytic cell forms of NAD(P)H oxidase are found extensively in the cardiovascular system. In the carotid body there is evidence that this NAD(P)H oxidase produces ROS that help regulate the chemotransduction pathways essential for neural control of ventilation. Recent reviews on the role of ROS in regulating neurorespiratory control at the level of the carotid body make clear that further research is needed for definitive description of these pathways [47, 48]. Non-phagocytic cell forms of NAD(P)H oxidase are found extensively in myocytes and fibroblasts and produce ROS critical to other intracellular signaling pathways [49].

Regulation of Mitochondrial Respiration

The roles of ROS and RNS in modulating ATP production are far from being fully elucidated. NO· has been shown to have concentration-dependent bimodal effects on mitochondrial respiration and the regulation of many other cellular processes. Low levels of NO· are associated with processes critical to cellular preservation such as regulating cGMP-mediated signaling, while high levels of NO· are associated with the disruption of cellular homeostasis and pathophysiologic effects [50]. NO· competes with O_2 at complex IV and thus reversibly inhibits the terminal acceptor of the electron transfer chain, thereby reducing ATP production [51, 52]. NO· can also react with O_2^- produced by complex IV to form peroxynitrite ($ONOO^-$). In the setting of reduced levels of intramitochondrial glutathione, this highly reactive compound can irreversibly bind to and inhibit complex I and reduce ATP production [53].

Mitochondrial antioxidant enzymes such as manganese superoxide dismutase (MnSOD), thioredoxin (TRX), and glutathione (GSH) are essential to the maintenance of redox homeostasis. Increased ROS/RNS production will inactivate, deplete or simply overcome antioxidant systems in the mitochondria leading to widespread damage to lipids, proteins, and nucleic acids. MtDNA is particularly susceptible to oxidative damage because of its close proximity to the site of production of ROS/RNS. O_2^- and NO· are highly labile and the damage they induce is diffusion-limited, thus the closer a potential target is to their production site the more vulnerable that target is to damage. All mtDNA encodes expressed genes. An oxidative modification or mutation is therefore more likely to cause a functional defect in mtDNA than in nuclear DNA, which contains non-coding elements. Since the mtDNA genes encode proteins of the electron transport chain, transfer RNA and ribosomal RNA, oxidative stress-induced mutations are highly likely to cause defects in the proteins and processes of the electron transport chain with a subsequent reduction in ETC function and possibly an increase in ROS and RNS production. The perpetual cycle of oxidative and nitrosative stress-induced transcriptional, translational, and post-translational defects, leading to increased ROS and RNS production, causing further defects in RNA and protein production, has been termed the mitochondrial catastrophe cascade and is one pathway to either mitochondrial apoptosis or to unregulated destruction. A counter-regulatory mechanism to maintain redox homeostasis is the ability of ROS and RNS to activate antioxidants, protecting against unmitigated oxidative and nitrosative damage.

This brief overview scarcely introduces the fundamental concepts of the modulation of cellular processes by ROS and RNS, their production, regulation, and clearance. As they are potent molecules that are rapidly produced in response to environmental changes, stimuli and metabolic needs of the cell, and are quickly cleared or neutralized and produced in close proximity to their sites of action, they can function as a nearly ideal signaling molecule or formidable toxins. It seems likely that current knowledge of the role of ROS and RNS in the maintenance of normal and critical cellular processes reflects just a small fraction of their regulatory effects and that the investigation of ROS and RNS as signaling molecules holds at least as much promise as the investigation of pathologic effects of oxidative and nitrosative stress. Fortunately, there are several excellent reviews of this topic for the interested reader [6, 54–57].

The Role of Reactive Oxygen Species and Reactive Nitrogen Species in Critical Illness

Sepsis

Despite advances in diagnosis, source control, supportive care and medical treatment, sepsis remains a common cause of morbidity and mortality in the pediatric intensive care unit with an estimated 42,000 cases of pediatric sepsis in the United States per year with attendant 10 % mortality [58]. The concept that oxidative and nitrosative stress are important in the pathogenesis of sepsis is not new [59–61]. Despite nearly two decades of research into oxidative and nitrosative stress in sepsis, knowledge on the subject still seems to be in the incipient phase and it would appear there is yet much to learn before therapies targeted to the control of these underlying processes can be successfully implemented. Studies of the pathogenesis, regulation and modulation of oxidative and nitrosative stress hold great promise for a clinical entity that is both common and deadly.

Vascular Dysregulation in Sepsis

The development of clinical sepsis is dependent upon the nuanced interaction of a myriad of host, pathogen, and environmental factors. One of the hallmarks of the disease is the development of multiple organ failure, including organs distant from the site of primary infection. One view of the cause of this organ failure has been that there is a maldistribution of blood flow in sepsis, with a loss of the peripheral autoregulation that normally ensures adequate perfusion of critical organs by directing blood flow to critical organs during times of stress and away from non-essential tissues.

Nitrosative stress and oxidative stress are thought to be key determinants of the endothelial dysfunction in septic shock. Both vasoconstrictor and vasodilator responses have been shown to be impaired in models of sepsis. As a result of decreased perfusing pressure due to altered arteriolar tone and microvascular plugging, individual organs fail due to an inadequate delivery of oxygen and substrate to meet the metabolic demands of the tissues, despite an overall normal to high cardiac output and oxygen carrying capacity. In fact, low tissue oxygenation levels have been documented in several animal models of early sepsis, supporting the hypothesis that organ failure in sepsis results from an inadequate oxygen delivery to individual tissues with normal or high oxygen extraction [62–64]. The phenomenon of catecholamine-resistant hypotension is not uncommon in the management of pediatric septic shock. This condition is also seen in mouse models of sepsis. A series of experiments using genetically engineered mice deficient in specific subtypes of NOS led to the conclusion that nNOS and iNOS but not eNOS are responsible for oxidative and nitrosative stress in sepsis [65]. Unlike their wild type counterparts, only iNOS knockout mice had preserved vasoconstrictor response to angiotensin II and norepinephrine in sepsis, while only nNOS knockouts had a preserved vasodilatory response. Despite preserved vascular tone, in this same set of experiments it was shown that capillary blood flow was not maintained in any NOS knockout strain in the septic state. However, knockout of a subunit of the ROS producing enzyme NADPH oxidase did preserve capillary blood flow in septic mice. Furthermore, in other experiments, infusion of a specific inhibitor of NADPH oxidase restored capillary blood flow in wild type mice after the induction of sepsis [66–68]. Taken together the data from this set of experiments would lead to the conclusion that vascular dysregulation and decreased organ perfusion in sepsis is a ROS-mediated disorder.

Microvascular plugging and disordered platelet, fibrin, and endothelial interactions are other contributors to tissue hypoxia in sepsis. As discussed in the preceding section on ROS and physiologic regulation, ROS induce a prothrombogenic state through (a) cell signaling pathways leading to altered gene transcription of endothelial cell adhesion molecules such as P-selectin [69, 70] (b) activation of redox sensitive pro-inflammatory enzymes such as phospholipase A2 and platelet activating factor, (c) oxidation and inactivation of tetrahydrobiopterin, a necessary cofactor for eNOS function [71, 72] and (d) inactivation of NO· [73–75]. Microvascular plugging and reduced capillary blood flow are important causes of tissue hypoxia due to the subsequent increase in the distance required for oxygen diffusion.

Many other examples of oxidative and nitrosative stress are found in the sepsis literature. Models of thermal injury plus tracheal instillation of bacteria have been shown to initiate a pathophysiologic profile closely resembling human ARDS and ALI with sepsis. In this model, injury is associated with increased markers of nitrosative and oxidative stress as well as hemodynamic and ventilatory changes characteristic of human sepsis [76, 77]. Early, selective inhibition of nNOS with subsequent inhibition of iNOS using highly specific antibodies attenuated hemodynamic abnormalities, hypoxia, fluid overload, tissue levels of lipid peroxidation products and normalized plasma nitrite/nitrate levels [78].

Cytopathic Hypoxia and Mitochondrial Dysfunction in Sepsis

An alternative explanation for the development of organ failure in septic shock is that there is a defect in oxygen utilization instead of oxygen delivery. Cytopathic hypoxia is a term applied to the paradigm that cellular and organ dysfunction occur in sepsis due to an inability of the cell to use oxygen and generate ATP. Also referred to as cellular dysoxia, this theory postulates that sepsis-induced organ dysfunction results from an acquired defect in oxidative phosphorylation and subsequent energetic failure of the cell. This concept is supported by observations of normal or elevated tissue PO_2s in skeletal muscle, ileal mucosa, and heart, as well as decreased oxygen extraction in mixed venous saturations or organ-specific venous return [64, 79–81].

Cytopathic hypoxia provides a rational explanation for the clinical experience that patients with severe sepsis can have profound but often reversible organ failure in sepsis without evidence of ultrastructural damage, ischemia, or necrosis. Recently this has even been hypothesized to be a regulated, adaptive response to severe sepsis that promotes survival through the process of metabolic hibernation. Some

intriguing literature on this subject can be found in recent publications [82–85].

As discussed in the preceding section on ROS and RNS and the regulation of mitochondrial respiration, free radicals are able to reduce mitochondrial oxidative phosphorylation. Patients and animals with severe sepsis have been shown to have significantly lower ATP concentrations, lower Complex I activity, elevated markers of lipid peroxidation, lower antioxidant (glutathione and thioredoxin) levels, and increased nitric oxide production that correlate with severity of illness and mortality [61, 86, 87].

ROS and Nuclear Factor kappa-B in Sepsis

An increase in superoxide production has been documented in in vitro, animal and human studies of sepsis. Although superoxide is itself a weak oxidant it can exert significant effects through stimulation of nuclear factor (NF)-kappa B. Activated NF-kappa B translocates to the nucleus where it binds to DNA and initiates transcription of proteins, particularly those required for immune and inflammatory regulation. ROS and NF-kappa B have been investigated in models of sepsis. Peripheral monocytes in endotoxin-injected mice had higher ROS, a reduction in the reduced glutathione pool, and increased NF-kappa B activity compared with controls [88]. In a study of patients with severe sepsis, increased activation of NF-kappa B was measured in peripheral neutrophils and monocytes with the highest values found in the patients that subsequently died [89]. This was corroborated in a subsequent study by the same group which demonstrated that treatment of septic patients with N-acetylcysteine, a clinically used antioxidant that inhibits NF-kappa B activation in vitro, reduced NF-kappa B activity in peripheral monocytes and that this reduction was associated with a reduction of the proinflammatory cytokine IL-8, but not with changes in other cytokines measured [90]. It would thus seem that oxidative regulation of NF-kappa B is an important element in the development of clinical sepsis [91].

Antioxidants in Sepsis

Oxidative stress in sepsis is an imbalance of pro-oxidant and antioxidant processes with a resultant excess of pro-oxidants that disrupt normal cell function. Not surprisingly, many models of sepsis and clinical studies have shown a reduction in antioxidant levels and activity. Superoxide dismutase (SOD) catalyzes the dismutation of superoxide into hydrogen peroxide and oxygen. Levels of the intramitochondrial form of SOD, MnSOD, were significantly elevated in patients with sepsis. Furthermore, patients that subsequently died had higher levels of mnSOD than survivors of sepsis [92, 93]. Thioredoxin (TRX) is a highly conserved antioxidant ubiquitous to plants, prokaryotes, and animals. Elevated levels of TRX have been demonstrated in patients with sepsis and septic shock. An excellent demonstration of the role that TRX may play in the modulation of oxidative stress is to be found in the animal experiments of Brenner et al. This group showed elevation of TRX in a cecal ligation and puncture (CLP) model of sepsis. Immediate post-surgical treatment with a neutralizing antibody to TRX markedly decreased survival in mice, while administration of exogenous TRX was associated with a significant survival benefit. Administration of TRX later in the course of sepsis decreased mortality from CLP but was not protective to the extent seen with early administration [94].

Therapies Targeting Oxidative and Nitrosative Stress in the Treatment of Sepsis

Specific treatments for severe sepsis remain elusive. A prospective, randomized, double blind placebo-controlled trial of 216 critically ill patients treated with the enteral antioxidants alpha-tocopherol and ascorbic acid (AA) demonstrated that this treatment resulted in a reduction in markers of lipid peroxidation and improved 28 day survival [95]. This corroborated earlier studies in which it was reported that the administration of alpha-tocopherol and AA resulted in clinical improvements in patients with trauma, sepsis, burns, and major surgeries [96, 97]. The potential role for the use of ascorbic acid in sepsis was recently the subject of a comprehensive review which presents evidence from in vitro and animal studies that ascorbic acid administration mitigates microvascular dysfunction in models of sepsis through eNOS mediated NO· production and scavenging of reactive oxygen species [98]. The implementation of the use of these agents in pediatric patients with sepsis requires further investigation.

The control of nitrosative stress in sepsis is another area of long-standing active research. Several agents that effect NOS have been studied. Methylene blue is a non-selective inhibitor of NO-stimulate cGMP activity. Nearly 20 years of investigation into the potential therapeutic role of this agent in septic shock has not demonstrated convincing clinical benefit. Small human studies have shown that the administration of methylene blue can reduce many of the cardiovascular abnormalities of septic shock [99, 100]. A multicenter, randomized placebo-controlled safety and efficacy trial of 312 ICU patients with septic shock showed that the use of a non-selective NOS inhibitor could reverse the cardiovascular derangements in these patients. Furthermore, treatment was associated with a significant increase in the proportion of subjects that had resolution of shock at 72 h post treatment, but not an increased 28 day survival [101]. However, another multicenter, randomized, placebo-controlled double-blind study of the administration of another non-selective NOS inhibitor to patients with septic shock was halted after nearly 800 patients were enrolled as an interim analysis showed a significantly higher mortality in the treatment group vs. control (59 % v. 49 % in the control

group) [102]. This was mirrored in a murine study of the administration of a non-selective NOS inhibitor which also showed a statistically significant increase in mortality in the treated versus untreated group [65]. The use of highly selective NOS inhibitors may be required to restore physiologic redox homeostasis.

More recently, a Phase II trial of a hemoglobin-based NO scavenger was shown to reverse many of the clinical effects and outcomes associated with septic shock without a need for increased medical interventions, indicating a lack of adverse effects [103]. Further demonstration of improved outcomes from well-designed clinical studies of patients treated with NO inhibitors will be needed for application to clinical practice.

Melatonin is a naturally occurring hormone with antioxidant properties that is secreted by the pineal gland [104, 105]. In distinction to adults, pediatric patients with sepsis have been demonstrated to maintain normal nocturnal secretion of melatonin. Interestingly non-survivors and those with more a more severe clinical picture had significantly higher levels of melatonin and significantly lower levels of the primary metabolite [106]. Although one may speculate that an inability to utilize melatonin is associated with a worse outcome in pediatric patients with sepsis the numbers are small and this data will need to be corroborated by other studies. Nonetheless, the concept of severe sepsis as a disorder of cellular antioxidant metabolism remains an intriguing area of investigation.

Mitochondrial-targeted antioxidants are a relatively recent development in the field of mitochondrial research [107–109]. One potential explanation for the disappointing results of large-scale clinical trials performed to test the use of non-specific antioxidants in sepsis is that these exogenously supplied compounds are unable to reach the intramitochondrial sites of maximal ROS and RNS production and effect. Mitochondria have a strong negative membrane potential, and cationic mitochondrial antioxidants such as MitoQ have been shown to accumulate within mitochondria [110]. Limited studies of these mitochondrial targeted antioxidants in in vitro and small animal models have demonstrated lower ROS generation and restoration of near normal mitochondrial membrane potential under experimental conditions relevant to sepsis, ischemia reperfusion, and aging [110–112]. A more recently developed class of targeted antioxidants uses small amino acid peptides to gain entry into the mitochondria. These have been shown to scavenge both reactive nitrogen and oxygen species. Although not yet tested in sepsis models, experimental data indicates beneficial effects in ischemia-reperfusion and other models [113, 114].

Over the last several years, a number of excellent reviews of oxidative and nitrosative stress in sepsis have been published [82–84, 115–122].

Traumatic Brain Injury and Epilepsy

Traumatic brain injury (TBI) is a common reason for ICU admission and remains a leading cause of childhood morbidity and mortality. Improved management of children with TBI requires a consideration of the role of reactive oxygen species and reactive nitrogen species in the pathogenesis, treatment and recovery phase of these injuries. The study of oxidative and nitrosative stress in TBI has led to some encouraging new treatment modalities with the potential for reducing long term morbidity in pediatric patients with TBI. Many of these are a long way from clinical use but others, with cerebral cooling being a prime example, are already being investigated in pediatric intensive care units.

Brain tissue is particularly susceptible to oxidative stress due to the particular composition of lipids, the high mitochondrial content in neural tissues, a robust rate of cerebral oxygen consumption and limited neural antioxidant stores. Traumatic brain injury (TBI) causes direct biochemical and structural alterations in neural tissue that can result in acute seizures and chronic epilepsy. The abnormal excitotoxicity and hypermetabolism that characterizes acute seizure activity results in an overproduction of superoxide [123], lower ratios of glutathione and other anti-oxidants [124–126], lipid oxidation [125], and mitochondrial DNA damage [127]. These findings from chemoconvulsant models of eplilepsy have been corroborated by recent human studies in which increased lipid oxidation products [128], decreased mitochondrial electron transport chain function [129], and reduced glutathione stores [130] were identified in patients with epilepsy. Oxidative modifications induced by excitotoxic damage can lead to neuronal loss through programmed death pathways or apoptotic pathways. The determination of the roles of ROS/RNS signaling pathways of preapoptosis will permit a novel approach to the improvement of outcomes in patients with epilepsy and TBI.

The role of ROS production in the pathogenesis of TBI has been further supported by experiments performed using mice deficient in the activity of the antioxidant enzyme superoxide dismutase (SOD). In a number of models of cerebral injury, SOD-deficient mice had increased seizure susceptibility, encephalopathy, neuronal cell injury, and shortened lifespan following an injurious intervention compared with wild-type mice subject to the same intervention [131–133]. Furthermore, over-expression or supplementation of SOD was protective against the development of neuronal injury [134–136]. Experimental TBI has been shown to activate both intrinsic and extrinsic pathways of apoptosis and there are some excellent reviews on the relationship between traumatic brain injury, epilepsy, reactive oxygen and nitrogen species, the modulation of oxidative stress, and neuronal apoptosis [11, 137–139].

Oxidative stress is thought to be a factor promoting the assembly of the mitochondrial permeability transition pore (mPTP) in neural tissue. Formation of the mPTP collapses the electron potential across the inner mitochondrial membrane, uncouples the electron transport chain, promotes further ROS production, and causes energetic failure and cell death [140]. Experiments such as this indicate that the development of neuronal apoptosis can be seen as a ROS/RNS-mediated, mPTP-dependent process.

Infants and young children are known to have particular vulnerabilities to traumatic brain injury and its sequelae. The child's proportionally larger cranial vault, less supportive bone and spine structures, more aqueous body tissues and dependence on caregivers for the identification and treatment of injury are but a few of the characteristics well known to the pediatric intensivist that render the young child more prone to adverse outcome from TBI. To this list should be added a developmental immaturity of systems for redox homeostasis in brain tissue including lower levels of the antioxidants metallothioneins [141, 142] and superoxide dismutases [143] that have been demonstrated in juvenile brains in humans and animals [144].

Therapies for Traumatic Brain Injury and Epilepsy

ROS and RNS have been shown to participate in the pathogenesis of traumatic brain injury and epilepsy. This has led to the investigation of means to manipulate oxidative and nitrosative stress as potential therapies. An early study using an infant rat model of the shaken baby syndrome demonstrated a significant increase in cortical lipid peroxidation products and histological damage associated with TBI. The administration of an antioxidant- lipid peroxidation inhibitor reduced the lipid peroxidation injury and hemorrhage but did not mitigate ultimate cortical atrophy [145]. Another study of an inhibitor of lipid peroxidation in TBI demonstrated a reduction in markers of oxidized lipids and nitrosative stress as well as an improvement in measures of mitochondrial function [126]. A more general therapeutic intervention of current great clinical interest to the pediatric intensivist, cerebral cooling, may possibly exert its therapeutic effect through the modulation of nitrosative and oxidative stress. In a rodent model of fluid percussive injury, animals randomized to the cerebral cooling group had higher antioxidant enzyme activities, lower levels of markers of lipid peroxidation, lower iNOS expression and lower markers of nitrosative stress when compared with animals receiving normothermic fluids. The hypothermic group also had smaller infarction zones and improved functional testing compared with normothermic animals [146]. Hypothermic treatment attenuated oxidative stress in children with severe TBI with preservation of CSF antioxidant levels and decreased protein oxidation [147]. However, a multi-center, randomized, Phase III trial of hypothermia in pediatric TBI was recently terminated at interim analysis due to futility [148]. Thus, the role of hypothermia in clinical TBI remains uncertain.

The role of oxidative and nitrosative stress in epilepsy is an additional area of active investigation. Some studies have used TBI as an inducer of epilepsy but many use chemical induction models which may have less relevance to pediatric seizures. Nonetheless, SOD-mimetics have demonstrated some success in animal models of encephalopathy and seizures [133, 149]. Promising results have been seen with therapies that inhibit the reactions of transition metals and ROS and the generation of O_2^-. The interaction of ROS and RNS with intracellular transition metals is a source of highly potent oxidizing molecules. Using a model of chemical-induced status epilepticus in the rat, synthetic iron chelators were used and resulted in improved outcomes as manifested by a reduction in markers of mitochondrial oxidative stress and mitochondrial DNA damage, as well as preservation of hippocampal cells structure [150].

The ketogenic diet has been used for years for the treatment of epilepsy, often with significant clinical improvement. The ketogenic diet promotes the production and utilization of ketones for metabolic substrate. It has also been shown to decrease production or ROS, improve mitochondrial redox state and activity as well as stimulate the synthesis of the endogenous antioxidant glutathione in rodent and human studies [151–154].

References

1. Fleming I, Busse R. Vascular cytochrome P450 in the regulation of renal function and vascular tone: EDHF, superoxide anions and blood pressure. Nephrol Dial Transplant. 2001;16:1309–11.
2. Puntarulo S, Cederbaum AI. Production of reactive oxygen species by microsomes enriched in specific human cytochrome P450 enzymes. Free Radic Biol Med. 1998;24:1324–30.
3. Bergendi L, Benes L, Durackova Z, Ferencik M. Chemistry, physiology and pathology of free radicals. Life Sci. 1999;65:1865–74.
4. Brand MD, Affourtit C, Esteves TC, et al. Mitochondrial superoxide: production, biological effects, and activation of uncoupling proteins. Free Radic Biol Med. 2004;37:755–67.
5. Dawson TM, Snyder SH. Gases as biological messengers: nitric oxide and carbon monoxide in the brain. J Neurosci. 1994;14:5147–59.
6. Droge W. Free radicals in the physiological control of cell function. Physiol Rev. 2002;82:47–95.
7. Halliwell B. Reactive oxygen species and the central nervous system. J Neurochem. 1992;59:1609–23.
8. Koopman WJ, Nijtmans LG, Dieteren CE, et al. Mammalian mitochondrial complex I: biogenesis, regulation, and reactive oxygen species generation. Antioxid Redox Signal. 2010;12:1431–70.
9. Koopman WJ, Verkaart S, Visch HJ, et al. Inhibition of complex I of the electron transport chain causes O2-. -mediated mitochondrial outgrowth. Am J Physiol Cell Physiol. 2005;288:C1440–50.
10. Orrenius S. Reactive oxygen species in mitochondria-mediated cell death. Drug Metab Rev. 2007;39:443–55.
11. Adam-Vizi V. Production of reactive oxygen species in brain mitochondria: contribution by electron transport chain and non-electron transport chain sources. Antioxid Redox Signal. 2005;7:1140–9.
12. Chen Q, Moghaddas S, Hoppel CL, Lesnefsky EJ. Ischemic defects in the electron transport chain increase the production of reactive oxygen species from isolated rat heart mitochondria. Am J Physiol Cell Physiol. 2008;294:C460–6.
13. Chen Q, Vazquez EJ, Moghaddas S, Hoppel CL, Lesnefsky EJ. Production of reactive oxygen species by mitochondria: central role of complex III. J Biol Chem. 2003;278:36027–31.
14. Lesnefsky EJ, Gudz TI, Moghaddas S, et al. Aging decreases electron transport complex III activity in heart interfibrillar mitochondria by alteration of the cytochrome c binding site. J Mol Cell Cardiol. 2001;33:37–47.
15. Moghaddas S, Hoppel CL, Lesnefsky EJ. Aging defect at the QO site of complex III augments oxyradical production in rat heart interfibrillar mitochondria. Arch Biochem Biophys. 2003;414:59–66.
16. Ceylan-Isik AF, Zhao P, Zhang B, Xiao X, Su G, Ren J. Cardiac overexpression of metallothionein rescues cardiac contractile dysfunction and endoplasmic reticulum stress but not autophagy in sepsis. J Mol Cell Cardiol. 2010;48:367–78.
17. Furchgott RF, Zawadzki JV. The obligatory role of endothelial cells in the relaxation of arterial smooth muscle by acetylcholine. Nature. 1980;288:373–6.
18. Bulteau AL, Szweda LI, Friguet B. Age-dependent declines in proteasome activity in the heart. Arch Biochem Biophys. 2002;397:298–304.
19. Friguet B, Stadtman ER, Szweda LI. Modification of glucose-6-phosphate dehydrogenase by 4-hydroxy-2-nonenal. Formation of cross-linked protein that inhibits the multicatalytic protease. J Biol Chem. 1994;269:21639–43.
20. Szweda PA, Friguet B, Szweda LI. Proteolysis, free radicals, and aging. Free Radic Biol Med. 2002;33:29–36.
21. Circu ML, Aw TY. Reactive oxygen species, cellular redox systems, and apoptosis. Free Radic Biol Med. 2010;48:749–62.
22. El-Agamey A, Lowe GM, McGarvey DJ, et al. Carotenoid radical chemistry and antioxidant/pro-oxidant properties. Arch Biochem Biophys. 2004;430:37–48.
23. Kojo S. Vitamin C: basic metabolism and its function as an index of oxidative stress. Curr Med Chem. 2004;11:1041–64.
24. Nakamura H, Nakamura K, Yodoi J. Redox regulation of cellular activation. Annu Rev Immunol. 1997;15:351–69.
25. Bolz SS, Vogel L, Sollinger D, et al. Nitric oxide-induced decrease in calcium sensitivity of resistance arteries is attributable to activation of the myosin light chain phosphatase and antagonized by the RhoA/Rho kinase pathway. Circulation. 2003;107:3081–7.
26. Grossini E, Molinari C, Mary DA, et al. Urocortin II induces nitric oxide production through cAMP and Ca2+ related pathways in endothelial cells. Cell Physiol Biochem. 2009;23:87–96.
27. Clark RH, Huckaby JL, Kueser TJ, et al. Low-dose nitric oxide therapy for persistent pulmonary hypertension: 1-year follow-up. J Perinatol. 2003;23:300–3.
28. Kinsella JP, Cutter GR, Walsh WF, et al. Early inhaled nitric oxide therapy in premature newborns with respiratory failure. N Engl J Med. 2006;355:354–64.
29. Rossaint R, Falke KJ, Lopez F, Slama K, Pison U, Zapol WM. Inhaled nitric oxide for the adult respiratory distress syndrome. N Engl J Med. 1993;328:399–405.
30. Rossaint R, Gerlach H, Schmidt-Ruhnke H, et al. Efficacy of inhaled nitric oxide in patients with severe ARDS. Chest. 1995;107:1107–15.
31. Rossaint R, Slama K, Steudel W, et al. Effects of inhaled nitric oxide on right ventricular function in severe acute respiratory distress syndrome. Intensive Care Med. 1995;21:197–203.
32. Walsh MC, Hibbs AM, Martin CR, et al. Two-year neurodevelopmental outcomes of ventilated preterm infants treated with inhaled nitric oxide. J Pediatr. 2010;156:556–61.e1.
33. Ambrosio G, Tritto I, Golino P. Reactive oxygen metabolites and arterial thrombosis. Cardiovasc Res. 1997;34:445–52.

34. Cerwinka WH, Cooper D, Krieglstein CF, Ross CR, McCord JM, Granger DN. Superoxide mediates endotoxin-induced platelet-endothelial cell adhesion in intestinal venules. Am J Physiol Heart Circ Physiol. 2003;284:H535–41.

35. Lewis MS, Whatley RE, Cain P, McIntyre TM, Prescott SM, Zimmerman GA. Hydrogen peroxide stimulates the synthesis of platelet-activating factor by endothelium and induces endothelial cell-dependent neutrophil adhesion. J Clin Invest. 1988; 82:2045–55.

36. Okayama N, Coe L, Oshima T, Itoh M, Alexander JS. Intracellular mechanisms of hydrogen peroxide-mediated neutrophil adherence to cultured human endothelial cells. Microvasc Res. 1999;57:63–74.

37. Schafer A, Alp NJ, Cai S, et al. Reduced vascular NO bioavailability in diabetes increases platelet activation in vivo. Arterioscler Thromb Vasc Biol. 2004;24:1720–6.

38. Dangel O, Mergia E, Karlisch K, Groneberg D, Koesling D, Friebe A. Nitric oxide-sensitive guanylyl cyclase is the only nitric oxide receptor mediating platelet inhibition. J Thromb Haemost. 2010;8:1343–52.

39. Loscalzo J. Nitric oxide insufficiency, platelet activation, and arterial thrombosis. Circ Res. 2001;88:756–62.

40. Cooper D, Stokes KY, Tailor A, Granger DN. Oxidative stress promotes blood cell-endothelial cell interactions in the microcirculation. Cardiovasc Toxicol. 2002;2:165–80.

41. Gregg D, de Carvalho DD, Kovacic H. Integrins and coagulation: a role for ROS/redox signaling? Antioxid Redox Signal. 2004;6:757–64.

42. Okayama N, Park JH, Coe L, et al. Polynitroxyl alphaalpha-hemoglobin (PNH) inhibits peroxide and superoxide-mediated neutrophil adherence to human endothelial cells. Free Radic Res. 1999;31:53–8.

43. Herkert O, Diebold I, Brandes RP, Hess J, Busse R, Gorlach A. NADPH oxidase mediates tissue factor-dependent surface procoagulant activity by thrombin in human vascular smooth muscle cells. Circulation. 2002;105:2030–6.

44. Decoursey TE, Ligeti E. Regulation and termination of NADPH oxidase activity. Cell Mol Life Sci. 2005;62:2173–93.

45. Keisari Y, Braun L, Flescher E. The oxidative burst and related phenomena in mouse macrophages elicited by different sterile inflammatory stimuli. Immunobiology. 1983;165:78–89.

46. Kuhns DB, Alvord WG, Heller T, et al. Residual NADPH oxidase and survival in chronic granulomatous disease. N Engl J Med. 2010;363:2600–10.

47. Gonzalez C, Lopez-Lopez JR, Obeso A, Perez-Garcia MT, Rocher A. Cellular mechanisms of oxygen chemoreception in the carotid body. Respir Physiol. 1995;102:137–47.

48. Weir EK, Archer SL. The role of redox changes in oxygen sensing. Respir Physiol Neurobiol. 2010;174:182–91.

49. Griendling KK, Sorescu D, Lassegue B, Ushio-Fukai M. Modulation of protein kinase activity and gene expression by reactive oxygen species and their role in vascular physiology and pathophysiology. Arterioscler Thromb Vasc Biol. 2000;20:2175–83.

50. Thomas DD, Ridnour LA, Isenberg JS, et al. The chemical biology of nitric oxide: implications in cellular signaling. Free Radic Biol Med. 2008;45:18–31.

51. Brown GC, Bolanos JP, Heales SJ, Clark JB. Nitric oxide produced by activated astrocytes rapidly and reversibly inhibits cellular respiration. Neurosci Lett. 1995;193:201–4.

52. Cleeter MW, Cooper JM, Darley-Usmar VM, Moncada S, Schapira AH. Reversible inhibition of cytochrome c oxidase, the terminal enzyme of the mitochondrial respiratory chain, by nitric oxide. Implications for neurodegenerative diseases. FEBS Lett. 1994;345:50–4.

53. Barker JE, Bolanos JP, Land JM, Clark JB, Heales SJ. Glutathione protects astrocytes from peroxynitrite-mediated mitochondrial damage: implications for neuronal/astrocytic trafficking and neurodegeneration. Dev Neurosci. 1996;18:391–6.

54. Acuna-Castroviejo D, Escames G, Leon J, Carazo A, Khaldy H. Mitochondrial regulation by melatonin and its metabolites. Adv Exp Med Biol. 2003;527:549–57.

55. Murphy MP. How mitochondria produce reactive oxygen species. Biochem J. 2009;417:1–13.

56. Turrens JF. Mitochondrial formation of reactive oxygen species. J Physiol. 2003;552:335–44.

57. Valko M, Leibfritz D, Moncol J, Cronin MT, Mazur M, Telser J. Free radicals and antioxidants in normal physiological functions and human disease. Int J Biochem Cell Biol. 2007;39:44–84.

58. Watson RS, Carcillo JA. Scope and epidemiology of pediatric sepsis. Pediatr Crit Care Med. 2005;6:S3–5.

59. Borrelli E, Roux-Lombard P, Grau GE, et al. Plasma concentrations of cytokines, their soluble receptors, and antioxidant vitamins can predict the development of multiple organ failure in patients at risk. Crit Care Med. 1996;24:392–7.

60. Cowley HC, Bacon PJ, Goode HF, Webster NR, Jones JG, Menon DK. Plasma antioxidant potential in severe sepsis: a comparison of survivors and nonsurvivors. Crit Care Med. 1996;24:1179–83.

61. Goode HF, Cowley HC, Walker BE, Howdle PD, Webster NR. Decreased antioxidant status and increased lipid peroxidation in patients with septic shock and secondary organ dysfunction. Crit Care Med. 1995;23:646–51.

62. Dyson A, Bryan NS, Fernandez BO, et al. An integrated approach to assessing nitroso-redox balance in systemic inflammation. Free Radic Biol Med. 2010;51:1137–45.

63. Dyson A, Singer M. Tissue oxygen tension monitoring: will it fill the void? Curr Opin Crit Care. 2010;17:281–9.

64. James PE, Madhani M, Roebuck W, Jackson SK, Swartz HM. Endotoxin-induced liver hypoxia: defective oxygen delivery versus oxygen consumption. Nitric Oxide. 2002;6:18–28.

65. Lange M, Hamahata A, Traber DL, Nakano Y, Traber LD, Enkhbaatar P. Specific inhibition of nitric oxide synthases at different time points in a murine model of pulmonary sepsis. Biochem Biophys Res Commun. 2010;404:877–81.

66. Lidington D, Li F, Tyml K. Deletion of neuronal NOS prevents impaired vasodilation in septic mouse skeletal muscle. Cardiovasc Res. 2007;74:151–8.

67. Wu F, Tyml K, Wilson JX. iNOS expression requires NADPH oxidase-dependent redox signaling in microvascular endothelial cells. J Cell Physiol. 2008;217:207–14.

68. Wu F, Wilson JX, Tyml K. Ascorbate protects against impaired arteriolar constriction in sepsis by inhibiting inducible nitric oxide synthase expression. Free Radic Biol Med. 2004;37:1282–9.

69. Ovechkin AV, Lominadze D, Sedoris KC, Robinson TW, Tyagi SC, Roberts AM. Lung ischemia-reperfusion injury: implications of oxidative stress and platelet-arteriolar wall interactions. Arch Physiol Biochem. 2007;113:1–12.

70. Secor D, Li F, Ellis CG, et al. Impaired microvascular perfusion in sepsis requires activated coagulation and P-selectin-mediated platelet adhesion in capillaries. Intensive Care Med. 2010;36: 1928–34.

71. Kanaya S, Ikeda H, Haramaki N, Murohara T, Imaizumi T. Intraplatelet tetrahydrobiopterin plays an important role in regulating canine coronary arterial thrombosis by modulating intraplatelet nitric oxide and superoxide generation. Circulation. 2001; 104:2478–84.

72. Tajima M, Sakagami H. Tetrahydrobiopterin impairs the action of endothelial nitric oxide via superoxide derived from platelets. Br J Pharmacol. 2000;131:958–64.

73. Begonja AJ, Teichmann L, Geiger J, Gambaryan S, Walter U. Platelet regulation by NO/cGMP signaling and NAD(P)H oxidase-generated ROS. Blood Cells Mol Dis. 2006;36:166–70.

74. Landmesser U, Dikalov S, Price SR, et al. Oxidation of tetrahydrobiopterin leads to uncoupling of endothelial cell nitric oxide synthase in hypertension. J Clin Invest. 2003;111:1201–9.

75. Kuzkaya N, Weissmann N, Harrison DG, Dikalov S. Interactions of peroxynitrite, tetrahydrobiopterin, ascorbic acid, and thiols: implications for uncoupling endothelial nitric-oxide synthase. J Biol Chem. 2003;278:22546–54.

76. Maybauer DM, Maybauer MO, Traber LD, et al. Effects of severe smoke inhalation injury and septic shock on global hemodynamics and microvascular blood flow in sheep. Shock. 2006;26:489–95.

77. Enkhbaatar P, Joncam C, Traber L, et al. Novel ovine model of methicillin-resistant Staphylococcus aureus-induced pneumonia and sepsis. Shock. 2008;29:642–9.

78. Lange M, Hamahata A, Traber DL, et al. Effects of early neuronal and delayed inducible nitric oxide synthase blockade on cardiovascular, renal, and hepatic function in ovine sepsis. Anesthesiology. 2010;113:1376–84.

79. Crouser ED, Julian MW, Dorinsky PM. Ileal VO(2)-O(2) alterations induced by endotoxin correlate with severity of mitochondrial injury. Am J Respir Crit Care Med. 1999;160:1347–53.

80. Boekstegers P, Weidenhofer S, Kapsner T, Werdan K. Skeletal muscle partial pressure of oxygen in patients with sepsis. Crit Care Med. 1994;22:640–50.

81. Schenkman KA, Arakaki LS, Ciesielski WA, Beard DA. Optical spectroscopy demonstrates elevated intracellular oxygenation in an endotoxic model of sepsis in the perfused heart. Shock. 2007;27:695–700.

82. Singer M. Cellular dysfunction in sepsis. Clin Chest Med. 2008; 29:655–60, viii–ix.

83. Levy RJ. Mitochondrial dysfunction, bioenergetic impairment, and metabolic down-regulation in sepsis. Shock. 2007;28:24–8.

84. Brealey D, Singer M. Mitochondrial dysfunction in sepsis. Curr Infect Dis Rep. 2003;5:365–71.

85. Azevedo LC. Mitochondrial dysfunction during sepsis. Endocr Metab Immune Disord Drug Targets. 2010;10:214–23.

86. Brealey D, Brand M, Hargreaves I, et al. Association between mitochondrial dysfunction and severity and outcome of septic shock. Lancet. 2002;360:219–23.

87. Escames G, Lopez LC, Ortiz F, et al. Attenuation of cardiac mitochondrial dysfunction by melatonin in septic mice. FEBS J. 2007;274:2135–47.

88. Victor VM, De la Fuente M. Immune cells redox state from mice with endotoxin-induced oxidative stress. Involvement of NF-kappaB. Free Radic Res. 2003;37:19–27.

89. Paterson RL, Galley HF, Dhillon JK, Webster NR. Increased nuclear factor kappa B activation in critically ill patients who die. Crit Care Med. 2000;28:1047–51.

90. Paterson RL, Galley HF, Webster NR. The effect of N-acetylcysteine on nuclear factor-kappa B activation, interleukin-6, interleukin-8, and intercellular adhesion molecule-1 expression in patients with sepsis. Crit Care Med. 2003;31:2574–8.

91. Abraham E. Nuclear factor-kappaB and its role in sepsis-associated organ failure. J Infect Dis. 2003;187 Suppl 2:S364–9.

92. Brenner T, Hofer S, Rosenhagen C, et al. Macrophage migration inhibitory factor (MIF) and manganese superoxide dismutase (MnSOD) as early predictors for survival in patients with severe sepsis or septic shock. J Surg Res. 2010;164:e163–71.

93. Brenner T, Rosenhagen C, Steppan J, et al. Redox responses in patients with sepsis: high correlation of thioredoxin-1 and macrophage migration inhibitory factor plasma levels. Mediat Inflamm. 2010;2010:985614.

94. Hofer S, Rosenhagen C, Nakamura H, et al. Thioredoxin in human and experimental sepsis. Crit Care Med. 2009;37:2155–9.

95. Crimi E, Liguori A, Condorelli M, et al. The beneficial effects of antioxidant supplementation in enteral feeding in critically ill patients: a prospective, randomized, double-blind, placebo-controlled trial. Anesth Analg. 2004;99:857–63, table of contents.

96. Galley HF, Howdle PD, Walker BE, Webster NR. The effects of intravenous antioxidants in patients with septic shock. Free Radic Biol Med. 1997;23:768–74.

97. Nathens AB, Neff MJ, Jurkovich GJ, et al. Randomized, prospective trial of antioxidant supplementation in critically ill surgical patients. Ann Surg. 2002;236:814–22.

98. Wilson JX. Mechanism of action of vitamin C in sepsis: ascorbate modulates redox signaling in endothelium. Biofactors. 2009; 35:5–13.

99. Juffermans NP, Vervloet MG, Daemen-Gubbels CR, Binnekade JM, de Jong M, Groeneveld AB. A dose-finding study of methylene blue to inhibit nitric oxide actions in the hemodynamics of human septic shock. Nitric Oxide. 2010;22:275–80.

100. Donati A, Conti G, Loggi S, et al. Does methylene blue administration to septic shock patients affect vascular permeability and blood volume? Crit Care Med. 2002;30:2271–7.

101. Bakker J, Grover R, McLuckie A, et al. Administration of the nitric oxide synthase inhibitor NG-methyl-L-arginine hydrochloride (546C88) by intravenous infusion for up to 72 hours can promote the resolution of shock in patients with severe sepsis: results of a randomized, double-blind, placebo-controlled multicenter study (study no. 144-002). Crit Care Med. 2004; 32:1–12.

102. Lopez A, Lorente JA, Steingrub J, et al. Multiple-center, randomized, placebo-controlled, double-blind study of the nitric oxide synthase inhibitor 546C88: effect on survival in patients with septic shock. Crit Care Med. 2004;32:21–30.

103. Kinasewitz GT, Privalle CT, Imm A, et al. Multicenter, randomized, placebo-controlled study of the nitric oxide scavenger pyridoxalated hemoglobin polyoxyethylene in distributive shock. Crit Care Med. 2008;36:1999–2007.

104. Escames G, Acuna-Castroviejo D, Lopez LC, et al. Pharmacological utility of melatonin in the treatment of septic shock: experimental and clinical evidence. J Pharm Pharmacol. 2006;58:1153–65.

105. Lowes DA, Almawash AM, Webster NR, Reid VL, Galley HF. Melatonin and structurally similar compounds have differing effects on inflammation and mitochondrial function in endothelial cells under conditions mimicking sepsis. Br J Anaesth. 2010;107:193–201.

106. Bagci S, Horoz O, Yildizdas D, Reinsberg J, Bartmann P, Mueller A. Melatonin status in pediatric intensive care patients with sepsis. Pediatr Crit Care Med. 2012;13(2):e120–3.

107. Sheu SS, Nauduri D, Anders MW. Targeting antioxidants to mitochondria: a new therapeutic direction. Biochim Biophys Acta. 2006;1762:256–65.

108. Szeto HH. Mitochondria-targeted peptide antioxidants: novel neuroprotective agents. AAPS J. 2006;8:E521–31.

109. Smith RA, Porteous CM, Coulter CV, Murphy MP. Selective targeting of an antioxidant to mitochondria. Eur J Biochem. 1999; 263:709–16.

110. Adlam VJ, Harrison JC, Porteous CM, et al. Targeting an antioxidant to mitochondria decreases cardiac ischemia-reperfusion injury. FASEB J. 2005;19:1088–95.

111. Lowes DA, Thottakam BM, Webster NR, Murphy MP, Galley HF. The mitochondria-targeted antioxidant MitoQ protects against organ damage in a lipopolysaccharide-peptidoglycan model of sepsis. Free Radic Biol Med. 2008;45:1559–65.

112. Skulachev VP. A biochemical approach to the problem of aging: "megaproject" on membrane-penetrating ions. The first results and prospects. Biochemistry (Mosc). 2007;72:1385–96.

113. Cho J, Won K, Wu D, et al. Potent mitochondria-targeted peptides reduce myocardial infarction in rats. Coron Artery Dis. 2007;18: 215–20.

114. Petri S, Kiaei M, Kipiani K, et al. Additive neuroprotective effects of a histone deacetylase inhibitor and a catalytic antioxidant in a transgenic mouse model of amyotrophic lateral sclerosis. Neurobiol Dis. 2006;22:40–9.

115. Andrades ME, Ritter C, Dal-Pizzol F. The role of free radicals in sepsis development. Front Biosci (Elite Ed). 2009;1:277–87.

116. Crouser ED. Mitochondrial dysfunction in septic shock and multiple organ dysfunction syndrome. Mitochondrion. 2004;4:729–41.

117. Exline MC, Crouser ED. Mitochondrial mechanisms of sepsis-induced organ failure. Front Biosci. 2008;13:5030–41.

118. Fink MP. Bench-to-bedside review: cytopathic hypoxia. Crit Care. 2002;6:491–9.

119. Huet O, Dupic L, Harrois A, Duranteau J. Oxidative stress and endothelial dysfunction during sepsis. Front Biosci. 2011;16:1986–95.

120. Protti A, Singer M. Bench-to-bedside review: potential strategies to protect or reverse mitochondrial dysfunction in sepsis-induced organ failure. Crit Care. 2006;10:228.

121. Berg RM, Moller K, Bailey DM. Neuro-oxidative-nitrosative stress in sepsis. J Cereb Blood Flow Metab. 2010;31:1532–44.

122. Dare AJ, Phillips AR, Hickey AJ, et al. A systematic review of experimental treatments for mitochondrial dysfunction in sepsis and multiple organ dysfunction syndrome. Free Radic Biol Med. 2009;47:1517–25.

123. Liang LP, Ho YS, Patel M. Mitochondrial superoxide production in kainate-induced hippocampal damage. Neuroscience. 2000;101:563–70.

124. Liang LP, Patel M. Seizure-induced changes in mitochondrial redox status. Free Radic Biol Med. 2006;40:316–22.

125. Tejada S, Roca C, Sureda A, Rial RV, Gamundi A, Esteban S. Antioxidant response analysis in the brain after pilocarpine treatments. Brain Res Bull. 2006;69:587–92.

126. Mustafa AG, Singh IN, Wang J, Carrico KM, Hall ED. Mitochondrial protection after traumatic brain injury by scavenging lipid peroxyl radicals. J Neurochem. 2010;114:271–80.

127. Waldbaum S, Liang LP, Patel M. Persistent impairment of mitochondrial and tissue redox status during lithium-pilocarpine-induced epileptogenesis. J Neurochem. 2010;115:1172–82.

128. Sudha K, Rao AV, Rao A. Oxidative stress and antioxidants in epilepsy. Clin Chim Acta. 2001;303:19–24.

129. Kunz WS, Kudin AP, Vielhaber S, et al. Mitochondrial complex I deficiency in the epileptic focus of patients with temporal lobe epilepsy. Ann Neurol. 2000;48:766–73.

130. Mueller SG, Trabesinger AH, Boesiger P, Wieser HG. Brain glutathione levels in patients with epilepsy measured by in vivo (1) H-MRS. Neurology. 2001;57:1422–7.

131. Kondo T, Reaume AG, Huang TT, et al. Reduction of CuZn-superoxide dismutase activity exacerbates neuronal cell injury and edema formation after transient focal cerebral ischemia. J Neurosci. 1997;17:4180–9.

132. Liang LP, Patel M. Mitochondrial oxidative stress and increased seizure susceptibility in Sod2(-/+) mice. Free Radic Biol Med. 2004;36:542–54.

133. Melov S, Doctrow SR, Schneider JA, et al. Lifespan extension and rescue of spongiform encephalopathy in superoxide dismutase 2 nullizygous mice treated with superoxide dismutase-catalase mimetics. J Neurosci. 2001;21:8348–53.

134. Murakami K, Kondo T, Epstein CJ, Chan PH. Overexpression of CuZn-superoxide dismutase reduces hippocampal injury after global ischemia in transgenic mice. Stroke. 1997;28:1797–804.

135. Pineda JA, Aono M, Sheng H, et al. Extracellular superoxide dismutase overexpression improves behavioral outcome from closed head injury in the mouse. J Neurotrauma. 2001;18:625–34.

136. Xu Y, Liachenko SM, Tang P, Chan PH. Faster recovery of cerebral perfusion in SOD1-overexpressed rats after cardiac arrest and resuscitation. Stroke. 2009;40:2512–8.

137. Robertson CL. Mitochondrial dysfunction contributes to cell death following traumatic brain injury in adult and immature animals. J Bioenerg Biomembr. 2004;36:363–8.

138. Slemmer JE, Shacka JJ, Sweeney MI, Weber JT. Antioxidants and free radical scavengers for the treatment of stroke, traumatic brain injury and aging. Curr Med Chem. 2008;15:404–14.

139. Waldbaum S, Patel M. Mitochondria, oxidative stress, and temporal lobe epilepsy. Epilepsy Res. 2010;88:23–45.

140. Sullivan PG, Rabchevsky AG, Waldmeier PC, Springer JE. Mitochondrial permeability transition in CNS trauma: cause or effect of neuronal cell death? J Neurosci Res. 2005;79:231–9.

141. Natale JE, Knight JB, Cheng Y, Rome JE, Gallo V. Metallothionein I and II mitigate age-dependent secondary brain injury. J Neurosci Res. 2004;78:303–14.

142. Suzuki K, Nakajima K, Otaki N, Kimura M. Metallothionein in developing human brain. Biol Signals. 1994;3:188–92.

143. Nishida A, Misaki Y, Kuruta H, Takashima S. Developmental expression of copper, zinc-superoxide dismutase in human brain by chemiluminescence. Brain Dev. 1994;16:40–3.

144. Bayir H, Kochanek PM, Kagan VE. Oxidative stress in immature brain after traumatic brain injury. Dev Neurosci. 2006;28:420–31.

145. Smith SL, Andrus PK, Gleason DD, Hall ED. Infant rat model of the shaken baby syndrome: preliminary characterization and evidence for the role of free radicals in cortical hemorrhaging and progressive neuronal degeneration. J Neurotrauma. 1998;15:693–705.

146. Kuo JR, Lo CJ, Chang CP, Lin MT, Chio CC. Attenuation of brain nitrostative and oxidative damage by brain cooling during experimental traumatic brain injury. J Biomed Biotechnol. 2010;2011:145214.

147. Bayir H, Adelson PD, Wisniewski SR, et al. Therapeutic hypothermia preserves antioxidant defenses after severe traumatic brain injury in infants and children. Crit Care Med. 2009;37:689–95.

148. Adelson PD, Wisniewski SR, Beca J, Brown SD, Bell M, Muizelaar JP, Okada P, Beers SR, Balasubramani GK, Hirtz D, Paediatric Traumatic Brain Injury Consortium. Comparison of hypothermia and normothermia after severe traumatic brain injury in children (Cool Kids): a phase 3, randomised controlled trial. Lancet Neurol. 2013;12(6):546–53.

149. Hinerfeld D, Traini MD, Weinberger RP, et al. Endogenous mitochondrial oxidative stress: neurodegeneration, proteomic analysis, specific respiratory chain defects, and efficacious antioxidant therapy in superoxide dismutase 2 null mice. J Neurochem. 2004;88:657–67.

150. Liang LP, Jarrett SG, Patel M. Chelation of mitochondrial iron prevents seizure-induced mitochondrial dysfunction and neuronal injury. J Neurosci. 2008;28:11550–6.

151. Kim do Y, Rho JM. The ketogenic diet and epilepsy. Curr Opin Clin Nutr Metab Care. 2008;11:113–20.

152. Milder JB, Liang LP, Patel M. Acute oxidative stress and systemic Nrf2 activation by the ketogenic diet. Neurobiol Dis. 2010;40:238–44.

153. Nazarewicz RR, Ziolkowski W, Vaccaro PS, Ghafourifar P. Effect of short-term ketogenic diet on redox status of human blood. Rejuvenation Res. 2007;10:435–40.

154. Jarrett SG, Milder JB, Liang LP, Patel M. The ketogenic diet increases mitochondrial glutathione levels. J Neurochem. 2008;106:1044–51.

Ischemia-Reperfusion Injury

Michael J. Hobson and Basilia Zingarelli

Abstract

Ischemia-reperfusion injury is common in many conditions in the intensive care unit. These clinical conditions include myocardial infarction, cerebral ischemia, stroke, solid organ transplantation, soft tissue flaps, extremity reimplantation, trauma, shock, or any other condition associated with low cardiac output or scarce oxygen utilization. While ischemia itself causes tissue damage, reperfusion may exacerbate this damage by inducing an inflammatory response and further contributing to tissue injury. Protection of tissues against injury by ischemia and reperfusion is, therefore, an issue of utmost clinical interest. This chapter provides a critical and comprehensive overview of the molecular and cellular mechanisms that lead to ischemia and reperfusion injury.

Keywords

Ischemia-reperfusion • Endothelial dysfunction • Neutrophils • Oxidative stress • Ischemic preconditioning

Introduction

Ischemia and reperfusion injury plays a critical role in several clinical conditions, including myocardial infarction, cerebral ischemia, stroke, solid organ transplantation, soft tissue flaps, extremity reimplantation, hemorrhagic and other cardiovascular shock conditions with low cardiac output. A dramatic reduction of oxygen supply may cause ischemia in a whole organ (global ischemia) or defined tissue territories (focal ischemia) and rapidly results in cell metabolic derangement, molecular alterations and dysfunction

M.J. Hobson, MD
Division of Critical Care Medicine,
Cincinnati Children's Hospital Medical Center,
3333 Burnet Avenue, Cincinnati, OH 45225, USA
e-mail: michael.hobson@cchmc.org

B. Zingarelli, MD, PhD (✉)
Division of Critical Care Medicine,
Cincinnati Children's Hospital Medical Center,
3333 Burnet Avenue, Cincinnati, OH 45229, USA
e-mail: basilia.zingarelli@cchmc.org

sequelae. If not reversed within a short period of time, the cellular dysmetabolism progresses to complete depletion of the energetic pools, accumulation of toxic substances and eventually to cell death. In all clinical conditions of ischemia, the main therapeutic intervention requires restoration of the blood flow (reperfusion) and/or recovery of the normal oxygen levels (re-oxygenation). Once perfusion is re-established tissue ischemia is generally reversed. However, a paradoxical injury process is elicited that can be simply characterized as an exaggerated inflammatory response leading to cellular death and organ dysfunction. Although the mechanisms underlying the phenomenon of ischemia and reperfusion injury have not been precisely defined, toxicity by reactive oxygen free radicals and oxidants, leukocyte-endothelial cell adhesion, and a marked inflammatory reaction have been implicated in the process of injury. The endothelium is damaged in the early minutes after reperfusion, i.e. before neutrophils accumulate and before tissue necrosis fully develops, and this suggests that endothelial injury is a crucial event in the post-ischemic inflammatory cascade. Neutrophil adherence to vascular endothelium is then an important event initiating further leukocyte activation

Table 24.1 Clinical conditions of cell hypoxia/ischemia

Reduction of DO₂		Increase of VO₂
Reduction of CaO₂	Reduction of CO	
Artery occlusion	Hypovolemic shock	Sepsis
Solid organ transplantation	Cardiogenic shock	Septic shock
Tissue and limb reimplantation	Cardiopulmonary bypass	
Severe hypotension	Congestive heart failure	
Hypobaric conditions	Dysrhythmias	
Drug-induced vasoconstriction		
Anemia		
Hemorrhage		

and release of cytodestructive agents (reactive species or enzymes), which in turn leads to amplification of the endothelial damage and to parenchyma or tissue injury.

Metabolic Derangements of Ischemia

Alteration of Oxygen Supply

Cells of all tissues undergo irreversible injury and death when deprived of oxygen and other nutrients. Oxygen delivery (DO₂) depends upon two variables: volume flow rate of blood (as determined by the cardiac output [CO]) and arterial oxygen content (CaO₂) [1]. Therefore, tissue *ischemia* may result as a consequence of arterial occlusion within the perfusion territory of an affected vessel or may be induced by insufficient tissue perfusion due to limited pump flow (Table 24.1). However, in some clinical conditions inadequate tissue energetic metabolism may derive by an increase in total body oxygen consumption (VO₂). For example, during septic shock, oxygenation of the splanchnic territory may be inadequate even in the presence of normal hepatic-splanchnic blood flow. This event is due to a major increase in metabolic demand and impaired oxygen extraction [2]. Tissue *hypoxia* may also occur as a result of reduced content or saturation of hemoglobin (i.e., severe anemia). In conditions of ischemia, energy failure develops rapidly and removal of toxic metabolites is often compromised. On the contrary, in conditions of hypoxia metabolic substrate delivery and energy production can continue and waste removal is maintained. Therefore, ischemia is a more deleterious event than hypoxia.

Energy Failure and Calcium Overload During Ischemia

Although quantitative and kinetic features of ischemic injury are different for each specialized cell type, several metabolic responses are shared (Fig. 24.1). Immediately upon ischemia, a time-dependent cascade of metabolic events occurs. The first event is a rapid depletion of intracellular adenosine triphosphate (ATP) stores and other high-energy phosphate compounds (such as creatine phosphate in the heart). The cell shifts from oxidative metabolism to an inefficient anaerobic glycolysis, producing only 2 mol of ATP/mol of glucose instead of the 38 mol of ATP normally produced during aerobic metabolism. This collapse of high-energy phosphate compounds impairs the energy-dependent cell processes, such as membrane ion pumps (Na⁺/H⁺ exchanger) and protein synthesis. Within seconds or minutes, these abnormalities become sufficiently severe to reduce cell function. For example, in the heart this metabolic derangement translates into reduction of the contractile force generated by actin-myosin cross-bridge formation; in the gut altered intestinal absorptive function is associated with translocation of bacteria from the intestine to the lymphatic vessels and blood stream.

Anaerobic glycolysis leads to glycogen depletion and lactate accumulation, which, in conjunction with increased inorganic phosphates from ATP hydrolysis, reduce intracellular and extracellular pH. Membrane depolarization and failure of ATP- dependent ion pumps leads to efflux of potassium and influx of sodium and calcium. Increase of intracellular sodium concentration is accompanied by water influx into the cell, leading to swelling of the cytoplasm and organelles, such as mitochondria and endoplasmic reticulum. At this point if oxygen supply is restored, cell injury is reversible. However if ischemia persists, cell injury may become irreversible. Increase of cytosol and mitochondrial concentration of calcium overcomes the cell calcium-exporting capacity. Mitochondria show amorphous matrix densities and granular dense bodies of calcium phosphate, which are considered the earliest sign of irreversible ischemic cell injury. Mitochondria play an important role in ischemic damage. Indeed, the excessive energy demand is likely to represent a crucial factor in the ensuing irreversible damage of cells, especially in cardiomyocytes, where the cell volume occupied by mitochondria is the greatest among all the cell types. A major role in the progression towards cell death might be attributed to the opening

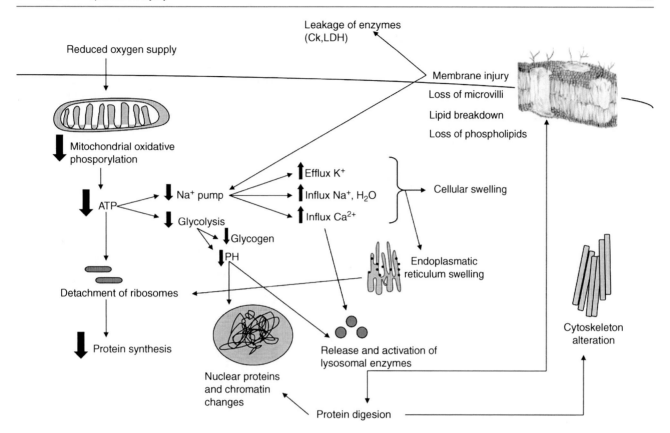

Fig. 24.1 Metabolic events and cellular derangement during ischemia. After reduction of oxygen supply, mitochondrial oxidative phosporylation is decreased with subsequent decrease in ATP generation and rate of glycolysis, and a progressive loss of glycogen content and decrease of protein synthesis. Accumulation of lactate and increased inorganic phosphates from ATP hydrolysis reduce intracellular and extracellular pH and cause membrane depolarization. This energy collapse impairs the membrane ion pumps resulting in increase of intracellular levels of Na^+, Ca^{2+} and influx of water, and decrease of intracellular levels of K^+. Water influx into the cell leads to swelling of the cytoplasm and organelles, such as mitochondria and endoplasmic reticulum, further impairing mitochondrial oxidative phosporylation and protein synthesis. The cytosol calcium overload causes activation of a number of enzymes (proteases, phospholipase, ATPase) and disrupts lysosomal membranes, further promoting the release of other acid hydrolases. Protein digestion by these lysosomal enzymes causes cellular damage at the cytoskeleton, nucleus and plasma membrane. After cell death, disruption of cell membrane leads to leakage of intracellular enzymes and proteins into the extracellular milieu such as creatine kinase (CK), lactate dehydrogenase (LDH) and others

of the *mitochondrial permeability transition pore*, which besides abolishing mitochondrial ATP production amplifies the damage by causing NAD^+ release.

The cytosol and mitochondrial calcium overload causes activation of a number of enzymes (proteases, phospholipase, ATPase), and disrupts mitochondrial and lysosomal membranes, further uncoupling mitochondrial oxidative phosphorylation and promoting the release of other acid hydrolases [3]. Cell death then occurs mainly by necrosis and is associated with widespread leakage of cellular enzymes or proteins across the cell membrane and into the plasma, which may provide important diagnostic tools of cell damage (such as the serum increase of creatine kinase and troponin levels for the diagnosis of myocardial infarction). However, apoptosis is also a major contributor of cell death and is activated by release of pro-apoptotic components from the altered mitochondria.

The Reperfusion Injury

Restoration of blood flow or oxygen supply is a mandatory therapeutic approach to resuscitate an ischemic tissue and can result in recovery of cell function if the cell is reversibly injured. Paradoxically, reoxygenation initiates a cascade of events that may lead to additional cell injury known as *reperfusion injury*. At least four major components contribute to reperfusion injury: oxidative and nitrosative stress, endothelial dysfunction, neutrophil activation and complement activation.

Oxidative and Nitrosative Stress

A delicate balance between intracellular oxidants and antioxidants likely influences many physiological functions of the cell. However, this balance is altered during reperfusion.

Fig. 24.2 Direct cellular injury by reactive oxygen and nitrogen species. Free radicals and oxidants may induce oxidation, carbonyl formation and nitrosylation, influencing the structure and function of many enzymes, proteins, lipids and DNA. DNA damage results in the activation of the nuclear enzyme poly (ADP-ribose) polymerase-1 (PARP-1), which causes depletion of the NAD$^+$ and ATP energetic pools and alteration of gene expression

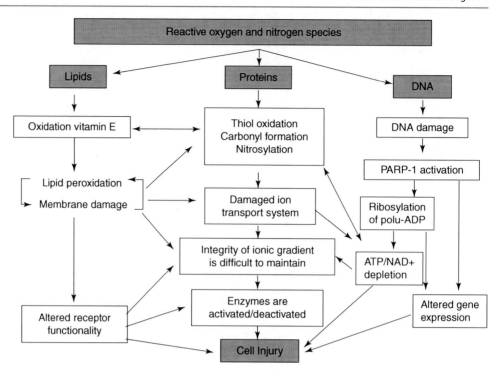

The restoration of oxygen supply to the ischemic tissue is responsible for a further cellular dysmetabolism since it induces the production of potent reactive species. Endothelial cells represent the first target of this event. The reactive species include reactive oxygen and nitrogen species such as superoxide (O_2^-), hydrogen peroxide (H_2O_2), oxidized lipoproteins, lipid peroxides, nitric oxide (NO) and peroxynitrite (ONOO) [4, 5]. Reactive species can be formed by several mechanisms; they can be produced by reduction of molecular oxygen in altered mitochondria; by enzymes such as xanthine oxidase (XO), NAD(P)H oxidase, cytochrome P450, nitric oxide synthetase (NOS) and cyclo-oxygenase (COX); and by auto-oxidation of catecholamines. Briefly, the production of oxyradicals starts early in the ischemic period in mitochondria with altered redox balance in endothelial or parenchymal cells and is further enhanced during reperfusion by a massive activation of XO in endothelial cells, and NAD(P)H oxidase in infiltrated neutrophils [4].

These reactive species mediate tissue injury by two main mechanisms: directly by inducing damage of important cellular macromolecules, and indirectly by activating signal transduction pathways, which are responsible for the production of inflammatory mediators and/or apoptotic mediators.

Direct Oxidative and Nitrosative Injury: Damage of Macromolecules, DNA and Activation of Poly (ADP-ribose) Polymerase-1 (PARP-1)

As highly reactive species, free radicals and oxidants induce oxidation of sulfhydryl groups and thioethers, as well as nitration and hydroxylation of aromatic compounds, thus influencing the structure and function of many enzymes, proteins, lipids and DNA [6, 7]. For instance, lipid peroxidation results in disruption of the cell membrane as well as the membranes of cellular organelles, and causes the release of highly cytotoxic products such as malondialdehyde. Modification of proteins by reactive oxygen and nitrogen species can cause inactivation of critical enzymes and can induce denaturation that renders proteins nonfunctional. For instance, tyrosine nitration induced by peroxynitrite or nitrogen derivatives may lead to dysfunction of superoxide dismutase and cytoskeletal actin [6]. Oxidation of sulfhydryl groups is responsible for the inhibition of critical mitochondrial enzymes [8] (Fig. 24.2).

Another important interaction occurs with nucleic acids, with the production of 8-hydroxydeoxyguanosine, 8-nitroguanine and the occurrence of DNA fragmentation [9]. The occurrence of DNA breakage results in the activation of the nuclear enzyme poly (ADP-ribose) polymerase-1 (PARP-1), which further amplifies tissue damage [10, 11] (Fig. 24.2). PARP-1 is a chromatin-associated nuclear enzyme, which possesses putative DNA repair function in eukaryotic cells. The enzyme is composed of three functional domains: an N-terminal DNA binding domain that binds to DNA strand breaks, a central automodification domain containing auto-poly (ADP-ribosyl)ation sites, and a C-terminal catalytic domain. Binding of the N-terminal domain to DNA nicks and breaks activates the C-terminal catalytic domain that, in turn, cleaves NAD$^+$ into ADP-ribose and nicotinamide. PARP-1 covalently attaches ADP-ribose to various nuclear proteins and PARP-1 itself and then extends the initial ADP-ribose group into a nucleic acid-like polymer, poly-(ADP)ribose. Extensive poly(ADP-ribosyl)ation can be induced by a wide variety of inflammatory stimuli including reactive species [12, 13]. Although poly(ADP-ribosyl)ation is an attempt of the cell to repair DNA, it appears that this process may be more harmful than beneficial. Once activated, in response to nicks and breaks in the strand DNA, PARP-1 initiates an energy consuming cycle, which rapidly depletes the intracellular NAD^+ and ATP energetic pools, slows the rate of glycolysis and mitochondrial respiration, and progresses to a loss of cellular viability postulated as a *suicide phenomenon* [13]. Several experimental reports have demonstrated that activation of PARP-1 is a major cytotoxic pathway of tissue injury in different pathologies associated with ischemia and reperfusion injury, and inflammation. Genetic deletion and pharmacological inhibition of PARP-1 has been shown to attenuate tissue injury in rodents after myocardial, cerebral and splanchnic infarction, cardiopulmonary bypass, sepsis, hemorrhagic shock, diabetes, and other conditions of inflammation [10–15]. In addition to the energetic failure, PARP-1 activation and poly(ADP-ribosyl)ation may also cause tissue damage by playing a role in gene expression. Experimental reports have suggested that PARP-1, by direct protein interaction and/or by poly(ADP-ribosyl)ation, alters the function of a variety of transcription factors, including the pro-inflammatory factors nuclear factor-κB (NF-κB) and activator protein-1 (AP-1), and the cytoprotective heat shock factor-1 (HSF-1), thus modulating the gene expression of several inflammatory mediators [12, 16, 17].

Clinical studies have reported that elevated plasma levels of the oxidative DNA adduct 8-hydroxydeoxyguanosine increase in adult patients with myocardial infarction and reperfusion during primary percutaneous coronary intervention and are associated with enhanced activation of PARP-1 in circulating leukocytes [18]. In a randomized, placebo-controlled, single-blind study in patients undergoing primary percutaneous coronary intervention, administration of a PARP inhibitor was safe and was associated with a trend of blunting inflammation [19].

Indirect Oxidative and Nitrosative Injury: The Interactive Role of Oxidants with Protein Kinases, Phosphatases and Transcription Factors

Another mechanism by which reactive oxygen and nitrogen species can induce tissue damage is via regulation of transcription pathways that regulate the pro-inflammatory profile of the cell. The exact intracellular molecular signaling mechanism of action of reactive oxygen and nitrogen species has not been completely characterized. However, it appears that reactive species may regulate cellular function through changes of critical thiol groups or aminoacid residues of mitogen-activated protein kinases and their regulatory

phosphatases, which are important components of an extensive network of interconnected signal transduction pathways [20, 21]. Mitogen-activated protein kinases mediate the transduction of extracellular signals from the receptor levels to the nuclear transcription factors. These kinases activate each other by sequential steps of phosphorylation; whereas their inactivation is mediated by phosphatases through dephosphorylation. At the downstream of this cascade, oxidant sensitive kinases include the extracellular signal-regulated kinase 1 and 2 (ERK 1/2), c-Jun amino-terminal kinase (JNK), P-38, and inhibitor κB kinase (IKK) [22]. Phosphorylation of ERK, JNK, P-38 and IKK activates nuclear proteins and transcription factors.

At the nuclear level, one critical transcription factor is NF-κB. NF-κB is ubiquitously found in all mammalian cells, and is central to the activation of several cytokines and inflammatory modulators in ischemia and reperfusion. NF-κB is usually present in the cytoplasm of the cell in an inactive state, bound to a related inhibitory protein known as inhibitor κBα (IκBα). A common pathway for the activation of NF-κB occurs when its inhibitor protein IκBα is phosphorylated by IKK [23]. Phosphorylated IκBα is targeted for rapid ubiquitination, and then degraded by the 26S proteasome. Degradation of IκBα unmasks the nuclear translocation sequence of NF-κB, allowing NF-κB to enter the nucleus, resulting in direct transcription of target genes [23].

Activator protein-1 (AP-1), another nuclear transcription factor, is also purportedly regulated by reactive species and is involved in the transcriptional expression of several genes involved in inflammation. AP-1 is a collective term referring to dimeric transcription factors commonly composed of c-Jun and c-Fos, or other activating subunits. AP-1 activation also requires phosphorylation of its subunits by JNK [24].

These signaling cascades are rapid and enable the cells to respond to environmental changes by inducing a prompt production of inflammatory mediators, such as cytokines, adhesion molecules, chemokines and metabolic enzymes, thus determining the functional outcome in response to stress. It is important to note that several of the inflammatory mediators, which are regulated by NF-κB (e.g., TNFα and IL-1), and/or AP-1 can in turn further activate these transcription factors, thus creating a self-maintaining inflammatory cycle that increases the severity and the duration of the inflammatory response [23–25] (Fig. 24.3). Activation of NF-κB and AP-1 has been demonstrated during reperfusion in ischemic brain, heart and liver and in conditions of sepsis and hemorrhagic shock in several experimental studies [16, 17, 26–28]. This data has been confirmed in humans, since nuclear translocation of NF-κB, in correlation with increase of AP-1 has been found in cardiac biopsies of adult patients with unstable angina [29]. Nuclear translocation of NF-κB has been found in myocardial tissue samples of infants and children with congenital heart disease before and after

Fig. 24.3 Activation of signal transduction pathways. Oxygen and nitrogen reactive species and several inflammatory mediators are potent stimuli for the activation of a cascade of mitogen-activated kinases. At the downstream of this cascade, the inhibitor κB kinase (IKK) phosphorylates inhibitor κB (IκBα) allowing its ubiquinitation and degradation. This event unmasks the nuclear factor-κB (NF-κB), which is free to translocate into the nucleus to initiate gene transcription. Similarly, once activated, c-Jun amino-terminal kinase (JNK) phosphorylates c-Jun allowing its dimerization with c-Fos, thus forming the transcription factor activator protein-1 (AP-1). Activation of both NF-κB and AP-1 induces production of inflammatory mediators, such as cytokines, adhesion molecules, enzymes (i.e., COX-2 and iNOS) and apoptotic modulators

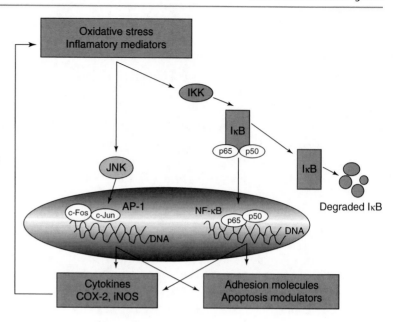

cardiopulmonary bypass, thus suggesting the contribution of inflammation to cardiac dysfunction [30]. The potential causative role of NF-κB activation in reperfusion injury is also supported by several studies in rodents demonstrating that pharmacological inhibitors of NF-κB exerts beneficial effects in models of myocardial ischemia and reperfusion injury, hemorrhagic shock and sepsis [23, 31]. These reports suggest that targeting nuclear transcription factors may represent an effective therapeutic approach in the treatment of ischemia and reperfusion. However, this hypothesis remains to be confirmed in human studies.

Sources of Reactive Oxygen and Nitrogen Species

Mitochondrial Production

The production of oxyradicals starts early in the ischemic period in mitochondria with altered redox balance. During ischemia, the metabolic reduction of the adenine nucleotide pool leaves the mitochondrial carrier in a more fully reduced state, which results in electron leakage from the respiratory chain. This increase in electron leakage reacts with residual molecular oxygen entrapped within the inner mitochondrial membrane, yielding to superoxide radical production. Re-introduction of oxygen with reperfusion re-energizes the mitochondria, but electron leakage further increases because of the ADP low content, enabling more reactions with molecular oxygen [4].

Xanthine Oxidase

The xanthine oxido-reductase enzyme system plays an important role in the catabolism of purine. It is mostly localized in the vascular endothelial, smooth muscle, and epithelial cells and exists in two interconvertible forms; xanthine

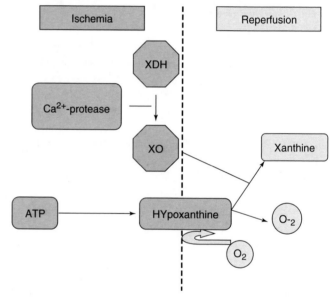

Fig. 24.4 Formation of superoxide anion (O_2^-) by xanthine oxidase (XO). During ischemia, xanthine dehydrogenase (XDH) is converted to XO by a Ca^{2+}-dependent protease. At the same time, ATP is degraded to hypoxanthine. During reperfusion, in the presence of large quantities of oxygen (O_2) and hypoxanthine, XO produces large amounts of O_2^-

dehydrogenase (XDH) and xanthine oxidase (XO) [32–34]. During ischemia, XDH is converted to the oxidase form by a protease activated by the intracellular overload of calcium. At the same time, ATP is degraded to hypoxanthine, which accumulates in the ischemic tissue. During reperfusion, with the presence of large quantities of molecular oxygen and high concentrations of hypoxanthine, XO yields to a burst of superoxide (Fig. 24.4). The xanthine oxido-reductase enzyme system has been shown to catalyze the reduction of nitrates and nitrites to nitrites and NO, respectively, thus also contributing to NO generation during ischemic conditions and during reperfusion [35, 36]. The hypothesis that generation of superoxide by XO may play a pathogenetic role in reperfusion injury has been supported by studies demonstrating that inactivation of XO with allopurinol ameliorates reperfusion-induced tissue damage in experimental animals and adult patients with myocardial infarction [37]. However, the role of XO in reperfusion injury in various organs is not fully confirmed. For example, there are no conclusive data to determine whether allopurinol has clinically important benefits for newborn infants with hypoxic-ischemic encephalopathy [38]. Furthermore, it appears that the conversion of XDH to XO is too slow to play a major role in the pathogenesis of ischemia and reperfusion injury in the liver [39]. The distribution of the XO among tissues varies variably with very low activity detected in the human heart, where it is located in the endothelium only, but not in the myocytes [40]. Interestingly, elevated plasma levels of XO have been reported in patients subjected to ischemia and reperfusion induced by limb tourniquets [41, 42], liver transplantation [43], or with small intestine infarct [44]. These circulating levels may bind to endothelial cells of distant sites and contribute to initiate oxidative damage in organs remote from the original ischemic tissue [34]. Therefore, because XO is present mainly in endothelial cells and as a circulating form in the plasma, XO-derived free radicals may play a role in mediating neutrophil adhesion by activating signal transduction pathways to the endothelium rather than directly inducing tissue damage.

Oxidative Burst from the Infiltrated Neutrophils: The NAD(P)H Oxidase

Secondary to endothelial activation, the local accumulation and activation of neutrophils significantly enhances local production of reactive oxygen species. Neutrophils contain the complex enzyme NAD(P)H oxidase which is a rich source of both superoxide and the potent oxidizing and chlorinating agent HOCl [4].

Nitric Oxide and Nitrosative Stress

Nitric oxide (NO) is a highly reactive gas and is synthesized from L-arginine by a family of enzymes known as NO synthase (NOS). Three isoforms of NOS have been identified: neuronal (nNOS or type 1), inducible (iNOS or type 2) and endothelial (eNOS or type 3) [45]. The eNOS and nNOS isoforms are constitutively expressed, calcium/calmodulin dependent, and produce low amount of NO. The iNOS isoform is a calcium/calmodulin-independent enzyme, which is responsible for a high output of NO and is expressed in almost every cell type in response to inflammatory cytokines and growth factors during diverse pathological conditions including sepsis, hemorrhagic shock, trauma and ischemia.

Under normal conditions, the constitutive forms of NOS release low concentrations of NO, which are critical to

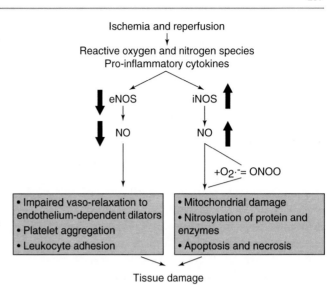

Fig. 24.5 Impairment of nitric oxide (NO) synthesis during ischemia and reperfusion. Oxygen and nitrogen reactive species and several inflammatory mediators may reduce NO production from the constitutive eNOS, thus impairing vascular relaxation to endothelium-dependent vasodilators and predisposing the endothelium to platelet aggregation and leukocyte adhesion. In severe ischemia and reperfusion high levels of NO may be produced by iNOS. Cytotoxic effects may be mediated directly by NO and/or indirectly by peroxynitrite, which is formed from the reaction of NO with superoxide. NO and peroxynitrite may inhibit the mitochondrial respiratory chain, induce nitrosylation of proteins and enzymes, and cause cell apoptosis and/or necrosis

normal physiology. For example, the nNOS-derived NO acts as a neurotransmitter and a second messenger. The eNOS-derived NO is the physiological mediator of vascular tone. Once formed by vascular endothelial cells, NO diffuses to adjacent smooth muscle cells and activates soluble guanylate cyclase, producing cGMP and reducing intracellular calcium concentration, thus resulting in vasodilatation. The endothelium-derived NO also scavenges oxygen free radicals, inhibits platelet aggregation and leukocyte adherence, and inhibits smooth muscle proliferation, thus maintaining normal tissue perfusion and vascular permeability. In the cardiomyocytes, under physiological conditions, both constitutive forms of NOS (type 1 and 3) have been described to release NO, which regulates cardiac function through direct effects on several aspects of cardiomyocyte contractility, from the fine regulation of excitation-contraction coupling (with positive inotropic and lusitropic effects) to modulation of (presynaptic and postsynaptic) autonomic signaling and mitochondrial respiration [45, 46].

It is well established that ischemia and reperfusion results in alteration of the NO pathway which may be summarized in two main events: (i) impairment of eNOS activity, and (ii) induction of iNOS (Fig. 24.5). After prolonged ischemia, and immediately at the onset of reperfusion, the burst of oxidants and the release of pro-inflammatory cytokines cooperate to reduce NO production from the constitutive eNOS, by scavenging effects and by reducing eNOS mRNA stability and expression, respectively [47–49]. Thus, reduction of NO release from the reperfusion-injured endothelium impairs vascular relaxation to endothelium-dependent vasodilators and predisposes the vascular endothelium to platelet aggregation and leukocyte adhesion. This early attenuation of endothelium-dependent vasodilatation has been considered a sensitive marker of endothelial dysfunction after ischemia and reperfusion in the heart and other vascular beds. Because of the very important effects of NO on vascular tone and thrombogenicity, drugs that can modulate NO levels have been used as therapeutic agents for the various angina syndromes for a long time and are also used in congestive heart failure and patients with left ventricular dysfunction. Nitrovasodilators, such as nitroprusside, that act by donating NO spontaneously, or glyceryl trinitrite and isosorbide dinitrate, that release NO after metabolic conversions, are able to activate guanylate cyclase and elevate cGMP in the vasculature, thus providing favorable hemodynamic effects, including vasodilatation, reduction of myocardial work, and reduction of oxygen consumption [50].

However, in severe ischemia and reperfusion high levels of NO are produced by iNOS and may be responsible for potentially noxious effects. Cytotoxic effects may be mediated directly by NO and/or indirectly by reactive NO-derived byproducts. In fact, when NO is produced in massive outburst, it reacts with superoxide to form the toxic oxidant peroxynitrite. Peroxynitrite causes oxidation of sulfhydryls, lipid peroxidation, RNA and DNA breakage [8, 9, 14], reacts with thiols, inhibits the mitochondrial respiratory chain by inactivating complexes I-III and induces nitration of tyrosine residues in proteins to form nitrotyrosine, thus altering protein structure and function. In the highly oxidative milieu of the reperfused tissue, in addition to peroxynitrite several other chemical reactions, involving nitrite, hypochlorous acid and peroxidases can induce tyrosine nitration and contribute to tissue damage [9]. Furthermore, NO can react with oxygen to yield other reactive intermediates. The nitrosative reactive species contribute then to cell dysfunction and death. The deleterious effects are mainly related to mitochondrial damage, collapse of the energetic capacity, and induction of apoptosis by releasing proteins from the mitochondria, and necrosis by lysis of plasma membrane [5–9]. However, the role of NO in ischemia and reperfusion injury is not completely known since several experimental studies with inhibitors of NO synthesis have reported controversial data [5]. It appears that multiple factors, such as NO concentration, redox status of the cell, NO-superoxide radical ratio, and length of ischemia will determine whether NO serves as a cytoprotective or cytotoxic agent. Certainly, in acute conditions of ischemia, small amounts of the endothelium-derived NO are important for the regulation of microvascular permeability and maintenance of local perfusion. On the contrary, in severe prolonged ischemia and reperfusion overproduction of NO may mediate deleterious effects.

Other Sources

It has been suggested that the ischemia and reperfusion-induced calcium overload activates phopholipases, which degrade cell membrane phospholipids releasing arachidonic acid [4]. Formation of prostaglandins and leukotrienes from arachidonic acid involves electron transfer that can initiate the formation of free radicals. Auto-oxidation of catecholamines may also contribute to oxygen free radicals, especially in ischemic myocardium, where catecholamines are released in abundance [4]. In ischemia-induced neurodegenerative disorders, the metabolism of dopamine produces reactive oxygen species (peroxide, superoxide, and hydroxyl radical), and a potent reactive quinone moiety [51]. However, the precise contribution of arachidonic acid metabolites and oxidation of catecholamines in reperfusion-induced oxidative stress is not completely known.

Alteration of Anti-oxidant Mechanisms

Decreased anti-oxidant activity may also contribute to the increase of reactive species. Under physiological conditions, several cellular mechanisms counterbalance the production of reactive species, including enzymatic and non-enzymatic pathways [52]. The enzymatic pathways are catalase and glutathione peroxidase, which coordinate the catalysis of hydrogen peroxide to water, and superoxide dismutase (SOD), which facilitate the formation of H_2O_2 from superoxide. The non-enzymatic pathways include intracellular anti-oxidants such as vitamins C, E, and β(beta)-carotene, ubiquinone, glutathione, lipoic acid, urate and cysteine. Thioredoxin and thioredoxin reductase form an additional redox regulatory system since they catalyze the regeneration of antioxidant molecules, such as ubiquinone (Q10), lipoic and ascorbic acid. However, these defense mechanisms fail when the reperfusion-induced robust generation of reactive species exceeds the cellular anti-oxidant activity [31]. In addition, intracellular levels of glutathione decline with a concomitant accumulation of the oxidized and inactive form of glutathione (GSSG). Maladaptative decreases of other non-enzymatic antioxidants may also occur. For instance, plasma levels of ascorbate [53] and atria levels of vitamin E are reduced in patients after cardiopulmonary bypass [31, 54]. Anti-oxidant capacity is also reduced in the plasma or in the venous effluent of reperfused myocardium in patients with short episodes of myocardial ischemia [55].

The Endothelial Dysfunction and Neutrophil Infiltration

The event of reperfusion is frequently associated with early endothelial dysfunction. The dysfunction appears to be triggered by the endothelial generation of a large burst of oxidant molecules

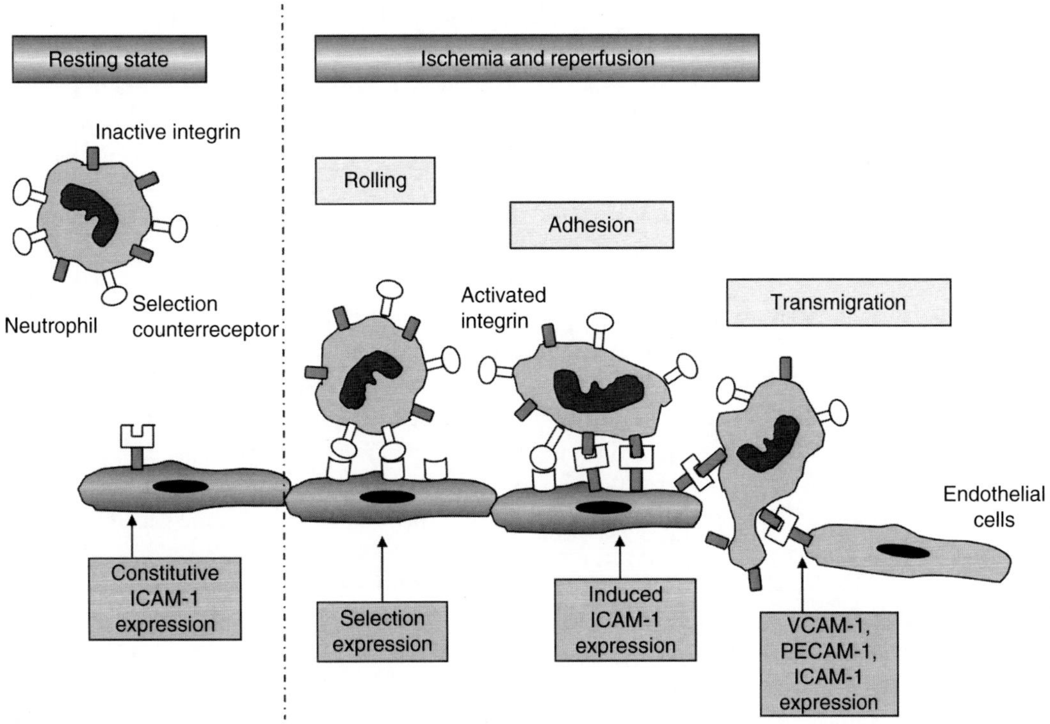

Fig. 24.6 Kinetics of neutrophil interaction with endothelium and infiltration into parenchymal tissue. During resting state no interaction exists between neutrophils and endothelium: the endothelium expresses low levels of intercellular adhesion molecule-1 (ICAM-1); whereas neutrophils express inactive integrins and low levels of selectin counter-receptors. After ischemia and reperfusion, a sequence of three complex steps coordinates neutrophil infiltration. The initial step is the *rolling* of neutrophils along the vessel wall and is promoted by selectins. The rolling neutrophils then become activated by local factors generated by the endothelium, resulting in their *adhesion* to the vessel wall. Finally, this firm attachment allows the *transmigration* of the neutrophil from the endothelium into the tissue. Adhesion and transmigration are mediated by the interaction of $\beta(beta)_2$- and $\beta(beta)_1$-integrins on the surface of neutrophils with immunoglobulin gene superfamily members, such as ICAM-1, VCAM-1 and PECAM-1

and amplified by accumulation of neutrophils into injured tissue. Secondary to oxidative stress and impairment of the NO pathways, vascular permeability increases and leads to edema formation and enhancement of interstitial pressure. When these detrimental changes occur in capillaries and arterioles, the local circulation of blood may be impaired, a phenomenon known as *no-reflow*. In the earliest stages of reperfusion after ischemia, neutrophils moving out of the circulation into inflamed tissue play a physiological role in the destruction of foreign antigens and remodeling of injured tissue. Nevertheless, neutrophils may augment damage to vascular and parenchymal cellular elements by the release of proteolytic enzymes (elastase, collagenase, cathepepsin, hyaluronidase), free radicals and proinflammatory mediators. Furthermore, neutrophils physically plug capillaries and small arterioles, thereby contributing to the no-reflow phenomenon and exacerbating the ischemic damage [56, 57].

Expression of Adhesion Molecules on Endothelial Surface: Loss of Endothelial Barrier Function

The localization of neutrophils to reperfused tissue after ischemia involves a sequence of three complex steps coordinated by endothelial adhesion molecules, which are recognized by specific receptors on the leukocyte membrane (Fig. 24.6). Three families of adhesion molecules have been identified: the selectins, the immunoglobulin gene superfamily and the integrins [58]. The initial interaction between leukocytes and endothelium is transient, resulting in the **rolling** of leukocytes along the vessel wall. Leukocyte rolling is promoted by the selectin family of adhesion glycoproteins, which are found on endothelial cells (P- and E-selectin), leukocytes (L-selectin), and platelets (P-selectin). P-selectin is constitutively expressed and located within Weibel-Palade bodies in the vascular endothelium and platelets. Therefore, it is rapidly translocated to the cell surface after exposure to hydrogen peroxide, peroxynitrite, thrombin, histamine or complement. E-selectin is synthetized after stimulation with pro-inflammatory cytokines (TNFα and IL-1) and expressed on the endothelial cells after several hours after ischemia and reperfusion injury. The corresponding ligands for selectins on the surface of the leukocyte are sialylated Lewis^x and A blood group antigens. In addition to endothelial cells, leukocytes also express a selectin (L-selectin), which participates in low affinity interactions with P- and E-selectin during the rolling phase [58, 59].

The rolling leukocytes then become activated by local factors generated by the endothelium, resulting in their arrest and *firm adhesion* to the vessel wall. The list of activating factors includes cytokines, chemoattractants (e.g., leukotriene B4, C5a, platelet activating factor) and chemoattractive chemokines, which bind to and activate integrins on leukocyte. Finally, this firm attachment allows the *transmigration or diapedesis* of the leukocyte from the endothelium into the tissue [59].

Firm adhesion and transmigration are mediated by the interaction of β_2- (also known as CD11/CD18) and β_1-integrins on the surface of leukocytes with immunoglobulin gene superfamily members expressed by endothelium [58]. The intercellular adhesion molecules (ICAMs), ICAM-1, ICAM-2 and ICAM-3, the vascular cellular adhesion molecule-1 (VCAM-1) and the platelet-endothelial cell adhesion molecule (PECAM) are members of the immunoglobulin superfamily. The CD11/CD18 family of integrins is the counter-receptor for ICAM-1 and ICAM-2, whereas VCAM-1 binds to the integrin *very late activation antigen-4* (VLA4 group/β_1-integrin) found on leukocytes [60].

ICAM-1 is constitutively expressed (at low levels) on the surface of endothelial cells and is responsible for the firm adhesion of neutrophils. Its surface expression is enhanced during inflammation in vivo on endothelial cells after exposure to oxidants or cytokines with maximal expression occurring within 4 h and persisting at least 24 h [60]. In addition to endothelial cells, ICAM-1 is also present on leukocyte, epithelial cells, cardiomyocytes and fibroblasts, thus contributing to the tissue margination of leukocytes [61].

VCAM-1 is not constitutively expressed on unstimulated endothelial cells. Exposure to inflammatory mediators or cytokines results in rapid upregulation. The VCAM-1 message levels reach a sustained high level by 2–3 h and gradually diminish over several days [60, 62]. Since VCAM-1 binds circulating monocytes and lymphocytes expressing the VLA4 group, the relatively delayed and sustained VCAM-1 response to cytokine may correspond to the switch to preferential adhesion and infiltration of mononuclear leukocytes typical of chronic inflammatory processes.

In this complex machinery of leukocyte trafficking, platelets also accumulates in the vessels resulting in further impairment of endothelial function and microcirculation. In fact, circulating platelets roll and adhere to the endothelium or subendothelial matrix using similar adhesion molecules and release substances that are able to cause further chemotaxis and migration of circulating leukocytes [63]. Since the abnormal sequestration of leukocytes is a central component in the development of reperfusion injury, therapeutic agents that block leukocyte-endothelial interactions, such as antibodies raised against adhesion molecules, have been used to inhibit the inflammatory response in a number of animal models of myocardial, splanchnic, cerebral, and liver reperfusion damage after ischemia [64]. In the clinical setting, however, very few studies have tested the efficacy of antibodies against adhesion molecules in organ transplantation, hemorrhagic shock and myocardial infarction with minor or unsatisfactory results [61, 64–67].

Loss of Endothelial Barrier: The Injury Vicious Cycle

Therefore, production of oxygen and nitrogen reactive species, endothelial injury, activation of neutrophil-attractive factors, and neutrophil infiltration (leading to further production of reactive species and proteolitycal enzymes) constitute a vicious cycle, which is ultimately responsible for endothelial and parenchymal injury. In the early phase of reperfusion (1–3 h after reperfusion), neutrophils are present mainly in the intravascular space (attached to the endothelium) and play an important role in the endothelial injury associated with reperfusion. At later stages, neutrophils emigrate into the tissues and exacerbate parenchymal damage. In this positive feedback cycle, reactive species activate a variety of oxidant processes, such as activation of signal transduction pathways, induction of peroxidation and DNA injury.

Complement Activation

The complement system is an important pathway of innate immune defense and inflammation [68]. It is composed of more than 30 plasma proteins, glycoproteins, soluble or membrane bound receptors. The complement system can be activated by three pathways: classical, lectin-binding and alternative pathway (Fig. 24.7). The classical pathway is initiated by antigen/antibody complex and/or inflammatory proteins such as C-reactive protein and serum amyloid protein. The alternative pathway is initiated by surface molecules containing carbohydrates and lipids. The lectin-binding pathway is initiated by the binding of mannose-binding lectin protein (MBL) resulting in activation of MLB-associated serine-proteases (MASPs). Data from numerous experimental animal studies of ischemia and reperfusion injury in different organ systems, as well as, clinical studies support the concept that activation of complement is a crucial pathogenetic event of tissue injury [69, 70]. All three pathways are activated in ischemia and reperfusion injury and seem to be involved in an organ-dependent manner [71]. Complement activation has been demonstrated in myocardial infarction, ischemia of the intestine, hindlimb, kidney, liver, hemorrhagic shock and sepsis. In the case of cardiopulmonary bypass procedure, contact of blood with artificial surfaces of the bypass equipment can also activate complement proteins. Under physiological conditions, endothelial cells contain proteins (decay accelerating factor and membrane cofactor protein), which protect against complement injury. However,

Fig. 24.7 Pathways of complement activation. The complement system can be activated by the classical, the lectin-binding and the alternative pathway. The classical pathway is initiated by immune complexes and/or inflammatory proteins such as C-reactive protein and serum amyloid. The lectin-binding pathway is initiated by the binding of mannose-binding lectin protein (MBL) resulting in activation of MLB-associated serine-proteases (MASPs). The alternative pathway is initiated by surface molecules of pathogens containing carbohydrates and lipids. All three pathways are activated in a unidirectional cascade of enzymatic reactions mediated by serine proteases leading to the formation of active factors. The three pathways converge at the generation of C3b and the terminal byproducts, C5a and the complex C5b-C59, also known as the terminal membrane attack complex (MAC), which mediate pro-inflammatory actions and cell lysis

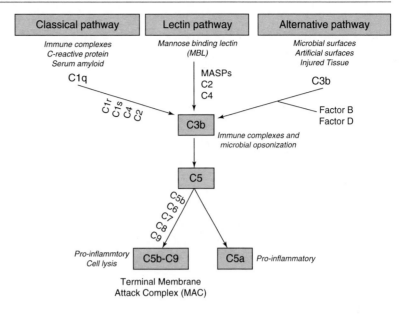

Table 24.2 Pro-inflammatory activities of C5a and MAC

Leukocyte activation	Platelet activation	Endothelial dysfunction	Other effects
Chemoattraction	Thromboxane release	Adhesion molecules expression	Cyclo-oxygenase and lipo-oxygenase activation
CD11b expression	P-selectin expression	Prothrombinase activation	PGDF release
Oxidative burst	von Willebrand factor and IIb/IIIa release	Reduction of NO	Cell lysis
Proteases release			
Histamine release	Prothrombinase activation		
Cytokine production			
Prostaglandin release			
Thromboxane release			

endothelial dysfunction during reperfusion may alter these protective mechanisms.

Complement activation results in a unidirectional cascade of enzymatic and biochemical reactions mediated by serine proteases leading to the formation of biologically active factors. In this cascade, the two terminal byproducts of complement activation, C5a and the complex C5b-C59, also known as the terminal membrane attack complex (MAC), are believed to mediate tissue injury. C5a is one of the most pro-inflammatory peptides with pleiotropic functions (Table 24.2). C5a serves as a powerful *chemoattractant* for neutrophils, monocytes and macrophages, where it binds on the C5aR receptor, and causes activation of adhesion molecules, thus increasing their adhesiveness and aggregation. C5a stimulates oxidative burst in neutrophils, the release of lysosomal enzymes and pro-inflammatory cytokines in macrophages and monocytes, and activates the coagulation pathway [69]. C5a can also bind to specific C5aR receptor in epithelial cells and activate the release of inflammatory mediators, such as cytokines [72]. C5a and MAC cause changes in the circulation and the vascular wall since they induce expression of adhesion molecules on endothelial cells and decrease the release of NO causing vasoconstriction [73, 74], thus amplifying the loss of vascular homeostasis and the endothelial dysfunction [71]. C5a and MAC activate platelets and favor the formation of procoagulant thrombin [69]. C3a and C5a, as well as C4a, also have *anaphylatoxin activity*. Anaphylatoxins cause increased vascular permeability, smooth muscle contraction, and mast cell degranulation.

The effects of complement inhibition have also been tested in several clinical trials. A recent systematic review and meta-analysis of trials using pexelizumab, a C5 complement monoclonal antibody, has reported that there is no clear benefit of adding pexelizumab to currently available therapies for ST elevation myocardial infarction. However, pexelizumab appears to reduce the risk of death in patients undergoing coronary artery bypass grafting [75].

Toll-Like Receptors and Damage Associated Molecular Patterns

Another class of molecules inherent in the regulation of ischemia-reperfusion injury is that of the toll-like receptors

(TLRs). Originally discovered for their role in the innate immune response to infection, TLRs recognize and bind an array of microbial molecular patterns, including peptides, lipopolysaccharide, and DNA [76]. Binding and activation of these receptors leads to recruitment of various intracellular adaptor molecules, and ultimately activation of the NF-κB pathway with subsequent pro-inflammatory cytokine production [77]. However, recent evidence suggests that endogenous tissue components released during stress or ischemia may also activate TLR-mediated pathways, thus implicating the role of TLRs in the pathogenesis of ischemia-reperfusion injury [78]. These endogenous signals have been termed danger-associated molecular patterns (DAMPs). Cellular necrosis and activation of extracellular matrix proteases in the ischemic tissue leads to release DAMPs into the surrounding environment [79]. Several possible DAMPs, which serve as TLR ligands, have been identified and include heat shock protein 60, cardiac myosin, and high-mobility group box 1 [79, 80].

TLR expression has been observed in all cellular components of ischemia-reperfusion injury, including leukocytes, endothelial cells, and cardiomyocytes [81]. Circulating TLRs may play a prominent role as well. Genetic deficiency of TLR2 and TLR4 has shown to decrease infarct size and improve cardiac function in animals subjected to myocardial ischemia-reperfusion [82]. These cardioprotective effects are also associated with reduced local and systemic levels of inflammatory cytokines [83, 84]. TLR receptors have also been implicated in the pathogenesis of renal and hepatic ischemia and reperfusion injury [85, 86]. Given the role of TLRs in the pathophysiology of ischemia and reperfusion injury, TLR antagonists have been tested as therapeutic agents in experimental studies; treatment with eritoran, a TLR4 specific antagonist, resulted in decreased infarct size and reduced NF-κB translocation in myocardial ischemia and reperfusion [87] and amelioration of post-reperfusion acute kidney injury [88]. Whether these antagonists may hold promising in the clinical setting is yet to be proven.

Matrix Metalloproteinases

Matrix metalloproteinases (MMP) comprise a class of zinc-dependent peptidases that have historically been recognized for their role in remodeling of the extracellular matrix in several biologic processes, including embryogenesis, wound healing, inflammation, and angiogenesis [89, 90]. Matrix metalloproteinases are further classified based on their particular proteolytic substrates, and currently there are 28 recognized enzymes. Ubiquitous to virtually all tissues, matrix metalloproteinases are synthesized as inactivated zymogens with an inhibitory pro-peptide domain that shields the zinc-containing catalytic site [89]. Various extracellular matrix proteases facilitate removal of the pro-peptide domain, thus allowing activation. In contrast, negative regulation of proteinase activity is predominantly under the control of four distinct tissue inhibitors of metalloproteinases (TIMP 1-4) [91].

Matrix metalloproteinases have been increasingly recognized as mediators of ischemia-reperfusion injury. For example, in hepatic ischemia and reperfusion, matrix metalloproteinase activation leads to disrupted tissue architecture and hepatic fibrosis [92]. Adult patients undergoing orthotopic liver transplant were shown to have elevated levels of MMP-9 5 min following graft reperfusion, and this rise correlated with elevated aspartate aminotransferase levels, suggesting a role for metalloproteinase-induced graft reperfusion injury [93]. Elevated MMP-9 expression has been found in renal allograft biopsies in pediatric and adult patients, where it is associated with signs of acute cellular rejection [94]. Elevated levels of MMP-8 and MMP-9 have also been described after cardiac surgery with cardiopulmonary bypass in children with congenital heart disease [95].

While matrix metalloproteinases have traditionally been viewed as active proteases in the extracellular matrix, recent evidence suggests that they also put forth prominent influence in the intracellular environment [89]. Oxidative stress, in particular, can upregulate intracellular MMP-2 and MMP-9 activity, and this has been shown to contribute to myocardial ischemia and reperfusion injury. The formation of reactive oxygen and nitrogen species upon reperfusion is a key step in the activation of these enzymes [96]. Activated MMP-2 within the cardiac myocyte has been shown to localize to the sarcomere and degrade cardiac troponin I [97] and to inversely correlate with cardiac mechanical dysfunction [98]. In a study of adult patients undergoing coronary artery bypass graft surgery, MMP-2 and -9 activity was increased in right atrial tissue biopsied after reperfusion from aortic cross-clamping; furthermore, MMP-2 levels were associated with worsened cardiac function following reperfusion [99]. The contribution of matrix metalloproteinases to ischemia and reperfusion injury is also influenced by a regulatory imbalance between the proteinases and their endogenous inhibitors TIMP-1 and TIMP-4, which are inactivated upon peroxynitrite formation [100, 101]. Several pharmacologic inhibitors of matrix metalloproteinases exist, including o-phenanthroline, GM-6001, batimastat and the tetracycline class of antibiotics [102]. To date, some studies have reported promising results with these inhibitors in the treatment of periodontal wound repair [103] and post-operatively following endovascular aortic aneurysm repair [104].

Cellular and Molecular Defenses Against Cell Injury

During ischemia and reperfusion, cellular and molecular defense mechanisms are also deployed in order to counteract the inflammatory response and reflect the attempt of the cell to adapt within the hypoxic and dysmetabolic environment. These cytoprotective mechanisms have generated particular interest in the research field, since they may provide a reasonable base for developing novel therapeutic approaches for reperfusion injury.

The Hypoxia-Inducible Factor-1 (HIF-1)

Deficiency of oxygen directly activates the nuclear transcription factor hypoxia-inducible factor-1 (HIF-1), which regulates gene expression of several mediators that render the cell capable to survive and function within a hypoxic environment. Under normoxic conditions, this factor is unstable and inactive; however, during hypoxia HIF-1 is stabilized and binds to the promoter regions of many cytoprotective genes. The list of genes includes genes for glucose transporters and glycolytic enzymes, thereby enhancing the capacity for anaerobic metabolism, and angiogenic growth factors for capillary formation and revascularization [105].

The Heat Shock Response

The heat shock response is a highly conserved cellular response to injury. This cellular defense mechanism is characterized by the increased expression of heat shock proteins (HSPs) that provide cytoprotection from inflammatory insults, including oxidative stress, viral infection, and ischemia-reperfusion injury. In eukaryotic cells, the production of HSPs is regulated at the nuclear level by the transcription heat shock factor-1 (HSF-1). Under physiological conditions, HSF-1 is a phosphorylated monomer located mainly in the cytoplasm. Activation of HSF-1 is induced by a variety of environmental stresses in the presence of elevated intracellular calcium and active protein kinases. Once activated, HSF-1 is translocated into the nucleus, forms trimers and binds to DNA to drive transcription of HSPs [106]. The function of HSPs has been linked to their role as molecular chaperones. These macromolecules bind to denatured or misfolded proteins, promoting their correct refolding, preservation or degradation [107]. Their cytoprotective mechanisms have been proven in several experimental studies. For instance, the HSP-70 directly protects against myocardial damage, improves metabolic recovery, and reduces infarct size in hearts of transgenic mice subjected to ischemia and reperfusion [107, 108]. Another important HSP is the HSP-32, also known as heme-oxygenase 1 (HO-1). The cytoprotective HO-1 has been documented as a successful therapeutic strategy in a number of transplantation models. The beneficial effect of HO-1 is mediated through an anti-oxidant mechanism. HO-1 removes a pro-oxidant (heme) while generating a putative anti-oxidant (bilirubin), carbon monooxide and iron ions [109].

The Reperfusion Injury Salvage Kinase (RISK) Pathway

Ischemia and reperfusion has also been shown to activate anti-apoptotic kinase signaling cascades, such as the kinases phosphoinositide-3 kinase (PI3K)-Akt and ERK 1/2, which have been implicated in cellular survival and referred as the reperfusion injury salvage kinase (RISK) pathways [110]. These kinases regulate cell proliferation, differentiation and survival. Although chronic activation of these pathways has been implicated in cardiac hypertrophy, activating these pro-survival kinases at the time of reperfusion or during ischemic preconditioning has been demonstrated to confer cardioprotection against reperfusion injury. The cardioprotective mechanism of Akt seems to be related to the targeting of apoptotic modulators. For example, Akt inhibits the pro-apoptotic proteins BAD and BAX, thus preventing the release of mitochondrial cytochrome c in response to an apoptotic stimulus and influences the activity of caspases [110].

Autophagy

As the intracellular environment becomes deranged during ischemia and reperfusion, cellular upregulation of autophagy may provide a protective response mechanism. Autophagy, or "self-digestion," involves the degradation of damaged cellular organelles by the formation of the autophagosome; a double-membrane vesicle, which encircles cellular debris and then fuses to the lysosome. The subsequent hydrolysis provides the cell new substrate for energy production and regeneration of healthy organelles [111]. Autophagy has been shown to play a role in the ischemia and reperfusion of several organs, including the heart, kidney, liver, and brain [112–115].

A basal level of autophagy exists for routine cellular maintenance, but the process may be upregulated in the face of starvation and stress [112]. Highly coordinated, interrelated signaling pathways serve to regulate autophagy. Numerous autophagy-specific genes, termed *Atg* genes, have critical functions in the initiation and progression of the autophagic pathway [116]. On the contrary, the mammalian target of rapamycin (mTOR) has negative regulatory influences on autophagy [117].

There are numerous triggers which upregulate autophagy during the pathophysiologic process of ischemia and reperfusion injury. The first and most logical stimulus is deprivation of cellular nutrients, including the depletion of high-energy phosphate stores [118]. Additional triggers include increased intracellular calcium, generation of reactive oxygen species, opening of the mitochondrial permeability transition pore, and endoplasmic reticulum stress [112].

While autophagy is known to be upregulated in response to ischemia and reperfusion, considerable debate exists as to whether this process is protective versus detrimental to the cell. Several autophagy-induced mechanisms advantageous to cellular survival have been outlined. The clearance of toxic protein aggregates and damaged mitochondria have been shown to provide a feedback mechanism for the synthesis of newer, more healthy organelles [119]. Furthermore, the breakdown products of autophagy can be employed for the generation of ATP, synthesis of proteins, and production of glutathione [119, 120]. Despite these apparent advantages, it may be that the consequences of autophagy during ischemia and reperfusion are dependent on various circumstances, including the phase of ischemia or reperfusion, the duration of ischemia, and the particular vascular bed involved [121]. A complex, dual role for autophagy in ischemia-reperfusion injury has also been proposed. For example, the induction of autophagy during myocardial ischemia enhanced myocyte survival; in contrast, upregulation of autophagy during the reperfusion phase worsened myocardial injury [118].

Resveratrol, a polyphenol found in grapes, wines, peanuts and fruits, has been of recent therapeutic interest due its anti-oxidant, anti-inflammatory properties and maintenance of mitochondrial function [122]. Resveratrol functions as a free-radical scavenger and has been shown to provide cardio-protection during myocardial ischemia and reperfusion by altering redox signaling pathways [123]. Current evidence also suggests that resveratrol protects against ischemia and reperfusion injury through induction of autophagy via inhibition of mammalian target of rapamycin (mTOR) [123].

Endogenous Hydrogen Sulfide Production

The endogenous gas hydrogen sulfide (H_2S) has struck recent interest for its potential role in ameliorating ischemia-reperfusion injury. Similar to nitric oxide and carbon monoxide, H_2S is a lipid soluble "gasotransmitter" with the ability to modulate intracellular targets after freely crossing the cellular membrane [124]. Production of H_2S comes from three separate enzymes: cystathionine ®(beta)-synthase, cystathionine ©(gamma)-lyase, and 3-mercaptopyruvate sulfur transferase. While previously labeled as a toxic compound, H_2S has now been shown to be endogenously produced at low levels within the body and has several important physiologic functions. For example, H_2S within the central nervous system functions as a neuromodulator [125]; intestinal H_2S induces smooth muscle relaxation within the splanchnic circulation [126].

Beyond its endogenous physiologic role, H_2S has also shown to be protective against ischemia and reperfusion injury in the heart, liver and kidneys in a variety of experimental studies [127–130]. Several cellular mechanisms account for the protective effects of this gas. Endogenous cerebral H_2S has been shown to act as a free radical scavenger, thereby inhibiting peroxynitrite within cerebral tissue [131]. In the setting of myocardial ischemia and reperfusion injury, several mechanisms are at work. Preconditioning with NaHS, serving as an H_2S donor, can lead to activation of the RISK pathway, thus protecting the myocyte from apoptosis [132]. Furthermore, H_2S-preconditioning in rat myocytes has been shown to reduce intracellular calcium [133]. Lastly, H_2S donors have the potential to reduce leukocyte infiltration into reperfused tissues by interrupting their interaction at the vascular endothelium [134]. Given these multiple mechanisms, H_2S may serve as a potential therapeutic target in ischemia and reperfusion injury. However, current difficulties in translating this molecule into a therapeutic application includes their potential to affect other enzyme systems, as well as its reduced selectivity to organs and its limited cell membrane permeability [135].

The Ischemic Preconditioning Response

Of particular biological and clinical relevance is the phenomenon known as *ischemic preconditioning response*. As noted originally in 1986 [136], multiple brief ischemic episodes (i.e., preconditioning) protect the heart from a subsequent sustained ischemic insult. Human clinical trials using ischemic preconditioning have been successfully carried out in the fields of cardiac, hepatic, and pulmonary surgery. Epidemiologic data exist to support the existence of preconditioning-induced neuroprotection in humans. Human skeletal muscle has been preconditioned experimentally, as have human proximal tubule renal cells. Additionally, preconditioning is not confined to one organ, but can also limit infarct size in remote, non-preconditioned organs (*remote preconditioning*). At present, there is no evidence for ischemic preconditioning occurring in the human intestine, although animal studies attest to the possibility [137, 138].

The protective effects of preconditioning occur in a well described bi-phasic kinetic. Tissue protection appears within minutes and lasts only 2–3 h (early phase or first window of protection), but reappears 24 h after the preconditioning stimulus (late phase or second window of protection) [139]. Within the early phase, cytoprotective mechanisms depend mainly on post-translational modifications of pre-existing cellular proteins. Late preconditioning is a genetic reprogramming of the organ that involves the simultaneous activation of multiple stress-responsive genes and *de novo* synthesis of several proteins, which ultimately results in the development of a protective phenotype. Sublethal ischemic insults release chemical signals (NO, adenosine, and reactive oxygen species) that trigger a series of signaling events (e.g., activation of protein kinases and NF-κB and culminates in increased synthesis of iNOS, COX-2, HO-1, SOD, and probably other cytoprotective proteins.

Conclusion

In clinical therapy of acute infarction of an organ or tissue, reperfusion has proven to be the only way to limit infarct size by restoring the fractional uptake of oxygen to maintain the rate of cellular oxidation. However, restoration of flow is accompanied by the detrimental manifestations of reperfusion injury, which influences the degree of recovery. Reperfusion injury refers to an extremely complex situation that had not occurred during the preceding ischemic period. The existence of such damage has clinical relevance, as it would imply the possibility of improving recovery with specific interventions applied only at the time of reperfusion. Therefore, knowledge of the precise sequence of biochemical and molecular events of reperfusion could lead to rational treatments designed to prevent or delay cell death. However, at the present time, there is no simple answer to the question of what determines cell death and the failure to recover cell function after reperfusion. The analysis of the current experimental data suggests the existence of a self-amplifying vicious cycle, which is governed by reactive species and involves cellular effectors (endothelial and parenchymal cells, neutrophils, platelets), inflammatory mediators and components of the coagulation and complement cascade. In this cycle, endogenous cytoprotective mechanisms also intervene to counter-act inflammation. As described throughout this chapter, the current experimental research has raised the exciting prospect that pharmacological intervention aimed to interrupt the various levels of this vicious cycle (such as the use of antioxidants, antibodies against adhesion molecules, inhibition of PARP-1 and NF-κB, induction of heat shock response, autophagy or ischemic preconditioning) may ameliorate cell dysfunction and prevent death. However, the predictability of in vivo experimentation in animals and its extrapolation to man is a function of the genetic kinship. Large clinical trials are needed to determine whether these novel therapeutic interventions may be beneficial to the patient.

References

1. Acierno LJ. Adolph Fick: mathematician, physicist, physiologist. Clin Cardiol. 2000;23:390–1.
2. Jakob SM. Clinical review: splanchnic ischaemia. Crit Care. 2002;6:306–612.
3. Taegtmeyer H, King LM, Jones BE. Energy substrate metabolism, myocardial ischemia, and targets for pharmacotherapy. Am J Cardiol. 1998;82:54K–60.
4. Ferrari R, Guardigli G, Mele D, Percoco GF, Ceconi C, Curello S. Oxidative stress during myocardial ischaemia and heart failure. Curr Pharm Des. 2004;10:1699–711.
5. Ferdinandy P, Schulz R. Nitric oxide, superoxide, and peroxynitrite in myocardial ischaemia-reperfusion injury and preconditioning. Br J Pharmacol. 2003;138:532–43.
6. Ischiropoulos H. Biological selectivity and functional aspects of protein tyrosine nitration. Biochem Biophys Res Commun. 2003;305:776–83.
7. Giordano FJ. Oxygen, oxidative stress, hypoxia, and heart failure. J Clin Invest. 2005;115:500–8.
8. Alvarez B, Radi R. Peroxynitrite reactivity with amino acids and proteins. Amino Acids. 2003;25:295–311.
9. Halliwell B. Free radicals, proteins and DNA: oxidative damage versus redox regulation. Biochem Soc Trans. 1996;24:1023–7.
10. Szabó C, Dawson VL. Role of poly(ADP-ribose) synthetase in inflammation and ischaemia-reperfusion. Trends Pharmacol Sci. 1998;19:287–98.
11. Zingarelli B. Importance of poly (ADP-ribose) polymerase activation in myocardial reperfusion injury. In: Szabó C, editor. Cell death: the role of poly (ADP-ribose) polymerase. Boca Raton: CRC Press LLC; 2000. p. 41–60.
12. D'Amours D, Desnoyers S, D'Silva I, Poirier GG. Poly(ADP-ribosyl)ation reactions in the regulation of nuclear functions. Biochem J. 1999;342:249–68.
13. Chiarugi A. Poly(ADP-ribose) polymerase: killer or conspirator? The 'suicide hypothesis' revisited. Trends Pharmacol Sci. 2002;23: 122–9.
14. Zingarelli B, O'Connor M, Wong H, Salzman AL, Szabó C. Peroxynitrite-mediated DNA strand breakage activates polyadenosine diphosphate ribosyl synthetase and causes cellular energy depletion in macrophages stimulated with bacterial lipopolysaccharide. J Immunol. 1996;156:350–8.
15. Zingarelli B, Salzman AL, Szabó C. Genetic disruption of poly (ADP-ribose) synthetase inhibits the expression of P-selectin and intercellular adhesion molecule-1 in myocardial ischemia/reperfusion injury. Circ Res. 1998;83:85–94.
16. Zingarelli B, Hake PW, O'Connor M, Denenberg A, Kong S, Aronow BJ. Absence of poly(ADP-ribose)polymerase-1 alters nuclear factor-κB activation and gene expression of apoptosis regulators after reperfusion injury. Mol Med. 2003;9:143–53.
17. Zingarelli B, Hake PW, O'Connor M, Denenberg A, Wong HR, Kong S, Aronow BJ. Differential regulation of activator protein-1 and heat shock factor-1 in myocardial ischemia and reperfusion injury: role of poly(ADP-ribose) polymerase-1. Am J Physiol Heart Circ Physiol. 2004;286:H1408–15.
18. Tóth-Zsámboki E, Horváth E, Vargova K, Pankotai E, Murthy K, Zsengellér Z, Bárány T, Pék T, Fekete K, Kiss RG, Préda I, Lacza Z, Gerö D, Szabó C. Activation of poly(ADP-ribose) polymerase by myocardial ischemia and coronary reperfusion in human circulating leukocytes. Mol Med. 2006;12:221–8.
19. Morrow DA, Brickman CM, Murphy SA, Baran K, Krakover R, Dauerman H, Kumar S, Slomowitz N, Grip L, McCabe CH, Salzman AL. A randomized, placebo-controlled trial to evaluate the tolerability, safety, pharmacokinetics, and pharmacodynamics of a potent inhibitor of poly(ADP-ribose) polymerase (INO-1001) in patients with ST-elevation myocardial infarction undergoing primary percutaneous coronary intervention: results of the TIMI 37 trial. J Thromb Thrombolysis. 2009;27:359–64.
20. Thannickal VJ, Fanburg BL. Reactive oxygen species in cell signaling. Am J Physiol Lung Cell Mol Physiol. 2000;279:L1005–28.
21. Yoshizumi M, Tsuchiya K, Tamaki T. Signal transduction of reactive oxygen species and mitogen-activated protein kinases in cardiovascular disease. J Med Invest. 2001;48:11–24.
22. Chang L, Karin M. Mammalian MAP kinase signalling cascades. Nature. 2001;410:37–40.

23. Zingarelli B, Sheehan M, Wong HR. Nuclear factor-κB as a therapeutic target in critical care medicine. Crit Care Med. 2003;31:S105–11.

24. Shaulian E, Karin M. AP-1 as a regulator of cell life and death. Nat Cell Biol. 2002;4:E131–6.

25. Karin M, Takahashi T, Kapahi P, Delhase M, Chen Y, Makris C, Rothwarf D, Baud V, Natoli G, Guido F, Li N. Oxidative stress and gene expression: the AP-1 and NF-κB connections. Biofactors. 2001;15:87–9.

26. Clemens JA, Stephenson DT, Dixon EP, Smalstig EB, Mincy RE, Rash KS, Little SP. Global cerebral ischemia activates nuclear factor-κB prior to evidence of DNA fragmentation. Brain Res Mol Brain Res. 1997;48:187–96.

27. Zwacka RM, Zhou W, Zhang Y, Darby CJ, Dudus L, Halldorson J, Oberley L, Engelhardt JF. Redox gene therapy for ischemia/reperfusion injury of the liver reduces AP1 and NF-κB activation. Nat Med. 1998;4:698–704.

28. Chang CK, Albarillo MV, Schumer W. Therapeutic effect of dimethyl sulfoxide on ICAM-1 gene expression and activation of NF-κB and AP-1 in septic rats. J Surg Res. 2001;95:181–7.

29. Valen G, Hansson GK, Dumitrescu A, Vaage J. Unstable angina activates myocardial heat shock protein 72, endothelial nitric oxide synthase, and transcription factors NF-κB and AP-1. Cardiovasc Res. 2000;47:49–56.

30. Mou SS, Haudek SB, Lequier L, Peña O, Leonard S, Nikaidoh H, Giroir BP, Stromberg D. Myocardial inflammatory activation in children with congenital heart disease. Crit Care Med. 2002;30: 827–32.

31. Marczin N, El-Habashi N, Hoare GS, Bundy RE, Yacoub M. Antioxidants in myocardial ischemia-reperfusion injury: therapeutic potential and basic mechanisms. Arch Biochem Biophys. 2003;420:222–36.

32. Hellsten-Westing Y. Immunohistochemical localization of xanthine oxidase in human cardiac and skeletal muscle. Histochemistry. 1993;100:215–22.

33. Harrison R. Structure and function of xanthine oxidoreductase: where are we now? Free Radic Biol Med. 2002;33:774–97.

34. Meneshian A, Bulkley GB. The physiology of endothelial xanthine oxidase: from urate catabolism to reperfusion injury to inflammatory signal transduction. Microcirculation. 2002;9: 161–75.

35. Godber BLJ, Doel JJ, Sapkota GP, Blake DR, Stevens CR, Eisenthal R, Harrison R. Reduction of nitrite to nitric oxide catalyzed by xanthine oxidoreductase. J Biol Chem. 2000;275:7757–63.

36. Li H, Samouilov A, Liu X, Zweier JL. Characterization of the magnitude and kinetics of xanthine oxidase-catalyzed nitrite reduction. Evaluation of its role in nitric oxide generation in anoxic tissues. J Biol Chem. 2001;276:24482–9.

37. Bulger EM, Maier RV. Antioxidants in critical illness. Arch Surg. 2001;136:1201–7.

38. Chaudhari T, McGuire W. Allopurinol for preventing mortality and morbidity in newborn infants with suspected hypoxic-ischaemic encephalopathy. Cochrane Database Syst Rev. 2008;2, CD006817.

39. Brass CA. Xanthine oxidase and reperfusion injury: major player or minor irritant? Hepatology. 1995;21:1757–60.

40. de Jong JW, van der Meer P, Nieukoop AS, Huizer T, Stroeve RJ, Bos E. Xanthine oxidoreductase activity in perfused hearts of various species, including humans. Circ Res. 1990;67:770–3.

41. Friedl HP, Smith DJ, Till GO, Thomson PD, Louis DS, Ward PA. Ischemia-reperfusion in humans. Appearance of xanthine oxidase activity. Am J Pathol. 1990;136:491–5.

42. Mathru M, Dries DJ, Barnes L, Tonino P, Sukhani R, Rooney MW. Tourniquet-induced exsanguination in patients requiring lower limb surgery. An ischemia-reperfusion model of oxidant and antioxidant metabolism. Anesthesiology. 1996;84:14–22.

43. Pesonen EJ, Linder N, Raivio KO, Sarnesto A, Lapatto R, Hockerstedt K, Makisalo H, Andersson S. Circulating xanthine oxidase and neutrophil activation during human liver transplantation. Gastroenterology. 1998;114:1009–15.

44. Terada LS, Dormish JJ, Shanley PF, Leff JA, Anderson BO, Repine JE. Circulating xanthine oxidase mediates lung neutrophil sequestration after intestinal ischemia-reperfusion. Am J Physiol. 1992;263:L394–401.

45. Bian K, Murad F. Nitric oxide (NO) – biogeneration, regulation, and relevance to human diseases. Front Biosci. 2003;8:d264–78.

46. Massion PB, Feron O, Dessy C, Balligand JL. Nitric oxide and cardiac function: ten years after, and continuing. Circ Res. 2003;93:388–98.

47. Ma XL, Weyrich AS, Lefer DJ, Lefer AM. Diminished basal nitric oxide release after myocardial ischemia and reperfusion promotes neutrophil adherence to coronary endothelium. Circ Res. 1993;72: 403–12.

48. de Frutos T, de Miguel Sanchez L, Farre J, Gomez J, Romero J, Marcos-Alberca P, Nunez A, Rico L, Lopez-Farre A. Expression of an endothelial-type nitric oxide synthase isoform in human neutrophils: modification by tumor necrosis factor-alpha and during acute myocardial infarction. J Am Coll Cardiol. 2001;37: 800–7.

49. Schulz R, Kelm M, Heusch G. Nitric oxide in myocardial ischemia/reperfusion injury. Cardiovasc Res. 2004;61:402–13.

50. Abrams J. Beneficial actions of nitrates in cardiovascular disease. Am J Cardiol. 1996;77:31C–7.

51. Stokes AH, Hastings TG, Vrana KE. Cytotoxic and genotoxic potential of dopamine. J Neurosci Res. 1999;55:659–65.

52. Nordberg J, Arner ES. Reactive oxygen species, antioxidants, and the mammalian thioredoxin system. Free Radic Biol Med. 2001;31:1287–312.

53. Ballmer PE, Reinhart WH, Jordan P, Buhler E, Moser UK, Gey KF. Depletion of plasma vitamin C but not of vitamin E in response to cardiac operations. J Thorac Cardiovasc Surg. 1994;108: 311–20.

54. Barsacchi R, Pelosi G, Maffei S, Baroni M, Salvatore L, Ursini F, Verunelli F, Biagini A. Myocardial vitamin E is consumed during cardiopulmonary bypass: indirect evidence of free radical generation in human ischemic heart. Int J Cardiol. 1992;37:339–43.

55. Buffon A, Santini SA, Ramazzotti V, Rigattieri S, Liuzzo G, Biasucci LM, Crea F, Giardina B, Maseri A. Large, sustained cardiac lipid peroxidation and reduced antioxidant capacity in the coronary circulation after brief episodes of myocardial ischemia. J Am Coll Cardiol. 2000;35:633–9.

56. Seal JB, Gewertz BL. Vascular dysfunction in ischemia-reperfusion injury. Ann Vasc Surg. 2005;19:572–84.

57. Rezkalla SH, Kloner RA. No-reflow phenomenon. Circulation. 2002;105:656–62.

58. Carlos TM, Harlan JM. Leukocyte-endothelial adhesion molecules. Blood. 1994;84:2068–101.

59. Lawrence MB, Springer TA. Leukocytes roll on a selectin at physiologic flow rates: distinction from and prerequisite for adhesion through integrins. Cell. 1991;65:859–73.

60. Malik AB, Lo SK. Vascular endothelial adhesion molecules and tissue inflammation. Pharmacol Rev. 1996;48:213–29.

61. Yonekawa K, Harlan JM. Targeting leukocyte integrins in human diseases. J Leukoc Biol. 2005;77:129–40.

62. Collins T, Read MA, Neish AS, Whitley MZ, Thanos D, Maniatis T. Transcriptional regulation of endothelial cell adhesion molecules: NF-κB and cytokine-inducible enhancers. FASEB J. 1995;9:899–909.

63. Gawaz M. Role of platelets in coronary thrombosis and reperfusion of ischemic myocardium. Cardiovasc Res. 2004;61:498–511.

64. Anaya-Prado R, Toledo-Pereyra LH, Lentsch AB, Ward PA. Ischemia/reperfusion injury. J Surg Res. 2002;105:248–58.

65. Rhee P, Morris J, Durham R, Hauser C, Cipolle M, Wilson R, Luchette F, McSwain N, Miller R. Recombinant humanized monoclonal antibody against CD18 (rhuMAb CD18) in traumatic hemorrhagic shock: results of a phase II clinical trial. Traumatic Shock Group. J Trauma. 2000;49:611–20.

66. Baran KW, Nguyen M, McKendall GR, Lambrew CT, Dykstra G, Palmeri ST, Gibbons RJ, Borzak S, Sobel BE, Gourlay SG, Rundle AC, Gibson CM, Barron HV, Limitation of Myocardial Infarction Following Thrombolysis in Acute Myocardial Infarction (LIMIT AMI) Study Group. Double-blind, randomized trial of an anti-CD18 antibody in conjunction with recombinant tissue plasminogen activator for acute myocardial infarction: Limitation of Myocardial Infarction Following Thrombolysis in Acute Myocardial Infarction (LIMIT AMI) study. Circulation. 2001;104:2778–83.

67. Faxon DP, Gibbons RJ, Chronos NA, Gurbel PA, Sheehan F, HALT-MI Investigators. The effect of blockade of the CD11/CD18 integrin receptor on infarct size in patients with acute myocardial infarction treated with direct angioplasty: the results of the HALT-MI study. J Am Coll Cardiol. 2002;40:1199–204.

68. Mastellos D, Morikis D, Isaacs SN, Holland MC, Strey CW, Lambris JD. Complement: structure, functions, evolution, and viral molecular mimicry. Immunol Res. 2003;27:367–86.

69. Guo RF, Ward PA. Role of C5a in inflammatory responses. Annu Rev Immunol. 2005;23:821–52.

70. Arumugam TV, Shiels IA, Woodruff TM, Granger DN, Taylor SM. The role of the complement system in ischemia-reperfusion injury. Shock. 2004;21:401–9.

71. Hart ML, Walsh MC, Stahl GL. Initiation of complement activation following oxidative stress. In vitro and in vivo observations. Mol Immunol. 2004;41:165–71.

72. Riedemann NC, Guo RF, Sarma VJ, Laudes IJ, Huber-Lang M, Warner RL, Albrecht EA, Speyer CL, Ward PA. Expression and function of the C5a receptor in rat alveolar epithelial cells. J Immunol. 2002;168:1919–25.

73. Park KW, Tofukuji M, Metais C, Comunale ME, Dai HB, Simons M, Stahl GL, Agah A, Sellke FW. Attenuation of endothelium-dependent dilation of pig pulmonary arterioles after cardiopulmonary bypass is prevented by monoclonal antibody to complement C5a. Anesth Analg. 1999;89:42–8.

74. Cable DG, Hisamochi K, Schaff HV. A model of xenograft hyperacute rejection attenuates endothelial nitric oxide production: a mechanism for graft vasospasm? J Heart Lung Transplant. 1999;18:177–84.

75. Testa L, Van Gaal WJ, Bhindi R, Biondi-Zoccai GG, Abbate A, Agostoni P, Porto I, Andreotti F, Crea F, Banning AP. Pexelizumab in ischemic heart disease: a systematic review and meta-analysis on 15,196 patients. J Thorac Cardiovasc Surg. 2008;136:884–93.

76. Liew FY, Xu D, Brint EK, O'Neill LA. Negative regulation of toll-like receptor-mediated immune responses. Nat Rev Immunol. 2005;5:446–58.

77. Fukata M, Vamadevan AS, Abreu MT. Toll-like receptors (TLRs) and Nod-like receptors (NLRs) in inflammatory disorders. Semin Immunol. 2009;21:242–53.

78. Kaczorowski DJ, Nakao A, McCurry KR, Billiar T. Toll-like receptors and myocardial ischemia/reperfusion, inflammation, and injury. Curr Cardiol Rev. 2009;5:196–202.

79. Krysko DV, Agostinis P, Krysko O, Garg AD, Bachert C, Lambrecht BN, Vandenabeel P. Emerging role of damage-associated molecular patterns derived from mitochondria in inflammation. Trends Immunol. 2011;32:157–64.

80. Tsung A, Sahai R, Tanaka H, Nakao A, Fink MP, Lotze MT, Yang H, Li J, Tracey KJ, Geller DA, Billiar TR. The nuclear factor HMGB1 mediates hepatic injury after murine liver ischemia-reperfusion. J Exp Med. 2005;201:1135–43.

81. Boyd JH, Mathur S, Wang Y, Bateman RM, Walley KR. Toll-like receptor stimulation in cardiomyocytes decreases contractility and initiates an NF-κB dependent inflammatory response. Cardiovasc Res. 2006;72:384–93.

82. Zhao P, Wang J, He L, Ma H, Zhang X, Zhu X, Dolence EK, Ren J, Li J. Deficiency in TLR4 signal transduction ameliorates cardiac injury and cardiomyocyte contractile dysfunction during ischemia. J Cell Mol Med. 2009;13:1513–25.

83. Sakata Y, Dong JW, Vallejo JG, Huang CH, Baker JS, Tracey KJ, Tacheuchi O, Akira S, Mann DL. Toll-like receptor 2 modulates left ventricular function following ischemia-reperfusion injury. Am J Physiol Heart Circ Physiol. 2007;292:H503–9.

84. Chong AJ, Shiamamoto, Hamptom CR, Takayama H, Spring DJ, Rothnie CL, Yada M, Pohlman TH, Verrier ED. Toll-like receptor 4 mediates ischemia/reperfusion injury of the heart. J Thorac Cardiovasc Surg. 2004;128:170–9.

85. Leemans JC, Stokman G, Claessen N, Rouschop KM, Teske GJ, Kirschning CJ, Akira S, van der Poll T, Weening JJ, Florquin S. Renal-associated TLR2 mediates ischemia/reperfusion injury in the kidney. J Clin Invest. 2005;115:2894–903.

86. Evankovich J, Billiar Tsung A. Toll-like receptors in hepatic ischemia/reperfusion and transplantation. Gastroenterol Res Pract. 2010;pii:537263.

87. Shimamoto A, Chung AJ, Yada M, Shomura S, Takayama H, Fleisig AJ, Agnew ML, Hampton CR, Rothnie CL, Spring DJ, Pohlman TH, Shimpo H, Verrier ED. Inhibition of Toll-like receptor 4 with eritoran attenuates myocardial ischemia-reperfusion injury. Circulation. 2006;114(1 suppl):I270–4.

88. Liu M, Gu M, Xu D, Lv Q, Zhang W, Wu Y. Protective effects of toll-like receptor 4 inhibitor eritoran on renal ischemia-reperfusion injury. Transplant Proc. 2010;42:1539–44.

89. Kandasamy AD, Chow AK, Ali MA, Schulz R. Matrix metalloproteinase-2 and myocardial oxidative stress injury: beyond the matrix. Cardiovasc Res. 2010;85:413–23.

90. Massova I, Kotra LP, Fridman R, Mobashery S. Matrix metalloproteinases; structures, evolution, and diversification. FASEB. 1998;12:1075–95.

91. Baker AH, Edwards DR, Murphy G. Metalloproteinase inhibitors: biological actions and therapeutic opportunities. J Cell Sci. 2002;115:3719–27.

92. Viappiani S, Sariahmetoglu M, Schulz R. The role of matrix metalloproteinase inhibitors in ischemia-reperfusion injury in the liver. Curr Pharm Des. 2006;12:2923–34.

93. Kuyvenhoven JP, Ringers J, Verspaget HW, Lamers CB, van Hoek B. Serum matrix metalloproteinase MMP-2 and MMP-9 in the late phase of ischemia and reperfusion injury in human orthotopic liver transplantation. Transplant Proc. 2003;35:2967–9.

94. Kitajima K, Koike J, Nozawa S, Yoshiike M, Takagi M, Chikaraishi T. Irreversible immunoexpression of matrix metalloproteinase-9 in proximal tubular epithelium of renal allografts with acute rejection. Clin Transplant. 2011;25:E336–44.

95. Hsia TY, McQuinn TC, Mukherjee R, Deardorff RL, Squires JE, Stroud RE, Crawford FA, Bradley SM, Reeves ST, Spinale FG. Effects of aprotinin or tranexamic acid on proteolytic/cytokine profiles in infants after cardiac surgery. Ann Thorac Surg. 2010;89:1843–52.

96. Okamoto T, Akaike T, Sawa T, Miyamoto Y, van der Vliet A, Maeda H. Activation of matrix metalloproteinases by peroxynitrite-induced protein S-glutathiolation via disulfide S-oxide formation. J Biol Chem. 2001;276:29596–602.

97. Wang W, Schulze CJ, Suarez-Pinzon WL, Dyck JR, Sawicki G, Schulz R. Intracellular action of matrix metalloproteinase-2 accounts for acute myocardial ischemia and reperfusion injury. Circulation. 2002;106:1543–9.

98. Cheung PY, Sawicki G, Wozniak M, Wang W, Radomski MW, Schulz R. Matrix metalloproteinase-2 contributes to ischemia-reperfusion injury in the heart. Circulation. 2000;101:1833–9.

99. Lalu MM, Pasini E, Schulze CJ, Ferrari-Vivaldi M, Ferrari-Vivaldi G, Bachetti T, Schulz R. Ischaemia-reperfusion injury activates

matrix metalloproteinases in the human heart. Eur Heart J. 2005;26:
27–35.

100. Frears ER, Zhang Z, Blake DR, O'Connell JP, Winyard PG.
Inactivation of tissue inhibitor of metalloproteinase-1 by peroxynitrite. FEBS Lett. 1996;381:21–4.

101. Donnini S, Monti M, Roncone R, Morbidelli L, Rocchigiani M,
Oliviero S, Casella L, Giachetti A, Schulz R, Ziche M.
Peroxynitrite inactivates human-tissue inhibitor of metalloprotein-
ase-4. FEBS Lett. 2008;582:1135–40.

102. Peterson JT. Matrix metalloproteinase inhibitor development and
the remodeling of drug discovery. Heart Fail Rev. 2004;9:63–79.

103. Gapski R, Hasturk H, Van Dyke TE, Oringer RJ, Wang S, Braun
TM, Giannobile WV. Systemic MMP inhibition for periodontal
wound repair: results of a multi-centre randomized-controlled
clinical trial. J Clin Periodontol. 2009;36:149–56.

104. Hackmann AE, Rubin BG, Sanchez LA, Geraghty PA, Thompson
RW, Curci JA. A randomized, placebo-controlled trial of doxycycline
after endoluminal aneurysm repair. J Vasc Surg. 2008;48:519–26.

105. Williams RS, Benjamin IJ. Protective responses in the ischemic
myocardium. J Clin Invest. 2000;106:813–8.

106. Stephanou A, Latchman DS. Transcriptional regulation of the heat
shock protein genes by STAT family transcription factors. Gene
Expr. 1999;7:311–9.

107. Knowlton AA, Sun L. Heat-shock factor-1, steroid hormones, and
regulation of heat-shock protein expression in the heart. Am J
Physiol Heart Circ Physiol. 2001;280:H455–64.

108. Okubo S, Wildner O, Shah MR, Chelliah JC, Hess ML, Kukreja
RC. Gene transfer of heat-shock protein 70 reduces infarct size in
vivo after ischemia/reperfusion in the rabbit heart. Circulation.
2001;103:877–81.

109. Abraham NG, Kappas A. Heme oxygenase and the cardiovascular-
renal system. Free Radic Biol Med. 2005;39:1–25.

110. Hausenloy DJ, Yellon DM. New directions for protecting the heart
against ischaemia-reperfusion injury: targeting the Reperfusion Injury
Salvage Kinase (RISK)-pathway. Cardiovasc Res. 2004;61:448–60.

111. Levine B, Kroemer G. Autophagy in the pathogenesis of disease.
Cell. 2008;132:27–42.

112. Dong Y, Undyala VV, Gottlieb RA, Mentzer Jr RM, Przyklenk K.
Autophagy: definition, molecular machinery, and potential role in
the myocardial ischemia-reperfusion injury. J Cardiovasc
Pharmacol Ther. 2010;15:220–30.

113. Isaka Y, Suzuki C, Abe T, Okumi M, Ichimaru N, Imamura R,
Kakuta Y, Matsui I, Takabatake Y, Rakugi H, Shimizu S, Takahara
S. Bcl-2 protects tubular epithelial cells from ischemia/reperfu-
sion injury by dual mechanisms. Transplant Proc. 2009;41:52–4.

114. Gotoh K, Lu Z, Morita M, Shibata M, Koike M, Waguri S, Dono
K, Doki Y, Kominami E, Sugioka A, Monden M, Uchiyama Y.
Participation of autophagy in the initiation of graft dysfunction
after rat liver transplantation. Autophagy. 2009;5:351–60.

115. Adhami F, Liao G, Morozov YM, Schloemer A, Schmithorst VJ,
Lorenz JN, Dunn RS, Vorhees CV, Wills-Karp M, Degen JL,
Davis RJ, Mizushima N, Rakic P, Dardzinski BJ, Holland SK,
Sharp FR. Cerebral ischemia-hypoxia induces intravascular coag-
ulation and autophagy. Am J Pathol. 2006;169:566–83.

116. Klionsky DJ. The molecular machinery of autophagy: unanswered
questions. J Cell Sci. 2005;118:7–18.

117. Ryter SW, Lee SJ, Smith A, Choi AM. Autophagy in vascular
disease. Proc Am Thorac Soc. 2010;7:40–7.

118. Matsui Y, Takagi H, Qu X, Abdellatif M, Sakoda H, Asano T, Levine
B, Sadoshima J. Distinct roles of autophagy in the heart during isch-
emia and reperfusion: roles of AMP-activated protein kinase and
Beclin 1 in mediating autophagy. Circ Res. 2007;100:914–22.

119. Rasbach KA, Schnellmann RG. Signaling of mitochondrial biogenesis following oxidant injury. J Biol Chem. 2007;282:2355–62.

120. Kanamori H, Takemura G, Marayuma G, Goto K, Tsujimoto A,
Ogina A, Li L, Kawamura I, Takeyama T, Kawaguchi T,
Nagashima K, Fujiwara T, Fujiwara H, Seishima M, Minatoguchi

S. Functional significance and morphological characterization of
starvation-induced autophagy in the adult heart. Am J Pathol.
2009;174:1705–14.

121. Takagi H, Matsui Y, Sadoshima J. The role of autophagy in mediating cell survival and death during ischemia and reperfusion in
the heart. Antioxid Redox Signal. 2007;9:1373–81.

122. Xi J, Wang H, Mueller RA, Norfleet EA, Xu Z. Mechanism for
resveratrol-induced cardioprotection against reperfusion injury
involves glycogen synthase kinase 3beta and mitochondrial permeability transition pore. Eur J Pharmacol. 2009;604:111–6.

123. Gurusamy N, Lekli I, Mukherjee S, Ray D, Ahsan MK,
Gherghiceanu M, Popescu LM, Das DK. Cardioprotection by resveratrol: a novel mechanism via autophagy involving the mTORC2
pathway. Cardiovasc Res. 2010;86:103–12.

124. Nicholson CK, Calvert JW. Hydrogen sulfide and ischemia-
reperfusion injury. Pharmacol Res. 2010;62:289–97.

125. Abe K, Kimura H. The possible role of hydrogen sulfide as an
endogenous neuromodulator. J Neurosci. 1996;16:1066–71.

126. Hosoki R, Matsuki N, Kimura H. The possible role of hydrogen
sulfide as an endogenous smooth muscle relaxant in synergy with
nitric oxide. Biochem Biophys Res Commun. 1997;237:527–31.

127. Johansen D, Ytrehus K, Baxter GF. Exogenous hydrogen sulfide
(H2S) protects against regional myocardial ischemia-reperfusion
injury—evidence for a role of K ATP channels. Basic Res Cardiol.
2006;101:53–60.

128. Bliksoen M, Kaljusto ML, Vaage J, Stenslokken KO. Effects of
hydrogen sulphide on ischaemia-reperfusion injury and ischaemic
preconditioning in the isolated, perfused rat heart. Eur J
Cardiothorac Surg. 2008;34:344–9.

129. Jha S, Calvert JW, Duranski MR, Ramachandran A, Lefer DJ.
Hydrogen sulfide attenuates hepatic ischemia-reperfusion injury:
role of antioxidant and antiapoptotic signaling. Am J Physiol
Heart Circ Physiol. 2008;295:H801–6.

130. Tripatara P, Patel NS, Collino M, Gallicchio M, Kieswich J,
Castiglia S, Benetti E, Stewart KN, Brown PA, Yaqoob MM,
Fantozzi R, Thiemermann C. Generation of endogenous hydrogen
sulfide by crystathionine gamma-lyase limits renal ischemia/reper-
fusion injury and dysfunction. Lab Invest. 2008;88:1038–48.

131. Whiteman M, Armstrong JS, Chu SH, Jia-Ling S, Wong BS,
Cheung NS, Halliwell B, Moore PK. The novel neuromodulator
hydrogen sulfide; an endogenous peroxynitrite "scavenger"?
J Neurochem. 2004;90:765–8.

132. Hu Y, Chen X, Pan TT, Neo KL, Lee SW, Khin ES, Moore PK,
Bian JS. Cardioprotection induced by hydrogen sulfide precondi-
tioning involves activation of ERK and PI3K/Akt pathways.
Pflugers Arch. 2008;455:607–16.

133. Pan TT, Neo KL, Hu LF, Yong QC, Bian JS. H2S preconditioning-
induced PKC activation regulates intracellular calcium handling
in rat cardiomyocytes. Am J Physiol Cell Physiol. 2008;294:
C169–77.

134. Zanardo RC, Brancaleone V, Distrutti E, Fiorucci S, Cirino G,
Wallace JL. Hydrogen sulfide is an endogenous modulator of
leukocyte-mediated inflammation. FASEB J. 2006;20:2118–20.

135. Li L, Moore PK. Putative biological roles of hydrogen sulfide in
health and disease: a breath of not so fresh air? Trends Pharmacol
Sci. 2008;29:84–90.

136. Murry CE, Jennings RB, Reimer KA. Preconditioning with ischemia: a delay of lethal cell injury in ischemic myocardium.
Circulation. 1986;74:1124–36.

137. Mallick IH, Yang W, Winslet MC, Seifalian AM. Ischemia-
reperfusion injury of the intestine and protective strategies against
injury. Dig Dis Sci. 2004;49:1359–77.

138. Pasupathy S, Homer-Vanniasinkam S. Surgical implications of
ischemic preconditioning. Arch Surg. 2005;140:405–10.

139. Stein AB, Tang XL, Guo Y, Xuan YT, Dawn B, Bolli R. Delayed
adaptation of the heart to stress: late preconditioning. Stroke.
2004;35:2676–9.

Part III

Resuscitation, Stabilization, and Transport of the Critically Ill or Injured Child

Vinay Nadkarni

Monica E. Kleinman and Meredith G. van der Velden

Abstract

Pediatric cardiac arrest is an infrequent but potentially devastating event. While return of spontaneous circulation (ROSC) is the immediate objective, the ultimate goal is survival with meaningful neurologic outcome. Once a perfusing rhythm is established, the pediatric cardiac arrest victim requires expert critical care to optimize organ function, prevent secondary injury, and maximize the child's potential for recovery. Common post-resuscitation conditions include acute lung injury, myocardial dysfunction, hepatic and renal insufficiency, and hypoxic-ischemic encephalopathy. This constellation is described by the term "post-cardiac arrest syndrome" and resembles the systemic inflammatory response seen in sepsis or major trauma. Children may have single organ failure or multi-organ dysfunction, and the need for critical care therapies may delay accurate evaluation of neurologic status and limit prognostic ability. Pediatric post-resuscitation therapies are not typically evidence-based given the paucity of randomized trials and heterogeneous nature of the patient population. Goals of care include normalizing physiologic and metabolic status, preventing secondary organ injury, and diagnosing and treating the underlying cause of the arrest. Therapeutic hypothermia has been shown to mitigate the severity of brain injury for adults following sudden arrhythmia induced cardiac arrest and neonates following resuscitation from hypoxic-ischemic encephalopathy at birth, but the role of targeted temperature control in pediatric post-arrest care is an area of active investigation. There is no single diagnostic test or set of criteria to accurately predict neurologic outcome, providing a challenging situation for critical care specialists and families alike.

Keywords

Resuscitation • Cardiac arrest • Critical care • Organ dysfunction • Post-cardiac arrest syndrome • Reperfusion • Brain injury

Introduction

The immediate objective of pediatric cardiopulmonary resuscitation is return of spontaneous circulation (ROSC), while the ultimate goal is survival with a favorable neurologic outcome. Once a perfusing rhythm is established, the pediatric cardiac arrest victim requires critical care focused to optimize organ function, prevent secondary injury, and maximize the child's potential for recovery. Common post-resuscitation conditions include acute lung injury, myocardial dysfunction, hepatic and renal insufficiency, and

M.E. Kleinman, MD (✉)
Division of Critical Care Medicine,
Department of Anesthesiology, Children's Hospital Boston,
300 Longwood Avenue, Bader 634, Boston, MA 02115, USA
e-mail: monica.kleinman@childrens.harvard.edu

M.G. van der Velden, MD
Department of Anesthesia, Children's Hospital Boston,
300 Longwood Avenue, Bader 634, Boston, MA 02115, USA
e-mail: meredith.vandervelden@childrens.harvard.edu

seizures/encephalopathy. The extent of neurologic injury may be initially difficult to assess due to multi-organ system failure following hypoxia-ischemia and reperfusion. In the pediatric intensive care unit (PICU), the most common cause of death following admission after cardiac arrest is hypoxic-ischemic encephalopathy [1, 2], which is also responsible for the most significant morbidity in survivors.

Considerations for post-resuscitation care are impacted by whether the resuscitation occurs out-of-hospital or in-hospital, since the epidemiology and etiology for pediatric cardiac arrest differ in these settings. Out-of-hospital arrest is more likely to be asphyxial in origin, in which cardiac arrest is the end result of progressive hypoxia and ischemia. Multiple cohort studies of out-of-hospital pediatric cardiac arrests have found that most were of respiratory origin [3–12]. A recent report from 11 North American sites participating in the Resuscitation Outcomes Consortium (ROC) found that the incidence of non-traumatic out-of-hospital cardiac arrest in patients <20 years of age was 8.04 per 100,000 person-years, and was significantly higher among infants than children or adolescents [5]. The initial cardiac rhythm was asystole or pulseless electrical activity (PEA) in 82 % of patients, and the most common etiology was an asphyxial event such as drowning or strangulation. In systematic reviews, trauma and sudden infant death syndrome remain the most common causes of pediatric out-of-hospital cardiac arrest [3, 13]. Survival ranges from 6.4 to 12 %, with rates of neurologically-intact survival of only 2.7–4 % [3–6, 13].

Pediatric cardiac arrest in the inpatient setting is more likely to be witnessed or to occur in a monitored setting, but a high proportion of patients have pre-existing co-morbidities [14]. Not surprisingly, the highest incidence of in-hospital pediatric cardiac arrest is in the PICU, affecting 1–6 % of patients admitted [15, 16]. Regardless, the outcome from in-hospital arrest is consistently better than for out-of-hospital events. A 2006 report of 880 pediatric inpatient arrests from a voluntary national registry found survival to hospital discharge was 27 %, while a 2009 review of 353 in-hospital cardiac arrests reported a survival to discharge rate of 48.7 % [17, 18]. The etiology of pediatric in-hospital arrest differs from out-of-hospital events in that cardiac conditions (including shock) are as likely as respiratory failure to be the immediate cause of the arrest (61–72 %) [12, 17]. Asystole and PEA account for 24–64 % of the initial cardiac rhythms. Interestingly, infants and children who are resuscitated from inpatient cardiac arrest have a high likelihood of favorable neurologic outcome, with results ranging from 63 to 76.7 % in two recent studies [17, 18].

Post-cardiac Arrest Syndrome

Recent advances in the understanding of pathophysiologic events following return of circulation have led to the description of the "post-cardiac arrest syndrome" [19].

This condition is characterized by myocardial dysfunction, neurologic impairment, and endothelial injury that resemble inflammatory conditions such as sepsis (capillary leak, fever, coagulopathy, vasodilation). The series of events during reperfusion can be divided into four phases: (1) immediate (first 20 min after ROSC); (2) early post-arrest (20 min through 6–12 h after resuscitation); (3) intermediate phase (6–12 h through 72 h post-arrest); and (4) recovery phase (beyond 72 h). Some experts have included a fifth phase, that of rehabilitation after discharge from an acute care setting (Fig. 25.1).

Pathophysiology of the Post-arrest Reperfusion State

The post-cardiac arrest syndrome results from two distinct but serial events – a period of ischemia, during which cardiac output and oxygen delivery are profoundly compromised, followed by a period of tissue and organ reperfusion. At the time of cardiac arrest, oxygen extraction increases in an effort to compensate for reduced delivery. As demand rapidly exceeds supply, tissue hypoxia triggers anaerobic metabolism and lactate production. At the cellular level, hypoxia limits oxidative phosphorylation and mitochondrial ATP production. As a result, ATP-dependent membrane functions such as maintenance of ion gradients begin to fail.

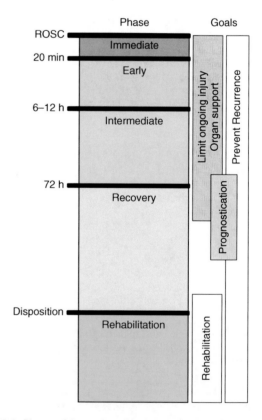

Fig. 25.1 Phases of the post-cardiac arrest syndrome (Reprinted from Neumar et al. [19]. With permission from Wolters Kluwer Health)

The resultant depolarization permits opening of voltage-dependent channels leading to entry of calcium, sodium, and water into the cell. Cellular injury and death follow, with tissues demonstrating high oxygen consumption at most risk.

Lopez-Herce et al. described the progression of physiologic and biochemical changes occurring in an infant swine model of asphyxial arrest [20]. At 10 min after discontinuation of mechanical ventilation, arterial pH had decreased from a median of 7.40 to 7.09, PaO_2 was unmeasurable, and $PaCO_2$ had increased from a median of 41 to 80 mmHg. Lactate increased from 0.8 to 5.7 mmol/L. After transient tachycardia and hypertension from increased systemic vascular resistance (SVR), progressive bradycardia and hypotension occurred with no measureable systemic blood pressure by 10 min. After 10 min, subjects were resuscitated with conventional CPR and one of four vasoconstrictor regimens (epinephrine alone, terlipressin alone, epinephrine + terlipressin, or no medications). ROSC was achieved in just over one-third of the animals within 20 min. Following ROSC, there was an initial brief recovery of cardiac index, SVR, and mean arterial pressure (MAP), followed by a progressive decline. Over the first 30 min after ROSC, arterial and venous pH increased but did not return to baseline, and lactate remained elevated.

Following ROSC, a complex cascade of biochemical events occurs as blood flow and oxygen delivery are restored. The major pathophysiologic processes include endothelial activation and formation of oxygen-free radicals. Endothelial activation by ischemia/reperfusion results in upregulation of inflammatory mediators (e.g., leukocyte adhesion molecules, procalcitonin, C-reactive protein, cytokines, TNF-α [alpha]) and downregulation of anti-inflammatory agents such as nitric oxide and prostacyclin [21–23]. Coupled with activation of the complement and coagulation cascades, this systemic response leads to capillary leak, intravascular coagulation, and impaired vasomotor regulation.

Although restoration of oxygen delivery is one objective of cardiopulmonary resuscitation, the post-resuscitation exposure of ischemic tissue to high concentrations of oxygen can be injurious due to generation of oxygen-free radicals. During ischemia, intracellular concentrations of hypoxanthine are increased; with the restoration of tissue oxygenation, hypoxanthine is converted to xanthine with oxygen radicals produced as a byproduct. Furthermore, ischemic tissue becomes depleted of natural anti-oxidant defenses such as nitric oxide, superoxide dismutase, glutathione peroxidase, and glutathione reductase. In an infant rat model of asphyxial arrest, animals resuscitated with 100 % oxygen during and after CPR showed decreased hippocampal reduced glutathione, increased activity of manganese superoxide dismutase, and increased cortical lipid peroxidation [24]. Reactive oxygen species have multiple negative effects and can modulate signaling molecules including protein kinases, transcription factors, receptors, and pro- and anti-apoptotic factors [25].

The use of anti-oxidant therapy or other inflammatory modulators to prevent or reduce the post-cardiac arrest syndrome is a promising area of research, primarily in animal models. Multiple agents have been studied including nitric oxide, N-acetylcysteine, erythropoietin, steroids, cyclosporine, ascorbic acid, trimetazidine and diazoxide [26–29].

Activation of the inflammatory cascade, with suppression of anti-inflammatory defense mechanisms, interferes with endothelial relaxation and promotes vasoconstriction and microvascular thrombosis. At the vital organ level this results in secondary ischemic injury [30]. In its most severe form, ischemia-reperfusion injury results in multiple organ system dysfunction (MODS), a common cause of delayed mortality following resuscitation from cardiac arrest. Individually, infants and children may demonstrate different patterns of organ injury, with neurologic and cardiac dysfunction most prevalent.

Post-resuscitation Care of the Respiratory System

Oxygenation and ventilation are key components of resuscitation from pediatric cardiac arrest. In the out-of-hospital setting, bag-mask ventilation is typically the initial airway management technique. Advanced life support teams may be trained and authorized to perform more invasive airway support such as supraglottic airway devices or tracheal intubation. Pre-hospital intubation for children with cardiac or respiratory arrest is an area of ongoing controversy. A large prospective randomized trial showed no difference in survival or neurologic outcome if children were intubated vs. ventilated via bag and mask for respiratory failure, respiratory arrest, or cardiac arrest. In the intubation group there was a high rate of failed intubations and unrecognized esophageal intubations. Critics of this study note that the EMS providers who participated in the study received 6 h of classroom and mannequin training, suggesting that the results could be partly attributed to lack of proficiency as opposed to the intervention itself [31].

If the infant or child was tracheally intubated during resuscitation, the first priority is to confirm appropriate tracheal tube position, patency, and security. Children who are intubated at a referring hospital prior to transport are more likely to have a right mainstem intubation than if they were intubated in a tertiary PICU (13.4 % vs. 3.9 %) [32]. Pre-hospital providers frequently select tracheal tubes that are either too large or too small for the patient's size [33]. A tracheal tube that is too small for the child may hinder adequate ventilation and oxygenation due to excessive glottic air leak and loss of tidal volume and end-expiratory pressure. Consideration should be given to reintubating the patient with a larger and/or a cuffed tracheal tube. A tracheal tube that is oversized, especially one with an inflated cuff, can injure the tracheal mucosa and increase the risk of complications such as subglottic stenosis. In addition to deflating the cuff, consideration should be given to replacing the tube under controlled circumstances with an age-appropriate size, weighing the risks and benefits of removing an existing airway. If a cuffed tracheal tube was used for intubation, cuff pressures should be measured and adjusted to the recommended level of ≤20 cm H_2O.

Regurgitation of gastric contents is common during cardiopulmonary resuscitation, leading to risk for aspiration. Reflux of acidic gastric material into the pharynx can occur even without active vomiting, especially when patients are in the supine position and have loss of lower esophageal sphincter tone. Regurgitation was reported in 20 % of adult patients who survived cardiac arrest and received bystander CPR, of whom 46 % had radiographic evidence of aspiration [34]. Aspiration of gastric contents or blood was documented on autopsy in 29 % of adult non-survivors after CPR [35]. Specific circumstances such as near-drowning are associated with a high incidence of regurgitation. Computerized tomography of the chest in drowning victims of multiple ages revealed evidence of pulmonary aspiration in 60 % of victims [36].

Bag-mask ventilations frequently result in gastric insufflation and distension and are the recommended initial technique for pediatric airway management during cardiac arrest [37]. The use of cricoid pressure, often advocated to reduce the risk of aspiration during positive-pressure ventilation and tracheal intubation, may not be as effective as once believed. Studies in anesthetized children suggest that the primary effect of cricoid pressure is to prevent gastric insufflation during mask ventilation, although there are no data about its efficacy during pediatric cardiac arrest [38, 39].

Following cardiac arrest, children are at risk for development of acute lung injury (ALI) and acute respiratory distress syndrome (ARDS) as a result of reperfusion injury of the lung and, potentially, pulmonary aspiration. ALI and ARDS are clinical diagnoses and are distinguished by the degree of impairment of oxygenation: a PaO_2/FiO_2 ratio of <300 denotes ALI, while a PaO_2/FiO_2 ratio of <200 is used to define ARDS [40]. ALI and ARDS are characterized by decreased lung compliance and increased alveolar-capillary permeability in the setting of a normal pulmonary arterial occlusion pressure, resulting in surfactant deactivation, pulmonary edema and infiltrates, and hypoxemia. True cardiogenic pulmonary edema is more likely to occur in adults after resuscitation from cardiac arrest, possibly related to the common precipitating factor of coronary artery occlusion and myocardial infarction with resultant depressed myocardial function.

The goals of mechanical ventilation in the pediatric patient after cardiac arrest include provision of adequate ventilation and oxygenation while minimizing the risk of ventilator-induced lung injury (barotrauma or volutrauma). Optimal ventilation and oxygenation parameters following resuscitation from pediatric cardiac arrest are unknown. In general, ventilation is considered acceptable if there is an adequate pH (≥7.30). Hyperventilation should be avoided to minimize the risk of further lung injury and to prevent secondary cerebral ischemia. Use of capnography for non-invasive assessment of ventilation may be misleading if there is increased dead space related to reduced pulmonary blood flow or parenchymal lung disease; in such situations arterial blood gas measurement is a more accurate method to measure $PaCO_2$.

Following return of spontaneous circulation, current American Heart Association guidelines recommend that the inspired oxygen concentration be progressively reduced based on pulse oximetry [37]. In the presence of a normal hemoglobin concentration, an arterial oxygen saturation of >94 % is typically sufficient for the infant or child post-arrest. In cases of severe anemia or hemorrhage, higher inspired oxygen concentrations may be appropriate until adequate oxygen carrying capacity is restored. Since an arterial oxygen saturation of 100 % could correspond with a PaO_2 anywhere between ~80 and 500 mmHg, pediatric resuscitation guidelines also recommend using 99 % as an upper limit for arterial oxygen saturation. Because the use of 100 % oxygen is a common default practice during intra- and interfacility transfer, whenever possible, providers should be advised to titrate FiO_2 to achieve the goal arterial oxygen saturations.

Exposure to high concentrations of oxygen may result in arterial hyperoxia, increasing the risk for oxygen free-radical formation and oxidative injury during reperfusion. Evidence from animal models and, more recently, human studies demonstrate that post-arrest hyperoxia worsens neurologic outcome [41–43]. Kilgannon et. al. reviewed >6,000 adult non-traumatic cardiac arrest patients who survived to hospital admission, and categorized them by the first PaO_2 obtained in the ICU. Patients who were hyperoxic, defined as a PaO_2 >300 mmHg, had a higher in-hospital mortality compared with patients who were normoxic (PaO_2 60–300 mmHg) or hypoxic (PaO_2 <60 mmHg). Even after controlling for multiple confounders, hyperoxia was an independent risk factor for mortality with an odds ratio of 1.8. The same investigators studied the relationship between post-resuscitation PaO_2 as a continuous variable and in-hospital mortality. Interestingly, the median post-resuscitation PaO_2 was 231 mmHg with an interquartile range of 149–349 mmHg. Using multivariable analysis, they demonstrated that for each 100 mmHg increase in PaO_2 during the first 24 h of admission there was a 24 % increase in mortality.

For patients with acute lung injury or ARDS, a lung protective strategy is typically employed using pressure-controlled ventilation. The components of a lung protective strategy include: (1) low tidal volumes (5–6 mL/kg), (2) limited plateau pressures (≤ 30 cm H_2O), (3) optimal PEEP to restore and maintain functional residual capacity, and (4) exposure to non-toxic concentrations of oxygen ($FiO_2 \leq 0.6$). A certain degree of respiratory acidosis is tolerated, an approach termed permissive hypercapnea. The level of hypercarbia that is acceptable may be influenced by other organ system concerns such as cerebral edema from hypoxic-ischemic brain injury. Cerebral blood vessel reactivity to carbon dioxide is preserved in comatose adult patients following cardiac arrest, so extremes of hypo- and hyperventilation should be avoided [44].

The initial maneuver for a patient with persistent hypoxemia is the escalation of PEEP in an effort to increase functional residual capacity and reduce intrapulmonary shunting. Those who remain hypoxemic or develop extrapulmonary air leak may be candidates for a trial of high frequency oscillatory ventilation (HFOV). Use of HFOV frequently requires neuromuscular blockade, however, which hampers ongoing neurologic assessment. Another therapeutic consideration is surfactant replacement therapy, which was found to decrease mortality in a recent meta-analysis of children with acute respiratory failure [45]. The optimal dosing, frequency, and duration of therapy have not been determined.

Post-resuscitation Care of the Cardiovascular System

Except for very brief episodes of cardiac arrest, most patients will demonstrate some impact of cardiac arrest on post-resuscitation circulatory status. Initial assessment should focus on the rate and rhythm, blood pressure, peripheral perfusion, and end-organ function (mental status, pupillary exam, urine output). An inappropriately slow heart rate associated with hypotension requires urgent treatment to prevent deterioration. Underlying causes of persistent bradycardia to consider include hypothermia, hypoxia, acidosis, electrolyte disturbances, hypoglycemia, toxins, or increased intracranial pressure. Appropriate management is directed at treating the suspected etiology and the use of pharmacologic agents to increase heart rate, such as adrenergic agents or vagolytic agents, or use of electrical pacing.

Tachycardia is commonly observed after resuscitation from cardiac arrest and may be multifactorial, resulting from use of β [beta]-adrenergic agents, early myocardial dysfunction, and cardiac rhythm disturbances. In general, tachycardia is well tolerated in infants and children, and treatment to control rate is indicated only if the patient has a tachyarrhythmia that results in hemodynamic compromise. Tachyarrhythmias should be managed according to the relevant treatment protocols depending on the type of rhythm and the patient's clinical status. Patients who are hypotensive in the setting of supraventricular or ventricular tachycardia should receive immediate synchronized cardioversion, with or without sedation depending on the level of consciousness [37]. If the patient is normotensive, pharmacologic therapy can be attempted while closely monitoring the patient's hemodynamic status. Other causes for tachyarrhythmias should also be considered, including central venous catheter position, electrolyte or metabolic derangements, hyperpyrexia, and adverse effects of adrenergic agents. Increased myocardial oxygen consumption associated with tachyarrhythmias may result in myocardial ischemia, and a 12-lead ECG may identify ST-segment changes or pre-excitation that could signal risk for further rhythm disturbances. Expert consultation with a pediatric cardiologist is recommended for guidance regarding anti-arrhythmic and other therapies.

Myocardial dysfunction occurs in most adults and children following resuscitation from cardiac arrest, a condition known as "myocardial stunning." Despite the restoration of myocardial blood flow and oxygen delivery, echocardiographic evidence of myocardial dysfunction typically persists for 24–48 h following resuscitation [46]. The pathophysiology of this reperfusion injury is characterized by cardiac tissue edema and decreased contractility with low cardiac index. Hemodynamic studies of children following near-drowning have demonstrated an increase in atrial and ventricular end-diastolic filling pressures as well as systemic and pulmonary vascular resistance [47]. In animal models, the degree of myocardial dysfunction is correlated with the duration of cardiac arrest and is more severe when cardiac arrest is due to ventricular fibrillation compared with asphyxia [48, 49]. Post-arrest troponin levels are inversely correlated with ejection fraction and survival in pediatric patients following resuscitation from cardiac arrest [50]. Pediatric animal studies suggest that the use of adult defibrillation doses leads to greater myocardial dysfunction and higher levels of troponin leak than attenuated pediatric doses [51].

The goals of hemodynamic support following resuscitation from cardiac arrest are to restore and maintain end-organ perfusion and oxygen delivery. Those children who are suspected of having inadequate preload due to volume loss may receive isotonic fluids in small boluses of 5–10 mL/kg, titrated to signs of improved hemodynamics such as resolving tachycardia and improved peripheral perfusion. Frequent reassessment after each fluid bolus is essential to avoid excessive increases in cardiac filling pressures that could lead to pulmonary edema and worsening gas exchange. Patients resuscitated from cardiac arrest in the setting of trauma or hemorrhage may benefit from resuscitation with blood products such as packed red blood cells to replete low blood volume and increase oxygen-carrying capacity. Optimization of preload is best accomplished using invasive monitoring in the critical care setting. Placement of a catheter with the tip in the SVC or IVC permits monitoring of central venous pressure to estimate right-sided filling

Table 25.1 Vasoactive agents for post-resuscitation myocardial dysfunction

	Type	Receptors	Physiologic effect	Dose range
Dopamine	Endogenous catecholamine	Dopaminergic agonist	Renal and splanchnic vasodilation	2–5 mcg/kg/min
		β [beta]-1 and -2 agonist	Positive inotropy and chronotropy	5–10 mcg/kg/min
		α [alpha]-agonist	Vasoconstriction	10–20 mcg/kg/min titrated to effect
Dobutamine	Synthetic catecholamine	β [beta]-1 and -2 with intrinsic α [alpha]-adrenergic agonist and antagonist activity	Positive inotropy and chronotropy; may cause systemic vasodilation	2–20 mcg/kg/min titrated to effect
Epinephrine	Endogenous catecholamine	β [beta]-1 and -2	Positive inotropy and chronotropy; vasodilation at low doses	Low dose: 0.1–0.3 mcg/kg/min;
		α [alpha]-1 and -2 agonist	At higher infusion rate causes potent vasoconstriction	High dose: 0.3–1 mcg/kg/min titrated to effect
Levosimendan	Calcium-sensitizer	Increases cardiac myocyte sensitivity to calcium; opens potassium channels on vascular smooth muscle	Positive inotropy, vasodilation ("inodilator")	Loading dose: 12–24 mcg/kg over 10 min; infusion: 0.1–0.2 mcg/kg/min
Milrinone	Phosphodiesterase type III (PDE III) inhibitor	No receptor; PDE III enzyme inhibition increases myocardial cAMP and intracellular calcium	Positive inotropy, vasodilation ("inodilator")	Load: 50–75 mcg/kg over 10–60 min; infusion: 0.5–0.75 mcg/kg/min
Norepinephrine	Endogenous catecholamine	β [beta]-1 and -2 agonist	Positive inotropy and chronotropy; vasoconstriction	0.1–2 mcg/kg/min titrated to effect
		α [alpha]-1 and -2 agonist		
Vasopressin	Endogenous posterior pituitary peptide hormone	V_1 (vascular smooth muscle), V_2 (renal)	Vasoconstriction, anti-diuresis	0.17–10 milliunits/kg/min (0.01–0.6 units/kg/h)

pressures. Femoral venous lines in the infrahepatic IVC have shown good correlation with right atrial filling pressures in cohorts of pediatric cardiac patients and critically ill children in the ICU setting even with changes in mean airway pressure and PEEP [52–55].

Inotropic and vasoactive infusions are the mainstay of therapy for post-arrest myocardial dysfunction. These agents improve cardiac output and oxygen delivery by increasing myocardial contractility and by either increasing or decreasing systemic vascular resistance. Despite the frequent use of vasoactive infusions for post-resuscitation myocardial support, to date there is no data to establish that such therapy improves patient outcome. The choice of agent depends on the individual patient's physiologic status and the presence or absence of hypotension. Most children with post-resuscitation myocardial dysfunction will have low cardiac output and high systemic vascular resistance and will benefit from medications that increase contractility and reduce afterload. If the patient is normotensive, inodilator drugs such as milrinone may improve cardiac output and end-organ perfusion with less myocardial oxygen cost compared with adrenergic inotropic agents. If the patient is hypotensive, afterload reduction is not likely to be tolerated and the use of agents with both inotropic and vasoconstrictive actions may be necessary to restore adequate end-organ perfusion pressure.

Medications used to manage post-arrest myocardial dysfunction are listed in Table 25.1, along with their primary hemodynamic effects. Most of the vasoactive agents listed have the potential to increase heart rate, either primarily or secondarily, which may limit their benefit due to associated increases in myocardial oxygen consumption. Among the adrenergic agents, significant tachycardia is less likely with norepinephrine. Use of milrinone may result in reflex tachycardia due to afterload reduction, which can generally be managed with judicious volume administration. The exclusive use of pure vasoconstrictor agents such as phenylephrine and vasopressin is not recommended for post-arrest myocardial dysfunction because these agents increase afterload without supporting contractility; however, for those patients who demonstrate refractory vasodilation in the post-arrest period, the use of vasopressin in conjunction with an inotropic agent may be beneficial [56]. Patients who remain hypotensive despite volume resuscitation and vasoactive infusions should be evaluated for adrenal insufficiency, which has been reported as a feature of the post-cardiac arrest syndrome.

Levosimendan is a relatively new inotropic agent that has been studied for treatment of congestive heart failure in adults. The drug acts as an inodilator by increasing myocardial sensitivity to calcium and by activation of peripheral vascular ATP-dependent potassium channels. Animal studies comparing levosimendan with dobutamine demonstrated a greater increase in left ventricular ejection fraction with levosimendan [57]. Several published case series of pediatric patients with post-cardiopulmonary bypass ventricular dysfunction describe improvement in cardiac output and decreased catecholamine requirements when levosimendan was utilized [58, 59].

The physiologic endpoints for post-resuscitation myocardial support are not well established for pediatric patients. Improved peripheral perfusion, normalization of heart rate, normotension, and adequate urine output are accepted clinical signs of improving cardiac function. Serum or whole blood lactate concentrations are laboratory markers of oxygen delivery and should improve as cardiac output normalizes unless there is impairment of oxygen utilization (as in sepsis) or reduced lactate metabolism (as in acute hepatic insufficiency). Echocardiography, while helpful in evaluating systolic function, is less reliable at demonstrating diastolic dysfunction and is of limited usefulness since it can only be performed at discrete points in time.

Placement of a central venous catheter with its tip in the superior vena cava allows the use of SVC oxygen saturations to assess the adequacy of oxygen delivery to the tissues. Proper measurement of $SvcO_2$ requires that co-oximetry be performed on a sample of venous blood from the SVC catheter to yield a measured (versus calculated) oxygen saturation. In the setting of normal arterial oxygen saturations and an adequate hemoglobin concentration, $SvcO_2$ reflects the adequacy of cardiac output. Normal $SvcO_2$ is between 70 and 80 %; an $SvcO_2$ <60 % is evidence for excess oxygen extraction in the setting of low cardiac output.

Patients with severe post-arrest myocardial dysfunction may also benefit from interventions to reduce oxygen consumption such as temperature control, sedation and analgesia, and neuromuscular blockade. If indicated by laboratory measurements, normalization of glucose, calcium, magnesium and phosphorous may also support myocardial contractility and prevent secondary cardiac arrhythmias [60].

Post-resuscitation Neurologic Management

Hypoxic-ischemic brain injury is one of the major factors contributing to mortality after cardiac arrest [1] and arguably the most important determinant of meaningful survival. Despite improved survival rates compared to adults [17], children resuscitated from cardiac arrest have a significant risk of mortality with a majority of survivors having poor neurological outcome [3–5, 12]. Post-cardiac arrest brain injury has been designated to describe the spectrum of neurologic dysfunction observed after cardiac arrest [19], the mitigation and management of which has become an intense focus of basic and clinical research [61].

Pathophysiology

The mechanisms of post-cardiac arrest brain injury are complex [62] and are at interplay with the other components of the post-cardiac arrest syndrome [19, 61]. However, despite extensive knowledge of the molecular mechanisms involved in hypoxic-ischemic injury, interventions to preserve affected neuronal cells remain elusive. Furthermore, the degree of injury itself depends on many factors including duration of cardiac arrest and patient age [63].

Ischemic neurologic injury is known to involve a three-part process [61]. During the initial phase of cessation of cerebral blood flow, oxygen, glucose and ATP are rapidly depleted from cellular stores [61, 64, 65] and toxic metabolites accumulate [65]. As a result, there is disruption of calcium homeostasis, glutamate release and neuronal hyperexcitability [61, 62, 66]. Elevation of intracellular calcium activates multiple enzymatic pathways resulting in further cell injury and death [61]. This occurs during conditions of total ischemia observed in cardiac arrest, as well as during the period of less severe ischemia accompanying effective cardiopulmonary resuscitation. While restoration of cerebral blood flow remains the foremost goal in management of cardiac arrest, there is compelling evidence that significant injury occurs upon brain reperfusion, resulting in a second phase of the injury process [63]. During the first few minutes after return of circulation there is hyperemia of the cerebral tissue [19], with associated lipid peroxidation, formation of oxygen free radicals, inflammatory injury and ongoing disruption of calcium homeostasis, glutamate release and enzymatic pathway activation. Apoptosis is a major consequence of injury during this stage [61]. Following the reperfusion stage is a period of cerebral hypoperfusion that can last for hours after resuscitation [67, 68]. Studies in adult patients have shown impaired cerebral autoregulation during this period [69, 70] with experimental pediatric animal models confirming these findings [71]. As a result, cerebral blood flow is dependent on systemic blood pressure so that avoidance of hypotension and efforts to minimize cerebral oxygen demands (e.g. sedation, seizure control, temperature control) are critical to avoid compounding neuronal injury [19, 69]. The exact cerebral blood flow required to optimize oxygen delivery is difficult to determine for any individual patient and likely changes over time [19]. Near-infrared spectroscopy (NIRS) is a non-invasive technology that has offered promise in determining individualized optimal cerebral blood flow to avoid cerebral hypoxia and ongoing neuronal ischemia [65, 72, 73].

Cerebral edema is also known to compromise cerebral oxygen delivery by elevating intracranial pressure [74] and reducing cerebral perfusion pressure. Within hours after the initial ischemic injury from cardiac arrest, the inflammatory process increases vascular permeability and disrupts the blood-brain barrier causing cerebral edema [62].

This pathophysiologic process, however, is not consistently associated with an increase intracranial pressure in the post-cardiac arrest patient [75, 76]. Furthermore, there is no data to support the use of routine intracranial pressure monitoring for management of the post-cardiac arrest patient [19].

Clinical Manifestations

Clinical manifestations of post-cardiac arrest brain injury in the critical care setting include disorders of arousal and consciousness, myoclonus, movement disorders, autonomic storms, neurocognitive dysfunction, seizures and brain death [19, 61, 77–79]. Of these, seizures represent an important manageable cause of secondary neuronal injury in the post-cardiac arrest patient. Seizures are known to increase cerebral metabolic demand and subsequent ischemic injury [80]. Seizures may be partial, generalized tonic-clonic or myoclonic [61], the latter of which has been associated with more severe cortical injury and worse prognosis [81, 82]. A prospective study of EEG monitoring in children undergoing therapeutic hypothermia after cardiac arrest reported an occurrence of electrographic seizures in 47 % of patients [83]. Studies of critically ill pediatric patients at risk of seizures from multiple diagnoses undergoing long-term video electroencephalography showed that seizures are relatively common in these patients [84, 85]. Most of these seizures were only detected by long-term EEG monitoring and missed by beside caregivers [85] and many of the suspected seizures by bedside staff were actually not epileptic seizures [84], both advocating a lower threshold for obtaining long-term EEG in patients at risk for seizures, including those in the post-cardiac arrest state. This coincides with the American Heart Association Guidelines recommending EEG evaluation in comatose adult patients after ROSC [86].

Management

Management of post-resuscitation brain injury involves therapies focused on preservation of cerebral blood flow and oxygen delivery and prevention of secondary brain injury by decreasing metabolic demand [62]. With regards to the former, the focus should be on avoidance of systemic arterial hypotension, avoidance of significant hypoxia with target oxygen saturation of 94 % or higher, ventilation to normocapnia, and management of cerebral edema [19, 62, 86]. Due to its effect on cerebral perfusion, the use of intentional hyperventilation should be reserved as temporizing rescue therapy in the setting of impending cerebral herniation [37]. With regards to the management of global cerebral edema in the post-cardiac arrest state, no trials exist to guide therapy in this specific population. Standard therapy involves promotion of venous drainage by elevation of the head of the bed to 30° and midline head position, avoidance of hypotonic fluid administration [87] and avoidance of hyperglycemia [62]. Animal models of cardiac arrest have demonstrated enhanced

cerebral blood flow after ROSC with use of hypertonic saline compared to normal saline, however, this is yet to be described in human studies [88].

Therapies directed at the prevention of secondary injury by decreasing metabolic demand include seizure control, analgesia, sedation and neuromuscular blockade, temperature control including therapeutic hypothermia and other neuroprotective measures. Prompt and aggressive treatment with conventional anti-convulsant regimens should be employed for seizure management in the post-resuscitation period. There have been no studies examining the role of prophylactic anti-convulsants; however, clinical and subclinical seizures should be treated aggressively with standard anti-convulsants such as benzodiazepines, fosphenytoin, levetiracetam, valproate and barbiturates [61], the latter of which may be needed for induction of pharmacologic coma for refractory seizures. All anti-convulsants should be used with vigilance towards managing the expected side effect of systemic hypotension and reduction in cerebral perfusion pressure.

There is no data to support routine use of sedation, analgesia or neuromuscular blockade to protect the brain from secondary injury in the post-cardiac arrest patient; however, some or all of the above may be required for safety and ease of mechanical ventilation and/or to facilitate achievement of therapeutic hypothermia (see below). Sedation and analgesia may reduce cerebral oxygen consumption and metabolic rate, improving matching of cerebral oxygen demand with supply. Propofol is not recommended for routine use as an anti-convulsant or sedative in pediatric patients due to the risk of propofol infusion syndrome [89, 90]. Use of pediatric sedation scales can be used to titrate sedative and analgesic medications [91, 92]. When neuromuscular blockade is necessary, use of EEG monitoring should be considered in order to detect masked seizure activity [19, 62].

Hyperthermia occurs commonly after neurological injury in humans and is associated with worse neurological outcomes [93–100] likely related to increased cerebral oxygen consumption and cellular destruction [101]. These findings have been documented in pediatric patients as well with temperatures ≥ 38 °C in the first 24 h after ROSC with associated unfavorable neurological outcome [102]. AHA guidelines recommend aggressive fever control with antipyretics and cooling devices in the post-resuscitation period [37, 86].

Beyond the clear recommendation for fever control in the post-cardiac arrest pediatric patient comes the question of use of therapeutic hypothermia. Therapeutic hypothermia is believed to work by reducing cerebral metabolism, suppressing neurological excitotoxicity, suppressing inflammation and vascular permeability, mitigating cell destructive enzymes and improving cerebral glucose metabolism [62, 64]. Mild induced hypothermia has been shown to improve neurological outcome in comatose adults after resuscitation from cardiac arrest associated with ventricular fibrillation [103, 104]. Similar outcomes were observed with hypothermia therapy in newborns with hypoxic-ischemic encephalopathy [105, 106]. With regards to the pediatric population, no prospective clinical trials have been published to date evaluating efficacy of therapeutic hypothermia in survivors of cardiac arrest, although a large multi-center trail is currently in progress [107–109]. A trial evaluating effect of therapeutic hypothermia on outcome after traumatic brain injury in pediatric patients showed no improvement in outcome with a trend towards increased mortality in the hypothermia group [110]. Retrospective studies of use of hypothermia after pediatric cardiac arrest have shown no benefit or harm, however, both called for a prospective, randomized trial to determine efficacy of therapeutic hypothermia after pediatric cardiac arrest [111, 112]. A feasibility trial of therapeutic hypothermia using a standard surface cooling protocol in pediatric patients after cardiac arrest showed feasibility and set the stage for future investigations of therapeutic hypothermia for cardiac arrest in children [113].

As therapeutic hypothermia is likely safe with temperatures in the range of 32–34 °C [114], the AHA recommends consideration of this intervention for children who remain comatose after resuscitation from cardiac arrest [87]. In spite of these recommendations, a survey of pediatric critical care providers demonstrated that therapeutic hypothermia was not widely used in this population and that the methods for utilization were variable [115]. Post-arrest hypothermia protocols, when initiated, should involve rapid initiation of cooling, continuous temperature monitoring and gradual rewarming. Side effects may include shivering, hemodynamic complications, electrolyte derangements, hyperglycemia, mild coagulopathy and risk of infection [62].

Numerous pharmacologic neuroprotective strategies have been proposed to improve neurological outcome after ischemic injury. No benefit has been observed in human trials involving barbiturates, glucocorticoids, calcium channel blockers, lidoflazine, benzodiazepines and magnesium sulfate [86, 116]. One trial showed improved survival and a trend towards improved neurologic outcome when coenzyme Q10 was used as an adjunct to therapeutic hypothermia [117].

Prognosis

For survivors of cardiac arrest, neurological prognosis is one of the most important factors guiding physicians and families in determining the appropriate level of care for the patient. Data that may be used when predicting outcome include historical features, clinical examination, neuroimaging, neurophysiologic studies and biochemical markers [118, 119]. In a report of the Quality Standards Subcommittee of the American Academy of Neurology, a practice parameter was created after systematic review of available evidence of neurological outcome in comatose adult survivors after

cardiopulmonary resuscitation for use in prognostication in such patients. Pupillary light response, corneal reflexes, motor responses to pain, myoclonic status epilepticus, serum neuron-specific enolase, and somatosenory evoked potential studies were shown to reliably assist in accurately predicting poor outcome. Notably, this practice parameter was not derived from patients treated with therapeutic hypothermia [118]. No similar report has been created for pediatric patients, however, a recent literature review of all available evidence in domains used to provide prognostic information in children with coma due to hypoxic ischemic encephalopathy, of which post-resuscitation brain injury would be included, suggests that abnormal exam signs (pupil reactivity and motor response), absent N_2O waves bilaterally on somatosensory evoked potentials, electrocerebral silence or burst suppression patterns on electroencephalogram, and abnormal magnetic resonance imaging with diffusion restriction in the cortex and basal ganglia are all individually highly predictive of poor outcome and when used in combination are even more predictive. This predictive accuracy can be improved by waiting 2–3 days after the event [119]. When evaluating prognostic indicators to predict neurologic outcome, attention should be paid to confounding factors that may affect the clinical neurological examination such as renal failure, liver failure, shock, metabolic acidosis and therapeutics such as sedatives, neuromuscular blockers and induced hypothermia [118].

Blood Glucose Management

Blood glucose derangements are common in adults and children after resuscitation from cardiac arrest. Studies in adult survivors of cardiac arrest demonstrated an association between post-arrest hyperglycemia and poor survival with unfavorable neurological outcomes [120–123]. Adult studies of out-of-hospital cardiac arrest survivors also observed worse outcomes with the administration of glucose-containing fluids during cardiopulmonary resuscitation [124]. A large retrospective registry report on adults with in-hospital cardiac arrest found an association with mortality if non-diabetic patients were either hyperglycemic or hypoglycaemic [125].

Recent studies in adults resuscitated from out-of-hospital cardiac arrest indicate that post-cardiac arrest patients may be treated optimally by maintaining blood glucose concentration below 8 mmol/L (144 mg/dL) [126–128]. Ninety survivors of out-of-hospital cardiac arrest due to ventricular fibrillation were cooled and randomized into two treatment groups: a strict glucose control group (SGC), with a blood glucose target of 4–6 mmol/L (72–108 mg/dL), and a moderate glucose control group (MGC), with a blood glucose target of 6–8 mmol/L (108–144 mg/dL). Both groups were treated with an insulin infusion for 48 h. Episodes of moderate hypoglycemia (<3.0 mmol/L or <54 mg/dL) occurred in 18 % of the SGC group and 2 % of the MGC group ($P=0.008$); however, there were no episodes of severe hypoglycemia (<2.2 mmol/L or <40 mg/dL). There was no difference in 30-day mortality between the groups ($P=0.846$).

Strict control of blood glucose to 4.4–6.1 mmol/L (80–110 mg/dL) with intensive insulin therapy reduced overall mortality in critically ill adults in a surgical ICU and appeared to protect the central and peripheral nervous systems [129, 130]. In a subsequent medical ICU study, however, the overall mortality was similar in both the intensive insulin and control groups [131]. Among those patients with a longer ICU stay (≥ 3 days), intensive insulin therapy reduced the mortality rate from 52.5 % (control group) to 43 % ($P=0.009$). However, use of intensive insulin therapy to maintain normoglycemia of 4.4–6.1 mmol/L (80–110 mg/dL) was associated with more frequent episodes of hypoglycemia and some have cautioned against its routine use in the critically ill [132, 133]. Finally, a large, multi-center trial of critically ill adults (NICE-SUGAR) showed an increase in 90-day mortality for patients who received tight glycemic control [134].

It is presently unknown if post-arrest hyperglycemia or administration of glucose in the peri-resuscitation period causes harm in children. A limited study in pediatric survivors of cardiac arrest demonstrated the occurrence of post-arrest hyperglycemia (mean blood glucose concentrations >150 mg/dL or >8.3 mmol/L) in more than two-thirds of children within the first 24 h after the arrest. Limited retrospective studies in critically ill, non-diabetic children indicate that hyperglycemia frequently occurs in these children and is independently associated with morbidity and mortality [135–137], but it unknown if the observed hyperglycemia is a surrogate marker of the severity of the child's illness injury rather than a cause of poor outcome. Two of these studies additionally demonstrated that hypoglycemia and increased glucose variability were also associated with higher mortality [137, 138].

To date there has been only one randomized controlled trial of insulin management in critically ill pediatric patients using a heterogenous group that was randomized to receive intensive insulin therapy vs. insulin for a threshold level of hyperglycemia [139]. The results of this study were favorable towards intensive insulin therapy, with shorter ICU stay, lower rates of secondary infection, and lower unadjusted 30-day ICU mortality. In the absence of specific pediatric data examining the efficacy and safety of intensive glycemic control following cardiac arrest, current recommendations are to target a normal range of blood glucose concentration.

Significant hyperglycemia is an indication for intravenous insulin infusion, although there is no consensus on a specific threshold for initiation of insulin. When using insulin in the post-resuscitation period, intensive blood glucose monitoring is essential to avoid hypoglycemia. Hypoglycemia poses a greater risk to the relatively immature pediatric brain compared with adults, especially in the setting of cardiac arrest with ischemia/reperfusion injury. The use of therapeutic hypothermia can further increase the risk for glucose derangements.

Acid-Base and Electrolyte Management

Acid-base and electrolyte abnormalities are commonly seen during and after recovery from cardiac arrest. These include, but are not limited to, metabolic acidosis, hyperkalemia, ionized hypocalcemia, and hypomagnesemia. Severe acidosis and other electrolyte disturbances may adversely affect cardiac function and vasomotor tone. Prompt recognition and correction of acid-base and electrolyte abnormalities in the post-arrest state is important to minimize the risk of arrhythmias and to support myocardial function.

Metabolic acidosis may be present prior to cardiac arrest as a result of inadequate oxygen delivery and is further exacerbated by tissue hypoxia and ischemia occurring during the low flow arrest state. Although metabolic acidosis may have widespread effects on cellular and organ function, the use of buffers during or immediately after pediatric cardiac arrest is generally not recommended. The administration of sodium bicarbonate leads to production of carbon dioxide and water; rapid diffusion of carbon dioxide may result in intracellular acidosis that is deleterious, especially to the brain. In addition, serum alkalosis shifts the oxyhemoglobin dissociation curve to the left, inhibiting oxygen delivery to the tissues.

The use of sodium bicarbonate in adults experiencing out-of-hospital cardiac arrest remains controversial [140–142]. While one large multi-center trial found that earlier and more frequent use of sodium bicarbonate was associated with higher early survival rates and better long-term outcome [141], other studies have shown no benefit from administration of sodium bicarbonate during and after cardiac arrest [143–145]. A prospective randomized controlled trial examined the use of buffer therapy (Tribonat) in the setting of cardiac arrest in adults and did not observe an improved outcome compared with saline [146]. There have been no prospective studies of the use of sodium bicarbonate during pediatric cardiac arrest, but two large retrospective studies of in and out-of-hospital arrests found an association between bicarbonate use and mortality [11, 18].

In general, management of post-arrest metabolic acidosis caused by increased lactate and other metabolic acids consists of restoring adequate tissue perfusion and oxygen delivery, while assuring adequate ventilation. Oxygen delivery is optimized by supporting cardiac output, as described in the previous section, and ensuring adequate oxygen content. An anion gap acidosis that does not improve in response to supportive care suggests an ongoing source of acid production such as ischemic bowel, or a respiratory chain disorder such as cyanide poisoning. Patients with a non-anion gap metabolic acidosis following cardiac arrest may be hyperchloremic from the use of large volumes of normal saline during resuscitation. Metabolic acidosis due to chloride administration is generally well tolerated and is associated with better outcomes than other forms of acidosis in critically ill patients [147, 148]. Treatment with bicarbonate is not usually indicated and the acidosis improves with restriction of chloride intake. There is limited evidence to support the use of buffer therapy in the post-resuscitation phase. Bicarbonate therapy may be indicated to manage renal tubular acidosis, characterized by a non-anion gap acidosis with elevated urine pH. There are specific conditions in which active correction of acidosis may by beneficial, such as the patient with pulmonary hypertension or the child with certain toxic ingestions (eg: tricyclic antidepressants). Continued alkalinization may also be considered for treatment of associated conditions such as rhabdomyolysis, hyperkalemia, and tumor lysis syndrome.

Prolonged cardiac arrest may be associated with ionized hypocalcemia, which appears to be time-dependent and perhaps related to intracellular sequestration of calcium [149, 150]. Hypocalcemia may also result from the rapid administration of blood products, which contain high concentrations of citrate that bind free calcium. Documented ionized hypocalcemia is an indication for treatment with exogenous calcium, as hypocalcemia negatively affects myocardial contractility and can contribute to post-arrest arrhythmias [151, 152]. Other indications for calcium administration include cardiac arrest in the setting of suspected or documented hyperkalemia or calcium-channel blocker overdose. Despite the potential benefits to of calcium for documented hypocalcemia, excess calcium administration may be harmful. During ischemia and reperfusion, calcium channels become more permeable, allowing influx of calcium. Increased intracellular calcium activates a number of secondary messengers leading to apoptosis and necrosis; indeed, intracellular calcium accumulation is thought to be the final common pathway for cell death [153]. A recent registry report of children experiencing in-hospital pediatric cardiac arrest observed that calcium use during resuscitation was associated with reduced survival to discharge and unfavorable neurologic outcome [154]. Given the retrospective nature of the study it is not possible to know if this association is based on effects of calcium or the use of calcium for patients who are unresponsive to other resuscitative measures. However, multiple adult studies, both randomized controlled trials and cohort studies, showed no benefit of calcium administration during cardiac arrest [155].

Magnesium is an important ion in cardiac conduction and plays a role in smooth and skeletal muscle tone. Magnesium is recommended for shock-refractory cardiac arrest due to the ventricular arrhythmia torsades de pointes, but there are conflicting data on its role in treating other rhythm disturbances. A pilot study of magnesium in adults with in-hospital cardiac arrest who were unresponsive to other measures demonstrated greater return of spontaneous circulation and more favorable neurologic outcome [156]; however, other studies have not demonstrated any difference in outcome [157, 158]. One randomized trial of magnesium administration in the post-resuscitation period found no benefit [159]. There have been no studies evaluating magnesium use during or after pediatric cardiac arrest.

Hyperkalemia following cardiac arrest may be secondary to metabolic acidosis as by hydrogen ions move intracellularly in exchange for potassium. This form of hyperkalemia responds readily to correction of acidosis and typically does not require other treatment. Hyperkalemia may also occur due to muscle or tissue injury related to the underlying cause of cardiac arrest such as trauma, prolonged seizures, or electrical shock. If life-threatening hyperkalemia requires treatment, the most effective methods to reduce serum concentration are the use of sodium bicarbonate and the infusion of insulin and glucose. These measures temporarily reduce extracellular potassium concentration but do not alter total body potassium; refractory hyperkalemia may require the use of hemodialysis for definitive correction. Resin binders and loop diuretics will also reduce potassium burden but their onset of action is more gradual. Calcium may be used to temporarily antagonize the adverse electrophysiologic effects of hyperkalemia by stabilizing myocyte membranes.

Immunologic Disturbances and Infection

Evidence of a "systemic inflammatory response syndrome" (SIRS) and endothelial activation triggered by whole-body ischemia and reperfusion in patients successfully resuscitated after cardiac arrest has been demonstrated in humans as early as 3 h after cardiac arrest [160]. Biochemical changes include a marked increase in plasma cytokines and soluble receptors such as interleukin-1ra (IL-1ra), interleukin-6 (IL-6), interleukin-8 (IL-8) [161, 162], interleukin-10 (IL-10), and soluble tumor necrosis factor receptor II, and were more pronounced in nonsurvivors. Additionally, plasma endotoxin was noted in about half of patients studied, possibly due to translocation through sites of intestinal ischemia and reperfusion damage [160, 163]. Studies have also shown increases in soluble intracellular adhesion molecule-1, soluble vascular-cell adhesion molecule-1 and P and E selectins suggesting neutrophil activation and endothelial injury [163–165], with additional studies demonstrating direct evidence of endothelial injury and inflammation with elevation of endothelial microparticles with the first 24 h after ROSC [166]. This inflammatory response from endothelial damage has been implicated in the vital organ dysfunction often witnessed after cardiac arrest [167]. Interestingly, in light of this immune activation, hyporesponsiveness of circulating leukocytes has also been noted in patients with cardiac arrest, a condition referred to as endotoxin tolerance. While possibly protective against overwhelming inflammation, endotoxin tolerance may contribute to immune paralysis with an increased risk of nosocomial infection [163].

Along with the possible immune dysfunction mentioned above, survivors of cardiac arrest have multiple risk factors for infection, including prolonged ICU stays, organ dysfunction, and invasive procedures [168]. Infectious complications in survivors of cardiac arrest are common [168–170] and have been associated with increased duration of mechanical ventilation and length of hospital stay [168, 169]. These infections may be even more frequent after therapeutic hypothermia [168]. Pneumonia is the most commonly reported infection [168–170] followed by bacteremia [168, 170] with *Staphylococcus* aureus being the most commonly isolated pathogen for all types of infection [168–170]. With regards to bacteremia, several studies have shown a significant proportion to be of intestinal origin, suggesting bacterial translocation from gut ischemia as a source [171, 172]. While there is no evidence to support the routine use of prophylactic antibiotics in critically ill survivors of cardiac arrest, vigilance for the possibility of infection and prompt evaluation and treatment are necessary to minimize further morbidity in this vulnerable population.

Coagulation Abnormalities

Studies in both animals and humans have shown marked activation of the coagulation cascade [173] without balanced activation of anti-thrombotic factors or endogenous fibrinolysis following cardiac arrest [174, 175]. Specifically, the profile of systemic coagulation abnormalities includes increased thrombin-antithrombin complexes, reduced antithrombin, protein C and protein S, activated thrombolysis (plasmin-antiplasmin complex) and inhibited thrombolysis (increased plasminogen activator inhibitor-1) [173]. In addition to alterations in the coagulation system, marked platelet activation occurs during and after cardiopulmonary resuscitation as evidenced by elevation of tissue-factor levels as well as low levels of tissue factor pathway inhibitor [176–179]. These hematologic derangements contribute to microcirculatory fibrin formation and microvascular thrombosis resulting in impairment of capillary perfusion and further organ and neurologic dysfunction [173, 179]. Furthermore, these changes are more prominent in those dying from early refractory shock and those with early inpatient mortality [173].

Therapeutic interventions directed at these hemostatic disorders have been reported in the literature. Thrombolytic therapy has been shown to improve cerebral microcirculatory perfusion in animal studies [180] and a meta-analysis suggested that thrombolysis during cardiopulmonary resuscitation can improve survival rate to discharge and neurological outcome [181]. However, a recent randomized clinical trial in adult patients showed no improvement in survival or neurological outcome with use of thrombolytic therapy in out-of-hospital cardiac arrest [182]. There are no studies examining the effects of cardiac arrest on the coagulation system in pediatric patients, making it difficult to recommend the routine use of heparin or thrombolytic therapies in this population.

Gastrointestinal Management

Gastrointestinal manifestations after cardiac arrest and cardiopulmonary resuscitation include those of a traumatic nature as well as those related to ischemic injury to the visceral organs. While traumatic injuries to the abdominal viscera following chest compressions are rare, case reports have described bowel injury [183], rupture and laceration of the liver [183, 184], gastric rupture [185], esophageal injury [186], splenic laceration and rupture [187] and injury to the biliary tract [188]. Awareness of the possibility of these rare but critical injuries is important in the post-cardiac arrest survivor.

With regards to ischemic injuries, the intra-abdominal organs seem to tolerate longer periods of ischemia than the heart and the brain [171]. With this in mind, however, mesenteric ischemia with injury to visceral organs has been well described, attributed to periods of no or low cardiac output as well as splanchnic vasoconstriction from use of vasoactive agents during resuscitation [189]. Associated complications include feeding intolerance, bacteremia related to bacterial translocation [172] and need for therapeutic intervention such as endoscopy [190] and bowel resection [191]. Reports have described gut dysfunction, endoscopic evidence of mucosal injury, transient hepatic dysfunction, colonic ischemia and necrosis, and acute pancreatitis, all of which may be consequences of mesenteric ischemia [171, 190–192]. Management of these injuries is largely supportive; in particular, intestinal ischemia is likely to be diffuse rather than focal, limiting the role for surgical intervention.

In addition to issues specifically related to cardiopulmonary resuscitation and the post-resuscitation syndrome, attention to general issues concerning gastrointestinal management in critically patients remains important. Early gut protection with proton pump inhibitors or H-2 blockers has been shown to decrease the risk of bleeding complications in critically ill adults [193] with less convincing evidence in children [194], but may be considered as part of routine intensive care in the post-cardiac arrest patient. Providing early enteral nutrition remains another important goal in the critically ill child [195, 196] with vigilance towards signs of feeding intolerance that may be related to gut dysfunction from mesenteric ischemia. The same precautions that are used for other critically ill patients with hypotension and hemodynamic instability apply when considering enteral nutrition in the post-cardiac arrest patient [197].

Acute Kidney Injury

Acute kidney injury (AKI) is common in adults following cardiac arrest [198], especially in patients with post-resuscitation cardiogenic shock [199]. Risk factors include duration of cardiac arrest, administration of vasoconstrictor agents, and pre-existing renal insufficiency [200, 201]. The use of therapeutic hypothermia may transiently delay recovery of renal function, but does not increase the incidence or renal failure or need for renal replacement therapy [202, 203]. There are no pediatric studies describing the incidence of AKI or to examine the role of renal replacement therapies following cardiac arrest. In general, the indications for renal replacement therapy in cardiac arrest survivors are the same as those used for other critically ill patients [204].

Endocrinologic Abnormalities

As the post-resuscitation state has been described as a "sepsis-like" syndrome [160], multiple studies have looked at the hormonal response to cardiac arrest. Relative adrenal insufficiency has been well described in critically ill children and adults, particularly those with systemic-inflammatory syndrome and vasopressor-dependent shock [205–207] with the dysfunction occurring at the level of the hypothalamus, pituitary and/or adrenal gland [207]. While a consensus on diagnostic criteria to define adrenal insufficiency in critical illness is lacking [205], the presence of adrenal insufficiency after cardiac arrest may be associated with poor outcome [208–214]. In spite of this, relative adrenal insufficiency may be under-evaluated in the post-cardiac arrest state in clinical practice [215]. Management of relative adrenal insufficiency in all critically ill patients involves the consideration of supplementation with corticosteroids. Studies evaluating the use of corticosteroids in adults with septic shock and relative adrenal insufficiency have been controversial [216, 217]. In patients with cardiac arrest, two small studies, one in animals and one in humans, demonstrated an improved rate of return of spontaneous circulation (ROSC) when subjects were treated with hydrocortisone during resuscitation [218, 219]. With regards to the post-resuscitation phase, a single trial investigating steroid therapy with vasopressin showed a survival benefit, however, interpretation of results specific to steroids was not possible [220]. There have been

no trials performed evaluating the use of corticosteroids alone in the post-resuscitation phase. Therefore, although relative adrenal insufficiency likely commonly exists after ROSC, there is not evidence to recommend routine use of corticosteroids in this patient population. A special consideration may need be taken in patients who have received etomidate as an induction agent prior to intubation, given its known adrenally suppressive effects [221].

Abnormalities in thyroid function have also been well described in critically ill patients following a variety of illnesses including trauma, sepsis, myocardial infarction, as well as following cardiopulmonary bypass and in brain death [222, 223]. These have been characterized as "euthyroid sick syndrome" and "non-thyroidal illness syndrome" [222] indicating an etiologic condition other than the thyroid axis itself. This state of abnormal thyroid homeostasis has also been demonstrated after cardiac arrest in both animals and humans [223–229] with alterations noted to be more pronounced after longer periods of resuscitation [226]. Controversy exists as to whether the thyroid function abnormalities noted in non-thyroidal illness syndromes, like cardiac arrest, represent an adaptive response that should be left alone or a maladaptive response that needs to be treated. As such, no convincing literature exists to support the restoration of normal serum thyroid hormone concentrations in critically ill patients with non-thyroidal illness syndromes [222]. In cardiac arrest specifically, animal studies have suggested that thyroid hormone replacement after cardiac arrest may improve cardiac output, oxygen consumption [224, 229] and neurologic outcome [225] with the type of thyroid hormone replacement being important [223], however, no human evidence suggests that routine replacement of thyroid hormone after cardiac arrest improves outcomes.

Conclusion

The relative infrequency of events and diverse etiologies of pediatric cardiac arrest have hampered the performance of randomized, controlled trials to assess intra- and post-cardiac arrest treatment strategies. For these reasons, many recommendations are based on animal studies, extrapolation from adult data, or expert consensus. Fortunately, several multi-center trials are in progress, so that post-resuscitation care guidelines are more likely to be evidence-based in the future.

References

1. Laver S, Farrow C, Turner D, Nolan J. Mode of death after admission to an intensive care unit following cardiac arrest. Intensive Care Med. 2004;30(11):2126–8.
2. Schindler MB, Bohn D, Cox PN, et al. Outcome of out-of-hospital cardiac or respiratory arrest in children. N Engl J Med. 1996; 335(20):1473–9.

3. Donoghue AJ, Nadkarni V, Berg RA, et al. Out-of-hospital pediatric cardiac arrest: an epidemiologic review and assessment of current knowledge. Ann Emerg Med. 2005;46(6):512–22.

4. Young KD, Gausche-Hill M, McClung CD, Lewis RJ. A prospective, population-based study of the epidemiology and outcome of out-of-hospital pediatric cardiopulmonary arrest. Pediatrics. 2004;114(1):157–64.

5. Atkins DL, Everson-Stewart S, Sears GK, et al. Epidemiology and outcomes from out-of-hospital cardiac arrest in children: the Resuscitation Outcomes Consortium Epistry-Cardiac Arrest. Circulation. 2009;119(11):1484–91.

6. Kitamura T, Iwami T, Kawamura T, et al. Conventional and chest-compression-only cardiopulmonary resuscitation by bystanders for children who have out-of-hospital cardiac arrests: a prospective, nationwide, population-based cohort study. Lancet. 2010;375(9723):1347–54.

7. Ong ME, Stiell I, Osmond MH, et al. Etiology of pediatric out-of-hospital cardiac arrest by coroner's diagnosis. Resuscitation. 2006;68(3):335–42.

8. Sirbaugh PE, Pepe PE, Shook JE, et al. A prospective, population-based study of the demographics, epidemiology, management, and outcome of out-of-hospital pediatric cardiopulmonary arrest. Ann Emerg Med. 1999;33(2):174–84.

9. Park CB, Shin SD, Suh GJ, et al. Pediatric out-of-hospital cardiac arrest in Korea: a nationwide population-based study. Resuscitation. 2010;81(5):512–7.

10. Kuisma M, Suominen P, Korpela R. Paediatric out-of-hospital cardiac arrests – epidemiology and outcome. Resuscitation. 1995;30(2):141–50.

11. Moler FW, Donaldson AE, Meert K, et al. Multicenter cohort study of out-of-hospital pediatric cardiac arrest. Crit Care Med. 2011;39(1):141–9.

12. Moler FW, Meert K, Donaldson AE, et al. In-hospital versus out-of-hospital pediatric cardiac arrest: a multicenter cohort study. Crit Care Med. 2009;37(7):2259–67.

13. Young KD, Seidel JS. Pediatric cardiopulmonary resuscitation: a collective review. Ann Emerg Med. 1999;33(2):195–205.

14. Reis AG, Nadkarni V, Perondi MB, Grisi S, Berg RA. A prospective investigation into the epidemiology of in-hospital pediatric cardiopulmonary resuscitation using the international Utstein reporting style. Pediatrics. 2002;109(2):200–9.

15. de Mos N, van Litsenburg RR, McCrindle B, Bohn DJ, Parshuram CS. Pediatric in-intensive-care-unit cardiac arrest: incidence, survival, and predictive factors. Crit Care Med. 2006;34(4):1209–15.

16. Parra DA, Totapally BR, Zahn E, et al. Outcome of cardiopulmonary resuscitation in a pediatric cardiac intensive care unit. Crit Care Med. 2000;28(9):3296–300.

17. Nadkarni VM, Larkin GL, Peberdy MA, et al. First documented rhythm and clinical outcome from in-hospital cardiac arrest among children and adults. JAMA. 2006;295(1):50–7.

18. Meert KL, Donaldson A, Nadkarni V, et al. Multicenter cohort study of in-hospital pediatric cardiac arrest. Pediatr Crit Care Med. 2009;10(5):544–53.

19. Neumar RW, Nolan JP, Adrie C, et al. Post-cardiac arrest syndrome: epidemiology, pathophysiology, treatment, and prognostication. A consensus statement from the International Liaison Committee on Resuscitation (American Heart Association, Australian and New Zealand Council on Resuscitation, European Resuscitation Council, Heart and Stroke Foundation of Canada, InterAmerican Heart Foundation, Resuscitation Council of Asia, and the Resuscitation Council of Southern Africa); the American Heart Association Emergency Cardiovascular Care Committee; the Council on Cardiovascular Surgery and Anesthesia; the Council on Cardiopulmonary, Perioperative, and Critical Care; the Council on Clinical Cardiology; and the Stroke Council. Circulation. 2008;118(23):2452–83.

20. Lopez-Herce J, Fernandez B, Urbano J, et al. Hemodynamic, respiratory, and perfusion parameters during asphyxia, resuscitation, and post-resuscitation in a pediatric model of cardiac arrest. Intensive Care Med. 2011;37(1):147–55.

21. Eltzschig HK, Collard CD. Vascular ischaemia and reperfusion injury. Br Med Bull. 2004;70:71–86.

22. Niemann JT, Rosborough JP, Youngquist S, et al. Cardiac function and the proinflammatory cytokine response after recovery from cardiac arrest in swine. J Interferon Cytokine Res. 2009;29(11):749–58.

23. Los Arcos M, Rey C, Concha A, Medina A, Prieto B. Acute-phase reactants after paediatric cardiac arrest. Procalcitonin as marker of immediate outcome. BMC Pediatr. 2008;8:18.

24. Walson KH, Tang M, Glumac A, et al. Normoxic versus hyperoxic resuscitation in pediatric asphyxial cardiac arrest: effects on oxidative stress. Crit Care Med. 2011;39(2):335–43.

25. Gore A, Muralidhar M, Espey MG, Degenhardt K, Mantell LL. Hyperoxia sensing: from molecular mechanisms to significance in disease. J Immunotoxicol. 2010;7(4):239–54.

26. Incagnoli P, Ramond A, Joyeux-Faure M, Pepin JL, Levy P, Ribuot C. Erythropoietin improved initial resuscitation and increased survival after cardiac arrest in rats. Resuscitation. 2009;80(6):696–700.

27. Minamishima S, Kida K, Tokuda K, et al. Inhaled nitric oxide improves outcomes after successful cardiopulmonary resuscitation in mice. Circulation. 2011;124(15):1645–53.

28. Charalampopoulos AF, Nikolaou NI. Emerging pharmaceutical therapies in cardiopulmonary resuscitation and post-resuscitation syndrome. Resuscitation. 2011;82(4):371–7.

29. Tsai MS, Huang CH, Tsai CY, et al. Ascorbic acid mitigates the myocardial injury after cardiac arrest and electrical shock. Intensive Care Med. 2011;37(12):2033–40.

30. Carden DL, Granger DN. Pathophysiology of ischaemia-reperfusion injury. J Pathol. 2000;190(3):255–66.

31. Gausche M, Lewis RJ, Stratton SJ, et al. Effect of out-of-hospital pediatric endotracheal intubation on survival and neurological outcome: a controlled clinical trial. JAMA. 2000;283(6):783–90.

32. Nishisaki A, Marwaha N, Kasinathan V, et al. Airway management in pediatric patients at referring hospitals compared to a receiving tertiary pediatric ICU. Resuscitation. 2011;82(4):386–90.

33. Easley RB, Segeleon JE, Haun SE, Tobias JD. Prospective study of airway management of children requiring endotracheal intubation before admission to a pediatric intensive care unit. Crit Care Med. 2000;28(6):2058–63.

34. Virkkunen I, Ryynanen S, Kujala S, et al. Incidence of regurgitation and pulmonary aspiration of gastric contents in survivors from out-of-hospital cardiac arrest. Acta Anaesthesiol Scand. 2007;51(2):202–5.

35. Lawes EG, Baskett PJ. Pulmonary aspiration during unsuccessful cardiopulmonary resuscitation. Intensive Care Med. 1987;13(6):379–82.

36. Christe A, Aghayev E, Jackowski C, Thali MJ, Vock P. Drowning-post-mortem imaging findings by computed tomography. Eur Radiol. 2008;18(2):283–90.

37. Kleinman ME, Chameides L, Schexnayder SM, et al. Part 14: pediatric advanced life support: 2010 American Heart Association Guidelines for Cardiopulmonary Resuscitation and Emergency Cardiovascular Care. Circulation. 2010;122(18 Suppl 3): S876–908.

38. Moynihan RJ, Brock-Utne JG, Archer JH, Feld LH, Kreitzman TR. The effect of cricoid pressure on preventing gastric insufflation in infants and children. Anesthesiology. 1993;78(4):652–6.

39. Salem MR, Wong AY, Mani M, Sellick BA. Efficacy of cricoid pressure in preventing gastric inflation during bag-mask ventilation in pediatric patients. Anesthesiology. 1974;40(1):96–8.

40. Wheeler AP, Bernard GR. Acute lung injury and the acute respiratory distress syndrome: a clinical review. Lancet. 2007; 369(9572):1553–64.

41. Balan IS, Fiskum G, Hazelton J, Cotto-Cumba C, Rosenthal RE. Oximetry-guided reoxygenation improves neurological outcome after experimental cardiac arrest. Stroke. 2006;37(12):3008–13.

42. Kilgannon JH, Jones AE, Parrillo JE, et al. Relationship between supranormal oxygen tension and outcome after resuscitation from cardiac arrest. Circulation. 2011;123(23):2717–22.

43. Kilgannon JH, Jones AE, Shapiro NI, et al. Association between arterial hyperoxia following resuscitation from cardiac arrest and in-hospital mortality. JAMA. 2010;303(21):2165–71.

44. Buunk G, van der Hoeven JG, Meinders AE. Cerebrovascular reactivity in comatose patients resuscitated from a cardiac arrest. Stroke. 1997;28(8):1569–73.

45. Duffett M, Choong K, Ng V, Randolph A, Cook DJ. Surfactant therapy for acute respiratory failure in children: a systematic review and meta-analysis. Crit Care. 2007;11(3):R66.

46. Kern KB, Hilwig RW, Rhee KH, Berg RA. Myocardial dysfunction after resuscitation from cardiac arrest: an example of global myocardial stunning. J Am Coll Cardiol. 1996;28(1):232–40.

47. Hildebrand CA, Hartmann AG, Arcinue EL, Gomez RJ, Bing RJ. Cardiac performance in pediatric near-drowning. Crit Care Med. 1988;16(4):331–5.

48. McCaul CL, McNamara P, Engelberts D, Slorach C, Hornberger LK, Kavanagh BP. The effect of global hypoxia on myocardial function after successful cardiopulmonary resuscitation in a laboratory model. Resuscitation. 2006;68(2):267–75.

49. Kamohara T, Weil MH, Tang W, et al. A comparison of myocardial function after primary cardiac and primary asphyxial cardiac arrest. Am J Respir Crit Care Med. 2001;164(7):1221–4.

50. Checchia PA, Sehra R, Moynihan J, Daher N, Tang W, Weil MH. Myocardial injury in children following resuscitation after cardiac arrest. Resuscitation. 2003;57(2):131–7.

51. Berg MD, Banville IL, Chapman FW, et al. Attenuating the defibrillation dosage decreases postresuscitation myocardial dysfunction in a swine model of pediatric ventricular fibrillation. Pediatr Crit Care Med. 2008;9(4):429–34.

52. Fernandez EG, Green TP, Sweeney M. Low inferior vena caval catheters for hemodynamic and pulmonary function monitoring in pediatric critical care patients. Pediatr Crit Care Med. 2004;5(1):14–8.

53. Chait HI, Kuhn MA, Baum VC. Inferior vena caval pressure reliably predicts right atrial pressure in pediatric cardiac surgical patients. Crit Care Med. 1994;22(2):219–24.

54. Murdoch IA, Rosenthal E, Huggon IC, Coutinho W, Qureshi SA. Accuracy of central venous pressure measurements in the inferior vena cava in the ventilated child. Acta Paediatr. 1994;83(5):512–4.

55. Reda Z, Houri S, Davis AL, Baum VC. Effect of airway pressure on inferior vena cava pressure as a measure of central venous pressure in children. J Pediatr. 1995;126(6):961–5.

56. Mayr V, Luckner G, Jochberger S, et al. Arginine vasopressin in advanced cardiovascular failure during the post-resuscitation phase after cardiac arrest. Resuscitation. 2007;72(1):35–44.

57. Huang L, Weil MH, Tang W, Sun S, Wang J. Comparison between dobutamine and levosimendan for management of postresuscitation myocardial dysfunction. Crit Care Med. 2005;33(3):487–91.

58. Egan JR, Clarke AJ, Williams S, et al. Levosimendan for low cardiac output: a pediatric experience. J Intensive Care Med. 2006;21(3):183–7.

59. Namachivayam P, Crossland DS, Butt WW, Shekerdemian LS. Early experience with Levosimendan in children with ventricular dysfunction. Pediatr Crit Care Med. 2006;7(5):445–8.

60. Yokoyama H, Julian JS, Vinten-Johansen J, et al. Postischemic [Ca2+] repletion improves cardiac performance without altering oxygen demands. Ann Thorac Surg. 1990;49(6):894–902.

61. Xiong W, Hoesch RE, Geocadin RG. Post-cardiac arrest encephalopathy. Semin Neurol. 2011;31(2):216–25.

62. Karanjia N, Geocadin RG. Post-cardiac arrest syndrome: update on brain injury management and prognostication. Curr Treat Options Neurol. 2011;13(2):191–203.

63. Neumar RW. Molecular mechanisms of ischemic neuronal injury. Ann Emerg Med. 2000;36(5):483–506.

64. Safar P, Behringer W, Bottiger BW, Sterz F. Cerebral resuscitation potentials for cardiac arrest. Crit Care Med. 2002;30(4 Suppl): S140–4.

65. Manole MD, Kochanek PM, Fink EL, Clark RS. Postcardiac arrest syndrome: focus on the brain. Curr Opin Pediatr. 2009;21(6):745–50.

66. White BC, Sullivan JM, DeGracia DJ, et al. Brain ischemia and reperfusion: molecular mechanisms of neuronal injury. J Neurol Sci. 2000;179(S 1–2):1–33.

67. Snyder JV, Nemoto EM, Carroll RG, Safar P. Global ischemia in dogs: intracranial pressures, brain blood flow and metabolism. Stroke. 1975;6(1):21–7.

68. Kagstrom E, Smith ML, Siesjo BK. Local cerebral blood flow in the recovery period following complete cerebral ischemia in the rat. J Cereb Blood Flow Metab. 1983;3(2):170–82.

69. Sundgreen C, Larsen FS, Herzog TM, Knudsen GM, Boesgaard S, Aldershvile J. Autoregulation of cerebral blood flow in patients resuscitated from cardiac arrest. Stroke. 2001;32(1):128–32.

70. Nishizawa H, Kudoh I. Cerebral autoregulation is impaired in patients resuscitated after cardiac arrest. Acta Anaesthesiol Scand. 1996;40(9):1149–53.

71. Manole MD, Foley LM, Hitchens TK, et al. Magnetic resonance imaging assessment of regional cerebral blood flow after asphyxial cardiac arrest in immature rats. J Cereb Blood Flow Metab. 2009;29(1):197–205.

72. Drayna PC, Abramo TJ, Estrada C. Near-infrared spectroscopy in the critical setting. Pediatr Emerg Care. 2011;27(5):432–9; quiz 440–2.

73. Orihashi K, Sueda T, Okada K, Imai K. Near-infrared spectroscopy for monitoring cerebral ischemia during selective cerebral perfusion. Eur J Cardiothorac Surg. 2004;26(5):907–11.

74. Paulson OB, Waldemar G, Schmidt JF, Strandgaard S. Cerebral circulation under normal and pathologic conditions. Am J Cardiol. 1989;63(6):2C–5.

75. Morimoto Y, Kemmotsu O, Kitami K, Matsubara I, Tedo I. Acute brain swelling after out-of-hospital cardiac arrest: pathogenesis and outcome. Crit Care Med. 1993;21(1):104–10.

76. Sakabe T, Tateishi A, Miyauchi Y, et al. Intracranial pressure following cardiopulmonary resuscitation. Intensive Care Med. 1987;13(4):256–9.

77. Young GB. Clinical practice. Neurologic prognosis after cardiac arrest. N Engl J Med. 2009;361(6):605–11.

78. Diamond AL, Callison RC, Shokri J, Cruz-Flores S, Kinsella LJ. Paroxysmal sympathetic storm. Neurocrit Care. 2005;2(3):288–91.

79. Hawker K, Lang AE. Hypoxic-ischemic damage of the basal ganglia. Case reports and a review of the literature. Mov Disord. 1990;5(3):219–24.

80. Krumholz A, Stern BJ, Weiss HD. Outcome from coma after cardiopulmonary resuscitation: relation to seizures and myoclonus. Neurology. 1988;38(3):401–5.

81. Hui AC, Cheng C, Lam A, Mok V, Joynt GM. Prognosis following postanoxic myoclonus status epilepticus. Eur Neurol. 2005;54(1):10–3.

82. Wijdicks EF, Parisi JE, Sharbrough FW. Prognostic value of myoclonus status in comatose survivors of cardiac arrest. Ann Neurol. 1994;35(2):239–43.

83. Abend NS, Topjian A, Ichord R, et al. Electroencephalographic monitoring during hypothermia after pediatric cardiac arrest. Neurology. 2009;72(22):1931–40.

84. Shahwan A, Bailey C, Shekerdemian L, Harvey AS. The prevalence of seizures in comatose children in the pediatric intensive care unit: a prospective video-EEG study. Epilepsia. 2010;51(7):1198–204.

85. Williams K, Jarrar R, Buchhalter J. Continuous video-EEG monitoring in pediatric intensive care units. Epilepsia. 2011;52(6): 1130–6.

86. Peberdy MA, Callaway CW, Neumar RW, et al. Part 9: post-cardiac arrest care: 2010 American Heart Association Guidelines for Cardiopulmonary Resuscitation and Emergency Cardiovascular Care. Circulation. 2010;122(18 Suppl 3):S768–86.

87. Kleinman ME, Srinivasan V. Postresuscitation care. Pediatr Clin North Am. 2008;55(4):943–67, xi.

88. Krep H, Breil M, Sinn D, Hagendorff A, Hoeft A, Fischer M. Effects of hypertonic versus isotonic infusion therapy on regional cerebral blood flow after experimental cardiac arrest cardiopulmonary resuscitation in pigs. Resuscitation. 2004;63(1):73–83.

89. Bray RJ. Propofol infusion syndrome in children. Paediatr Anaesth. 1998;8(6):491–9.

90. Iyer VN, Hoel R, Rabinstein AA. Propofol infusion syndrome in patients with refractory status epilepticus: an 11-year clinical experience. Crit Care Med. 2009;37(12):3024–30.

91. Ista E, van Dijk M, Tibboel D, de Hoog M. Assessment of sedation levels in pediatric intensive care patients can be improved by using the COMFORT "behavior" scale. Pediatr Crit Care Med. 2005;6(1):58–63.

92. Curley MA, Harris SK, Fraser KA, Johnson RA, Arnold JH. State Behavioral Scale: a sedation assessment instrument for infants and young children supported on mechanical ventilation. Pediatr Crit Care Med. 2006;7(2):107–14.

93. Natale JE, Joseph JG, Helfaer MA, Shaffner DH. Early hyperthermia after traumatic brain injury in children: risk factors, influence on length of stay, and effect on short-term neurologic status. Crit Care Med. 2000;28(7):2608–15.

94. Takino M, Okada Y. Hyperthermia following cardiopulmonary resuscitation. Intensive Care Med. 1991;17(7):419–20.

95. Hickey RW, Kochanek PM, Ferimer H, Graham SH, Safar P. Hypothermia and hyperthermia in children after resuscitation from cardiac arrest. Pediatrics. 2000;106(1 Pt 1):118–22.

96. Zeiner A, Holzer M, Sterz F, et al. Hyperthermia after cardiac arrest is associated with an unfavorable neurologic outcome. Arch Intern Med. 2001;161(16):2007–12.

97. Langhelle A, Tyvold SS, Lexow K, Hapnes SA, Sunde K, Steen PA. In-hospital factors associated with improved outcome after out-of-hospital cardiac arrest. A comparison between four regions in Norway. Resuscitation. 2003;56(3):247–63.

98. Diringer MN, Reaven NL, Funk SE, Uman GC. Elevated body temperature independently contributes to increased length of stay in neurologic intensive care unit patients. Crit Care Med. 2004;32(7):1489–95.

99. Takasu A, Saitoh D, Kaneko N, Sakamoto T, Okada Y. Hyperthermia: is it an ominous sign after cardiac arrest? Resuscitation. 2001;49(3):273–7.

100. Greer DM, Funk SE, Reaven NL, Ouzounelli M, Uman GC. Impact of fever on outcome in patients with stroke and neurologic injury: a comprehensive meta-analysis. Stroke. 2008;39(11):3029–35.

101. Fink EL. Global warming after cardiac arrest in children exists. Pediatr Crit Care Med. 2010;11(6):760–1.

102. Bembea MM, Nadkarni VM, Diener-West M, et al. Temperature patterns in the early postresuscitation period after pediatric inhospital cardiac arrest. Pediatr Crit Care Med. 2010;11(6):723–30.

103. Mild therapeutic hypothermia to improve the neurologic outcome after cardiac arrest. N Engl J Med. 2002;346(8):549–56.

104. Bernard SA, Gray TW, Buist MD, et al. Treatment of comatose survivors of out-of-hospital cardiac arrest with induced hypothermia. N Engl J Med. 2002;346(8):557–63.

105. Gluckman PD, Wyatt JS, Azzopardi D, et al. Selective head cooling with mild systemic hypothermia after neonatal encephalopathy: multicentre randomised trial. Lancet. 2005;365(9460):663–70.

106. Shankaran S, Laptook AR, Ehrenkranz RA, et al. Whole-body hypothermia for neonates with hypoxic-ischemic encephalopathy. N Engl J Med. 2005;353(15):1574–84.

107. Baltagi S, Fink EL, Bell MJ. Therapeutic hypothermia: ready… fire…aim? How small feasibility studies can inform large efficacy trials. Pediatr Crit Care Med. 2011;12(3):370–1.

108. Sloniewsky D. Pediatric patients with out-of hospital cardiac arrest: is therapeutic hypothermia for them? Crit Care Med. 2011;39(1):218–9.

109. Koch JD, Kernie SG. Protecting the future: neuroprotective strategies in the pediatric intensive care unit. Curr Opin Pediatr. 2011;23(3):275–80.

110. Hutchison JS, Ward RE, Lacroix J, et al. Hypothermia therapy after traumatic brain injury in children. N Engl J Med. 2008;358(23):2447–56.

111. Fink EL, Clark RS, Kochanek PM, Bell MJ, Watson RS. A tertiary care center's experience with therapeutic hypothermia after pediatric cardiac arrest. Pediatr Crit Care Med. 2010;11(1):66–74.

112. Doherty DR, Parshuram CS, Gaboury I, et al. Hypothermia therapy after pediatric cardiac arrest. Circulation. 2009;119(11):1492–500.

113. Topjian A, Hutchins L, DiLiberto MA, et al. Induction and maintenance of therapeutic hypothermia after pediatric cardiac arrest: efficacy of a surface cooling protocol. Pediatr Crit Care Med. 2011;12(3):e127–35.

114. Hutchison JS, Doherty DR, Orlowski JP, Kissoon N. Hypothermia therapy for cardiac arrest in pediatric patients. Pediatr Clin North Am. 2008;55(3):529–44, ix.

115. Haque IU, Latour MC, Zaritsky AL. Pediatric critical care community survey of knowledge and attitudes toward therapeutic hypothermia in comatose children after cardiac arrest. Pediatr Crit Care Med. 2006;7(1):7–14.

116. Weigl M, Tenze G, Steinlechner B, et al. A systematic review of currently available pharmacological neuroprotective agents as a sole intervention before anticipated or induced cardiac arrest. Resuscitation. 2005;65(1):21–39.

117. Damian MS, Ellenberg D, Gildemeister R, et al. Coenzyme Q10 combined with mild hypothermia after cardiac arrest: a preliminary study. Circulation. 2004;110(19):3011–6.

118. Wijdicks EF, Hijdra A, Young GB, Bassetti CL, Wiebe S. Practice parameter: prediction of outcome in comatose survivors after cardiopulmonary resuscitation (an evidence-based review): report of the Quality Standards Subcommittee of the American Academy of Neurology. Neurology. 2006;67(2):203–10.

119. Abend NS, Licht DJ. Predicting outcome in children with hypoxic ischemic encephalopathy. Pediatr Crit Care Med. 2008;9(1):32–9.

120. Mullner M, Sterz F, Binder M, Schreiber W, Deimel A, Laggner AN. Blood glucose concentration after cardiopulmonary resuscitation influences functional neurological recovery in human cardiac arrest survivors. J Cereb Blood Flow Metab. 1997;17(4):430–6.

121. Longstreth Jr WT, Inui TS. High blood glucose level on hospital admission and poor neurological recovery after cardiac arrest. Ann Neurol. 1984;15(1):59–63.

122. Calle PA, Buylaert WA, Vanhaute OA. Glycemia in the postresuscitation period. The Cerebral Resuscitation Study Group. Resuscitation. 1989;17(Suppl):S181–8; discussion S199–206.

123. Longstreth Jr WT, Diehr P, Cobb LA, Hanson RW, Blair AD. Neurologic outcome and blood glucose levels during out-of-hospital cardiopulmonary resuscitation. Neurology. 1986;36(9):1186–91.

124. Longstreth Jr WT, Copass MK, Dennis LK, Rauch-Matthews ME, Stark MS, Cobb LA. Intravenous glucose after out-of-hospital cardiopulmonary arrest: a community-based randomized trial. Neurology. 1993;43(12):2534–41.

125. Beiser DG, Carr GE, Edelson DP, Peberdy MA, Hoek TL. Derangements in blood glucose following initial resuscitation from in-hospital cardiac arrest: a report from the national registry of cardiopulmonary resuscitation. Resuscitation. 2009;80(6):624–30.

126. Oksanen T, Skrifvars MB, Varpula T, et al. Strict versus moderate glucose control after resuscitation from ventricular fibrillation. Intensive Care Med. 2007;33(12):2093–100.

127. Sunde K, Pytte M, Jacobsen D, et al. Implementation of a standardised treatment protocol for post resuscitation care after out-of-hospital cardiac arrest. Resuscitation. 2007;73(1):29–39.

128. Losert H, Sterz F, Roine RO, et al. Strict normoglycaemic blood glucose levels in the therapeutic management of patients within 12 h after cardiac arrest might not be necessary. Resuscitation. 2008;76(2):214–20.

129. Van den Berghe G, Schoonheydt K, Becx P, Bruyninckx F, Wouters PJ. Insulin therapy protects the central and peripheral nervous system of intensive care patients. Neurology. 2005;64(8):1348–53.

130. van den Berghe G, Wouters P, Weekers F, et al. Intensive insulin therapy in the critically ill patients. N Engl J Med. 2001;345(19):1359–67.

131. Van den Berghe G, Wilmer A, Hermans G, et al. Intensive insulin therapy in the medical ICU. N Engl J Med. 2006;354(5):449–61.

132. Marik PE, Varon J. Intensive insulin therapy in the ICU: is it now time to jump off the bandwagon? Resuscitation. 2007;74(1):191–3.

133. Watkinson P, Barber VS, Young JD. Strict glucose control in the critically ill. BMJ. 2006;332(7546):865–6.

134. Finfer S, Chittock DR, Su SY, et al. Intensive versus conventional glucose control in critically ill patients. N Engl J Med. 2009;360(13):1283–97.

135. Srinivasan V, Spinella PC, Drott HR, Roth CL, Helfaer MA, Nadkarni V. Association of timing, duration, and intensity of hyperglycemia with intensive care unit mortality in critically ill children. Pediatr Crit Care Med. 2004;5(4):329–36.

136. Faustino EV, Apkon M. Persistent hyperglycemia in critically ill children. J Pediatr. 2005;146(1):30–4.

137. Wintergerst KA, Buckingham B, Gandrud L, Wong BJ, Kache S, Wilson DM. Association of hypoglycemia, hyperglycemia, and glucose variability with morbidity and death in the pediatric intensive care unit. Pediatrics. 2006;118(1):173–9.

138. Hirshberg E, Larsen G, Van Duker H. Alterations in glucose homeostasis in the pediatric intensive care unit: hyperglycemia and glucose variability are associated with increased mortality and morbidity. Pediatr Crit Care Med. 2008;9(4):361–6.

139. Vlasselaers D, Milants I, Desmet L, et al. Intensive insulin therapy for patients in paediatric intensive care: a prospective, randomised controlled study. Lancet. 2009;373(9663):547–56.

140. Bar-Joseph G, Abramson NS, Jansen-McWilliams L, et al. Clinical use of sodium bicarbonate during cardiopulmonary resuscitation – is it used sensibly? Resuscitation. 2002;54(1):47–55.

141. Bar-Joseph G, Abramson NS, Kelsey SF, Mashiach T, Craig MT, Safar P. Improved resuscitation outcome in emergency medical systems with increased usage of sodium bicarbonate during cardiopulmonary resuscitation. Acta Anaesthesiol Scand. 2005;49(1):6–15.

142. Vukmir RB, Katz L. Sodium bicarbonate improves outcome in prolonged prehospital cardiac arrest. Am J Emerg Med. 2006;24(2):156–61.

143. Stiell IG, Wells GA, Hebert PC, Laupacis A, Weitzman BN. Association of drug therapy with survival in cardiac arrest: limited role of advanced cardiac life support drugs. Acad Emerg Med. 1995;2(4):264–73.

144. van Walraven C, Stiell IG, Wells GA, Hebert PC, Vandemheen K. Do advanced cardiac life support drugs increase resuscitation rates from in-hospital cardiac arrest? The OTAC Study Group. Ann Emerg Med. 1998;32(5):544–53.

145. Dybvik T, Strand T, Steen PA. Buffer therapy during out-of-hospital cardiopulmonary resuscitation. Resuscitation. 1995;29(2):89–95.

146. Bjerneroth G. Alkaline buffers for correction of metabolic acidosis during cardiopulmonary resuscitation with focus on Tribonat – a review. Resuscitation. 1998;37(3):161–71.

147. Scheingraber S, Rehm M, Sehmisch C, Finsterer U. Rapid saline infusion produces hyperchloremic acidosis in patients undergoing gynecologic surgery. Anesthesiology. 1999;90(5):1265–70.

148. Brill SA, Stewart TR, Brundage SI, Schreiber MA. Base deficit does not predict mortality when secondary to hyperchloremic acidosis. Shock. 2002;17(6):459–62.

149. Gando S, Igarashi M, Kameue T, Nanzaki S. Ionized hypocalcemia during out-of-hospital cardiac arrest and cardiopulmonary resuscitation is not due to binding by lactate. Intensive Care Med. 1997;23(12):1245–50.

150. Urban P, Scheidegger D, Buchmann B, Barth D. Cardiac arrest and blood ionized calcium levels. Ann Intern Med. 1988;109(2):110–3.

151. Niemann JT, Cairns CB. Hyperkalemia and ionized hypocalcemia during cardiac arrest and resuscitation: possible culprits for post-countershock arrhythmias? Ann Emerg Med. 1999;34(1):1–7.

152. American Heart Association Guidelines for Cardiopulmonary Resuscitation and Emergency Cardiovascular Care. Circulation. 2005;112(24 Suppl):IV1–203.

153. Cheung JY, Bonventre JV, Malis CD, Leaf A. Calcium and ischemic injury. N Engl J Med. 1986;314(26):1670–6.

154. Srinivasan V, Morris MC, Helfaer MA, Berg RA, Nadkarni VM. Calcium use during in-hospital pediatric cardiopulmonary resuscitation: a report from the National Registry of Cardiopulmonary Resuscitation. Pediatrics. 2008;121(5):e1144–51.

155. Neumar RW, Otto CW, Link MS, et al. Part 8: adult advanced cardiovascular life support: 2010 American Heart Association Guidelines for Cardiopulmonary Resuscitation and Emergency Cardiovascular Care. Circulation. 2010;122(18 Suppl 3):S729–67.

156. Miller B, Craddock L, Hoffenberg S, et al. Pilot study of intravenous magnesium sulfate in refractory cardiac arrest: safety data and recommendations for future studies. Resuscitation. 1995;30(1):3–14.

157. Allegra J, Lavery R, Cody R, et al. Magnesium sulfate in the treatment of refractory ventricular fibrillation in the prehospital setting. Resuscitation. 2001;49(3):245–9.

158. Thel MC, Armstrong AL, McNulty SE, Califf RM, O'Connor CM. Randomised trial of magnesium in in-hospital cardiac arrest. Duke Internal Medicine Housestaff. Lancet. 1997;350(9087):1272–6.

159. Longstreth Jr WT, Fahrenbruch CE, Olsufka M, Walsh TR, Copass MK, Cobb LA. Randomized clinical trial of magnesium, diazepam, or both after out-of-hospital cardiac arrest. Neurology. 2002;59(4):506–14.

160. Adrie C, Adib-Conquy M, Laurent I, et al. Successful cardiopulmonary resuscitation after cardiac arrest as a "sepsis-like" syndrome. Circulation. 2002;106(5):562–8.

161. Ito T, Saitoh D, Fukuzuka K, et al. Significance of elevated serum interleukin-8 in patients resuscitated after cardiopulmonary arrest. Resuscitation. 2001;51(1):47–53.

162. Mussack T, Biberthaler P, Kanz KG, et al. Serum S-100B and interleukin-8 as predictive markers for comparative neurologic outcome analysis of patients after cardiac arrest and severe traumatic brain injury. Crit Care Med. 2002;30(12):2669–74.

163. Adrie C, Laurent I, Monchi M, Cariou A, Dhainaou JF, Spaulding C. Postresuscitation disease after cardiac arrest: a sepsis-like syndrome? Curr Opin Crit Care. 2004;10(3):208–12.

164. Geppert A, Zorn G, Karth GD, et al. Soluble selectins and the systemic inflammatory response syndrome after successful cardiopulmonary resuscitation. Crit Care Med. 2000;28(7):2360–5.

165. Gando S, Nanzaki S, Morimoto Y, Kobayashi S, Kemmotsu O. Out-of-hospital cardiac arrest increases soluble vascular endothelial adhesion molecules and neutrophil elastase associated with endothelial injury. Intensive Care Med. 2000;26(1):38–44.

166. Fink K, Schwarz M, Feldbrugge L, et al. Severe endothelial injury and subsequent repair in patients after successful cardiopulmonary resuscitation. Crit Care. 2010;14(3):R104.

167. Adams JA. Endothelium and cardiopulmonary resuscitation. Crit Care Med. 2006;34(12 Suppl):S458–65.

168. Mongardon N, Perbet S, Lemiale V, et al. Infectious complications in out-of-hospital cardiac arrest patients in the therapeutic hypothermia era. Crit Care Med. 2011;39(6):1359–64.

169. Gajic O, Festic E, Afessa B. Infectious complications in survivors of cardiac arrest admitted to the medical intensive care unit. Resuscitation. 2004;60(1):65–9.

170. Tsai MS, Chiang WC, Lee CC, et al. Infections in the survivors of out-of-hospital cardiac arrest in the first 7 days. Intensive Care Med. 2005;31(5):621–6.

171. Cerchiari EL, Safar P, Klein E, Diven W. Visceral, hematologic and bacteriologic changes and neurologic outcome after cardiac arrest in dogs. The visceral post-resuscitation syndrome. Resuscitation. 1993;25(2):119–36.

172. Gaussorgues P, Gueugniaud PY, Vedrinne JM, Salord F, Mercatello A, Robert D. Bacteremia following cardiac arrest and cardiopulmonary resuscitation. Intensive Care Med. 1988;14(5):575–7.

173. Adrie C, Monchi M, Laurent I, et al. Coagulopathy after successful cardiopulmonary resuscitation following cardiac arrest: implication of the protein C anticoagulant pathway. J Am Coll Cardiol. 2005;46(1):21–8.

174. Bottiger BW, Motsch J, Bohrer H, et al. Activation of blood coagulation after cardiac arrest is not balanced adequately by activation of endogenous fibrinolysis. Circulation. 1995;92(9):2572–8.

175. Gando S, Kameue T, Nanzaki S, Nakanishi Y. Massive fibrin formation with consecutive impairment of fibrinolysis in patients with out-of-hospital cardiac arrest. Thromb Haemost. 1997;77(2):278–82.

176. Bottiger BW, Bohrer H, Boker T, Motsch J, Aulmann M, Martin E. Platelet factor 4 release in patients undergoing cardiopulmonary resuscitation – can reperfusion be impaired by platelet activation? Acta Anaesthesiol Scand. 1996;40(5):631–5.

177. Gando S, Nanzaki S, Morimoto Y, Kobayashi S, Kemmotsu O. Tissue factor and tissue factor pathway inhibitor levels during and after cardiopulmonary resuscitation. Thromb Res. 1999;96(2):107–13.

178. Gando S, Kameue T, Nanzaki S, Igarashi M, Nakanishi Y. Platelet activation with massive formation of thromboxane A2 during and after cardiopulmonary resuscitation. Intensive Care Med. 1997;23(1):71–6.

179. Bottiger BW, Martin E. Thrombolytic therapy during cardiopulmonary resuscitation and the role of coagulation activation after cardiac arrest. Curr Opin Crit Care. 2001;7(3):176–83.

180. Fischer M, Bottiger BW, Popov-Cenic S, Hossmann KA. Thrombolysis using plasminogen activator and heparin reduces cerebral no-reflow after resuscitation from cardiac arrest: an experimental study in the cat. Intensive Care Med. 1996;22(11):1214–23.

181. Li X, Fu QL, Jing XL, et al. A meta-analysis of cardiopulmonary resuscitation with and without the administration of thrombolytic agents. Resuscitation. 2006;70(1):31–6.

182. Bottiger BW, Arntz HR, Chamberlain DA, et al. Thrombolysis during resuscitation for out-of-hospital cardiac arrest. N Engl J Med. 2008;359(25):2651–62.

183. Ziegenfuss MD, Mullany DV. Traumatic liver injury complicating cardio-pulmonary resuscitation. The value of a major intensive care facility: a report of two cases. Crit Care Resusc. 2004;6(2):102–4.

184. Meron G, Kurkciyan I, Sterz F, et al. Cardiopulmonary resuscitation-associated major liver injury. Resuscitation. 2007; 75(3):445–53.

185. Reiger J, Eritscher C, Laubreiter K, Trattnig J, Sterz F, Grimm G. Gastric rupture – an uncommon complication after successful cardiopulmonary resuscitation: report of two cases. Resuscitation. 1997;35(2):175–8.

186. Krischer JP, Fine EG, Davis JH, Nagel EL. Complications of cardiac resuscitation. Chest. 1987;92(2):287–91.

187. Stallard N, Findlay G, Smithies M. Splenic rupture following cardiopulmonary resuscitation. Resuscitation. 1997;35(2):171–3.

188. Ladurner R, Kotsianos D, Mutschler W, Mussack T. Traumatic pneumobilia after cardiopulmonary resuscitation. Eur J Med Res. 2005;10(11):495–7.

189. Prengel AW, Lindner KH, Wenzel V, Tugtekin I, Anhaupl T. Splanchnic and renal blood flow after cardiopulmonary resuscitation with epinephrine and vasopressin in pigs. Resuscitation. 1998;38(1):19–24.

190. L'Her E, Cassaz C, Le Gal G, Cholet F, Renault A, Boles JM. Gut dysfunction and endoscopic lesions after out-of-hospital cardiac arrest. Resuscitation. 2005;66(3):331–4.

191. Stockman W, De Keyser J, Brabant S, et al. Colon ischaemia and necrosis as a complication of prolonged but successful CPR. Resuscitation. 2006;71(2):260–2.

192. Piton G, Barbot O, Manzon C, et al. Acute ischemic pancreatitis following cardiac arrest: a case report. JOP. 2010;11(5):456–9.

193. Cook DJ, Reeve BK, Guyatt GH, et al. Stress ulcer prophylaxis in critically ill patients. Resolving discordant meta-analyses. JAMA. 1996;275(4):308–14.

194. Reveiz L, Guerrero-Lozano R, Camacho A, Yara L, Mosquera PA. Stress ulcer, gastritis, and gastrointestinal bleeding prophylaxis in critically ill pediatric patients: a systematic review. Pediatr Crit Care Med. 2010;11(1):124–32.

195. Mehta NM. Approach to enteral feeding in the PICU. Nutr Clin Pract. 2009;24(3):377–87.

196. Mehta NM, Compher C. A.S.P.E.N. Clinical Guidelines: nutrition support of the critically ill child. JPEN J Parenter Enteral Nutr. 2009;33(3):260–76.

197. McClave SA, Chang WK. Feeding the hypotensive patient: does enteral feeding precipitate or protect against ischemic bowel? Nutr Clin Pract. 2003;18(4):279–84.

198. Domanovits H, Mullner M, Sterz F, et al. Impairment of renal function in patients resuscitated from cardiac arrest: frequency, determinants and impact on outcome. Wien Klin Wochenschr. 2000;112(4):157–61.

199. Chua HR, Glassford N, Bellomo R. Acute kidney injury after cardiac arrest. Resuscitation. 2012;83(6):721–7.

200. Domanovits H, Schillinger M, Mullner M, et al. Acute renal failure after successful cardiopulmonary resuscitation. Intensive Care Med. 2001;27(7):1194–9.

201. Mattana J, Singhal PC. Prevalence and determinants of acute renal failure following cardiopulmonary resuscitation. Arch Intern Med. 1993;153(2):235–9.

202. Zeiner A, Sunder-Plassmann G, Sterz F, et al. The effect of mild therapeutic hypothermia on renal function after cardiopulmonary resuscitation in men. Resuscitation. 2004;60(3):253–61.

203. Knafelj R, Radsel P, Ploj T, Noc M. Primary percutaneous coronary intervention and mild induced hypothermia in comatose survivors of ventricular fibrillation with ST-elevation acute myocardial infarction. Resuscitation. 2007;74(2):227–34.

204. Lameire N, Van Biesen W, Vanholder R. Acute renal failure. Lancet. 2005;365(9457):417–30.

205. Annane D, Maxime V, Ibrahim F, Alvarez JC, Abe E, Boudou P. Diagnosis of adrenal insufficiency in severe sepsis and septic shock. Am J Respir Crit Care Med. 2006;174(12):1319–26.

206. Hebbar KB, Stockwell JA, Leong T, Fortenberry JD. Incidence of adrenal insufficiency and impact of corticosteroid supplementation in critically ill children with systemic inflammatory syndrome and vasopressor-dependent shock. Crit Care Med. 2011;39(5):1145–50.

207. Menon K, Ward RE, Lawson ML, Gaboury I, Hutchison JS, Hebert PC. A prospective multicenter study of adrenal function in critically ill children. Am J Respir Crit Care Med. 2010;182(2):246–51.

208. Pene F, Hyvernat H, Mallet V, et al. Prognostic value of relative adrenal insufficiency after out-of-hospital cardiac arrest. Intensive Care Med. 2005;31(5):627–33.

209. Schultz CH, Rivers EP, Feldkamp CS, et al. A characterization of hypothalamic-pituitary-adrenal axis function during and after human cardiac arrest. Crit Care Med. 1993;21(9):1339–47.

210. Kim JJ, Hyun SY, Hwang SY, et al. Hormonal responses upon return of spontaneous circulation after cardiac arrest: a retrospective cohort study. Crit Care. 2011;15(1):R53.

211. Kim JJ, Lim YS, Shin JH, et al. Relative adrenal insufficiency after cardiac arrest: impact on postresuscitation disease outcome. Am J Emerg Med. 2006;24(6):684–8.

212. Lindner KH, Strohmenger HU, Ensinger H, Hetzel WD, Ahnefeld FW, Georgieff M. Stress hormone response during and after cardiopulmonary resuscitation. Anesthesiology. 1992;77(4):662–8.

213. Ito T, Saitoh D, Takasu A, Kiyozumi T, Sakamoto T, Okada Y. Serum cortisol as a predictive marker of the outcome in patients resuscitated after cardiopulmonary arrest. Resuscitation. 2004;62(1):55–60.

214. Hekimian G, Baugnon T, Thuong M, et al. Cortisol levels and adrenal reserve after successful cardiac arrest resuscitation. Shock. 2004;22(2):116–9.

215. Miller JB, Donnino MW, Rogan M, Goyal N. Relative adrenal insufficiency in post-cardiac arrest shock is under-recognized. Resuscitation. 2008;76(2):221–5.

216. Annane D, Sebille V, Charpentier C, et al. Effect of treatment with low doses of hydrocortisone and fludrocortisone on mortality in patients with septic shock. JAMA. 2002;288(7):862–71.

217. Sprung CL, Annane D, Keh D, et al. Hydrocortisone therapy for patients with septic shock. N Engl J Med. 2008;358(2):111–24.

218. Smithline H, Rivers E, Appleton T, Nowak R. Corticosteroid supplementation during cardiac arrest in rats. Resuscitation. 1993;25(3):257–64.

219. Tsai MS, Huang CH, Chang WT, et al. The effect of hydrocortisone on the outcome of out-of-hospital cardiac arrest patients: a pilot study. Am J Emerg Med. 2007;25(3):318–25.

220. Mentzelopoulos SD, Zakynthinos SG, Tzoufi M, et al. Vasopressin, epinephrine, and corticosteroids for in-hospital cardiac arrest. Arch Intern Med. 2009;169(1):15–24.

221. Payen JF, Dupuis C, Trouve-Buisson T, et al. Corticosteroid after etomidate in critically ill patients: a randomized controlled trial. Crit Care Med. 2012;40(1):29–35.

222. Bello G, Paliani G, Annetta MG, Pontecorvi A, Antonelli M. Treating nonthyroidal illness syndrome in the critically ill patient: still a matter of controversy. Curr Drug Targets. 2009;10(8): 778–87.

223. Whitesall SE, Mayor GH, Nachreiner RF, Zwemer CF, D'Alecy LG. Acute administration of T3 or rT3 failed to improve outcome following resuscitation from cardiac arrest in dogs. Resuscitation. 1996;33(1):53–62.

224. D'Alecy LG. Thyroid hormone in neural rescue. Thyroid. 1997;7(1):115–24.

225. Facktor MA, Mayor GH, Nachreiner RF, D'Alecy LG. Thyroid hormone loss and replacement during resuscitation from cardiac arrest in dogs. Resuscitation. 1993;26(2):141–62.

226. Iltumur K, Olmez G, Ariturk Z, Taskesen T, Toprak N. Clinical investigation: thyroid function test abnormalities in cardiac arrest associated with acute coronary syndrome. Crit Care. 2005;9(4): R416–24.

227. Longstreth Jr WT, Manowitz NR, DeGroot LJ, et al. Plasma thyroid hormone profiles immediately following out-of-hospital cardiac arrest. Thyroid. 1996;6(6):649–53.

228. Wortsman J, Premachandra BN, Chopra IJ, Murphy JE. Hypothyroxinemia in cardiac arrest. Arch Intern Med. 1987;147(2):245–8.

229. Zwemer CF, Whitesall SE, Nachreiner RF, Mayor GH, D'Alecy LG. Acute thyroid hormone administration increases systemic oxygen delivery and consumption immediately following resuscitation from cardiac arrest without changes in thyroid-stimulating hormone. Resuscitation. 1997;33(3):271–80.

Predicting Outcomes Following Resuscitation

Akira Nishisaki

Abstract

Outcomes of pediatric resuscitation depend on the location, pre-arrest and arrest variables including quality of CPR. Out-of-hospital cardiac arrest has poorer survival and neurological outcomes due to the longer period of no-flow time, as well as the underlying etiologies of out-of-hospital cardiac arrest that are themselves associated with poor outcomes (e.g. Sudden Infant Death Syndrome or drowning). In contrast, more than 90 % of in-hospital pediatric cardiac arrests are witnessed or monitored, and CPR is provided. Half of in-hospital pediatric cardiac arrest victims are successfully resuscitated to return of spontaneous circulation and a quarter will survive to discharge. Sixty-five percent of survived children had favorable neurological outcomes. Pre-arrest and arrest variables are highly associated with survival and neurological outcomes. However, these pre-arrest and arrest variables tend to have a high false positive rate for predicting poor neurological outcomes. There are no reliable predictors of outcome in children. High quality of CPR is associated with short term survival outcomes. For post-arrest variables, absence of pupillary exams after 48 h is predictive for poor neurological outcome when therapeutic hypothermia is not induced. EEG finding with mild slowing and rapid improvement are associated with good outcomes, while burst suppression, electrocerebral silence, and lack of reactivity are associated with poor outcome. Somatosensory evoked potentials (SSEPs) are much less influenced by drugs, and resistant to environmental noise artifacts in contrast to bedside EEG. Bilateral absence of the N20 components in SSEPs is consistently associated with poor neurological outcomes. Serum neuron-specific enolase (NSE) and S-100B protein have been evaluated as prognostic indicators. NSE had higher discriminative ability for poor neurological outcomes compared to S100-B protein. For patients receiving therapeutic hypothermia, absence or extensor motor responses after achievement of normothermia is predictive for poor neurological outcomes. Neurological finding during therapeutic hypothermia is not reliable.

Keywords

Cardiac arrest • Outcome • Prediction • Pediatric cerebral performance scale (PCPC) • Pediatric overall performance scale (POPC) • Electroencephalography (EEG) • Somatosensory evoked potentials (SSEPs) • Neuron-specific enolase (NSE) • S-100B • Therapeutic hypothermia

A. Nishisaki, MD, MSCE
Department of Anesthesiology and Critical Care Medicine,
The Children's Hospital of Philadelphia,
34th Street and Civic Center Blvd., CHOP Main 8NE Suite 8566,
Philadelphia, PA, USA
e-mail: nishisaki@email.chop.edu

D.S. Wheeler et al. (eds.), *Pediatric Critical Care Medicine*,
DOI 10.1007/978-1-4471-6362-6_26, © Springer-Verlag London 2014

Introduction

Outcomes of pediatric cardiac arrest are quite different in out-of-hospital cardiac arrest versus in-hospital cardiac arrest. Out-of-hospital cardiac arrest is associated with markedly worse outcomes, due to the longer period of no-flow time, as well as the underlying etiologies of out-of-hospital cardiac arrest that are themselves associated with poor outcomes (e.g. Sudden Infant Death Syndrome: SIDS, or drowning). In addition, many out-of-hospital cardiac arrests are unwitnessed, and less than half of children suffering an out-of-hospital cardiac arrest receive bystander Cardiopulmonary resuscitation (CPR). In contrast, more than 90 % of in-hospital pediatric cardiac arrests are witnessed or monitored, and CPR is provided by healthcare providers.

Out-of-Hospital Cardiac Arrest

The overall incidence of non-traumatic pediatric out-of-hospital cardiac arrest reported in a recently published, multi-center, population-based study in the U.S. is approximately 8.04 per 100,000 pediatric person-years (95 % CI: 7.27–8.81) [1]. The survival to hospital discharge in this study was only 6.4 % of all arrests, which is significantly higher than the reported rates of survival in adult out-of-hospital cardiac arrests (adult: 4.5 %, p = 0.03). The age of the patient at the time of cardiac arrest appears to play an important role in outcome, as the survival rate for infants was 3.3 % – significantly lower compared to both children (<12 years of age, 9.1 %) and adolescents (12–19 years of age, 8.9 %) [1]. Another population-based study showed the rate of return of spontaneous circulation among out-of-hospital pediatric cardiac arrest victims was 26 %, with a 1-month survival of 8 % [2]. In this study, neurologically-favorable outcome, defined as Glasgow-Pittsburgh Cerebral Performance Category scale (1 = good performance, 2 = moderate disability, 3 = severe cerebral disability, 4 = coma/vegetative state, 5 = death) of 1–2 or no change from baseline was observed in 3 % of all non-traumatic out-of-hospital pediatric cardiac arrest victims. Finally, a meta-analysis showed 12 % of out-of-hospital cardiac arrest victims survived to discharge, and only 33 % of survivors had intact neurological survival at discharge [3]. Collectively, these studies confirm the results of older studies that out-of-hospital cardiac arrest remains associated with poor (some investigators would even say "dismal") outcome.

In-Hospital Cardiac Arrest

Approximately half of in-hospital pediatric cardiac arrest victims are successfully resuscitated to return of spontaneous circulation [4]. A report from the National Registry of Cardiopulmonary Resuscitation (NRCPR) showed that more than 90 % of in-hospital cardiac arrests are witnessed or monitored, and the majority (65 %) occurred in an intensive care unit setting. The survival-to-discharge rate of in-hospital pediatric cardiac arrest was higher in children than adults (27 % vs. 18 %, adjusted Odds ratio = 2.29, 95 % CI, 1.95–2.68). Perhaps more importantly, 65 % of survived children had favorable neurological outcomes [4]. Collectively, these studies suggest that while the outcome from in-hospital cardiac arrest remains poor, it is much better compared to reported outcomes from out-of-hospital cardiac arrests [5, 6].

Classifying Outcomes Following Resuscitation

The outcome measures of pediatric cardiopulmonary arrest are challenging. Currently, international consensus-based reporting guidelines (the so-called Utstein templates) are commonly used [7]. While the "gold standard" outcome is the neurological function after hospital discharge, defining and reporting this measure is often practically difficult and expensive. Therefore, several surrogate outcome measures have been used including Sustained ROSC (Return of Spontaneous or Sustained Circulation), Survival after arrest >24 h, Survival to hospital discharge, Functional outcome (Pediatric Overall Performance Scale: POPC), Neurological outcome (Pediatric Cerebral Performance Scale: PCPC) (Table 26.1). Since many children who experience in-hospital cardiac arrest have underlying neurological conditions, it is practical to include a change in PCPC as a neurological outcome. Many studies define good neurological outcomes as the PCPC 1 or 2, or no change in PCPC at the time of discharge compared to pre-arrest condition [5].

Predicting Outcomes Following Resuscitation

Prognostic tools for predicting outcome for children who have suffered a cardiac arrest would be extremely helpful to the bedside clinician. This information is used by family and care providers to determine the appropriate level of care offered and provided to each patient. For example, the family may opt not to pursue tracheostomy and limit or withdraw technological support if the child's neurological prognosis seems poor with vegetative state. Therefore overly positive or negative prognostification should be avoided. When the literature is reviewed, it is crucial to examine the degree of informational bias (self-fulfilling prophesy). This occurs when the neurological prognosis of a patient is predicted poor and subsequently the life- sustaining therapy is withheld, while the true hypothetical outcome would have been otherwise. To minimize this effect, we need to evaluate the diagnostic characteristics of each

Table 26.1 Pediatric cerebral performance category scale (PCPC)

Score	Category	Description
1	Normal	Age-appropriate level of functioning; preschool child developmentally appropriate; school-age child attends regular classes
2	Mild disability	Able to interact at an age-appropriate level; minor neurological disease that is controlled and does not interfere with daily functioning (eg, seizure disorder); preschool child may have minor developmental delays but more than 75 % of all daily living developmental milestones are above the 10th percentile; school-age child attends regular school, but grade is not appropriate for age, or child is failing appropriate grade because of cognitive difficulties
3	Moderate disability	Below age-appropriate functioning; neurological disease that is not controlled and severely limits activities; most activities of preschool child's daily living developmental milestones are below the 10th percentile; school-age child can perform activities of daily living but attends special classes because of cognitive difficulties and/or has a learning deficit
4	Severe disability	Preschool child's activities of daily living milestones are below the 10th percentile, and child is excessively dependent on others for provision of activities of daily living; school-age child may be so impaired as to be unable to attend school; school-age child is dependent on others for provision of activities of daily living; abnormal motor movements for both preschool and school-age child may include nonpurposeful, decorticate, or decerebrate responses to pain
5	Coma/ vegetative state	Coma; unawareness
6	Death	

Worst level of performance for any single criterion is used for categorizing. Deficits are scored *only* if they result from a neurological disorder. Assessments are done from medical records or interview with caretaker

Table 26.2 Pre-arrest, arrest and post-arrest variables associated with neurological outcomes

		Good outcome	Poor outcome
Pre-arrest	Age	Infant (only in-hospital cardiac arrest)	
	Causes of cardiac arrest	Respiratory failure	Trauma
		Cardiac (post-operative)	Septic shock Hematological/ oncological
Arrest	First monitored rhythm	Ventricular fibrillation Pulseless ventricular tachycardia Bradycardia	Asystole
	Location of cardiac arrest	In-hospital	Out-of-hospital
	Witnessed?	Witnessed	Unwitnessed
	Bystander CPR	Performed	Not performed
	Duration of no flow time (time from cardiac arrest to the initiation of chest compression)	Short	Long
	Quality of CPR	Good	Poor
	Duration of chest compression	Short	Long
	Doses of epinephrine	Equal or less than two doses	More than two doses
Post-arrest	Temperature		Hyperthermia
	Blood pressure	Hypertension	Hypotension
	Inotrope		Requires inotrope support
	Serum lactate level		High
	Serum glucose level		Hyperglycemia

predictor (pre-arrest and arrest variables, neurological exam findings, and neurological tests) closely.

List of Predictors (Pre-arrest, Arrest, Post-arrest)

From large pediatric studies, pre-arrest and arrest variables are highly associated with survival and neurological outcomes. However, it should be noted that these pre-arrest and arrest variables tend to have a high false positive rate for predicting poor neurological outcomes, similar to adult studies [8]. The current resuscitation literature clearly states that there are no reliable predictors of outcome in children [7–9]. For instance, while the duration of CPR is highly associated with survival outcomes, several studies have documented neurologically intact survival after prolonged in-hospital CPR [10, 11]. It is also important to

emphasize that high quality of CPR is associated with short term survival outcomes. There are several variables, then, that can impact outcome. Table 26.2 shows pre-arrest and arrest variables associated with survival and neurological outcomes [5, 6, 12, 13].

Neurological Diagnostic Studies for Prognostification

There are several limitations to using neurological studies to determine prognosis after cardiac arrest. Sedation and paralysis are often required for management of post-cardiac arrest patients for physiologic stability or cerebral protection by preventing agitation or shivering which increases cerebral metabolic rate. This iatrogenic sedation and paralysis affects both the accuracy and reproducibility of the neurologic examination and the bedside EEG. Cerebral imaging studies such as CT or MRI require transport of unstable patients to radiology suites and are often not feasible. In addition, there is limited data correlating findings on these studies with long-term neurologic outcome. More recently therapeutic hypothermia is more widely accepted after cardiac arrest, and the effect of induced hypothermia on neurological exam or neurophysiologic studies (EEGs, SSEPs) are still under investigation.

Neurologic Exam

In large adult studies with prospective data collection, absence of pupillary response [Likelihood ratio 10.2 (95 % CI: 1.8–48.6)], absence of corneal reflex [Likelihood ratio 12.9 (95 % CI: 2.0–68.7)] at 24 h after the cardiac arrest were highly predictive for poor neurological outcome defined by Cerebral performance categories 3 or higher (severe cerebral disability, coma, vegetative state or death). Absence of a motor response [Likelihood ratio 9.2 (95 % CI: 2.1–49.4)] at 72 h was also highly predictive for poor neurological outcome [14]. Each component of coma assessment has moderate to substantial, but not complete level of agreement among raters regardless of disciplines. Glasgow coma scale or combined various neurological findings have not yielded additional predictive value in most studies. It is noteworthy that the motor component of the GCS score is more useful and accurate than the GCS sum score. The American Academy of Neurology published a practice parameter in 2006 [8] that stated the prognosis is invaluably poor in comatose patients with absent pupillary or corneal reflexes from 1 to 3 days after cardiac arrest, or absent or extensor motor responses (Motor component of the GCS less than 3) 3 days after cardiac arrest. Myoclonus status epilepticus, defined as spontaneous, repetitive, unrelenting, generalized multifocal myoclonus involving the face, limbs, and axial musculature in comatose patients) is associated with poor outcome with a 0 % (95 % CI: 0–8.8 %) false positive rate on day 1.

There are significantly fewer pediatric studies available. One small study with 57 consecutive children with hypoxic ischemic encephalopathy showed absence of pupillary response at 24 h and absence of spontaneous ventilation at 24 h were both 100 % predictive for poor neurological outcome – defined as severe disability, vegetative state or death (Positive predictive value = 100 %) [15]. In another pediatric study with 102 children with severe brain injury including both traumatic brain injury and HIE, the initial pupillary exam in the ICU had limited predictive value for neurological outcomes [16]. Specifically, the presence of initial pupillary response was 67 % (95 % CI: 53–78 %) predictive for favorable neurological outcome, and bilaterally absent pupillary response was 78 % (95 % CI: 58–91 %) predictive for unfavorable outcomes. In their subset of HIE patients (n = 36), the absence of bilateral pupillary exam at the last exam in the ICU (from 48 h up to 9 days after ICU

admission, the majority of examinations were performed on day 3–7) was 100 % predictive for unfavorable outcomes. The motor responses, however, had limited predictive value. Absence of bilateral motor responses was 93 % sensitive, 50 % specific for poor neurological outcomes defined as severe disability, vegetative or death.

Neurophysiologic Studies

In adult studies, the EEG literature is confounded by different classification systems and variable intervals of recordings after CPR. In general, generalized suppression to ≤20 microvolts, burst-suppression pattern with generalized epileptiform activity, or generalized periodic complexes on a flat background are associated with outcomes no better than persistent vegetative states [8]. In pediatric studies, similar findings are documented in a series of in-hospital cardiac arrest patients who survived at least 24 h [13, 15, 17]. In general, mild slowing and rapid improvement are associated with good outcomes, while burst suppression, electrocerebral silence, and lack of reactivity are associated with poor outcome. In one study, discontinuous activity defined as intervals of very low amplitude activity and bursts, spikes and epileptiform discharges had 100 % (95 % CI: 56–100 %) positive predictive value for poor neurological outcomes (severe disability, vegetative state or death) [15]. Another study, however, reported one infant who had burst and suppression pattern on EEG and had favorable outcomes [17]. Several other studies evaluated the reactivity of EEG to stimulation and identified it has moderate positive predictive value. The absence of reactivity in EEG, however, does not consistently indicate poor outcomes [15]. The prognostic accuracy (i.e. false positive rate) has not been established for those 'malignant' EEG patterns in both adults and children. Furthermore EEG is sensitive to drugs often administered to critically ill children after cardiac arrest. This limits the clinical use of EEG findings as prognosticators.

Somatosensory evoked potentials (SSEPs) are much less influenced by drugs, and resistant to environmental noise artifacts. Sufficient data in adults have demonstrated that absence of the N20 components are consistently associated with poor neurological outcomes. In one large adult multicenter study with 301 patients comatose at 72 h after CPR, 136 (45 %) had at least one bilateral absence of N20 on SSEPs. All of those had poor neurological outcomes (persistent coma or death at 1 month), with positive predictive value of 100 % (97 % CI: 97–100 %) [18]. In children, this finding is consistent across several studies: i.e. no children with hypoxic ischemic encephalopathy with absence of bilateral N20 had good neurological outcomes [15, 19–21]. However, it is important to note that the sensitivity is much lower: i.e. the presence of bilateral N20 does not predict favorable neurological outcomes. One study demonstrated high specificity for both good and poor neurological outcomes when SSEPs are used in combination with motor examination [20]. Brainstem auditory evoked potentials (BAEPs) and visual evoked potentials (VEPs) have been also evaluated in the past, however, their role in predicting neurological outcomes are less clear. In summary there is good evidence for abnormal SSEPs (absence of bilateral N20) being highly specific for poor neurological outcome. Prediction is best achieved by combining motor examination and SSEPs together.

Biomarkers

Serum neuron-specific enolase (NSE), S-100B protein, and creatine kinase brain isoenzyme (CKBB) in CSF (cerebrospinal fluid) have been evaluated as prognostic indicators for patients after CPR. NSE is a gamma isomer of enolase located in neurons and neuroectodermal cells. Elevation of NSE indicates neuronal injury. S-100B protein is a calcium-binding astroglial protein. CKBB is present in both neurons and astrocytes. The existing adult literature documents high positive predictive value of NSE within 72 h (100 %, 95 % CI: 97–100 %) for poor neurological outcome in a large cohort of patients using a priori defined cutoff (>33 mcg/L) [18]. An abnormal level was most commonly seen after 48 h of cardiac arrest. In the same study, an elevated serum S-100B protein level with cutoff of 0.7 mcg/L within 72 h also showed high positive predictive value for poor neurological outcome, but not 100 % (98 %, 95 % CI:93–99 %). CKMB in CSF had only a modest positive predictive value (median 85 %).

Topjian et al. evaluated the predictive value of the serum NSE and S-100B protein in children after cardiac arrest [22]. Poor neurological outcome was defined as PCPC change ≥2 from pre-arrest to post-arrest discharge. NSE level was significantly higher among children with poor neurological outcomes at 48, 72 and 96 h after arrest. A level of 51 mcg/L or higher at 48 h had 50 % sensitivity and 100 % specificity for poor outcomes. Interestingly, S-100B level was not different between good and poor outcome groups at any time points up to 96 h. Consistent with adult studies, NSE had higher discriminative ability for poor neurological outcomes compared to S100-B protein.

Neuroimaging

Neuroimaging has been explored as a modality for prognostication after cardiac arrest. There is general consensus that computed tomography (CT) may take 24 h to develop findings consistent with HIE (cerebral edema identified by poor gray white matter differentiation). The prognostic value of CT scan for poor neurological outcome is not well defined in both adult and children after cardiac arrest. Magnetic resonance imaging (MRI) has been identified useful especially when diffuse cortical signal changes on diffusion-weighted imaging (DWI) or fluid-attenuated inversion recovery (FLAIR) are used.

In children with hypoxemic coma, abnormal brain MRI with DWI and FLAIR showed high sensitivity but moderate specificity for poor neurological outcome. In one study with children with hypoxic coma from various etiologies, the positive predictive value of the abnormal MRI for poor neurological outcome was 82 % from their initial MRI studies. The false negative rate was 4 %, indicating that small number of patients with normal MRI results may still experience poor neurological outcome [23]. MRIs obtained during 4–7 days after the injury demonstrated higher accuracy with positive predictive value for poor prognosis (92 %) and negative predictive value (100 %), compared to MRI during 1–3 days (positive predictive value 100 %, negative predictive value 50 %). A similar finding was observed in children after drowning [24]. MR Spectroscopy to detect tissue cerebral hypoxia by measuring elevation of lactate, glutamine and glutamate and decrease in N-acetylaspartate (NAA) may also have capability to predict outcomes, however, we currently have insufficient evidence [13, 24]. In summary, a normal MRI after 3 days is a reasonably accurate predictor of good neurological outcome. Abnormal MRI results, however, do not necessarily indicate poor outcomes.

Other Important Considerations

The use of therapeutic hypothermia for cerebral protection presents yet another challenge for predicting neurological outcomes of CPR survivors. A typical therapeutic hypothermia protocol involves sedatives and paralytic use to prevent shivering that can potentially increase cerebral metabolic rate. Abend and colleagues recently published the predictive value of motor and pupillary responses in children treated with therapeutic hypothermia after cardiac arrest [25]. In their study, children who had return of spontaneous circulation had therapeutic hypothermia for 24 h followed by 12–24 h of rewarming to normothermia (36.5°C). Poor neurological outcome was defined as Pediatric Cerebral Performance Category score of 4–6. The positive predictive value of the absent motor function for poor neurological outcomes reached 100 % at 24 h after normothermia was achieved. The positive predictive value of absent pupillary response for poor neurological outcomes reached 100 % by the end of hypothermia phase. The earlier exams soon after the resuscitation or at 1 h after achievement of hypothermia (<34°C) had lower positive predictive value. This finding is consistent with an adult study demonstrating that the poor neurological exam (absence of brainstem reflex, motor response, or presence of myoclonus) are not as specific for poor neurological outcomes in patients with induced hypothermia after cardiac arrest [26].

Hypothermia suppresses EEG activities and increase latencies of the cortical responses in SSEPs. Two adult studies showed bilateral absence of N20 in SSEPs during hypothermia universally indicated poor neurological outcome [26, 27]. The study mentioned above by Abend and colleagues reported the incidence of seizures are high (47 %) in children after cardiac arrest with therapeutic hypothermia targeted at 34°C [28]. Interestingly no patients had seizure within 6 h after EEG monitoring was initiated. Seizure was observed at the end of cooling phase or more commonly during the rewarming phase. The EEG background characteristics during the hypothermia phase were predictive for neurological outcomes; specifically the burst suppression pattern was associated with poor neurological outcomes while slowing/attenuation was associated with better neurological outcomes. Seizure activity was also associated with more abnormal background, and associated with worse outcomes. As the therapeutic hypothermia after pediatric cardiac arrest is being utilized more often, we expect more knowledge accumulation regarding the accuracy of predictors of neurological outcomes in the next 5–10 years.

Conclusion

Outcomes of pediatric resuscitation depend on the location, pre-arrest and arrest variables including quality of CPR. Out-of-hospital cardiac arrest has poorer survival and neurological outcomes. Absence of pupillary exams after 48 h is predictive for poor neurological outcome when therapeutic hypothermia is not induced. For patients receiving therapeutic hypothermia, absence or extensor motor responses after achievement of normothermia is predictive for poor neurological outcomes. Neurological finding during therapeutic hypothermia is not reliable. Bilateral absence of the N20 components in SSEPs is consistently associated with poor neurological outcomes in children with normothermia.

References

1. Atkins DL, Everson-Stewart S, Sears GK, Daya M, Osmond MH, Warden CR, Berg RA, Resuscitation Outcomes Consortium Investigators. Epidemiology and outcomes from out-of-hospital cardiac arrest in children: the resuscitation outcomes consortium epistry-cardiac arrest. Circulation. 2009;119:1484–91.
2. Nitta M, Iwami T, Kitamura T, Nadkarni VM, Berg RA, Shimizu N, Ohta K, Nishiuchi T, Hayashi Y, Hiraide A, Tamai H, Kobayashi M, Morita H, Utstein Osaka Project. Age-specific differences in outcomes after out-of-hospital cardiac arrests. Pediatrics. 2011;128: e812–20.
3. Donoghue AJ, Nadkarni V, Berg RA, Osmond MH, Wells G, Nesbitt L, Stiell IG, CanAm Pediatric Cardiac Arrest Investigators. Out-of-hospital pediatric cardiac arrest: an epidemiologic review and assessment of current knowledge. Ann Emerg Med. 2005;46:512–22.
4. Nadkarni VM, Larkin GL, Peberdy MA, Carey SM, Kaye W, Mancini ME, Nichol G, Lane-Truitt T, Potts J, Ornato JP, Berg RA, National Registry of Cardiopulmonary Resuscitation Investigators.

5. Moler FW, Meert K, Donaldson AE, Nadkarni V, Brilli RJ, Dalton HJ, Clark RS, Shaffner DH, Schleien CL, Statler K, Tieves KS, Hackbarth R, Pretzlaff R, van der Jagt EW, Levy F, Hernan L, Silverstein FS, Dean JM, Pediatric Emergency Care Applied Research Network. In-hospital versus out-of-hospital pediatric cardiac arrest: a multicenter cohort study. Crit Care Med. 2009;37:2259–67.
6. Moler FW, Donaldson AE, Meert K, Brilli RJ, Nadkarni V, Shaffner DH, Schleien CL, Clark RS, Dalton HJ, Statler K, Tieves KS, Hackbarth R, Pretzlaff R, van der Jagt EW, Pineda J, Hernan L, Dean JM, Pediatric Emergency Care Applied Research Network. Multicenter cohort study of out-of-hospital pediatric cardiac arrest. Crit Care Med. 2011;39:141–9.
7. Jacobs I, Nadkarni V, Bahr J, Berg RA, Billi JE, Bossaert L, Cassan P, et al. Cardiac arrest and cardiopulmonary resuscitation outcome reports: update and simplification of the Utstein templates for resuscitation registries: a statement for healthcare professionals from a task force of the International Liaison Committee on Resuscitation. Circulation. 2004;110:3385–97.
8. Wijdicks EF, Hijdra A, Young GB, Bassetti CL, Wiebe S, Quality Standards Subcommittee of the American Academy of Neurology. Practice parameter: prediction of outcome in comatose survivors after cardiopulmonary resuscitation (an evidence-based review): report of the Quality Standards Subcommittee of the American Academy of Neurology. Neurology. 2006;67:203–10.
9. Kleinman ME, Chameides L, Schexnayder SM, Samson RA, Hazinski MF, Atkins DL, Berg MD, de Caen AR, Fink EL, Freid EB, Hickey RW, Marino BS, Nadkarni VM, Proctor LT, Qureshi FA, Sartorelli K, Topjian A, van der Jagt EW, Zaritsky AL. Part 14: pediatric advanced life support: 2010 American Heart Association guidelines for cardiopulmonary resuscitation and emergency cardiovascular care. Circulation. 2010;122:S876–908.
10. Morris MC, Wernovsky G, Nadkarni VM. Survival outcomes after extracorporeal cardiopulmonary resuscitation instituted during active chest compressions following refractory in-hospital pediatric cardiac arrest. Pediatr Crit Care Med. 2004;5:440–6.
11. Raymond TT, Cunnyngham CB, Thompson MT, Thomas JA, Dalton HJ, Nadkarni VM, American Heart Association National Registry of CPR Investigators. Outcomes among neonates, infants, and children after extracorporeal cardiopulmonary resuscitation for refractory inhospital pediatric cardiac arrest: a report from the National Registry of Cardiopulmonary Resuscitation. Pediatr Crit Care Med. 2010;11:362–71.
12. Meert KL, Donaldson A, Nadkarni V, Tieves KS, Schleien CL, Brilli RJ, Clark RS, Shaffner DH, Levy F, Statler K, Dalton HJ, van der Jagt EW, Hackbarth R, Pretzlaff R, Hernan L, Dean JM, Moler FW, Pediatric Emergency Care Applied Research Network. Multicenter cohort study of in-hospital pediatric cardiac arrest. Pediatr Crit Care Med. 2009;10:544–53.
13. Abend NS, Licht DJ. Predicting outcome in children with hypoxic ischemic encephalopathy. Pediatr Crit Care Med. 2008;9:32–9.
14. Booth CM, Boone RH, Tomlinson G, Detsky AS. Is this patient dead, vegetative, or severely neurologically impaired? Assessing outcome for comatose survivors of cardiac arrest. JAMA. 2004;291: 870–9.
15. Mandel R, Martinot A, Delepoulle F, Lamblin MD, Laureau E, Vallee L, Leclerc F. Prediction of outcome after hypoxic-ischemic encephalopathy: a prospective clinical and electrophysiologic study. J Pediatr. 2002;141:45–50.
16. Carter BG, Butt W. A prospective study of outcome predictors after severe brain injury in children. Intensive Care Med. 2005;31:840–5.
17. Nishisaki A, Sullivan 3rd J, Steger B, Bayer CR, Dlugos D, Lin R, Ichord R, Helfaer MA, Nadkarni V. Retrospective analysis of the prognostic value of electroencephalography patterns obtained in

First documented rhythm and clinical outcome from in-hospital cardiac arrest among children and adults. JAMA. 2006;295:50–7.

pediatric in-hospital cardiac arrest survivors during three years. Pediatr Crit Care Med. 2007;8:10–7.

18. Zandbergen EG, Hijdra A, Koelman JH, Hart AA, Vos PE, Verbeek MM, de Haan RJ, PROPAC Study Group. Prediction of poor outcome within the first 3 days of postanoxic coma. Neurology. 2006;66:62–8.

19. Carter BG, Taylor A, Butt W. Severe brain injury in children: long-term outcome and its prediction using somatosensory evoked potentials (SEPs). Intensive Care Med. 1999;25:722–8.

20. Carter BG, Butt W. Are somatosensory evoked potentials the best predictor of outcome after severe brain injury? A systematic review. Intensive Care Med. 2005;31:765–75.

21. Carrai R, Grippo A, Lori S, Pinto F, Amantini A. Prognostic value of somatosensory evoked potentials in comatose children: a systematic literature review. Intensive Care Med. 2010;36:1112–26.

22. Topjian AA, Lin R, Morris MC, Ichord R, Drott H, Bayer CR, Helfaer MA, Nadkarni V. Neuron-specific enolase and S-100B are associated with neurologic outcome after pediatric cardiac arrest. Pediatr Crit Care Med. 2009;10:479–90.

23. Christophe C, Fonteyne C, Ziereisen F, Christiaens F, Deltenre P, De Maertelaer V, Dan B. Value of MR imaging of the brain in children with hypoxic coma. AJNR Am J Neuroradiol. 2002;23: 716–23.

24. Dubowitz DJ, Bluml S, Arcinue E, Dietrich RB. MR of hypoxic encephalopathy in children after near drowning: correlation with quantitative proton MR spectroscopy and clinical outcome. AJNR Am J Neuroradiol. 1998;19:1617–27.

25. Abend NS, Topjian AA, Kessler S, Gutierrez-Colina AM, Berg R, Nadkarni V, Dlugos DJ, Clancy RR, Ichord RN. Outcome prediction by motor and pupillary responses in children treated with therapeutic hypothermia after cardiac arrest. Pediatr Crit Care Med. 2012;13(1):32–8.

26. Rossetti AO, Oddo M, Logroscino G, Kaplan PW. Prognostication after cardiac arrest and hypothermia: a prospective study. Ann Neurol. 2010;67:301–7.

27. Tiainen M, Kovala TT, Takkunen OS, Roine RO. Somatosensory and brainstem auditory evoked potentials in cardiac arrest patients treated with hypothermia. Crit Care Med. 2005;33: 1736–40.

28. Abend NS, Topjian A, Ichord R, Herman ST, Helfaer M, Donnelly M, Nadkarni V, Dlugos DJ, Clancy RR. Electroencephalographic monitoring during hypothermia after pediatric cardiac arrest. Neurology. 2009;72:1931–40.

Basic Management of the Pediatric Airway

Derek S. Wheeler

Abstract

The primary goal of basic airway management is to provide support and stabilization of the airway in a timely manner. Acute airway obstruction is common in critically ill children. Early recognition and management of acute airway obstruction represents one of the basic foundations of critical care medicine. Anatomical differences between pediatric and adult patients render children more susceptible to acute airway compromise. It is therefore important to recognize and understand these differences as they may have an impact on the success of airway management.

Keywords

Tracheal intubation • Endotracheal tube • Rapid sequence intubation • Airway management • Airway positioning • Nasal airway • Oral airway • Chin lift • Triple maneuver

Introduction

The primary goal of basic airway management is to provide support and stabilization of the airway in a timely manner. Acute airway obstruction is common in critically ill children. Early recognition and management of acute airway obstruction represents one of the basic foundations of critical care medicine. Anatomical differences between pediatric and adult patients render children more susceptible to acute airway compromise. It is therefore important to recognize and understand these differences as they may have an impact on the success of airway management.

D.S. Wheeler, MD, MMM
Division of Critical Care Medicine, Cincinnati Children's Hospital Medical Center, University of Cincinnati College of Medicine, 3333 Burnet Avenue, Cincinnati, OH 45229-3039, USA
e-mail: derek.wheeler@cchmc.org

Developmental Anatomy and Physiology of the Pediatric Airway

The upper airway is a vital part of the respiratory tract and consists of the nose, paranasal sinuses, pharynx, larynx, and extra-thoracic trachea. The structural complexity of the upper airway reflects its diverse functions, which include phonation, olfaction, humidification and warming of inspired air, preservation of airway patency, and protection of the airways [1, 2]. The pediatric airway is markedly different from the adult airway [3–6]. These differences are most dramatic in the infant's airway and become less important as the child grows – the upper airway assumes the characteristics of the adult airway by approximately 8 years of age. Anatomic features which differ between children and adults include (i) a proportionally larger head and occiput (relative to body size), causing neck flexion and leading to potential airway obstruction when lying supine; (ii) a relatively larger tongue, decreasing the size of the oral cavity; (iii) decreased muscle tone, resulting in passive obstruction of the airway by the tongue; (iv) a shorter, narrower, horizontally positioned, softer epiglottis; (v) cephalad and anterior position of the larynx; (v) shorter, smaller, narrower trachea; and (vi) funnel-shaped versus cylindrical airway, such that the narrowest

D.S. Wheeler et al. (eds.), *Pediatric Critical Care Medicine*,
DOI 10.1007/978-1-4471-6362-6_27, © Springer-Verlag London 2014

a   **b**

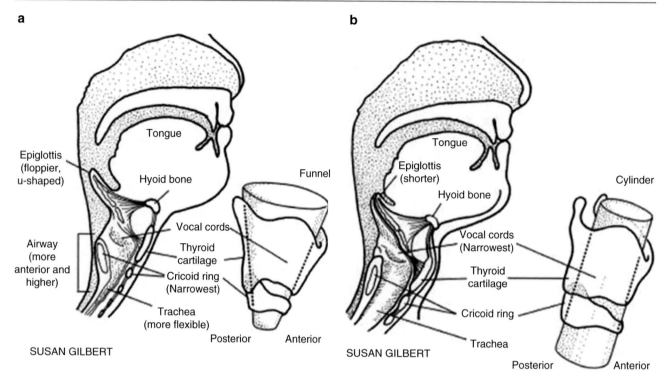

Fig. 27.1 Anatomic differences between the pediatric (**a**) and adult (**b**) airway (Reprinted from George et al. [255]. With permission from Center for Pediatric Emergency Medicine)

portion of the airway is located at the level of the cricoid cartilage (Fig. 27.1).

The first and perhaps most obvious difference is that the pediatric airway is much smaller in diameter and shorter in length compared to that of the adult. For example, the length of the trachea changes from approximately 4 cm in neonates to approximately 12 cm in adults, and the tracheal diameter varies from approximately 3 mm in the premature infant to approximately 25 mm in the adult [4, 6]. According to Hagen-Poiseuille's law, the change in air flow resulting from a reduction in airway diameter is directly proportional to the airway radius elevated to the fourth power:

$$Q = (\Delta P \pi r^4) / (8 \eta L) \qquad (27.1)$$

where Q is flow, ΔP is the pressure gradient from one end of the airway to the other end, r is the radius of the airway, η is the viscosity of the air, and L is the length of the airway. Therefore, increasing the length of the airway (L), increasing the viscosity of the air (η), or decreasing the radius of the airway will reduce laminar air flow. Changing the airway radius, however, has the greatest effect on flow. Small amounts of edema will therefore have a greater effect on the caliber of the pediatric airway compared to the adult airway, resulting in a greater increase in airway resistance (Fig. 27.2).

Aside from these size differences, the pediatric airway demonstrates several additional unique features as intro-

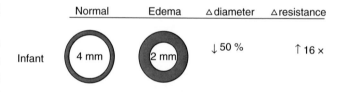

Fig. 27.2 Age-dependent effects of a reduction in airway caliber on the airway resistance and airflow. Normal airways are represented on the *left*, edematous airways are represented on the *right*. According to Hagen-Poiseuille's law, airway resistance is inversely proportional to the radius of the airway to the *fourth power* when there is laminar flow and to the *fifth power* when there is turbulent flow. One mm of circumferential edema will reduce the diameter of the airway by 2 mm, resulting in a 16-fold increase in airway resistance in the pediatric airway (cross-sectional area reduced by 75 % in the pediatric airway). Note that turbulent air flow (such as occurs during crying) in the child would increase the resistance by 32-fold

duced above [3–6]. For example, the larynx is located relatively cephalad in the neck with the inferior margin of the cricoid cartilage residing at approximately the level of C2–C3 in infants compared to C4–C5 in adults. This elevated position brings the epiglottis and palate in close proximity, thus making the infant an obligate nose breather in the first few weeks to months of life, which has potential clinical significance for various congenital abnormalities of the nasal airway. Infants are at greater risk of upper airway obstruction as nasal breathing doubles the resistance to airflow [6]. In addition, the nares are much smaller in children and can account for nearly 50 % of the total resistance of the airways. The nares are easily obstructed by secretions, edema, blood, or even an ill-fitting facemask, all of which can significantly increase the work of breathing. The tongue, which is large relative to the size of the oral cavity, more easily apposes the palate and represents one of the more common causes of upper airway obstruction in unconscious infants and children. A jaw-thrust maneuver or placement of either an oral or nasal airway will lift the tongue and relieve the obstruction in this situation (see below).

Direct laryngoscopy and tracheal intubation requires the alignment of three axes: the oral axis, the pharyngeal axis, and the laryngotracheal (variably known as the tracheal axis or laryngeal axis in certain publications) axis (Fig. 27.3). Normally, the oral axis is perpendicular to the laryngotracheal axis and the pharyngeal axis is positioned at an angle of 45° to the laryngotracheal axis. Placement of a folded towel beneath the occiput will flex the neck onto the chest, thereby aligning the pharyngeal and laryngotracheal axes. With proper extension of the atlanto-occipital joint, i.e. head extension and neck flexion (*sniff position*) these three axes are superimposed to establish the necessary line of visualization for optimal tracheal intubation (although proper airway positioning via the *sniff position* is somewhat controversial, as discussed further below). The cephalad position of the infant's larynx effectively shortens the length over which these three axes are superimposed, thereby creating more of an acute angle between the base of the tongue and the glottic opening. The glottic opening appears *anterior* such that adequate visualization may be difficult during direct laryngoscopy. The occiput is much larger in children compared to adults, leading to hyperflexion of the neck on the chest. A neck or shoulder roll will facilitate adequate visualization of the glottic opening during laryngoscopy. In addition, straight laryngoscope blades are often used in infants and young children to better visualize the airway during tracheal intubation.

The epiglottis is short, narrow, and angled posteriorly away from the long axis of the trachea and may be difficult to control via vallecular suspension with a curved laryngoscope blade. A straight laryngoscope blade is preferable to a curved laryngoscope blade in this situation. The adult vocal cords lie perpendicular to the laryngotracheal axis, while the infant's vocal cords are angled in an anterior-caudal position (the anterior attachments are more inferior compared to the posterior attachments). The tracheal tube can therefore become caught on the anterior commissure during passage through the glottic opening. Simple rotation of the tracheal tube will usually allow the tube to pass in this situation.

The narrowest portion of the pediatric airway is located below the level of the vocal cords at the cricoid cartilage, whereas the narrowest portion of the adult airway is at the level of the vocal cords (Fig. 27.4). The pediatric airway is

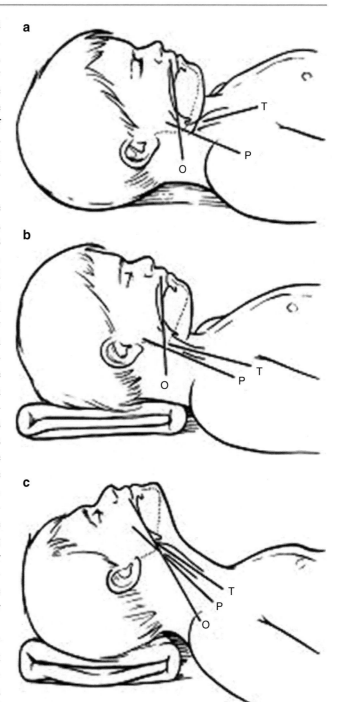

Fig. 27.3 Correct positioning of the child more than 2 years of age for ventilation and tracheal intubation. (**a**) With the patient on a flat surfacem the oral (*O*), pharyngeal (*P*), and tracheal (*T*) axes pass through three divergent planes. (**b**) A folded sheet or towel placed under the occiput of the head aligns the pharyngeal and tracheal axes. (**c**) Extension of the atlanto-occipital joint results in alignment of the oral, pharyngeal, and tracheal axes (Reprinted from Coté et al. [4]. With permission from Elsevier)

funnel-shaped as a result, compared to the cylindrical shape of the adult airway (Fig. 27.5). This anatomical configuration is one reason why uncuffed tracheal tubes can be used

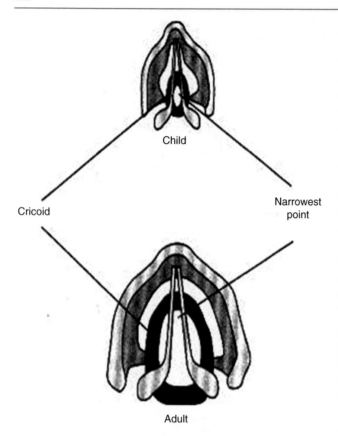

Fig. 27.4 The narrowest portion of the pediatric airway is at the cricoid cartilage vs the vocal cords in the adult

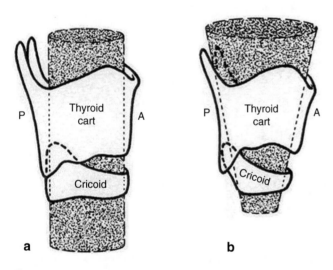

Fig. 27.5 Configuration of the adult (**a**) and the infant (**b**) larynx. Note the *cylindrical shape* of the adult larynx. The infant larynx is *funnel shaped* because of a narrow cricoid cartilage. *A* indicates anterior, *P* Posterior (Reprinted from Coté et al. [4]. With permission from Elsevier)

glottic opening, and cuffed tracheal tubes are essential to provide for adequate ventilation and protection from aspiration. The subglottic airway is completely encircled by the cricoid cartilage and is restricted in its ability to freely expand in diameter. In addition, the subglottic airway contains loosely attached connective tissue that can rapidly expand with inflammation and edema, leading to dramatic reductions in airway caliber (see again, Fig. 27.2). Children are at significant risk for viral laryngotracheobronchitis (croup) or post-extubation stridor, especially when an oversized tracheal tube is used or the cuff is overinflated. Young children are also at risk for acquired subglottic stenosis when exposed to prolonged or recurrent tracheal intubation.

The newborn trachea is soft and six times more compliant than that of the adult trachea. The transverse muscles are arranged uniformly, but longitudinal smooth muscles vary throughout the entire tracheal length. The musculature of the lower half of the trachea is more developed and functions to preserve stability of the tracheal lumen. Tracheal growth progresses throughout childhood into puberty. After puberty, the C-shaped cartilaginous tracheal rings do not expand, such that tracheal growth is the result of further growth of the tracheal musculature and soft tissue [3–6].

Basic Airway Management

Stabilization of the airway is of primary importance during the initial resuscitation of the critically ill or injured child. No matter what the cause or underlying condition, further attempts at resuscitation or treatment will fail without proper control of the airway. The goals of airway management are threefold: (i) relieve anatomic obstruction, (ii) prevent aspiration of gastric contents, and (iii) promote adequate gas exchange.

Positioning

Emergency management of the airway proceeds in a sequential order and begins with proper positioning of the head and protection of the cervical spine- all critically injured children have cervical spine injury until proven otherwise. Collapse of the tongue and soft tissues leads to obstruction of the upper airway and is the most common cause of airway obstruction in children. The *triple airway maneuver* is a simple method of relieving airway obstruction in this scenario and includes (i) proper head positioning while avoiding neck flexion (*head tilt maneuver* or *sniff position* – although the *head tilt* should be avoided whenever cervical spine injury is suspected), (ii) anterior displacement of the mandible (*jaw thrust maneuver*), and (iii) placement of an oral airway (Figs. 27.6 and 27.7) [7].

effectively in infants and children in that an effective seal will often form between the tracheal tube and the ring-like cricoid cartilage. Conversely, in adults, the circular tracheal tube will not form a good seal through the trapezoid-shaped

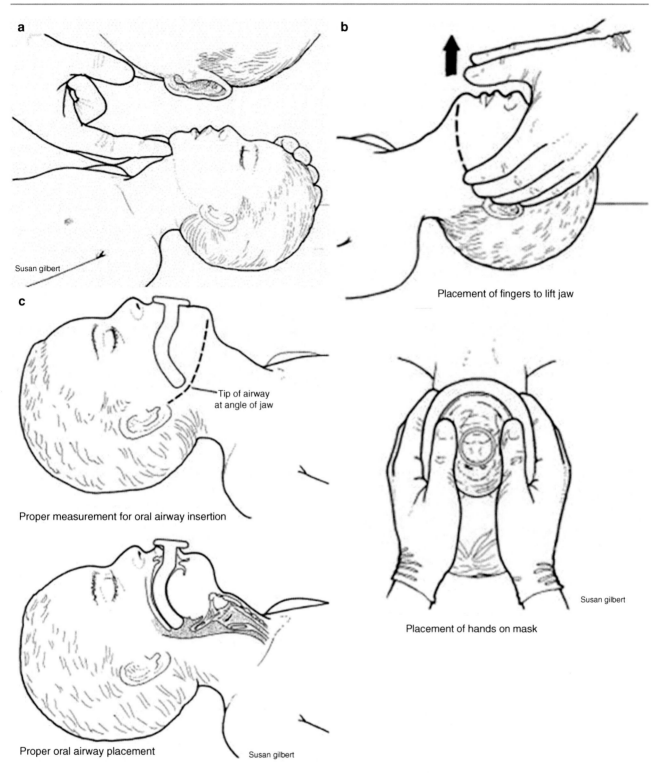

a

Susan gilbert

b

Placement of fingers to lift jaw

c

Tip of airway
at angle of jaw

Proper measurement for oral airway insertion

Placement of hands on mask

Susan gilbert

Proper oral airway placement   Susan gilbert

Fig. 27.6 The *triple airway maneuver*. (**a**) Head tilt-chin lift. (**b**) Jaw-thrust. (**c**) Placement of an oral airway (Reprinted from George et al. [255]. With permission from Center for Pediatric Emergency Medicine)

As discussed above, proper alignment of the three axes (the oral axis, the pharyngeal axis, and the laryngotracheal axis) by placing the patient in the so-called *sniff position* has been a widely accepted practice since the late 1800s [8].

Some authors have questioned the theory that the *sniff position* offers the best alignment of these three axes [7, 9–13] (Figs. 27.8 and 27.9). Notably, these investigations have all been performed in adults, and given the stark differences

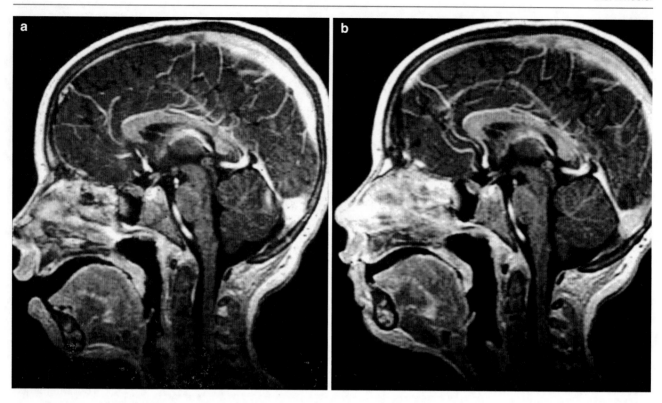

Fig. 27.7 Midline sagittal magnetic resonance imaging before (**a**) and after (**b**) chin lift. Note that the diameter of the pharyngeal airway is enlarged (Reprinted from Von Ungern-Sternberg et al. [7]. With permission from John Wiley & Sons, Inc)

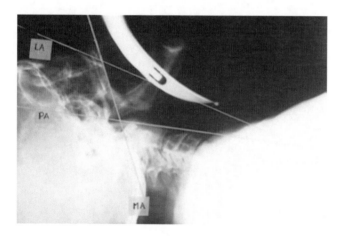

Fig. 27.8 Intubation in sniffing position. *LA* laryngeal axis (i.e., laryngotracheal axis), *MA* mouth axis, *PA* pharyngeal axis (Reprinted from Borron et al. [9]. With permission from Wolter Kluwers Health)

between the pediatric and adult airway, it is difficult to translate these findings to children. In addition, several other studies [14] have shown that the *sniff position* is the preferred position for optimal airway management. However, some general comments may be helpful. Because of the larger relative size of the occiput in infants and young children, head elevation with the use of a pillow or pad placed beneath the head is usually not necessary for optimal visualization

(Fig. 27.10) [14–16]. As children get older, head elevation with the use of a pillow or pad may be required, though the exact age at which this should be instituted is not known [14]. Suffice it to say that the ideal position for direct laryngoscopy and tracheal intubation for any particular patient may not be known in advance. The "sniff position" is perhaps a useful starting point, with adjustment and repositioning as required.

Airway Adjuncts

Airway adjuncts such as the oral airway and nasopharyngeal airway help to relieve obstruction of the airway by lifting the tongue from the soft tissues of the posterior pharynx. Oral airways consist of a flange, a short bite-block segment, and a curved body made of hard plastic that is designed to fit over the back of the tongue, thereby relieving airway obstruction and providing a conduit for airflow and for suctioning of the oropharynx. Proper sizing of the oral airway is imperative, as an incorrectly sized (either too long or too short) oral airway may exacerbate airway obstruction (Fig. 27.11). Sizes generally range from 4 to 10 cm in length (Guedel sizes 000–4). An oral airway is inserted by depressing the tongue with a blade/tongue depressor and following the curve of the tongue. Another commonly described method in which the

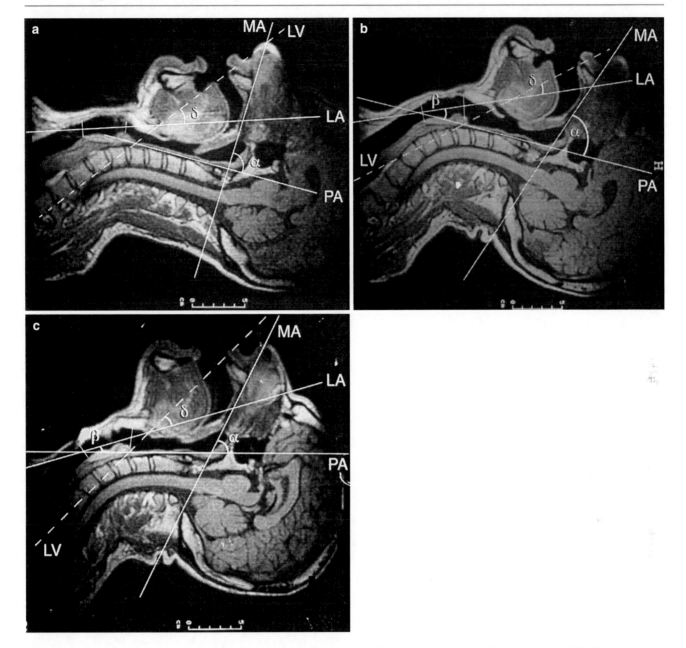

Fig. 27.9 Magnetic resonance imaging showing alignment of the three axes (*MA* mouth axis, *LA* laryngotracheal axis, *PA* pharyngeal axis) during (**a**) Neutral position, (**b**) Simple head extension, and (**c**) "Sniffing" position (Reprinted from Adnet et al. [10]. With permission from Wolter Kluwers Health)

oral airway is inserted with its concave side facing the palate and then rotating it to follow the curve of the tongue may damage the oral mucosa and/or teeth and should be avoided. Oral airways are poorly tolerated in children with an intact gag reflex and are therefore contraindicated in awake or semiconscious children.

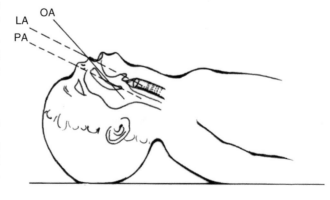

Fig. 27.10 Optimal head position for direct laryngoscopy in infants (*OA* oral axis or mouth axis, *LA* laryngotracheal axis, *PA* pharyngeal axis). No head elevation is required (Reprinted from El-Orbany et al. [14]. With permission from Wolter Kluwers Health)

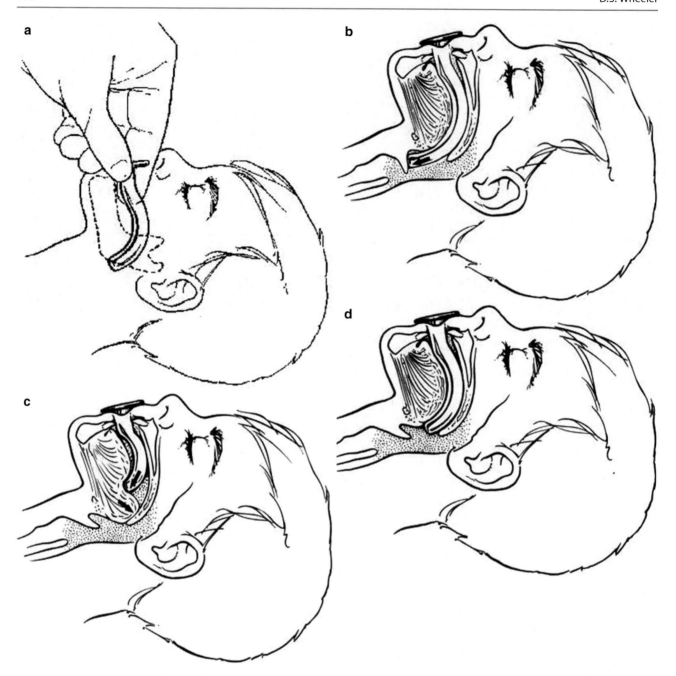

Fig. 27.11 (**a**) Proper oral airway selection. An airway of the proper size should relieve obstruction caused by the tongue without damaging laryngeal structures. The appropriate size can be estimated by holding the airway next to the child's face – the tip of the airway should end just cephalad to the angle of the mandible (*broken line*), resulting in proper alignment with the glottic opening. An oral airway that is either too large (**b**) or too short (**c**) may exacerbate obstruction of the airway. (**d**) Conversely, a correctly sized oral airway will lift the tongue off the posterior wall of the oropharynx, relieving airway obstruction (Reprinted from Coté et al. [4]. With permission from Elsevier)

A nasopharyngeal airway (*nasal trumpet*) should be used if the patient is semi-conscious, as use of the oral airway can lead to vomiting and potential aspiration of gastric contents in this scenario. The nasopharyngeal airway consists of a soft, rubber tube that is designed to pass through the nasal alae and beyond the base of the tongue, thereby relieving airway obstruction (Fig. 27.12) and providing a conduit for airflow. An appropriately sized nasopharyngeal airway extends from the nares to the tragus of the ear and should be of the largest diameter possible – it should pass relatively easy through the nasal alae with lubrication. The nasopharyngeal airway should not cause blanching of the nasal alae – if blanching occurs, the airway is too large. Nasopharyngeal airways are available in sizes 12–36 F, with a 12 F airway

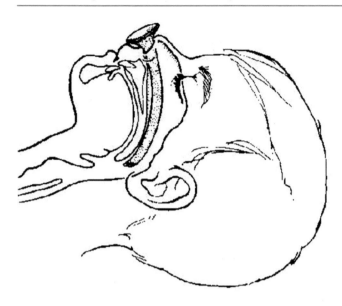

Fig. 27.12 The proper nasopharyngeal airway length is approximately equal to the distance from the tip of the nose to the tragus of the ear (Reprinted from Coté et al. [4]. With permission from Elsevier)

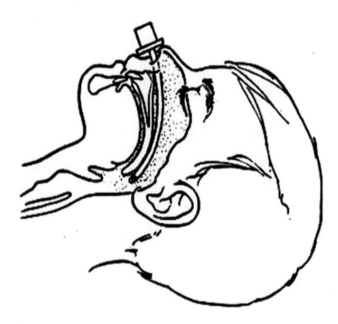

Fig. 27.13 A shortened, cut-off tracheal tube may also be used as a nasopharyngeal airway

(closely approximating a 3-mm tracheal tube) easily fitting through the nasal passages and nasopharynx of a full term newborn. A shortened tracheal tube is an acceptable substitute if a nasopharyngeal airway is not readily available (Fig. 27.13). The nasopharyngeal airway is lubricated and passed through the nasal passages perpendicular to the plane of the face and gently so as to avoid laceration of friable lymphoid tissue and subsequent bleeding. The use of nasopharyngeal airways is contraindicated in children with coagulopathies, CSF leaks, or basilar skull fractures.

Tracheal Intubation

Indications

If all of the above measures fail to stabilize the airway, tracheal intubation should be performed in an expeditious manner (Table 27.1). The most common indication for tracheal intubation in the PICU is acute respiratory failure. Acute respiratory failure is conceptually defined as an inadequate exchange of O_2 and CO_2 resulting in an inability to meet the body's metabolic needs. Clinical criteria, arbitrarily set at a PaO_2 <60 mmHg (in the absence of congenital heart disease) and a $PaCO_2$ >50 mmHg, are not rigid parameters, but rather serve as a context in which to interpret the clinical scenario. Failure of the anatomic elements involved in gas exchange – the conducting airways, the alveoli, and the pulmonary circulation – results in disordered gas exchange and is clinically manifested as hypoxemia (hypoxic respiratory failure). Failure of the respiratory pump – the thorax, respiratory muscles, and nervous system –results in an inability to effectively pump air into and out of the lungs, thereby leading to hypoventilation and subsequent hypercarbia (hypercarbic respiratory failure). While there are clear consequences of dysfunction of each these components, each also interacts significantly with the other. Therefore, failure of one frequently is followed by failure of the other.

Other common indications for tracheal intubation in the PICU include upper airway obstruction, e.g. epiglottitis, croup, airway trauma, etc.; neuromuscular weakness leading to neuromuscular respiratory failure, e.g. Guillain-Barre syndrome, myasthenia gravis, Duchenne muscular dystrophy, etc.; central nervous system disease, resulting in the loss of protective airway reflexes and inadequate respiratory drive, e.g. head trauma, stroke, etc.; and cardiopulmonary arrest. Importantly, tracheal intubation in the latter situation provides an avenue for administration of resuscitation medications (the medications that may be administered via the tracheal tube are easily recalled by the mnemonic, *LEAN* = *L*idocaine; *E*pinephrine; *A*tropine; *N*aloxone) when vascular access is unavailable. Tracheal intubation may become necessary in children with impaired mucociliary clearance (e.g., secondary to inhalation injury, prolonged tracheal intubation, etc.) or copious, thick, tenacious respiratory secretions as a means for aggressive pulmonary toilet and frequent suctioning. Tracheal intubation may also provide a means for administration of therapeutic gases (e.g., carbon dioxide, nitrogen, inhaled nitric oxide) in order to manipulate pulmonary vascular resistance in children with pulmonary hypertension or cyanotic congenital heart disease with single ventricle physiology.

Children with hemodynamic instability (e.g., shock, low cardiac output syndrome following cardiopulmonary bypass, etc.) may also benefit from early tracheal intubation and mechanical ventilation. Agitation and excessive work of

Table 27.1 Indications for tracheal intubation

Respiratory failure (defined in terms of either inadequate oxygenation or ventilation)
Upper airway obstruction
Shock or hemodynamic instability
Neuromuscular weakness with progressive respiratory compromise
Absent protective airway reflexes
Inadequate respiratory drive
Cardiac arrest (for emergency drug administration)

Table 27.2 Anatomic factors associated with a difficult airway

Small mouth, limited mouth opening or short interincisor distance
Short neck or limited neck mobility
Mandibular hypoplasia
High, arched and narrow palate
Poor mandibular translation
Poor cervical spine mobility
Obesity
Mucopolysaccharidoses

breathing increase oxygen consumption, which may lead to cardiovascular collapse in the face of an already compromised oxygen delivery. The excessive oxygen consumption often associated with the shock state has been compared by some investigators to running an 8-min mile, 24 h a day, 7 days a week [17]. For example, Aubier and colleagues [18] induced cardiogenic shock in dogs via cardiac tamponade and noted that the arterial pH was significantly lower and the lactate concentration significantly higher in dogs who were spontaneously breathing, as compared to dogs that were mechanically ventilated. Using this same model, these investigators studied respiratory muscle and organ blood flow using radioactively labelled microspheres in order to assess the influence of the working respiratory muscles on the regional distribution of blood flow when arterial pressure and cardiac output were lowered. Blood flow to the respiratory muscles increased significantly during cardiac tamponade in spontaneously breathing dogs – diaphragmatic flow, in fact, increased to 361 % of control values – while it decreased in dogs that were mechanically ventilated. More importantly, while the arterial blood pressure and cardiac output were comparable in the two groups, blood flow distribution during cardiac tamponade was quite different. The respiratory musculature received 21 % of the cardiac output in spontaneously breathing dogs, compared with only 3 % in the dogs that were mechanically ventilated. Blood flows to the liver, brain, and quadriceps muscles were significantly higher during tamponade in the dogs that were mechanically ventilated compared with the dogs who were spontaneously breathing [19]. These findings have been further corroborated in experimental models of septic shock [20] and clinical studies involving adults with cardiorespiratory disease [21] and critical illness [22, 23]. Therefore, with the judicious and careful use of sedation, neuromuscular blockade, tracheal intubation, and mechanical ventilatory support, a large fraction of the cardiac output used by the working respiratory muscles can be made available for perfusion of other vital organs during the low cardiac output state [18–23].

Assessment and Preparation

Resuscitation of any critically ill or injured child is chaotic even under ideal circumstances, and emergency airway man-

agement is often fraught with difficulties. Prior preparation and appropriate training of personnel therefore assumes vital importance [24]. The appropriate equipment and medications should be prepared well in advance [25]. Ideally, all of the necessary equipment for basic and advanced airway management should be readily accessible in an easily identifiable, central location in the PICU. Many PICUs keep all of the necessary airway equipment in specialized *airway carts* (similar to the *crash cart*) or *airway rolls* that can be brought to the bedside in an emergency.

The American Society of Anesthesiology defines a *difficult airway* by the presence of anatomic and/or clinical factors that complicate either mask ventilation or tracheal intubation by an experienced physician [26]. A *difficult intubation* is defined by the need for more than three tracheal intubation attempts or attempts lasting greater than 10 min [26]. Notably, this definition was developed specifically for the operating room scenario – most critically ill patients probably would not tolerate an intubation attempt lasting greater than 10 min. *Difficult ventilation* is defined as the inability of a trained physician to maintain the oxygen saturation >90 % with bag-valve-mask ventilation at an FIO_2 of 1.0 [26]. Some children (e.g., children with neuromuscular disease, cerebral palsy, obstructive sleep apnea, etc.) are dependent upon coordinated tone of the upper airway muscles to maintain a patent airway and are very sensitive to sedation, anesthesia, and neuromuscular blockade, resulting in significant difficulty with mask ventilation. The inability to mask ventilate has considerably more implications than does failure to tracheally intubate, as subsequent management options are limited (see below). Importantly, there is tremendous overlap between anatomic factors that predict a *difficult airway*, *difficult intubation*, and *difficult ventilation* (Table 27.2). In one study as many as 15 % of difficult intubations were also associated with difficult mask ventilation [27]. Fortunately, however, difficult intubations are relatively uncommon, even in children, with an estimated incidence between 2 and 4 %. Inability to mask ventilate has an even lower incidence, 0.02–0.001 % [28].

A number of quick, easy techniques have been proposed to predict a *difficult airway*. Unfortunately, a recent retrospective analysis suggested that performing this kind of

Fig. 27.14 Samsoon and Young modification of the Mallampati airway classification

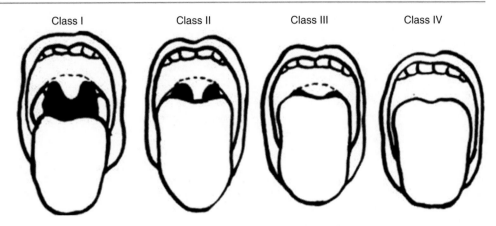

Class I   Class II   Class III   Class IV

airway assessment was not feasible in 70 % of critically ill adults [29]. An airway assessment may be even more difficult in children, as most of the reported techniques require cooperation on the part of the patient [5, 30, 31]. Moreover, most studies demonstrate that these bedside techniques have both poor inter-observer agreement and positive predictive value [32, 33]. Regardless, whenever feasible, an airway assessment should be performed so that problems with either bag-valve-mask ventilation or tracheal intubation can be anticipated and prepared for in advance.

Generally, in the absence of any obvious airway abnormality or specific syndrome associated with a difficult airway (see below), most difficult airways can be recognized by performing the following three maneuvers: (i) oropharyngeal examination, (ii) assessment of atlanto-occipital joint mobility, and (iii) assessment of the potential displacement area. These three tests correctly predict a difficult airway in adults virtually 100 % of the time. However, these three tests may not be applicable to the pediatric patient as they require cooperation on the part of the patient. The relative size of the oral cavity is assessed by asking the child to open his or her mouth. The Mallampati classification system [34], as modified by Samsoon and Young [35] classifies the degree of airway difficulty based upon the ability to visualize the faucial pillars, soft palate, and uvula (Fig. 27.14). A Mallampati class of I or II predicts a relatively easy airway, while a Mallampati class > II predicts an increased difficulty with adequate visualization of the airway during laryngoscopy. Critically ill patients with altered mental status or children may be unable to cooperate with this kind of assessment, though evaluation of the oropharyngeal airway with a tongue blade may be feasible and worthwhile [5, 30, 36]. Cormack and Lehane [37] proposed a classification system based upon the ability to visualize the glottic opening during laryngoscopy, though this type of assessment is probably more useful as a means to facilitate communication of the degree of difficulty between providers and not as a screening tool for predicting a difficult airway at the bedside. The interincisor distance can also be assessed at this time – an interincisor distance less than two fingertips in breadth can be associated with a difficult airway [5, 38]. Decreased range of motion at the atlanto-occipital joint leads to poor visualization of the glottis during laryngoscopy. Cervical spine immobilization with a C-collar may also limit atlanto-occipital joint extension, leading to a potentially difficult airway. Finally, if three fingers in adolescents, two fingers in children, and one finger in infants can be placed between the anterior ramus of the mandible and the hyoid bone, the so-called *potential displacement area*, adequate visualization of the glottis during laryngoscopy usually will be successful (Fig. 27.15). If the *potential displacement area* is too small, excessive extension of the neck will only shift the larynx into a more *anterior* position [38]. The *BURP* maneuver (*b*ack, *u*p, and *r*ightward *p*ressure on the laryngeal cartilage) displaces the larynx in three directions, (i) posteriorly against the cervical vertebra, (ii) superiorly as possible, and (iii) laterally to the right and may improve visualization of the glottic opening in this situation (Fig. 27.15) [39, 40].

Several malformation syndromes are associated with a difficult airway based upon the presence of a few notable anatomic features:

1. *Macroglossia*: A large tongue in children with Beckwith-Wiedemann syndrome or Trisomy 21 (Down syndrome) may be difficult to control and make visualization of the glottis during laryngoscopy difficult. Mask ventilation under these circumstances may also be difficult and frequently requires placement of an oral or nasal airway. A curved laryngoscope blade may be more appropriate in this scenario.

2. *Mandibular hypoplasia*: Mandibular hypoplasia is frequent in children with the Pierre-Robin sequence (see below), Crouzon disease, Goldenhar syndrome, and Treacher-Collin syndrome. Mandibular hypoplasia forces the tongue posteriorly in the oropharynx and hinders visualization of the glottis during larnygoscopy. Alternative techniques, including use of a laryngeal mask airway (LMA), light wand, or fiberoptic bronchoscope are frequently required in these children and should be readily available.

Fig. 27.15 (**a**) Diagram of airway, demonstrating *potential displacement area* for tracheal intubation. (**b**) Laryngoscopy with displacement of the tongue and soft tissue into the *potential displacement area*. (**c**) BURP maneuver, determining the optimal external laryngeal manipulation with the free (*right*) hand ((**a**, **b**) Reprinted from Berry [256]. With permission from Elsevier, (**c**) Reprinted from Benumof [257]. With permission from Elsevier)

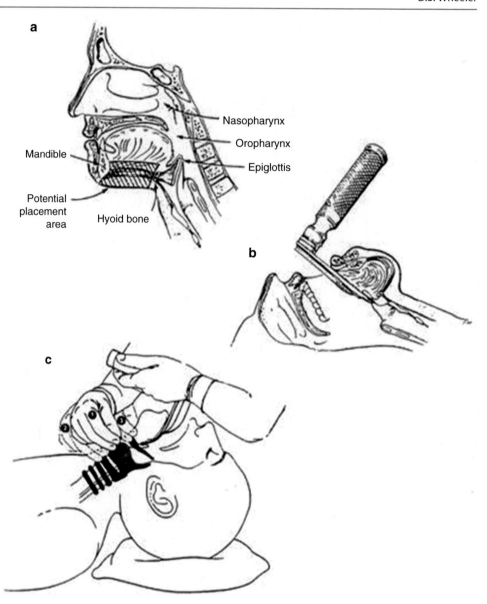

3. *Limited cervical motion*: Limited atlanto-occipital range of motion is frequently found in children with Goldenhar syndrome and Klippel-Feil syndrome, thereby limiting an adequate line of sight to the glottis due to failure of the three axes (discussed above) to align. Other disease processes such as juvenile rheumatoid arthritis and neuromuscular scoliosis also can result in limited cervical spine mobility. Children with Trisomy 21 or trauma, on the other hand, have atlanto-occipital instability, and cervical spine precautions should be followed.
4. *Mucopolysaccharidoses*: Children with the mucopolysaccharidoses often have difficult airways due to a number of factors.

Specific points regarding management of the difficult pediatric airway are discussed in great detail in the following chapter.

Equipment

All the necessary equipment for airway management must be available at the bedside before any attempts at tracheal intubation are made! At a minimum, this list includes (i) a source of oxygen (either wall or tank) with the necessary tubing, ventilation bag (either a self-inflating or standard anesthesia bag, appropriately sized), and mask (appropriately sized); (ii) a source of suction (either portable suction or wall suction) and appropriate suction catheters (preferably the rigid, wide-bore *tonsil tip* or Yankauer suction catheters); (iii) laryngoscope and proper-sized blade with a well-functioning light; (iv) tracheal tubes of the anticipated size, plus the next size largest and smallest (see below); (v) stylet; (vi) a means of securing the tracheal tube. Additional items include oral airways, nasopharyngeal airways, and a Magill forceps.

Table 27.3 Suggested laryngoscope sizes based on patient weight

Child's weight (kg)	Laryngoscope
0–3	Miller 0
3–5	Miller 0, 1
5–12	Miller 1
12–20	Macintosh 2
20–30	Macintosh 2, Miller 2
>30	Macintosh 3, Miller 2

Laryngoscope blades are available in several different shapes and sizes, but are usually classified into straight (e.g., Miller, Phillips, Wis-Hipple) versus curved (e.g., Macintosh) blades. Straight blades are preferable to curved blades in neonates, infants, and young children due to the relatively cephalad position of the glottis, the large tongue (relative to the size of the oral cavity), and the large, floppy epiglottis which may be difficult to control with a curved blade (see above). Perhaps the most important consideration for selection of the laryngoscope blade is its length (Table 27.3) – shorter blades make visualization of the glottis difficult, while longer blades make it difficult to avoid direct pressure on the upper lip, teeth, and gums. The laryngoscope should be checked for proper functioning and adequate illumination prior to use.

The appropriate size for the tracheal tube is based on the child's age. Generally, a 3.0 or 3.5 mm tracheal tube should be used in term infants, while a 4.0 mm tracheal tube should be used for infants older than 6–8 months of age. Beyond 8 months of age, the appropriate size for the tracheal tube can be determined according to the following rule:

$$\text{Tracheal tube}\left(\text{mm i.d.}\right) = \frac{\text{Age}\left(\text{y}\right)}{4} + 4 \qquad (27.2)$$

The outside diameter of the tracheal tube usually approximates the diameter of the child's little finger. It is important to note that this rule is only a starting guideline, and different sized tubes (one size smaller AND one size larger) should be readily available during attempts at tracheal intubation. The tracheal tube should pass through the glottis easily and with minimal force, and the presence of a minimal air leak heard around the tracheal tube with inflating pressures of 20–30 cmH$_2$O will assure adequate perfusion of the tracheal mucosa and lessen the risk of tissue necrosis, edema, scarring, and postextubation stridor. Importantly, children with a history of subglottic stenosis or other airway anomalies may require a smaller size tube than predicted by age criteria. In addition, children with Trisomy 21 generally require trachel tubes at least two sizes smaller than predicted by age [41].

Historically, uncuffed tubes have been generally recommended for children less than 8 years of age. A prolonged period of tracheal intubation and a poorly fitted tracheal tube are significant risk factors for damage to the tracheal mucosa

regardless of whether the tracheal tube is cuffed or uncuffed. Cuffed tracheal tubes may have significant advantages over uncuffed tracheal tubes, including better control of air leakage and decreased risk of aspiration and infection in mechanically ventilated children, and are being used with greater frequency in this age group, especially when high inflation pressures are required to provide adequate oxygenation and ventilation in the setting of severe acute lung disease. The available data suggests that there is no difference in the incidence of post-extubation stridor in children who were tracheally intubated with cuffed tubes as compared to those who received uncuffed tubes [42–46]. A good rule-of-thumb is that whenever a cuffed tube is used, a half size smaller tube from what would normally be used (based on the rule above) should be selected.

A malleable, yet rigid stylet may be inserted into the tracheal tube in order to shape the tube to the desired configuration (e.g., *hockey stick*) before attempting tracheal intubation. However, the tip of the stylet must not protrude beyond the distal tip of the tracheal tube, in order to minimize the potential of airway trauma. In addition, the stylet should be lubricated with a water-soluble lubricant prior to insertion into the tracheal tube in order to facilitate its easy removal once the tracheal tube has been placed.

Airway Pharmacology

Laryngoscopy and tracheal intubation are commonly associated with profound physiologic disturbances that may adversely affect the critically ill or injured child. In addition to pain and anxiety, laryngoscopy causes an increase in blood pressure and heart rate [47–50], though decreased heart rate and hypotension may be more common in infants as a consequence of their increased parasympathetic tone [49]. Hypoxia and hypercarbia are also common, especially in children with impending respiratory failure. Children are at even greater risk compared to adults for significant hypoxemia during attempts at tracheal intubation, given their higher resting oxygen consumption and lower functional residual capacity (FRC) [50–52]. Laryngoscopy and tracheal intubation increase intracranial pressure (which may exacerbate intracranial hypertension in children with head injury or lead to intracranial hemorrhage in children with coagulopathies or vascular malformations), intraocular pressure, and intragastric pressure (further compounding the risk of regurgitation and aspiration of gastric contents) [50, 53, 54]. Tracheal intubation may also provoke bronchospasm, especially in children with asthma. The use of appropriate pre-induction agents or adjuncts, induction agents, and neuromuscular blockade may modify these physiologic responses and lessen the potential for adverse effects related to laryngoscopy and tracheal intubation. It is extremely important to remember

Table 27.4 Pre-induction agents used for tracheal intubation

Agent	Indication	Dose	Comments
Oxygen	Prevent hypoxia during laryngoscopy	100 % oxygen	
Atropine	Prevent bradycardia during larygoscopy and administration of succinylcholine	0.01–0.02 mg/kg IV (minimum dose of 0.1 mg)	Probably not necessary in children >1 year of age
Glycopyrrolate	Prevent bradycardia and decrease oral secretions	3–5 mcg/kg IV	
Lidocaine	Blunt the increase in ICP during laryngoscopy	1–1.5 mg/kg IV	Administered 3–5 min prior to laryngscopy
Fentanyl	Blunt the increase in HR and BP during laryngoscopy	2–3 µg/kg IV	
Vecuronium	*Defasciculating dose*	0.01 mg/kg IV	Prevents muscle soreness and pain as well as the increase in ICP, intragastric, and intraocular pressure following succinylcholine
Rocuronium	*Defasciculating dose*	0.05 mg/kg IV	See above
Esmolol	Blunt the increase in HR and BP during laryngoscopy	2 mg/kg IV (adult studies)	Rarely used in children
			Use with caution in hemodynamically unstable patients
			May precipitate bronchospasm

that attenuation of these normal responses following tracheal intubation may unmask hemodynamic instability leading to, at times, profound hypotension [55].

Pre-induction Agents

Several pre-induction agents are commonly used for tracheal intubation in critically ill or injured children, including cholinergic antagonists, lidocaine, opioids, β-adrenergic antagonists, and non-depolarizing neuromuscular blocking agents (NDNMBs) (Table 27.4). Cholinergic antagonists such as atropine (0.01–0.02 mg/kg IV, with a minimum dose of 0.1 mg) and glycopyrrolate (3–5 mcg/kg IV) may be administered in order to prevent bradycardia (especially in critically ill infants with high parasympathetic tone) and decrease oral secretions. Succinylcholine also causes bradycardia, especially in infants and young children [56–58]. Atropine is usually recommended when using succinylcholine in children less than 1 year of age, though the use of atropine in older children is more controversial and frequently not necessary [59–62]. Lidocaine (1–1.5 mg/kg IV) may be administered 3–5 min before laryngoscopy and tracheal intubation in order to blunt the associated hypertensive response and increase in intracranial pressure. Unfortunately, strong evidence to suggest that this practice improves neurological outcome is not available [63–65]. Topical lidocaine may be just as effective as intravenous lidocaine in blunting the physiologic response to laryngoscopy [66], and lidocaine is probably not necessary if an induction agent such as propofol (see below) is used. Fentanyl (2–3 µg/kg IV) or the synthetic opioids (e.g., sufentanil, alfentanil, or remifentanil), which are all derivatives of fentanyl, have also been used to blunt the physiologic response to laryngoscopy and tracheal intubation [67–69]. Fentanyl is also commonly used as an induction agent and is discussed further below. Esmolol is a rapid-onset, short-acting, cardioselective β-adrenergic antagonist that is frequently used in adults to attenuate the tachycardia and hypertension resulting from laryngoscopy and tracheal intubation [66, 68, 70]. Esmolol, either alone or in combination with fentanyl may be more effective than either lidocaine or fentanyl [67, 71–76], and the combination of fentanyl and esmolol may be particularly effective in this situation. However, caution should be exercised as there are currently no reports on the use of esmolol as a pre-induction agent for tracheal intubation in children. Most adult studies use an esmolol dose of 2 mg/kg IV administered 1–2 min prior to laryngoscopy. Esmolol is contraindicated in children with reactive airways disease or asthma and is probably contraindicated in situations where hemodynamic instability could be anticipated. Finally, some protocols recommend the use of a *defasiculating dose* of NDNMB prior to the use of succinylcholine – this is discussed further below.

Induction Agents

There are a variety of anxiolytic, analgesic, and sedative agents commonly used to facilitate tracheal intubation (Table 27.5). An ideal induction agent induces unconsciousness predictably with a rapid onset of action, short duration of action, and few side effects. Unfortunately, the ideal induction agent doesn't exist! While the choice of which induction agent to use in any given situation depends primarily on individual physician preference and comfort, there are some important caveats to bear in mind. One particular agent may be appropriate in a given clinical scenario and entirely inappropriate in another. The induction agent should be therefore selected based upon the particular clinical scenario with the goal of rapid induction and minimal adverse effects (Table 27.6).

Thiopental is a short-acting barbiturate with a rapid onset of action (10–20 s) at the recommended dose of 2–3 mg/kg

Table 27.5 Commonly used induction agents used for tracheal intubation

Agent	Dose	Onset	Recovery (min)	Indications	Precautions
Thiopental	2–3 mg/kg IV	10–20 s	15–30	Status epilepticus	Bronchospasm
				Isolated head trauma (with normal hemodynamics)	Hypotension
Etomidate	0.15–0.3 mg/kg IV	30–60 s	3–5	Trauma shock (?)	Causes adrenal suppression
					Decreases seizure threshold
Ketamine	1–2 mg/kg IV	1–2 min	5–10	Status asthmaticus	May increase ICP (?)
Propofol	2–4 mg/kg IV	30–60 s	3–5	Isolated head trauma	Hypotension
				Status epilepticus	
Midazolam	0.1–0.2 mg/kg IV	3–5 min	20–30		Hypotension
Fentanyl	5–10 μg/kg IV	30–60 s	10–15		Rarely used as the sole agent
					Rigid chest syndrome

Table 27.6 Suggested induction agents for specific clinical scenarios

Status epilepticus	Isolated head trauma	Shock	Head trauma + shock	Status asthmaticus
Propofol -or- midazolam	Propofol -or- midazolam	Etomidate (?) -or- ketamine	Etomidate	Ketamine

IV. Thiopental decreases cerebral oxygen consumption and effectively reduces ICP [77, 78], making it an ideal induction agent for children with closed head injury [79–83]. Its hemodynamic side effects (potent vasodilation, venodilation, and myocardial depression at higher doses) limited its use in children with hypotension. Additional side effects included histamine release, with subsequent hypotension or bronchospasm, coughing, and laryngospasm. Unfortunately, the drug was removed from the market by its manufacturer due to its use in executions by lethal injection in the United States [84].

Etomidate (0.3 mg/kg IV) is another agent that decreases cerebral oxygen consumption and hence ICP, but without significant detrimental effects on either the heart or systemic vascular resistance, making it a good alternative to thiopental in children with closed head injury and hypotension [85]. Etomidate lacks analgesic effects and should be administered in conjunction with an opioid such as fentanyl. Etomidate does cause adrenal suppression [86–91] and should not be used for long-term sedation in the PICU. Some experts have further suggested that etomidate should not be used for induction for tracheal intubation in critically ill patients [92–96]. Etomidate appears to cause adrenal suppression for at least 12–24 h following a single dose [90, 92, 97–99], though some investigators have questioned the clinical significance of these effects [100, 101]. Indeed, in several recent studies, the effects of etomidate on the adrenal axis were not associated with worse outcomes (prolonged length of stay, increased mortality) [102–105]. In addition, while a meta-analysis of studies in which etomidate was used in critically ill patients with sepsis did show an association with increased mortality [106], the results of another meta-analysis which included studies in which etomidate was used in all critically ill patients (not just those with sepsis) did not [107]. Given the ongoing controversy, one approach would be to reserve etomidate for hemodynamically unstable patients without sepsis. Another approach would be to recognize that etomidate can cause adrenal suppression and to treat accordingly when it is used in critically ill children who are at risk for hemodynamic compromise. Finally, etomidate does cause myoclonic activity and may lower the seizure threshold in children with either CNS pathology or epilepsy [108].

The benzodiazepines (midazolam, lorazepam, and diazepam) are potent anxiolytics and amnestics, but lack analgesic properties, and are therefore commonly co-administered with a narcotic such as morphine or fentanyl (see below). Midazolam (0.1–0.2 mg/kg IV) has a relatively rapid onset of action (3–5 min) and shorter duration of action (20–30 min) and is more frequently used in this setting than either lorazepam or diazepam. Midazolam does have some effects on reducing ICP [109–111], though clearly propofol and etomidate are superior in this regard. Midazolam may reduce mean arterial blood pressure (MAP), thereby lowering cerebral perfusion pressure (CPP), as CPP = MAP–ICP [110] and should be used with caution in children with hemodynamic instability [112–115]. The hemodynamic effects may be more pronounced in newborns and infants [112, 114], so particular caution should be exercised in this patient population.

Morphine (0.1–0.2 mg/kg IV) causes profound histamine release and potential hypotension or exacerbation of bronchospasm and is generally not used as an induction agent for tracheal intubation [116, 117]. Fentanyl is approximately 180× more potent than morphine and does not cause histamine release, but may cause chest wall rigidity when large doses are administered rapidly [118–122]. Opioid-induced chest wall rigidity may be reversed with IV naloxone or neuromuscular blockade [117, 123]. While largely devoid of significant cardiovascular side effects, hypotension can occasionally occur with the use of fentanyl [124–126]. The dose required for induction of anesthesia [doses as high as 30–150 μg/kg IV have been reported in the literature) is much higher compared to the dose required for analgesia alone [116, 117, 124, 125, 127], though reports on the use of fentanyl for tracheal intubation in the critically ill or injured are relatively limited [128]. For these reasons, fentanyl is probably better utilized as either a pre-induction agent (see above) or as an adjunct to another induction agent.

Ketamine is a phencyclidine (PCP) derivative that has potent amnestic, analgesic, and sympathomimetic properties. It is generally considered a dissociative anesthetic agent and acts by selectively inhibiting the cerebral cortex and thalamus while stimulating the limbic system [116, 117]. While ketamine has direct negative inotropic effects [129, 130], systemic blood pressure is preserved, primarily through increased sympathetic stimulation [116, 117, 131]. The hemodynamic safety of ketamine in children with congenital heart disease is well established [132–135]. Critically ill patients have rarely been known to respond to ketamine with profound hypotension due to the depletion of endogenous catecholamines [131, 136, 137], otherwise ketamine is widely considered the induction agent of choice in hemodynamically unstable patients [116, 117], including those with cardiac tamponade [138, 139]. Ketamine is also a potent bronchodilator (related to its sympathomimetic effects) and has been used therapeutically in children with status asthmaticus [140–143] and is also the induction agent of choice for laryngoscopy and tracheal intubation of children with reactive airways disease or asthma [144]. Contrary to common belief, while spontaneous ventilation is preserved in most children, larger doses may precipitate laryngospasm or apnea. Ketamine also increases cerebral blood flow and ICP and should be used with caution in children with closed head injury and high ICP, though recently these concerns have been questioned [145–150]. Ketamine was historically felt to be contraindicated in patients with pulmonary hypertension, as it was thought that it could increase pulmonary vascular resistance and provoke a pulmonary hypertensive crisis. Recent studies, however, support the use of ketamine in this patient population [134, 151–155]. Additional side effects of ketamine include hypersalivation and emergence dysphoria and/or hallucinations. Emergence dysphoria and hallucinations can usually be mitigated with concomitant administration of benzodiazepines. Given all of the potential advantages of ketamine, and in light of the potential disadvantages of etomidate discussed above, several investigators have suggested that ketamine should be considered the induction agent of choice in all hemodynamically unstable patients [156]. To that end, a multicenter, randomized, controlled trial comparing ketamine to etomidate for tracheal intubation in critically ill adults showed that ketamine was at least as effective as etomidate, without the undesirable side effect of adrenal insufficiency [157].

Propofol (2–4 mg/kg IV) is an induction agent with a rapid onset of action (30–60 s) and short duration of action (3–5 min) that is frequently used for rapid sequence intubation in adults [116, 117, 158]. Propofol reduces ICP and decreases cerebral metabolism and effectively attenuates the hemodynamic response to direct laryngoscopy and tracheal intubation [116, 117, 158]. Propofol is a potent vasodilator and venodilator, and to some extent has negative inotropic effects, thereby limiting its use to patients with stable hemodynamics [116, 117, 158].

While there are certainly other sedative agents available that have been used during tracheal intubation, the ones discussed are by far the most common induction agents used in the critical care setting [144, 159]. For example, in a recently published multicenter registry of tracheal intubation in the PICU, the three most common induction agents were fentanyl, midazolam, and ketamine, which were used in 63, 57, and 23 % of 1,715 tracheal intubations performed, respectively. Interestingly, etomidate was used in only 1.5 % of tracheal intubations [159]. The important points to keep in mind are to select an induction agent that is appropriate to the clinical setting and understand its potential adverse effects.

Neuromuscular Blocking Agents (NMBs)

Several excellent reviews are available on the pharmacology of neuromuscular blocking agents [79–81, 116, 117, 160–164]. In addition, the reader is referred to the chapter on neuromuscular blockade later in this textbook. Non-depolarizing neuromuscular blockers (NDNMB) act by competitively inhibiting the interaction of ACh with its receptor on the motor end-plate. Neuromuscular transmission requires the binding of two ACh molecules (one ACh molecule binds to each alpha subunit), thus even if only one binding site is occupied by a NDNMB, ACh activation is effectively inhibited. However, approximately 90–95 % of the ACh receptors must be blocked before neuromuscular transmission is completely inhibited [160]. The diaphragm is more densely populated with ACh receptors compared to other muscles, so the diaphragm may continue to function even after the muscles of the hands and upper airway have been effectively paralyzed [160]. The NDNMB (Table 27.7) are all highly water-soluble, positively-charged quarternary ammonium compounds commonly subdivided into two main classes. The benzylisoquinolones include mivacurium, atracurium, cis-atracurium, doxacurium, and d-tubocurarine. All of these compounds, with the exception of mivacurium, are degraded by a non-enzymatic chemical process called Hofmann elimination at physiologic pH and temperature, and are therefore commonly used in children with renal insufficiency or liver failure. Mivacurium, on the other hand, is metabolized by plasma cholinesterase. The aminosteroids include pancuronium, vecuronium, and rocuronium. These compounds are metabolized in the liver

Table 27.7 Neuromuscular blocking agents used for tracheal intubation

Agent	Class	Dose	Onset	Recovery (min)	Comments
Succinylcholine	DNMB	1–2 mg/kg IV	60 s	5–10	See adverse reactions Table 27.8
		2–4 mg/kg IM	3–4 min		
Atracurium	NDNMB	0.6 mg/kg IV	2–3 min	20–30	Hofmann degradation
					Histamine release
Cis-atracurium	NDNMB	0.1 mg/kg IV	2–3 min	25–40	Hofmann degradation
Rocuronium	NDNMB	0.6 mg/kg IV	60 s	25–35	Hepatobiliary excretion
Mivacurium	NDNMB	0.1 mg/kg IV	2–3 min	15–30	Degraded by plasma cholinesterase
Vecuronium	NDNMB	0.1 mg/kg IV	60–120 s	20–40	Hepatobiliary and renal excretion
Pancuronium	NDNMB	0.1 mg/kg IV	2–3 min	60–120	Tachycardia common

Table 27.8 Succinylcholine, its side effects and relative contraindications

Side effect	Mechanism
Muscle soreness/pain	Fasciculations due to initial depolarization of the NMJ (may be prevented with the use of a defasciculating dose, typically one-tenth dose of a NDNMB, e.g. 0.01 mg/kg vecuronium)
Hyperkalemia	SCh will typically raise serum K^+ 0.5–1 mEq/L due to initial depolarization of the NMJ (serious and life-threatening hyperkalemia may occur with renal failure or when extrajunctional AChR are upregulated (crush injury, burns, disuse atrophy, muscular dystrophy)
	Contraindications:
	1. Pre-existing hyperkalemia
	2. Acute renal failure or chronic renal insufficiency
	3. History of trauma, burns, crush injury (at risk period occurs between 48 h and 120 days of post-injury)
	4. Disuse atrophy, neuromuscular diseases (e.g. Duchenne's muscular dystrophy)
Malignant hyperthermia (syndrome characterized by unremitting muscle rigidity, hyperthermia, hypercapnia, and metabolic acidosis)	Mechanism not completely understood
	Contraindicated in patients with family history of malignant hyperthermia
Increased intraocular pressure	Contraction of extraocular muscles during initial depolarization of NMJ (may be prevented with "defasciculating dose")
	Contraindications:
	1. Glaucoma
	2. Open globe injury
Increased intracranial pressure	Fasciculations and muscle rigidity (may be prevented with "defasciculating dose")
	Use with caution in patients with head injury
Increased intragastric pressure	Contraction of abdominal muscles (may be prevented with "defasciculating dose")
	Use with caution in patients with full stomach (increased risk of aspiration)
Prolonged neuromuscular blockade	Plasma pseudocholinesterase deficiency (liver disease, pregnancy, h/o oral contraceptive use, familial pseudocholinesterase deficiency)

and excreted in the urine and bile. Duration of neuromuscular blockade may therefore be prolonged in patients with either renal or hepatic disease. The choice of which NDNMB to use in any given situation depends primarily on individual physician preference and comfort. However, caution should be exercised when using the longer-acting NDNMBs if a difficult airway and/or difficult intubation is anticipated –these drugs should not be used in children who may be difficult to ventilate with bag-valve-mask ventilation.

Succinylcholine (SCh), is the only depolarizing NMB currently available for clinical use and was introduced into clinical practice in 1951. SCh consists of two acetylcholine molecules joined together. SCh binds to the AChR and produces initial depolarization and muscle contraction, which is observed clinically as fasciculations. However, the AChR remains in an inactive state and muscle relaxation occurs (phase I block). Neuromuscular blockade persists until SCh is hydrolyzed to succinate and choline by plasma pseudocholinesterase, which occurs much more slowly than the breakdown of ACh by true AChE. Further exposure of the NMJ to SCh may result in a prolonged state of muscle relaxation that cannot be reliably reversed pharmacologically (phase II block). The duration of blockade may also be increased if there is a decrease in endogenous pseudocholinesterase (e.g., familial pseudocholinesterase deficiency, hepatic disease). SCh has numerous side effects that have limited its use in routine clinical settings (Table 27.8). In addition to the receptors localized to the NMJ, SCh will also occupy other nicotinic, cholinergic receptors located throughout the body. For example, administration of SCh to infants may produce vagally mediated bradycardia, and for this reason, most clinicians will administer atropine prior to SCh in this patient population. SCh also produces initial contraction of the extraocular muscles, which may lead to increased intraocular pressure. Similarly, SCh may also produce increased intracranial pressure. Many physicians recommend the use of a *defasciculating dose*, or one-tenth of the intubation dose of a NDNMB such as vecuronium prior to administering SCh [79–81, 116, 117]. Theoretically, the use of a *defasciculating dose* prevents the muscle soreness and pain, as well as the increase in intracranial, intragastric, and intraocular pressure following administration of SCh. However, the available evidence that such a protocol improves outcome is limited [165].

Given the long list of potential adverse effects, succinylcholine is falling out of favor in the PICU. In the multicenter database registry mentioned above [159], rocuronium was the most common NMB used (56 %), followed by vecuronium (25 %), and cisatracurium (8.2 %). Succinylcholine was used in only 0.8 % of all intubations. Several studies have shown that rocuronium is clinically equivalent to succinylcholine for tracheal intubation, though with a longer recovery time [166–169]. However, some studies still suggest that succinylcholine provides quicker and more favorable intubation conditions than rocuronium [170–172]. Given that few studies have been performed in children, rocuronium would appear to be an acceptable alternative to succinylcholine for the majority of tracheal intubations performed in the PICU. In cases where a faster recovery time is desirable (potentially difficult airway, difficult bag-valve-mask ventilation, etc.) and in the absence of contraindications, succinylcholine may be the preferable NMB agent.

Oral Tracheal Intubation

Oxygen should be administered to all critically ill and/or injured children in the highest possible concentration and regardless of the measured oxygen saturation until an initial assessment of cardiorespiratory status is completed. Breathing 100 % oxygen for 2–3 min creates a nitrogen washout that will fill ventilated alveoli with oxygen, and under most conditions an alveolar oxygen tension of 663 mmHg yields an adequate reservoir to provide sufficient oxygen delivery following the onset of apnea that occurs following sedation and neuromuscular blockade [173, 174]. This oxygen reservoir theoretically permits adequate oxygenation of blood circulating through the pulmonary blood vessels for up to 3 or 4 min following the onset of apnea [175]. However, infants and young children, in particular, have a high metabolic rate or oxygen consumption (7 mL/kg/

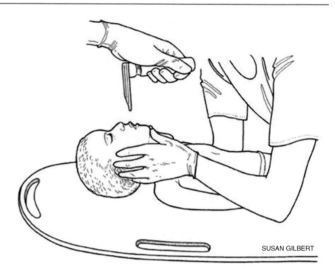

Fig. 27.16 Manual in-line stabilization of the cervical spine during tracheal intubation (Reprinted from George et al. [255]. With permission from Center for Pediatric Emergency Medicine)

min in children compared to 3 mL/kg/min in adults) [173, 175] and will develop hypoxia faster than adults. Once this oxygen reservoir is used up, arterial oxygen saturation will decrease precipitously after the onset of apnea.

Heart rate, blood pressure, and oxygen saturation should be monitored continuously during attempts at tracheal intubation, as mechanical stimulation of the airway may induce bradyarrhythmias, particularly in neonates and infants (see above). If either hypoxemia or bradycardia occurs, tracheal intubation should be interrupted and the child should be ventilated at FIO$_2$ 1.00 via bag-valve-mask ventilation. Immediately prior to laryngoscopy, the child is positioned (*sniff position* as described above, with manual cervical spine stabilization if cervical spine injury is suspected) (Fig. 27.16), and pre-induction medications are administered, as clinically indicated. Once all preparations have been made, the appropriate induction agents and NMB are administered. The laryngoscope is held in the left hand, and the blade is inserted into the right side of the mouth following the natural contour of the pharynx to the base of the tongue (Fig. 27.17). Control of the tongue is achieved by sweeping the proximal end of the blade to the midline, thereby moving the tongue towards the middle of the mouth, providing a channel along the right side of the mouth for visualization of the airway and passage of the tracheal tube. The tip of a curved blade is inserted into the vallecula, thereby lifting the epiglottis and visualizing the glottis by vallecular suspension. In contrast, the tip of a straight blade is used to lift the epiglottis directly in order to visualize the glottis (Fig. 27.18). Once the blade is positioned correctly, traction is exerted in the direction of the long axis of the laryngoscope handle – the laryngoscope blade must not be used as a lever and the teeth/gums are not to be used as the

Fig. 27.17 Operator's view of the glottis during laryngoscopy (**a**) with subsequent placement of the tracheal tube (**b**) (Reprinted from George et al. [255]. With permission from Center for Pediatric Emergency Medicine)

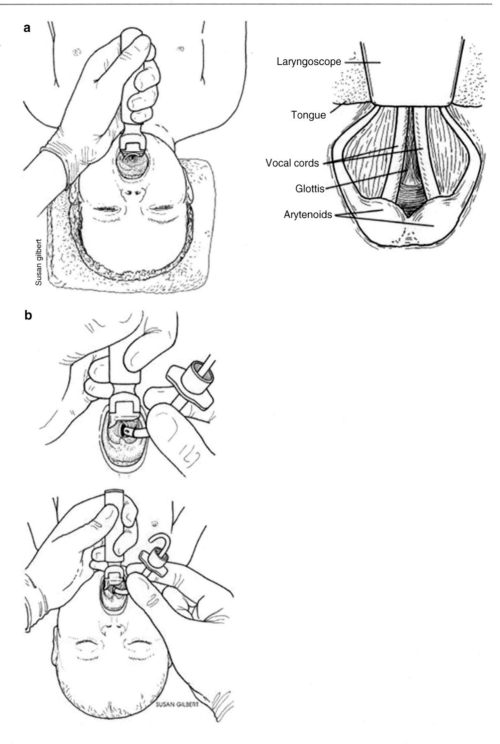

Susan gilbert

a

Laryngoscope

Tongue

Vocal cords

Glottis

Arytenoids

b

SUSAN GILBERT

fulcrum! It is frequently helpful to have a second provider place a slight amount of traction on the corner of the mouth to enable better visualization of the airway. The *BURP* maneuver [39, 40] may be used to further facilitate visualization of the glottic opening (see again, Fig. 27.15). However, the *BURP* maneuver may worsen visualization of the glottic opening when used in conjunction with cricoid pressure [176]. Alternatively, a laryngeal lift [177] or mandibular advancement (i.e., jaw-thrust maneuver) [178] maneuver can

be performed to better visualize the glottic opening. The utility of cricoid pressure has been questioned, as undue or improperly applied force may cause complete loss of adequate visualization of the glottis [179–181]. The tracheal tube is inserted from the right corner of the mouth and not down the barrel of the laryngoscope blade. The tracheal tube is then passed through the vocal cords under direct visualization. The black glottic marker of the tube is placed at the level of the vocal cords. Alternatively, when a cuffed tracheal

a

b

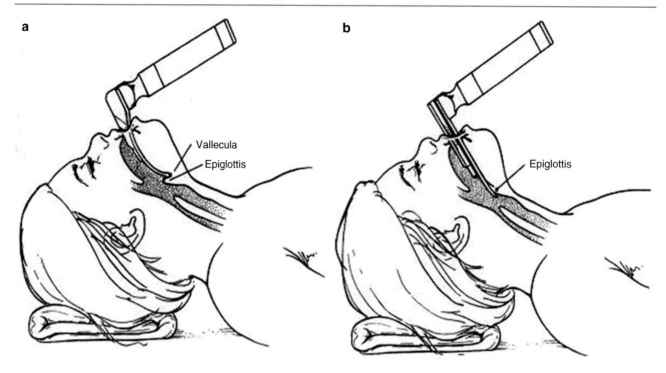

Fig. 27.18 Position of laryngoscope blade when using (**a**) a curved blade versus (**b**) a straight blade. A straight blade may also be used in the same manner as a curved blade, i.e., its tip is placed in the vallecula – this is a matter of preference and experience. (**a**) The tip of the curved laryngoscope blade is positioned in the vallecula and is used to *lift* the

epiglottis via vallecular suspension in order to visualize the glottic opening. (**b**) The tip of the straight laryngoscope blade is used to directly *lift* the epiglottis in order to visualize the glottic opening (Reprinted from George et al. [255]. With permission from Center for Pediatric Emergency Medicine)

tube is used, the cuff is placed just below the vocal cords. The depth of insertion of the tracheal tube is also commonly estimated either by multiplying the inside diameter of the tube by 3, or by using the following formula:

$$\text{Depth of insertion}\,(\text{cm}) = \frac{\text{Age}\,(y)}{2} + 12 \qquad (27.3)$$

Immediately following tracheal intubation, the correct position of the tracheal tube is confirmed by observation for symmetrical chest movements, auscultation of equal breath sounds over each axilla and not over the abdomen, and documentation of end-tidal CO_2 [182–184]. Capnometry/capnography is the most reliable and most valid way to confirm tracheal intubation [182] and is the now widely viewed as the standard of care. A chest radiograph should be obtained to document proper position with the distal tip of the tracheal tube above the carina in the mid-trachea (Fig. 27.19).

Nasal Tracheal Intubation

Under the vast majority of circumstances, oral tracheal intubation is preferred for emergency management of the airway. However, nasotracheal intubation is generally more comfortable for semi-conscious children, causes less stimulation of the gag reflex, and is more easily secured, especially in chil-

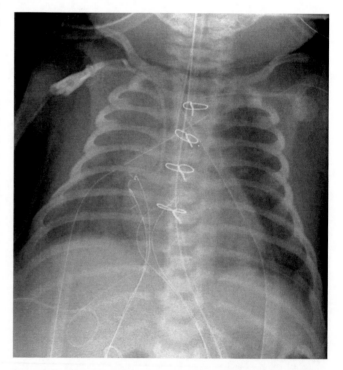

Fig. 27.19 Chest radiograph demonstrating proper position of the tracheal tube, with the tip located midway between the thoracic inlet and the carina

dren with copious oral secretions or saliva. In addition, oral tracheal tubes are more easily kinked or bitten. Nasotracheal tubes appear to be safe for use in neonates, infants, and children [185–188], though some studies suggest an increased risk of nosocomial sinusitis and pneumonia associated with nasotracheal intubation [189–191]. Anecdotally, we have found that the use of nasotracheal tubes decreases the risk of unplanned or accidental extubation, which may be associated with an increased risk of nosocomial pneumonia [192–195]. The available literature appears to support this contention [196–198]. Nevertheless, nasotracheal intubation is technically more challenging than orotracheal intubation and may be more time-consuming. For these reasons, whenever nasotracheal intubation is preferred in a critically ill infant or child, it should generally follow orotracheal intubation in order to facilitate adequate oxygenation and ventilation until a nasotracheal airway is established. The nasotracheal route is contraindicated in the presence of a coagulopathy, maxillofacial trauma, and basilar skull fractures.

A topical vasoconstricting agent such as 0.25 % phenylephrine or 0.05 % oxymetazoline may minimize the risk of bleeding. The nare is anesthetized and lubricated with lidocaine jelly, and a tracheal tube the same diameter as the oral tube is gentle passed through the nare and advanced along the floor of the nasal cavity into the nasopharynx. The oral tracheal tube is placed in the left-hand corner of the mouth while an assistant continues applying positive pressure ventilation. The oral and nasal tracheal tubes are visualized with the laryngoscope – the oral tracheal tube may need to be moved away from the nasal tracheal tube using the Magill forceps. The tip of the nasal tracheal tube is grasped with the Magill forceps and positioned directly above the cords, anterior to the oral tracheal tube. As the assistant removes the oral tracheal tube, the nasal tracheal tube is gently advanced through the vocal cords – the Magill forceps should not be used to advance the tracheal tube through the vocal cords, as this may cause trauma to the glottis. Several methods of estimating the depth of insertion of nasotracheal tubes have been described [199–201], though the following formula works well in children up to 4 years of age [200]:

$$\text{Depth of insertion (in cm)} = 10.5 + (\text{weight, in kg}) / 2 \quad (27.4)$$

Complications of nasotracheal intubation include bleeding, adenoid injury, sinusitis, and trauma to the nasal turbinates, nasal septum, or nares (e.g., pressure necrosis) [187, 202].

Rapid Sequence Intubation (RSI)

Unlike elective tracheal intubation performed in the operating room suite, critically ill or injured children should be assumed to have a full stomach, placing them at risk for regurgitation and aspiration of gastric contents. Trauma, pain, anxiety, and critical illness all reduce gastric emptying, such that regardless of when the child last ate, he or she is still considered to have a full stomach. Rapid sequence intubation (RSI) should be performed to decrease the risk of aspiration in these situations. The keys to successful RSI can be easily recalled by the *six P's*: preparation, preoxygenation, premedication, paralysis, passage of the tracheal tube, and postintubation care [83, 116, 117, 162]. Preparation is paramount to a smooth, safe, and successful tracheal intubation. If possible, an *AMPLE* history is obtained (A = Allergies; M = Medications; P = Past medical history; L = Last meal; E = Existing circumstances). A directed physical examination should be performed, with particular attention to the anatomy of the upper airway. All the necessary medications and equipment is assembled at the child's bedside (see above).

Pre-oxygenation or nitrogen wash-out is performed via the administration of 100 % oxygen via a tight-fitting face mask without positive pressure ventilation. Pre-oxygenation creates a reservoir of oxygen in the lung that limits hypoxemia during subsequent attempts at tracheal intubation (see above). Premedication consists of the administration of both premedication (e.g. lidocaine, atropine, etc.) and induction agents, and the combination of medications should be tailored specifically to the clinical circumstance. Sellick's maneuver (cricoid pressure) is employed immediately prior to sedation and neuromuscular blockade in order to compress the upper esophagus between the cricoid cartilage and the cervical vertebral column and should be maintained until proper placement of the tracheal tube is confirmed [203]. Sellick's maneuver prevents the passive regurgitation of gastric contents [204–206], though excessive cricoid pressure may worsen airway obstruction or interfere with visualization of the glottis during laryngoscopy, as reviewed above.

A rapid-acting, short duration NMB is administered next. Succinycholine provides safe and effective neuromuscular blockade for the majority of patients, though rocuronium or high-dose vecuronium (0.25–0.3 mg/kg) are acceptable alternatives if there are contraindications or concerns regarding the use of succinycholine. Pre-treatment with a defasciculating dose of a NDNMB may prevent the muscle fasciculations (and the subsequent pain and soreness that result) associated with succinylcholine, though again the available evidence supporting this practice is relatively limited [79–81, 83, 116, 117, 159, 162, 207–210]. Typically, one-tenth of the normal dose of a NDNMB is administered 1–3 min before administering succinylcholine (e.g. vecuronium, one-tenth of 0.1 mg/kg/dose = 0.01 mg/kg defasciculating dose). Priming, on the other hand, entails the administration of a smaller dose (again, typically one-tenth the normal dose) of a NDNMB administered 3–5 min prior to the full dose of the same NDNMB. Priming is thought to shorten the time of onset of neuromuscular blockade, though again evidence suggesting any real clinical benefits or improvements in outcome is limited.

Once the child is relaxed, laryngoscopy and intubation are performed (see above). If laryngoscopy is not immediately successful and the child's oxygen saturation begins to fall, assisted ventilation is administered via bag-valve-mask ventilation with cricoid pressure. Tracheal intubation is confirmed by direct visualization of the tracheal tube passing through the glottis, auscultation of the chest and abdomen (breath sounds auscultated in both axilla and not the epigastric area), and detection of end-tidal CO_2. A chest radiograph is the final method of verification of proper placement of the tracheal tube and should be obtained with the head and neck in the midline, neutral position. Flexion and extension of the neck moves the tracheal tube towards the carina (flexion, *chin moves down*) and away from the carina (extension, *chin moves up*), respectively [211, 212]. After proper placement of the tracheal tube is verified, a long-acting sedative should be administered.

The importance of RSI should be emphasized. RSI, when performed properly, provides superior, safer intubating conditions compared to either nasotracheal or oral tracheal intubation performed with sedation alone [79–81, 83, 116, 117, 162]. However, RSI is not necessary and provides no additional advantages in children with cardiopulmonary arrest. Finally, RSI should be performed with caution, if at all, in children who are dependent upon their own upper airway musculature to maintain adequate airway patency. In these cases, neuromuscular blockade may impair the ability to visualize the airway during laryngoscopy, and more importantly, it may prevent, impair, or even preclude the ability to provide adequate oxygenation and ventilation with bag-valve-mask ventilation.

Complications of Tracheal Intubation

Complications following tracheal intubation are variable. Excluding failed tracheal intubation, right main bronchus intubation, and esophageal intubation, immediate complications include hemodynamic derangements in response to laryngoscopy (described above) such as bradycardia, dysrhythmias, and hypertension, as well as hypoxia, aspiration, subluxation of the cervical spine (especially in children with either a congenital deformity of the cervical spine or children with traumatic injury to the cervical spine), loss of teeth, injury to the lips and gingivae, and injury to the airway. Postobstructive pulmonary edema (POPE) frequently occurs following the relief of upper airway obstruction [213–222]. POPE, also known as negative pressure pulmonary edema, is believed to result from the excessive negative pressures required to inhale against an upper airway obstruction, resulting in increased venous return, increased right ventricular preload, and increased pulmonary blood volume. In addition, the negative intrathoracic pressure during inspiration leads to

increased left ventricular afterload. These factors tend to favor the development of pulmonary edema. While frequently asymptomatic, POPE may cause hypoxia, increased work of breathing, and shortness of breath. Treatment, though rarely required, includes administration of supplemental oxygen, positive pressure ventilation, and diuretics. Once the child is initially stabilized, further management depends on the degree of obstruction and the etiology. The child should be admitted to the PICU where constant supervision and airway intervention can take place immediately, if required.

Most late complications of tracheal intubation (e.g. post-extubation stridor and in rare instances, acquired subglottic stenosis) occur due to incorrect tracheal tube size [223, 224], traumatic or multiple intubations [225], and inadequate sedation/analgesia resulting in excessive up and down movement of the tracheal tube [223, 226–228]. The *air-leak test* is a poor predictor of extubation success, though it may predict the presence of post-extubation stridor with some degree of accuracy [229, 230]. The use of corticosteroids in the prevention and/or treatment of post-extubation stridor is advocated by many pediatric intensivists, though there is very little evidence to support the universal use of corticosteroids at this time [230–233]. The most serious late complication of tracheal intubation is acquired subglottic stenosis, though several studies support the safety of tracheal intubation (rather than early tracheotomy) in children requiring long-term ventilatory support due to burns, botulism, acute lung disease, and prematurity [234–236].

Tracheal Extubation

A trial of extubation is appropriate when the conditions which resulted in tracheal intubation are no longer present. However, extubation failure is associated with significant morbidity, including an increased incidence of ventilator-associated pneumonia, an increased length of stay in both the ICU and hospital, and an increased risk of mortality [237–240]. Specific, concrete guidelines and objective criteria regarding when to attempt tracheal extubation are lacking, and unfortunately, adult weaning indexes based upon direct measurements of pulmonary function have been applied to children with only varied success [241–249]. General recommendations include (i) reversal of the disease process which prompted tracheal intubation (e.g., resolution of hypoxemic respiratory failure, improvement in mental status, etc.); (ii) presence of an intact cough and gag reflex (i.e. ability to maintain and protect the airway); (iii) acceptable oxygenation and ventilation on minimal mechanical ventilatory support; (iv) appropriate neurological status (generally, either a GCS >8 or spontaneous eye-opening and the ability to follow simple commands); and (v) hemodynamic stability. In children who were tracheally intubated secondary to upper airway obstruction, the presence

Table 27.9 Reversal agents

Agent	Dose	Onset (min)	Duration (h)
Neostigmine	0.025–0.1 mg/kg IV	3–5	1–2
Pyridostigmine	0.1–0.25 mg/kg IV	3–5	2–3

These agents should be administered either in conjunction with (neostigmine) or after (pyridostigmine) atropine, 0.01–0.02 mg/kg IV (minimum dose of 0.1 mg) or glycopyrrolate, 3–5 mcg/kg IV

of an audible leak around the tracheal tube is also a criterion for extubation. Finally, adequate reversal of neuromuscular blockade must be present – adequate reversal is generally assumed by either the ability to sustain a head lift or, in an infant, a leg lift. While the use of pharmacologic agents to reverse either sedation or neuromuscular blockade may be occasionally necessary (Table 27.9), reliance on these medications to *make a child ready for extubation* is fraught with danger and should be summarily avoided.

It is a common practice to hold nasogastric feedings for 4–6 h prior to an attempt at extubation, though a recent study showed that continuous transpyloric feeding during tracheal extubation was safe and improved the delivery of more optimal nutrition [250]. Sedation during weaning from mechanical ventilation towards extubation may be difficult. For example, the need for continued sedation to prevent an uncontrolled or accidental extubation often conflicts with the desire to decrease sedation to the point where a child is awake enough to attempt extubation. Anecdotally, we and others have found that the use of a short-acting agent such as propofol or dexmedetomidine facilitates opioid or benzodiazepine withdrawal during the peri-extubation period (Wheeler DS, unpublished data) [251–254]. Typically, dexmedetomidine or propofol is initiated as the dosage of opioid and benzodiazepine infusions are rapidly de-escalated, usually approximately 6–12 h prior to a trial of extubation. Children are then generally extubated shortly after the propofol or dexmedetomidine is discontinued. We have also extubated children while maintaining a *plane of sedation and analgesia* with low-dose dexmedetomidine (Wheeler DS, unpublished data). Finally, corticosteroids (dexamethasone, 0.5 mg/kg/dose IV every 6 h, beginning 12 h prior to extubation and continued for the first 12 h following extubation) are occasionally administered during the peri-extubation period in an attempt to minimize post-extubation stridor, though again there is scant evidence to support this practice.

References

1. Brown OE. Structure and function of the upper airway. In: Westmore RF, Muntz HR, McGill TJI, editors. Pediatric otolaryngology. Principles and practice pathways. New York: Thieme Medical Publishers; 2000. p. 679–88.
2. Healy GB. Introduction to disorders of upper airway. In: Westmore RF, Muntz HR, McGill TJI, editors. Pediatric otolaryngology. Principles and practice pathways. New York: Thieme Medical Publishers; 2000. p. 763–74.
3. Eckenhoff J. Some anatomic considerations of the infant larynx influencing endotracheal anesthesia. Anesthesiology. 1951;12:401–10.
4. Coté CJ, Ryan JF, Tordes ID, Groudsouzian NG, editors. A practice of anesthesia for infants and children. 2nd ed. Philadelphia: WB Saunders; 1993.
5. McNiece WL, Dierdorf SF. The pediatric airway. Semin Pediatr Surg. 2004;13:152–65.
6. Dickison AE. The normal and abnormal pediatric upper airway. Recognition and management of obstruction. Clin Chest Med. 1987;8:583–96.
7. Von Ungern-Sternberg BS, Erb TO, Reber A, Frei FJ. Opening the upper airway – airway maneuvers in pediatric anesthesia. Pediatr Anesth. 2005;15:181–9.
8. Greenland KB, Eley V, Edwards MJ, Allen P, Irwin MG. The origins of the sniffing position and the three axes alignment theory for direct laryngoscopy. Anaesth Intensive Care. 2008;36:23–7.
9. Borron SW, Lapostolle F, Lapandry C. The three axis alignment theory and the "sniffing position": perpetuation of an anatomic myth? Anesthesiology. 1999;91:1964–5.
10. Adnet F, Borron SW, Dumas JL, Lapostolle F, Cupa M, Lapandry C. Study of the "sniffing position" by magnetic resonance imaging. Anesthesiology. 2001;94:83–6.
11. Adnet F, Baillard C, Borron SW, Denantes C, Lefebvre L, Galinski M, Martinez C, Cupa M, Lapostolle F. Randomized study comparing the "sniffing position" with simple head extension for laryngoscopic view in elective surgery patients. Anesthesiology. 2001;95:836–41.
12. Rao SL, Kunselman AR, Schuler HG, DesHarnais S. Laryngoscopy and trachea intubation in the head-elevated position in obese patients: a randomized, controlled, equivalence trial. Anesth Analg. 2008;107:1912–8.
13. Lebowitz PW, Shay H, Straker T, Rubin D, Bodner S. Shoulder and head elevation improves laryngoscopic view for tracheal intubation in nonobese as well as obese individuals. J Clin Anesth. 2012;24:104–8.
14. El-Orbany M, Woehlick H, Salem MR. Head and neck position for direct laryngoscopy. Anesth Analg. 2011;113:103–9.
15. Motoyama EK, Gronert BJ, Fine GF. Induction of anesthesia and maintenance of the airway in infants and children. In: Motoyama EK, Davis PJ, editors. Smith's anesthesia for infants and children. 7th ed. Philadelphia: Mosby Elsevier; 2005. p. 338–47.
16. Vialet R, Nau A. Effect of head posture on pediatric oropharyngeal structures: implications for airway management in infants and children. Curr Opin Anaesthesiol. 2009;22:396–9.
17. Cipolle MD, Pasquale MD, Cerra FB. Secondary organ dysfunction: from clinical perspectives to molecular mediators. Crit Care Clin. 1993;9:261–98.
18. Aubier M, Viires N, Syllie G, Mozes R, Roussos C. Respiratory muscle contribution to lactic acidosis in low cardiac output. Am Rev Resp Dis. 1982;126:648–52.
19. Viires N, Sillye G, Aubier M, Rassidakis A, Roussos C. Regional blood flow distribution in dog during induced hypotension and low cardiac output. Spontaneous breathing versus artificial ventilation. J Clin Invest. 1983;72:935–47.
20. Hussain SN, Roussos C. Distribution of respiratory muscle and organ blood flow during endotoxic shock in dogs. J Appl Physiol. 1985;59:1802–8.
21. Field S, Kelly SM, Macklem PT. The oxygen cost of breathing in patients with cardiorespiratory disease. Am Rev Resp Dis. 1982;126:9–13.
22. Manthous CA, Hall JB, Kushner R, Schmidt GA, Russo G, Wood LD. The effect of mechanical ventilation on oxygen consumption in critically ill patients. Am J Respir Crit Care Med. 1995;151:210–4.

23. Marik PE, Kaufman D. The effects of neuromuscular paralysis on systemic and splanchnic oxygen utilization in mechanically ventilated patients. Chest. 1996;109:1038–42.

24. Nakayama DK, Gardner MJ, Rowe MI. Emergency endotracheal intubation in pediatric trauma. Ann Surg. 1990;211:218–23.

25. Brenner BE, Kauffman J. Response to cardiac arrests in a hospital setting: delays in ventilation. Resuscitation. 1996;31:17–23.

26. American Society of Anesthesiologists. Practice guidelines for management of the difficult airway: a report by the American Society of Anesthesiologists Task Force on Management of the Difficulty Airway. Anesthesiology. 1993;78:597–602.

27. Williamson JA, Webb RK, Szekely S, Gillies ER, Dreosti AV. The Australian incident monitoring study. Difficult intubation: an analysis of 2000 incident reports. Anaesth Intensive Care. 1993;21:602–7.

28. Kopp VJ, Bailey A, Calhoun PE, et al. Utility of the Mallampati classification for predicting difficult intubation in pediatric patients. Anesthesiology. 1995;83:3A1147 (abstract).

29. Levitan RM, Everett WW, Ochroch EA. Limitations of difficult airway prediction in patients intubated in the emergency department. Ann Emerg Med. 2004;44:307–13.

30. Frei FJ, Ummerhofer W. Difficult intubation in paediatrics. Paediatr Anaesth. 1996;6:251–63.

31. Yentis SM. Predicting difficult intubation – worthwhile exercise or pointless ritual? Anaesthesia. 2002;57:105–9.

32. Rosenstock C, Gillesberg I, Gatke MR, Levin D, Kristensen MS, Rasmussen LS. Inter-observer agreement of tests used for prediction of difficult laryngoscopy/tracheal intubation. Acta Anaesthesiol Scand. 2005;49:1057–62.

33. Shiga T, Wajima Z, Inoue T, Sakamoto A. Predicting difficult intubation in apparently normal patients: a meta-analysis of bedside screening test performance. Anesthesiology. 2005;103:429–37.

34. Mallampati SR. Clinical signs to predict difficult tracheal intubation (hypothesis). Can Anaesth Soc J. 1983;30:316–7.

35. Samsoon GL, Young JR. Difficult tracheal intubation: a retrospective study. Anaesthesia. 1987;42:487–90.

36. Duchynski R, Brauer K, Hutton K, Jones S, Rosen P. The quick look airway classification. A useful tool in predicting the difficult out-of-hospital intubation: experience in an air medical transport program. Air Med J. 1998;17:46–50.

37. Cormack RS, Lehane J. Difficult tracheal intubation in obstetrics. Anaesthesia. 1984;39:1105–11.

38. Westhorpe RN. The position of the larynx in children and its relationship to the ease of intubation. Anaesth Intensive Care. 1987;15:384–8.

39. Knill RL. Difficult laryngoscopy made easy with a "BURP"! Can J Anaesth. 1993;40:279–82.

40. Takahata O, Kubota M, Mamiya K, et al. The efficacy of the "BURP" maneuver during a difficult laryngoscopy. Anesth Analg. 1997;84:419–21.

41. Shott SR. Down syndrome: analysis of airway size and a guide for appropriate intubation. Laryngoscope. 2000;110:585–92.

42. Newth CJ, Rachman B, Patel N, Hammer J. The use of cuffed versus uncuffed endotracheal tubes in pediatric intensive care. J Pediatr. 2004;144:333–7.

43. Silver GM, Freiburg C, Halerz M, Tojong J, Supple K, Gamelli RL. A survey of airway and ventilator management strategies in North American pediatric burn units. J Burn Care Rehabil. 2004;25:435–40.

44. Deakers TW, Reynolds G, Stretton M, Newth CJ. Cuffed endotracheal tubes in pediatric intensive care. J Pediatr. 1994;125:57–62.

45. Khine HH, Corddry DH, Kettrick RG, Martin TM, McCloskey JJ, Rose JB, et al. Comparison of cuffed and uncuffed endotracheal tubes in young children during general anesthesia. Anesthesiology. 1997;86:627–31.

46. Fine GF, Borland LM. The future of the cuffed endotracheal tube. Paediatr Anaesth. 2004;14:38–42.

47. Wycoff CC. Endotracheal intubation: effects on blood pressure and pulse rate. Anesthesiology. 1960;21:153–8.

48. Tomori Z, Widdicombe JG. Muscular, bronchomotor, and cardiovascular reflexes elicited by mechanical stimulation of the respiratory tract. J Physiol. 1969;200:25–49.

49. Marshall TA, Deeder R, Pai S, Berkowitz GP, Austin TL. Physiologic changes associated with endotracheal intubation in preterm infants. Crit Care Med. 1984;12:501–3.

50. Thompson AE. Pediatric airway management. In: Fuhrman BP, Zimmerman J, editors. Pediatric critical care medicine. St. Louis: Mosby; 1998. p. 106–25.

51. Hardman JG, Wills JS, Aitkenhead AR. Factors determining the onset and course of hypoxemia during apnea: an investigation using physiologic modelling. Anesth Analg. 2000;90:619–24.

52. Hardman JG, Wills JS. The development of hypoxaemia during apnoea in children: a computational modelling investigation. Br J Anaesth. 2006;97:564–70.

53. Jaber S, Amraoui J, Lefrant J-Y, Arich C, Cohendy R, Landreau L, et al. Clinical practice and risk factors for immediate complications of endotracheal intubation in the intensive care unit: a prospective, multiple-center study. Crit Care Med. 2006;34:2355–61.

54. Jaber S, Jung B, Corne P, Sebbane M, Muller L, Changques G, et al. An intervention to decrease complications related to endotracheal intubation in the intensive care unit: a prospective, multiple-center study. Intensive Care Med. 2010;36:248–55.

55. Horak J, Weiss S. Emergency management of the airway: new pharmacology and the control of comorbidities in cardiac disease, ischemia, and valvular heart disease. Crit Care Clin. 2000;16:411–27.

56. Leigh MD, McCoy DD, Belton KM, et al. Bradycardia following IV administration of succinylcholine chloride to infants and children. Anesthesiology. 1957;18:698–702.

57. Stoelting RK, Petersson C. Heart-rate slowing and junctional rhythm following IV succinylcholine with and without intramuscular atropine pre-anesthetic medication. Anesth Analg. 1975;54:705–9.

58. Craythorne NWB, Turndoff H, Dripps RD. Changes in pulse rate and rhythm associated with the use of succinylcholine in anesthetized patients. Anesthesiology. 1960;21:465–70.

59. Blanc VF. Atropine and succinylcholine: beliefs and controversies in paediatric anaesthesia. Can J Anaesth. 1995;42:1–7.

60. McAuliffe G, Bissonnette B, Boutin C. Should the routine use of atropine before succinylcholine in children be reconsidered? Can J Anaesth. 1995;42:724–9.

61. Parnis SJ, van der Walt JH. A national survey of atropine use by Australian anaesthesiologists. Anaesth Intensive Care. 1994;22:61–5.

62. Shorten GD, Bissonnette B, Hartley E, Nelson W, Carr AS. It is not necessary to administer more than 10 mcg of atropine to older children before succinylcholine. Can J Anaesth. 1995;42:8–11.

63. Splinter WM. Intravenous lidocaine does not attenuate the haemodynamic response of children to laryngoscopy and tracheal intubation. Can J Anaesth. 1990;37:440–3.

64. Lev R, Rosen P. Prophylactic lidocaine use preintubation: a review. J Emerg Med. 1994;12:499–506.

65. Robinson N, Clancy M. In patients with head injury undergoing rapid sequence intubation, does pretreatment with intravenous lignocaine/lidocaine lead to an improved neurological outcome? A review of the literature. Emerg Med J. 2001;18:453–7.

66. Kovac AL. Controlling the hemodynamic response to laryngoscopy and endotracheal intubation. J Clin Anesth. 1996;8:63–79.

67. Feng CK, Chan KH, Liu KN, et al. A comparison of lidocaine, fentanyl, and esmolol for attenuation of cardiovascular response to laryngoscopy and tracheal intubation. Acta Anaesthesiol Sin. 1996;34:61–7.

68. Wadbrook PS. Advances in airway pharmacology: emerging trends and evolving controversy. Emerg Med Clin North Am. 2000;18:767–88.

69. Pathak D, Slater RM, Ping SS, et al. Effects of alfentanil and lidocaine on the hemodynamic response to laryngoscopy and tracheal intubation. J Clin Anesth. 1990;2:81–5.

70. Figueredo E, Garcia-Fuentes EM. Assessment of the efficacy of esmolol on the haemodynamic changes induced by laryngoscopy and tracheal intubation: a meta-analysis. Acta Anaesthesiol Scand. 2001;45:1011–22.

71. Helfman SM, Gold MI, DeLisser EA, Herrington CA. Which drug prevents tachycardia and hypertension associated with tracheal intubation: lidocaine, fentanyl, or esmolol? Anesth Analg. 1991;72:482–6.

72. Singh H, Vichitvejpaisal P, Gaines GY, White PF. Comparative effects of lidocaine, esmolol, and nitroglycerin in modifying the hemodynamic response to laryngoscopy and intubation. J Clin Anesth. 1995;7:5–8.

73. Kindler CH, Schumacher PG, Schneider MC, Urwyler A. Effects of intravenous lidocaine and/or esmolol on hemodynamic responses to laryngoscopy and intubation: a double-blind, controlled, clinical trial. J Clin Anesth. 1996;8:491–6.

74. Atlee JL, Dhamee MS, Olund TL, George V. The use of esmolol, nicardipine, or their combination to blunt hemodynamic changes after laryngoscopy and tracheal intubation. Anesth Analg. 2000;90:280–5.

75. Levitt MA, Dresden GM. The efficacy of esmolol versus lidocaine to attenuate the hemodynamic response to intubation in isolated head trauma patients. Acad Emerg Med. 2001;8:19–24.

76. Chung KS, Sinatra RS, Halevy JD, Paige D, Silverman DG. A comparison of fentanyl, esmolol, and their combination for blunting the haemodynamic responses during rapid-sequence intubation. Can J Anaesth. 1992;39:774–9.

77. Shapiro HM, Galindo A, Wyte SR, Harris AB. Rapid intraoperative reduction of intracranial pressure with thiopentone. Br J Anaesth. 1998;81:798–803.

78. Kofke WA, Dong ML, Bloom M, Policare R, Janosky J, Sekhar L. Transcranial Doppler ultrasonography with induction of anesthesia for neurosurgery. J Neurosurg Anesthesiol. 1994;6:89–97.

79. Yamamoto LG, Yin GK, Britten AG. Rapid sequence anesthesia induction for emergency intubation. Pediatr Emerg Care. 1990;6:200–13.

80. Nakayama DK, Waggoner T, Venkataraman ST, Gardner M, Lynch JM, Orr RA. The use of drugs in emergency airway management in pediatric trauma. Ann Surg. 1992;216:205–11.

81. Gerardi MJ, Sacchetti AD, Cantor RM, et al. Rapid-sequence intubation of the pediatric patient. Pediatric Emergency Medicine Committee of the American College of Emergency Physicians. Ann Emerg Med. 1996;28:55–74.

82. Silber SH. Rapid sequence intubation in adults with elevated intracranial pressure: a survey of emergency medicine residency programs. Am J Emerg Med. 1997;15:263–7.

83. Sagarin MJ, Chiang V, Sakles JC, et al. Rapid sequence intubation for pediatric emergency airway management. Pediatr Emerg Care. 2002;18:417–23.

84. Koppel N. Execution drug halt raises ire of doctors. Wall Street Journal, January 25, 2011. http://online.wsj.com/article/SB1000142405274870 4279704576102380584250672.html?KEYWORDS=koppel. Accessed 22 Jul 2013.

85. Batjer HH. Cerebral protective effects of etomidate: experimental and clinical aspects. Cerebrovasc Brain Metab Rev. 1993;5:17–32.

86. Wagner RL, White PF. Etomidate inhibits adrenocortical function in surgical patients. Anesthesiology. 1984;61:647–51.

87. Fragen RJ, Shanks CA, Molteni A, Avram MJ. Effects of etomidate on hormonal responses to surgical stress. Anesthesiology. 1984;61:652–6.

88. Wanscher M, Tonnesen E, Huttel M, Larsen K. Etomidate infusion and adrenocortical function. A study in elective surgery. Acta Anaesthesiol Scand. 1985;29:483–5.

89. Moore RA, Allen MC, Wood PJ, Rees LH, Sear JW. Peri-operative endocrine effects of etomidate. Anaesthesia. 1985;40:124–30.

90. Duthie DJ, Fraser R, Nimmo WS. Effect of induction of anaesthesia with etomidate on corticosteroid synthesis in man. Br J Anaesth. 1985;57:156–9.

91. Preziosi P, Vacca M. Adrenocortical suppression and other endocrine effects of etomidate. Life Sci. 1988;42:477–89.

92. Oglesby AJ. Should etomidate be the induction agent of choice for rapid sequence intubation in the emergency department? Emerg Med J. 2004;21:655–9.

93. Annane D. ICU physicians should abandon the use of etomidate! Intensive Care Med. 2005;31:325–6.

94. Jackson Jr WL. Should we use etomidate as an induction agent for endotracheal intubation in patients with septic shock? A critical appraisal. Chest. 2005;127:1031–8.

95. den Brinker M, Joosten KF, Liem O, et al. Adrenal insufficiency in meningococcal sepsis: bioavailable cortisol levels and impact of interleukin-6 levels and intubation with etomidate on adrenal function and mortality. J Clin Endocrinol Metab. 2005;90:5110–7.

96. Cohan P, Wang C, McArthur DL, et al. Acute secondary adrenal insufficiency after traumatic brain injury: a prospective study. Crit Care Med. 2005;33:2358–66.

97. Absalom A, Pledger D, Kong A. Adrenocortical function in critically ill patients 24h after a single dose of etomidate. Anaesthesia. 1999;54:861–7.

98. Hildreth AN, Meija VA, Maxwell RA, Smith PW, Dart BW, Barker DE. Adrenal suppression following a single dose of etomidate for rapid sequence induction: a prospective randomized study. J Trauma. 2008;65:573–9.

99. Schenarts CL, Burton JH, Riker RR. Adrenocortical dysfunction following etomidate induction in emergency department patients. Acad Emerg Med. 2001;8:1–7.

100. Sokolove PE, Price DD, Okada P. The safety of etomidate for emergency rapid sequence intubation of pediatric patients. Pediatr Emerg Care. 2000;16:18–21.

101. Guldner G, Schultz J, Sexton P, Fortner C, Richmond M. Etomidate for rapid-sequence intubation in young children: hemodynamic effects and adverse events. Acad Emerg Med. 2003;10:134–9.

102. Tekwani KL, Watts HF, Rzechula KH, Sweis RT, Kulstad EB. A prospective observational study of the effect of etomidate on septic patient mortality and length of stay. Acad Emerg Med. 2009;16:11–4.

103. Tekwani KL, Watts HF, Sweis RT, Rzechula KH, Kulstad EB. A comparison of the effects of etomidate and midazolam on hospital length of stay in patients with suspected sepsis: a prospective, randomized study. Ann Emerg Med. 2010;56:481–9.

104. Banh KV, James S, Hendey GW, Snowden B, Kaups K. Single-dose etomidate for intubation in the trauma patient. J Emerg Med. 2012;43:e277–82.

105. McPhee LC, Badawi O, Fraser GL, Lerwick PA, Riker RR, Zuckerman IH, et al. Single-dose etomidate is not associated with increased mortality in ICU patients with sepsis: analysis of a large electronic ICU database. Crit Care Med. 2013;41:774–83.

106. Chan CM, Mitchell AL, Shorr AF. Etomidate is associated with mortality and adrenal insufficiency in sepsis: a meta-analysis. Crit Care Med. 2012;40:2945–53.

107. Hohl CM, Kelly-Smith CH, Yeung TC, Sweet DD, Doyle-Waters M, Schulzer M. The effect of a bolus dose of etomidate on cortisol levels, mortality, and health services utilization: a systematic review. Ann Emerg Med. 2010;56:105–13.

108. Bergen JM, Smith DC. A review of etomidate for rapid sequence intubation in the emergency department. J Emerg Med. 1997;15:221–30.

109. Forster JA, Juge O, Morel D. Effects of midazolam on cerebral blood flow in human volunteers. Anesthesiology. 1982;56:453–5.

110. Papazian L, Albanese J, Thirion X, Perrin G, Durbec O, Martin C. Effect of bolus doses of midazolam on intracranial pressure and cerebral perfusion pressure in patients with severe head injury. Br J Anaesth. 1993;71:267–71.

111. Sanchez-Izquierdo-Riera JA, Caballero-Cubedo RE, Perez-Vela JL, et al. Propofol versus midazolam: safety and efficacy for sedating the severe trauma patient. Anesth Analg. 1998;86:1219–24.

112. Burtin P, Daoud P, Jacqz-Aigrain E, Mussat P, Moriette G. Hypotension with midazolam and fentanyl in the newborn. Lancet. 1991;337:1545–6.

113. Davis DP, Kimbro TA, Vilke GM. The use of midazolam for prehospital rapid-sequence intubation may be associated with a dose-related increase in hypotension. Prehosp Emerg Care. 2001;5:163–8.

114. Ng E, Klinger G, Shah V, Taddio A. Safety of benzodiazepines in newborns. Ann Pharmacother. 2002;36:1150–5.

115. Choi YF, Wong TW, Lau CC. Midazolam is more likely to cause hypotension than etomidate in emergency department rapid sequence intubation. Emerg Med J. 2004;21:700–2.

116. McAllister JD, Gnauck KA. Rapid sequence intubation of the pediatric patient: fundamentals of practice. Pediatr Clin North Am. 1999;46:1249–84.

117. Reynolds SF, Heffner J. Airway management of the critically ill patient: rapid-sequence intubation. Chest. 2005;127:1397–412.

118. Wells S, Williamson M, Hooker D. Fentanyl-induced chest wall rigidity in a neonate: a case report. Heart Lung. 1994;23:196–8.

119. MacGregor DA, Bauman LA. Chest wall rigidity during infusion of fentanyl in a two-month-old infant after heart surgery. J Clin Anesth. 1996;8:251–4.

120. Bennet JA, Abrams JT, Van Riper DF, Horrow JC. Difficult or impossible ventilation after sufentanil-induced anesthesia is caused primarily by vocal cord closure. Anesthesiology. 1997;87:1070–4.

121. Fahnenstich H, Steffan J, Kau N, Bartmann P. Fentanyl-induced chest wall rigidity and laryngospasm in preterm and term infants. Crit Care Med. 2000;28:836–9.

122. Muller P, Vogtmann C. Three cases with different presentation of fentanyl-induced muscle rigidity – a rare problem in intensive care of neonates. Am J Perinatol. 2000;17:23–6.

123. Caspi J, Klausner JM, Safadi T, et al. Delayed respiratory depression following fentanyl anesthesia for cardiac surgery. Crit Care Med. 1988;16:238–40.

124. Stanley TH, Webster LR. Anesthetic requirements and cardiovascular effects of fentanyl-oxygen and fentanyl-diazepam-oxygen anesthesia in man. Anesth Analg. 1978;57:411–6.

125. Shupak RC, Harp JR, Stevenson-Smith W, et al. High dose fentanyl for neuroanesthesia. Anesthesiology. 1983;58:579–82.

126. Chudnofsky CR, Wright SW, Dronen SC, et al. The safety of fentanyl use in the emergency department. Ann Emerg Med. 1989;18:635–9.

127. Bailey PL, Wilbrink J, Zwanikken P, et al. Anesthetic induction with fentanyl. Anesth Analg. 1985;64:48–53.

128. Taylor I, Marsh DF. Fentanyl is not best anaesthetic induction agent in rapid sequence intubation. BMJ. 1998;317:1386.

129. Gelissen HP, Epema AH, Henning RH, Krijnen HJ, Hennis PJ, den Hertog A. Inotropic effects of propofol, thiopental, midazolam, etomidate, and ketamine on isolated human atrial muscle. Anesthesiology. 1996;84:397–403.

130. Kawakubo A, Fujigaki T, Uresino H, Zang S, Sumikawa K. Comparative effects of etomidate, ketamine, propofol, and fentanyl on myocardial contractility in dogs. J Anesth. 1999;13:77–82.

131. White PF, Way WL, Trevor AJ. Ketamine-its pharmacology and therapeutic uses. Anesthesiology. 1982;56:119–36.

132. Reich DL, Silvay G. Ketamine: an update on the first twenty-five years of clinical experience. Can J Anaesth. 1989;36:186–97.

133. Morray JP, Lynn A, Stamm SJ, Herndon PS, Kawabori I, Stevenson JG. Hemodynamic effects of ketamine in children with congenital heart disease. Anesth Analg. 1984;63:895–9.

134. Hickey PR, Hansen DD, Cramolin GM, Vincent RN, Lang P. Pulmonary and systemic hemodynamic responses to ketamine in infants with normal and elevated pulmonary vascular resistance. Anesthesiology. 1985;62:287–93.

135. Oklu E, Bulutcu FS, Yalcin Y, Ozbeck U, Cakali E, Bayindir O. Which anesthetic agent alters the hemodynamic status during pediatric catheterization? Comparison of propofol versus ketamine. J Cardiothorac Vasc Anesth. 2003;17:686–90.

136. Wong DH, Jenkins LC. The cardiovascular effects of ketamine in hypotensive rats. Can Anaesth Soc J. 1975;22:339–48.

137. Dewhirst E, Frazier WJ, Leder M, Fraser DD, Tobias JD. Cardiac arrest following ketamine administration for rapid sequence intubation. J Intensive Care Med. 2013;28:375–9.

138. Stanley TH, Weidauer HE. Anesthesia for the patient with cardiac tamponade. Anesth Analg. 1973;52:110–4.

139. Kaplan JA, Bland Jr JW, Dunbar RW. The perioperative management of pericardial tamponade. South Med J. 1976;69:417–9.

140. Rock MJ, Reyes de la Rocha S, L'Hommedieu CS, Truemper E. Use of ketamine in asthmatic children to treat respiratory failure refractory to conventional therapy. Crit Care Med. 1986;14:514–6.

141. Nehama J, Pass R, Bechtler-Karsch A, Steinberg C, Notterman DA. Continuous ketamine infusion for the treatment of refractory asthma in a mechanically ventilated infant: case report and review of the pediatric literature. Pediatr Emerg Care. 1996;12:294–7.

142. Youssef-Ahmed MZ, Silver P, Nimkoff L, Sagy M. Continuous infusion of ketamine in mechanically ventilated children with refractory bronchospasm. Intensive Care Med. 1996;22:972–6.

143. Petrillo TM, Fortenberry JD, Linzer JF, Simon HK. Emergency department use of ketamine in pediatric status asthmaticus. J Asthma. 2001;38:657–64.

144. Bano S, Akhtar S, Zia N, Khan UR, Haq AU. Pediatric endotracheal intubations for airway management in the emergency department. Pediatr Emerg Care. 2012;28:1129–31.

145. Bourgoin A, Albanese J, Wereszczynski N, Charbit M, Vialet R, Martin C. Safety of sedation with ketamine in severe head injury patients: comparison with sufentanil. Crit Care Med. 2003;31:711–7.

146. Himmelseher S, Durieux ME. Revising a dogma: ketamine for patients with neurological injury? Anesth Analg. 2005;101:524–34.

147. Bar-Joseph G, Guilburd Y, Tamir A, Guilburd JN. Effectiveness of ketamine in decreasing intracranial pressure in children with intracranial hypertension. J Neurosurg Pediatr. 2009;4:40–6.

148. Filanovsky Y, Miller P, Kao J. Myth: ketamine should not be used as an induction agent for intubation in patients with head injury. CJEM. 2010;12:154–7.

149. Michalczyk K, Sullivan JE, Berkenbosch JW. Pretreatment with midazolam blunts the rise in intracranial pressure associated with ketamine sedation for lumbar puncture in children. Pediatr Crit Care Med. 2013;14:e149–55.

150. Chang LC, Raty SR, Ortiz J, Bailard NS, Mathew SJ. The emerging use of ketamine for anesthesia and sedation in traumatic brain injuries. CNS Neurosci Ther. 2013;19:390–5.

151. Lee TS, Hou X. Vasoactive effects of ketamine on isolated rabbit pulmonary arteries. Chest. 1995;107:1152–5.

152. Maruyama K, Maruyama J, Yokochi A, Muneyuki M, Miyasaka K. Vasodilatory effects of ketamine on pulmonary arteries in rats with chronic hypoxic pulmonary hypertension. Anesth Analg. 1995;80:786–92.

153. Williams GD, Philip BM, Chu LF, Boltz MG, Kamra K, Terwey H, et al. Ketamine does not increase pulmonary vascular resistance in children with pulmonary hypertension undergoing sevoflurane anesthesia and spontaneous ventilation. Anesth Analg. 2007;105:1578–84.

154. Munro HM, Felix DE, Nykanen DG. Dexmedetomidine/ketamine for diagnostic cardiac catheterization in a child with idiopathic pulmonary hypertension. J Clin Anesth. 2009;21:435–8.

155. Williams GD, Maan H, Ramamoorthy C, Kamra K, Bratton SL, Bair E, et al. Perioperative complications in children with pulmonary hypertension undergoing general anesthesia with ketamine. Paediatr Anaesth. 2010;20:28–37.

156. Scherzer D, Leder M, Tobias JD. Pro-con debate: etomidate or ketamine for rapid sequence intubation in pediatric patients. J Pediatr Pharmacol Ther. 2012;17:142–9.

157. Jabre P, Combes X, Lapostolle F, Dhaouadi M, Ricard-Hibon A, Vivien B, et al. Etomidate versus ketamine for rapid sequence intubation in acutely ill patients: a multicenter randomized controlled trial. Lancet. 2009;374:293–300.

158. Wilbur K, Zed PJ. Is propofol an optimal agent for procedural sedation and rapid sequence intubation in the emergency department? CJEM. 2001;3:302–10.

159. Nishisaki A, Turner DA, Brown 3rd CA, Walls RM, Nadkarni VM. A National Emergency Airway Registry for Children: landscape of tracheal intubation in 15 PICUs. Crit Care Med. 2013;41:874–85.

160. Gronert BJ, Brandom BW. Neuromuscular blocking drugs in infants and children. Pediatr Clin North Am. 1994;41:73–90.

161. Martin LD, Bratton SL, O'Rourke PP. Clinical uses and controversies of neuromuscular blocking agents in infants and children. Crit Care Med. 1999;27:1358–68.

162. Zelicof-Paul A, Smith-Lockridge A, Schnadower D, et al. Controversies in rapid sequence intubation in children. Curr Opin Pediatr. 2005;17:355–62.

163. Doobinin KA, Nakagawa TA. Emergency department use of neuromuscular blocking agents in children. Pediatr Emerg Care. 2000;16:441–7.

164. Brandom BW, Fine GF. Neuromuscular blocking drugs in pediatric anesthesia. Anesthesiol Clin North Am. 2002;20:45–58.

165. Clancy M, Halford S, Walls R, Murphy M. In patients with head injuries who undergo rapid sequence intubation using succinylcholine does pretreatment with a competitive neuromuscular blocking agent improve outcome? A literature review. Emerg Med J. 2001;18:373–5.

166. Nelson JM, Morell RC, Butterworth 4th JF. Rocuronium versus succinylcholine for rapid-sequence induction using a variation of the timing principle. J Clin Anesth. 1997;9:317–20.

167. Mazurek AK, Rae B, Hann S, Kim JI, Catro B, Cote CJ. Rocuronium versus succinylcholine: are they equally effective during rapid-sequence induction of anesthesia? Anesth Analg. 1998;87:1259–62.

168. Andrews JI, Kumar N, van den Brom RH, Olkkola KT, Roest GJ, Wright PM. A large simple randomized trial of rocuronium versus succinylcholine in rapid-sequence induction of anaesthesia along with propofol. Acta Anaesthesiol Scand. 1999;43:4–8.

169. Mencke T, Knoll H, Schreiber JU, Echternach M, Klein S, Noeldge-Schomburg G, et al. Rocuronium is not associated with more vocal cord injuries than succinylcholine after rapid-sequence induction: a randomized, prospective, controlled trial. Anesth Analg. 2006;102:943–9.

170. Perry JJ, Lee J, Wells G. Are intubation conditions using rocuronium equivalent to those using succinylcholine? Acad Emerg Med. 2002;9:813–23.

171. Sluga M, Ummenhofer W, Studer W, Siegemund M, Marsch SC. Rocuronium versus succinylcholine for rapid sequence induction of anesthesia and endotracheal intubation: a prospective, randomized trial in emergent cases. Anesth Analg. 2005;101:1356–61.

172. Perry JJ, Lee JS, Sillberg VA, Wells GA. Rocuronium versus succinylcholine for rapid sequence induction intubation. Cochrane Database Syst Rev 2008;(2):CD002788.

173. O'Rourke PP, Crone RK. The respiratory system. In: Gregory G, editor. Pediatric anesthesia. 2nd ed. New York: Churchill Livingstone; 1989. p. 63–91.

174. Berthoud M, Read DH, Norman J. Preoxygenation: how long? Anaesthesia. 1983;38:96–102.

175. McGowan P, Skinner A. Preoxygenation: the importance of a good face mask seal. Br J Anaesth. 1995;75:777–8.

176. Snider DD, Clarke D, Finucane BT. The "BURP" maneuver worsens the glottic view when applied in combination with cricoid pressure. Can J Anaesth. 2005;52:100–4.

177. Krantz MA, Poulos JG, Chaouki K, Adamek P. The laryngeal lift: a method to facilitate endotracheal intubation. J Clin Anesth. 1993;5:297–301.

178. Tamura M, Ishikawa T, Kato R, Isono S, Nishino T. Mandibular advancement improves the laryngeal view during direct laryngoscopy performed by inexperienced physicians. Anesthesiology. 2004;100:598–601.

179. Ho AM, Wong W, Ling E, Chung DC, Tay BA. Airway difficulties caused by improperly applied cricoid pressure. J Emerg Med. 2001;20:29–31.

180. Smith CE, Boyer D. Cricoid pressure decreases ease of tracheal intubation using fiberoptic laryngoscopy (WuScope System). Can J Anaesth. 2002;49:614–9.

181. Haslam N, Parker L, Duggan JE. Effect of cricoid pressure on the view at laryngoscopy. Anaesthesia. 2005;60:41–7.

182. Grmec S. Comparison of three different methods to confirm tracheal tube placement in emergency intubation. Intensive Care Med. 2002;28:701–4.

183. Erasmus PD. The use of end-tidal carbon dioxide monitoring to confirm endotracheal tube placement in adult and paediatric intensive care units in Australia and New Zealand. Anaesth Intensive Care. 2004;32:672–5.

184. Cumming C, McFadzean J. A survey of the use of capnography for the confirmation of correct placement of tracheal tubes in pediatric intensive care units in the UK. Paediatr Anaesth. 2005;15:591–6.

185. Orlowski JP, Ellis NG, Amin NP, Crumrine RS. Complications of airway intrusion in 100 consecutive cases in a pediatric ICU. Crit Care Med. 1980;8:324–31.

186. McMillan DD, Rademake AW, Buchan KA, Reid A, Machin G, Sauve RS. Benefits of orotracheal and nasotracheal intubation in neonates requiring ventilatory assistance. Pediatrics. 1986;77:39–44.

187. Black AE, Hatch DJ, Nauth-Misir N. Complications of nasotracheal intubation in neonates, infants, and children: a review of 4 years' experience in a children's hospital. Br J Anaesth. 1990;65:461–7.

188. Holzapfel L, Chevret S, Madinier G, et al. Influence of long-term oro- or nasotracheal intubation on nosocomial maxillary sinusitis and pneumonia: results of a prospective, randomized, clinical trial. Crit Care Med. 1993;21:1132–8.

189. Deutschman CS, Wilton P, Sinow J, et al. Paranasal sinusitis associated with nasotracheal intubation: a frequently unrecognized and treatable source of sepsis. Crit Care Med. 1986;14:111–4.

190. Salord F, Gaussorgues P, Marti-Flich J, et al. Noscomial maxillary sinusitis during mechanical ventilation: a prospective comparison of orotracheal versus the nasotracheal route for intubation. Intensive Care Med. 1990;16:390–3.

191. Bach A, Boehrer H, Schmid H, Geiss HK. Noscomial sinusitis in ventilated patients. Nasotracheal versus orotracheal intubation. Anaesthesia. 1992;47:335–9.

192. Bonten M, Kollef MH, Hall JB. Risk factors for ventilator-associated pneumonia: from epidemiology to patient management. Healthc Epidemiol. 2004;38:1141–9.

193. Elward A, Warren D, Fraser V. Ventilator-associated pneumonia in pediatric intensive care unit patients: risk factors and outcomes. Pediatrics. 2002;109:758–64.

194. Rowin M, Patel V, Christenson J. Pediatric intensive care unit nosocomial infections: epidemiology, sources and solutions. Crit Care Clin. 2003;19:473–87.

195. Fayon M, Tucci M, Lacroix J, et al. Nosocomial bacterial pneumonia and tracheitis in pediatric intensive care: a prospective study. Am J Respir Crit Care Med. 1997;155:162–9.

196. Scott PH, Elgen H, Moye LA, Georgitis J, Laughlin JJ. Predictability and consequences of spontaneous extubation in a pediatric ICU. Crit Care Med. 1985;13:228–32.

197. Little LA, Koenig JC, Newth CJL. Factors affecting accidental extubations in neonatal and pediatric intensive care patients. Crit Care Med. 1990;18:163–5.

198. Chevron V, Menard JF, Richard JC, Girault C, Leroy J, Bonmarchand G. Unplanned extubation: risk factors of development and predictive criteria for reintubation. Crit Care Med. 1998;26:1049–53.

199. Freeman JA, Fredricks BJ, Best CJ. Evaluation of a new method for determining tracheal tube length in children. Anaesthesia. 1995;50:1050–2.

200. de la Sierra Antona M, Lopez-Herce J, Ruperez M, Garcia C, Garrido G. Estimation of the length of nasotracheal tube to be introduced in children. J Pediatr. 2002;140:772–4.

201. Elwood T, Stillions DM, Woo DW, Bradford HM, Ramamoorthy C. Nasotracheal intubation: a randomized trial of two methods. Anesthesiology. 2002;96:51–3.

202. Gowdar K, Bull MJ, Schreiner KL, Lemons JA, Gresham EL. Nasal deformities in neonates. Their occurrence in those treated with nasal continuous positive airway pressure and nasal endotracheal tubes. Am J Dis Child. 1980;134:954–7.

203. Sellick BA. Cricoid pressure to control the regurgitation of stomach contents during induction of anaesthesia. Lancet. 1961;2:404–6.

204. Salem MR, Wong AY, Fizzotti GF. Efficacy of cricoid pressure in preventing aspiration of gastric contents in paediatric patients. Br J Anaesth. 1972;44:401–4.

205. Salem MR, Wong AY, Mani M, Sellick BA. Efficacy of cricoid pressure in preventing gastric inflation during bag-mask ventilation in pediatric patients. Anesthesiology. 1974;40:96–8.

206. Moynihan RJ, Brock-Utne JG, Archer JH, Feld LH, Kreitzman TR. The effect of cricoid pressure on preventing gastric insufflation in infants and children. Anesthesiology. 1993;78:652–6.

207. Koenig KL. Rapid-sequence intubation of head trauma patients: prevention of fasciculations with pancuronium versus minidose succinylcholine. Ann Emerg Med. 1992;21:929–32.

208. Rubin MA, Sadovnikoff N. Neuromuscular blocking agents in the emergency department. J Emerg Med. 1996;14:193–9.

209. Motamed C, Choquette R, Donati F. Rocuronium prevents succinylcholine-induced fasciculations. Can J Anaesth. 1997;44:1262–8.

210. Martin R, Carrier J, Pirlet M, et al. Rocuronium is the best nondepolarizing relaxant to prevent succinylcholine fasciculations and myalgia. Can J Anaesth. 1998;45:521–5.

211. Sugiyama K, Yokoyama K. Displacement of the endotracheal tube causes by change of head position in pediatric anesthesia: evaluation by fiberoptic bronchoscopy. Anesth Analg. 1996;82:251–3.

212. Olufolabi AJ, Charlton GA, Spargo PM. Effect of head posture on tracheal tube position in children. Anaesthesia. 2004;59:1069–72.

213. Galvis AG, Stool SE, Bluestone CD. Pulmonary edema following relief of acute upper airway obstruction. Ann Otol. 1980;80:124–8.

214. Sofer, Bar-Ziv J, Scharf SM. Pulmonary edema following relief of upper airway obstruction. Chest. 1984;86:401–3.

215. Kanter RK, Watchko JF. Pulmonary edema associated with upper airway obstruction. Am J Dis Child. 1984;38:356–8.

216. Barin ES, Stevenson IF, Donnelly GL. Pulmonary oedema following acute upper airway obstruction. Anaesth Intensive Care. 1986;14:54–7.

217. Warner LO, Beach TP, Martino JD. Negative pressure pulmonary oedema secondary to airway obstruction in an intubated infant. Can J Anaesth. 1988;35:507–10.

218. Oudjhane K, Bowen A, Oh KS, Young LW. Pulmonary edema complicating upper airway obstruction in infants and children. Can Assoc Radiol J. 1992;43:278–82.

219. Deepika K, Kenaan CA, Barrocas AM, Fonseca JJ, Bikazi GB. Negative pressure pulmonary edema after acute upper airway obstruction. J Clin Anesth. 1997;9:403–8.

220. Sofer S, Baer R, Gussarsky Y, Lieberman A, Bar-Ziv J. Pulmonary edema secondary to chronic upper airway obstruction. Hemodynamic study in a child. Intensive Care Med. 1984;10:317–9.

221. McConkey PP. Postobstructive pulmonary oedema – a case series and review. Anaesth Intensive Care. 2000;28:72–6.

222. Ringold S, Klein EJ, Del Beccaro MA. Postobstructive pulmonary edema in children. Pediatr Emerg Care. 2004;20:391–5.

223. Contencin P, Narcy P. Size of endotracheal tube and neonatal acquired subglottic stenosis. Study Group for Neonatology and Pediatric Emergencies in the Parisian Area. Arch Otolaryngol Head Neck Surg. 1993;119:815–9.

224. Easley RB, Segeleon JE, Haun SE, Tobias JD. Prospective study of airway management of children requiring endotracheal intubation before admission to a pediatric intensive care unit. Crit Care Med. 2000;28:2058–63.

225. Ehrlich PF, Seidman PS, Atallah O, Haque A, Helmkamp J. Endotracheal intubations in rural pediatric trauma patients. J Pediatr Surg. 2004;39:1376–280.

226. Supance JS, Reilly JS, Doyle WJ, Bluestone CD, Hubbard J. Acquired subglottic stenosis following prolonged endotracheal intubation. A canine model. Arch Otolaryngol. 1982;108:727–31.

227. Pashley NR. Risk factors and the prediction of outcome in acquired subglottic stenosis in children. Int J Pediatr Otorhinolarngol. 1982;4:1–6.

228. Wiel E, Vilette B, Darras JA, Scherpereel P, Leclerc F. Laryngotracheal stensosi in children after intubation. Report of five cases. Paediatr Anaesth. 1997;7:415–9.

229. Mhanna MJ, Zamel YB, Tichy CM, Super DM. The "air leak" test around the endotracheal tube, as a predictor of postextubation stridor, is age dependent in children. Crit Care Med. 2002;30:2639–43.

230. Foland JA, Super DM, Dahdah NS, Mhanna MJ. The use of the air leak test and corticosteroids intubated children: a survey of pediatric critical care fellowship directors. Respir Care. 2002;47:662–6.

231. Saleem AF, Bano S, Haque A. Does prophylactic use of dexamethasone have a role in reducing post extubation stridor and reintubation in children? Indian J Pediatr. 2009;76:555–7.

232. McCaffrey J, Farrell C, Whiting P, Dan A, Bagshaw SM, Delaney AP. Corticosteroids to prevent extubation failure: a systematic review and meta-analysis. Intensive Care Med. 2009;35:977–86.

233. Khemani RG, Randolph A, Markovitz B. Steroids for post extubation stridor: pediatric evidence is still inconclusive. Intensive Care Med. 2010;36:1276–7.

234. Wohl DL, Tucker JA. Infant botulism: considerations for airway management. Laryngoscope. 1992;102:1251–4.

235. Anderson TD, Shah UK, Schreiner MS, Jacobs IN. Airway complications of infant botulism: ten-year experience with 60 cases. Otolaryngol Head Neck Surg. 2002;126:234–9.

236. Kadilak PR, Vanasse S, Sheridan RL. Favorable short- and long-term outcomes of prolonged translaryngeal intubation in critically ill children. J Burn Care Rehabil. 2004;25:262–5.

237. Torres A, Gatell JM, Aznar E, et al. Re-intubation increases the risk of nosocomial pneumonia in patients needing mechanical ventilation. Am J Respir Crit Care Med. 1995;152:137–41.

238. Epstein SK, Ciubotaru RL, Wong JB. Effect of failed extubation on the outcome of mechanical ventilation. Chest. 1997;112:186–92.

239. Esteban A, Alia I, Gordo F, et al. Extubation outcome after spontaneous breathing trials with T-tube or pressure support ventilation. Am J Respir Crit Care Med. 1997;156:459–65.

240. Khan N, Brown A, Venkataraman ST. Predictors of extubation success and failure in mechanically ventilated infants and children. Crit Care Med. 1996;24:1568–79.

241. El-Khatib MF, Baumeister B, Smith PG, Chatburn RL, Blumer JL. Inspiratory pressure/maximal inspiratory pressure: does it

predict successful extubation in critically ill infants and children? Intensive Care Med. 1996;22:264–8.

242. Baumeister BL, El-Khatib MF, Smith PG, Blumer JL. Evaluation of predictors of weaning from mechanical ventilation in pediatric patients. Pediatr Pulmonol. 1997;24:344–52.

243. Farias JA, Alia I, Esteban A, Golubicki AN, Olazarri FA. Weaning from mechanical ventilation in pediatric intensive care patients. Intensive Care Med. 1998;24:1070–5.

244. Thiagarajan RR, Bratton SL, Martin LD, Brogan TV, Taylor D. Predictors of successful extubation in children. Am J Respir Crit Care Med. 1999;160:1562–6.

245. Manczur TI, Greenough A, Pryor D, Rafferty GF. Assessment of respiratory drive and muscle function in the pediatric intensive care unit and prediction of extubation failure. Pediatr Crit Care Med. 2000;1:124–6.

246. Hubble CL, Gentile MA, Tripp DS, Craig DM, Meliones JN, Cheifetz IM. Deadspace to tidal volume ratio predicts successful extubation in infants and children. Crit Care Med. 2000;28:2034–40.

247. Manczur TI, Greenough A, Pryor D, Raffert GF. Comparison of predictors of extubation from mechanical ventilation in children. Pediatr Crit Care Med. 2000;1:28–32.

248. Venkataraman ST, Khan N, Brown A. Validation of predictors of extubation success and failure in mechanically ventilated infants and children. Crit Care Med. 2000;28:2991–6.

249. Farias JA, Alia I, Retta A, et al. An evaluation of extubation failure predictors in mechanically ventilated infants and children. Intensive Care Med. 2002;28:752–7.

250. Lyons KA, Brilli RJ, Wieman RA, Jacobs BR. Continuation of transpyloric feeding during weaning of mechanical ventilation and tracheal extubation in children: a randomized, controlled trial. JPEN J Parenter Enter Nutr. 2002;26:209–13.

251. Sheridan RL, Keaney T, Stoddard F, Enfanto R, Kadillack P, Breault L. Short-term propofol infusion as an adjunct to extubation in burned children. J Burn Care Rehabil. 2003;24:356–60.

252. Finkel JC, Elrefai A. The use of dexmedetomidine to facilitate opioid and benzodiazepine detoxification in an infant. Anesth Analg. 2004;98:1658–9.

253. Finkel JC, Johnson YJ, Quezado ZM. The use of dexmedetomidine to facilitate acute discontinuation of opioids after cardiac transplantation in children. Crit Care Med. 2005;33:2110–2.

254. Teng SN, Kaufman J, Czaja AS, Friesen RH, da Cruz EM. Propofol as a bridge to extubation for high-risk children with congenital cardiac disease. Cardiol Young. 2011;21:46–51.

255. Foltin GL, Tunik MG, Cooper A, Markenson D, Treiber M, Phillips R, Karpeles T, editors. Teaching resource for instructors in prehospital pediatrics. New York: Center for Pediatric Emergency Medicine; 1998.

256. Berry FA, editor. Anesthetic management of difficult and routine pediatric patients. 2nd ed. London: Churchill Livingstone; 1990. p. 173.

257. Benumof JL, editor. Airway management: principles and practice. St. Louis: Mosby-Yearbook, Inc; 1996. p. 268.

Pediatric Difficult Airway Management: Principles and Approach in the Critical Care Environment

28

Paul A. Stricker, John Fiadjoe, and Todd J. Kilbaugh

Abstract

Airway management in the child with anatomic features that preclude effective airway management using standard techniques requires an approach tailored to the individual child's anatomy and physiology. Optimal management necessitates careful planning, effective communication, additional equipment, qualified personnel, and appropriate medications. Therefore, training of personnel, implementation of decision algorithms, and acquisition of appropriate equipment are institutional elements that are essential in facilitating the optimal care of these children. This chapter discusses the salient principles in developing an effective approach to difficult airway management in the pediatric intensive care setting. In addition, a selection of devices useful in pediatric difficult airway management is presented. Finally, institutional systems-based considerations for difficult airway management in the critically ill child are discussed. Pediatric difficult airway management in the intensive care environment presents a wide range of challenges. Children in whom airway management is expected to be difficult are often unable to cooperate with awake airway management techniques that are often the primary approach in adult patients. The availability of a variety of indirect laryngoscopes has significantly increased the intensivist's ability to safely manage many of these children in the ICU. Successful airway management in these children requires careful planning, preparation, and often multidisciplinary cooperation.

Keywords

Pediatric • Difficult Airway • Ventilation • Oxygenation • Intubation • Tracheostomy • Rapid Sequence • Laryngoscopy • LMA • Bronchoscopy

P.A. Stricker, MD
Department of Anesthesiology and Critical Care Medicine,
The Children's Hospital of Philadelphia and the Perelman School
of Medicine at the University of Pennsylvania, 34th Street
and Civic Center Boulevard, Philadelphia, PA 19104, USA
e-mail: strickerp@email.chop.edu

J. Fiadjoe, MD
Department of Anesthesiology and Critical Care Medicine,
Children's Hospital of Philadelphia,
34th & Civic Center Blvd, Philadelphia, PA 19104, USA
e-mail: fiadjoe@email.chop.edu

T.J. Kilbaugh, MD (✉)
Department of Anesthesiology and Critical Care Medicine,
Children's Hospital of Philadelphia,
34th Civic Center Blvd, Philadelphia, PA 19147, USA
e-mail: kilbaugh@email.chop.edu

Introduction

The management of the child in whom a standard approach to airway management is difficult presents significant challenges in the intensive care setting. From a physiologic perspective, healthy children and infants have higher oxygen consumption rates, reduced functional residual capacity (FRC), and elevated closing volumes compared to adults. These physiologic characteristics result in rapid oxyhemoglobin desaturation following apnea. Coexistent critical illness (increased oxygen consumption, pulmonary impairment) exacerbates intolerance of apnea and hypoventilation. The clinical impact of these variables on airway management is that there is relatively little time to

D.S. Wheeler et al. (eds.), *Pediatric Critical Care Medicine*,
DOI 10.1007/978-1-4471-6362-6_28, © Springer-Verlag London 2014

secure the airway, especially with apneic intubation techniques.

Airway management in the child with anatomic features that preclude effective airway management using standard techniques requires an approach tailored to the individual child's anatomy and physiology. Optimal management necessitates careful planning, effective communication, additional equipment, qualified personnel, and appropriate medications. Therefore, training of personnel, implementation of decision algorithms, and acquisition of appropriate equipment are institutional elements that are essential in facilitating the optimal care of these children. This chapter discusses the salient principles in developing an effective approach to difficult airway management in the pediatric intensive care setting. In addition, a selection of devices useful in pediatric difficult airway management is presented. Finally, institutional systems-based considerations for difficult airway management in the critically ill child are discussed.

What Is a Difficult Airway?

According to the report by the American Society of Anesthesiologists (ASA) Task Force on Management of the Difficult Airway, a standardized definition of the difficult airway cannot be identified in the literature [1]. The definition suggested by this task force is "The clinical situation in which a conventionally trained anesthesiologist experiences difficulty with face mask ventilation of the upper airway, difficulty with tracheal intubation, or both [1]." As such, the difficult airway is not a single entity or disease state, but a clinical endpoint associated with a wide variety of diseases and conditions (Table 28.1). While there are certain characteristics that predict a difficult airway (Table 28.2), there are many cases in which a difficult airway is unexpected. The extant literature on difficult airway management is replete

Table 28.1 Conditions associated with difficult airway management in children

Cornelia de Lange syndrome	Noonan syndrome	Cri-du-chat
Robin sequence	Klippel-Feil syndrome	Treacher Collin's syndrome
Goldenhar syndrome	TMJ ankylosis	Hunter's syndrome
Arthrogryposis multiplex congenital	Hurler's syndrome	San Fillipo's syndrome
Scleroderma	Hemifacial microsomia	Cervical spine injury
Dystrophic epidermolysis bullosa	Trismus	Cystic hygroma
Nager's syndrome	Epiglottitis	Angioedema
Beckwith-Wiedemann	Fibrodysplasia ossificans progressiva	Presence of halo or other external craniofacial hardware

Table 28.2 Physical examination findings associated with difficult airway management

Micrognathia	Limited mouth opening
Prominent maxillary incisors	Decreased cervical range of motion
Non-compliant submandibular tissues	Increased neck circumference

with cases series and case reports describing various techniques that have been effective in specific scenarios by specific providers. However, owing to the myriad of clinical conditions associated with the difficult airway in children and its relatively low incidence, systematic studies to determine the optimal management are lacking.

Principles of Difficult Airway Management: The ASA Difficult Airway Algorithm

The conduct of prospective randomized clinical trials evaluating various management strategies is problematic, and in general, the approach to the airway must be tailored to the individual patient and the available resources. In 1993, the American Society of Anesthesiologists (ASA) Task Force on Management of the Difficult Airway published a set of practice guidelines for difficult airway management [2]. An update to these guidelines was subsequently published in 2013 [1]. Due in large part to the paucity of high level evidence in the literature, these guidelines were developed based on the available literature and expert opinion/consensus to provide rational guidance to practitioners. The algorithm included in these guidelines (Fig. 28.1) has come to be the bedrock for clinical decision-making in difficult airway management. It is important to note that this algorithm was developed to provide a framework for population management; it *does not* describe specifics of individual patient management. Furthermore, the algorithm represents guidelines that while widely adopted do not necessarily represent standard of care, especially in pediatrics. The following section has been derived and adapted from the ASA Difficult Airway Algorithm [1].

Basic Management Problems

Identification of what fundamental elements of airway management are likely to pose problems is the first step in the process of difficult airway management. Identifying anticipated problems prior to intervention is crucial to allow for proper planning (determination of venue, acquisition of necessary equipment and medication, and expert consultation) and promotes successful and safe patient care. The potential for five primary problems should be considered: difficult ventilation, difficult intubation, difficult supraglottic airway placement, difficulty with cooperation, and difficult tracheostomy.

Fig. 28.1 American Society of Anesthesiologist difficult airway algorithm (Reprinted from [1]. With permission from Wolter Kluwers Health)

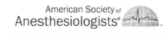

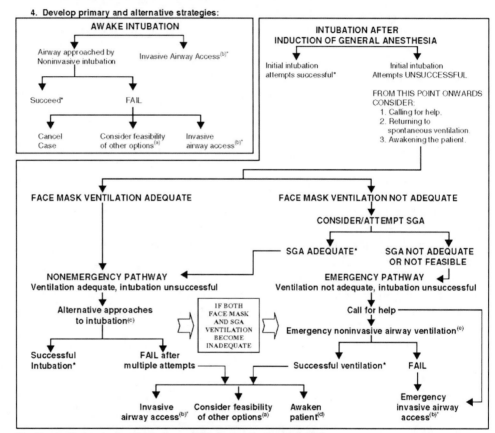

American Society of
Anesthesiologists®

DIFFICULT AIRWAY ALGORITHM

1. **Assess the likelihood and clinical impact of basic management problems:**
   - Difficulty with patient cooperation or consent
   - Difficult mask ventilation
   - Difficult supraglottic airway placement
   - Difficult laryngoscopy
   - Difficult intubation
   - Difficult surgical airway access

2. **Actively pursue opportunities to deliver supplemental oxygen throughout the process of difficult airway management.**

3. **Consider the relative merits and feasibility of basic management choices:**
   - Awake intubation *vs.* intubation after induction of general anesthesia
   - Non-invasive technique *vs.* invasive techniques for the initial approach to intubation
   - Video-assisted laryngoscopy as an initial approach to intubation
   - Preservation *vs.* ablation of spontaneous ventilation

4. **Develop primary and alternative strategies:**

*Confirm ventilation, tracheal intubation, or SGA placement with exhaled CO_2

a. Other options include (but are not limited to): surgery utilizing face mask or supraglottic airway (SGA) anesthesia (e.g., LMA, ILMA, laryngeal tube), local anesthesia infiltration or regional nerve blockade. Pursuit of these options usually implies that mask ventilation will not be problematic. Therefore, these options may be of limited value if this step in the algorithm has been reached via the Emergency Pathway.

b. Invasive airway access includes surgical or percutaneous airway, jet ventilation, and retrograde intubation.

c. Alternative difficult intubation approaches include (but are not limited to): video-assisted laryngoscopy, alternative laryngoscope blades, SGA (e.g., LMA or ILMA) as an intubation conduit (with or without fiberoptic guidance), fiberoptic intubation, intubating stylet or tube changer, light wand, and blind oral or nasal intubation.

d. Consider re-preparation of the patient for awake intubation or canceling surgery.

e. Emergency non-invasive airway ventilation consists of a SGA.

Difficult Ventilation

The ability to deliver effective ventilation of the upper airway by facemask is of critical importance, and should be emphasized to trainees and in continuing medical education. Patients who present challenges to facemask ventilation represent an extremely high-risk group of patients. If difficult facemask ventilation is identified by physical exam findings (such as patients who have had head and neck irradiation, patients with upper airway space occupying lesions, burn patients with neck contractures) [3] or by history, expert consultation is strongly advised. The Han scale (Table 28.3) is a simple and useful tool for defining difficult facemask

Table 28.3 Han scale for grading ease of facemask ventilation

Grade	Description
1	Ventilated by mask
2	Ventilated by mask with oral airway/adjuvant with or without muscle relaxant
3	Difficult ventilation (inadequate, unstable, or requiring two providers) with or without muscle relaxant
4	Unable to mask ventilate with or without muscle relaxant

ventilation [4]. Using a definition of difficult ventilation as a 3 or 4 on this scale, the incidence of difficult facemask ventilation has been reported in adults as being anywhere from 1.4 to 2.2 % [5, 6]. The only available study that assessed the incidence of difficult mask ventilation in children reported a similar incidence of 2.1 % in *non-obese* children [7].

Difficult Intubation

The majority of patients who are identified as being "difficult intubations" are in fact patients in whom glottic exposure with direct laryngoscopy is difficult. Thankfully, many (but not all) patients in whom direct laryngoscopy is difficult can be readily managed with an alternative device. A good example is the child with cervical spine immobility who presents no challenges to facemask ventilation and is readily managed with indirect (video) laryngoscopy. Difficult direct laryngoscopy is not the only reason patients may be classified as being difficult to intubate; abnormal tracheal anatomy in some patients may make tracheal tube passage difficult. Such patients require a similarly carefully planned management approach. Intensivists should suspect a difficult direct laryngoscopy in patients with obvious craniofacial anomalies such as micrognathia, hemifacial microsomia, and less obvious findings such as microtia, inability to open the mouth, and cervical spine immobility.

Difficult Supraglottic Airway Insertion/Placement

The development and release into clinical practice of the LMA (laryngeal mask airway) by Dr. Archie Brain in 1985 revolutionized airway management. Subsequent development of second generation devices that allow for gastric drainage tube insertion has further improved the utility of these devices. More recently, supraglottic airway devices with design features that facilitate their use as conduits for tracheal intubation have further expanded the functionality of this group of airway devices. Consequently, identification of those patients in whom supraglottic airway use is not feasible can be critically important as these devices can provide life-saving ventilation in patients difficult to ventilate by facemask.

Difficulty with Patient Cooperation

Securing the airway in the awake or lightly sedated patient is regarded by many as the safest approach to airway management. Adults, adolescents, and older children with sufficient adaptability and coping skills are able to cooperate with airway management techniques while awake or mildly sedated. However, most pediatric patients lack the requisite understanding and coping skills for these techniques to be effective, and therefore require relatively deep levels of sedation or anesthesia. Furthermore, critical illness may limit a child's physiologic reserve and interfere with a child's ability to cooperate with awake/lightly sedated techniques. The ASA guidelines acknowledge this particular challenge in pediatrics, where it is stated that "airway management in the uncooperative or pediatric patient may require an approach (e.g. intubation attempts after induction of general anesthesia) that might not be regarded as the primary approach in a cooperative patient [1]."

Difficult Tracheostomy

Performance of a tracheostomy or emergent cricothyrotomy may be the best primary means of securing the airway in some children. However, even elective tracheostomies are difficult to perform in small children, even by experienced pediatric surgeons. In fact, some children have anatomic abnormalities (flexed/fused neck or very short neck) that make a tracheostomy nearly impossible to perform. Anticipation of difficult tracheostomy may mandate expert consultation and interdisciplinary planning of what airway management strategy to pursue and which venue (ICU vs. operating room) is the best location to attempt airway management.

Basic Management Choices

The ASA algorithm next instructs practitioners to consider three basic management choices: awake intubation vs. intubation attempts after the induction of general anesthesia, non-invasive vs. invasive technique for initial approach to intubation, and whether to preserve or ablate spontaneous ventilation.

Awake Intubation vs. Anesthetized Intubation

An awake or lightly sedated approach to tracheal intubation is often regarded as the safest strategy because conscious control of breathing (respiratory drive) is not impaired and protective airway reflexes are preserved. Awake intubation requires anesthesia of the pharynx/nasopharynx and upper airway and requires specific training. This technique also requires a cooperative patient, which is often a barrier in pediatrics. Another important barrier to the use of this technique in infants and small children is the weight-based limitation of local anesthetic dosages to achieve airway anesthesia. This makes awake/sedated approaches more difficult in children, and consequently compared with adults, difficult pediatric airways are more commonly managed under deep sedation or anesthesia. Although anesthesiologists are trained in difficult airway skills, most do not have subspecialty training in pediatrics and for many it is an infrequent event to secure a difficult pediatric airway and the set of skills required is different from an adult difficult airway. For the intensivist directing a transport of a critically ill child with a difficult airway to a higher level of care at a specialized pediatric center from a center without pediatric anesthesiologists, this should be taken into account in the medical decision making for a safe and effective transport of a critically ill child.

Non-invasive vs. Invasive Technique for Initial Approach to Intubation

In some cases, the optimal initial technique may be invasive. Invasive techniques include tracheostomy (surgical or percutaneous) and cricothyrotomy. It is fortunately rare that these techniques are required. In these cases expert consultation with an otolaryngologist and anesthesiologist is a necessity; further discussion is beyond the scope of this text.

Preservation vs. Ablation of Spontaneous Ventilation

Spontaneous ventilation can be ablated by sedative/hypnotic agents as well as by administration of muscle relaxants. It is important to emphasize that the administration of muscle relaxant medications should be accompanied by hypnotic agents in most patients. In managing the difficult airway, the ASA guidelines implore practitioners to "actively pursue opportunities to deliver supplemental oxygen throughout the process of difficult airway management." One of the principal advantages of preservation of spontaneous ventilation is gas exchange, which helps maintain oxygen saturation during intubation attempts. Additionally, spontaneously breathing patients may have preserved upper airway muscle tone to help maintain airway patency. However, there are some pitfalls with maintaining spontaneous ventilation. An inadequate level of anesthesia or sedation can interfere with the intubation attempt, as the child may cough or gag, the child may have inadequate jaw relaxation, or the child may develop laryngospasm.

Ablation of spontaneous ventilation with neuromuscular blockade is advantageous in some scenarios. With neuromuscular blockade the advantages are that the patient is motionless and does not cough, the jaw is relaxed, and laryngospasm is not a risk. Some of the potential disadvantages of neuromuscular blockade are essentially the opposites of the advantages spontaneous ventilation—namely that there is potential for upper airway soft tissue collapse with loss of the ability to ventilate, and arterial desaturation during prolonged intubation attempts. Another disadvantage is that manual positive pressure ventilation may result in gastric insufflation, causing compromised ventilation (through abdominal competition) and/or regurgitation of gastric contents. This can be particularly problematic in infants and smaller children where an inflated stomach can significantly reduce functional residual capacity.

Preparation

The most important aspect for successful management of the difficult airway is adequate preparation. This cannot be emphasized enough. Failure to secure the airway is often related to inadequate preparation, which may be in the form of inadequate planning, backup equipment, or available personnel. Performing a thorough history and physical examination with attention to the airway informs the consideration of the basic management problems and management choices described above. This is especially helpful during the postoperative hand-off from anesthesia providers to intensive care team members following surgical procedures. A critical aspect of the transition of care should be description of bag-mask ventilation and intubation, including: view of larynx, equipment used, personnel required, and number of attempts. With or without this information, intensivists should quickly develop a detailed management plan once the decision is made to secure the airway. This plan should address four components:

1. A primary and secondary plan to maintain oxygenation and ventilation throughout the intubation process
2. A primary and secondary plan for intubation
3. Additional personnel and expert consultation
4. A rescue plan for a cannot ventilate/cannot intubate scenario

A suggested algorithm for decision-making in the management of the anticipated difficult airway is presented in Fig. 28.2. While developing primary and backup strategies is crucial, of equal importance is ensuring that the equipment, medications, and appropriate personnel are ready and immediately available to implement them. Once sedatives/hypnotic agents or muscle relaxants have been given, the ability to set up and troubleshoot equipment is limited. A selection of suggested equipment and medications that should be available during any intubation attempt in the ICU is presented in Table 28.4.

Venue

Selection of the optimal venue for managing the airway of a critically ill child is dynamic and must take into account a wide range of patient-specific variables. When consulted, anesthesiologists and otolaryngologists often prefer to

Fig. 28.2 A decision-making guide for management of the anticipated difficult pediatric airway

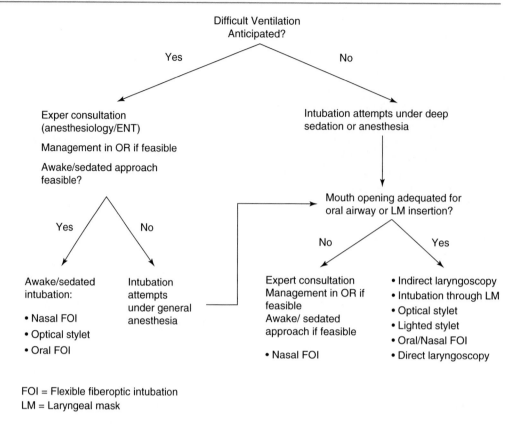

FOI = Flexible fiberoptic intubation
LM = Laryngeal mask

Table 28.4 Suggested bedside equipment and medications for tracheal intubation in the ICU

Ventilation adjuncts:

　Facemasks- expected size and a size larger and smaller

　Oral airways- expected size and a size larger and smaller

　Nasopharyngeal airways- expected size and a size larger and smaller

　Laryngeal mask airway- expected size and a size larger and smaller

Tracheal tubes:

　Full complement of cuffed pediatric size tubes (3.0–8.0 mm I.D.)

　Uncuffed pediatric tubes (2.5–5.0 mm I.D.)

　Tracheal tube stylets in sizes for use in various tube sizes

Medications:

　Atropine

　Succinylcholine

　Non-depolarizing muscle relaxant (e.g. vecuronium)

　Sedative/hypnotic (e.g. Midazolam, propofol, ketamine, dexmedetomidine)

　Opioid (e.g. fentanyl)

　Oxymetazoline spray (nasal intubations)

Laryngoscopes:

　Standard laryngoscope with full complement of curved and straight blades

　Indirect laryngoscope with appropriate size blade

Miscellaneous items:

　Water-based lubricant jelly

　Tongue depressor

　Functioning suction

manage the airway in the operating room environment. However, this requires patient transport, which is time consuming and may interfere with delivery of concomitant medical management. The risks of transporting unstable patients often outweigh the benefits of having consultants manage the airway in their most familiar environment. Also, the increasing availability and more widespread use of indirect laryngoscopy in the intensive care setting have made this environment appropriate for difficult airway management in many cases. To this end, an appropriately equipped difficult airway cart should be readily available in the ICU. Suggested contents of such a cart are described later in this chapter. Having a difficult airway cart in the ICU ensures that critical equipment is available to care for patients who cannot be transported to the operating room.

Determination of the preferred venue for airway management requires close multidisciplinary coordination led by the intensive care team. In making this decision, one caveat to consider is when an infant or child is at high risk for the need of a surgical airway. Often this is difficult to predict; however, if the multidisciplinary team has time and transport is possible our institution prefers to attempt these intubation in an operating room with proper lighting, table, and surgical assistants. This may provide a significant advantage to surgeons to quickly and safely obtain a surgical airway.

Table 28.5 Comparison of three sedation regimens for airway management

	Midazolam/ fentanyl	High-dose dexmedetomidine	Ketamine
Sedation	++	+	++
Analgesia	++	+	+++
Amnesia	++	±	+++
Reversible	Yes	No	No
Clinician familiarity	+++	±	++
Pt responsive to commands	+	+	No
Respiratory drive	–	++	+
Adjuncts required	No	±	No

Pharmacologic Management

Sedation for Intubation with Spontaneous Ventilation Maintained

The goals of sedation for tracheal intubation with spontaneous ventilation are to provide patient comfort (sedation, analgesia, and amnesia), maintain hemodynamic stability, maintain airway patency and breathing, maintain oxyhemoglobin saturation, and provide satisfactory conditions for intubation. There is a paucity of evidence supporting one regimen over another. A comparison of four different sedation regimens in terms of various desirable properties is presented in Table 28.5

Benzodiazepine and Opiates

The combination of a benzodiazepine and an opiate is one the most commonly used regimen in pediatric patients. One report of this technique describes a series of children with difficult intubation sedated with midazolam (0.05 mg/kg) and remifentanil (0.75 mcg/kg bolus over 60 s followed by an infusion of 0.075 mcg/kg), topical anesthesia was applied to the airway and all patients were intubated successfully while maintaining spontaneous ventilation throughout [8]. Remifentanil should be titrated slowly as apnea and muscle rigidity are a known consequences of higher doses (3 mcg/ kg) [9]. Advantages of this regimen are that it provides sedation, analgesia, and amnesia. Also, physicians and nurses are familiar with administration of these agents, and antagonists are available in the event of excessive effect. However, respiratory drive can be profoundly impaired, and these drugs may cause hemodynamic compromise by decreasing sympathetic tone when given in combination and high dosage.

Dexmedetomidine

Dexmedetomidine, an alpha-2-agonist, has been used in adults to facilitate tracheal intubation [10, 11] and has been used as the sole anesthetic in infants undergoing bronchoscopy [12]. Demedetomidine use in pediatric difficult airway management has also been reported [13–15]. It should be noted that this is an "off-label" use of dexmedetomidine. The utility of this agent in the critical care environment as part of a difficult intubation regimen remains understudied. Dexmedetomidine has several favorable qualities that make it potentially useful in the pediatric ICU. First, dexmedetomidine provides sedation and analgesia, while preserving respiratory drive. Second, pediatric intensivists are increasingly familiar with its administration. Potential limitations are that it is not reversible, may cause hemodynamic effects (bradycardia, hypertension) [16] that may not be tolerated in a critically ill child. A common dosing scheme is to administer 1 mcg/kg followed by an infusion of 0.5–7 mcg/kg/h. While this may achieve satisfactory sedation, many children will require higher doses (3 mcg/kg bolus followed by an infusion of 2 mcg/kg/h) similar to what has been reported for sedation for radiologic imaging studies in children [17]. To achieve satisfactory conditions for airway management, dexmedetomidine has been combined with topically administered lidocaine [14], small incremental doses of ketamine (0.25 mg/kg) [18], or midazolam [19] titrated to effect.

Ketamine

Ketamine is attractive for use an agent for sedation for airway management due to its ability as a standalone agent to provide sedation, profound analgesia, and amnesia, while usually preserving respiratory drive [20]. However, there is no antagonist available and the dissociative anesthetic state produced by ketamine precludes effective communication with the child. In many scenarios ketamine preserves blood pressure and hemodynamics by acting as a sympathomimetic promoting catecholamine release, however in critically ill patients with catecholamine depleted states hemodynamic compromise may occur [21].

Neuromuscular Blockade

Neuromuscular blockade may be useful to create optimal intubating conditions and may improve the ability to deliver manual ventilation by facemask [5, 22, 23]. As described above, administration of muscle relaxants may carry the risk of worsening ventilation in some patients which could result in a catastrophic "cannot intubate, cannot ventilate" situation, making the use of neuromuscular blockade for difficult airway management controversial. Changes to this debate may be on the horizon, and practice will evolve as the drugs we use evolve. A new cyclodextrin agent, Sugammadex, has been developed which gives the ability to rapidly reverse profound neuromuscular blockade from rocuronium and vecuronium [24, 25]. This agent binds to these non-depolarizing neuromuscular blockers with reversal of clinical effect. If this medication becomes commercially available in the US, as it has in parts of Europe, many clinicians may reconsider how they approach the question of whether or not to administer these neuromuscular blocking drugs in patients with an anticipated difficult airway.

Succinylcholine

In the absence of the availability to reverse profound neuromuscular blockade from non-depolarizing agents, one of the risks of administering these drugs is that it commits the patient to non-reversible clinical effect for at least 20 min depending on the class of the agent. If neuromuscular blockade is considered as part of plan to manage a pediatric difficult airway, then the short acting depolarizing neuromuscular blocker succinylcholine may be a reasonable option due to the fact that it has a relatively short time to functional recovery of the diaphragm and airway reflexes of 8–10 min [26]. In 1994, the U.S. Food and Drug Administration applied a black box warning stating that succinylcholine is contraindicated for use in routine pediatric airway management, recommending its use be reserved for emergency intubations and when there is a need to immediately secure the airway. However, the need to secure the airway in the critically ill child with an anticipated difficult airway does not constitute "routine" airway management, and in the absence of specific contraindications, the use of succinylcholine in this setting is acceptable and may be advantageous. Furthermore, the possibility of giving succinylcholine should be considered since it is a primary treatment of laryngospasm which may develop and complicate attempts at tracheal intubation in the sedated and spontaneously breathing child.

Airway Management Equipment

Ventilation Adjuncts

The ability to deliver or maintain effective ventilation is of prime importance throughout the process of difficult airway management. In fact, the feature that divides the ASA difficult airway algorithm into the "non-emergency" and "emergency" pathways is the determination of adequacy of ventilation. In the case where the initial intubation attempt has failed but ventilation remains adequate, it is important to call for help rather than perseverating with the intubation technique that has initially failed. *Proper technique and continual training for facemask ventilation is crucial for success.* Upper airway obstruction should initially be managed with a chin lift/jaw thrust and extension of the neck (when not contraindicated) combined with positive airway pressure [27–29]. In contrast to the plethora of tools that are available for tracheal intubation, the tools that are available to help

ventilate children are limited to the oral airway, the nasal airway, the modified nasal trumpet, two-person two-handed mask ventilation, and the laryngeal mask (and other supraglottic airways).

Oral Airways

Insertion of an oral airway frequently relieves airway obstruction. The proper size is selected by holding the airway next to the child's face—the proper sized airway has its distal tip lying just beyond the angle of the mandible when the proximal end is held by the mouth. Oral airways are in general poorly tolerated by awake or lightly sedated children and may trigger unwanted events, such as: coughing, vomiting, and laryngospasm.

Nasopharyngeal Airways

Insertion of a nasopharyngeal airway is better tolerated in awake or lightly sedated children. The proper sized airway has its distal tip lying 2–3 cm inferior to the space between the angle of the mandible and the tragus. The most common complication of insertion is epistaxis, which may complicate subsequent intubation attempts by impairing visualization. The risk of epistaxis and its severity can be reduced by administration of topical vasoconstrictors (phenylephrine, oxymetazoline) to the nasal mucosa prior to insertion.

Modified Nasopharyngeal Airway

A standard nasopharyngeal airway can be modified by inserting the 15 mm adaptor from an endotracheal tube into the proximal opening. This modified nasopharyngeal airway is a useful ventilation adjunct; it can be connected to a bag-valve device and used to deliver positive pressure ventilation when the opposite naris and mouth are held closed [30, 31]. Alternatively, this device can be connected to a mapleson circuit and used to deliver supplemental oxygen and continuous positive airway pressure.

Two-Person, Two-Handed Ventilation

Converting from a single provider ventilation technique to a two-person, two-handed technique can result in dramatic improvement in the effectiveness of manual ventilation. Converting to this technique helps improve mask seal, optimizes head/jaw position, and should be among the primary steps taken to manage inadequate or suboptimal facemask ventilation. It is critical to understand that children requiring a two-person two-handed technique should be regarded as being difficult to ventilate [4, 5].

Laryngeal Mask and Supraglottic Airways

The laryngeal mask airway was initially introduced into clinical practice in 1985 [32], and pediatric versions became available soon thereafter. The laryngeal mask airway represents one of the most important airway management tools available and has changed the approach to rescue ventilation and management of difficult airways. Insertion of the laryngeal mask mimics the path of a food bolus. The index finger of the dominant hand is placed at the junction of the lubricated deflated mask and its airway tube, and the tip of the mask is pressed cranially along the hard palate and is advanced along the palate until the tip rests at the upper esophageal inlet. Correct technique is important to ensure adequate placement and to minimize complications. Insertion of this device is quickly learned with a high success rate even for novices [33, 34]. Effective ventilation is often delivered even when the position is suboptimal [35]. According to the ASA difficult airway algorithm, insertion of a laryngeal mask is the first step that should be considered or attempted should ventilation become difficult or inadequate. It is important that pediatric intensivists be facile with placement of these devices and this skill should be part of continuing medical education for pediatric ICU staff. A number of variations of the original Laryngeal Mask Airway (LMA North America, San Diego CA, USA) have become available. Available data does not show that one version is far superior to another in the pediatric population. Practitioners should trial different variations to find the one they feel most comfortable with for the use in critically ill children in their institution. In addition to being tremendously valuable as ventilation adjuncts, laryngeal masks can be used as conduits for fiberoptic intubation [36–40], and have become indispensible in difficult airway algorithms in most institutions including our own. Some laryngeal masks, such as the air-Q (Mercury Medical, Clearwater FL, USA) have been designed specifically for use as intubation conduits. Blind intubation through a laryngeal mask is not recommended [41, 42] because the epiglottis frequently overlies the laryngeal aperture of the laryngeal mask [35] and would be traumatized with blind tube insertion, which could lead to edema, glottic obstruction, and compromised ventilation.

Tracheal Intubation Tools

In the past, equipment appropriate for the management of difficult tracheal intubation in children was limited. In recent years there has been a proliferation of devices to manage the difficult airway. Many of the devices that were originally developed for use in adults are now available in pediatric sizes. Presented below is an overview and discussion of some of the various devices available for use in children with attention to the advantages and limitations of each.

Direct Laryngoscopy

There are situations in which it is reasonable to attempt intubation by direct laryngoscopy in the child in whom a difficult intubation is suspected. It is vital in these situations that failure of direct laryngoscopy is anticipated and backup strategies have been readied accordingly. When difficult direct laryngoscopy is anticipated and an attempt at direct laryngoscopy is planned, the laryngoscopy should be performed by the most skilled laryngoscopist available to limit the number of attempts. Laryngoscopy attempts should not be made by a novice in a child with a known or suspected difficult airway. The number of attempts should be limited (one or two), as repeated attempts may create edema or bleeding which can lead to difficulty with ventilation and may also make subsequent intubation attempts more difficult. Direct laryngoscopy may be a reasonable initial approach in the child where direct laryngoscopy is suspected to be difficult but there is no history to confirm difficulty, facemask ventilation is not expected to be problematic, and intubation by an alternative means can be readily accomplished. Another situation where an initial intubation approach using direct laryngoscopy would be appropriate may be in a child who was previously difficult but the interval history suggests that intubation by direct laryngoscopy is feasible, and facemask ventilation is not expected to be problematic. Direct laryngoscopy should not be attempted when a recent direct laryngoscopy by an experienced laryngoscopist was difficult. Likewise, if the history and physical examination are highly predictive of failed direct laryngoscopy, there is no value in attempting direct laryngoscopy to prove this. In this situation, direct laryngoscopy is only likely to confound subsequent intubation attempts and should be avoided. A right retro- molar approach to direct laryngoscopy is a reasonable technique in some scenarios to attempt when standard direct laryngoscopy fails. The blade is inserted in the extreme corner of the mouth thereby shortening the distance to the larynx and minimizing the intrusion of maxillary structures into the line of sight. If this technique has not been attempted and practiced on a regular basis, it should not be attempted.

Flexible Bronchoscope

The flexible bronchoscope is undoubtedly the most versatile intubation instrument available and remains an indispensable tool for difficult airway management. While this is the most versatile tool, the flexible bronchoscope has some drawbacks. First, it is not an intuitive device to use, and it takes a lot of practice to acquire and maintain the skill set required for its use. This alone makes it an impractical tool for many pediatric intensivists, and underlines the necessity of team approach with pediatric anesthesiologists in approaching difficult airways. Furthermore, the presence of fogging, blood and secretions can make intubation difficult. Also, bronchoscopes are expensive, they require specific protocols for cleaning, and they break easily when improperly handled. These limitations have in large part created a demand for alternative devices. It should be remembered, however, that the flexible bronchoscope is the *only* intubation tool that can be used in certain scenarios, such as in children with severely limited mouth opening.

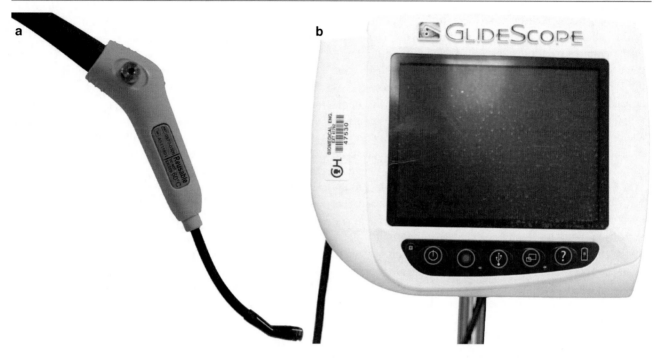

Fig. 28.3 (a) Glidescope Cobalt. A reusable video baton that delivers an image to a portable monitor. The video baton inserts into different sized curved plastic disposable laryngoscopy blades. Various sizes of the disposable blade are available, and are suitable for use in neonates through adults. (b) Glidescope Cobalt video screen

Video/Indirect Laryngoscopes

Video and indirect laryngoscopes (also known as optical laryngoscopes) have become attractive devices for airway management in large part because the mechanical skill set they employ is similar to what is used for direct laryngoscopy, making them intuitive to use. The principal advantage of these devices in managing the difficult airway is that a direct line-of-sight (from the eye to the glottis) does not need to be achieved, and so many of the anatomic obstacles to achieving visualization of the glottis with direct laryngoscopy (such as cervical immobility, retrognathia) are circumvented and excellent glottic exposure can be readily achieved. Furthermore, because direct line-of-sight visualization is not needed, intubations with indirect laryngoscopes can be performed with little or no neck extension, making them attractive for use in cases of cervical instability. While tracheal intubation using indirect laryngoscopy has many advantages, it is not without limitations. Importantly, each device has a minimum amount of mouth opening that is required, and as such these devices cannot be used if mouth opening is severely restricted. Although they can be used to facilitate nasotracheal intubation, they function best for oral intubations. As with any optical device, fogging, blood, and secretions can make visualization problematic. Finally, while the mechanical skill set is similar to direct laryngoscopy, it is important to recognize that it is a different skill set, and although glottic visualization may be readily achieved, tracheal tube passage may still prove difficult. It is the dexterity of movement to manipulate the endotracheal tube to the glottis opening and into the trachea that often requires the most practice and skill to successfully intubate a child with a difficult airway using indirect laryngoscopy. There are several indirect laryngoscopes available is sizes appropriate for infants and children. A discussion of a selection of these devices follows below.

Bullard Laryngoscope

The Bullard Laryngoscope was introduced into clinical practice in 1989 by Dr. Roger Bullard, an obstetric anesthesiologist who is the father of modern indirect laryngoscopy. The Bullard Laryngoscope has a low profile metal blade that delivers an image from near the blade tip to an eyepiece through a combination of fiber optics and mirrors. It has an incorporated metal stylet that the tracheal tube is loaded onto which directs the tube toward the field of view as the tube is advanced. While this device is not currently in widespread use, it is important to mention since all of the other modern indirect laryngoscopes are essentially variations on Dr. Bullard's device; his innovation was the starting point for the devices available today.

Glidescope Cobalt

The Glidescope Cobalt (Verathon, Bothwell, WA, USA) is a video laryngoscope that has a reusable video baton that delivers an image to a portable monitor (Fig. 28.3). The video baton inserts into different sized curved plastic disposable laryngoscopy blades. Various sizes of the disposable blade are available, and are suitable for use in neonates through adults. A smaller baton is required for the smaller pediatric blades. The incorporated light source of this device warms the clear plastic blade which helps prevent fogging. Another advantage is the portability of the device- it is relatively lightweight and comes on a stand that can be quickly moved where it is needed. Setup is simple, and it is intuitive to use. There have been a few validation studies evaluating the Glidescope for use in normal pediatric airways [43–45], and a number of case reports describing its use in difficult pediatric airways [46–48]. As with other methods of indirect laryngoscopy, the use of the glidescope may be precluded in patients with limited mouth opening. In addition, despite the ease with which a satisfactory view of the larynx can be achieved, practice is necessary to develop the skills to advance the tube into the trachea.

Storz Video Laryngoscope

The Storz Direct Coupled Interface (DCI) Video laryngoscope (Karl Storz GmbH, Tuttlingen, Germany) is a video device that integrates fiberoptics and a lens into a metal blade with the shape of conventional Miller and Macintosh blades. The blade connects to a device-specific camera, which transmits the fiberoptic image from near the tip of the blade to a video monitor. One advantage of these video laryngoscope blades is that they can be used for direct laryngoscopy; therefore, if the direct laryngoscopy view is poor the operator can convert to using the video monitor view. This is particularly useful in children who are suspected but not known to be difficult to intubate by direct laryngoscopy. Unlike many other video systems the Storz Miller 1 video laryngoscope allows documentation of the direct laryngoscopy grade prior to intubating using video guidance. There have been a number of studies looking at the Storz Video Laryngoscope in children with normal airways [49, 50], with the results generally showing improved laryngoscopic views with slightly longer intubation times. The Storz Miller 1 video laryngoscope has also been shown to improve laryngoscopy grade and intubation success in a difficult airway manikin model [51]. The Storz Video Laryngoscope is a useful adjunct in the management of the difficult infant airway, and at our center is a popular tool to rescue infants in whom direct laryngoscopy has failed.

Airtraq

The Airtraq Optical Laryngoscope (Prodol Meditec S.A., Vizcaya, Spain) is an excellent example of a modern device incorporating improvements of the innovative features of the Bullard laryngoscope (Fig. 28.4). It is an optical laryngoscope that has a curved, low profile blade. Along the side of the device is a channel that the tube is loaded into that directs it towards the center of the field of view when it is advanced.

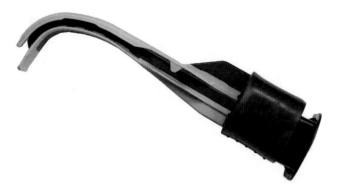

Fig. 28.4 Airtraq Optical Laryngoscope. An optical laryngoscope that has a curved, low profile blade. Along the side of the device is a channel that the tube is loaded into that directs it towards the center of the field of view

A magnified wide-angle image from near the tip of the device is delivered to the eyepiece from the lens using prisms and mirrors; there are no fiberoptics. The incorporated light source warms the lens, which makes fogging less of a problem. Guidance of the endotracheal tube using the airtraq is different from other video laryngoscopes without a channel in that it requires the manipulation of the entire device to direct tube. The Airtraq is the only optical laryngoscope that is completely disposable. Furthermore, each unit is relatively inexpensive, it is as portable as a standard laryngoscope, it requires minimal setup, and it can be purchased and stored without need for maintenance. All of these properties make the airtraq particularly attractive for use in intensive care units, emergency rooms, and for use by specialized transport teams. The Airtraq is available in pediatric and infant sizes. While there are models without the tube-directing channel that can be used for nasotracheal intubations, however for difficult airway management this device is best used for orotracheal intubation.

Optical Stylets

Optical stylets are rigid metal stylets onto which a tracheal tube is loaded that deliver an image from the stylet's tip to an eyepiece through fiber optics. The optical stylet can be a useful adjunct in the management of routine and difficult pediatric intubations [15, 52–54]. It is an uncomplicated tool that is easily learned, portable, and simple to prepare. There are presently two commercially available pediatric sized models available in the U.S.- the Shikani Optical Stylet (Clarus Medical, Minneapolis, MN, USA) and the Storz Bonfils (Karl Storz GmbH, Tuttlingen, Germany) (Fig. 28.5). Many find navigation of the tip of an optical stylet to be more intuitive than navigation with a flexible bronchoscope. With optical stylet intubation, the tip of the stylet is positioned at the glottic inlet and the tracheal tube is then advanced off of the stylet into the trachea. Because these devices are rigid they can be used to displace soft tissue. Like indirect

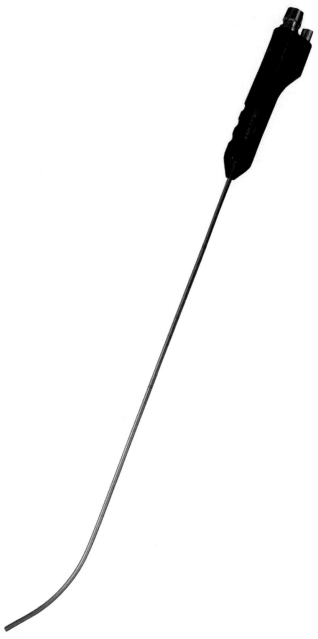

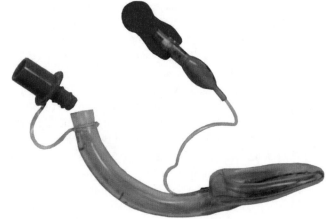

Fig. 28.6 Air-Q Laryngeal mask airway specifically designed for use as conduits for tracheal intubation

Laryngeal Masks as Intubation Conduits

Laryngeal masks continue to have an important place in the management of the challenging pediatric airway. They are useful both as ventilation adjuncts and as conduits for tracheal intubation. Since the development of the original laryngeal mask airway, there has been a proliferation of new supraglottic airway devices for use in adults and children. While some models fail to offer significant design improvements, others have improved on the original design by Dr. Brain [55], making specific modifications to facilitate pediatric use. Some of these, such as the Air-Q (LMA North America, San Diego CA, USA) (Fig. 28.6) have been specifically designed for use as conduits for tracheal intubation. Laryngeal masks remain a critically important adjunct in the airway management of the infants and neonates. One advantage to using a laryngeal mask as an intubation conduit is that ventilation is readily established between and even during intubation attempts. Intubation through a laryngeal mask should be performed under fiberoptic guidance only. Blind intubation through a laryngeal mask is not recommended in children [41, 42]. The use of a laryngeal mask as an intubation conduit likely requires expert consultation; the nuanced skill set for performing this technique requires practice to acquire and maintain.

The Air-Q (Mercury Medical) is a curved laryngeal mask that has unique characteristics that facilitate fiberoptic intubation with cuffed endotracheal tubes in infants and neonates without the need to performing additional maneuvers. The airway tube is wide enough to accommodate the pilot balloon of standard endotracheal tubes and the length is shortened to facilitate the removal of the mask after tracheal intubation. The 15 mm adapter on the airway tube is detachable which facilitates passage of the pilot balloon of a cuffed tube following fiberoptic intubation through the device. As with other laryngeal masks, it is easy to insert and position and full glottic visualization is readily achieved when the fiberoptic bronchoscope is advanced to the laryngeal

Fig. 28.5 Storz Bonfils. Optical stylets are rigid metal stylets onto which a tracheal tube is loaded that deliver an image from the stylet's tip to an eyepiece through fiber optics

laryngoscopes, intubation can be performed without extending the neck. These devices are portable, and are relatively inexpensive, and they can be used on patients of all ages. Limitations include the learning curve with these devices, and visualization problems due to fogging, blood, and secretions in the airway may make intubation difficult. Other disadvantages include a short optical depth of field and the potential for impaired visualization from fogging and secretions. Finally, when not used with a camera and video display, the operator may lose sight of position in the airway when his/her attention is directed through the eyepiece.

aperture of the device. The manufacturer supplies a stabilizer bar that is used to stabilize the tracheal tube as the air-Q is removed. The air-Q is a useful adjunct in management of difficult pediatric airway management that addresses several issues that can make the use of laryngeal masks as intubation conduits in the smallest patients challenging.

The Unanticipated Difficult Airway

When an airway proves unexpectedly difficult, the degree of preparation discussed above has often not been done. Nonetheless, practitioners should have alternative plans for airway management every time an intubation is planned, including plans for managing unexpected difficulties. All of the appropriate ventilation adjuncts should be available, and an alternative plan for tracheal intubation other than direct laryngoscopy should be in place. Failure at initial intubation attempts should trigger escalation of care in the form of calling for help and readying additional equipment. Simulation offers an attractive approach to preparing for managing an unexpected difficult airway. Deficiencies of equipment and institutional preparedness as well as provider decision-making skills can be identified and addressed, allowing for potential patient harm to be averted.

Systems Management

Safe and effective difficult pediatric airway management is fostered by the presence of a number of institutional factors. These include (but are not limited to) the dedication of adequate institutional resources toward the acquisition and maintenance of appropriate equipment, implementation of management algorithms and triggers for escalation of care, and educational activities to develop and maintain the skills required for the care of these children.

In terms of equipment, a pediatric difficult airway cart should be available in several critical locations at any institution managing critically ill children, and we suggest that all carts are identical in equipment and placement. Suggested contents of a pediatric difficult airway cart are listed in Table 28.6.

Escalation of care should be discussed at individual institutions and specific protocols put into place for critical situations. An example of an escalation of care trigger might be that a policy is implemented whereby three failed intubation attempts using direct laryngoscopy mandates a call for help, reassessment of the intubation strategy, and use of an alternative intubation device. Institutions should also have in place mechanisms to ensure providers acquire and maintain the requisite skills. For example, simulation programs can help foster an effective nursing and physician team approach for airway management in the ICU. Development

Table 28.6 Suggested contents of a pediatric difficult airway cart

Ventilation adjuncts:
Facemasks, sizes neonate-adult
Oral airways, sizes – expected neonate-adult
Nasopharyngeal airways- sizes 12 French- 34 French
Laryngeal mask airway- Full complement of sizes
Tracheal tubes:
Full complement of cuffed pediatric size tubes (3.0–8.0 mm I.D.)
Uncuffed pediatric tubes (2.5–5.0 mm I.D.)
Tracheal tube stylets in sizes for use in various tube sizes
Medications:
2 % Lidocaine
Viscous lidocaine
Oxymetazoline spray
Laryngoscopes:
Standard laryngoscope with full complement of curved and straight blades
Indirect laryngoscope with appropriate size blade
Specialized equipment:
Airway exchange catheters, full complement of sizes
14 Gauge angiocatheters
Jet ventilator
Emergency cricothyrotomy kit (small pediatric and adult sizes)
Carbon dioxide detection devices
Surgical tracheostomy tray
Miscellaneous items:
Malleable atomizers
Syringes
14–16 Gauge angiocatheters
Water-based lubricant jelly
Tongue depressors

and maintenance of skill set with specific devices can be achieved through simulation and semi-elective use in patients without cardiopulmonary compromise requiring intubation for procedures or regular rotation/experience in the operating room. In larger pediatric hospitals, difficult airway teams able to respond to critical situations should be defined, available, and easily triggered into action. Pediatric anesthesiologists and otolaryngologists are integral members of these teams for development, training, and implementation.

Tracheal Extubation in the Child with a Difficult Airway

Tracheal extubation of a child with a difficult airway can be challenging in terms of resources, location, and personnel. First, it is not practical and likely not necessarily safe to extubate every child in the operating room. It is up to the intensivists in coordination with members of the difficult airway team (anesthesia, ENT) to determine the optimal location. There are several advantages to extubation of a child with a difficult airway in the operating room, including: equipment availability (including room for equipment), adjustable operating room bed, proper/adjustable lighting, surgical team availability and comfort. Disadvantages include: timing (OR availability), resource utilization, transport of a critically ill patient, and transfer of care of a critically ill patient to a new team. If the intensive care team decides to extubate the trachea of a child with a difficult airway in the ICU, it is important for the team to have plans in place to deal with the known problems and the unforeseen problems that may have developed since the initial intubation. The first step in planning for the extubation of a difficult airway is to review the records of previous intubations, and if possible to have a direct discussion with the team members who performed the previous intubations about technique, equipment, and potential pitfalls. Second, is to plan for potential changes in anatomy and physiology that may have taken place since the initial intubation: airway edema, laryngotracheal injury, cardiopulmonary dysfunction, and ongoing neurologic injury. A difficult airway cart should be readily available, appropriate medications available for reintubation and cardiopulmonary support, and team members trained and facile with the pediatric difficult airway. A final important consideration is the time of day to attempt the extubation of a difficult airway. While some failures may occur immediately post-extubation due to laryngotracheal or neurologic dysfunction, many extubations fail several hours later due to ongoing cardiopulmonary compromise. This should be taken into account based on resources available (especially at night) that can deal with a pediatric patient in respiratory distress and a difficult airway, a potentially lethal combination.

Conclusion

Pediatric difficult airway management in the intensive care environment presents a wide range of challenges. Children in whom airway management is expected to be difficult are often unable to cooperate with awake airway management techniques that are often primary approach in adult patients. The availability of a variety of indirect laryngoscopes has significantly increased the intensivist's ability to safely manage many of these children in the ICU. Successful airway management in these children requires careful planning, preparation, and often multidisciplinary cooperation.

References

1. Practice guidelines for management of the difficult airway: an updated report by the American Society of Anesthesiologists Task Force on Management of the Difficult Airway. Anesthesiology. 2013;118(2):251–70.
2. Practice guidelines for management of the difficult airway. A report by the American Society of Anesthesiologists Task Force on Management of the Difficult Airway. Anesthesiology. 1993;78(3):597–602.
3. Rutledge C. Difficult mask ventilation in 5-year-old due to submental hypertrophic scar: a case report. AANA J. 2008;76(3):177–8.
4. Han R, Tremper K, Kheterpal S, O'Reilly M. Grading scale for mask ventilation. Anesthesiology. 2004;101(1):267.
5. Kheterpal S, Han R, Tremper K, Shanks A, Tait A, O'Reilly M, Ludwig T. Incidence and predictors of difficult and impossible mask ventilation. Anesthesiology. 2006;105(5):885–91. doi:00000542-200611000-00007 [pii].
6. Kheterpal S, Martin L, Shanks A, Tremper K. Prediction and outcomes of impossible mask ventilation: a review of 50,000 anesthetics. Anesthesiology. 2009;110(4):891–7.
7. Tait A, Voepel-Lewis T, Burke C, Kostrzewa A, Lewis I. Incidence and risk factors for perioperative adverse respiratory events in children who are obese. Anesthesiology. 2008;108(3):375–80.
8. Erden V, Yangtin Z, Erkalp K, Delatioglu H. Conscious sedation for difficult intubation in children. Anaesth Intensive Care. 2009;37(5):863.
9. Choong K, AlFaleh K, Doucette J, Gray S, Rich B, Verhey L, Paes B. Remifentanil for endotracheal intubation in neonates: a randomised controlled trial. Arch Dis Child Fetal Neonatal Ed. 2010;95(2):F80–4. doi:10.1136/adc.2009.167338. 95/2/F80 [pii].
10. Abdelmalak B, Makary L, Hoban J, Doyle DJ. Dexmedetomidine as sole sedative for awake intubation in management of the critical airway. J Clin Anesth. 2007;19(5):370–3. doi:10.1016/j.jclinane.2006.09.006. S0952-8180(07)00088-8 [pii].
11. Bergese SD, Khabiri B, Roberts WD, Howie MB, McSweeney TD, Gerhardt MA. Dexmedetomidine for conscious sedation in difficult awake fiberoptic intubation cases. J Clin Anesth. 2007;19(2):141–4. doi:10.1016/j.jclinane.2006.07.005. S0952-8180(06)00310-2 [pii].
12. Shukry M, Kennedy K. Dexmedetomidine as a total intravenous anesthetic in infants. Paediatr Anaesth. 2007;17(6):581–3. doi:10.1111/j.1460-9592.2006.02171.x. PAN2171 [pii].
13. Sukhupragarn W, Churnchongkolkul W. Glidescope intubation after failed fiberoptic intubation. Paediatr Anaesth. 2010;20(9):901–2. doi:10.1111/j.1460-9592.2010.03373.x. PAN3373 [pii].
14. Stricker P, Fiadjoe J, McGinnis S. Intubation of an infant with Pierre Robin sequence under dexmedetomidine sedation using the Shikani Optical Stylet. Acta Anaesthesiol Scand. 2008;52(6):866–7.
15. Shukry M, Hanson R, Koveleskie J, Ramadhyani U. Management of the difficult pediatric airway with Shikani Optical Stylet. Paediatr Anaesth. 2005;15(4):342–5.
16. Mason KP, Zurakowski D, Zgleszewski S, Prescilla R, Fontaine PJ, Dinardo JA. Incidence and predictors of hypertension during high-dose dexmedetomidine sedation for pediatric MRI. Paediatr Anaesth. 2010;20(6):516–23. doi:10.1111/j.1460-9592.2010.03299.x. PAN3299 [pii].
17. Mason KP, Zurakowski D, Zgleszewski SE, Robson CD, Carrier M, Hickey PR, Dinardo JA. High dose dexmedetomidine as the sole sedative for pediatric MRI. Paediatr Anaesth. 2008;18(5):403–11. doi:10.1111/j.1460-9592.2008.02468.x. PAN2468 [pii].
18. Iravani M, Wald SH. Dexmedetomidine and ketamine for fiberoptic intubation in a child with severe mandibular hypoplasia. J Clin Anesth. 2008;20(6):455–7. doi:10.1016/j.jclinane.2008.03.012. S0952-8180(08)00189-X [pii].
19. Jooste EH, Ohkawa S, Sun LS. Fiberoptic intubation with dexmedetomidine in two children with spinal cord impingements. Anesth Analg. 2005;101(4):1248. doi:10.1213/01.ANE.0000173765.94392.80. 101/4/1248 [pii].
20. Canet J, Castillo J. Ketamine: a familiar drug we trust. Anesthesiology. 2012;116(1):6–8. doi:10.1097/ALN.0b013e31823da398.
21. Christ G, Mundigler G, Merhaut C, Zehetgruber M, Kratochwill C, Heinz G, Siostrzonek P. Adverse cardiovascular effects of ketamine infusion in patients with catecholamine-dependent heart failure. Anaesth Intensive Care. 1997;25(3):255–9.

22. Warters RD, Szabo TA, Spinale FG, DeSantis SM, Reves JG. The effect of neuromuscular blockade on mask ventilation. Anaesthesia. 2011;66(3):163–7. doi:10.1111/j.1365-2044.2010.06601.x.

23. Calder I, Yentis S, Patel A. Muscle relaxants and airway management. Anesthesiology. 2009;111(1):216–7. doi:10.1097/ALN.0b013e3181a9728b. 00000542-200907000-00048 [pii].

24. Kopman AF. Sugammadex: a revolutionary approach to neuromuscular antagonism. Anesthesiology. 2006;104(4):631–3. doi:00000542-200604000-00003 [pii].

25. de Boer HD, Driessen JJ, Marcus MA, Kerkkamp H, Heeringa M, Klimek M. Reversal of rocuronium-induced (1.2 mg/kg) profound neuromuscular block by sugammadex: a multicenter, dose-finding and safety study. Anesthesiology. 2007;107(2):239–44. doi:10.1097/01.anes.0000270722.95764.37 00000542-200708000-00010 [pii].

26. Donati F. The right dose of succinylcholine. Anesthesiology. 2003;99(5):1037–8.

27. Reber A, Wetzel SG, Schnabel K, Bongartz G, Frei FJ. Effect of combined mouth closure and chin lift on upper airway dimensions during routine magnetic resonance imaging in pediatric patients sedated with propofol. Anesthesiology. 1999;90(6):1617–23.

28. Reber A, Paganoni R, Frei FJ. Effect of common airway manoeuvres on upper airway dimensions and clinical signs in anaesthetized, spontaneously breathing children. Br J Anaesth. 2001;86(2):217–22.

29. Meier S, Geiduschek J, Paganoni R, Fuehrmeyer F, Reber A. The effect of chin lift, jaw thrust, and continuous positive airway pressure on the size of the glottic opening and on stridor score in anesthetized, spontaneously breathing children. Anesth Analg. 2002;94(3):494–9.

30. Beattie C. The modified nasal trumpet maneuver. Anesth Analg. 2002;94(2):467–9.

31. Holm-Knudsen R, Eriksen K, Rasmussen L. Using a nasopharyngeal airway during fiberoptic intubation in small children with a difficult airway. Paediatr Anaesth. 2005;15(10):839–45.

32. Brain AI, McGhee TD, McAteer EJ, Thomas A, Abu-Saad MA, Bushman JA. The laryngeal mask airway. Development and preliminary trials of a new type of airway. Anaesthesia. 1985;40(4):356–61.

33. Brimacombe J. The advantages of the LMA over the tracheal tube or facemask: a meta-analysis. Can J Anaesth. 1995;42(11):1017–23.

34. Abdi W, Dhonneur G, Amathieu R, Adhoum A, Kamoun W, Slavov V, Barrat C, Combes X. LMA supreme versus facemask ventilation performed by novices: a comparative study in morbidly obese patients showing difficult ventilation predictors. Obes Surg. 2009;19(12):1624–30. doi:10.1007/s11695-009-9953-0.

35. Von Ungern-Sternberg BS, Wallace CJ, Sticks S, Erb TO, Chambers NA. Fibreoptic assessment of paediatric sized laryngeal mask airways. Anaesth Intensive Care. 2010;38(1):50–4.

36. Selim M, Mowafi H, Al-Ghamdi A, Adu-Gyamfi Y. Intubation via LMA in pediatric patients with difficult airways. Can J Anaesth. 1999;46(9):891–3.

37. Johnson C, Sims C. Awake fibreoptic intubation via a laryngeal mask in an infant with Goldenhar's syndrome. Anaesth Intensive Care. 1994;22(2):194–7.

38. Fiadjoe J, Stricker P, Kovatsis P, Isserman R, Harris B, McCloskey J. Initial experience with the air-Q as a conduit for fiberoptic tracheal intubation in infants. Paediatr Anaesth. 2010;20(2):205–6.

39. Muraika L, Heyman J, Shevchenko Y. Fiberoptic tracheal intubation through a laryngeal mask airway in a child with Treacher Collins syndrome. Anesth Analg. 2003;97(5):1298–9.

40. Asai T, Nagata A, Shingu K. Awake tracheal intubation through the laryngeal mask in neonates with upper airway obstruction. Paediatr Anaesth. 2008;18(1):77–80.

41. Auden S, Lerner G. Blind intubation via the laryngeal mask: a word of caution. Paediatr Anaesth. 2000;10(4):452.

42. Fiadjoe JE, Stricker PA, Kovatis P. Blind intubation through the air-Q laryngeal mask in children - a word of caution. Paediatr Anaesth. 2010;20(9):900–1. doi:10.1111/j.1460-9592.2010.03363.x. PAN3363 [pii].

43. Hirabayashi Y, Otsuka Y. Early clinical experience with GlideScope video laryngoscope in 20 infants. Paediatr Anaesth. 2009;19(8):802–4.

44. Kim J, Na H, Bae J, Kim D, Kim H, Kim C, Kim S. GlideScope video laryngoscope: a randomized clinical trial in 203 paediatric patients. Br J Anaesth. 2008;101(4):531–4.

45. Redel A, Karademir F, Schlitterlau A, Frommer M, Scholtz L, Kranke P, Kehl F, Roewer N, Lange M. Validation of the GlideScope video laryngoscope in pediatric patients. Paediatr Anaesth. 2009;19(7):667–71.

46. Bishop S, Clements P, Kale K, Tremlett M. Use of GlideScope Ranger in the management of a child with Treacher Collins syndrome in a developing world setting. Paediatr Anaesth. 2009;19(7):695–6.

47. Eaton J, Atiles R, Tuchman J. GlideScope for management of the difficult airway in a child with Beckwith-Wiedemann syndrome. Paediatr Anaesth. 2009;19(7):696–8.

48. Viola L, Fiadjoe JE, Stricker PA, Maxwell LG. Video laryngoscopy in infants: one device does not fit all. Paediatr Anaesth. 2011;21(9):987–9. doi:10.1111/j.1460-9592.2011.03612.x.

49. Vlatten A, Aucoin S, Litz S, Macmanus B, Soder C. A comparison of the STORZ video laryngoscope and standard direct laryngoscopy for intubation in the pediatric airway-a randomized clinical trial. Paediatr Anaesth. 2009;19(11):1102–7.

50. Macnair D, Baraclough D, Wilson G, Bloch M, Engelhardt T. Pediatric airway management: comparing the Berci-Kaplan Video Laryngoscope with direct laryngoscopy. Paediatr Anaesth. 2009;19(6):577–80.

51. Fiadjoe JE, Stricker PA, Hackell RS, Salam A, Gurnaney H, Rehman MA, Litman RS. The efficacy of the Storz Miller 1 video laryngoscope in a simulated infant difficult intubation. Anesth Analg. 2009;108(6):1783–6. doi:10.1213/ane.0b013e3181a1a600. 108/6/1783 [pii].

52. Jansen A, Johnston G. The Shikani Optical Stylet: a useful adjunct to airway management in a neonate with popliteal pterygium syndrome. Paediatr Anaesth. 2008;18(2):188–90.

53. Weiss M, Hartmann K, Fischer J, Gerber A. Video-intuboscopic assistance is a useful aid to tracheal intubation in pediatric patients. Can J Anaesth. 2001;48(7):691–6.

54. Gravenstein D, Liem E, Bjoraker D. Alternative management techniques for the difficult airway: optical stylets. Curr Opin Anaesthesiol. 2004;17(6):495–8.

55. Brain AI. The laryngeal mask-a new concept in airway management. Br J Anaesth. 1983;55(8):801–5.

Central Venous Vascular Access

29

Jennifer Kaplan, Matthew F. Niedner, and Richard J. Brilli

Abstract

In children, central venous catheters are most often used for cardiovascular monitoring, emergency vascular access, intermittent blood removal for laboratory analysis, fluid and drug administration, plasmapheresis, hemodialysis, and long-term chemotherapy. This chapter provides an overview of choices in central venous access sites, describes central venous catheterization techniques, and delineates associated risks and complications. Decisions regarding the "best" site for central venous cannulation depend upon patient specific clinical variables, risk of complications, operator experience, future vascular access needs, and projected length of time the catheter will remain in place. In 2011, the Centers for Disease Control (CDC) published updated recommendations regarding the selection, insertion, maintenance, and discontinuation of central lines. This guideline deserves review by practitioners who insert and/or maintain central venous lines in children (see Table 29.1). The femoral vein is the most common site for central venous access in children. This site may have the lowest insertion risk profile and a high degree of operator experience across multiple specialties. In adult patients, IJ and subclavian vessels are preferred sites because the rates of infection and deep venous thrombosis may be less than that found with femoral venous catheterization, however in children these differences are less clear. In children, operator experience and need for minimal sedation when placing femoral catheters, are important drivers in site choice. The subclavian vein is the preferred route for long-term venous access in children because it is easily inserted via the tunneled approach, is well tolerated, and is associated with few complications. Standard landmark insertion techniques

J. Kaplan, MD, MS
Division of Critical Care Medicine, Department of Pediatrics,
Cincinnati Children's Hospital Medical Center,
University of Cincinnati College of Medicine,
3333 Burnet Avenue, Cincinnati, OH 45229, USA
e-mail: jennifer.kaplan@cchmc.org

M.F. Niedner, MD
Pediatric Intensive Care Unit, Division of Critical Care Medicine,
Department of Pediatrics, University of Michigan Medical Center,
Mott Children's Hospital, F-6894 Mott #0243,
1500 East Medical Center Dr, Ann Arbor, MI 48109-0243, USA
e-mail: mniedner@med.umich.edu

R.J. Brilli, MD (✉)
Division of Critical Care Medicine, Department of Pediatrics,
Nationwide Children's Hospital, The Ohio State University
College of Medicine, 700 Children's Drive,
Columbus, OH 43205, USA
e-mail: rbrilli@nationwidechildrens.org

D.S. Wheeler et al. (eds.), *Pediatric Critical Care Medicine*,
DOI 10.1007/978-1-4471-6362-6_29, © Springer-Verlag London 2014

still apply however the role of ultrasound guided CVC placement is growing in popularity and is recommended by some regulatory groups. Inexperienced operators may benefit most from ultrasound guided insertion. Pediatric providers should use their judgment about when to apply this important adjunct for line placement.

Keywords

Central Line • Percutaneous Venous Access • Central Venous Access • Central Line Placement • Vascular Access

Introduction

Percutaneous central venous access is a common procedure performed in emergency departments (ED) and intensive care units. In adults, in the United States, approximately three million central venous catheters are placed annually, resulting in 15 million central venous catheter (CVC) days in ICUs each year [1, 2]. Like adults, critically ill children often require central venous catheter placement. These catheters are used for cardiovascular monitoring, emergency vascular access during crisis situations, intermittent blood removal for laboratory analysis, fluid and drug administration, plasmapheresis, hemodialysis, and long-term chemotherapy [3–7]. Chiang et al., in a retrospective review of ED admissions over 5 years, reported that among all patients who required placement of a central venous catheter, 20 of 121 patients (17 %) had the catheter placed as a result of a cardiac or respiratory arrest, 78 patients (64 %) had catheters placed for lack of peripheral access, and 23 patients (19 %) had catheters placed for inadequate or unstable peripheral access [5]. Multiple sites using varied techniques have been described for obtaining central venous access in children. Each site and access method has associated risks and benefits. This chapter will provide an overview of choices in central venous access sites, describe standard techniques for central venous catheterization, and delineate associated risks and complications. Other methods of venous access, such as intraosseous access, venous cut down, or peripherally inserted central catheters, will not be part of this review because they are well outlined in other standard references [7]. Catheter related blood stream infections and catheter related thrombosis are the subject of other chapters in this textbook and will be only briefly discussed here.

Choice of Sites and Type of Catheter

There are multiple sites available for central venous catheterization in children. These sites include the femoral, subclavian, internal and external jugular, and axillary veins. Recently peripherally inserted central catheters (PICCs) have been used more frequently to obtain central venous access. PICCs are usually inserted into the basilic or cephalic veins and then advanced into the central circulation. Decisions regarding the "best" site for central venous cannulation depend upon multiple patient specific clinical variables, risk of complications, operator experience, future vascular access needs, and projected length of time the catheter will remain in place [8–11]. Practitioners who insert central lines should be familiar with the existing evidence to minimize untoward complications associated with these invasive devices. In 2011, the Centers for Disease Control (CDC) published updated recommendations regarding the selection, insertion, maintenance, and discontinuation of central lines [12]. The CDC guideline provides exhaustive recommendations pertaining to the maintenance care of catheters and their attachment devices, all focused upon infection prevention. Most of these recommendations pertain to nursing practice and are beyond the scope of this chapter. However, Table 29.1 summarizes the CDC recommendations most relevant to practitioners who insert central venous catheters. Much of this information is not new and some recommendations are derived from adult patients with central lines and therefore may have limited value to the pediatric practitioner. A couple of items deserve specific mention. A category 1A recommendation is to avoid the use of the subclavian vein for percutaneous access in patients with advanced kidney disease or those receiving chronic hemodialysis. This recommendation is intended to prevent subclavian vein stenosis and preserve the use of the subclavian vein for future access needs. Another item pertains to the recommendation to use new sterile gloves when handling the new catheter during guidewire exchange (Category II recommendation) and a 1B recommendation to use guidewire exchange to replace a malfunctioning catheter if there is no evidence of infection.

The femoral vein is the most common site for central venous access in children, especially in the emergency setting [5]. This site may have the lowest insertion risk profile and a high degree of operator experience across multiple specialties, hence its frequent use. In a cohort of 121 ED patients who required central venous access, 101 (83 %) had CVC placement in the femoral vein, 12 (10 %) had the catheter placed in the subclavian vein, and 7 (6 %) in the internal jugular vein [5]. Clinical variables that may impact the choice of site for cannulation include the coagulation status of the patient, whether the patient is breathing spontaneously or via mechanical ventilation, and the severity of the patient's respiratory illness. For example, patients with a significant

Table 29.1 Centers for disease control's recommendations for the selection, insertion, and removal of central lines

Category IA: strongly recommended for implementation and strongly supported by well-designed experimental, clinical or epidemiologic studies

Educate healthcare personnel re central line indications, proper insertion/maintenance practices, and infection control measures to prevent intravascular catheter-related infections

Periodically assess knowledge of and adherence to proper central line practices for all involved personnel

Designate only trained personnel who demonstrate competence for insertion/maintenance of central lines

Achieve skin antisepsis at the insertion site with a chlorhexidine-alcohol product

Employ maximal sterile barrier precautions during central line insertion, including sterile gloves

Avoid subclavian site if advanced kidney disease or chronic hemodialysis (to avoid subclavian vein stenosis)

Use antibiotic -impregnated central lines if the catheter is expected to remain in place >5 days if, after successful implementation of a comprehensive strategy to reduce rates of CLABSI, the CLABSI rate is not decreasing

Category IB: strongly recommended for implementation and supported by some experimental, clinical, or epidemiologic studies and a strong theoretical rationale; or an accepted practice (e.g. aseptic technique) supported by limited evidence

Maintain aseptic technique for the insertion and care of intravascular catheters

Hand hygiene should be performed before and after palpating catheter insertion sites as well as before and after inserting, replacing, accessing, repairing, or dressing a central line

Select a central line with the fewest number of ports/lumens essential for patient management

Use a guidewire exchange to replace a malfunctioning temporary catheter if no evidence of infection is present

Do not routinely replace nor exchange over a guidewire central lines to prevent catheter-related infections

When adherence to aseptic technique cannot be ensured (e.g., medical emergency), replace as soon as possible

Use ultrasound guidance to place central lines – if this technology is available and inserter trained in its use

Use a chlorhexidine-impregnated sponge dressing for temporary short-term catheters if the CLABSI rate is not decreasing despite adherence to basic prevention measures, including education and training, appropriate use of chlorhexidine for skin antisepsis, and maximum sterile barrier precautions

Category II: suggested for implementation and supported by suggestive clinical or epidemiologic studies or a theoretical rational

In adults, use an upper-extremity site for catheter insertion; replace a catheter inserted in a lower extremity site to an upper extremity site as soon as possible

Use new sterile gloves before handling the new catheter when guidewire exchanges are performed

Use a sutureless securement device to reduce the risk of infection for intravascular catheters

Use prophylactic antimicrobial lock solution in patients with long term catheters who have a history of multiple CRBSI despite optimal maximal adherence to aseptic technique

Do not remove CVCs or PICCs on the basis of fever alone. Use clinical judgment regarding the appropriateness of removing the catheter if infection is evidenced elsewhere or if a noninfectious cause of fever is suspected

Remove umbilical catheters as soon as possible when no longer needed or when any sign of vascular insufficiency to the lower extremities is observed. Optimally, umbilical artery catheters should not be left in place >5 days. Umbilical venous catheters should be removed as soon as possible when no longer needed, but can be used up to 14 days if managed aseptically

coagulopathy may be at greater risk from inadvertent arterial puncture, especially if the access site does not easily allow for direct pressure to the artery. This could make subclavian venipuncture higher risk compared to the femoral approach. For patients breathing spontaneously (less likely to hold still for the procedure) or those requiring high ventilator settings, the risk of an unplanned pneumothorax associated with the subclavian or internal jugular approach could make the femoral vein the preferred site. Subclavian and internal jugular sites may have lower catheter maintenance risks including lower infection rates compared to the femoral vein and thus may be preferred when central venous access is performed electively and the duration of cannulation is expected to be prolonged [2, 13]. Additionally, vein caliber can limit the size of catheter that can be inserted. This is of particular concern for infants and toddlers where lower extremity vessels are disproportionally smaller compared to above the diaphragm vessels. If a large-caliber vessel is required for flow-dependent extracorporeal therapies (e.g., CRRT, ECMO), then site selection may be determined by the necessary cannula size.

Femoral Venous Catheterization

Demographic and Historical Data

Studies from the 1950s reported high complication rates from femoral vein cannulation and as a result femoral venous access fell out of favor [14]. Today, femoral vein catheterization is frequently used in critically ill children because of its relatively low risk profile and high insertion success rate, in a variety of clinical settings.

Indications and Contraindications for Placement

Femoral veins are excellent central venous access sites in critically ill children. The femoral veins are attractive because they are perceived as a simple site for percutaneous insertion, especially by inexperienced operators and the cannulation can often be performed with minimal supplemental sedation. This is particularly important in children who are not receiving mechanical ventilation at the time of catheter placement. In addition, risks of life-threatening complications at the time of insertion are reduced because of easy compressibility of local vessels (femoral artery) and the remote location from the lung. The femoral vessels are also preferred if there are relative or absolute contraindications to accessing the jugular or subclavian veins. For example, in patients at risk for intracranial hypertension, placement of central venous catheters in the jugular or subclavian veins may precipitate vascular thrombosis, which could create obstruction to cerebral venous drainage and potentially life threatening increases in intracranial hypertension. In this clinical setting, a femoral venous catheter may be preferred [8]. In addition, patients with severe respiratory failure who require high mechanical ventilatory pressures may be at increased risk should a pneumothorax develop during the placement of a cervicothoracic central venous catheter. In this setting the femoral site may be preferred as well. In patients with a recognized coagulopathy, the femoral site is preferable because direct compression of the femoral vessels can occur, especially in the event of inadvertent puncture of the femoral artery [8]. Multiple studies demonstrate that femoral vein catheterization is a rapid and safe route for obtaining intravenous access in patients requiring massive intravenous fluid infusions or following cardiac arrest [4, 15, 16]. Furthermore, the femoral artery provides an easily recognized landmark to facilitate straightforward catheter insertion.

Some clinical situations warrant placement of central venous catheters at sites other than the femoral vein. Trauma to the lower extremity, pelvis, or inferior vena cava is a relative contraindication for femoral vein catheterization [8]. In addition, bulky abdominal tumors, inferior vena cava, common iliac, or femoral thrombosis, abdominal hematomas, venous anomalies and prior pelvic radiation are associated with increased risk of complications from femoral venous catheter placement [17].

In adult patients, practitioners have traditionally avoided femoral CVC placement because of concerns about the risk of deep venous thrombosis, excess infectious risks compared to other sites, and potentially inaccurate central venous pressure measurements derived from the femoral vessels [18–21]. While the jury may still be out in the adult critical care community regarding the use femoral catheters, evidence in children suggests a safer risk profile for femoral catheters than is observed in adults, especially when catheters are used for short periods of time [22, 23]. Perceived ease of insertion combined with a low insertion risk profile, often make the femoral vessels the preferred site in children [23, 24]. In adults and children, there is a wide range of reported rates for venous thrombosis associated with central venous catheters (1–60 %), however the thrombosis rates in children, are not significantly different between the femoral vessels and cervicothoracic vessels [25, 26]. Furthermore, in children, infectious complications associated with femoral venous catheters are similar and in one report less than that reported for cervicothoracic central venous catheters [27–29]. Finally, multiple studies have demonstrated that

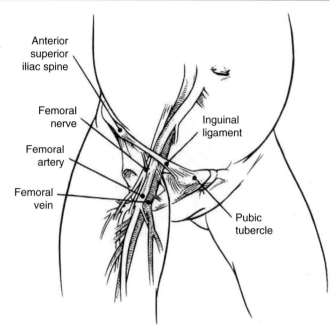

Fig. 29.1 Femoral Vein Anatomy (Source: PALS Provider Manual © 1997, American Heart Association, Inc)

in the absence of elevated intraabdominal pressures and even in the presence of high mechanical ventilatory support, central venous pressure measurements derived from femoroiliac veins are similar to measurements obtained from cervicothoracic veins and may accurately predict right atrial pressures [30–33].

Anatomy

The femoral vein lies in the femoral sheath, medial to the femoral artery immediately below the inguinal ligament (Fig. 29.1). The femoral triangle is an anatomic region of the upper thigh with the boundaries including the inguinal ligament cephalad, sartorius muscle laterally, and adductor longus muscle medially. The contents of the femoral triangle from lateral to medial are the femoral nerve, femoral artery and femoral vein. The femoral sheath lies within the femoral triangle and includes the femoral artery, femoral vein and lymph nodes. The femoral vein runs superficially in the thigh approaching the inguinal ligament in the femoral triangle. The vein dives steeply in a posterior direction, superior to the inguinal ligament, as it becomes the iliac vein. The femoral vein lies medial to the femoral artery in the femoral sheath inferior to the inguinal ligament. In patients with a palpable pulse, the femoral vein can be located just medial to the femoral arterial pulse inferior to the inguinal ligament. In pulseless patients, the femoral artery can be assumed to be at a point half-way along a line drawn from the pubic tubercle to the anterior superior iliac spine, at a level 1–2 cm inferior to the inguinal ligament. The femoral vein is located 0.5–1.5 cm medial to the center of the femoral artery, depending upon the size of the patient [34].

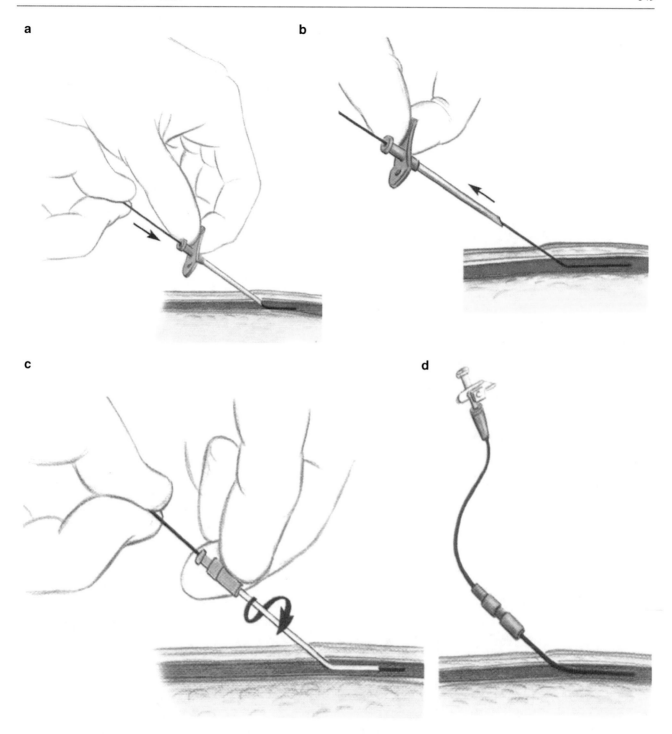

Fig. 29.2 Seldinger Technique for central venous catheter insertion. (**a**) Insert needle into the target vessel and pass the flexible end of the guidewire into the vessel. (**b**) Remove the needle, leaving the guidewire in place. (**c**) Using a twisting motion, advance the catheter into the ves- sel. (**d**) Remove the guidewire, and connect the catheter to an appropri- ate flow device or monitoring device (Source: PALS Provider Manual © 2002, American Heart Association, Inc)

Insertion Technique

Femoral vein insertion should be performed using the Seldinger technique [35]. The Seldinger technique was first described by Sven Seldinger in 1953 and enabled practitio- ners to insert a large size catheter over a guidewire that was placed in the vein by venipuncture with a small size needle (Fig. 29.2). The femoral site should be prepared and draped as for any surgical procedure and in non-emergent clinical situations, using full sterile barrier (Fig. 29.3) [36]. The optimal position of the leg can vary according to the prefer- ence of the operator – some prefer slight external rotation at the hip and others prefer full "frog leg" external rotation. The location of the femoral vein is 0.5–2 cm inferior to the inguinal ligament, just medial to the femoral artery. Because the overlying skin in the inquinal region, especially in babies, is often slack and redundant, it can be important to develop a method to maintain traction on the skin while palpating for the arterial pulse and then maintaining this traction while inserting the needle (Fig. 29.4a, b). The syringe should be held at a 30–45° angle from the skin, aimed cephalad over the femoral vein site. Some operators approach the vessel from the side maintaining traction on the skin

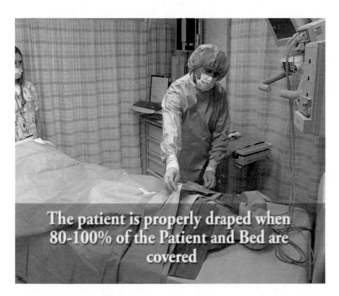

Fig. 29.3 Full sterile barrier during elective insertion of central venous catheter

and palpating the pulse with the opposite hand (Fig. 29.5), while others approach the vessel directly (Fig. 29.4b). Most operators locate the vein and obtain venous blood flashback by advancing the needle/syringe at a 30° angle toward the ischial ramus while withdrawing the syringe plunger, creating negative pressure within the syringe (Fig. 29.5). If venous blood is not returned, the needle/syringe should be slowly withdrawn, pulling back constantly on the plunger. If the vein is not located, redirect the needle searching from medial to lateral until the vein is located. To avoid lacerating the vessels, the needle should be withdrawn to the skin surface prior to changing direction. Puncture of the vein is indicated by blood return (flashback in the syringe) while advancing or slowly withdrawing the needle. An alternative method to locate the vein is to advance the needle/syringe over the vein site toward the ischial ramus to a depth of 1–2 cm without negative pressure in the syringe and then withdraw the needle applying negative pressure to the syringe, thus obtaining venous blood flashback on the withdrawal of the needle. The advantage of this method is that it allows the operator to firmly rest the hand on the thigh during needle/syringe withdrawal, which allows the operator to freeze when venous blood flashback occurs. This is especially important in small infants where the cross-sectional area of the needle and that of the vein are similar in size and as a result it is easy for the needle to move outside the lumen of the vessel as the syringe is gently removed from the needle. By freezing the operator's hand in position, this method allows for greater success with guidewire placement (Fig. 29.6). Kanter et al. demonstrated by use of ultrasound that the greatest probability of successful puncture of the

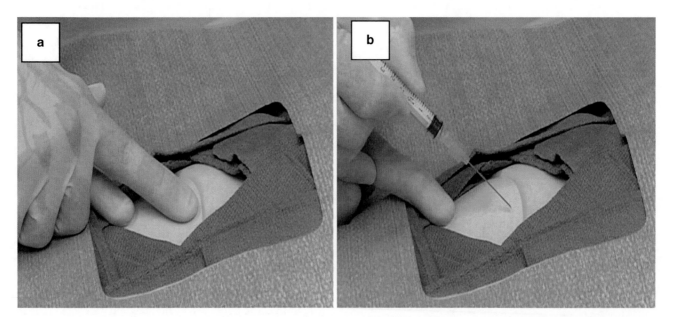

Fig. 29.4 (**a**) Palpation of femoral pulse with traction on redundant skin. (**b**) Skin traction is maintained as initial skin puncture occurs. The needle is advanced through the vessel and venous flashback occurs as the needle is withdrawn using negative pressure on the syringe

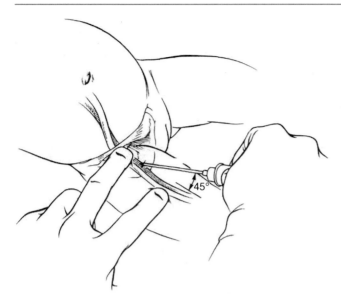

Fig. 29.5 One approach to the femoral vessel – needle and syringe advanced at 45° angle to the skin (Source: PALS Provider Manual © 1997, American Heart Association, Inc)

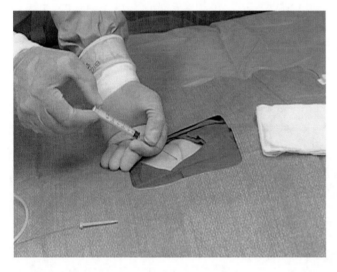

Fig. 29.6 Operator's hand resting on infant's thigh allowing the hand to freeze when venous flashback occurs

femoral vein was located 4–5 mm medial to the femoral artery pulse [37]. In addition, if it is assumed that entry into the central half of the vein will result in successful catheterization, successive attempts 5 mm and 6 mm medial to the pulse would result in cumulative successful insertion in 53 and 61 %, respectively, with no arterial punctures. A third attempt 4 mm medial to the pulse further increases cumulative success to 78 %, but the arterial puncture rate would increase to 3 %. Ultrasound guided central venous puncture is becoming common practice in adults and may increase insertion success rates and reduce insertion complication rates, especially for inexperienced operators or in difficult

access patients such as obese patients, patients with poor arterial pulses, or those with partial vessel thrombosis [38].

As described by Seldinger, after observing blood return, the syringe is disconnected from the needle hub and the guidewire is advanced through the needle and into the vein. It is important to leave part of the wire in view at all times. The advancement of the wire should be smooth without meeting any resistance. If resistance occurs during guidewire advancement, it is possible the wire is meeting a previously unrecognized thrombus, is advancing into the subcutaneous tissue, or most likely is advancing into the ascending lumbar veins which drain into the common iliac veins proximal to the femoral vein. Once the wire is in good position, remove the needle over the wire, holding the guidewire in place. Make a small ¼ to ½cm skin incision at the site of entry of the guidewire into the skin. Be certain that the bevel of the scalpel blade is away from the guidewire. Hold the dilator near its tip and advance the dilator over the guidewire into the femoral vein. The dilator should be advanced using a gentle boring motion. Holding the guidewire in place, remove the dilator while applying light pressure to the femoral site, as bleeding is likely to occur when the dilator is removed. Place the catheter over the guidewire and insert into the femoral vessel. Once the catheter is inserted, remove the guidewire and aspirate blood through the catheter to ascertain placement and patency of the catheter. Secure the catheter in place and cover with a sterile dressing.

Important warnings to consider during cannulation of the femoral vein include: (1) puncture of the femoral artery requires application of direct pressure for 5–10 min or until hemostasis is achieved; (2) never push the guidewire or catheter against resistance, properly placed guidewires float freely; (3) the guidewire can be sheared off if pulled out of the needle against resistance, if resistance is met on withdrawal of the guidewire, pull out the needle and the guidewire simultaneously; (4) the guidewire should remain in view at all times because guidewires have remained in vessels or have floated into the central circulation when not properly monitored (Fig. 29.7).

Confirmation of Placement

Confirmation of proper CVC position is required after placement of all CVCs. A post-procedure x-ray is the initial and usually only confirmatory test needed after femoral vein catheter insertion [39]. Some have questioned the value of confirmatory x-rays for uncomplicated placement of femoral venous catheters, however unsuspected catheter tip placement in the ascending lumbar veins can occur with potentially serious consequences, especially if such placement is unrecognized [40]. Several clinical variables can alert the clinician to possible improper femoral catheter placement: (1) guidewire that meets resistance during advancement - suspect ascending lumbar placement or thrombosis; (2) bright red blood or arterial pulsation when vessel puncture takes place – suspect arterial placement; (3) catheter tip on x-ray that points too

cephalad – suspect ascending lumbar placement (Fig. 29.8); (4) catheter tip on x-ray that crosses the midline from the right groin position or tip that is too cephalad from the left – suspect arterial placement (Fig. 29.9). If the location of the catheter tip is in question a dye study should be performed to confirm proper placement in the vascular bed (Figs. 29.8b and 29.9b). Placing a transducer on the end of the catheter or sending blood from the catheter for blood gas determination may help distinguish arterial from venous placement.

Complications and Risks

Femoral venous catheterization in children is generally regarded as safe, but as with all central venous catheters, complications do occur. In a prospective study evaluating femoral vascular catheterization in children, Venkataraman et al. reported that 74 of 89 (83 %) femoral venous catheterizations had no complications during catheter insertion and the other 15 (17 %) had either minor bleeding or hematomas at the insertion site [6]. During 13 of these femoral vein catheterizations, there was inadvertent puncture of the femoral artery. Overall catheterization success rate was 94.4 %. Less experienced operators required significantly more attempts (2.6 ± 1.5) to attain success than experienced operators (1.5 ± 0.5). Forty-five (51 %) patients were ≤1 year of age. The median duration of catheterization was 5 days

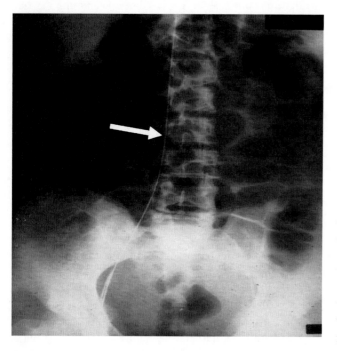

Fig. 29.7 Guidewire left in right femoral vein hemodialysis catheter (*arrow*)

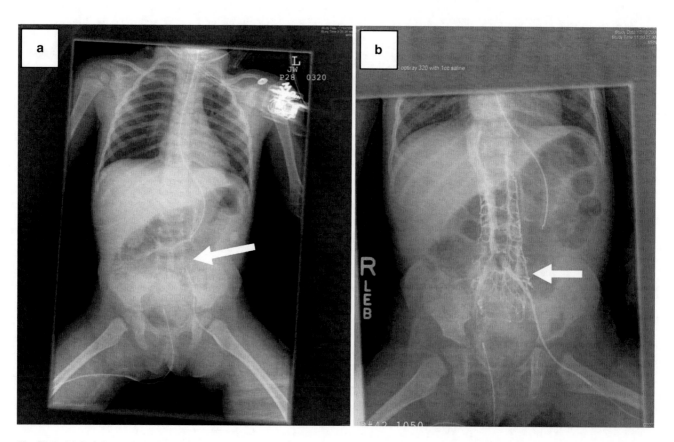

Fig. 29.8 (**a**) Left femoral venous catheter tip pointing cephalad. (**b**) Dye confirmation of ascending lumbar catheter placement

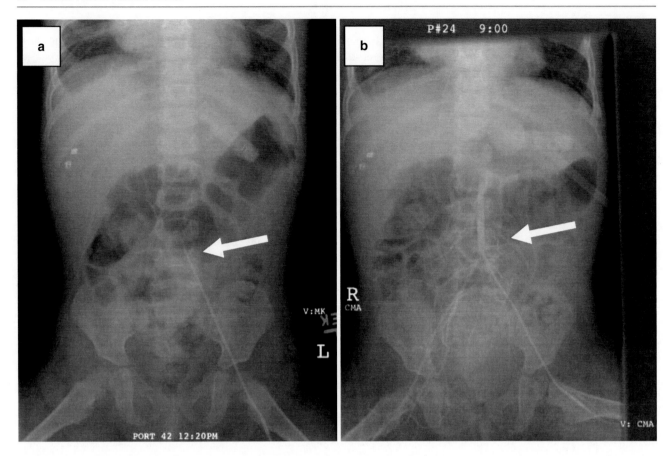

Fig. 29.9 (**a**) Left femoral catheter considered venous in patient with low blood pressure and marginal oxygenation. (**b**) Dye study (*aortagram*) confirming unexpected arterial placement

with 21 % as ≤3 days duration, 43 % as 4–7 days, 26 % as 7–14 days, and 10 % as >14 days. Long-term complications were uncommon. Sixty-eight patients had no long-term complications, eight had leg swelling (all <1 year of age) and 11 patients had either suspected or confirmed catheter related blood stream infection. Kanter also examined the safety and effectiveness of femoral central venous catheter insertion [8]. This prospective observational study included 29 pediatric patients who underwent attempted percutaneous femoral venous catheter placement. Femoral catheterization was successful in 86 % of patients attempted. Arterial puncture was the only significant complication of insertion, occurring in 14 % of patients and was not associated with adverse sequelae. The most significant complication associated with indwelling femoral central venous catheters was leg swelling or documented thrombosis, which occurred in 11 % of 74 critically ill patients during a 4 year period of observation. Lastly, Stenzel et al. prospectively reviewed complication rates over a 45 month period for percutaneously placed femoral and non-femoral central venous catheters [29]. Of the 395 catheters placed during this time period, 41 % were femoral. The mean duration of catheterization was 8.9 days. No complications occurred during femoral catheter insertion.

Of the 162 femoral catheters, nine non-infectious complications occurred, which included four thromboses, one vessel perforation, one embolism, one catheter discontinuity, and two bleeding episodes. Stenzel concluded, "Femoral venous catheterization offers practical advantages for central venous access over other sites. The low incidence of complications in this study suggests that the femoral vein is the preferred site in most critically ill children when central venous catheterization is indicated."

Subclavian Vein Catheterization

Demographic and Historical Data

The infraclavicular approach to subclavian vein catheterization was originally introduced in 1952 [41]. Supraclavicular approaches to the subclavian vein have been described but have not gained wide popularity as the primary approach for subclavian vein catheterization, though complication rates between the two approaches are similar [42]. Groff and Ahmed were among the first to describe their experience with subclavian vein catheterization in children [43]. They reported upon 28 patients all less than 1 year of age (20 newborns plus eight infants less than 6 months of age). Complications included one hemothorax, one pneumothorax, and two hydrothoraces. They concluded that subclavian catheterization in children was safe. More recently, Venkataraman et al. described their experience with infraclavicular subclavian catheterization placement by nonsurgeons in 100 consecutive patients [10]. One-third of their patients were less than 1 year of age. The overall success rate was 92 % and even under emergency conditions the success rate was 89 %. Minor complications were few and included bleeding at the site, hematomas, and self-limited premature ventricular beats. There were six major complications, four pneumothoraces, and two catheter related blood stream infections. Others have concluded that subclavian vein catheterization in children, even under emergency conditions, is safe and is associated with few major complications, especially when performed by experienced operators [11, 44, 45].

Indications

In adult patients, internal jugular and subclavian vessels are preferred sites for central venous catheterization because the rates of infection and deep venous thrombosis appear less than that found with femoral central venous catheterization, however in children these differences are less clear [2]. Furthermore, in children, operator experience and need for minimal sedation when placing femoral catheters, are important drivers of the decision process regarding which vessel is preferred. For long-term central venous access, the subclavian vein has long been the preferred route for central venous access in children because it is easily inserted via the tunneled approach, is well tolerated, and is associated with few complications [46]. For elective or emergency percutaneous central venous access in children, the subclavian vein can be catheterized safely as described previously, however some specific clinical situations may further guide the decision to use this vessel. In obese or edematous patients, the clavicle can act as an easily identifiable landmark to assist in vessel cannulation, thus making the subclavian vein the preferred approach [47]. In patients with shock, the subclavian vein may be preferred because it is less likely to collapse than the internal jugular vein. The subclavian approach is not ideal in uncooperative patients, especially non intubated children, in patients with abnormal chest anatomy, patients with previous clavicular fracture, or those with bleeding diathesis [48]. In the event of unplanned subclavian artery puncture during catheterization attempts, patients with significant coagulopathy may be at greater risk because it is difficult to apply direct compression to the artery. Lastly, some report that the technique for subclavian vein catheterization is not enhanced using ultrasound guidance, whereas femoral and internal

jugular vein catheterization success rates and complication rates can be improved using ultrasound guidance [49, 50]. Using ultrasound guidance, Gualtieri et al., were able to demonstrate increased success rates for subclavian vein catheterization, especially for less experienced operators [51]. They also reported no major complications.

For cervicothoracic central vein catheterization, controversy exists regarding which vessel is preferred – internal jugular or subclavian veins. No pediatric specific data exists which compares the rates of success and complications for these two approaches, however a recent systemic review has been published for adult patients [52]. Pooled data from 17 reports from 1982 to 1999 were analyzed which included nearly 2,000 jugular catheters and 2,500 subclavian catheters. Despite the many potential problems routinely associated with such a large data aggregation from multiple reports, some conclusions can be derived. Arterial punctures occurred with greater frequency with the internal jugular approach; however catheter malposition was significantly more common with subclavian vein catheterization. If rapid and correct catheter tip position is required (patient in shock requiring inotropes or hemodynamic monitoring), the jugular approach is preferred. There was no difference in the incidence of hemothorax, pneumothorax, or vessel occlusion between the two approaches. Data was too disparate to draw firm conclusions regarding comparative catheter related infection rates. Operator success rates were not reported in this review.

Anatomy

The subclavian vein begins as a continuation of the axillary vein at the lateral border of the first rib, crosses over the first rib, and passes in front of the anterior scalene muscle (Fig. 29.10). The anterior scalene muscle separates the subclavian vein from the subclavian artery (Fig. 29.10b). The vein continues behind the medial third of the clavicle where it is immobilized by small attachments to the rib and clavicle. At the medial border of the anterior scalene muscle and behind the sternocostoclavicular joint, the subclavian vein combines with the internal jugular to form the innominate or brachiocephalic vein.

Insertion Technique

The patient is positioned in a supine, head-down position of at least 15–30° (Fig. 29.11). A rolled towel or sandbag is placed under the shoulders longitudinally between the scapulae. Jung et al. demonstrated that tilting the head toward the catheterization side appears to reduce the incidence of catheter malposition during the right infraclavicular subclavian approach in infants [53]. Introduce the needle 1 cm below the junction of the middle and medial thirds of the clavicle

Fig. 29.10 (a) Clavicular landmarks and vascular anatomy. (b) Sagittal view: Course of subclavian artery and vein between boney structures and anterior scalenus muscle (Reprinted from Novak and Venus [47]. With permission from Lippincott Williams & Wilkins)

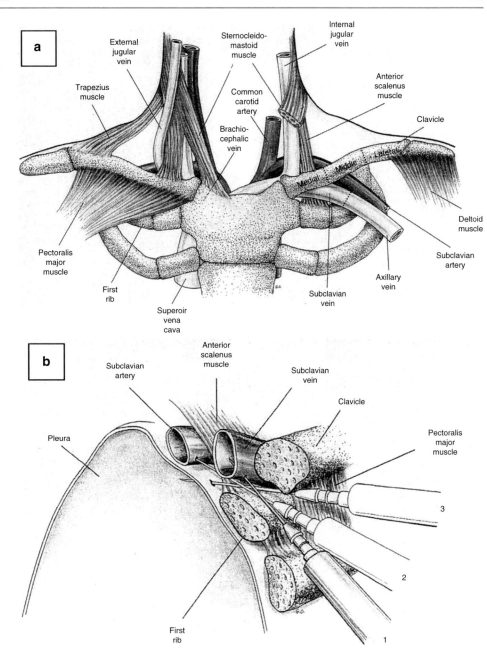

(Fig. 29.11b). The sternal notch acts as a landmark to direct insertion of the needle. The syringe and needle should be held parallel to the frontal plane just beneath the posterior aspect of the clavicle or "marched down" the clavicle to avoid puncturing the pleura or subclavian artery. The bevel of the needle should be oriented caudally as the vein is entered to minimize catheter tip malposition. In children, especially infants, blood "flashback" into the syringe may occur either during advancement or withdrawal of the needle/syringe, therefore it is important to withdraw the needle slowly and always with negative pressure exerted on the syringe hub. Upon entering the subclavian vein, using the Seldinger technique, a guidewire is placed through the needle to lie in the anticipated area of the superior vena cava. The catheter should be appropriately anchored to the skin and a sterile dressing placed over the site.

Proper patient position, especially in children, is an important factor that can impact successful subclavian vein catheterization. Land et al. demonstrated that when the shoulder is in neutral position the subclavian vein is overlapped by the medial third of the clavicle, thereby allowing this segment of the bone to serve as a landmark for insertion [54]. These results were confirmed by Tan et al. who demonstrated through anatomic dissection that infraclavicular subclavian venipuncture should be performed with the shoulders in a neutral position and slightly retracted, hence the vertical

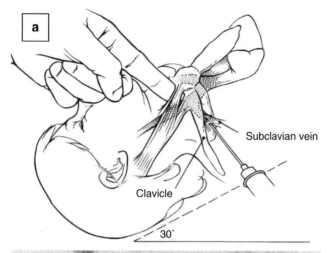

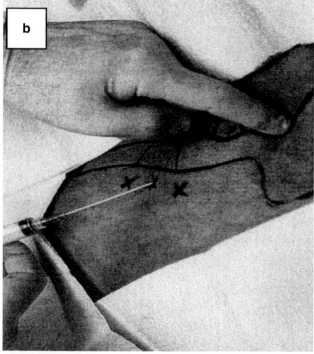

Fig. 29.11 (**a**) Subclavian vein anatomy – infraclavicular approach (Source: PALS Provider Manual © 1997, American Heart Association, Inc). (**b**) Medial infraclavicular approach (Reprinted from Novak and Venus [47]. With permission from Lippincott Williams & Wilkins)

placement of a small towel or sandbag between the scapulae will allow the shoulders to fall back into a proper position and facilitate vessel cannulation [55].

Confirmation of Placement

Significant morbidity and mortality exists with malposition of central venous catheters. Case reports demonstrate cardiac tamponade and perforation secondary to CVC insertion and catheter migration [56, 57]. A retrospective case review in children demonstrates a mortality rate of 34 % for CVC-related pericardial effusions [58]. Furthermore the Food and Drug Administration (FDA) states "the catheter tip should not be placed in or allowed to migrate into the heart" and recommends that CVC tips be positioned outside of the right atrium, preferably in the distal superior vena cava [1]. Andropoulos describes a formula for catheter insertion length that predicts positioning of the catheter tip above the right atrium 97 % of the time [59]. His report derives the formula by analyzing 452 right internal jugular and subclavian catheterizations in infants undergoing open heart surgery. The correct length of catheter insertion (cm) = (height in cm/10) – 1 for patients ≤ 100 cm in height and (height in cm/10) – 2 for patients >100 cm in height. This author has had anecdotal success in predicting proper catheter tip placement by using a "paper tape measure" to determine the distance on the chest surface from the proposed insertion site to the sternal-manubrium junction, which approximates the superior vena cava – right atrial junction.

After subclavian vein catheterization, confirmation of catheter tip placement is usually done by chest radiography however controversy exists regarding the necessity for post-procedural chest radiographs following cervicothoracic central venous catheter placement. McGee et al. described the results of a prospective, randomized, multicenter trial in adults and found that using conventional insertion techniques, the initial position of the catheter tip was in the heart in 47 % of 112 catheterizations [60]. Gladwin et al. demonstrated that the incidence of axillary vein or right atrial catheter malposition from internal jugular venous catheterization was 14 % [61]. The positive predictive value of a decision rule based on a questionnaire designed to detect potential mechanical complications and malpositioned catheters was 15 %. The sensitivity and specificity of the decision rule for detecting complications and malpositions was 44 and 55 %, respectively. This suggests that clinical factors alone do not reliably identify malpositioned catheters. Others report that chest radiography may not be necessary to confirm proper catheter placement if: (1) the procedure is performed by an experienced operator; (2) the procedure is "straightforward"; and (3) the operator requires <3 or 4 needle passes to access the vessel [62–64]. In children, no current "official" data driven recommendations exist regarding post-procedure chest radiography, however this author has observed many unexpected catheter tip placements, even in straightforward procedures, such that post-procedure chest radiography seems warranted. Figure 29.12 depicts several catheters wherein the malposition was not clinically evident and was discovered only at the time of confirmatory chest radiograph.

Complications

Reported complications from subclavian venipuncture include failure to locate the vein, puncture of the subclavian

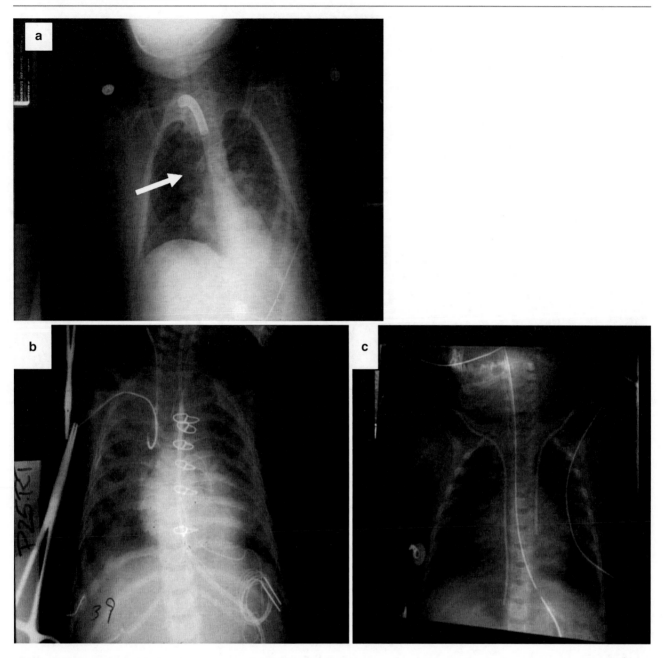

Fig. 29.12 Malpositioned subclavian catheters: (**a**) Catheter tip against lateral wall of superior vena cava (SVC). (**b**) Catheter curled in SVC. (**c**) Catheter through RA into IVC in patient with bilateral vena cavae

artery, catheter misplacement, pneumothorax, mediastinal hematoma, hemothorax, injury to adjacent nerve structures, and cannulation of the thoracic duct when cannulating the left subclavian vein. The incidences of these complications vary from 0.5 to 12 % [49, 52, 65, 66]. In general, life-threatening mechanical complications (tension pneumothorax, hemothorax) are uncommon in adults and children, occurring in <3 % of catheter insertions [10, 19, 44, 49]. In the report by Mansfield, complications occurred in greater than 25 % of those patients wherein catheterization was unsuccessful [49]. In adults, the overall failure rate of subclavian vein catheterization ranges from 10 to 19 % and is primarily dependent upon operator experience [67]. Where controversy once existed, more studies are being published which suggest that ultrasound-guided subclavian vein cannulation is the preferred method based upon data showing lower complication rates, shorter time to access, and fewer attempts to achieve vessel cannulation [49, 51, 68]. Additional discussion will follow in the section pertaining to ultrasound guided central venous cannulation.

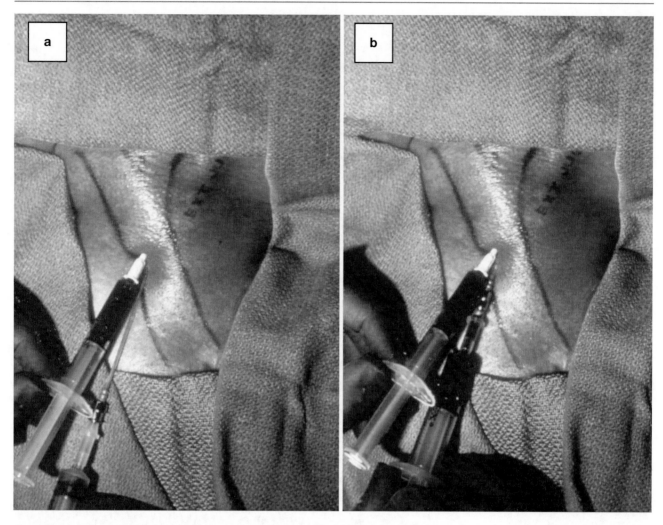

Fig. 29.13 "Finder needle" technique for IJV catheterization – anterior approach. (**a**) Small bore "finder needle" in place at apex of the triangle created by the clavicle and the sternal and clavicular bellies of the SCM and insertion of a large bore needle along the same trajectory. (**b**) Finder needle and large bore needle in place

Internal Jugular Vein Catheterization

Demographic: Historical Data: Indications for Placement

English et al. were the first to describe the safety and efficacy of internal jugular vein (IJV) catheterization in children [69]. They reported upon a series of 85 infants and children and found a 91 % success rate of catheterization and reported few complications using the medial approach to the vein. Prince et al. expanded upon the IJV experience in children and reported an overall catheterization success rate of 77 %. They also reported three patients with local hematomas at the site of insertion when the carotid artery was punctured [70]. They attributed their low rate of complications to the use of a small gauge "finder needle" to locate the vein and avoid unnecessary probing for the vein location (Fig. 29.13). Hall and colleagues described their success with two approaches

(posterior and medial) to IJV catheterization in children [71]. Successful catheterization occurred in >90 % of attempts and multiple attempts did not increase complication rates. The only complications were three arterial punctures. In this series, the IJV approach was used successfully in 20 patients who required resuscitation.

Internal jugular vein catheterization is associated with a high rate of successful catheter placement. Non-emergent catheterizations are successful in more than 90 % of patients. Use of the IJV for emergency catheterization during cardiopulmonary resuscitation is more difficult primarily because management of the airway, including tracheal intubation and bag ventilation, make access to the neck less available and identification of surface landmarks for catheter insertion more difficult. IJV cannulation is often considered when other central vascular approaches are less desirable, such as in the presence of coagulation abnormalities or chest trauma. The low incidence of pneumothorax makes the IJV

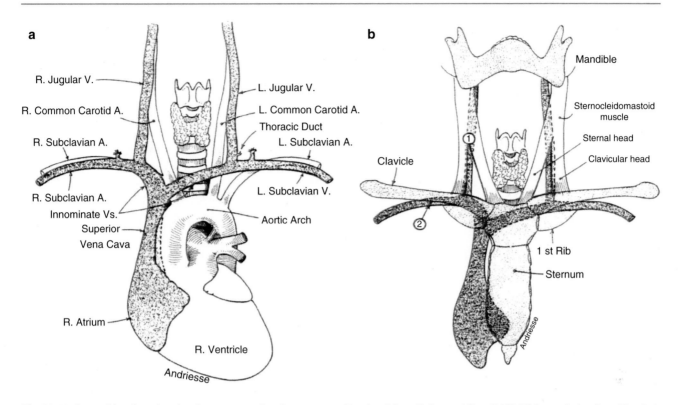

Fig. 29.14 Internal jugular vein related structures and surface anatomy (Reprinted from Todres and Cote [122]. With permission from Elsevier)

preferable in patients with significant pulmonary disease and lung hyperinflation (pleural dome elevated in the thorax) such as patients receiving high levels of positive pressure mechanical ventilatory support to treat respiratory failure. In addition, for patients with significant coagulation dysfunction, the IJV is favored because local compression of the vein or carotid artery is possible, whereas this is not an option with subclavian vein catheterization. The right IJV is also an optimal insertion site during emergency transvenous pacing, since it facilitates passage of the pacemaker through the tricuspid valve. In addition the right IJV may be preferred because of the position of the pleural dome, the absence of the thoracic duct, and the less acute angle at the junction of the IJV and innominate vein [47]. Cervical trauma with swelling or anatomic distortion at the insertion site may make IJV catheterization difficult or relatively contraindicated [72]. In adults, significant carotid artery disease is a relative contraindication to IJV catheterization.

Anatomy

The internal jugular vein emerges from the base of the skull through the jugular foramen, and enters the carotid sheath anterior and lateral to the carotid artery (Fig. 29.14).

The internal jugular vein usually runs beneath the triangle formed by the sternal and clavicular heads of the sternoclei-domastoid muscle (SCM) as it approaches the underside of clavicle. The caliber of the IJV increases as it approaches the clavicle. The vein is closer to the skin surface at the level of the clavicle as well. Beneath the clavicle the right internal jugular vein joins the subclavian vein to form the innominate vein, which continues in a straight path to the superior vena cava. The left internal jugular vein joins the left subclavian vein at nearly a right angle; consequently any catheter inserted into the left IJV must negotiate this turn [73] (Fig. 29.15d). The carotid artery usually lies medial and posterior to the IJV in the carotid sheath. In children positioned with their head in the neutral position, Roth et al. demonstrated that the IJV was most often found antero-lateral and anterior (54 and 24 %, respectively) in relation to the carotid artery [74]. The stellate ganglion and the cervical sympathetic trunk lie medial and posterior to the IJV. Near the junction of the IJV and the subclavian vein is the pleural dome, with the left pleural dome slightly more cephalad than the right. The lymphatic duct is adjacent to the junction of the left IJV and innominate vein. Anatomic variation of the IJV is common and clinical maneuvers can significantly affect vessel dynamics (vessel caliber). These variations can have an important impact upon success rates for IJV catheterization. Using ultrasound, Mallory et al. determined that palpation of the carotid artery decreases the IJV lumen cross-sectional area [75]. He suggests that when attempting IJV cannulation, a mental note should be made regarding

Fig. 29.15 Cervicothoracic catheter placement –
catheter tip malpositions: (**a**, **b**) Catheter tips striking
lateral wall of superior vena cava – vessel erosion risk.
(**c**) Ventricular placement. (**d**) Short left IJV catheter
striking innominate vein wall – vessel erosion risk. (**e**)
Short right subclavian catheter striking lateral wall of
innominate vein – vessel erosion risk (Reprinted from
Todres and Cote [122]. With permission from Elsevier)

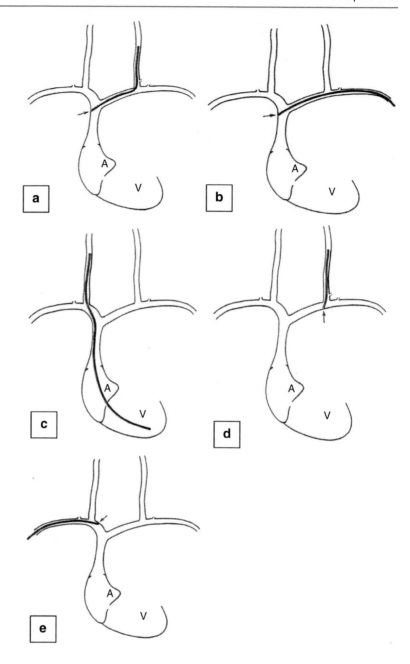

the position of the carotid artery; however the artery should
not be palpated during actual needle/syringe insertion.
Maneuvers that increase the cross-sectional area and internal
diameter of the IJV include: (1) Trendelenburg position with
a 15–30° of head-down tilt; (2) the valsalva maneuver; and
(3) retracting the skin over the vein in a direction opposite
to the direction of the advancing needle. In addition, clinical
conditions which increase right atrial pressures also increase
the vessel lumen cross-sectional area. In another report
locating the position of the IJV by ultrasound demonstrated,
in adults, that in 3 % of patients studied the IJV lumen did
not increase in response to valsalva, in 1 % the IJV lumen
was >1 cm lateral to the carotid artery, in 2 % the IJV was

positioned medially over the carotid artery, and in 5 % the
IJV was positioned outside the area which is predicted by
surface landmarks [76]. Suk et al. reported that using a skin
traction method using tape to stretch and secure the skin in
the cephalad and caudal positions increased the ultrasound-
measured cross-sectional area of the IJV by 40 % in infants
and 34 % in children [77].

Insertion Technique

Detailed step by step videos on the placement of central
venous catheters and the use of ultrasound guidance have

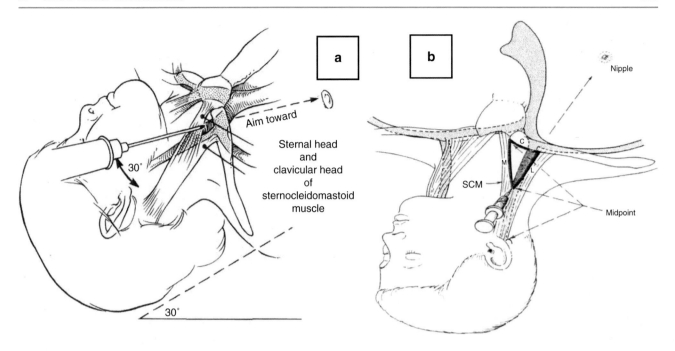

Fig. 29.16 Internal jugular vein anatomy: (**a**) Medial approach (Source: PALS Provider Manual © 1997, American Heart Association, Inc). (**b**) Medial approach with triangle between bellies of SCM (Reprinted from Todres and Cote [122]. With permission from Elsevier)

been published [78, 79]. Here we detail the insertion technique using the surface landmark method. The patient is positioned in Trendelenburg position (unless contraindicated, such as with elevated intracranial pressure) with head down 15–30°. For the medial approach (Fig. 29.16) the two bellies of the SCM should be palpated by placing the index finger in the triangle created by the clavicle and the sternal and clavicular bellies of the SCM. Retract the skin cephalad to the insertion site prior to inserting the needle into the skin. This may increase the vessel lumen cross-sectional area. During actual venipuncture, avoid trying to retract the carotid artery medially and away from the IJV as this is likely to decrease the IJV lumen diameter. For the medial approach, the approximate insertion site is one half the distance along a line from the sternal notch to the mastoid prominence. Insert the needle at an angle about 20–30° above the plane of the skin. Advance the needle while applying slight negative pressure on the syringe. Venous flashback indicating venipuncture may occur during needle advancement or withdrawal, therefore if unsuccessful during advancement then the needle should be withdrawn slowly. The needle should be completely removed from the skin prior to redirecting to avoid vessel laceration. This is particularly important in small infants. Before attempting to place the guidewire (Seldinger technique), it is important to demonstrate free flow of "blue" blood into the syringe. Do not try to place the wire if blood cannot be easily withdrawn, if the blood in the syringe is pulsating, or if the blood is obviously very oxygenated (bright red). Gently twist the syringe off the needle hub, maintain the needle in the same position and always occlude the needle hub with your finger

to prevent air aspiration. The guidewire should be advanced without meeting any resistance. Resistance to wire advancement usually means the lumen of the needle is now outside the vessel. In this case, the wire can be removed and needle position slightly adjusted. If in trying to remove the wire, resistance is encountered, this can mean the wire is bent near the needle bevel. In this case the wire and needle should be removed together. This reduces the risk of shearing off the end of the wire. Once the guidewire is successfully advanced, the needle can be removed while holding the guidewire in place. Be careful not to advance the guidewire to its full length as cardiac arrhythmias may occur. Make a small ¼–½ cm skin incision at the site of entry of the guidewire into the skin. Be certain that the bevel of the scalpel blade is away from the guidewire. Hold the dilator near its tip and advance the dilator over the guidewire into the IJV. The dilator should not be fully advanced as its purpose is to dilate the subcutaneous tissue and make a hole in the vessel. Holding the guidewire in place, remove the dilator while applying light pressure to site. Place the catheter over the guidewire and insert into the IJV. Once the catheter is inserted, remove the guidewire and aspirate blood through the catheter to ascertain placement and patency of the catheter. Secure the catheter in place.

Posterior and anterior approaches to the IJV can also be used. These have similar success rates for cannulation and because the insertion sites are higher (more cephalad) in the neck, these approaches may carry lower risk of pneumothorax. Figures 29.16 and 29.17 depict all three approaches.

Some have suggested that using a "finder needle" to locate the IJV both reduces the incidence of carotid artery puncture

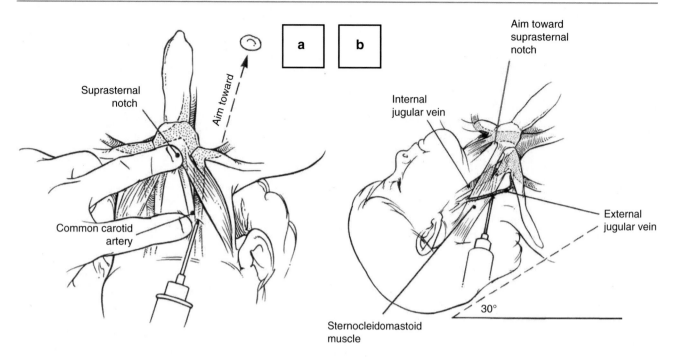

Fig. 29.17 Alternative approaches to IJV catheterization: (**a**) Anterior. (**b**) Posterior (Source: PALS Provider Manual © 1997, American Heart Association, Inc)

and if advertent arterial puncture occurs, the smaller bore "finder needle" will cause less damage to the arterial wall and reduce the sequelae that might occur from carotid artery hematoma. Figure 29.13 demonstrates first finding the IJV with a small bore needle and then advancing the larger bore needle along the same trajectory as the "finder needle." Alternatively, the finder needle can be removed and the large bore introducer needle advanced in the same plane as the initial finder needle. This technique may be most useful in obese patients with poor surface landmarks or in patients with coagulopathy wherein puncture of the artery may be more problematic than usual.

Confirmation of Placement

Optimal location of a catheter in the internal jugular vein is in the superior vena cava near the junction with the right atrium, but not in it. Chest radiography is commonly used to confirm the position of the central venous catheter tip. Clinical controversy regarding the need for post procedure chest radiography is similar to that described for subclavian vein catheterization. As reported previously, Gladwin found that 14 % of IJV catheter tips were malpositioned in a series of 107 consecutive adult patients [61]. Given the risk of unrecognized catheter malposition, which because of small patient size, may be greater in children than adults, post procedure chest radiography is warranted even in patients who are clinically unchanged post procedure.

Complications

Other than complications related to catheter maintenance (infections and thrombosis), complications related to catheter insertion are uncommon. Arterial puncture is the most common complication and is usually easily resolved with direct pressure to the punctured vessel. Nicolson reported an 8 % incidence of arterial puncture but minimal sequelae from the arterial puncture because she used the finder needle technique to avoid puncturing the artery with the large bore needle that is needed to pass the guidewire [80, 81]. Arterial puncture is significantly more common with IJV catheterization than with subclavian vein catheterization, with a reported incidence of 2–11 % in adults [52, 73, 82]. Pneumothorax or hemothorax are rare complications with an average incidence of 0–0.2 % [27, 76, 83, 84].

Catheter tip malposition is a frequent complication of all central venous catheters and IJV catheters are no exception. As previously described, dysrhythmias, pericardial tamponade, and mediastinal effusions have been reported when stiff plastic catheters erode through thin vessel walls [58, 85, 86]. Figure 29.18 depicts several IJV catheter malpositions in children. Figure 29.18b shows a short left IJV catheter with its tip at the IJV – innominate junction. Subsequent chest radiograph reveals a widened mediastinum filled with lipid as a result of vessel erosion by the catheter and extravasation of parenterally administered lipid into the mediastinum (Fig. 29.18c). Figures 29.19 and 29.15 depict both correctly positioned and malpositioned cervicothoracic catheters. Malpositioned catheters are at high risk for vessel erosion.

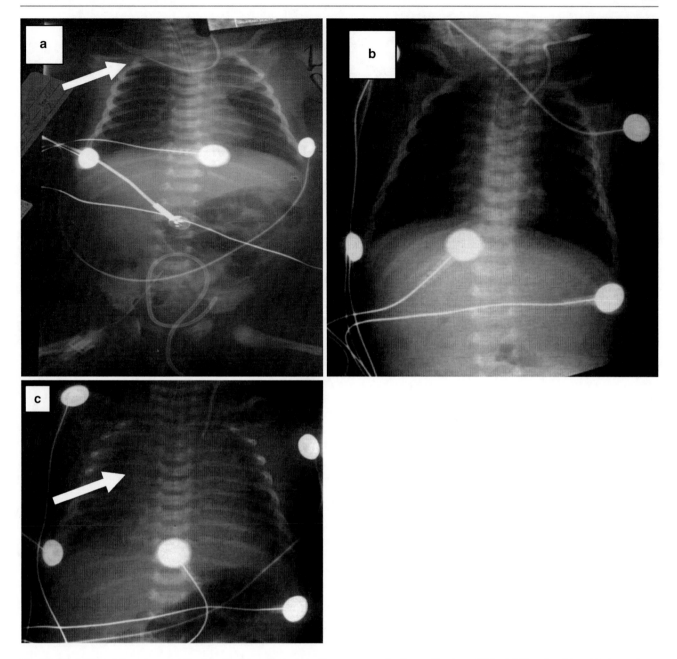

Fig. 29.18 (a) Left IJV catheter malposition in right subclavian vein – no recognized complications. (b) Left IJV malpositioned in innominate vein. (c) Catheter erodes through vessel wall – widened mediastinum with lipid extravasation

Axillary Vein Catheterization

Demographic and Historical Data: Indications for Use

The axillary vein is an alternative, and less commonly discussed, access site for central venous catheterization in children. A percutaneous approach to axillary vein catheterization was first described in 1981 and a modified technique further described in very low birth weight infants [87, 88]. These reports demonstrated a high success rate for cannulation with minimal complication rates. Oriot's report included axillary vein catheterization in 226 neonates with only nine failures [88]. In a few patients, non-persisting extrasystoles occurred during catheter insertion but disappeared with correct positioning of the catheter. No intrathoracic complications were noted. Metz reported on a cohort of 47 critically ill children (age 14 days to 9 years) who underwent 52 separate attempts at axillary vein catheterization. His reported success rate for cannulation was 79 % [89]. The most common reasons the axillary vein was used included: (1) poor alternative access sites; (2) need for hyperalimentation; (3) need for central

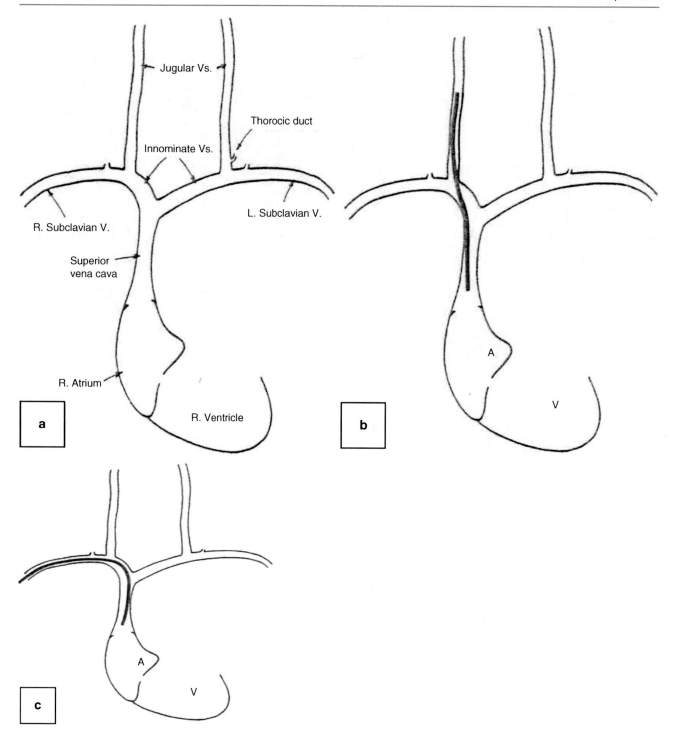

Fig. 29.19 Cervicothoracic catheter placement – proper catheter tip positions: (**a**) Normal vascular anatomy. (**b**) Right IJV. (**c**) Right subclavian vein (Reprinted from Todres and Cote [122]. With permission from Elsevier)

venous pressure monitoring; and (4) preservation of femoral vessels for cardiac catheterization.

Martin has recently reported his experience with single lumen axillary catheters placed in 60 adults in a surgical intensive care unit [90]. Insertion complications were infrequent and deep venous upper extremity thrombosis occurred in 11 % of the patients. He concluded that because the thrombosis rates were similar between axillary vein and cervicothoracic catheters, the axillary vein offered an attractive alternative when other sites were unavailable.

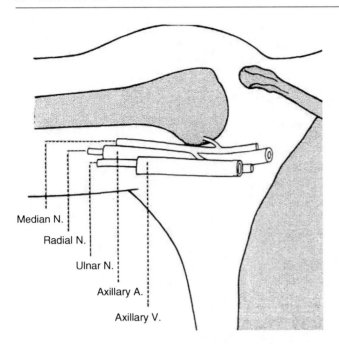

Fig. 29.20 Axillary vein anatomy (Reprinted from Metz et al. [89]. With permission from American Academy of Pediatrics)

Anatomy

The axillary vein begins at the junction of the basilic and brachial veins running medial, anterior and caudal to the axillary artery. In the chest at the lateral border of the first rib it becomes the subclavian vein. The artery and vein lie within the axillary fascia and the brachial plexus runs between the artery and vein (Fig. 29.20).

Technique

Catheter insertion is accomplished with the child placed in the Trendelenburg position, if not contraindicated, and the arm abducted between 100° and 130°. The position of the axillary artery is determined by palpation while retracting the redundant axillary skin with the opposite hand. The vein is punctured parallel and inferior to the artery as described by Gouin [91]. A 22-gauge short Teflon catheter can be used to cannulate the vein as if inserting a peripheral venous catheter. Alternatively, a thin-walled needle appropriate for the central venous catheter use can be used to obtain venous flashback. The needle/syringe should be inserted using negative pressure on the syringe hub. Once venous blood is obtained, the syringe is carefully disconnected from the needle and the guidewire inserted as per standard Seldinger technique. The axillary vein in children is very mobile in the axillary soft tissue and the greatest challenge to cannulation is fixing the vein in position so that the needle can enter the vessel. Firm traction of the redundant skin can help with this issue.

Complications

Complications associated with axillary vein insertion include failed cannulation, catheter malposition, arterial puncture, transient paresthesia, pneumothorax and axillary hematoma [92, 93]. The frequency of complications reported by Metz in a pediatric cohort is low – with complications of insertion occurring in 3.8 % – one pneumothorax and one hematoma [89]. Four additional complications occurred while the catheter was in place and these included venous stasis of the arm, venous thrombosis of the subclavian vein proximal to the catheter tip, parenteral nutrition infiltration secondary to catheter dislodgment, and one catheter-related infection.

The axillary vein route has a lower rate of successful cannulation and results in higher incidence of catheter malposition and arterial puncture when compared with IJV catheterization, however the IJV route had a greater risk of pneumothorax [93]. Axillary vein catheter insertion success was 84 %, which is lower than IJV catheterization. Martin concluded that this rate of success was acceptable when other sites are less unavailable.

Ultrasound-Guided Central Vein Catheterization: The New Standard?

Traditionally percutaneous insertions of CVCs have been performed by utilizing anatomic surface landmarks. Recently, bedside use of Doppler ultrasound has been used to facilitate vessel visualization. In some settings, the use of ultrasound increases catheter placement success rates, especially for novice operators, and reduces complications. Doppler ultrasound assist with catheter placement was first reported in 1984 [94]. Gualtieri et al. demonstrated in a prospective, randomized study that subclavian vein catheterization was successful in 23 of 25 (92 %) attempts using ultrasound guidance compared to 12 of 27 (44 %) using conventional landmark techniques [51]. In the hands of less experienced operators, ultrasound guidance improves subclavian vein cannulation success and in high-risk patients with obesity or coagulopathy, the use of ultrasound improved cannulation success with fewer significant complications [95].

In adults, multiple reports have shown that ultrasound guided central venous access is associated with decreased number of attempts, higher access success rates, and fewer catheter insertion related complications compared to surface landmark techniques [50, 96–98]. A randomized, controlled clinical trial in adults compared the overall success rate for IJV cannula placement by comparing dynamic (real-time) ultrasound, static ultrasound and surface anatomical landmarks. The odds for successful cannulation using dynamic ultrasound was 54 (95 % CI 6.6–44.0) times higher compared to landmark methodology [38]. Recently, Fragou et al.

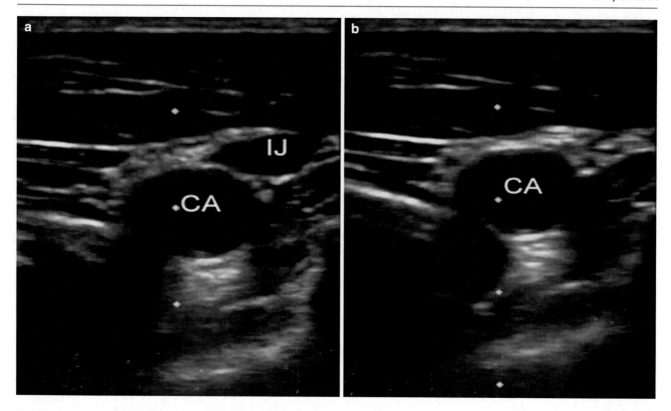

Fig. 29.21 Ultrasound image of internal jugular (*IJ*) vein and carotid artery (*CA*) with the ultrasound probe lightly touching the skin (**a**) and with gentle pressure compressing the IJ vein but maintaining the diameter of the CA (**b**)

compared ultrasound-guided infraclavicular subclavian vein cannulation to landmark methodology and found significantly shorter access time, fewer attempts, and complications in the ultrasound group compared to the landmark group. Catheter misplacement was not different between groups. They suggest that ultrasound-guided subclavian vein cannulation should be the method of choice [68].

Similar findings regarding the benefits of ultrasound guidance have been demonstrated in pediatric patients. The success rate for IJ catheter placement in infants prior to cardiac surgery was 100 % in the ultrasound group compared with a 77 % success rate in the group who underwent catheter placement by landmarks only [99]. In a separate study, Verghese also demonstrated that US-guidance for IJ catheter placement led to quicker cannulation times and fewer attempts [100]. In a recent meta-analysis, Sigaut et al. analyzed five clinical trials that compared ultrasound guidance to anatomical landmarks during IJV access in pediatric patients [101]. The authors found that ultrasound guidance had no effect on the rate of complications or IJV failure rate. However, in this study, four of the five studies were performed in cardiac surgery patients and therefore the results may not be generalizable to the heterogeneous pediatric intensive care unit population.

Prospective clinical data on the use of ultrasound guidance in the general PICU population is limited. Froehlich et al. performed a prospective study in a quaternary multidisciplinary pediatric intensive care unit [102]. The overall success rate and time to success of CVC placement was not significantly different between the landmark and ultrasound groups. However, 40 % (37/93) of the patients in the landmark group required four or more attempts compared with only 20 % (24/119) of the patients in the ultrasound group. The number of inadvertent arterial punctures was less in the ultrasound group compared with the landmark group, and all arterial punctures occurred at the femoral site. A national survey of the use of bedside ultrasound in pediatric critical care was recently conducted by Lambert et al. [103]. Seventy percent of responders stated they currently use bedside ultrasound. Pediatric ICUs with greater than 12 beds, greater than 1,000 yearly admissions, and university-based institutions with either a pediatric critical care medicine fellowship or a cardiovascular thoracic surgery program were more likely to use bedside ultrasound for CVC placement. The preferred site for bedside ultrasound was "almost always" or "frequently" the IJV. Importantly, formal training on bedside ultrasound use occurred in 20 % of ultrasound using responders. Figure 29.21 depicts IJV and carotid artery images as observed using ultrasound guidance.

The advantages associated with ultrasound guided central venous catheter placement include detection of anatomic variations and exact vessel location, avoidance of central veins with pre-existing thrombosis that may prevent successful central venous catheter placement, and guidance of both guidewire and catheter placement after initial needle insertion. The greatest benefit for use of ultrasound guidance may occur for the inexperienced operator and for all operators in high-risk clinical situations. The results from randomized controlled clinical trial in adults, comparing success rates for catheterization and complication rates were so compelling in favor of real-time ultrasound guided placement of percutaneous central venous catheters that some have called ultrasound guidance the "new standard of care" [36, 104].

In summary, the use of ultrasound guided CVC placement in pediatrics occurs commonly and should be in the arsenal available to all practitioners who place central catheters. These authors believe that the data in children pertaining to ultrasound use is sufficient to require that it be available for bedside use, but not sufficient to require its use in all circumstances. Clinicians should continue to use their judgment about when to apply this important adjunct for line placement. Furthermore inexperienced operators and physicians in training may benefit the most from the use of bedside ultrasound during CVC placement.

Complications Associated With Central Venous Catheter Placement

Central venous catheters are associated with numerous complications, some minor and others life-threatening. These complications are primarily related to mechanical complications at the time of catheter insertion or complications that occur during maintenance of the catheter. Catheter associated blood stream infections and catheter related thrombosis are major complications that occur during catheter maintenance and have been the subject of excellent recent reviews and are topics of other chapters in this text [105, 106]. They will not be the subject of this review. Furthermore, mechanical complications associated with insertion have been previously discussed under the heading for each type of catheterization and the reader is referred to those sections. A brief summary will be included here.

A retrospective review of over 1,400 central venous catheters placed in children demonstrated that age, sex, type of catheter, primary disease, indication for placement, level of physician training, and operator experience were not associated with increased complication risks [22]. Conversely, in a study by Sznajder et al. the complication rate for inexperienced physicians was double the rate of more experienced physicians when performing central venous catheter insertion [67].

Pneumothorax

In children, pneumothorax is reported as a complication in 1–2 % of CVC insertions placed by surgical staff surgical and in 4 % of patients when performed by nonsurgical staff [10, 22, 107]. More recent data indicates that a pneumothorax occurred in only two out of 156 patients (1.2 %) who underwent central venous catheter placement by pediatricians skilled in emergency procedures [108].

Arterial Puncture

Using classic Seldinger technique arterial puncture occurs during central venous catheter insertion in 1.5–15 % [8–10, 22, 94, 109]. Merrer et al. demonstrated that catheter insertion during the night was significantly associated with the occurrence of mechanical complications including arterial puncture [19].

Catheter Malposition: Femoral Catheters

It is important to determine catheter placement because malposition of central venous catheters can result in both morbidity and mortality [40, 110]. Malposition of femoral catheters in the ascending lumbar vein is an infrequent complication but if left in place can result in tetraplegia. Zenker et al. reviewed contrast radiographs taken immediately after insertion of 44 transfemoral catheters in a neonatal intensive care unit [40]. Malposition of catheters in the left ascending lumbar vein was detected in two newborns. Paravertebral malposition has been previously reported in neonates [111–113]. These reports demonstrate that catheter position was initially misinterpreted or assessed inadequately until the onset of complications. In newborns, the vertebrolumbar and azygous systems represent an extensive, highly variable, intercommunicating network in which alterations in pressure and flow direction may occur. The large capacity of the lumbar veins and the vertebral plexus can compensate for occlusion of the inferior vena cava. Use of catheters misplaced in this posterior system can give rise to retroperitoneal, peritoneal or spinal epidural fluid extravasation [98, 114, 115]. Ultrasonography, lateral radiography, or venogram is required in cases in which the location of the catheter tip is in question. Catheters in the ascending lumbar vein or vertebral plexus should be removed immediately. Warning signs that may indicate catheter malposition include: (1) loss of blood return on aspiration; (2) subtle lateral deviation, or "hump," of the catheter at the level of L4 or L5 on frontal abdominal radiographs in catheters placed from the left side (Fig. 29.8); (3) a catheter path directly overlying the vertebral column rather than the expected path to the right of midline for a catheter in the inferior vena cava; (4) resistance to guidewire advancement during insertion [96]. A lateral abdominal radiograph may confirm the posterior position of the catheter, however this author has found that a venogram (injecting dye directly into the catheter – Fig. 29.8) is the best method to confirm proper placement of these catheters.

Catheter Malposition and Post Procedure Chest Radiographs: Cervicothoracic Catheters

As noted previously, Fig. 29.15 depicts cervicothoracic catheter malpositions that are potentially hazardous. Three recent reports describing experience in adult patients conclude that a postprocedure chest radiograph is unnecessary in the asymptomatic patient after IJV catheterization when using fluoroscopy or ultrasound during catheter placement [116–118]. Similar recommendations are made for subclavian vein approach. A study in adults focusing on the subclavian vein catheterization concluded that postprocedure chest radiograph has minimal benefit and is not necessary, unless the patient shows sign of clinical deterioration post procedure [119]. Others have advocated that a postprocedure chest x-ray may be omitted in cases after line placement when experienced clinicians use good technique and good clinical judgment [61, 120]. In pediatrics little data driven recommendations are available, however Janik reports that routine chest x-ray is not indicated after uneventful central venous catheter insertion when monitored with concurrent fluoroscopy [121]. These recommendations were based on a low rate of complications of 1.6 %. In addition, all children who had pulmonary complications displayed signs and symptoms suggestive of impaired respiratory function. This recommendation may not be relevant to the pediatric ICU setting where catheters are rarely placed with fluoroscopic guidance. In the ICU, these authors recommend chest radiography after all percutaneously placed central venous catheters, regardless of post procedure clinical status.

References

1. Food and Drug Administration: precautions with central venous catheters. FDA Taskforce. FDA Drug Bulletin. 1989. p. 15–6.
2. O'Grady NP, Alexander M, Dellinger EP, et al. Guidelines for the prevention of intravascular catheter-related infections. Pediatrics. 2002;110(5):e51.
3. Abraham E, Shapiro M, Podolsky S. Central venous catheterization in the emergency department. Crit Care Med. 1983;11:515–7.
4. Getzen LC, Pollak EW. Short-term femoral vein catheterization – a safe alternative venous access? Am J Surg. 1979;138:876–8.
5. Chiang VW, Baskin MN. Uses and complications of central venous catheters inserted in a pediatric emergency department. Pediatr Emerg Care. 2000;16(4):230–2.
6. Venkataraman ST, Thompson AE, Orr RA. Femoral vascular catheterization in critically ill infants and children. Clin Pediatr. 1997;36:311–9.
7. Vascular access. In: Zaritsky AL, Nadkarni V, Hickey R, et al., editors. PALS provider manual. Dallas: American Heart Association; 2002. p. 155–72.
8. Kanter RK, Zimmerman JJ, Strauss RH, Stoeckel KA. Central venous catheter insertion by femoral vein: safety and effectiveness for the pediatric patient. Pediatrics. 1986;77(6):842–7.
9. Durbec O, Viviand X, Potie F, et al. A prospective evaluation of the use of femoral venous catheters in critically ill adults. Crit Care Med. 1997;25:1986–9.
10. Venkataraman ST, Orr RA, Thompson AE. Percutaneous infraclavicular subclavian vein catheterization in critically ill infants and children. J Pediatr. 1988;113(3):480–5.
11. Finck C, Smith S, Jackson R, et al. Percutaneous subclavian central venous catheterization in children younger than one year of age. Am Surg. 2002;68:401–6.
12. Centers for Disease Control and Prevention. Guidelines for the prevention of intravascular catheter-related infections. 2011. www.cdc.gov/hicpac/BSI/BSI-guidelines-2011.html. Accessed Oct 2011.
13. Niedner MF, Huskins WC, Colantuoni E, et al. Epidemiology of central line associated bloodstream infections in the pediatric intensive care unit. Infect Control Hosp Epidemiol. 2011;32:1200–8.
14. Moncrief JA. Femoral catheters. Ann Surg. 1958;147:166–72.
15. Swanson RS, Uhlig PN, Gross PL, McCabe CJ. Emergency intravenous access through the femoral vein. Ann Emerg Med. 1984;13(4):244–7.
16. Goldstein AM, Weber JM, Sheridan RL. Femoral venous access is safe in burned children: an analysis of 224 catheters. J Pediatr. 1997;130(3):442–6.
17. Nidus B, Speyer J, Bottino J, et al. Repeated femoral vein cannulation for administration of chemotherapeutic agents. Ca Treat Rep. 1983;67:186.
18. Bansmer G, Keith D, Tesluk H. Complication following use of indwelling catheters of the inferior vena cava. JAMA. 1958;167:1606–11.
19. Merrer J, De Jonghe B, Golliot F, Lefrant JY, Raffy B, Barre E, et al. Complications of femoral and subclavian venous catheterization in critically ill patients: a randomized controlled trial. JAMA. 2001;286(6):700–7.
20. Seneff MG, Rippe JM. Central venous catheters. In: Rippe JM, Irwin RS, Alpert JS, et al., editors. Intensive care medicine. Boston: Little Brown; 1985. p. 16–33.
21. McIntyre KM, Lewis AJ, editors. Textbook of advance cardiac life support. Dallas: American Heart Association; 1990.
22. Smyrnios NA, Irwin RS. The jury on femoral vein catheterization is still out. Crit Care Med. 1997;25:1943–6.
23. de Jonge RC, Polderman KH, Gemke RJ. Central venous catheter use in the pediatric patient: mechanical and infectious complications. Pediatr Crit Care Med. 2005;6:329–39.
24. Johnson EM, Saltzman DA, Suh G, Dahms RA, Leonard AS. Complications and risks of central venous catheter placement in children. Surgery. 1998;124:911–6.
25. Beck C, Dubois J, Grignon A, Lacroix J, David M. Incidence and risk factors of catheter-related deep vein thrombosis in a pediatric intensive care unit: a prospective study. J Pediatr. 1998;133(2):237–41.
26. Jacobs B, Brilli R, Babcock D. High incidence of vascular thrombosis after placement of subclavian & internal jugular venous catheters in children. Crit Care Med. 1999;27:A29.
27. Casado-Flores J, Barja J, Martino R, et al. Complications of central venous catheterization in critically ill children. Pediatr Crit Care Med. 2001;2:57–62.
28. Richards M, Edwards J, Culver D, et al. Nosocomial infections in pediatric intensive care units in the United States. National Nosocomial Infections Surveillance System. Pediatrics. 1999;103:103–9.
29. Stenzel JP, Green TP, Fuhrman BP, et al. Percutaneous femoral venous catheterizations: a prospective study of complications. J Pediatr. 1989;114:411–5.
30. Fernendez E, Green T, Sweeney M. Low inferior vena caval catheters for hemodynamic and pulmonary function monitoring in pediatric critical care patients. Ped Crit Care Med. 2004;5:14–8.
31. Lloyd R, Donnerstein R, Berg R. Accuracy of central venous pressure measurement from the abdominal inferior vena cava. Pediatrics. 1992;89:506–8.

32. Ho K, Joynt G, Tan P. A comparison of central venous pressure and common iliac venous pressure in critically ill mechanically ventilated patients. Crit Care Med. 1998;26:461–4.

33. Dillon P, Columb M, Hume D. Comparison of superior vena caval and femoroiliac venous pressure measurements during normal and inverse ratio ventilation. Crit Care Med. 2001;29:37–9.

34. Tribett D, Brenner M. Peripheral and femoral vein cannulation. In: Venus B, Mallory D, editors. Problems in critical care – vascular access. Philadelphia: JB Lippincott; 1988. p. 266–85.

35. Seldinger SI. Catheter replacement of the needle in percutaneous arteriography; a new technique. Acta Radiol. 1953;39(5): 368–76.

36. Raad I, Hohn D, Gilbreath B, et al. Prevention of central venous catheter-related infection by using maximal sterile barrier precautions during insertion. Infect Control Hosp Epidemiol. 1994;15: 231–8.

37. Kanter R, Gorton J, Palmieri K, et al. Anatomy of femoral vessels in infants and guidelines for venous catheterization. Pediatrics. 1989;83:1020–2.

38. Milling T, Rose J, Briggs W, et al. Randomized, controlled clinical trial of point-of-care limited ultrasonography assistance of central venous cannulation: the Third Sonography Outcomes Assessment Program (SOAP-3) Trial. Crit Care Med. 2005;33:1764–9.

39. Otto C. Central venous pressure monitoring. In: Blitt C, Hines R, editors. Monitoring in anesthesia and critical care medicine. 3rd ed. New York: Churchill Livingston; 1995. p. 173–212.

40. Zenker M, Rupprecht T, Hofbeck M, et al. Paravertebral and intraspinal malposition of transfemoral central venous catheters in newborns. J Pediatr. 2000;136(6):837–40.

41. Aubaniac R. L'injection intraveineuse sous-claviculaire. Presse Med. 1952;60:1656–9.

42. Sterner S, Plummer D, Clinton I, et al. A comparison of the supraclavicular approach and the infraclavicular approach for subclavian vein catheterization. Ann Emerg Med. 1986;15:421–4.

43. Groff S, Ahmed N. Subclavian vein catheterization in the infant. J Ped Surg. 1974;9:171–4.

44. Casado-Flores J, Valdivielso-Serna A, Perez-Jurado L, et al. Subclavian vein catheterization in critically ill children: analysis of 322 cannulations. Intensive Care Med. 1991;17:350–4.

45. McGovern T, Brandt B. Percutaneous infraclavicular subclavian venous access in infants and children. Contemp Surg. 1994;45(6): 335–9.

46. Stovroff M, Teague W. Intravenous access in infants and children. Pediatr Clin N Am. 1998;45:1373–93.

47. Novak R, Venus B. Clavicular approaches for central vein cannulation. In: Venus B, Mallory D, editors. Problems in critical care – vascular access. Philadelphia: JB Lippincott; 1988. p. 242–65.

48. Kaye W, Dubin H. Vascular cannulation. In: Civetta J, Taylor W, Kirby R, editors. Critical care. 1st ed. Philadelphia: JB Lippincott; 1988. p. 211–25.

49. Mansfield PF, Hohn DC, Fornage BD, et al. Complications and failures of subclavian-vein catheterization. N Engl J Med. 1994;331: 1735–8.

50. Randolph AG, Cook DJ, Gonzales CA, et al. Ultrasound guidance for placement of central venous catheters: a meta-analysis of literature. Crit Care Med. 1996;24:2053–8.

51. Gualtieri E, Deppe S, Sipperly M, et al. Subclavian venous catheterization: greater success rate for less experienced operators using ultrasound guidance. Crit Care Med. 1995;23(4):692–7.

52. Ruesch S, Walder B, Tramer MR. Complications of central venous catheters: internal jugular versus subclavian access – a systematic review. Crit Care Med. 2002;30(2):454–60.

53. Jung C, Bahk J, Kim M, et al. Head position for facilitating the superior vena caval placement of catheters during right subclavian approach in children. Crit Care Med. 2002;30:297–9.

54. Land RE. Anatomic relationships of the right subclavian vein. A radiologic study pertinent to percutaneous subclavian venous catheterization. Arch Surg. 1971;102(3):178–80.

55. Tan BK, Hong SW, Huang MH, Lee ST. Anatomic basis of safe percutaneous subclavian venous catheterization. J Trauma. 2000; 48(1):82–6.

56. van Engelenburg K, Festen C. Cardiac tamponade: a rare but life-threatening complication of central venous catheters in children. J Pediatr Surg. 1998;33(12):1822–4.

57. Beattie PG, Kuschel CA, Harding JE. Pericardial effusion complicating a percutaneous central venous line in a neonate. Acta Paediatr. 1993;82(1):105–7.

58. Nowlen TT, Rosenthal GL, Johnson GL, et al. Pericardial effusion and tamponade in infants with central catheters. Pediatrics. 2002;110:137–42.

59. Andropoulos D, Bent S, Skjonsby B, et al. The optimal length of insertion of central venous catheters for pediatric patients. Anesth Analg. 2001;93:883–6.

60. McGee W, Ackerman B, Rouben L, et al. Accurate placement of central venous catheters: a prospective, randomized, multicenter trial. Crit Care Med. 1993;21:1118–23.

61. Gladwin MT, Slonim A, Landucci DL, et al. Cannulation of the internal jugular vein: is postprocedural chest radiography always necessary? Crit Care Med. 1999;27(9):1819–23.

62. Bailey S, Shapiro S, Mone M, et al. Is immediate chest radiograph necessary after central venous catheter placement in a surgical intensive care unit? Am J Surg. 2000;180:517–22.

63. Puls L, Twedt C, Hunter J, et al. Confirmatory chest radiographs after central line placement: are they warranted? South Med J. 2003;96:1138–41.

64. Lessnau K. Is chest radiography necessary after uncomplicated insertion of a triple-lumen catheter in the right internal jugular vein, using the anterior approach? Chest. 2005;127:220–3.

65. Conces D, Holden R. Aberrant locations and complications in initial placement of subclavian vein catheters. Arch Surg. 1984;119:293–5.

66. Defalque R, Gletcher M. Neurological complications of central venous cannulation. J Parenter Enter Nutr. 1988;12:406–9.

67. Sznajder J, Zveibil F, Bitterman H, et al. Central vein catheterization: failure and complication rates by three percutaneous approaches. Arch Intern Med. 1986;146(2):259–61.

68. Fragou M, Gravvanis A, Dimitriou V, et al. Real-time ultrasound-guided subclavian vein cannulation versus the landmark method in critical care patients: a prospective randomized study. Crit Care Med. 2011;39:1607–12.

69. English I, Frew R, Pigott J, et al. Percutaneous catheterization of the internal jugular vein. Anaesthesia. 1969;24:521–31.

70. Prince S, Sullivan R, Hackel A. Percutaneous catheterization of the internal jugular vein in infants and children. Anesthesiology. 1976;44:170–4.

71. Hall D, Geefhuysen J. Percutaneous catheterization of the internal jugular vein in infants and children. J Ped Surg. 1977;12: 719–22.

72. Wyte S, Barker W. Central venous catheterization: internal jugular approach and alternatives. In: Roberts J, Hedges J, editors. Clinical procedures in emergency medicine. Philadelphia: WB Saunders; 1985. p. 321–32.

73. McGee W, Mallory D. Cannulation of the internal and external jugular veins. In: Venus B, Mallory D, editors. Problems in critical care – vascular access. Philadelphia: JB Lippincott; 1988. p. 217–41.

74. Roth B, Marciniak B, Engelhardt T, Bissonnette B. Anatomic relationship between the internal jugular vein and the carotid artery in preschool children – an ultrasonographic study. Pediatr Anesth. 2008;18:752–6.

75. Mallory D, Shawker T, Evans R, et al. Effects of clinical maneuvers on sonographically determined internal jugular vein size during venous cannulation. Crit Care Med. 1990;18:1269–73.

76. Denys B, Uretsky B. Anatomical variations of internal jugular vein location: impact on central venous access. Crit Care Med. 1991;19:1516–9.

77. Suk E, Kim D, Kil H, Kweon TD. Effects of skin traction on cross-sectional area of the internal jugular vein in infants and young children. Anesth Intensive Care. 2010;38:342–5.

78. Graham A, Ozment C, Tegtmeyer K, Lai S, Braner D. Videos in clinical medicine. Central venous catherization. N Engl J Med. 2007;356:e21.

79. Ortega R, Song M, Hansen CJ, Barash P. Videos in clinical medicine. Ultrasound-guided internal jugular vein cannulation. N Engl J Med. 2010;362:e57.

80. Nicolson S, Sweeney M, Moore R, et al. Comparison of internal and external jugular cannulation of the central circulation in the pediatric patient. Crit Care Med. 1985;13:747–9.

81. Jobes D, Schwartz A, Greenhow D, et al. Safer jugular vein cannulation: recognition of arterial puncture and preferential use of the external jugular route. Anesthesiology. 1983;59:353.

82. Vaughan RW, Weygandt GR. Reliable percutaneous central venous pressure measurement. Anesth Analg. 1973;52:709–16.

83. Johnson F. Internal jugular vein catheterization. N Y State J Med. 1978;78(14):2168–71.

84. Brinkman A, Costley D. Internal jugular venipuncture. JAMA. 1973;223:182–3.

85. Daniels S, Hannon D, Meyer R, et al. Paroxysmal supraventricular tachycardia: a complication of jugular central venous catheters in neonates. AJDC. 1984;138:474–5.

86. Smith-Wright D, Green T, Lock J, et al. Complications of vascular catheterization in critically ill children. Crit Care Med. 1984;12:1015–7.

87. Meignier M, Nicolas F. [Perfusion by axillary approach in the child (author's transl)]. Ann Pediatr (Paris). 1981;28:291–2.

88. Oriot D, Defawe G. Percutaneous catheterization of the axillary vein in neonates. Crit Care Med. 1988;16:285–6.

89. Metz R, Lucking S, Chaten F, et al. Percutaneous catheterization of the axillary vein in infants and children. Pediatrics. 1990;85:531–3.

90. Martin C, Viviand X, Saux P, et al. Upper-extremity deep vein thrombosis after central venous catheterization via the axillary vein. Crit Care Med. 1999;27:2626–9.

91. Gouin F, Martin C, Saux P. Central and pulmonary artery catheterizations via the axillary vein. Acta Anaesth Scand. 1985;81:27–9.

92. Taylor B, Yellowlees I. Central venous cannulation using the infraclavicular axillary vein. Anesthesiology. 1990;72:55–8.

93. Martin C, Eon B, Auffray J, et al. Axillary or internal jugular central venous catheterization. Crit Care Med. 1990;18:400–2.

94. Legler D, Nugent M. Doppler localization of the internal jugular vein facilitates central venous cannulation. Anesthesiology. 1984; 60:481–2.

95. Gilbert T, Seneff M, Becker R. Facilitation of internal jugular venous cannulation using an audio-guided Doppler ultrasound vascular access device: results from a prospective, dual-center, randomized, crossover clinical study. Crit Care Med. 1995; 23:60–5.

96. Miller A, Roth B, Mills T, et al. Ultrasound guidance versus the landmark technique for the placement of central venous catheters in the emergency department. Acad Emerg Med. 2002;9:800–5.

97. Keenan S. Use of ultrasound to place central lines. J Crit Care. 2002;17:126–37.

98. Hind D, Calvert N, McWilliams R, et al. Ultrasonic locating devices for central venous cannulation: meta-analysis. BMJ. 2003;327:361.

99. Verghese S, Magill W, Patel R, et al. Ultrasound-guided internal jugular venous cannulation in infants: a prospective comparison with the traditional palpation method. Anesthesiology. 1999;91:71–7.

100. Verghese S, Magill W, Patel R, et al. Comparison of three techinques for internal jugular vein cannulation in infants. Paediatr Anaesth. 2000;10:505–11.

101. Sigaut S, Skhiri A, Stany I, et al. Ultrasound guided internal jugular vein access in children and infant: a meta-analysis of published studies. Paediatr Anaesth. 2009;19:1199–206.

102. Froehlich C, Rigby M, Rosenberg E, et al. Ultrasound-guided central venous catheter placement decreases complications and decreases placement attempts compared with the landmark technique in patients in a pediatric intensive care unit. Crit Care Med. 2009;37:1090–6.

103. Lambert R, Boker J, Maffei F. National survey of bedside ultrasound use in pediatric critical care. Pediatr Crit Care Med. 2011;12:655–9.

104. Feller-Kopman D. Ultrasound guided central venous catheter placement: the new standard of care ? Crit Care Med. 2005; 33:1875–6.

105. Rowin M, Patel V, Christenson J. Pediatric intensive care unit nosocomial infections: epidemiology, sources and solutions. Crit Care Clin – Pediatric Crit Care. 2003;19(3):473–88.

106. Jacobs B. Central venous catheter occlusion and thrombosis. Crit Care Clin – Pediatric Crit Care. 2003;19:489–514.

107. Gauderer M, Stellato T. Subclavian broviac catheters in children – technical considerations in 146 consecutive placements. J Pediatr Surg. 1985;20:402–5.

108. Citak A, Karabocuoglu M, Ucsel R, et al. Central venous catheters in pediatric patients-subclavian venous approach as the first choice. Pediatr Int. 2002;44:83–6.

109. Conz P, Dissegna D, Rodighiero M, et al. Cannulation of the internal jugular vein: comparison of the classic Seldinger technique and an ultrasound guided method. J Nephrol. 1997;10:311–3.

110. Lavandosky G, Gomez R, Montes J. Potentially lethal misplacement of femoral central venous catheters. Crit Care Med. 1996;24:893–6.

111. Bass W, Lewis D. Neonatal segmental myoclonus associated with hyperglycorrhachia. Pediatr Neurol. 1995;13:77–9.

112. Lussky R, Trower N, Fisher D, et al. Unusual misplacement sites of percutaneous central venous lines in the very low birth weight neonate. Am J Perinatol. 1997;14:63–7.

113. Kelly M, Finer N, Dunbar L. Fatal neurologic complication of parenteral feeding through a central vein catheter. Am J Dis Child. 1984;138:352–3.

114. Odaibo F, Fajardo CA, Cronin C. Recovery of intralipid from lumbar puncture after migration of saphenous vein catheter. Arch Dis Child. 1992;67:1201–3.

115. Bonadio W, Losek J, Melzer-Lange M. An unusual complication from a femoral venous catheter. Pediatr Emerg Care. 1988;4:27–9.

116. Lucey B, Varghese JC, Haslam P, et al. Routine chest radiographs after central line insertion: mandatory postprocedural evaluation or unnecessary waste of resources? Cardiovasc Intervent Radiol. 1999;22:381–4.

117. Guth A. Routine chest X-rays after insertion of implantable long-term venous catheters: necessary or not? Am Surg. 2001;67:26–9.

118. Chang T, Funaki B, Szymski G. Are routine chest radiographs necessary after image-guided placement of internal jugular central venous access devices? Am J Roentgenol. 1998;170:335–7.

119. Burn P, Skewes D, King D. Role of chest radiography after the insertion of a subclavian vein catheter for ambulatory chemotherapy. Can Assoc Radiol J. 2001;52:392–4.

120. Molgaard O, Nielsen M, Handberg B, et al. Routine X-ray control of upper central venous lines: is it necessary? Acta Anaesthesiol Scand. 2004;48:685–9.

121. Janik J, Cothren C, Janik J, et al. Is a routine chest x-ray necessary for children after fluoroscopically assisted central venous access? J Pediatr Surg. 2003;38:1199–202.

122. Todres D, Cote C. Procedures. In: Cote C, Ryan J, Todres D, Goudsouzian N, editors. A practice of anesthesia for infants and children. 2nd ed. Philadelphia: WB Saunders; 1993. p. 508.

Shock

Derek S. Wheeler and Joseph A. Carcillo Jr.

Abstract

Shock is one of the most frequently diagnosed, yet poorly understood disorders in the pediatric intensive care unit (PICU). Shock is defined by an imbalance between oxygen and substrate delivery versus metabolic demand (oxygen consumption is often used as a surrogate of metabolic demand). The epidemiology, pathophysiology, and management of critically ill children with shock are distinctly different from that in critically ill adults. Early recognition of the features of shock leads to early treatment and better outcomes.

Keywords

Shock • Sepsis • Septic shock • Distributive shock • Obstructive shock • Hypovolemic shock • Cardiogenic shock • Neurogenic shock • Anaphylactic shock • Compensated shock • Uncompensated shock • Irreversible shock • Fluid resuscitation

Historical Perspective

Shock is one of the most frequently diagnosed, yet poorly understood disorders in the pediatric intensive care unit (PICU). The very definition of what constellation of physical signs and symptoms comprise *shock* remains controversial, in part due to the vast array of disorders that cause shock in critically ill and injured children (Table 30.1). Webster's Dictionary defines *shock* as *any sudden disturbance or agitation of the mind or emotions* [1]. Indeed, at one time in history, shock was thought to be due to a "nervous condition" and was treated with all manner of treatments, such as stimulants, depressants, and even electrical shock therapy [2]. A more appropriate and contemporary definition, however,

D.S. Wheeler, MD, MMM (✉)
Division of Critical Care Medicine, Cincinnati Children's Hospital Medical Center, University of Cincinnati College of Medicine, 3333 Burnet Avenue, Cincinnati, OH 45229-3039, USA
e-mail: derek.wheeler@cchmc.org

J.A. Carcillo Jr., MD
Pediatric Intensive Care Unit,
Children's Hospital of Pittsburgh of UPMC,
4401 Forbes Avenue, FP 2118, Pittsburgh, PA 15224, USA
e-mail: carcillo@ccm.upmc.edu

would define *shock* as *a sudden disturbance or agitation of the body's normal homeostasis*. Obtaining a more accurate, scientific definition of the clinical state known as shock has become increasingly difficult with the recognition of the complexity of the biochemical and molecular perturbations of the shock state.

Although Hippocrates was perhaps the first to describe the constellation of signs and symptoms of shock, the French surgeon Henri Francois Le Dran is widely credited with the first use of the medical term *shock* (literally translated from the French verb *choquer*) in 1737 in his textbook, *A Treatise of Reflections Drawn from Experience with Gunshot Wounds* [3]. Le Dran had used the term to describe *a sudden impact or jolt*, and by happenstance, a mistranslation by the English physician Clare in 1743 introduced the term into the English language to describe the sudden deterioration of a patient's condition following major trauma [4]. The term was further popularized by the English physician, Edwin A. Morris, who used the term in his article *A practical treatise on shock after operations and injuries* in 1867 [5]. Samuel Gross called shock *the rude unhinging of the machinery of life* in 1872 [6]. John Warren called shock *a momentary pause in the act of death* in 1895 [7]. Blalock defined shock as *a peripheral circulatory failure, resulting from a discrepancy in the size of*

D.S. Wheeler et al. (eds.), *Pediatric Critical Care Medicine*,
DOI 10.1007/978-1-4471-6362-6_30, © Springer-Verlag London 2014

Table 30.1 Common causes of shock in children

Hypovolemic shock

Fluid and electrolye losses

Vomiting

Diarrhea

Nasogastric tube drainage renal losses (via excessive urinary output)

Diuretic administration

Diabetes mellitus

Diabetes insipidus

Adrenal insufficiency

Fever

Heat stroke

Excessive sweating

Water deprivation

Sepsis

Burns

Pancreatitis

Small bowel obstruction

Hemorrhage

Trauma

Fractures

Spleen laceration

Liver laceration

Major vessel injury

Intracranial bleeding (especially neonates)

Hastrointestinal bleeding

Surgery

Cardiogenic shock

Myocarditis

Cardiomyopathy

Myocardial ischemia (e.g. kawasaki's disease, anomalous origin of the left coronary artery, etc)

Ventricular outflow tract obstruction

Acute dysrhythmias

Post cardiopulmonary bypass

Obstructive shock

Tension pneumothorax

Cardiac tamponade

Pulmonary embolism

Distributive shock

Sepsis

Anaphylaxis

Neurogenic shock

the vascular bed and the volume of the intravascular fluid in 1940 [8]. Finally, the famed physiologist Carl Wiggers offered the following definition in 1942: *Shock is a syndrome resulting from a depression of many functions but in which reduction of the effective circulating blood volume is of basic importance and in which impairment of the circulation steadily progresses until it eventuates into a state of irreversible circulatory failure* [9].

While all of these descriptions are appropriate, shock is very simply placed in economic terms as supply not matching demand, in that there is an inadequate delivery

of oxygen and metabolic substrates to meet the metabolic demands of the cells and tissues of the body. We now recognize Gross' *machinery of life* as the mechanisms that assure adequate oxygen delivery and utilization at the cellular level. Inadequate oxygen delivery results in cellular hypoxia, anaerobic metabolism and resultant lactic acidosis, activation of the host inflammatory response, and eventual vital organ dysfunction. Left untreated, shock leads to progressively worsening organ dysfunction and eventually organ failure and subsequent death.

Shock is a clinical diagnosis and is characterized by hyoperfusion of several organ systems. The initial diagnosis is often based upon the clinical presence of tachycardia, decreased urine output, mottled skin, and altered levels of consciousness. Shock may occur with a decreased, normal, or even increased cardiac output as well as a decreased, normal, or increased blood pressure [10, 11]. Just as important, shock may occur in the scenario of globally decreased tissue perfusion, as in the case with profound hypotension, or decreased regional tissue perfusion.

Hypovolemic shock, the most common cause of shock in children [10], has been described in the medical literature for over 150 years. For example, a pandemic of cholera claimed more than 23,000 lives in England during 1831 [12]. The accepted treatment at that time was blood-letting, which not surprisingly often failed. A 22 year-old medical graduate of Edinburgh University named William O'Shaughnessy was the first to note that the blood from patients suffering from cholera had *lost a large portion of its water* and later suggested a novel treatment by returning the blood to its *natural specific gravity* by replacing its *deficient saline*. O'Shaughnessy sent a letter to the *Lancet* [13] that included the following description of terminal cholera: *On the floor, before the fireplace. . .lay a girl of slender make and juvenile height; with the face of a superannuated hag. She uttered no moan, gave expression of no pain, … The colour of her countenance was that of lead – a silver blue, ghastly tint; her eyes were sunk deep into the sockets, as though they had been driven in an inch behind their natural position; her mouth was squared; her features flattened; her eyelids black; her fingers shrunk, bent, and inky in their hue. All pulse was gone at the wrist, and a tenacious sweat moistened her bosom. In short, Sir, that face and form I never can forget, were I to live to beyond the period of man's natural age.* O'Shaughnessy offers a highly accurate and classic portrayal of the late stages of uncompensated and irreversible shock. However, it was Thomas Latta who followed O'Shaughnessy's advice and first attempted intravenous fluid resuscitation in 1832. Ironically, William O'Shaughnessy received a knighthood for his work on the electric telegraph and not for his work on cholera, and Thomas Latta died a relative unknown less than 1 year after his classic observations [14].

The modern era of pediatric shock did not begin until much later, when intravenous therapy replaced subcutaneous therapy as a means of fluid resuscitation during the 1960s and 1970s. Deaths associated with diarrheal disease in the U.S. decreased from 67 per 100,000 infants to 23 per 100,000 infants following the widespread use of metal intravenous catheters, with a further reduction from 23 to 2.6 per 100,000 infants noted by 1985 associated with the use of plastic intravenous catheters [15]. Thomas et al. [15] reviewed data from the Vital Statistics of the United States from 1960 to 1991 and noted an eightfold reduction in the mortality rate from hypovolemic shock from 1/1,000 infants in 1960 to 0.12/1,000 infants in 1991. Significantly, the steepest decrease in mortality occurred during the decade between 1975 and 1985 coinciding with implementation of IV fluid therapy using plastic catheters in children. While numerous factors are responsible for this decline, the development of pediatric critical care medicine as a subspecialty, along with the aggressive use of intravenous fluids has certainly contributed substantially to this profound reduction in mortality and undoubtedly represents one of modern pediatric medicine's great accomplishments.

Although significant progress has been made in elucidating the molecular and cellular basis of shock, morbidity and mortality from shock remain unacceptably high. For example, Watson and colleagues evaluated a U.S. population sample for all-cause mortality in children in 1995 and noted that the two leading causes of death were trauma and severe sepsis [16]. Orr and colleagues evaluated a 5,000 patient database of children referred from the community setting to five separate pediatric hospitals in 2000 [17]. Shock, defined in this report by the presence of either hypotension or a capillary refill >2 s was the leading cause of death in these children, regardless of trauma status. Although head trauma was more common among patients who died, shock at the outside community hospital was a major predictor of subsequent death. Of major concern, only 7 % of the 5,000 patients were referred for a diagnosis of *shock*, yet more than 40 % of these children did, in fact, meet prospectively defined criteria for the diagnosis of shock. Community physicians were more likely to refer these children for respiratory distress when shock was present, even though the presence of shock was a significant risk factor for subsequent mortality. Therefore, despite the dramatic advances in the care of children with shock over the last 50 years, shock remains both common and often underappreciated in children transported to tertiary care pediatric hospitals.

A Brief Overview of Cellular Respiration and the Cellular Basis of Shock

Adenosine triphosphate (ATP) is the energy currency of the cell – therefore, shock is a state of acute energy failure in which there is insufficient ATP production to support systemic cellular function. During stress and periods of increased energy demand, glucose is produced from glycogenolysis and gluconeogenesis. Fat metabolism is the secondary source of energy in this scenario. Long chain fatty acids are oxidized and carnitine is utilized to shuttle acetyl coenzyme A (acetyl CoA) into mitochondria. Protein catabolism can also contribute acetyl CoA to the Krebs cycle for energy production. Aerobic metabolism provides 20 times more energy than anaerobic metabolism. Glucose is oxidized to pyruvate via glycolysis (also called the Embden-Meyerhof pathway), generating only two molecules of ATP in the process. When oxygen supply is adequate, pyruvate enters the mitochondria and is converted to acetyl CoA by the pyruvate dehydrogenase enzyme complex, after which it is completely oxidized to CO_2 and H_2O via the Kreb's cycle (also known as the tricarboxylic acid or citric acid cycle) and oxidative phosphorylation, generating a *net* total of 36–38 mol of ATP for every mole of glucose. Conversely, when oxygen supply is inadequate, pyruvate is reduced by NADH and lactate dehydrogenase to lactate, a relatively inefficient process that generates considerably less ATP.

Cells do not have the means to store oxygen and are therefore dependent upon a continuous supply that closely matches the changing metabolic needs that are necessary for normal metabolism and cellular function. If oxygen supply is not aligned with these metabolic requirements, hypoxia will ensue, eventually resulting in cellular injury and/or death. As defined above, shock is a state characterized by an inadequate delivery of oxygen and metabolic substrates to meet the metabolic demands of the cells and tissues of the body. Alterations in cellular function and structure result directly from the consequent derangements in cellular metabolism and energy production. Eventually, these derangements lead to cellular necrosis, with subsequent release of proteolytic enzymes and other toxic products which produce a systemic inflammatory response.

In practical terms, using this operational definition, a state of shock may result from inadequate oxygen delivery, inadequate substrate delivery (*glycopenia*), or mitochondrial dysfunction (*cellular dysoxia*). Oxygen delivery to the cells and tissues is dependent primarily upon three factors: (i) hemoglobin concentration (Hb), (ii) cardiac output (CO), and (iii) the relative proportion of oxyhemoglobin, i.e. percent oxygen saturation (SaO_2). Oxygen is transported in the blood combined with hemoglobin, though a relatively small amount is freely dissolved in the plasma fraction of the blood. When fully saturated, each gram of hemoglobin can carry approximately 1.34 mL of oxygen at normal body temperature, such that the oxygen content of arterial blood is determined by Eq. 30.1.

$$CaO_2(g\,O_2/mL)$$
$$= (Hb \times 1.34 \times SaO_2) + (0.003 \times PaO_2) \quad (30.1)$$

Oxygen delivery (DO$_2$) is therefore determined by Eq. 30.2.

$$DO_2 = CO \times CaO_2 \qquad (30.2)$$

It can easily be shown that one of the most important elements of CaO$_2$ (and hence, tissue oxygen delivery) is the arterial hemoglobin concentration. While oxygen delivery from the left ventricle is linearly related to the hemoglobin concentration, capillary flow may be impaired at an extremely high hematocrit due to increased viscosity of the blood. The optimal hemoglobin concentration to maximize tissue oxygen delivery appears to be around 10 g/dL.

Generally, more oxygen is delivered to the cells of the body than the cells actually require for normal metabolism. However, a low cardiac output (*stagnant hypoxia*), low hemoglobin concentration (*anemic hypoxia*), or low hemoglobin saturation (*hypoxic hypoxia*) will result in inadequate delivery of oxygen unless a compensatory change occurs in any of the other factors. Finally, even when oxygen delivery and glucose delivery is adequate, shock may occur as a result of mitochondrial dysfunction. For example, cyanide poisons the oxidative phosphorylation chain preventing production of ATP. *Cellular dysoxia* (also known as *cytopathic hypoxia*) may theoretically occur from one or a combination of several mechanisms, including diminished delivery of a key substrate (e.g., pyruvate) to the Kreb's cycle, inhibition of a key enzyme involved in either the Kreb's cycle or the electron transport chain, or uncoupling of oxidative phosphorylation. One additional mechanism is through activation of the mitochondrial DNA repair enzyme, poly (ADP-ribose) synthetase, or PARS, which is also commonly known as poly (ADP-ribose) polymerase, or PARP, in which more NAD$^+$ is consumed than ATP is being produced [18–20].

As stated above, under resting conditions, given a normal distribution of cardiac output, global oxygen delivery (Eq. 30.2) is more than adequate to meet the total oxygen requirements of the tissues needed to maintain aerobic metabolism, referred to as oxygen consumption (VO$_2$). This excess delivery or *oxygen reserve* serves as a buffer, such that a modest reduction in oxygen delivery is more than adequately compensated by increased extraction of the delivered oxygen, without any significant reduction in oxygen consumption. During stress or vigorous exercise, oxygen consumption markedly increases, as does oxygen delivery. Therefore, in the majority of circumstances, the metabolic demands of the cells and tissues of the body dictate the level of oxygen delivery. However, very little oxygen is stored in the cells and tissues of the body. Therefore, as oxygen delivery falls with critical illness, oxygen extraction must necessarily increase to meet metabolic demands, and oxygen consumption remains relatively constant (i.e., *delivery-independent*). However, there is a critical level of oxygen delivery ("critical DO$_2$") at which the body's compensatory

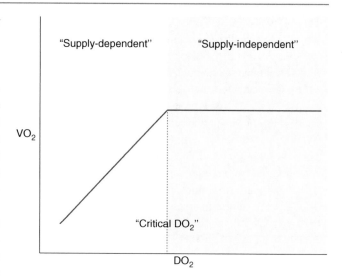

Fig. 30.1 The oxygen delivery – oxygen consumption relationship. See text for explanation

mechanisms are no longer able to keep up with metabolic needs (i.e. the point at which oxygen extraction is maximal). Once oxygen delivery falls below this level, oxygen consumption must also fall and is said to become *supply-dependent* (Fig. 30.1). This point also corresponds to the so-called anaerobic threshold, the point at which aerobic metabolism shifts to anaerobic metabolism and lactate production increases significantly.

Theoretically, oxygen delivery can be augmented by increasing either the cardiac output or the arterial oxygen content.

$$DO_2 = CO \times \left[\left(Hb \times 1.34 \times SaO_2 \right) + \left(0.003 \times PaO_2 \right) \right] \ (30.3)$$

However, in clinical practice, global oxygen delivery (as calculated mathematically by the equations above) is not necessarily a true reflection of what occurs at the local tissue capillary beds. Regional oxygen delivery may therefore significantly differ between different tissue capillary beds, such that increasing <u>global</u> oxygen delivery has relatively little effect on augmenting oxygen delivery to different tissue capillary beds (Table 30.2) [21]. This may be one reason (among many) that efforts to improve outcomes by increasing oxygen delivery to supranormal levels have almost universally failed [22–27].

In years past, a so-called pathologic supply-dependency was believed to exist in association with certain disease processes (e.g., sepsis, ARDS, etc.). Early experimental models of sepsis [28–30] and clinical data [31] reported that the critical oxygen extraction ratio was lower than normal during these critical illnesses; that is oxygen consumption became *delivery-dependent* at a higher critical DO2 in critically ill patients. This observation implied an intrinsic defect at the cellular level in oxygen extraction. However, most of the

Table 30.2 Differences in regional blood flow and oxygen consumption at rest

Regional circulation	% Cardiac output	% VO$_2$
Cerebral	13	20
Coronary	4	11
Renal	19	7
GI tract and liver	24	25
Skeletal muscle	21	30
Skin	9	2
Other	10	5

subsequent clinical data on which this concept of a pathologic supply-dependency was based is suspect due to the fact that most of the studies determined oxygen consumption (VO2) using the Fick equation (Eq. 30.4). As can be readily observed, Eqs. 30.3 and 30.4 share several common variables.

$$VO_2 = CO \times \left(\begin{array}{l} Hb \times 1.34 \times (SaO_2 - SvO_2) \\ +0.003 \times (PaO_2 - PvO_2) \end{array} \right) \quad (30.4)$$

The potential for computation error arises because the measurements of these variables in the calculation of DO$_2$ and VO$_2$ result in a mathematical coupling of measurement errors in the shared variables resulting in false correlation between oxygen delivery and consumption. In order to avoid potential mathematical coupling, oxygen consumption and delivery should be determined independent of each other. Studies in which VO$_2$ was directly measured (rather than calculated using the Fick principle) largely have disproved this pathologic supply dependency hypothesis [32–36]. The true answer, given the stark differences in regional circulation (that are likely compounded during critical illness) probably lies somewhere in the middle. In other words, augmenting oxygen delivery is undoubtedly one of the first and foremost priorities in the management of critically ill children, though until better methods and techniques are available to monitor regional differences in oxygen delivery and consumption, focusing on supranormal levels of oxygen delivery or attempts at titrating therapy to the so-called critical DO$_2$ (i.e. by titrating therapy until oxygen consumption no longer increases, such that the patient is on the supply-independent portion of the oxygen delivery/oxygen consumption curve) is unwarranted.

Differences Between Pediatric Shock and Adult Shock

Children are not small adults is an oft repeated axiom in the subspecialty of pediatric critical care medicine. The developmental differences between children and adults have very important implications on the pathophysiology and management of shock and have been reviewed extensively [37–40]. Age-specific differences in hemoglobin concentration and composition, heart rate, stroke volume, blood pressure, pulmonary vascular resistance, systemic vascular resistance, metabolic rate, glycogen stores, and protein mass are the basis for many age-specific differences in the cardiovascular and metabolic responses to shock [15, 37, 41–43]. For example, newborns have a higher hemoglobin concentration (mostly fetal hemoglobin) but low total blood volumes. They also have the highest total body water composition (Fig. 30.2). Newborns have comparatively higher heart rates, lower stroke volumes, near systemic pulmonary artery blood pressures, and higher metabolic rates with high energy needs, but the lowest glycogen stores and protein mass for glucose production [15, 43].

At birth, the normal newborn transitions from fetal to neonatal circulation when inhalation of oxygen reduces pulmonary vascular resistance and allows blood to flow through the lungs, rather than bypass the lungs through the patent ductus arteriosus. When pulmonary circulation is firmly established, the ductus arteriosus closes and newborn circulation is assured. In the presence of shock, acidosis prevents the ductus arteriosus from closing and elevated pulmonary vascular resistance persists. If untreated, persistent pulmonary hypertension results in right ventricular failure with septal bowing and inadequate cardiac output from the left ventricle. Resuscitation of the newborn with shock therefore requires meticulous attention to maintaining (i) adequate heart rates with chronotropes (newborns predominantly have high parasympathetic tone and do not fully develop sympathetic vesicles until the age of 6 months), (ii) blood volume (the newborn only has approximately one cup (approximately 80 mL/kg) of blood [44], and (iii) newborn circulation (using pulmonary vasodilators such as inhaled nitric oxide, and reversing metabolic acidosis). In addition, glucose infusion rates of 8 mg/kg/min or higher are often necessary to prevent hypoglycemia in the presence of low glycogen and protein gluconeogenesis stores. Newborns with refractory shock respond well to extracardiac support life support (ECLS) because mortality is uniformly caused by low cardiac output with high pulmonary and/or systemic vascular resistance.

Neonates, infants, and young children also have high systemic vascular resistance and vasoactive capacity, such that hypotension is a very late sign of shock (Fig. 30.3). This is a survival mechanism designed to counterbalance the limited cardiac reserve of the young. For example, neonates and infants, in particular, have relatively decreased left ventricular mass compared to adults [45, 46], as well as an increased ratio of type I collagen (decreased elasticity) to type III collagen (increased elasticity) [47]. In addition, the myocardium in neonates and infants functions at a relatively high contractile state, even at baseline [48, 49], such that neonates and infants have a relatively limited capacity to increase stroke

Fig. 30.2 Total body water (*TBW*), which consists of the intracellular (*ICF*) and extracellular (*ECF*) fluid compartments, as a percentage of body weight decreases rapidly with age. The ECF compartment consists of the plasma volume (5 % TBW) and the interstitial volume (15 % TBW). The ECF volume decreases rapidly during the first year of life, while the ICF volume remains relatively constant. Fluid losses usually affect either the interstitial or intracellular compartments. Infants have a proportionately higher ratio of ECF to ICF, which predisposes them to rapid fluid losses. For example, 10 % dehydration in a 6 month-old child weighing 7-kg is equivalent to approximately 700 mL, which is roughly one-tenth the total volume loss required to produce the same degree of dehydration in a 70-kg adult (approximately 7,000 mL fluid loss) [15]

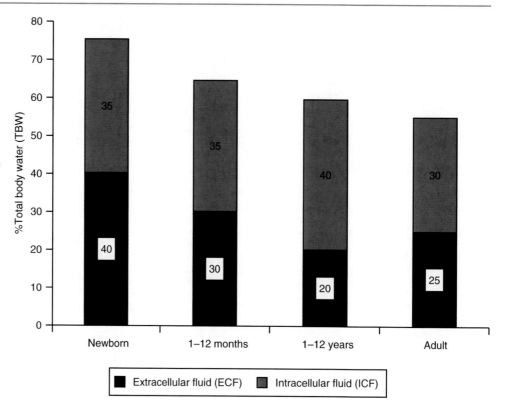

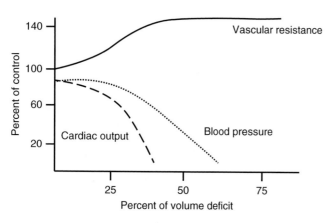

Fig. 30.3 As shown in the figure, children may lose up to approximately 25 % of the blood volume before they become hypotensive. As cardiac output falls, systemic vascular resistance increases, so that mean arterial blood pressure remains constant. Recall that by Hagen-Poiseuille's law (analogous to Ohm's law of electrical current flow), the fluid flow (Q) through a system is related to the pressure drop aross the system divided by the resistance of the system. In other words, Q (cardiac output) = MAP/SVR. Similarly, MAP = Q × SVR. If Q decreases and SVR increases, MAP remains constant

volume during stress [46, 49, 50]. Neonates and infants are therefore critically dependent upon an increase in heart rate to generate increased cardiac output during stress. However, coronary artery (and hence, myocardial) perfusion occurs to the greatest degree during diastole and is directly proportional to the difference between diastolic blood pressure and

left atrial pressure, and inversely proportional to the heart rate (as an indirect measure of diatolic filling time). Under conditions of hypovolemia, an adult can easily double the heart rate from 70 to 140 beats per minute (bpm) to maintain an adequate cardiac output (cardiac reserve); however, the newborn or infant cannot double heart rate from 140 to 280 bpm or 120 to 240 bpm respectively, because these heart rates will not allow adequate coronary artery perfusion. Indeed supraventricular tachycardia with heart rates of 240 bpm or higher frequently lead to inadequate cardiac filling and subsequent poor tissue perfusion. During states of shock, newborns, infants, and children compensate by peripheral vasoconstriction to maintain adequate perfusion to the heart, brain, and kidney, and hypotension is an extremely late and poor prognostic sign.

These differences between pediatric and adult shock are perhaps best illustrated by a now classic study by Ceneviva and colleagues [51]. These investigators categorized 50 children with (in this case) fluid-refractory septic shock according to hemodynamic state, based upon hemodynamic data obtained with the Pulmonary Artery (PA) catheter, into one of three possible cardiovascular derangements (i) a hyperdynamic state characterized by a high cardiac output (>5.5 L/min/m² BSA) and low systemic vascular resistance (<800 dyn s/cm⁵) (classically referred to as *warm shock*); (ii) a hypodynamic state characterized by low cardiac output (<3.3 L/min/m² BSA) and low systemic vascular resistance (SVR); or (iii) a hypodynamic state characterized by low cardiac output and high SVR (>1,200 dyn s-cm⁵) (classically referred to as *cold shock*). Importantly, hemodynamic data was obtained following aggressive fluid resuscitation (minimum 60 mL/kg fluid in the first hour, with pulmonary capillary wedge pressure >8 mmHg). In contrast to adults in which the early stages of septic shock is characterized by a high cardiac output and low SVR, most of these children were in a hypodynamic state characterized by low cardiac output and high systemic vascular resistance (cold shock) and required the addition of vasodilators to decrease SVR, increase CI, and improve peripheral perfusion [51]. Children with low cardiac output (as defined by a cardiac index less than 2.0 L/min/m² BSA) had the highest risk of mortality. These findings have been confirmed in multiple studies using a variety of methods to measure cardiac output and vascular resistance [52–58]. Collectively, these studies all point to the fact that hypotension in children is a very late sign that portends a poor prognosis. Moreover, children more commonly present with cold shock, as opposed to warm shock. Early recognition and appropriate treatment (guided to the relevant hemodynamic derangements) of children with shock is therefore crucial.

Pathophysiology of Shock

Hemodynamic Relationships in Shock

An understanding of the relationship between flow (i.e. cardiac output), perfusion pressure (i.e. mean arterial blood pressure [MAP] – central venous pressure [CVP]), and vascular resistance (systemic vascular resistance, or SVR) is vital to the understanding of the pathophysiology of shock. Hagen-Poiseuille's Law (analogous to Ohm's Law of electrical flow) states that flow (i.e. cardiac output) is directly proportional to the pressure difference (MAP-CVP), i.e. perfusion pressure (or driving pressure) divided by the resistance.

$$CO = \Delta P / R = \left(MAP - CVP\right) / SVR \qquad (30.5)$$

Under ideal laminar flow conditions, in which vascular resistance is independent of flow and pressure, the relationship between pressure, flow, and resistance is shown by Fig. 30.4. In other words, an increase in resistance will decrease blood flow at any given perfusion pressure (and vice versa). At any given blood flow, an increase in resistance will increase the perfusion pressure (and vice versa). This relationship does not hold under conditions of turbulent (or pulsatile) flow, as turbulence decreases the flow at any given pressure according to Hagen-Poiseuille's Law.

The perfusion pressure may be a more important determinant of flow than blood pressure alone. According to

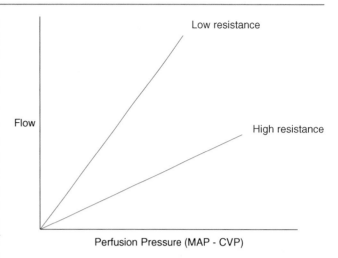

Fig. 30.4 The relationship between pressure, flow, and resistance

Eq. 30.5, one can theoretically have a normal MAP but no forward flow (CO), e.g. if CVP is equal to MAP (which would of course be rare and catastrophic). Conceptually, however, when fluid resuscitation is used to improve blood pressure, the increase in MAP must be greater than the concomitant increase in CVP. If the increase in MAP is less than the increase in CVP then the perfusion pressure is actually reduced, and hence cardiac output is reduced. Inotropic agents, and not additional fluid resuscitation, are indicated to improve cardiac output in this scenario. Understanding this relationship helps guide the management of *blood flow* reflected as cardiac output. Cardiac output can be decreased when perfusion pressure (MAP-CVP) is decreased, but it can also be decreased when the perfusion pressure (MAP-CVP) is normal and vascular resistance is increased (by Eq. 30.5). Hence, children with normal blood pressure can have inadequate cardiac output because systemic vascular tone is too high. Cardiac output can be improved in this scenario with the use of inotropes, vasodilators, and volume loading. The cardiovascular pathophysiology of shock can therefore be attributed either to reduced cardiac output, reduced perfusion pressure (MAP-CVP or DBP-CVP), or both. Reduced cardiac output is caused either by reduced heart rate or reduced stroke volume caused by hypovolemia (inadequate preload), decreased contractility (insufficient inotropy), or excess vascular resistance (increased afterload). Reduced perfusion pressure can be caused by reduced MAP or increased CVP.

Compensatory Mechanisms in Shock

Following the onset of hemodynamic dysfunction, several homeostatic compensatory mechanisms (summarized in Table 30.3) are initiated in an attempt to maintain end organ perfusion and function. Many of these compensatory mechanisms can be clinically recognized during the early stages

Table 30.3 Compensatory responses to the shock state

1. Mechanisms to maintain effective circulating blood volume

  (a) Decreased venous capacitance (via venoconstriction)

    Increased sympathetic tone

    Release of epinephrine from the adrenal medulla

    Increased angiotensin II (activation of the renin-angiotensin-aldosterone axis)

    Increased circulating vasopressin via release from the posterior pituitary gland

  (b) Decreased renal fluid losses

    Decreased Glomerular Filtration Rate (GFR)

    Increased aldosterone release (activation of the renin-angiotensin-aldosterone axis)

    Increased vasopressin release from the posterior pituitary gland

  (c) Fluid redistribution to the vascular space

    Starling effect (fluid redistribution from the interstitial space)

    Osmotic effect (fluid redistribution from the intracellular space)

2. Mechanisms to maximize cardiac performance

  (a) Increase heart rate

    Increased sympathetic tone

    Release of epinephrine from the adrenal medulla

  (b) Increase contractility

    Increased sympathetic tone

    Release of epinephrine from the adrenal medulla

  (c) Increased Frank-Starling mechanism (increased preload = increased cardiac output)

    Decreased venous capacitance (see above)

    Decreased renal losses of fluid (see above)

    Fluid redistribution to the vascular space (see above)

3. Mechanisms to maintain preferential perfusion to the vital organs (*dive reflex*)

  (a) Extrinsic regulation of systemic arterial tone

  (b) Autoegulation of vital organs (brain, heart, kidneys)

4. Mechanisms to optimize conditions for oxygen unloading

  (a) Increased concentration of red blood cell 2,3-DPG

  (b) Tissue acidosis (Bohr Effect)

  (c) Decreased Tissue PO_2

of shock. The progression of shock is commonly divided into three phases: compensated, uncompensated, and irreversible shock [10, 11] (Table 30.4). During compensated shock, oxygen delivery to the brain, heart, and kidney is often maintained at the expense of *less vital* organs. Signs and symptoms of the shock state, though often subtle, may be apparent even at this early stage. Notably, hypotension is not a feature during this stage – rather, increased peripheral vascular tone and increased heart rate maintain a normal cardiac output and a normal blood pressure. As shock progresses to the *uncompensated stage*, the body's compensatory mechanisms eventually contribute to the further progression of the shock state (e.g., blood is shunted away from the skin, muscles, and gastrointestinal tract in order to maintain perfusion of the brain, heart, and kidneys, leading to ischemia in these vascular beds with subsequent release

of toxic substances, further perpetuating the shock state). Cellular function deteriorates further, culminating in end-organ dysfunction. The *terminal* or *irreversible stage* of shock implies irreversible organ injury, especially of the vital organs (brain, heart, and kidneys). Intervention at this late stage is unsuccessful, and death occurs even if therapeutic intervention restores cardiovascular measurements such as heart rate, blood pressure, cardiac output, and oxygen saturation to normal.

Functional Classification of Shock

Hinshaw and Cox [44] proposed a classification scheme for shock in 1972 that is still relevant today. The four major categories of shock include (i) hypovolemic shock (shock as a consequence of inadequate circulating volume), (ii) obstructive shock (shock caused by obstruction of blood flow to and from the heart), (iii) cardiogenic shock (shock caused by primary pump failure), and (iv) distributive shock (shock caused by maldistribution of the circulating volume) (Table 30.5). Notably, distributive shock encompasses septic shock, anaphylactic shock, and neurogenic shock (all subtypes of vasodilatory shock) [59]. This classification scheme is relatively arbitrary, especially when viewed in the context that different features of each category may be present at the same time (e.g. septic shock is often characterized by manifestations of hypovolemic shock, cardiogenic shock, and distributive shock). However, this kind of simplistic view of the different types of shock can provide valuable information about the pathophysiological alterations involved, and knowledge of these pathophysiological alterations can then be used to guide appropriate management.

Hypovolemic Shock

Hypovolemic shock is the most common cause of shock in children and claims the lives of millions of children each year worldwide [10, 15, 60–63]. Diarrheal illnesses leading to dehydration and hypovolemic shock account for as many as 30 % of all deaths in infants and young children worldwide. Dengue shock syndrome (DSS) is another important cause of hypovolemic shock worldwide [64, 65]. Nearly 8,000 children less than 5 years of age die every day from dehydration and hypovolemic shock [60, 61, 66]. While diarrheal illnesses are an important cause of hypovolemic shock in children in developing nations, hypovolemic shock is an important problem that affects children in the U.S. and other developed nations as well [67]. For example, hypovolemic shock accounts for nearly 10 % of all hospital admissions and 300 annual deaths in children younger than 5 years of age in the U.S. alone [60, 68].

Table 30.4 Stages of shock

Organ system	Compensated shock	Uncompensated shock	Irreversible shock
Central nervous system	Agitation Anxiety ↓ Lethargy Somnolence	Altered mental status Hypoxic-ischemic injury	Hypoxic-ischemic injury and cell necrosis
Heart	Tachycardia	Tachycardia ↓ Bradycardia	Myocardial ischemia Cell necrosis
Lungs	Tachypnea Increased WOB	Acute respiratory failure	Acute respiratory failure
Kidneys	Oliguria ↑ urinary osmolality ↑ urinary sodium $FE_{Na} < 1$	Acute tubular necrosis Acute renal failure	Tubular necrosis
Gastrointestinal tract	Ileus Feeding intolerance Stress gastritis	Pancreatitis Acalculous cholecystitis GI bleeding Gut translocation	GI bleeding Sloughing
Liver	Centrilobular injury Elevated transaminases	Centrilobular necrosis *Shock liver*	Hepatic failure
Hematologic	Endothelial activation Platelet activation (Pro-coagulant, hypofibrinolytic)	DIC	DIC
Metabolic	Glycogenolysis Gluconeogensis Lipolysis Proteolysis	Glycogen depletion Hypoglycemia	Hypoglycemia
Immune system	Immunoparalysis	Immunoparalysis	Immunoparalysis

Table 30.5 Classification of shock

Type of shock	Preload	Afterload	Contractility
Hypovolemic	↓	↑	N
Cardiogenic	↑	↑	↓
Obstructive	↓	↑	N
Distributive	↑, ↓, or N	↓	↑

Traumatic injuries are the leading cause of mortality in children and adolescents. While closed-head injuries account for the vast majority of these deaths, hemorrhagic shock accounts for a significant number of deaths in children on an annual basis. Blunt trauma is more common in children, which differs from penetrating trauma in that multiple organs are often involved, occult injury is common, and progressive organ damage is frequent due to continued hemorrhage, edema, or ischemia. Blunt trauma associated with motor vehicle accidents is especially common in the pediatric age group. While penetrating trauma secondary to gunshot or stab wounds is more common in adolescents, these injuries account for a small percentage of all pediatric injuries even in urban trauma centers [69]. Regardless, recent statistics suggest that the incidence of penetrating trauma is increasing in the pediatric population [70, 71].

The source of blood loss in hemorrhagic shock may be external and readily identifiable. For example, the scalp is highly vascular and lacerations in this area can account for a significant amount of blood loss in children. More commonly, however, the source of blood loss is internal and requires a high index of suspicion. Intra-abdominal injuries (e.g. spleen laceration, liver laceration, etc.) and long-bone fractures can result in significant blood loss. For example, an occult femur fracture may result in the loss of up to 500–1,000 mL of blood into the soft tissues of the thigh, though isolated femur fractures rarely cause hemorrhagic shock in children [72–74].

As discussed above, children appear to be at a greater risk for hypovolemic shock compared to adults due to a number of important age-specific physiological differences. For example, total body water (TBW) as a percentage of body weight decreases rapidly with age. Based on such an analysis, it would seem logical to assume that children, due to their relatively greater percentage of TBW, would be protected against dehydration; unfortunately, this is not the case. TBW consists of the intracellular (ICF) and extracellular

Table 30.6 Clinical signs and symptoms of dehydration in children

% Dehydration

Sign/symptom	Mild (4–5 %)	Moderate (6–9 %)	Severe (≥10 %)
General appearance	Thirsty, restless, alert	Thirsty, drowsy, postural hypotension	Drowsy, limp, cold, mottled
Peripheral pulses	Normal rate and strength	Rapid and weak	Rapid, thready, occasionally not palpable
Respirations	Normal	Deep, rapid	Deep, rapid
Anterior fontanelle	Normal, flat	Sunken	Very sunken
Skin turgor	Pinch retracts quickly	Pinch retracts slowly	Pinch retracts very slowly ("tenting")
Capillary refill	Normal (<2 s)	Prolonged (3–4 s)	Very prolonged (>4 s)
Eyes	Normal, tearing	Sunken, dry	Very sunken, dry
Mucous membranes	Moist	Dry	Very dry
Blood pressure	Normal	Normal (low-range)	Hypotension

Table 30.7 Classification of hemorrhagic shock in children

	Class I	Class II	Class III	Class IV
Blood loss (%)	<15 %	15–25 %	26–39 %	>40 %
Cardiovascular	Normal to ↑ HR	↑ HR	↑↑ HR	↑↑↑ HR
	Normal blood pressure	Normal blood pressure	Hypotension	Profound hypotension
	Normal pulses	Diminished peripheral pulses	Thready peripheral pulses	Absent peripheral pulses
				Thready central pulses
Respiratory	Normal rate	Tachypnea	Moderate tachypnea	Severe tachypnea
CNS	Slightly anxious	Irritable, confused, combative	Diminished response to pain	Coma
Skin	Warm, pink	Cool extremities	Cool extremities	Cold extremities
		Mottling	Mottling	Pallor
			Pallor	Cyanosis
	Normal cap refill	Delayed cap refill	Prolonged cap refill	
Kidneys	Normal urine output	Oligurua	Oligura	Anuria
		Increased urine specific gravity	Increased BUN	
Acid-base	Normal pH	Normal pH	Metabolic acidosis	Metabolic acidosis

(ECF) fluid compartments. The ECF compartment consists of the plasma volume (5 % TBW) and the interstitial volume (15 % TBW). The ECF volume decreases rapidly during the first year of life, while the ICF volume remains relatively constant. However, fluid losses usually affect either the interstitial or intracellular compartments. Experimental models utilizing radio-labeled albumin demonstrate that the percentage of body weight lost is directly proportional to the percentage of plasma volume lost (e.g., children who lose 5 % of their body weight have lost approximately 5 % of their plasma volume) [75]. It is useful to quantify the amount of dehydration based upon clinical signs and symptoms or the percentage of weight loss (Table 30.6). Finally, the total amount of fluid loss required to produce shock is significantly less in children compared to adults. For example, 10 % dehydration, indicative of moderate dehydration by most accounts, in a 6 month-old child weighing 7-kg (approximately 700 mL fluid loss) is one-tenth the total volume loss required to produce the same degree of dehydration in a 70-kg adult (approximately 7,000 mL fluid loss) [15].

The total blood volume is usually estimated as 7–8 % of the total body weight, or 70–80 mL/kg. Loss of up to 15 % of the total blood volume (Class I shock as defined by the American College of Surgeons) usually results in minimal signs and symptoms (Table 30.7). Heart rate may increase to maintain adequate cardiac output, though blood pressure is usually maintained in the normal range. Hypotension, in fact, is a relatively late sign of hypovolemic shock. Compensatory mechanisms such as an increased heart rate and peripheral vascular resistance can maintain a normal blood pressure even in the face of a 30–40 % loss of the total blood volume. Hypotension, therefore, defines a state of *uncompensated shock* and is a relatively late and ominous finding in the critically ill or injured child.

Obstructive Shock

Obstructive shock is caused by a mechanical obstruction of blood flow to and/or from the heart. Common causes of obstructive shock include tension pneumothorax, cardiac tamponade, and pulmonary embolism, which are discussed in greater detail in subsequent chapters. Also included in this category are the congenital heart lesions characterized by left-sided obstruction (e.g., critical aortic stenosis, coarctation of the aorta, interrupted aortic arch, hypoplastic left heart syndrome) or right-sided obstruction (e.g., tricuspid atresia, pulmonary stenosis, Ebstein's anomaly, etc. – which impair systemic venous return to the right side of the heart and hence result in diminished preload to the left side of the heart), which are also discussed in greater detail elsewhere in the textbook.

Tension Pneumothorax

A pneumothorax is defined as an accumulation of air in the pleural space. A tension pneumothorax occurs due to the progressive accumulation of air in the pleural space, leading to shift of the mediastinum to the contralateral hemithorax and subsequent compression (and total collapse) of the contralateral lung and great vessels, compromising both cardiovascular and respiratory function. Whether the air enters the pleural space through a defect in the chest wall, a lacerated or ruptured bronchus, or a ruptured alveolus, a one-way valve effect is created such that air enters during inhalation, but cannot exit during exhalation. Accumulation of air continues until the intrathoracic pressure of the affected hemithorax equilibrates with atmospheric pressure. At this point, the accumulation of pressure within the thorax leads to depression of the ipsilateral hemi-diaphragm and displacement of the mediastinum (and associated great vessels) towards the contralateral hemi-thorax. While the superior vena cava (SVC) is able to move to some extent, the inferior vena cava (IVC) is relatively fixed within the diaphragm and will be compressed. As two-thirds of the venous return in older children and adults comes from below the diaphragm [76], compression of the IVC leads to a drastic and profound reduction in venous return to the heart, leading to cardiovascular collapse and signs and symptoms of obstructive shock. Decompression of the pneumothorax via needle thoracentesis or thoracostomy tube placement will improve symptoms and is therefore the treatment of choice.

Pulmonary Embolism

Pulmonary embolism (PE) is uncommonly diagnosed in children and is often only discovered on autopsy [77–80]. In fact, approximately 50 % of patients who have fatal PE are not diagnosed until autopsy. However, PE occurs more frequently in children than commonly assumed [81, 82], and unfortunately, PE is frequently fatal and difficult to diagnose. The clinical presentation often is confusing, perhaps compounded by the fact that very few pediatricians have a lot of experience with this disorder. Results of screening tests, such as oxygen saturation, electrocardiography, and chest radiography, may be normal. Thus, a high index of clinical suspicion is necessary.

A massive PE has a profound impact upon gas exchange and hemodynamics. Obstruction to flow through the pulmonary artery results in increased deadspace ventilation (i.e., affected lung segments are ventilated but not perfused), which is observed clinically as a substantial decrease in the end-tidal CO_2 ($ETCO_2$) that no longer reflects arterial PCO_2. A widened alveolar-to-arterial gradient, (A-a) PO_2 is present in most children as well. The mechanism for hypoxemia is somewhat controversial, though several mechanisms likely play a role. For example, an intracardiac right-to-left shunt through a patent foramen ovale may occur as right atrial pressure increases and eventually exceeds that of left atrial pressure. In addition, V/Q mismatching is compounded by the accompanying fall in cardiac output that results from massive PE, leading to mixed venous desaturation. PE increases the right ventricular (RV) afterload, resulting in an increase in the RV end-diastolic volume (EDV). The increase in RVEDV adversely affects left ventricular hemodynamics through ventricular interdependence. Specifically, the interventricular septum bows into the left ventricle (LV) and impairs diastolic filling, resulting in decreased LV preload and subsequent hypotension. The diagnosis, pathophysiology, and management of PE are discussed elsewhere in the textbook.

Cardiac Tamponade

The pericardium is relatively non-compliant, such that the accumulation of a small amount of fluid (usually less than 200 mL) is sufficient to produce cardiac tamponade. However, chronic accumulation of fluid may accumulate with little to no hemodynamic derangements as the pericardium slowly stretches to accommodate the excess volume. The therapeutic implications of an acute versus chronic pericardial fluid accumulation are also important. For example, removal of even a small volume of pericardial fluid from an acute effusion or hemopericardium will decrease the intra-pericardial pressure significantly and relieve symptoms of cardiac tamponade. Conversely, due to the change in the pericardial compliance curves, a large volume of pericardial fluid from a symptomatic, chronic effusion will need to be removed to attain comparable relief of tamponade.

Cardiac tamponade is produced by compression of the heart by accumulation of pericardial fluid beyond a certain threshold. The true *filling pressure* of the heart is represented by the myocardial transmural pressure (i.e., intracardiac pressure minus intra-pericardial pressure). Therefore, as intra-pericardial pressure rises, the *filling pressure* of the heart decreases and stroke volume falls. The body attempts to compensate for the increase in intra-pericardial pressure (and hence transmural pressure) by increasing systemic central venous pressure and pulmonary venous pressure, so that the left and right ventricular filling pressures are higher than the intra-pericardial pressure. Left and right atrial pressures increase and equilibrate as the intra-pericardial pressure rises. Though this equalization of atrial pressures is often touted as a hallmark of cardiac tamponade, it is more commonly observed with inflammation-induced etiologies and should not be relied on as a pathognomonic sign of tamponade in the post-operative cardiac patient [83, 84].

Pericardiocentesis is the lifesaving procedure of choice for children with cardiac tamponade. Medical stabilization with fluid resuscitation and inotropic support is temporary at best and somewhat controversial as fluid resuscitation may precipitate (i.e. in the case of low-pressure tamponade) or worsen tamponade physiology, especially in children who are either normovolemic or hypervolemic. In the latter scenario, fluid administration will increase intracardiac pressures further, hence increasing intrapericardial pressures and worsening tamponade [85–89]. The pathophysiology, diagnosis, and management of cardiac tamponade are discussed in greater detail later in the textbook.

Left Ventricular Outflow Tract Obstruction

While not commonly considered in the category of obstructive shock, there are several congenital heart defects that result in left ventricular outflow tract obstruction (LVOT) which produce signs and symptoms of obstructive shock. These include lesions such as critical aortic stenosis, critical coarctation of the aorta, interrupted aortic arch, and hypoplastic left heart syndrome (which includes mitral stenosis or atresia, as well as aortic stenosis or atresia), among others [90, 91]. These lesions all present in the neonatal period, as once the ductus arteriosus closes, there is no longer any egress for oxygenated blood to get from the heart to the rest of the body. Successful resuscitation of these patients requires early recognition, so that the proper therapy can be initiated. Fluid resuscitation and vasoactive medications are only temporizing measures – relief of obstruction by opening up the ductus arteriosus with prostaglandin E_1 (PGE_1) is lifesaving. However, PGE_1 can also cause systemic vasodilation [92, 93], which can result in profound hypotension in the face of a fixed LVOT, where the heart cannot increase output to compensate. Fluid resuscitation and initiation of vasoactive medications are therefore just as important as starting the PGE_1. Once the patient has been stabilized, palliation or repair via cardiac catheterization or surgery is the definitive treatment. The diagnosis, pathophysiology, and management of LVOT are discussed elsewhere in the textbook.

Right-sided Obstructive Lesions

Right-sided obstructive lesions, such as tricuspid atresia, Ebstein's anomaly, pulmonic stenosis, etc. all produce significant cyanosis due to inadequate pulmonary blood flow. However, these lesions also decrease preload back to the left side of the heart, which again results in signs and symptoms of obstructive shock. The diagnosis, pathophysiology, and management of these lesions are discussed elsewhere in the textbook.

Cardiogenic Shock

Cardiogenic shock is the term used to describe inadequate oxygen delivery resulting from depressed stroke volume as a result of myocardial failure. The generation of an adequate stroke volume as it relates to the contractile apparatus of the myocyte is reviewed in detail later in this textbook. However, suffice it to say that calcium (Ca^{2+}) homeostasis is paramount to this physiologic process as it facilitates both systolic contraction (inotropy) and diastolic relaxation (lusitropy). Following depolarization, Ca^{2+} enters the myocyte via voltage-gated, L-type channels. This increase in intracellular Ca^{2+} triggers further release of Ca^{2+} from the sarcoplasmic reticulum (SR) via ryanodine receptors. Ca^{2+} then binds to the myofilament troponin C to cause contraction. Following contraction, Ca^{2+} is removed from the intracellular space back into the SR by a series of Ca^{2+}-regulating proteins including: SR Ca^{2+}-ATPase, SERCA and phospholamban. Importantly, phospholamban is subject to functional regulation on the basis of its phosphorylation state modulated by kinases (e.g. protein kinase C, cAMP-protein kinase, Ca^{2+}-calmodulin kinase) and phosphatases (e.g. PP1) [94]. In its phosphorylated form, phospholamban dissociates from SERCA resulting in increased uptake of intracellular Ca^{2+} into the SR causing myocyte relaxation as well as having a subsequent positive inotropic effect. This mechanism is also utilized by β_1-adrenergic receptor agonists, which lead to G-protein-coupled receptor activation of adenylate cyclase resulting in elevation in cAMP levels, activation of PKA, and subsequent phosphorylation of phospholamban – thus having a positive inotropic effect. Also related to this pathway, type III phosphodiesterases hydrolyze cAMP to terminate the activation process. Thus, type III phosphodiesterase inhibitors (e.g. milrinone) prevent the breakdown of cAMP thereby augmenting both contraction and relaxation and may have a synergistic effect of prolonging the inotropic effect of β_1-agonists. In addition, there is mounting evidence that the β_1-adrenergic receptor pathway is dysfunctional in certain settings (e.g. sepsis) [95], so that while the use of β_1-receptor agonists to augment inotropy may be unsuccessful, the use of non-receptor-based phosphodiesterase inhibition may be a preferred pharmacologic approach [96].

Among the myriad of diseases that are associated with abnormal myocardial function (Table 30.8), a variety of mechanisms may be responsible for contractile dysfunction including: circulating myocardial depressant factors, myofilament insensitivity to Ca^{2+}, apopotosis and/or necrosis, uncoupling of myocyte mitochondrial energy production and/or β-receptor down-regulation/dysfunction. However, regardless of the underlying pathology, the characteristic mechanical defect in cardiogenic shock is a marked reduction in contractility that shifts the left ventricular end-systolic pressure-volume curve to the right. As a result, at a similar

Table 30.8 Common precipitating causes of cardiogenic shock

Infectious:

Viral myocarditis (coxsackie a and b, adenovirus, other enteroviruses)

Bacterial (fulminant) myocarditis(gram negative and gram positive sepsis)

Rickettsial

Protozoal

Metabolic:

Storage diseases (glycogen storage disease, mucopolysaccharidoses)

Carnitine deficiency

Acidosis

Hypocalcemia

Inflammatory diseases:

Kawasaki's disease

Rheumatic fever

Systemic lupus erythematous

Juvenile rheumatoid arthritis

Hypoxic-ischemic injury:

Perinatal asphyxia

Near-drowning

Post-cardiopulmonary bypass

Asphyxia/near-sids

Myocardial infarction/anamolous left coronary artery

Toxicities:

Anthracyclines

Sulfonamides

Calcium channel blockers

β-Receptor blockers

Thyrotoxicosis

Cardiac-related causes:

Dysrhythmias:

Bradycardia

Supraventricular tachycardia

Ventricular tachycardia

Cardiomyophathies:

Idiopathic dilated cardiomyopathy

Familial dilated cardiomyopathy

Increased afterload:

Aortic stenosis

Coarctation of the aorta

Hypertrophic cardiomyopathy

Coarctation of the aorta

Malignant hypertension/pheochromocytoma

Neuromuscular disorders:

Duchenne muscular dystrophy

Spinal muscular atrophy

degree of afterload or systolic pressure, the ventricle ejects less stroke volume per beat resulting in a substantially increased end-systolic volume. In order to compensate for the diminished stroke volume, the curvilinear diastolic pressure-volume curve also shifts to the right, reflecting a decrease in diastolic compliance or lusitropy so that the increased diastolic filling is ultimately coupled with an increase in LV end-diastolic pressure (LVEDP). Thus, this compensatory mechanism to enhance cardiac output increases LVEDP with a concomitant cost of both increased myocardial oxygen demand and the development of signs of congestive heart failure (e.g. pulmonary edema, hepatomegaly, jugular venous distention, pedal edema) commonly observed in this setting. The diagnosis, pathophysiology, and management of cardiogenic shock is discussed elsewhere in the textbook.

Distributive Shock

Distributive shock, as the name implies, results from abnormalities in vasomotor tone that lead to the maldistribution of a normally effective blood volume and flow. Peripheral vasodilation and shunting can lead to a state of *relative hypovolemia*. In other words, peripheral vasodilation increases venous capacitance, resulting in a decrease in the effective mean circulatory filling pressure (P_{mcf}). P_{mcf} is defined as the mean pressure that exists in the vascular system if the cardiac output stops and the pressure within the vascular system is allowed to equilibrate. P_{mcf} is dependent upon the volume of blood in the vascular system and the smooth muscle tone of the venous system (i.e., venous capacitance) [97–101]. Distributive shock arises from a variety of disorders and encompasses various states of shock arising from anaphylaxis (*anaphylactic shock*), central nervous system injury (which includes *neurogenic shock*), and *sepsis*.

Anaphylaxis refers to a systemic, immediate hypersensitivity reaction that is potentially life-threatening and characterized by the onset of signs and symptoms within seconds to minutes following exposure to the offending agent (e.g. insect envenomation, medication, food, etc.), involvement of multiple organ systems, and involvement of systems distant from the site of exposure. While the true incidence of anaphylaxis is difficult to define, it is certainly not uncommon and the most frequent causes of anaphylaxis are foods, hymenoptera stings and medications. Anaphylaxis is caused by the release of mediators from mast cells and basophils. Antigen bridging of IgE antibodies bound to FcεRI (high affinity IgE) receptors on the cell surface leads to the aggregation of the receptors and activation of an enzymatic cascade initiating mediator release. Mast cells and basophils are concentrated near exposed mucosal surfaces, such as the lung and the gastrointestinal tract, and as such, children with anaphylaxis will typically present with signs and symptoms affecting these organ systems (wheezing, respiratory distress, vomiting, hives, etc.). While several mediators are released from the mast cell and basophil, including histamine, platelet activating factor (PAF), and the leukotrienes (the so-called *slow-reacting substances of anaphylaxis*), histamine is the most important mediator of anaphylaxis. Intramuscular administration of epinephrine is the mainstay of the treatment of anaphylaxis. Additional adjunctive therapies include the administration of systemic corticosteroids and parenteral antihistamines. The diagnosis, pathophysiology, and management of anaphylaxis and anaphylactic shock are discussed elsewhere in the textbook.

Neurogenic shock results from autonomic dysfunction occurring secondary to injury to the spinal cord. Loss of peripheral vascular tone and subsequent increased venous capacitance lead to a relative hypovolemia due to expansion of the vascular space (i.e. an increase in P_{mcf}). Children with neurogenic shock often fail to improve with fluid resuscitation but instead respond to treatment with selective alpha-adrenergic vasoactive infusions. Importantly, *spinal shock* refers to the acute loss of sensation accompanied by motor paralysis and the loss of spinal muscle reflexes that occurs following a spinal cord injury (usually transection of the spinal cord). Some of the spinal muscle reflexes gradually recover over time, and the patient eventually becomes exhibits hyperreflexia. While neurogenic shock often occur concomitant with spinal shock, the two are distinct entities and should not be confused.

Septic shock is the last sub-category of distributive shock. As mentioned above, patients with septic shock exhibit many of the features of the other types of shock, including hypovolemic shock (both an absolute and relative fluid deficit are often observed), cardiogenic shock (due to the presence of circulating cardiac depressant factors), and finally, distributive shock. For this reason, septic shock is often placed in a category all of its own. The diagnosis, pathophysiology, and management of septic shock are discussed elsewhere in the textbook.

Diagnosis of Shock

Shock is primarily a clinical diagnosis. The diagnosis is relatively straightforward in the latter stages of shock, as in a child who is lethargic, ashen, gray, tachypneic, cold, and hypotensive (see *the superannuated hag* above). Unfortunately, intervention at this stage (i.e. irreversible shock) is unlikely to be successful. The diagnosis of shock requires a high index of suspicion. Early recognition and timely, aggressive intervention is paramount. Important historical clues in the infant are poor feeding, slow weight gain, sweating with feeds and fussiness, whereas an older child may complain of sleep difficulties (orthopnea), excessive fatigue, exercise limitations, chronic cough and palpitations. Family history of congenital heart disease, metabolic disease and autoimmune disease, along with medication exposure and infectious disease exposure should be ascertained. The presence of tachycardia, tachypnea, gallop, rales, jugular

venous distention, hepatomegaly and extremity edema are consistent with congestive heart failure. As discussed above, the body's compensatory mechanisms will maintain adequate function of the vital organs (*compensatory stage* of shock) for a time so that frank hypotension remains both a late and ominous sign.

In its final stages, uncompensated shock can be characterized by the presence of anion gap acidosis. An anion gap >16 mEq/L can be used as a surrogate marker for ATP depletion and energy failure. When oxygen delivery is inadequate, anaerobic metabolism occurs through glycolysis with pyruvate being converted to lactate and lactic acid, which is largely responsible for the anion gap. *Glycopenic* shock can be diagnosed when an anion gap exists in the presence of hypoglycemia (inadequate substrate), hyperglycemia (insulin resistance), or euglycemia (inadequate substrate + insulin resistance). When glucose utilization is inadequate, the anion gap is caused by organic acid intermediates produced by catabolism of protein and or fat to fuel the Krebs cycle.

It cannot be over-emphasized that early recognition of shock is critical as time-sensitive, early reversal of clinical signs of shock has been shown to influence outcomes in critically ill patients. In adults, Rivers and colleagues [102] demonstrated the importance of early goal-directed therapies, which maintain not only blood pressure but also oxygen delivery, in improving outcome [102–107]. In this study, adults presenting to the emergency department in severe sepsis or septic shock were randomized early on to receive either therapies directed at achieving normal blood pressure or therapies directed towards achieving not only normal blood pressure but also a superior vena cava (SVC) oxygen saturation ≥70 %. In this latter arm, investigators used packed red blood cell transfusion (for patients with a hemoglobin less than 10 g/dL to reverse *anemic shock*) and/or fluids and inotropic support (to reverse *ischemic shock*) if the SVC saturation remained less than 70 %. The theory behind this approach is based on the concept of oxygen delivery reviewed above in which DO_2 depends on oxygen carrying capacity (hemoglobin), oxygen content of arterial blood (percent oxyhemoglobin plus dissolved oxygen), and cardiac output. Thus, if the hemoglobin and arterial oxygen saturation are normal, then cardiac output predominantly determines oxygen delivery. As cardiac output decreases and metabolic demands remain the same, the mitochondria extract more oxygen to maintain a similar amount of energy production; therefore, the oxygen saturation of blood returning to the heart (normally ~75 %) decreases. Rivers et al. [102] observed that patients in the first arm attained a normal blood pressure but had an average SVC oxygen saturation of only 65 %. In contrast, those in the second treatment arm received more blood transfusions, fluid resuscitation, and inotrope use to both maintain normal blood pressure and achieve an SVC saturation >70 %. Of note, this early (within 6 h), goal-directed (SVC saturation >70 %) therapy resulted in a nearly 50 % reduction in mortality. In a second analysis of this study, the authors evaluated patients who had shock characterized by tachycardia and decreased SVC O_2 saturation with normal or high blood pressure. Interestingly, these patients had higher mortality rates than those patients presenting with hypotension. When this group of patients with tachycardia, low SVC O_2 saturation, and normotension were evaluated by treatment arms, those who received therapies directed towards a goal SVC O_2 saturation >70 % had reduced multiple organ failure and mortality. The authors described this type of shock without hypotension as *cryptic* or *ischemic* shock. *Ischemic* shock without hypotension can be represented by the following equation: Decreased cardiac output = (normal or high mean arterial pressure – central venous pressure)/ increased systemic vascular resistance. Their data suggests that reversal of this normotensive *ischemic* shock can reduce organ failure and mortality. De Oliviera and colleagues also demonstrated similar findings in a randomized interventional trial in children with septic shock. In the control arm, therapies were directed to normalizing capillary refill time and blood pressure. In the interventional arm, therapies were also directed to maintaining an SVC O_2 sat >70 %. This intervention resulted in the use of more fluid resuscitation, blood tranfusions, and intrope and vasodilator infusions, as well as a reduction in mortality from 39 to 12 % [108].

Emergency departments place central lines for measurement of SVC oxygen saturations less frequently in children than in adults making a corresponding study in children unlikely, though the feasibility of this approach in adults has been confirmed by multiple studies [109–114]. However, in a similar manner, a recent landmark study showed that the predominant factor that reduces mortality and neurologic morbidity in children transported to tertiary care pediatric hospitals is the reversal of shock through early recognition and resuscitation in the referring emergency department [115]. In this study, Han and colleagues examined early goal directed therapy for neonatal and pediatric shock in community hospital emergency departments, using prolonged capillary refill >2 s as a practical though inferior surrogate marker of decreased SVC O_2 saturation. In all patients with shock, both mortality and morbidity increased with the following progression of clinical signs: tachycardia alone → hypotension with normal capillary refill → prolonged capillary refill without hypotension → and finally, the combination of prolonged capillary refill with hypotension (which carried the highest mortality risk). Reversal of these clinical signs in the emergency department reduced mortality and morbidity by more than 50 % and each hour that passed without reversal of hypotension or reduction in capillary refill was associated with a twofold increased odds ratio of death. Thus, the ability to both

recognize and reverse shock in children may be the most important lessons to be learned in the practice of pediatric critical care medicine.

Therapeutic Endpoints of Resuscitation in Pediatrics

Traditional Endpoints

Resuscitation to clinical goals remains the first priority in the management of shock. Children should be resuscitated to normal mental status, normal pulse quality proximally and distally, equal central and peripheral temperatures, capillary refill <2 s, and urine output >1 mL/kg/h. Many of these clinical features of shock lack interrater reliability and validity, especially when used as "stand alone" therapeutic endpoints [116–121]. However, serial examination of multiple clinical features by the same clinician can be used to effectively identify and monitor children with shock [122]. Because 20 % of blood flow goes to both the brain and the kidney, clinical assessment of the function of these two organs can be informative and a normal mental status and urine output generally suggest adequately compensated oxygen delivery. However, the clinician should not necessarily be reassured by a normal mental status, as altered mental status is a very late sign of shock. Distal pulse quality, temperature, and capillary refill reflect systemic vascular tone and cardiac output. Normal capillary refill and toe temperature assures a cardiac index greater than 2.0 L/min/m^2 and superior vena cava oxygen saturation $\geq$70 % [123]. Fluid resuscitation should be monitored using a combination of physical exam findings (palpation of the liver edge, increasing tachypnea, onset of basilar rales on auscultation, etc.) in addition to monitoring tools (central venous or atrial pressures) as surrogate indicators of when fluid resuscitation has likely been adequate and it is necessary to initiate inotropic therapy. The predictive hemodynamic response to a fluid bolus can often be ascertained by applying gentle but constant pressure over the liver in the right upper quadrant to provide an *auto transfusion* while assessing the immediate hemodynamic response in terms of heart rate and blood pressure changes. The recent studies referenced above add support to the concept that titrating resuscitation to simple clinical parameters is likely to be as effective as utilizing advanced hemodynamic parameters such as SVC O_2 saturation.

Normal heart rate and perfusion pressure for age (MAP-CVP) should be the initial hemodynamic goals. Fluid resuscitation can be monitored by observing the effects on heart rate and MAP-CVP. The heart rate should decrease and MAP-CVP increase when fluid resuscitation is effective. In contrast, the heart rate may increase and MAP-CVP will narrow if too much fluid is given. The *shock index* (HR/SBP)

Fig. 30.5 (**a**) Max Harry Weil's "5-2 Rule" for CVP-titrated Fluid Management. A volume of 50, 100, or 200 mL of fluid (depending upon the initial CVP) is administered through a peripheral intravenous catheter over 10 min. If at any time during the administration of this fluid the CVP rises by more than 5 cmH₂O, the infusion should be stopped. Following the infusion, the "5-2" rule is applied. If the CVP has risen by more than 2 cm, but less than 5 cm, the patient should be monitored at 10 min intervals. If the CVP has risen by more than 2 cm and remains elevated, no additional fluid is administered. If the CVP has declined to within 2 cm of the initial value, another fluid challenge (again, the amount will depend upon the CVP) is administered. (**b**) Max Harry Weil's "7-3" Rule for PAOP-titrated Fluid Management. A volume of 50, 100, or 200 mL of fluid (depending upon the initial PAOP) is administered through a peripheral intravenous catheter over 10 min. If at any time during the administration of this fluid the PAOP rises by more than 7 cmH₂O, the infusion should be stopped. Following the infusion, the "7-3" rule is applied. If the PAOP has risen by more than 3 cm, but less than 7 cm, the patient should be monitored at 10 min intervals. If the PAOP has risen by more than 3 cm and remains elevated, no additional fluid is administered. If the PAOP has declined to within 3 cm of the initial value, another fluid challenge (again, the amount will depend upon the PAOP) is administered (Reprinted from Weil and Henning [130]. With permission from Wolters Kluwer Health)

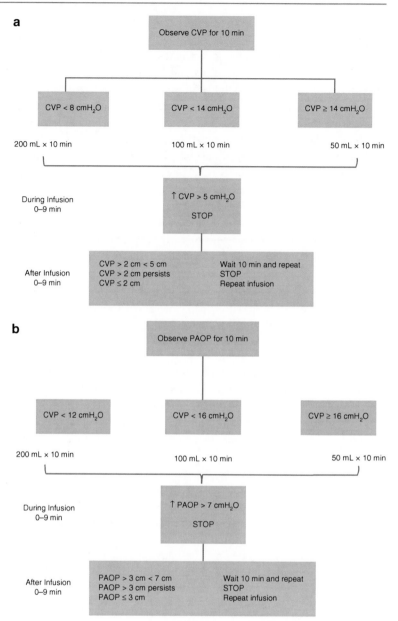

Cardiac Filling Pressures

Both the right-sided cardiac filling pressures (central venous pressure, CVP; right atrial pressure) and left-sided cardiac filling pressures (pulmonary artery occlusion pressure, PAOP, also known as the wedge pressure and/or [107, 124–128] can also be used to assess the effectiveness of fluid and inotrope therapy. If the applied therapy (e.g. preload or inotropy) increases the stroke volume, then the heart rate will decrease and systolic blood pressure will increase resulting in a lower shock index value. However, if stroke volume does not improve with resuscitation then heart rate will not decrease, systolic blood pressure will not increase, and shock index will not improve.

pulmonary capillary wedge pressure; left atrial pressure) have also been used as therapeutic endpoints of resuscitation [118, 129]. For example, Max Harry Weil developed a resuscitation protocol based upon CVP and PAOP in the early days of critical care medicine (Fig. 30.5) [130]. Importantly, the site in which CVP is measured (femoral vein, internal jugular vein, subclavian vein) does not matter, as the CVP measured in the femoral vein appears to adequately approximate right atrial pressure in children, particularly in the absence of intra-abdominal pathology [131–135]. Unfortunately, the vast majority of clinical studies have shown that CVP does not reliably or accurately predict fluid responsiveness in critically ill patients [136, 137]. In addition, a meta-analysis of 13 randomized clinical trials showed that invasive hemodynamic monitoring with the pulmonary artery catheter (PAC) increased overall mortality in critically ill patients [138]. Finally, a multi-center, randomized clinical trial comparing PAC-guided therapy versus central venous catheter (CVC)-guided therapy in critically ill adults with acute lung injury showed that use of the PAC increased complications and hospital costs without improving outcome [139, 140]. However, it should be noted that CVP was used as a resuscitation end-point in the Early Goal-Directed Therapy trial of severe sepsis/septic shock [102], as well as the Surviving Sepsis Campaign [113, 114]. Therefore, it would seem that cardiac filling pressures should not be used as the sole therapeutic endpoint of resuscitation, but as part of an entire set of resuscitation endpoints. Importantly, there are few (if any) randomized, controlled trials of CVP- or PAOP-titrated fluid management in critically ill children with shock, and any current recommendations are based upon anecdotal experience and translation from adult studies.

Venous Oximetry and Near-Infrared Spectroscopy

In the era of early goal-directed therapy, an increasing number of pediatric intensivists are placing superior vena cava (SVC) central venous catheters in order to monitor SVC oxygen saturation (SVC O_2). Due to the increased relative size and weight of the head versus the body in infants and young children, blood flow through the SVC comprises a much larger percentage of total cardiac output compared to the inferior vena cava (IVC) [76], perhaps making SVC O_2 an ideal therapeutic endpoint in children. The SVC O_2 (directly measured via co-oximetry) has a reasonable correlation with the mixed venous oxygen saturation [141]. There is a commercially available central venous catheter (PediaSat Oximetry Catheter, Edwards Life Sciences, Irvine, CA) with a sensor on the tip that continuously measures SVC O_2 [142–145]. However, there remains some question as to the accuracy of these catheters, particularly at lower SVC O_2 (<70 %), which would be when such a catheter would be most useful [143, 144, 146]. In addition, the growing use of near-infrared spectroscopy (NIRS) in the Cardiac Intensive Care Unit (CICU) population has led to a few studies using this technology in older children with shock (In Vivo Optical Spectroscopy, INVOS System, Somanetics, Troy, MI) [147–151]. However, further studies are necessary before the use of these devices can be considered standard monitoring tools in the PICU. The data supporting using SVC O_2 saturation as a therapeutic endpoint in critically ill children is limited [108]. Nevertheless, targeting a SVC O_2 saturation to >70 % is an oft quoted goal. Similar to the approach in adults, the critically ill child in shock should be transfused if the hemoglobiin is sub-optimal and if normalized, then inotropes and vasodilators can be used to improve cardiac output until the SVC saturation is >70 %.

$AVDO_2$

An additional target sometimes used by clinicians is to maintain a normal arterial to venous oxygen content difference, the so-called $AVDO_2$. The $AVDO_2$ can be calculated as follows:

$$CaO_2 = (1.39 \times Hgb) \times art.saturation + (PaO_2 \times 0.003)$$
$$= ml\ O_2 / 100\ ml\ blood$$
$$(30.6)$$

$$CvO_2 = (1.39 \times Hgb) \times ven.saturation + (PvO_2 \times 0.003)$$
$$= ml\ O_2 / 100\ ml\ blood$$
$$(30.7)$$

$$AVDO_2\ (ml\ O_2 / 100\ ml\ blood) = CaO_2 - CvO_2 \quad (30.8)$$

Typical normal values (Hgb = 14, paO_2 90 and SaO_2 = 100 %, pvO_2 40 and SvO_2 = 75 %) would show an average difference of usually less than 5 ml O_2/ 100 ml blood which corresponds to a saturation difference of 25 %. When the $AVDO_2$ is greater than 5, suggesting increased oxygen extraction because of inadequate oxygen delivery (i.e. an oxygen deficit), then cardiac output should be increased with inotrope and vasodilator therapy until the $AVDO_2$ returns to the normal range. The $AVDO_2$ is most accurately determined when the venous saturation is measured in the pulmonary artery. In these circumstances, cardiac output can be measured using either the pulmonary artery catheter and thermodilution or PICCO as reviewed in the chapter on Hemodynamic Monitoring, later in this textbook. In this setting, a typical goal cardiac index is ≥2.5 L/min/m² in cardiogenic shock and between 3.5 and 6.0 L/min/m² in septic shock. Furthermore, with the aid of either a pulmonary artery catheter (to measure the capillary wedge pressure as an estimate of LVEDP) or a left atrial catheter (as commonly provided by the cardiac surgeon), these surrogates of LVEDP can be trended to that value at which the best cardiac output can be achieved. For example, higher filling pressures may be required to attain the required end diastolic volume to achieve optimal stroke volume in a non-compliant, post-operative myocardium that can be determined during the wean from cardiopulmonary bypass.

Lactate

Many clinicians use lactate as a serum measure of anaerobic metabolism [152–155]; however, lactate can be elevated by a number of conditions in the absence of shock, including metabolic disorders, lymphoproliferative disorders, liver failure, and sepsis. Following lactate levels has been most useful in the setting of pre-operative and post-operative cardiogenic shock (although levels can be increased even in the absence of the low flow state). For these patients, mortality risk increases as serum lactate levels rise above 2.0 mmol/L. More helpful may be trending the change in lactate, as it has been shown that a change in lactate level of ≥ 0.75 mmol/L per hour was associated with worse outcomes and was superior to predicting a poor outcome (89 % sensitivity, 100 % specificity and a 100 % positive predictive value) as compared to single worse values [156]. When used as a hemodynamic goal, a diminishing value over time with an ultimate value <2.0 mmol/L is generally the target (i.e. lactate clearance). Interestingly, a recent multi-center, randomized, non-inferiority clinical trial in adults with septic shock suggested that targeting lactate clearance is at least comparable to targeting SVC O_2 ≥ 70 % [157]. A follow-up analysis of this same study showed that achieving the SVC O_2 target (≥ 70 %) without achieving the lactate clearance target (≥ 10 %) was more strongly associated with mortality, compared to achieving the lactate clearance target without achieving the SVC O_2 target [158]. In other words, if only one of these targets is achieved, failure to achieve the lactate clearance target has a worse prognosis. Global targets (i.e. superior vena cava oxygen saturation, mixed venous oxygen saturation, etc.) may not truly reflect regional targets (lactate clearance, NIRS, etc.) [159]. Lastly, a substantial number of patients in this trial never developed increased lactate levels, which has also been observed in critically ill children with severe sepsis and septic shock [108]. More studies testing lactate clearance as a therapeutic endpoint of resuscitation, especially in critically ill children, are required.

Management of Shock

Fluid Therapy

Fluid therapy is the hallmark of shock resuscitation in infants and children. In this context, intravenous fluid boluses are used to reverse the hypovolemic state and optimize contractility based on the principle of the Starling curve. Approximately 8 % of the total blood volume is contained within the arterial side, 70 % in the venous side, and 12 % in the capillary beds. The total blood volume in a baby is approximately 80–85 mL/kg, and decreases slightly (to 65–75 mL/kg) in the infant or child. Rapid resuscitation is often necessary to restore circulating volume. Rapid fluid boluses in increments of 20 mL/kg minimally up to 60 mL//kg [160] may be required to restore intravascular volume. However, if the patient has capillary leak syndrome as may occur in septic shock, then quite large volumes (up to and at times exceeding 100 mL/kg) may be needed in the first several hours.

Either crystalloids (e.g. 0.9 % normal saline or lactated ringers) or colloids (e.g. 5 % albumin) can be used to restore intravascular volume. While it appears that less colloid fluids may be needed than crystalloid fluids (as colloid fluids redistribute to the extravascular space more slowly), a large, multi-center, randomized, controlled trial demonstrated no differences among outcomes in adults resuscitated with normal saline as compared to 4 % albumin [161]. Of note, in a subgroup analysis there was a suggestion that 4 % albumin was more effective in patients with sepsis/septic shock when compared to crystalloid, though this nearly 5 % mortality reduction did not reach statistical significance [161]. Of interest, there are a growing number of studies showing that colloids may be better in critically ill children [162–168]. Even more compelling are the results of the FEAST study, a randomized, controlled trial in which children presenting with a severe febrile illness at the time of admission to the hospital (in Uganda, Kenya, or Tanzania) received either 20–40 mL/kg 5 % albumin, 20–40 mL/kg 0.9 % saline, or no fluid bolus. There were no differences in mortality at 48 h between the saline (110/1,047 children, 10.5 %) and albumin (111/1,050 children, 10.6 %) groups, though mortality was lowest (76/1,044 children, 7.3 %) in the control group that did not receive a fluid bolus. These results were consistent across all sub-group analyses [169]. A follow-up analysis of these results showed that excess mortality occurred as a result of cardiovascular collapse and not fluid overload (pulmonary edema, neurologic deterioration, etc.) [170]. Hence use of fluid resuscitation in the severe anemia/ high cardiac output malaria populations found in Sub-Saharan Africa is deleterious in part because further hemodilution exacerbates anemia and decreases rather than increases oxygen delivery. In contrast, fluid resuscitation in the capillary leak/ hypovolemia populations found in the UK and Netherlands meningococcemia belt and in the Southeast Asia Dengue belt is beneficial because increased ventricular filling improved cardiac output and oxygen delivery. With these caveats in mind, the usual practice in most PICUs in the US is to initiate volume resuscitation for hypovolemic patients with crystalloid fluids as a first line and follow with colloid if needed.

Rapid bolus of volume employing a push technique not only restores intravascular volume, but may also *turn off* expression of inflammation and coagulation genes. Numerous studies have shown that rapid and aggressive volume resuscitation within the first hour, improves survival not only in animal models, but more importantly in humans with shock. Fluid administration should be judicious, however, in neonates and children with cardiogenic failure from cardiomyopathy or congenital heart disease, as lower myocardial compliance often results in less volume need to achieve optimal stroke volume as predicted by Starling curves. Conversely, these children may be pushed off the Starling curve in the setting of over-aggressive fluid administration. Because of this, titrating in volume boluses as low as 5–10 mL/kg is often done while carefully monitoring the trend of CVP, LAP, PAOP, MAP and mixed venous saturation in these patients.

Blood Products

Transfusion with packed red blood cells (PRBC) is absolutely crucial in children with anemia and shock. Mitochondria cannot extract the last 20 % of oxygen bound to hemoglobin. Under normal conditions the mitochondria typically extract 25 % of oxygen bound to hemoglobin. This is reflected clinically by a mixed venous oxygen saturation of 75 % in a healthy patient with an arterial blood oxygen saturation of 100 %. In a child with 10 g/dL hemoglobin, only 8 g/dL is available for extraction as 20 % cannot be extracted. Thus, 2.5 g/dL is used for oxygen extraction, leaving a surplus of 5.5 g/dL of hemoglobin. In states of hemolysis, anemic shock can develop as surplus hemoglobin is lost (i.e. drops below 5 g/dL). Mortality rates are known to increase as the hemoglobin drops below 6 g/dL in various settings including hemorrhagic shock. The FEAST trial demonstrated this harmful effect [169]. Transfusion of blood is lifesaving in these circumstances. Whole blood is available in some parts of the world, while packed red blood cells are available in other parts of the world. The usual hemoglobin concentration of packed red blood cells is 20 g/dL. Since the blood volume of the child ranges from 65 to 85 mL/kg based on age, 10 mL/kg of packed red cells should increase the hemoglobin concentration by approximately 2 g/dL. Blood can be rapidly infused in patients with life threatening hemolytic anemia, however, furosemide may be needed to prevent fluid overload if hypovolemia is not a concurrent challenge.

The optimal hematocrit in critically ill patients with shock remains a matter of debate. There is no question that a restrictive transfusion strategy is safe in critically ill children in the PICU who are hemodynamically stable [171]. However, the optimal transfusion threshold for hemodynamically unstable children in the PICU is less certain [172]. An early study by Crowell and Smith based on an in vitro model of the microcirculation suggested that the optimal hematocrit is >30 % [173]. The blood viscosity increased substantially and reduced blood flow through glass capillaries of fixed diameter as the hematocrit increased. Based on their results, these investigators calculated that the hematocrit for optimal oxygen delivery was around 30 %. Experimental evidence in animals has further suggested that viscosity begins to compromise blood flow at hematocrits approaching 40–45 % [172]. Again, it is interesting to note that one of the therapeutic endpoints in the EGDT trial was a hematocrit of 30 % [102].

Vasoactive Medications

There are several different vasoactive medications (Table 30.9) that are commonly used in the PICU [174]. These are routinely placed into different categories based upon their principal hemodynamic effect. Inotropic agents (inotropes) are used to increase contractility and as a result, stroke volume and cardiac output. Most of the inotropic agents are adrenergic receptor agonists and include both endogenously produced catecholamines (e.g. dopamine,

Table 30.9 Vasoactive pharmacologic agents commonly used in the management of pediatric shock

Agent	Dose range	Comments
Dopamine[a, b, c]	3–5 µg/kg/min	*Renal-dose dopamine* (primarily dopaminergic agonist activity); increases renal and mesenteric blood flow, increases natriuresis and urine output
	5–10 µg/kg/min	Inotropic (β_1 agonist) effects predominate; increases cardiac contractility, heart rate, and blood pressure
	10–20 µg/kg/min	Vasopressor (α_1 agonist) effects predominate; increases peripheral vascular resistance and blood pressure
Dobutamine[a, b]	5–10 µg/kg/min	Inotropic effects (β_1 agonist) predominate; increases contractility and reduces afterload
Epinephrine[a, b]	0.03–0.1 µg/kg/min	Inotropic effects (β_1 and β_2 agonist) predominate, increases contractility and heart rate; may reduce afterload to a slight extent via β_2 effects
	0.1–1 µg/kg/min	Vasopressor effects (α_1 agonist) predominate; increases peripheral vascular resistance and blood pressure
Norepinephrine[a, b]	0.1–1 µg/kg/min	Potent vasopressor (α_1 and β_1 agonist); increases heart rate, contractility, and peripheral vascular resistance; absent β_2 effect distinguishes it from epinephrine
Phenylephrine[a, b, d]	0.1–0.5 µg/kg/min	Potent vasopressor with primarily α_1 agonist effects; indicated in tetralogy of Fallot hypercyanotic spells (*tet spells*)
Vasopressin[a, b, e]	0.0003–0.002 units/kg/min (0.018–0.12 units/kg/h)	Vasopressor (via V_1) without inotrope activity; may be indicated in refractory shock
Nitroglycerin[a, d, f]	0.5–3 µg/kg/min	Dose dependent venodilator and vasodilator (cGMP mediated)

(continued)

Table 30.9 (continued)

Agent	Dose range	Comments
Nitroprusside[a, g]	0.5–3 µg/kg/min	Systemic arterial vasodilator (c GMP mediated)
Inamrinone[a, h]	0.75 mg/kg I.V. bolus over 2–3 min followed by maintenance infusion 5–10 µg/kg/min	Inodilator (Type III phosphodiesterase inhibitor); increases cardiac output via increased contractility and afterload reduction
Milrinone[a, i]	50 µg/kg administered over 15 min followed by a continuous infusion of 0.5–0.75 µg/kg/min	Inodilator (Type III phosphodiesterase inhibitor); increases cardiac output via increased contractility and afterload reduction
Prostaglandin E_1 (PGE$_1$)[j]	0.3–0.1 µg/kg/min	Maintains patent ductus arteriosus (cAMP effect)

[a]Correct volume depletion prior to starting infusion

[b]Extravasation may produce tissue necrosis (as a general recommendation, should be administered via central venous access). Treatment with subcutaneous administration of phentolamine as follows:

   Neonates: infiltrate area with a small amount (e.g., 1 mL) of solution (made by diluting 2.5–5 mg in 10 mL of preservative free NS) within 12 h of extravasation; do not exceed 0.1 mg/kg or 2.5 mg total

   Infants, children, and adults: infiltrate area with a small amount (eg, 1 mL) of solution (made by diluting 5–10 mg in 10 mL of NS) within 12 h of extravasation; do not exceed 0.1–0.2 mg/kg or 5 mg total

[c]Dopamine has exhibited nonlinear kinetics in children (dose changes may not achieve steady-state for approximately 1 h, compared to 20 min in adults)

[d]Exhibits rapid tachyphylaxis (dose may need to be increased with time to achieve same clinical effect)

[e]Dose not well established in children or adults; abrupt discontinuation of infusion may result in hypotension (gradually taper dose to discontinue the infusion); May be associated with profound peripheral vasoconstriction (leading to tissue ischemia)

[f]May cause profound hypotension in volume-depleted patients; nitroglycerin adsorbs to plastics; I.V. must be prepared in glass bottles and special administration sets intended for nitroglycerin (nonpolyvinyl chloride) must be used

[g]Converted to cyanide by erythrocyte and tissue sulfhydryl group interactions; cyanide is converted in the liver by the enzyme rhodanase to thiocyanate (thiocyanate levels should be monitored)

[h]Metabolized in the liver; causes thrombocytopenia (may be dose-related); milrinone is now preferred agent

[i]Metabolized in the kidney; relatively long half-life (use with caution in children with hemodynamic instability)

[j]Dose may be decreased once the ductus arteriosus has opened with very little change in therapeutic effects; may cause hypotension, apnea, cutaneous flushing

epinephrine, and norepinephrine) as well as synthetic analogs (e.g. dobutamine). The exceptions to this pharmacologic mechanism are agents that inhibit type III phosphodiesterase (e.g. inamrinone, milrinone, and enoximone), resulting in elevated cAMP, as well as those agents that increase sensitivity of the myofilament to calcium (e.g. levosimendan). Vasodilators are used to decrease systemic vascular resistance (recall again that CO = MAP/SVR, so that by reducing SVR, CO will increase). The most commonly used vasodilators are nitroprusside and nitroglycerin. Vasopressors are used to increase systemic vascular resistance, in order to increase perfusion pressure (discussed above). Most of the currently available vasopressors are adrenergic receptor agonists (e.g., dopamine, epinephrine, norepinephrine, phenylephrine).

Inotropes

Most of the currently available inotropes act through either direct stimulation of the adrenergic receptors or through inhibition of phosphodiesterases to increase cAMP. Adrenergic receptors fall into three categories: α-adrenergic, β-adrenergic and dopaminergic (DA) receptors. The receptors responsible for inotropic stimulation are the β_1-adrenoreceptors located on the myocardium, while the β_2-receptors exist on the vascular and bronchial smooth muscle and mediate vaso- and broncho- dilation, respectively. α-adrenoreceptors include the α_1 subtype located on peripheral vasculature and stimulation mediates smooth muscle

contraction and thus, vasopressor effects (discussed below). Following their initial descriptions α_2-receptors were identified on the presynaptic terminals of sympathetic nerves and stimulation inhibited norepinephrine release. They have also been identified on postsynaptic smooth muscle where stimulation results in contraction, though the contribution of this mechanism to vasopressor effects of adrenergic agonists is not fully known [175]. From a pharmacokinetic standpoint, nearly all the inotropes used clinically are cleared by first-order kinetics, such that changes in infusion rates linearly correlate to plasma concentrations, making them practical to titrate to clinical effect. In addition, the adrenergic receptor agonists are rapidly metabolized by circulating catechol-O-methyltransferase (COMT) followed by deamination (via monoamine oxidase) or sulfoconjugation (by phenolsulfotransferase) such that effective half-life of these agents is on the order of minutes. Therefore, these agents are preferably administered via continuous infusion – most commonly via a central venous catheter. Of note, the phosphodiesterase inhibitors are cleared by the kidneys (requiring dosage adjustments in renal failure) and possess a half-life estimated to be 45–60 min.

Dopamine

Historically, the mainstay of inotropic therapy in pediatrics has been dopamine which is the immediate precursor in the catecholamine biosynthetic pathway. Because of its unique properties of being able to stimulate dopaminergic (0–3 µg/

kg/min), β-adrenergic (3–10 µg/kg/min) and α-adrenergic receptors (>10 µg/kg/min) in a dose-dependent manner, some clinicians refer to this agent as an *inovasopressor*, as both inotropic and vasopressor activity can be observed with escalating dosage. The pharmacologic effect of dopamine is derived from two relatively equipotent properties – direct agonist stimulation of the receptors and indirect release of norepinephrine from the sympathetic vesicles. Because infants less than 6 months have been considered to not possess their full number of sympathetic vesicles (corroborated in studies of immature animals), it has been suggested that there is a relative age-specific insensitivity to the drug, such that increased infusion rates may be necessary [176]. However, this data remains controversial in that Seri et al. [177] have demonstrated clear physiologic responses to normal dopamine infusion rates (3–7 µg/kg/min) in premature infants. Relative *dopamine insensitivity* can also be observed in older children and adults who may have exhausted endogenous catecholamine reserves because of prolonged stress responses prior to reaching the clinical care setting.

When infused at 3–10 µg/kg/min, dopamine increases cardiac contractility and cardiac output with only modest effects on heart rate and systemic vascular resistance. Because of its general effectiveness and the vast familiarity and experience with this agent, dopamine has remained the first line inotropic agent for *fluid refractory* shock. Infusion rates can be increased gradually in order to titrate its inotropic effect to the goals outlined above. Surveys of common practice suggest that while infusion rates as high as 40 µg/kg/min have been reported, most clinicians stop escalating at 20 µg/kg/min and choose instead to add a second vasoactive agent. It should also be noted that dopamine administration through a peripheral intravenous catheter is not any safer compared to other vasoactive medications, as is commonly believed.

Because of the imprecise ability to differentiate infusion rates mediating strictly inotropic effects from vasopressor effects during the transition from β to α-adrenergic receptor stimulation, some clinicians express concern for the use of dopamine alone in cardiogenic shock. Though relatively few studies have been performed, it has been suggested that because dopamine alone increases not only mean arterial blood pressure, but also pulmonary capillary wedge pressure and myocardial oxygen extraction, clinicians consider adding a vasodilator (e.g. dobutamine) as the combination may be more beneficial than dopamine alone in this setting [178]. Another major effect of dopamine is to selectively increase renal and splanchnic perfusion. However, the ascribed renal protective effect of *renal-dose* dopamine has not been substantiated in several large clinical trials designed to examine this possible benefit and more likely to be related to modest improvements in cardiac output associated with even low infusion rates [179].

Dopamine, similar to most inotropic agents, will worsen ventilation/perfusion matching such that intrapulmonary shunt increases and as a result, PaO_2 may decrease. In addition, dopamine also inhibits prolactin secretion [180], which may have adverse results on the host immune response [181]. Finally, dopamine has been shown to increase VO_2 and oxygen extraction to a greater extent than the improvements observed in cardiac output and DO_2 in critically ill children following the Norwood procedure [182]. As an interesting aside, a multicenter, cohort study in critically ill adults with sepsis noted that patients who were treated with dopamine had a higher mortality compared to those who were treated with other agents [183]. Moreover, a meta-analysis of studies comparing dopamine to norepinephrine in critically ill adults with severe sepsis/septic shock again showed that dopamine increases mortality [184]. However, while the evidence against dopamine is growing, dopamine remains the first-line vasoactive medication in many PICUs.

Dobutamine

Dobutamine is an inotropic agent synthetically derived from the catecholamine parent structure that possesses mixed β-receptor agonist activities. Thus, dobutamine possesses both chronotropic and inotropic properties mediated through $β_1$-adrenergic receptor stimulation as well as modest vasodilating effects related to its $β_2$-adrenergic receptor agonist property. The limitation of vasodilating effects relate to its preparation as a racemic mixture where the (+) isomer has potent effects at the β-receptor and modest α adrenergic antagonist effects, but conversely the (−) isomer is a selective $α_1$-adrenergic receptor agonist mediating vasoconstrictor effects [185]. In addition, it has been observed that at infusion rates >10 µg/kg/min, dobutamine can lead to significant afterload reduction and at times hypotension. This is thought to occur because dobutamine at this infusion rate may possess $α_2$ agonist effects which inhibit release of norepinephrine from the pre-synaptic terminals to further reduce vascular tone. Similar to dopamine, there may be an age-specific insensitivity to dobutamine in children. Perkin and co-workers demonstrated that children under the age of 2 years have a reduced response to dobutamine [186]. Despite these complex properties, the primary hemodynamic effects are to increase contractility, most often with little change in the heart rate or mean arterial blood pressure despite substantial increases in cardiac output. Because of these properties, dobutamine is most commonly indicated in the clinical setting that necessitates increasing inotropy without augmenting systemic vascular resistance, as occurs most commonly with pure cardiogenic shock (e.g. myocarditis). In these cases, dobutamine will increase stroke volume while decreasing central venous pressure and often improves the ratio between myocardial oxygen supply and demand. However, a growing body of evidence suggests that inotropic agents, such as dobutamine and milrinone increase long-term mortality in patients with heart failure, leading many experts to recommend against their use in this setting [187–190].

Epinephrine

Epinephrine is the endogenous circulating neurohormone released from the adrenal medulla during stress which possesses β_1, β_2, α_1, and α_2 adrenergic receptor agonist activity. It is a commonly used adjuvant inotrope for patients who fail to respond adequately to dopamine therapy or are too hypotensive to tolerate the vasodilating effects of inodilators such as dobutamine or milrinone. Adults and children who are resistant to either dopamine or dobutamine therapy will frequently respond to epinephrine. At the lower dosage or infusion rates (0.03 toward 0.1–0.3 μg/kg/min, so called *low dose epinephrine*) its β-adrenergic effects predominate such that it is principally an inotropic agent. Based on this principal, epinephrine has become an increasingly utilized second-line inotropic agent in the setting of low cardiac output states (e.g. post-cardiopulmonary bypass). The α-adrenergic effect on increasing systemic vascular resistance becomes more prominent as the epinephrine infusion rate approaches and exceeds 0.3 μg/kg/min, in which case it is sometimes described as an *inovasopressor*. Though epinephrine can mediate splanchnic vasoconstriction and theoretically lead to intestinal ischemia, this adverse effect is thought to be less significant in the critical care setting as it is countered by significant augmentation of cardiac output [191]. Patients with heart failure and increased systemic vascular resistance may be harmed by higher dosage epinephrine unless it is concomitantly administered with a vasodilator or inodilator. Non-cardiac related effects of epinephrine include increasing plasma glucose levels, increasing fatty acid levels, and increased renin activity with a concomitant decrease in serum potassium and aldosterone levels.

Norepinephrine

While norepinephrine is classically considered to be a vasopressor, it does have mixed α-adrenergic and β-adrenergic effects. Again, these effects are dose-dependent. Norepinephrine is an endogenous neurotransmitter in the sympathetic nervous system. At lower doses (typically on the order of 0.01–0.05 μg/kg/min), norepinephrine can improve contractility and hence cardiac output via its β_1-adrenergic effects. At higher doses, it is almost a pure α-adrenergic agonist with primarily vasopressor effects.

Phosphodiesterase Inhibitors

The phosphodiesterase (PDE) inhibitors are a class of drugs called bipyridines which mediate both inotropy and vasodilation, and as a result are often referred to as *inodilators*. These agents mediate their effects by preventing hydrolysis of cAMP (Type III PDE inhibitorsI, e.g. milrinone, amrinone,

enoximone, or pentoxyfilline) and/or cGMP (Type V PDE inhibitors, e.g. sildenafil, dipyrimadole, or pentoxyfilline). When type III PDE inhibitors are administered alone, the increase in cAMP improves contractility and also causes vasodilation of pulmonary and systemic arterial vasculature resulting in decreased ventricular afterload. Unique to this class of agents, PDE inhibitors improve ventricular relaxation (so called *lusitropic property*). This effect is mediated by decreased breakdown of cAMP resulting in activation of protein kinase A which subsequently phosphorylates the sarcoplasmic reticulum protein, phospholamban. This phosphorylation modulates the activation of sarcoplasmic reticulum ATPase (SERCA) resulting in more rapid uptake of cytosolic calcium thus facilitating more rapid and improved myocyte relaxation [192, 193]. As a result of these pharmacologic properties, the main hemodynamic effects of PDE inhibitors are to decrease both systemic and pulmonary vascular resistances, decrease filling pressures, and substantially augment cardiac output, most often with very little change in heart rate. Other effects noted with the use of PDE inhibitors include coronary artery dilation, thus there is little change in myocardial oxygen consumption, and putative anti-inflammatory effects which have made it an attractive option in fluid-resuscitated, low cardiac output shock as most commonly occurs in pediatric septic shock [96]. Finally, it is notable that PDE inhibitors mediate their effects independent of β-adrenergic receptor ligation. It has become increasingly appreciated that β-receptor down-regulation (e.g. in congestive heart failure), signaling disruption (e.g. in sepsis), and polymorphisms all may affect the manner by which this receptor-based pharmacologic mechanism can be utilized clinically, so that PDE inhibitors may provide superior clinical effects in these settings.

The interaction of PDE inhibitors with concomitant inotropes, vasodilators, and even vasopressors can be used to therapeutic advantages in patients with a variety of forms of shock. For example, epinephrine can remain a potent and relatively pure inotrope at higher dosages when combined with a type III PDE inhibitor that will prevent breakdown of cAMP produced by β_1 and β_2 adrenergic stimulation such that increased cAMP inhibits the usual effects of epinephrine-mediated α_1 adrenergic stimulation. In a similar manner, norepinephrine may be a more effective inotrope while maintaining vasopressor effectiveness, when administered with a Type III PDE inhibitor. The hydrolysis of norepinephrine-mediated β_1-receptor cAMP production is inhibited so that increased cAMP improves both contractility and relaxation. In addition, norepinephrine-mediated α_1 and α_2 adrenergic effects remain unopposed because milrinone possesses no specific β_1 receptor activity and therefore has minimal vasodilatory effect in the face of potent α-adrenergic vasoconstriction. In a related manner, the type V PDE inhibitors (e.g. sildenafil, dipyridamole) may potentiate the pulmonary vasodilator effects of inhaled nitric oxide.

As alluded to above, one major challenge posed by the use of currently licensed PDE inhibitors is their relatively prolonged half-life as compared to catecholamines and nitrosovasodilators. Although the latter agents are eliminated within minutes, PDE inhibitors are not eliminated for hours. Milrinone is primarily bound to plasma proteins (~75 %) and predominantly eliminated by the kidney while inamrinone is predominantly eliminated by the liver, thus, this half-life elimination is even more important in the setting of organ failure. When untoward side effects are encountered (e.g. hypotension), these drugs should be discontinued immediately. Of note, norepinephrine has been reported as being an effective antidote for these toxicities. As mentioned above, norepinephrine, on the basis of its α_1 and β_1, but not β_2 adrenergic activity will increase blood pressure via vasoconstriction (α_1 effect) and cardiac output (β_1 effect), but not exacerbate the vasodilatory effect of the phosphodiesterase inhibitor.

Other Agents

Of historic note, isoproterenol was an important and commonly used inodilator that possesses both β_1 and β_2 adrenergic activity. It used to be considered an important drug in the treatment of heart block, refractory status asthmaticus, and pulmonary hypertensive crises with right ventricular failure although its unfavorable safety profile with regards to increasing myocardial oxygen demand resulting in ischemic injury has substantially tempered its use over the past decade. Levosimendan represents a relatively newer class of *inodilators* which sensitizes calcium binding in the actin-tropomyosin complex to improve contractility, while simultaneously hyperpolarizing potassium channels to cause vasodilation [194]. There is a growing body of literature on levosimendan use in critically ill children [195–202]. However, at the time of this writing, levosimendan is not available in the United States. Calcium chloride infusions have also been used as inotropic agents, though there are limited studies in children and adults [203–205]. Some of the unique developmental differences in excitation-contraction coupling in the pediatric myocardium are importantly considered here. The relative immaturity of intracellular calcium regulation (T tubules, sarcoplasmic reticulum, L-type Ca^{2+} channels) causes alterations in the normal mechanisms leading to the Ca^{2+}-induced Ca^{2+} release (CICR) that triggers excitation-contraction coupling, such that the neonatal myocardium is more dependent upon extracellular calcium versus intracellular calcium for contractility compared to the mature heart [206–210]. These developmental differences also explain the extreme sensitivity of neonates to calcium channel antagonists [207]. Tri-iodothyronine is also an effective inotropic agent which has long been used to preserve cardiac function in patients who are brain dead and have low T_3 levels [211].

A randomized controlled trial in neonates showed that use of tri-iodothyronine as a post cardiac surgery inotrope improved outcomes [212, 213].

Vasodilators

Vasodilators (Table 30.9) are used to reduce either pulmonary or systemic vascular resistance and improve cardiac output. The *nitrosovasodilators* depend on release of nitrosothiols (nitric oxide donor) to activate soluble guanylate cyclase and release cGMP. Sodium nitroprusside is both a systemic and pulmonary vasodilator. In the setting of a failing myocardium, careful titration of nitroprusside to achieve lower afterload may improve cardiac output even though changes in blood pressure may not be observed. The usual starting infusion rate is on the order of 0.5–1 µg/kg/min. Nitroglycerin has a somewhat selective dose-dependent effect in that at <1 µg/kg/min it is a coronary artery vasodilator, 1 µg/kg/min it provides pulmonary vasodilation, and at 3 µg/kg/min it mediates systemic vasodilation. Inhaled nitric oxide is a selective pulmonary vasodilator which can be started at 5 PPM (see chapter on nitric oxide later in this textbook) when needed to afterload the RV or decrease PVR. Prostaglandins (PG) increase cAMP levels to provide potent systemic and pulmonary vasodilation. Prostacyclin (PGI_2) can be started at 3 ng/kg/min and an increasing experience with this agent suggests that continuous infusions are necessary to maintain its effect. Numerous PGI_2 analogs continue to be developed (e.g. treprostinil, iloprost, and beraprost sodium); however, their role in hemodynamic support of the critically ill child remain incompletely defined [214].

Alpha-adrenergic antagonists also have a role as vasodilators. Phentolamine, which is a competitive antagonist, has been used in combination with epinephrine or norepinephrine to offset the alpha-adrenergic effects and facilitate the beta-adrenergic effects of these agents. Phenoxybenzamine has also been used for afterload reduction in neonates with single ventricle physiology [215, 216]. Phenoxybenzamine binds to and inhibits the alpha-adrenergic receptor through covalent modification so it possesses a very long half-life elimination making its routine use uncommon in the PICU setting.

Vasopressors

In the setting of distributive shock, low SVR results in significant hypotension and as a result inadequate organ perfusion pressure. Thus, principal pharmacologic agents indicated in anaphylactic, neurogenic, and vasodilatory (warm) septic shock include those mediating vasoconstrictive effects, so-called *vasopressors* (Table 30.9). As reviewed above, a number of the agents that provide inotropic support at lower infusion rates via β-adrenergic stimulation, transition to providing vasopressor activity as a result of α-adrenergic agonism at escalating infusion rates. For example, titration upwards of dopamine (>10 μg/kg/min) and epinephrine (>0.3 μg/kg/min) infusion rates increase SVR. Without the concomitant increase in inotropy provided by these agents, a simple escalation in afterload will increase blood pressure, but at the expense of less stroke volume and greater ventricular work. In a similar manner, norepinephrine, which possesses predominantly α-adrenergic stimulation, also possesses β-receptor activity so that it can be effective for dopamine-resistant shock on the basis of both inotropic and vasopressor activity. As a result, dopamine and norepinephrine may have their greatest role in the maintenance of adequate perfusion pressure in children with shock.

Phenylephrine

Different from these *mixed* agonists, phenylephrine is a pure α-adenergic receptor agonist that can be effectively titrated to augment systemic afterload. Because of this property, one of its principal roles in pediatrics historically has been for reversal of *tet spells* (hypercyanotic spells) in children with tetralogy of Fallot. Infants and children with tetralogy of Fallot have a thickened infundibulum which spasms and causes right to left blood flow through the ventricular septal defect, which substantially reduces pulmonary blood flow and leads to life-threatening hypoxemia. Therapies used to treat this *spell* include oxygen and morphine to relax the infundibulum, and knee-to-chest positioning to increase afterload and help generate left to right flow across the ventricular septal defect. When these maneuvers fail, phenylephrine is implemented to increase systemic arterial vasoconstriction resulting to left to right shunting and perfusion of the lung. Because phenylephrine has no beta-adrenergic effects it does not increase heart rate and hence the heart is better able to fill.

Vasopressin

Vasopressin is being used more frequently for catecholamine-refractory shock in children [217–221]. Vasopressin is usually administered only in physiologic doses and is thought to improve blood pressure not only through interaction with the vasopressin receptor and the phospholipase C second messenger system, but also by increasing release of ACTH and subsequent cortisol release. This vasopressor should also be used with caution because it can reduce cardiac output in children with poor cardiac function. A multicenter, randomized, placebo-controlled trial in critically ill children of low-dose vasopressin (0.0005–0.002 U/kg/min) showed no benefit [222]. Aside from this clinical trial and several smaller case series, there has not been sufficient experience or clinical studies performed as of yet to fully determine the role of either low-dose, hormonal-level dosing or higher vasoconstrictive dosing of vasopressin in various forms of shock. In current clinical practice, it is most commonly instituted in catecholamine-resistant, refractory, vasodilatory shock, though earlier indications may be identified by ongoing studies.

Hydrocortisone

Clinical use of hydrocortisone in shock has also been re-examined in recent years. Centrally and peripherally-mediated adrenal insufficiency is increasingly common in the pediatric intensive care setting [223–225]. Many children are being treated for chronic illnesses with corticosteroids with subsequent pituitary-adrenal axis suppression. Many children have central nervous system anomalies and acquired illnesses. Some children have purpura fulminans and Waterhouse-Friedrichsen Syndrome [226]. Other investigators have reported reduced cytochrome P450 activity and decreased endogenous production of cortisol and aldosterone in some children. Interestingly, adrenal insufficiency can present with low cardiac output and high systemic vascular resistance or with high cardiac output and low systemic vascular resistance. The diagnosis should be considered in any child with catecholamine-resistant vasodilatory shock. The dose recommended for stress dosing of methylprednisolone is 2 mg/kg follow by the same dose over 24 h, but practice varies greatly among intensivists [227]. Central or peripheral adrenal insufficiency may be diagnosed in adequately volume resuscitated infants or children who require epinephrine or norepinephrine infusions for shock, and have a baseline cortisol level <18 mg/dL [228].

When considering the dose of hydrocortisone to be used for patients with shock it is important to understand two concepts. First, hydrocortisone must be multiplied by 6 to be glucocorticoid equivalent to methylprednisone and by 30 to be glucocorticoid equivalent to dexamethasone dosing. The use of methylprednisone at 2 mg/kg as a loading dose and then 1 mg/kg every 6 h is equivalent to 30 mg/kg of hydrocortisone in glucocorticoid equivalent dosing. The use of 0.5 mg/kg of dexamethasone every 6 h is equivalent to 60 mg/kg/day of hydrocortisone in glucocorticoid equivalent dosing. Neither methylprednisone nor dexamethasone has any mineralocorticoid effect; however, hydrocortisone has both glucocorticoid and mineralocorticoid effect. For this reason hydrocortisone is generally recommended over methylprednisone or dexamethasone for adrenal insufficiency. Second, cortisol levels differ during stress and shock so efforts to treat patients with adrenal insufficiency should be directed to achieving these levels. During surgical stress, cortisol levels increase to 30 μg/dL range. However, during acute shock cortisol levels can reach 150–300 µg/dL. Hydrocortisone infusion at 2 mg/kg/day (50 mg/m² B.S.A./day) will achieve serum cortisol levels in the range of 20–30 µg/dL, whereas infusions at 50 mg/kg/day can achieve levels of up to 150 µg/dL. Unfortunately, the majority of clinical data examining the role of corticosteroids in improving outcome in shock are derived from adult studies. Importantly, a multicenter, randomized, controlled trial of stress-dose hydrocortisone in critically ill adults with severe sepsis/septic shock failed to show any improvement in outcomes [229]. Adrenal insufficiency and its treatment is discussed in great detail elsewhere in this textbook.

Extra-Corporeal Life Support (ECLS)

In patients who remain in shock (cardiac index <2.0 L/m² B.S.A./min) despite use of the above therapies, extra-cardiac mechanical support has been associated with up to a 50 % survival in children and 80 % survival in newborns. These forms of cardiac support include the veno-arterial extracorporeal membrane oxygenation, the left ventricular assist device, and the aortic balloon counter pulsation device. ECMO is commonly used in smaller children. Veno-venous ECMO could be considered but only in the unusual occurrence when shock is due to ventilator-associated (high intrathoracic pressure) cardiac dysfunction. Veno-arterial ECMO is successful when shock is due to cardiac dysfunction. Typical criteria for this use includes a CI <2.0 L/m² B.S.A./min or the need for more than 1 µg/kg/min of epinephrine with on-going evidence of inadequate tissue perfusion. Larger children can be managed with mechanical assist devices. These modalities are discussed in greater detail elsewhere in this text.

Conclusion

Shock is a common time-sensitive cause of death in critically ill children with excellent outcome when appropriately recognized and treated. Early recognition and implementation of goal-directed therapies attains best outcomes. Therapies should be directed to timely reversal of anemia, hypoxia, ischemia, and glycopenia. Fluids and inotropes should be used to reverse hypotension and decrease capillary refill to <2 s within 1 h of clinical presentation. Adrenal shock should be recognized and treated with hydrocortisone. Long term goals after the first hour are maintenance of normal cardiac output, blood pressure, and $SVCO_2$ saturation >70 %. Appropriate glucose infusion rates should be delivered and insulin used to reverse hyperglycemia. Fluids, inotropes, vasodilators, vasopressors, hydrocortisone, thyroid, and extra-cardiac mechanical support devices may be required to accomplish this goal.

References

1. Neufeldt V, Guralnik B, editors. Webster's new world dictionary of American English. 3rd ed. New York: Simon and Schuster, Inc; 1988.
2. Manji RA, Wood KE, Kumar A. The history and evolution of circulatory shock. Crit Care Clin. 2009;25:1–29.
3. LeDran HF. A treatise, or reflections drawn from practice on gunshot wounds. London: J. Clarke & Co; 1737.
4. Mello PMVC, Sharma VK, Dellinger RP. Shock: an overview. Semin Respir Crit Care Med. 2004;25:619–28.
5. Morris EA. A practical treatise on shock after operations and injuries. London: Hardwicke; 1867.
6. Gross SG, editor. A system of surgery: pathological, diagnostic, therapeutic, and operative. Philadelphia: Lea and Febiger; 1872.
7. Warren JC. Surgical pathology and therapeutics. Philadelphia: W.B. Saunders; 1895.
8. Blalock A, editor. Principles of surgical care, shock, and other problems. St Louis: CV Mosby; 1940.
9. Wiggers CJ. Present status of shock problem. Physiol Rev. 1942;22:74–123.
10. Perkin RM, Levin DL. Shock in the pediatric patient. Part I. J Pediatr. 1982;101:163–9.
11. Perkin RM, Levin DL. Shock in the pediatric patient, part II: therapy. J Pediatr. 1982;101:319–32.
12. Baskett TF. William O'Shaughnessy, Thomas Latta, and the origins of intravenous saline. Resuscitation. 2002;55:231–4.
13. O'Shaughnessy WB. The cholera in the North of England. Lancet. 1831;1:401–4.
14. MacGillivray ND. Latta of Leith: pioneer in the treatment of cholera by intravenous saline solution. J R Coll Physicians Edinb. 2006;36:80–5.
15. Thomas NJ, Carcillo JA. Hypovolemic shock in the pediatric patient. New Horiz. 1998;6:120–9.
16. Watson RS, Carcillo JA, Linde-Zwirble WT, Clermont G, Lidicker J, Angus DC. The epidemiology of severe sepsis in children in the United States. Am J Respir Crit Care Med. 2003;167:695–701.
17. Orr RA, Kuch B, Carcillo J, Han Y. Shock is under-reported in children transported for respiratory distress: a multi-center study. Crit Care Med. 2003;31:A18 (abstract).
18. Szabo C. In: Evans TW, Fink MP, editors. Cytopathic hypoxia in circulatory shock: the role of poly (ADP-Ribose) synthetase activation. New York: Springer; 2002.
19. Fink MP. Cytopathic hypoxia. Mitochondrial dysfunction as mechanism contributing to organ dysfunction in sepsis. Crit Care Clin. 2001;17:219–37.
20. Cairns CB. Rude unhinging of the machinery of life: metabolic approaches to hemorrhagic shock. Curr Opin Crit Care. 2001;7:437–43.
21. Fahey JT, Lister G, editors. Oxygen demand, delivery, and consumption. St. Louis: Mosby, Inc.; 1998.
22. Timmins AC, Hayes M, Yau E, Watson JD, Hinds CJ. The relationship between cardiac reserve and survival in critically ill patients receiving treatment aimed at achieving supranormal oxygen delivery and consumption. Postgrad Med J. 1992;68 Suppl 2:S34–40.
23. Hayes MA, Yau EH, Timmins AC, Hinds CJ, Watson D. Response of critically ill patients to treatment aimed at achieving supranormal oxygen delivery and consumption. Relationship to outcome. Chest. 1993;103:886–95.
24. Gattinoni L, Brazzi L, Pelosi P, Latini R, Tognoni G, Pesenti A, et al. A trial of goal-oriented hemodynamic therapy in critically ill patients. SvO2 Collaborative Group. N Engl J Med. 1995;333:1025–32.
25. Velmahos GC, Demetriades D, Shoemaker WC, Chan LS, Tatevossian R, Wo CC, et al. Endpoints of resuscitation of critically injured patients: normal or supranormal? A prospective randomized trial. Ann Surg. 2000;232:409–18.

26. McKinley BA, Kozar RA, Cocanour CS, Valdivia A, Sailors RM, Ware DN, et al. Normal versus supranormal oxygen delivery goals in shock resuscitation: the response is the same. J Trauma. 2002;53:825–32.

27. Balogh Z, McKinley BA, Cocanour CS, Kozar RA, Valdivia A, Sailors RM, et al. Supranormal trauma resuscitation causes more cases of abdominal compartment syndrome. Arch Surg. 2003;138:637–43.

28. Nelson DP, Samsel RW, Wood LDH, Schumaker PT. Pathologic supply dependence of systemic and intestinal O2 uptake during endotoxemia. J Appl Physiol. 1988;64:2410–9.

29. Nelson DP, Beyer C, Samsel RW, Wood LDH, Schumaker PT. Pathologic supply dependence of O2 uptake during bacteremia in dogs. J Appl Physiol. 1987;63:1487–9.

30. Cain SM, Curtis SE. Experimental models of pathologic oxygen supply dependency. Crit Care Med. 1991;19:603–12.

31. Russell JA, Phang PT. The oxygen delivery/consumption controversy: approaches to management of the critically ill. Am J Respir Crit Care Med. 1994;149:533–7.

32. Hanique G, Dugernier T, Laterre PF, Dougnac A, Roeseler J, Reynaert MS. Significance of pathologic oxygen supply dependency in critically ill patients: comparison between measured and calculated methods. Intensive Care Med. 1994;20:12–8.

33. Steltzer H, Hiesmayr M, Mayer N, Krafft P, Hammerle AF. The relationship between oxygen delivery and uptake in the critically ill: is there a critical or optimal therapeutic value? A meta-analysis. Anaesthesia. 1994;49:229–36.

34. De Backer D, Moraine JJ, Berre J, Kahn RJ, Vincent JL. Effects of dobutamine on oxygen consumption in septic patients. Direct versus indirect indeterminations. Am J Respir Crit Care Med. 1994;150:95–100.

35. Phang PT, Cunningham KF, Ronco JJ, Wiggs BR, Russell JA. Mathematical coupling explains dependence of oxygen consumption on oxygen delivery in ARDS. Am J Respir Crit Care Med. 1994;150:318–23.

36. Yu M, Burchell S, Takiguchi SA, McNamara JJ. The relationship of oxygen consumption measured by indirect calorimetry to oxygen delivery in critically ill patients. J Trauma. 1996;41:41–50.

37. Wynn J, Cornell TT, Wong HR, Shanley TP, Wheeler DS. The host response to sepsis and developmental impact. Pediatrics. 2010;125:1031–41.

38. Wheeler DS, Zingarelli B, Wong HR. Children are not small adults. Open Inflamm. 2011;4:4–15.

39. Aneja R, Carcillo J. Differences between adult and pediatric septic shock. Minerva Anestesiol. 2011;77:986–92.

40. Wheeler DS, Basu RK. Pediatric shock: an overview. Open Pediatr Med. 2013;7:2–9.

41. Carcillo JA. Pediatric septic shock and multiple organ failure. Crit Care Clin. 2003;19:413–40.

42. Watson RS, Carcillo JA. Scope and epidemiology of pediatric sepsis. Pediatr Crit Care Med. 2005;2005:S3–5.

43. Carcillo JA, Wheeler DS, Kooy NW, Shanley TP, editors. Shock. London: Springer; 2007.

44. Hinshaw LB, Cox BG, editors. The fundamental mechanisms of shock. New York: Plenum Press; 1972.

45. Ichihashi K, Ewert P, Welmitz G, Lange P. Changes in ventricular and muscle volumes of neonates. Pediatr Int. 1999;41:8–12.

46. Joyce JJ, Dickson PI, Qi N, Noble JE, Raj JU, Baylen BG. Normal right and left ventricular mass development during early infancy. Am J Cardiol. 2004;93:797–801.

47. Marijianowski MM, van der Loos CM, Mohrschladt MF, Becker AE. The neonatal heart has a relatively high content of total collage and type I collagen, a condition that may explain the less compliant state. J Am Coll Cardiol. 1994;23:1204–8.

48. Crepaz R, Pitscheider W, Radetti G, Gentili L. Age-related variation in left ventricular myocardial contractile state expressed by the stress velocity relation. Pediatr Cardiol. 1998;19:463–7.

49. Luce WA, Hoffman TM, Bauer JA. Bench-to-bedside review: developmental influences on the mechanisms, treatment and outcomes of cardiovascular dysfunction in neonatal versus adult sepsis. Crit Care. 2007;11:228.

50. Rowland DG, Gutgesell HP. Non-invasive assessment of myocardial contractility, preload, and afterload in healthy newborn infants. Am J Cardiol. 1995;75:818–21.

51. Ceneviva G, Paschall JA, Maffei F, Carcillo JA. Hemodynamic support in fluid refractory pediatric septic shock. Pediatrics. 1998;102:e19.

52. Reynolds EM, Ryan DP, Sheridan RL, Doody DP. Left ventricular failure complicating severe pediatric burn injuries. J Pediatr Surg. 1995;30:264–70.

53. Pollack MM, Fields AI, Ruttiman UE. Distributions of cardiopulmonary variables in pediatric survivors and nonsurvivors of septic shock. Crit Care Med. 1985;13:454–9.

54. Parr GV, Blackstone EH, Kirklin JW. Cardiac performance and mortality early after intracardiac surgery in infants and young children. Circulation. 1975;51:867–74.

55. Pollack MM, Fields AI, Ruttiman UE. Sequential cardiopulmonary variables of infants and children in septic shock. Crit Care Med. 1984;12:554–9.

56. Mercier J-C, Beaufils F, Hartmann J-F, Azema D. Hemodynamic patterns of meningococcal shock in children. Crit Care Med. 1988;16:27–33.

57. Feltes TF, Pignatelli R, Kleinart S, Mariscalco MM. Quantitated left ventricular systolic mechanics in children with septic shock utilizing noninvasive wall-stress analysis. Crit Care Med. 1994;22:1647–58.

58. Brierley J, Peters MJ. Distinct hemodynamic patterns of septic shock at presentation to pediatric intensive care. Pediatrics. 2008;122:752–9.

59. Landry DW, Oliver JA. The pathogenesis of vasodilatory shock. N Engl J Med. 2001;345:588–95.

60. King CK, Glass R, Bresce JS, Duggan C. Managing acute gastroenteritis among children. MMWR Recomm Rep. 2003;52:1–16.

61. Black RE, Morris SS, Bryce J. Where and why are 10 million children dying every year? Lancet. 2003;361:2226–34.

62. Carcillo JA, Tasker RC. Fluid resuscitation of hypovolemic shock: acute medicine's great triumph for children. Intensive Care Med. 2006;32:958–61.

63. Hobson MJ, Chima RS. Pediatric hypovolemic shock. Open Pediatr Med. 2013;7 Suppl 1:10–5.

64. Hung NT. Fluid management for dengue in children. Paediatr Int Child Health. 2012;32 Suppl 1:39–42.

65. Wills BA, Nguyen MD, Ha TL, Dong TH, Tran TN, Le TT, et al. Comparison of three fluid solutions for resuscitation in dengue shock syndrome. N Engl J Med. 2005;353:877–89.

66. Duggan C, Santosham M, Glass RI. The management of acute diarrhea in children. MMWR Recomm Rep. 1992;41:1–20.

67. Fisher JD, Nelson DG, Beversdorf H, Satkowiak LJ. Clinical spectrum of shock in the pediatric emergency department. Pediatr Emerg Care. 2010;26:622–5.

68. Glass RI, Lew JF, Gangarosa RE, LeBaron CW, Ho MS. Estimates of morbidity and mortality rates for diarrheal diseases in American children. J Pediatr. 1991;118:S27–33.

69. Morgan IWM, O'Neill J,JA. Hemorrhagic and obstructive shock in pediatric patients. New Horiz. 1998;6:150–4.

70. Fraga AM, Fraga GP, Stanley C, Costantini TW, Coimbra R. Children at danger: injury fatalities among children in San Diego County. Eur J Epidemiol. 2010;25:211–7.

71. Schecter SC, Betts J, Schecter WP, Victorino GP. Pediatric penetrating trauma: the epidemic continues. J Trauma Acute Care Surg. 2012;73:721–5.

72. Anderson WA. The significance of femoral fractures in children. Ann Emerg Med. 1982;11:174–7.

73. Barlow B, Niemirska M, Gondhi R, et al. Response to injury in children with closed femur fractures. J Trauma. 1987;27:429–30.

74. Lynch JM, Gardner MJ, Gains B. Hemodynamic significance of pediatric femur fractures. J Pediatr Surg. 1996;31:1358–61.

75. Czaczkes JW. Plasma volume as an index of total fluid loss. Am J Dis Child. 1962;102:190–3.

76. Salim MA, DiSessa TG, Arheart KL, Alpert BS. Contribution of superior vena caval flow to total cardiac output in children: a doppler echocardiographic study. Circulation. 1995;92:1860–5.

77. Babyn PS, Gahunia HK, Massicote P. Pulmonary thromboembolism in children. Pediatr Radiol. 2005;35:258–74.

78. Truitt AK, Sorrells DL, Halvorson E, Starring J, Kurkchubasche AG, Tracy TFJ, et al. Pulmonary embolism: which pediatric trauma patients are at risk? J Pediatr Surg. 2005;40:124–7.

79. Dijk FN, Curtin J, Lord D, Fitzgerald DA. Pulmonary embolism in children. Paediatr Respir Rev. 2013;13:112–22.

80. Van Ommen CH, Peters M. Acute pulmonary embolism in childhood. Thromb Res. 2006;118:13–25.

81. Stein PD, Kayali F, Olson RE. Incidence of venous thromboembolism in infants and children: data from the National Hospital Discharge Survey. J Pediatr. 2004;145:563–5.

82. Chan AK, Deveber G, Monagle P, Brooker LA, Massicotte PM. Venous thrombosis in children. J Thromb Haemost. 2003;1:1443–55.

83. Shabetai R, Fowler NO, Guntheroth WG. The hemodynamics of cardiac tamponade and constrictive pericarditis. Am J Cardiol. 1970;26:480–9.

84. Reddy PS, Curtiss EI, Uretsky BF. Spectrum of hemodynamics changes in cardiac tamponade. Am J Cardiol. 1990;66:1487–91.

85. Cogswell TL, Bernath GA, Keelan J,MH, Wann LS, Klopfenstein HS. The shift in the relationship between intrapericardial fluid pressure and volume induced by acute left ventricular pressure overload during cardiac tamponade. Circulation. 1986;74:173–80.

86. Gascho JA, Martins JB, Marcus ML, Kerber RE. Effects of volume expansion and vasodilators in acute pericardial tamponade. Am J Physiol. 1981;240:H49–53.

87. Spodick DH. Current concepts: acute cardiac tamponade. N Engl J Med. 2003;349:684–90.

88. Spodick DH. In: Caturelli G, editor. Medical treatment of cardiac tamponade. Rome: TIPAR Poligrafica; 1991.

89. Hashim R, Frankel H, Tandon M, Rabinovici R. Fluid resuscitation-induced cardiac tamponade. J Trauma. 2002;53:1183–4.

90. Marino BS, Bird GL, Wernovsky G. Diagnosis and management of the newborn with suspected congenital heart disease. Clin Perinatol. 2001;28:91–136.

91. Colletti JE, Homme JL, Woodridge DP. Unsuspected neonatal killers in emergency medicine. Emerg Med Clin North Am. 2004;22:929–60.

92. Heymann MA, Clyman RI. Evaluation of alprostadil (prostaglandin E1) in the management of congenital heart disease in infancy. Pharmacotherapy. 1982;2:148–55.

93. Kramer HH, Sommer M, Rammos S, Krogmann O. Evaluation of low dose prostaglandin E1 treatment for ductus dependent congenital heart disease. Eur J Pediatr. 1995;154:700–7.

94. Luo W, Grupp IL, Harrer J. Targeted ablation of the phospholamban gene is associated with markedly enhanced myocardial contractility and loss of beta-agonist stimulation. Circ Res. 1994;75:401–9.

95. Bernardin G, Strosberg AD, Bernard A, Mattei M, Marullo S. Beta-adrenergic receptor-dependent and -independent stimulation of adenylate cyclase is impaired during severe sepsis in humans. Intensive Care Med. 1998;24:1315–22.

96. Barton P, Garcia J, Kouatli A, Kitchen L, Zorka A, Lindsay C, et al. Hemodynamic effects of i.v. milrinone lactate in pediatric patients with septic shock. A prospective, double-blinded, randomized, placebo-controlled, interventional study. Chest. 1996;109: 1302–12.

97. Rothe CF. Mean circulatory filling pressure: its meaning and measurement. J Appl Physiol. 1993;74:499–509.

98. Parkin WG. Volume state control – a new approach. Crit Care Resusc. 1999;1:311–21.

99. Peters J, Mack GW, Lister G. The importance of the peripheral circulation in critical illness. Intensive Care Med. 2001;27:1446–58.

100. Jansen JR, Maas JJ, Pinsky MR. Bedside assessment of mean systemic filling pressure. Curr Opin Crit Care. 2010;16:231–6.

101. Henderson WR, Griesdale DE, Walley KR, Sheel AW. Clinical review: Guyton – the role of mean circulatory filling pressure and right atrial pressure in controlling cardiac output. Crit Care. 2010;14:243.

102. Rivers E, Nguyen B, Havstad S, Ressler J, Muzzin A, Knoblich B, et al. Early goal-directed therapy in the treatment of severe sepsis and septic shock. N Engl J Med. 2001;345:1368–77.

103. Rivers EP, Nguyen HB, Huang DT, Donnino M. Early goal-directed therapy. Crit Care Med. 2004;32:314–5; author reply 5.

104. Rivers EP. Early goal-directed therapy in severe sepsis and septic shock: converting science to reality. Chest. 2006;129:217–8.

105. Natanson C, Danner RL. Early goal-directed therapy reduced mortality and multiorgan dysfunction in severe sepsis or septic shock. ACP J Club. 2002;136:90.

106. Nguyen HB, Corbett SW, Menes K, Cho T, Daugharthy J, Klein W, et al. Early goal-directed therapy, corticosteroid, and recombinant human activated protein C for the treatment of severe sepsis and septic shock in the emergency department. Acad Emerg Med. 2006;13:109–13.

107. Rhodes A, Bennett ED. Early goal-directed therapy: an evidence-based review. Crit Care Med. 2004;32:S448–50.

108. de Oliveira CF, de Oliveira DS, Gottschald AF, Moura JD, Costa GA, Ventura AC, et al. ACCM/PALS haemodynamic support guidelines for paediatric septic shock: an outcomes comparison with and without monitoring central venous oxygen saturation. Intensive Care Med. 2008;34:1065–75.

109. Shapiro NI, Howell MD, Talmor D, Lahey D, Ngo L, Buras J, et al. Implementation and outcomes of the Multiple Urgent Sepsis Therapies (MUST) protocol. Crit Care Med. 2006;34:1025–32.

110. Trzeciak S, Dellinger RP, Abate NL, Cowan RM, Stauss M, Kilgannon JH, et al. Translating research to clinical practice: a 1-year experience with implementing early goal-directed therapy for septic shock in the emergency department. Chest. 2006;129:225–32.

111. Kortgen A, Niederprum P, Bauer M. Implementation of an evidence-based "standard operating procedure" and outcome in septic shock. Crit Care Med. 2006;34:943–9.

112. Ferrer R, Artigas A, Levy MM, Blanco J, Gonzalex-Diaz G, Garnacho-Montero J, et al. Improvement in process of care and outcome after a multicenter severe sepsis educational program in Spain. JAMA. 2008;299:2294–303.

113. Levy MM, Artigas A, Phillips GS, Rhodes A, Beale R, Osborn T, et al. Outcomes of the surviving sepsis campaign in intensive care units in the USA and Europe: a prospective cohort study. Lancet Infect Dis. 2012;12:919–24.

114. Levy MM, Dellinger RP, Townsend SR, Linde-Zwirble WT, Marshall JC, Bion J, et al. The surviving sepsis campaign: results of an international guideline-based performance improvement program targeting severe sepsis. Crit Care Med. 2010;38:367–74.

115. Han YY, Carcillo JA, Dragotta MA, Bills DM, Watson RS, Westerman ME, et al. Early reversal of pediatric-neonatal septic shock by community physicians is associated with improved outcome. Pediatrics. 2003;112:793–9.

116. Tibby SM, Hatherill M, Murdoch IA. Capillary refill time and core-peripheral temperature gap as indicators of haemodynamic status in paediatric intensive care patients. Arch Dis Child. 1999;80:163–6.

117. Otieno H, Were E, Ahmed I, Charo E, Brent A, Maitland K. Are bedside features of shock reproducible between different observers? Arch Dis Child. 2004;89:977–9.

118. Tisherman SA, Barie P, Bokhari F, Bonadies J, Daley B, Diebel L, et al. Clinical practice guideline: endpoints of resuscitation. J Trauma. 2004;57:898–912.

119. Leonard PA, Beattie TF. Is measurement of capillary refill time useful as part of the initial assessment of children? Eur J Emerg Med. 2004;11:158–63.

120. Roland D, Clarke C, Borland ML, Pascoe EM. Does a standardised scoring system of clinical signs reduce variability between doctors' assessments of the potentially dehydrated child? J Paediatr Child Health. 2010;46:103–7.

121. Lobos AT, Lee S, Menon K. Capillary refill time and cardiac output in children undergoing cardiac catheterization. Pediatr Crit Care Med. 2012;13:136–40.

122. Gorelick MH, Shaw KN, Murphy KO. Validity and reliability of clinical signs in the diagnosis of dehydration in children. Pediatrics. 1997;99:E6.

123. Raimer PL, Han YY, Weber MS, Annich GM, Custer JR. A normal capillary refill time <2 seconds is associated with superior vena cava oxygen saturation of >70 %. J Pediatr. 2011;158:968–72.

124. Rady MY, Smithline HA, Blake H, Nowak R, Rivers E. A comparison of the shock index and conventional vital signs to identify acute, critical illness in the emergency department. Ann Emerg Med. 1994;24:685–90.

125. Rady MY, Rivers EP, Martin GB, Smithline HA, Appelton T, Nowak RM. Continuous central venous oximetry and shock index in the emergency department: use in the evaluation of clinical shock. Am J Emerg Med. 1992;10:538–41.

126. Birkhahn RH, Gaeta TJ, Terry D, Bove JJ, Tloczkowski J. Shock index in diagnosing early acute hypovolemia. Am J Emerg Med. 2005;23:323–6.

127. Rady MY, Nightingale P, Little RA, Edwards JD. Shock index: a re-evaluation in acute circulatory failure. Resuscitation. 1992;23:227–34.

128. Rappaport LD, Deakyne S, Carcillo JA, McFann K, Sills MR. Age- and sex-specific normal values for shock index in National Health and Nutrition Examination Survey 1999–2008 for ages 8 years and older. Am J Emerg Med. 2013;31:838–42.

129. Bajwa EK, Malhotra A, Thompson BT. Methods of monitoring shock. Semin Respir Crit Care Med. 2004;25:629–44.

130. Weil MH, Henning RJ. New concepts in the diagnosis and fluid treatment of circulatory shock. Anesth Analg. 1979;58:124–32.

131. Murdoch IA, Rosenthal E, Huggon IC, Coutinho W, Qureshi SA. Accuracy of central venous pressure measurements in the inferior vena cava in the ventilated child. Acta Paediatr. 1994;83:512–4.

132. Chait HI, Kuhn MA, Baum VC. Inferior vena caval pressure reliably predicts right atrial pressure in pediatric cardiac surgical patients. Crit Care Med. 1994;22:219–24.

133. Nahum E, Dagan O, Sulkes J, Schoenfeld T. A comparison between continuous central venous pressure measurement from right atrium and abdominal vena cava or common iliac vein. Intensive Care Med. 1996;22:571–4.

134. Walsh JT, Hildick-Smith DJR, Newell SA, Lowe MD, Satchithananda DK, Shapiro LM. Comparison of central venous and inferior vena caval pressures. Am J Cardiol. 2000;85:518–20.

135. Fernandez EG, Green TP, Sweeney M. Low inferior vena caval catheters for hemodynamic and pulmonary function monitoring in pediatric critical care patients. Pediatr Crit Care Med. 2004;5:14–8.

136. Marik PE, Baram M, Vahid B. Does central venous pressure predict fluid responsiveness? A systematic review of the literature and the tale of seven mares. Chest. 2008;134:172–8.

137. Marik PE, Cavallazi R. Does the central venous pressure predict fluid responsiveness? An updated meta-analysis and a plea for some common sense. Crit Care Med. 2013;41:1774–81.

138. Shah MR, Hasselblad V, Stevenson LW, Binanay C, O'Connor CM, Sopko G, et al. Impact of the pulmonary artery catheter in critically ill patients: meta-analysis of randomized clinical trials. JAMA. 2005;294:1664–70.

139. Clermont G, Kong L, Weissfeld LA, Lave JR, Rubenfeld GD, Roberts MS, et al. The effect of pulmonary artery catheter use on costs and long-term outcomes of acute lung injury. PLoS One. 2011;6:e22512.

140. Wheeler AP, Bernard GR, Thompson BT, Schoenfeld D, Wiedemann HP, de Boisblanc B, et al. Pulmonary-artery versus central venous catheter to guide treatment of acute lung injury. N Engl J Med. 2006;354:2213–24.

141. Perez AC, Eulmesekian PG, Minces PG, Schnitzler EJ. Adequate agreement between venous oxygen saturation in right atrium and pulmonary artery in critically ill children. Pediatr Crit Care Med. 2009;10:76–9.

142. Spenceley N, Skippen P, Krahn G, Kissoon N. Continuous central venous saturation monitoring in pediatrics: a case report. Pediatr Crit Care Med. 2008;9:e13–6.

143. Baulig W, Bettex D, Burki C, Schmitz A, Spielmann N, Woitzek K, et al. The PediaSat continuous central SvO2 monitoring system does not reliably indicate state or course of central venous oxygenation. Eur J Anaesthesiol. 2010;27:720–5.

144. Baulig W, Spielmann N, Zaiter H, Lijovic T, Bettex D, Burki C, et al. In-vitro evaluation of the PediaSat continuous central venous oxygenation monitoring system. Eur J Anaesthesiol. 2010;27:289–94.

145. Ranucci M, Isgro G, De La Torre T, Romitti F, De Benedetti D, Carlucci C, et al. Continuous monitoring of central venous oxygen saturation (Pediasat) in pediatric patients undergoing cardiac surgery: a validation study of a new technology. J Cardiothorac Vasc Anesth. 2008;22:847–52.

146. Kissoon N, Spenceley N, Krahn G, Milner R. Continuous central venous oxygen saturation monitoring under varying physiological conditions in an animal model. Anaesth Intensive Care. 2010;38:883–9.

147. Ginther R, Sebastian VA, Huang R, Leonard SR, Gorney R, Guleserian KJ, et al. Cerebral near-infrared spectroscopy during cardiopulmonary bypass predicts superior vena cava oxygen saturation. J Thorac Cardiovasc Surg. 2011;142:359–65.

148. Marimon GA, Dockery WK, Sheridan MJ, Agarwal S. Near-infrared spectroscopy cerebral and somatic (renal) oxygen saturation correlation to continuous venous oxygen saturation via intravenous oximetry catheter. J Crit Care. 2012;27:e13–8.

149. Ranucci M, Isgro G, De La Torre T, Romitti F, Conti D, Carlucci C. Near-infrared spectroscopy correlates with continuous superior vena cava oxygen saturation in pediatric cardiac surgery patients. Pediatr Anaesth. 2008;18:1163–9.

150. Hanson SJ, Berens RJ, Havens PL, Kim MK, Hoffman GM. Effect of volume resuscitation on regional perfusion in dehydrated pediatric patients as measured by two-site near-infrared spectroscopy. Pediatr Emerg Care. 2009;25:150–3.

151. Ghanayem NS, Wernovsky G, Hoffman GM. Near-infrared spectroscopy as a hemodynamic monitor in critical illness. Pediatr Crit Care Med. 2011;12:S27–32.

152. Hatherill M, McIntyre AG, Wattie M, Murdoch IA. Early hyperlactatemia in critically ill children. Intensive Care Med. 2000;26:314–8.

153. Ramakrishna B, Graham SM, Phiri A, Mankhambo L, Duke T. Lactate as a predictor of mortality in Malawian children with WHO-defined pneumonia. Arch Dis Child. 2012;97:336–42.

154. Scott HF, Donoghue AJ, Gaieski DF, Marchese RF, Mistry RD. The utility of early lactate testing in undifferentiated pediatric systemic inflammatory response syndrome. Acad Emerg Med. 2012;19:1276–80.

155. Shah A, Guyette F, Suffoleto B, Schultz B, Quintero J, Predis E, et al. Diagnostic accuracy of a single point-of-care prehospital serum lactate for predicting outcomes in pediatric trauma patients. Pediatr Emerg Care. 2013;29:715–9.

156. Charpie JR, Dekeon MK, Goldberg CS, Mosca RS, Bove EL, Kulik TJ. Serial blood lactate measurements predict early outcome

after neonatal repair or palliation for complex congenital heart disease. J Thorac Cardiovasc Surg. 2000;120:73–80.

157. Jones AE, Shapiro NI, Trzeciak S, Arnold RC, Claremont HA, Kline JA. Lactate clearance vs central venous oxygen saturation as goals of early sepsis therapy: a randomized clinical trial. JAMA. 2010;303:739–46.

158. Puskarich MA, Trzeciak S, Shapiro NI, Arnold RC, Heffner AC, Kline JA, et al. Prognostic value and agreement of achieving lactate clearance or central venous oxygen saturation goals during early sepsis resuscitation. Acad Emerg Med. 2012;19:252–8.

159. Napoli AM, Machan JT, Forcada A, Corl K, Gardiner F. Tissue oxygenation does not predict central venous oxygen saturation in emergency department patients with severe sepsis and septic shock. Acad Emerg Med. 2010;17:349–52.

160. Carcillo JA, Davis AL, Zaritsky A. Role of early fluid resuscitation in pediatric septic shock. JAMA. 1991;266:1242–5.

161. Investigators. TSS. A comparison of albumin and saline for fluid resuscitation in the intensive care unit. JAMA. 2004;350:2247–56.

162. Ngo NT, Cao XT, Kneen R, Willis B, Nguyen VM, Nguyen TQ, et al. Acute management of dengue shock syndrome: a randomized double-blind comparison of 4 intravenous fluid regimens in the first hour. Clin Infect Dis. 2001;32:204–13.

163. Upadhyay M, Singhi S, Murlidharan J, Kaur N, Majumdar S. Randomized evaluation of fluid resuscitation with crystalloid (saline) and colloid (polymer from degraded gelatin in saline) in pediatric septic shock. Indian Pediatr. 2005;42:223–31.

164. Akech S, Gwer S, Idro R, Fegan G, Eziefula AC, Newton CR, et al. Volume expansion with albumin compared to gelofusine in children with severe malaria: results of a controlled trial. PLoS Clin Trials. 2006;15:e21.

165. Akech S, Ledermann H, Maitland K. Choice fluids for resuscitation in children with severe infection and shock: systematic review. BMJ. 2010;341:c4416.

166. Akech SO, Jemutai J, Timbwa M, Kivaya E, Boga M, Fegan G, et al. Phase II trial on the use of Dextran 70 or starch for supportive therapy in Kenyan children with severe malaria. Crit Care Med. 2010;38:1630–6.

167. Akech SO, Karisa J, Nakamya P, Boga M, Maitland K. Phase II trial of isotonic fluid resuscitation in Kenyan children with severe malnutrition and hypovolaemia. BMC Pediatr. 2010;10:71.

168. Maitland K, Pamba A, English M, Peshu N, Marsh K, Newton C, et al. Randomized trial of volume expansion with albumin or saline in children with severe malaria: preliminary evidence of albumin benefit. Clin Infect Dis. 2005;40:538–45.

169. Maitland K, Kiguli S, Opoka RO, Engoru C, Olupot-Olupot P, Akech SO, et al. Mortality after fluid bolus in African children with severe infection. N Engl J Med. 2011;364:2483–95.

170. Maitland K, George EC, Evans JA, Kiguli S, Olupot-Olupot P, Akech SO, et al. Exploring mechanisms of excess mortality with early fluid resuscitation: insights from the FEAST trial. BMC Med. 2013;11:68.

171. Lacroix J, Hebert PC, Hutchison JS, Hume HA, Tucci M, Ducruet T, et al. Transfusion strategies for patients in pediatric intensive care units. N Engl J Med. 2007;356:1609–19.

172. Istaphanous GK, Wheeler DS, Lisco SJ, Shander A. Red blood cell transfusion in critically ill children: a narrative review. Pediatr Crit Care Med. 2011;12:174–83.

173. Crowell JW, Smith EE. Determinant of the optimal hematocrit. J Appl Physiol. 1967;22:501–4.

174. Hollenberg SM. Vasoactive drugs in circulatory shock. Am J Respir Crit Care Med. 2011;183:847–55.

175. van Swieten PA, Timmermans PBMWM. Cardiovascular alpha-2 receptors. J Mol Cell Cardiol. 1983;15:717–33.

176. Stopfkuchen H, Racke K, Schworer H, Queisser-Luft A, Vogel K. Effects of dopamine infusion on plasma catecholamines in preterm and term infants. Eur J Pediatr. 1991;150:503–6.

177. Seri I, Abassi S, Wood DC, Gerdes JS. Regional hemodynamic effects of dopamine in the sick preterm neonate. J Pediatr. 1998;133:728–34.

178. Richard C, Ricome JL, Rimailho A, Bottineau G, Auzepy P. Combined hemodynamic effects of dopamine and dobutamine in cardiogenic shock. Circulation. 1983;67:620–6.

179. Bellomo R, Chapman M, Finfer S, Hickling K, Myburgh J. Low-dose dopamine in patients with early renal dysfunction: a placebo-controlled randomised trial. Australian and New Zealand Intensive Care Society (ANZICS) Clinical Trials Group. Lancet. 2000;356:2139–43.

180. Jones D, Bellomo R. Renal-dose dopamine: from hypothesis to paradigm to dogma to myth and, finally, superstition? J Intensive Care Med. 2005;20:199–211.

181. Felmet KA, Hall MW, Clark RS, Jaffe R, Carcillo JA. Prolonged lymphopenia, lymphoid depletion, and hypoprolactinemia in children with nosocomial sepsis and multiple organ failure. J Immunol. 2005;174:3765–72.

182. Li J, Zhang G, Holtby H, Humpi T, Caldarone CA, Van Arsell GS, et al. Adverse effects of dopamine on systemic hemodynamic status and oxygen transport in neonates after the Norwood procedure. J Am Coll Cardiol. 2006;48:1859–64.

183. Sakr Y, Reinhart K, Vincent JL, Sprung CL, Moreno R, Ranieri VM, et al. Does dopamine administration in shock influence outcome? Results of the Sepsis Occurrence in Acutely Ill Patients (SOAP) study. Crit Care Med. 2006;34:589–97.

184. De Backer D, Aldecoa C, Njimi H, Vincent JL. Dopamine versus norepinephrine in the treatment of septic shock: a meta-analysis. Crit Care Med. 2012;40:725–30.

185. Ruffolo RJ. Review: the pharmacology of dobutamine. Am J Med Sci. 1987;294:244–8.

186. Perkin RM, Levin DL, Webb R, Aquino A, Reedy J. Dobutamine: a hemodynamic evaluation in children with shock. J Pediatr. 1982;100:977–83.

187. Bayram M, De Luca L, Massie MB, Gheorghiade M. Reassessment of dobutamine, dopamine, and milrinone in the management of acute heart failure syndromes. Am J Cardiol. 2005;19:47G–58.

188. Hodt A, Steine K, Atar D. Medical and ventilatory treatment of acute heart failure: new insights. Cardiology. 2006;106:1–9.

189. Mebazaa A, Gheorghiade M, Pina IL, Harjola VP, Hollenberg SM, Follath F, et al. Practical recommendations for prehospital and early in-hospital management of patients presenting with acute heart failure syndromes. Crit Care Med. 2008;36:S129–39.

190. Jefferies JL, Hoffman TM, Nelson DP. Heart failure treatment in the intensive care unit in children. Heart Fail Clin. 2010;6:531–58.

191. Coffin LHJ, Ankeney JL, Beheler EM. Experimental study and clinical use of epinephrine for treatment of low cardiac output syndrome. Circulation. 1966;33:178–85.

192. Monrad ES, McKay RG, Baim DS, Colucci WS, Fifer MA, Heller GV, et al. Improvement in indexes of diastolic performance in patients with congestive heart failure treated with milrinone. Circulation. 1984;70:1030–7.

193. Haghighi K, Gregory KN, Kranias EG. Sarcoplasmic reticulum Ca-ATPase-phospholamban interactions and dilated cardiomyopathy. Biochem Biophys Res Commun. 2004;322:1214–22.

194. Toller WG, Levosimendan SC. A new inotropic and vasodilator agent. Anesthesiology. 2006;104:556–69.

195. Turanlahti M, Boldt T, Palkama T, Antila S, Lehtonen L, Pesonen E. Pharmacokinetics of levosimendan in pediatric patients evaluated for cardiac surgery. Pediatr Crit Care Med. 2004;5:457–62.

196. Braun JP, Schneider M, Dohmen P, Dopfmer U. Successful treatment of dilative cardiomyopathy in a 12-year-old girl using the calcium sensitizer levosimendan after weaning from mechanical biventricular assist support. J Cardiothorac Vasc Anesth. 2004;18:772–4.

197. Egan JR, Clarke AJ, Williams S, Cole AD, Ayer J, Jacobe S, et al. Levosimendan for low cardiac output: a pediatric experience. J Intensive Care Med. 2006;21:183–7.

198. Namachivayam P, Crossland DS, Butt WW, Shekerdemian LS. Early experience with levosimendan in children with ventricular dysfunction. Pediatr Crit Care Med. 2006;7:445–8.

199. Momeni M, Rubay J, Matta A, Rennotte MT, Veyckemans F, Poncelet AJ, et al. Levosimendan in congenital cardiac surgery: a randomized, double-blind clinical trial. J Cardiothorac Vasc Anesth. 2011;25:419–24.

200. Suominen PK. Single-center experience with levosimendan in children undergoing cardiac surgery and in children with decompensated heart failure. BMC Anesthesiol. 2011;11:11–8.

201. Lechner E, Hofer A, Leitner-Peneder G, Freynschlag R, Mair R, Weinzettel R, et al. Levosimendan versus milrinone in neonates and infants after corrective open-heart surgery: a pilot study. Pediatr Crit Care Med. 2012;13:542–8.

202. Ebade A, Khalil MA, Mohamed AK. Levosimendan is superior to dobutamine as an inodilator in the treatment of pulmonary hypertension for children undergoing cardiac surgery. J Anesth. 2013;27:334–49.

203. Zaloga GP, Strickland RA, Butterworth JF, Mark LJ, Mills SA, Lake CR. Calcium attenuates epinephrine's beta-adrenergic effects in postoperative heart surgery patients. Circulation. 1990;81:196–200.

204. Royster RL, Butterworth JF, Prielipp RC, Robertie PG, Kon ND, Tucker WY, et al. A randomized, blinded, placebo-controlled evaluation of calcium chloride and epinephrine for inotropic support after emergence from cardiopulmonary bypass. Anesth Analg. 1992;74:3–13.

205. Murdoch IA, Qureshi SA, Huggon IC. Perioperative haemodynamic effects of an intravenous infusion of calcium chloride in children following cardiac surgery. Acta Paediatr. 1994;83:658–61.

206. Wibo M, Bravo G, Godfraind T. Postnatal maturation of excitation-contraction coupling in rate ventricle in relation to the subcellular localization and surface density of 1,4-dihydropyridine and ryanodine receptors. Circ Res. 1991;68:662–73.

207. Brillantes AM, Bezprozvannaya S, Marks AR. Developmental and tissue-specific regulation of rabbit skeletal and cardiac muscle calcium channels involved in excitation-contraction coupling. Circ Res. 1994;75:503–10.

208. Escobar AL, Ribeiro-Costa R, Villalba-Galea C, Zoghbi ME, Perez CG, Meija-Alvarez R. Developmental changes of intracellular Ca2+ transients in beating rat hearts. Am J Physiol Heart Circ Physiol. 2004;286:H971–8.

209. Huang J, Xu L, Thomas M, Whitaker K, Hove-Madsen L, Tibbits GF. L-type Ca2+ channel function and expression in neonatal rabbit ventricular myocytes. Am J Physiol Heart Circ Physiol. 2006;290:H2267–76.

210. Huang J, Hove-Madsen L, Tibbits GF. Ontogeny of the Ca2 + − induced Ca2+ release in rabbit ventricular myocytes. Am J Physiol. 2008;294:C516–25.

211. Taniguchi S, Kitamura S, Kawachi K, Doi Y, Aoyama N. Effects of hormonal supplements on the maintenance of cardiac function in potential donor patients after cerebral death. Eur J Cardiothorac Surg. 1992;6:96–102.

212. Bettendorf M, Schmidt KG, Grulich-Henn J, Ulmer HE, Heinrich UE. Tri-iodothyronine treatment in children after cardiac surgery: a double-blind, randomised, placebo-controlled study. Lancet. 2000;356:529–34.

213. Dimmick S, Badawi N, Randell T. Thyroid hormone supplementation for the prevention of morbidity and mortality in infants undergoing cardiac surgery. Cochrane Database Syst Rev. 2004;(3):CD004220

214. Howard LS, Morrell NW. New therapeutic agents for pulmonary vascular disease. Paediatr Respir Rev. 2005;6:285–91.

215. Motta P, Mossad E, Toscana D, Zestos M, Mee R. Comparison of phenoxybenzamine to sodium nitroprusside in infants undergoing surgery. J Cardiothorac Vasc Anesth. 2005;19:54–9.

216. Tweddel JS, Hoffman GM, Fedderly RT, Berger S, Thomas JPJ, Ghanayem NS, et al. Phenoxybenzamine improves systemic oxygen delivery after the Norwood procedure. Ann Thorac Surg. 1999;67:161–8.

217. Delmas A, Leone M, Rousseau S, Albanese J, Martin C. Clinical review: vasopressin and terlipressin in septic shock patients. Crit Care. 2005;9:212–22.

218. Rosenzweig EB, Starc TJ, Chen JM, Cullinane S, Timchak DM, Gersony WM, et al. Intravenous arginine-vasopressin in children with vasodilatory shock after cardiac surgery. Circulation. 1999;100:II182–6.

219. Liedl JL, Meadow W, Nachman J, Koogler T, Kahana MD. Use of vasopressin in refractory hypotension in children with vasodilatory shock: five cases and a review of the literature. Pediatr Crit Care Med. 2002;3:15–8.

220. Lechner E, Dickerson HA, Fraser CDJ, Chang AC. Vasodilatory shock after surgery for aortic valve endocarditis: use of low-dose vasopressin. Pediatr Cardiol. 2004;25:558–61.

221. Vasudevan A, Lodha R, Kabra SK. Vasopressin infusion in children with catecholamine-resistant septic shock. Acta Paediatr. 2005;94:380–3.

222. Choong K, Bohn D, Fraser DD, Gaboury I, Hutchison JS, Joffe AR, et al. Vasopressin in pediatric vasodilatory shock: a multicenter randomized controlled trial. Am J Respir Crit Care Med. 2009;180:632–9.

223. Pizarro CF, Troster EJ, Damiani D, Carcillo JA. Absolute and relative adrenal insufficiency in children with septic shock. Crit Care Med. 2005;33:855–9.

224. den Brinker M, Joosten KF, Liem O, de Jong FH, Hop WC, Hazelzet JA, et al. Adrenal insufficiency in meningococcal sepsis: bioavailable cortisol levels and impact of interleukin-6 levels and intubation with etomidate on adrenal function and mortality. J Clin Endocrinol Metab. 2005;90:5110–7.

225. Hatherill M, Tibby SM, Hilliard T, Turner C, Murdoch IA. Adrenal insufficiency in septic shock. Arch Dis Child. 1999;80:51–5.

226. Adem PV, Montgomery CP, Husain AN, Koogler TK, Arangelovich V, Humilier M, et al. Staphylococcus aureus sepsis and the Waterhouse-Friderichsen syndrome in children. N Engl J Med. 2005;353:1245–51.

227. Benken ST, Hutson TK, Gardiner RL, Wheeler DS. A single-center review of prescribing trends and outcomes of corticosteroid replacement therapy in critically ill children with septic shock. Open Crit Care Med. 2010;3:51–6.

228. Hebbar KB, Stockwell JA, Leong T, Fortenberry JD. Incidence of adrenal insufficiency and impat of corticosteroid supplementation in critically ill children with systemic inflammatory response syndrome and vasopressor-dependent shock. Crit Care Med. 2011;39:1145–50.

229. Sprung CL, Annane D, Keh D, Moreno R, Singer M, Freivogel K, et al. Hydrocortisone therapy for patients with septic shock. N Engl J Med. 2008;358:111–24.

Acute Respiratory Failure

Kyle J. Rehder, Jennifer L. Turi, and Ira M. Cheifetz

Abstract

Acute respiratory failure is a common diagnosis among critically ill children and a leading cause of morbidity, mortality, and health care expenditures in the pediatric critical care setting. This chapter examines the anatomic, developmental, and physiologic characteristics that place infants and children at risk for respiratory failure. Respiratory failure may commonly present as hypoxemia and/or hypercarbia, but may be caused by a wide array of disease processes. As such, the varied etiologies of pediatric acute respiratory failure are reviewed, including upper and lower airway obstruction, causes of hypoventilation, ventilation perfusion inequality, and diffusion impairment. The chapter concludes with a discussion of evaluation of respiratory failure and a summary of key treatment principles, including lung-protective strategies.

Keywords

Acute Respiratory Failure • Mechanical Ventilation • Hypoxemia • Hypercarbia

Introduction

Acute respiratory failure is a major cause of morbidity and mortality in the pediatric critical care setting, accounting for approximately 50 % of admissions to pediatric intensive care unit (PICUs) [1]. While the possible etiologies of respiratory failure are highly variable (ranging from infectious etiologies, such as pneumonia, sepsis, and bronchiolitis to neurologic etiologies, such as traumatic brain injury, seizures, and stroke), many of these potential causes are included within the top ten leading causes of death among children [2, 3]. For example, in infants, two common causes of acute respiratory failure – neonatal respiratory distress syndrome and sudden

K.J. Rehder, MD (✉) • J.L. Turi, MD
I.M. Cheifetz, MD, FCCM, FAARC
Division of Pediatric Critical Care Medicine,
Department of Pediatrics, Duke Children's Hospital,
DUMC 3046, Erwin Road, Durham, NC 27710, USA
e-mail: kyle.rehder@duke.edu; jennifer.turi@duke.edu;
ira.cheifetz@duke.edu

infant death syndrome – account for more than 40 % of total mortality [2].

Developmental differences in children contribute to the prevalence and severity of respiratory failure in this age group. Children have reduced elastic recoil of their alveoli, which can result in increased alveolar collapse in the presence of altered pulmonary compliance. In addition, they have fewer alveoli and less *collateral ventilation* channels (Fig. 31.1) to allow ventilation distal to an obstructed airway [4]. The chest wall of an infant has greater compliance as compared to an older child or adult due to more horizontally aligned ribs, which make it more difficult to generate a greater negative intrathoracic pressure in the presence of decreased pulmonary compliance. The relatively weak cartilaginous support of the airways in children compared to adults may lead to dynamic compression (and subsequent airway obstruction) in disease processes associated with high expiratory flow rates and increased airway resistance (e.g. asthma, bronchiolitis). Finally, the airway of a child is significantly narrower than that of an adult, which can contribute greatly to the development of increased airway resistance as well as airway obstruction due to secretions.

D.S. Wheeler et al. (eds.), *Pediatric Critical Care Medicine*,
DOI 10.1007/978-1-4471-6362-6_31, © Springer-Verlag London 2014

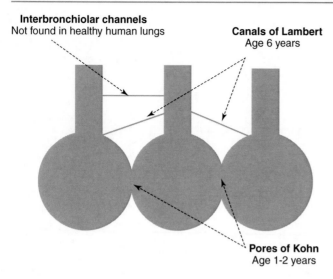

Interbronchiolar channels
Not found in healthy human lungs

Canals of Lambert
Age 6 years

Pores of Kohn
Age 1-2 years

Fig. 31.1 Collateral ventilation. The adult lung contains anatomic channels that allow for collateral ventilation distal to an obstructed airway. These channels include (1) interalveolar channels (pores of Kohn), (2) bronchiole-alveolar channels (canals of Lambert), and (3) interbronchiolar channels. The pores of Kohn appear at around 1–2 years of age, while the canals of Lambert appear at around 6 years of age. Notably, interbronchiolar channels develop pathologically and are not found in healthy human lungs in either children or adults. Infants and children are therefore at a greater risk for atelectasis and consequent ventilation-perfusion mismatch due to airway obstruction

The numerous etiologies of respiratory failure in infants and children reflect the multiple levels of involvement of the respiratory system and its integration with other organ systems. Thus, the management of acute respiratory failure in the pediatric critical care setting is a great challenge and requires a thorough understanding of the physiology and potential dysfunction of the various components of the respiratory system.

Definition

Respiratory failure is defined as an inadequate exchange of oxygen (i.e. hypoxemic respiratory failure) and carbon dioxide (i.e. hypercarbic respiratory failure) to meet the body's metabolic needs. Clinical criteria, arbitrarily set at a PaO_2 <60 mmHg and a $PaCO_2$ >50 mmHg, are not rigid parameters, but rather serve as a context in which to interpret the entire clinical scenario. Failure of the respiratory system may occur due to inadequate air movement, insufficient gas diffusion at the alveolus, and/or poor pulmonary blood flow. Maintaining adequate respiratory function requires proper functioning of the conducting airways, alveoli, pulmonary circulation, and the respiratory pump, comprised of the thorax, respiratory musculature, and nervous system. While there are clear consequences of dysfunction of each these components, each also interacts significantly with the

others. Therefore, failure of one frequently is followed by failure of another, leading to progressive hypoxemia and/or hypercarbia.

Etiologies of Respiratory Failure

Upper Airway Obstruction

As compared to adolescents and adults, infants and children are at risk for upper airway obstruction for a variety of anatomic reasons, including relatively large adenoids, tonsils, and tongues and relatively small mandibles and subglottic airways. These anatomic differences may be exaggerated by a host of genetic/congenital syndromes associated with upper airway anomalies. Upper airway obstruction is discussed in more detail elsewhere in this textbook.

One important anatomic difference between children and adults is the relative caliber of the pediatric versus adult airway. Poiseuille's law demonstrates amplified airway resistance with relatively small changes in airway diameter, such that the change in air flow is directly proportional to the airway radius elevated to the fourth power:

$$Q = \left(\Delta P \pi r^4\right)/8\eta L$$

where Q is flow, ΔP is the pressure gradient across the length of the airway, r is the radius of the airway, η is the viscosity of the air, and L is the length of the airway. Therefore, while increasing the length of the airway (L) or the viscosity of the air (η) will reduce laminar air flow, decreasing the airway radius will have a much more drastic effect. In conditions of turbulent air flow, airway resistance is inversely proportional to the airway radius to the fifth power (r^5). Hence, small amounts of edema will have a greater effect on the caliber of the pediatric airway compared to the adult airway, resulting in a greater increase in airway resistance (Fig. 31.2). This is particularly important in young children and infants, whose airways are not only naturally smaller, but who also have cone-shaped, rather than cylindrical, laryngeal anatomy [5]. This places the narrowest portion of small child's upper airway at the level of the cricoid ring, rather than at the glottis, as in adults. The susceptibility to edema of the soft tissues at the cricoid ring places these children at greater risk for upper airway obstruction secondary to infection, such as laryngotracheobronchitis (croup) [6].

Due to the higher compliance of the chest wall, children are also less equipped to compensate for the increased resistance from upper airway obstruction. Respiratory failure may occur as a result of increased work of breathing, elevated metabolic demand, and/or poor gas exchange. While respiratory failure may initially present as gradual hypoxemia or hypercarbia, it may also rapidly progress to acute respiratory collapse once respiratory muscles become overly fatigued.

| Normal | Edema | Δ diameter | Δ resistance |

Infant 4 mm 2 mm ↓50 % ↑16×

Adult 8 mm 6 mm ↓25 % ↑3×

Fig. 31.2 Age-dependent effects of a reduction in airway caliber on the airway resistance and airflow. Normal airways are represented on the left (*top*, infants; *bottom*, adults), edematous airways are represented on the right. According to Poiseuille's law, airway resistance is inversely proportional to the radius of the airway to the *fourth power* when there is laminar flow and to the *fifth power* when there is turbulent flow. One mm of circumferential edema will reduce the diameter of the airway by 2 mm, resulting in a 16-fold increase in airway resistance in the pediatric airway versus a threefold increase in the adult (cross-sectional area reduced by 75 % in the pediatric airway versus a 44 % decrease in the adult airway). Note that turbulent air flow (such as occurs during crying) in the child would increase the resistance by 32-fold

Lower Airway Obstruction

Given the extensive surface area of the numerous small peripheral airways, the upper airway provides the maximum level of resistance in adults. However, in children less than 6 years old, whose lung growth is not yet complete, resistance is greatest in the lower airways. Therefore, diseases affecting the smaller airways can significantly increase airway resistance and work of breathing.

As with upper airway obstruction, the lower airways of children are highly susceptible to slight changes in airway diameter. Therefore, children's airway resistance is easily affected by edema and bronchospasm associated with diseases such as asthma, bronchiolitis, and cystic fibrosis. Initially, the patient is unable to completely expel air, as airways can collapse from positive intrapleural pressure generated during forced expiration (Fig. 31.3). The inability to fully exhale leads to air trapping and hyperinflation of the lungs.

Hyperinflation may compromise respiratory muscle function by altering chest wall geometry. An increase in functional residual capacity (FRC) above the normally predicted value decreases elastic recoil of the chest wall and shortens muscle fiber length. At shorter muscle fiber lengths, adequate alveolar ventilation will require more energy, as each muscle contraction will generate less force [7]. Furthermore, hyperinflation flattens the diaphragm, decreasing its ability to efficiently generate pressure and facilitate thoracic expansion [8]. Hyperinflation likewise alters the spatial arrangement of the diaphragmatic muscle fibers, such that contraction of the fibers now arranged in series and perpendicular to the chest wall will result in paradoxical inward movement of the thorax [9].

Dynamic collapse of the lower airways (e.g., tracheo- and bronchomalacia) is also more common in children than

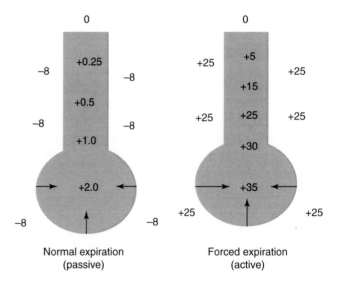

Note: Elastic recoil of alveolus is + 10 cmH$_2$O!!

Fig, 31.3 Dynamic compression in children. The cartilaginous support of the conducting airways will have spread to its most distal point, the segmental bronchus, by the 12th week of gestation. After birth, the cartilaginous support of the conducting airways increases throughout the remainder of childhood. The relative weakness of the cartilaginous support in the infant compared to the adult may lead to dynamic compression in situations associated with high expiratory flow rates and increased airway resistance (e.g., bronchiolitis, asthma, or even crying). During a forced expiration, intrapleural pressure becomes more positive with respective to atmospheric pressure. There is a point along the airway that the intrapleural pressure (pressure outside the airway) will be equal to the pressure inside the airway (i.e. transmural pressure gradient is zero). Past this point, the transmural pressure gradient becomes negative, and the airway begins to collapse

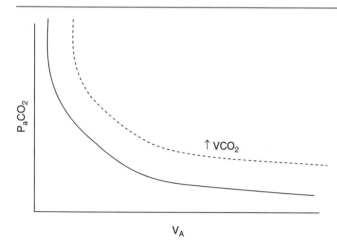

Fig. 31.4 Relationship of P_aCO_2 to alveolar ventilation (V_A). As V_A increases, P_aCO_2 decreases. As CO_2 production (VCO_2) increases, this relationship is shifted upward and to the right

adults due to the immature cartilaginous support of the airways. This typically presents as expiratory and/or inspiratory lower airways obstruction and is often exacerbated during times of illness, especially viral infections. It is important to distinguish malacia from lower airway obstruction secondary to bronchospasm, as the treatments for bronchospasm will relax airway musculature and may worsen the dynamic compression seen with malacia.

In severe cases of lower airway obstruction, functional hypoventilation and resultant hypercarbia is observed secondary to decreased expiratory air flow. The resultant hypercarbia from lower airway obstruction may be coupled with hypoxia if air flow is disrupted to a great degree, if significant atelectasis is present, or when coupled with alveolar disease (e.g., RSV bronchiolitis / pneumonitis). In the most severe of cases, the airway becomes so constricted that air flow may cease during both inspiration and expiration.

Hypoventilation

Decreased alveolar ventilation results in inadequate removal of CO_2 from the alveoli, leading to an increased alveolar carbon dioxide concentration (P_ACO_2), and subsequently, an increased arterial carbon dioxide concentration (P_aCO_2). In steady state, CO_2 elimination must be balanced by CO_2 production, such that $PaCO_2$ is directly proportional to the quantity of CO_2 produced (VCO_2) and inversely proportional to alveolar ventilation (V_A) (Fig. 31.4).

$$PaCO_2 = (VCO_2 * K) / V_A$$

While minute ventilation (V_E) is the product of tidal volume (V_t) and respiratory frequency, alveolar ventilation is determined by the difference between total minute ventilation

and the degree of both anatomic and physiologic dead space ventilation (V_D).

$$V_E = V_t * frequency$$

$$V_A = V_E - V_D$$

Therefore, CO_2 balance will be altered with changes to minute ventilation and/or alterations in the quantity of physiologic dead space.

Homeostasis of carbon dioxide balance is primarily controlled by altering minute ventilation, through changes in tidal volume and respiratory frequency. Adequate respiration requires signals from the central nervous system to be transferred via the spinal cord, peripheral nerves, and neuromuscular junction to the respiratory muscles. The action of these muscles on the chest wall generates negative intrathoracic pleural pressure to allow inspiration. Expiration then follows, using the energy stored during the preceding inspiratory phase as elastic recoil. Ventilation can become ineffective in the presence of an inadequate ventilatory drive, altered chest wall structure or muscle function, or compromised pulmonary mechanics.

Hypercarbia related to an inadequate control of the ventilatory drive can result from dysfunction centrally, at the level of the brainstem, or more peripherally at the spinal or peripheral nerve pathways. Failure of the central drive of respiration is most commonly due to sedative, narcotic, or hypnotic drugs. Less commonly, hypoventilation may result from brainstem injuries at the level of the mid-to-lower brainstem or from abnormal autonomic regulation of breathing at the level of the central nervous system with little on no response to hypercapnia [4]. The inability of a patient to effectively respond to CO_2 can be congenital, as seen in central hypoventilation syndrome or inborn errors of metabolism (e.g., pyruvate dehydrogenase deficiency), or acquired as a result of posterior fossa tumors, infection (e.g., encephalitis), or severe hypoxic-ischemic injury. Alternatively, other brain injuries or lesions, some intoxications, and hepatic encephalopathy can lead to a significantly increased respiratory drive (i.e., hyperventilation) and eventual ventilatory failure [10].

Significant hypoventilation will secondarily result in hypoxemia with decreased O_2 delivery to the alveoli given the indirect relationship of P_AO_2 to P_ACO_2 via the alveolar gas equation:

$$P_AO_2 = F_iO_2 (P_{atm} - P_{H2O}) - (P_aCO_2 / RQ)$$

where P_{atm} is the atmospheric pressure, P_{H2O} is the vapor pressure of water (usually estimated at 47 mmHg at 37°C), and RQ is the respiratory quotient (usually estimated at 0.8). In the absence of other causes, clinically significant hypoxemia (i.e. PaO_2 <60 mmHg) does not occur under normal conditions – breathing ambient air at sea level – until a P_ACO_2

greater than 72 mmHg is attained. Hypoventilation does not change the A-a gradient, and hypoxemia caused by hypoventilation can be easily corrected with supplemental O_2.

In addition to alterations in alveolar ventilation, CO_2 elimination can be greatly affected by altered dead space ventilation, characterized by the amount of ventilation that does not participate in gas exchange. Physiologic dead space is comprised of anatomic dead space – a fixed volume representing the gas volume in the conducting airways – and alveolar dead space, representing the volume of gas that reaches the alveoli but does not participate in gas exchange secondary to inadequate perfusion. The volume of physiologic dead space can be estimated by comparing the arterial pCO_2 with the end tidal pCO_2 (P_ECO_2) [4]:

$$V_D = \left(P_aCO_2 - P_ECO_2\right) * V_E / P_aCO_2$$

$$V_D / V_t = \left(P_aCO_2 - P_ECO_2\right) / P_aCO_2$$

The normal Vd/Vt ratio is <0.3 for both infants and adults. An increase in this ratio signifies an increase in dead space ventilation and will generally necessitate an increase in minute ventilation to avoid the subsequent development of hypercarbia and hypoxemia.

Respiratory Muscle Insufficiency

Effective ventilation requires that the inspiratory muscles be able to generate sufficient force to overcome the resistive and elastic loads imposed by the airways and lung parenchyma, respectively. The primary muscle of inspiration, the diaphragm, is typically involved in hypercarbia associated with disordered respiratory muscle function. Normally, contraction of the diaphragm draws air into the lungs both by its piston like caudal displacement and elevation of the lower ribs as the muscle contracts against the relatively noncompressible abdomen. In addition, the transverse diameter of the thorax can increase due to the coupling of the upper and lower ribs [11]. The diaphragm has a significant level of reserve, with only approximately 10–15 % of its motor units being active during rest [12]. This allows the diaphragm to respond to increased levels of work for prolonged periods of time.

During increased inspiratory effort, the sternocleidomastoid, scalene and intercostal muscles are recruited to augment inspiration by orienting the ribs in a more horizontal direction, thus further increasing the transverse diameter of the thorax. Both the diaphragm and accessory inspiratory muscles are less effective in children less than 2 years of age because the chest wall is more compliant and the ribs are in a more horizontal position at rest [11]. While abdominal muscles are typically considered expiratory muscles, they also serve to augment inspiration by decreasing end-expiratory lung volume below FRC to assist inspiration by the outward elastic recoil of the chest wall during the subsequent inspiration [10]. In addition, expiratory muscles may serve to elevate the diaphragm to achieve a more optimal muscle fiber length for maximal contraction [11].

Excessive work of breathing can fatigue the respiratory muscles, resulting in an inability to generate the increased pleural pressure required to maintain an adequate alveolar ventilation in the face of increased requirements [7]. Muscle fatigue occurs when the energy supply is no longer adequate to meet demand, whether because of increased demand, increased resistive forces (e.g., large airway obstruction, asthma), increased elastic loads (e.g., edema), or decreased energy supply. Blood flow to the diaphragm and other inspiratory muscles is determined by cardiac output, perfusion pressure, oxygen carrying capacity of the blood, and the ability of the muscles to increase perfusion in response to increased demand. Decreased blood flow to these muscles will decrease substrate delivery.

With increased activity, the diaphragm requires approximately 10–20 times greater oxygen delivery to meet its metabolic demands [13, 14]. Factors that impair oxygen delivery to the muscles, such as hypoxemia, anemia or decreased cardiac output, can increase the onset of fatigue [15]. Ventilatory muscle function can likewise be affected by metabolic and nutritional disturbances. Decreased levels of potassium, phosphorous, magnesium, or calcium can result in decreased muscle strength [10], while malnutrition can markedly reduce the strength and endurance of respiratory muscles [16]. Similarly, a number of drugs that are capable of altering metabolism can impair muscle function. These include aminoglycosides and calcium-channel blockers that can interfere with neuromuscular transmission and corticosteroids that may promote muscle atrophy [17].

Muscle weakness, or the fixed inability to generate an adequate inspiratory force, is determined by the adequacy of neuronal drive, innervation, neuromuscular transmission and fiber type distribution as well as length-tension and force-velocity relationships [10]. Given the reduction in force generated by a weak muscle, it will require more energy to perform a given amount of work [9]. Once respiratory muscle strength is below 50 % of its predicted value, ventilator pump failure is likely to occur, with the severity of CO_2 retention proportionate to the degree of weakness [18]. Respiratory muscles are susceptible to weakness from disseminating neuromuscular disorders, spinal cord injuries, muscular dystrophies, Guillain-Barre, and myasthenia gravis [19]. Other factors that decrease the ability of a muscle to generate maximal force, such as atrophy, immaturity, or disease, predispose the muscle to developing fatigue.

Elevated airway resistance or reduced compliance of the respiratory system will increase respiratory work load and can greatly contribute to ventilatory failure either alone or in conjunction with other factors. In the absence of a disorder of the central drive for respiration, ventilatory failure can be seen as an imbalance between respiratory work load and ventilatory strength and endurance. While the presence of depressed respiratory drive, flail chest, or neuromuscular disease may precipitate hypercarbia, more frequently, they exacerbate hypercarbia in the presence of poor pulmonary compliance or increased airway resistance. Gas exchange can also be adversely affected by non-pulmonary factors, leading to increased respiratory workload. Decreased cardiac output, increased oxygen extraction, and/or abnormal hemoglobin will each negatively impact mixed venous saturations and may drastically increase the respiratory effort needed to maintain adequate gas exchange.

Ventilation/Perfusion (V/Q) Inequality

The most common etiology for hypoxemia in the pediatric critical care setting is the unequal matching of alveolar ventilation to capillary perfusion (Fig. 31.5a–d). When ventilation and perfusion are unequally distributed, the lung cannot transfer oxygen and carbon dioxide as effectively. Resultant hypercarbia may follow hypoxemia, but as CO_2 diffuses approximately 20 times more readily than O_2 across aqueous tissues, hypercarbia will not appear until significant inequality is present.

The efficiency of alveolar ventilation depends on the regional distribution of the inhaled gas as determined by gravitational factors and the compliance and resistance of the lung unit. The effect of gravity on the thorax creates an intrapleural pressure gradient that distributes gas to the alveoli heterogeneously. Thus, the greater gravitational pressure at the base of the lung generates less intrapleural pressure and so expands these alveoli less. This creates a seeming paradox in the normal lung, where lower volume alveoli have greater compliance and are more easily inflated then higher volume alveoli because they are situated on the steeper segment of the pressure-volume curve (Fig. 31.6) [20]. Increased ventilation in the dependent lung regions follows.

Both perfusion and ventilation of the lung increase significantly from the apex to the base, though perfusion increases at a far more rapid rate due to the relative increased density of blood compared to air [20]. Therefore, while the average ventilation/perfusion ratio is equal throughout the entire lung, there is greater ventilation to perfusion at the apex; while at the base, blood flow is in excess of ventilation (Fig. 31.7). This unequal matching of ventilation and perfusion results in the development of an alveolar-arterial PO_2 difference (A-aO_2) with a normal A-a gradient of approximately 5 mmHg in a young adult.

In the presence of alveolar disease, edema and inflammation worsen compliance and exaggerate the intrapleural pressure gradient. As intrapleural pressure exceeds alveolar pressure, atelectasis or closure of lung units in dependent lung regions will occur during a portion of tidal ventilation. This inverts the normal distribution of ventilation causing the apex of the lung to receive improved ventilation. While there are significant changes in the distribution of alveolar ventilation, perfusion is less affected. Perfusion continues to be greatest at the base of the lungs, such that poorly ventilated lung units continue to be perfused. Well oxygenated blood from regions of high V/Q mix with poorly oxygenated blood from regions of low V/Q resulting in an increased A-a gradient.

In children less than 6 years of age, the reduced elastic recoil of the lungs frequently lowers functional residual capacity (FRC) below the closing volume of the alveoli. Therefore, dependent lung regions may close during exhalation, and non-dependent regions will be preferentially ventilated [21]. Inhomogeneous ventilation increases as pulmonary compliance worsens and the portions of lung below the closing volume increases. Alveolar ventilation may be further altered by increased airway resistance as seen in croup, bronchiolitis and asthma.

Despite the smaller lung size in children, pulmonary arterial pressure is very similar to that of adults. This allows the pressure in the pulmonary capillaries to remain greater than alveolar pressure more consistently, resulting in more continuous perfusion of the entire lung. Subsequently, in the child with normal lungs, there is less V/Q inequality.

In a spontaneously breathing patient, a normal $PaCO_2$ can frequently be maintained at the expense of increased ventilation. The elevated CO_2 from lower V/Q units will stimulate increased alveolar ventilation, so that the $PaCO_2$ does not rise. If alveolar ventilation cannot increase secondary to muscle weakness, lung disease, or increased sedation, then V/Q inequality will also result in an elevated $PaCO_2$.

Breathing 100 % oxygen ($F_iO_2 = 1.0$) will correct hypoxemia due solely to V/Q inequality, by replacing alveolar nitrogen with O_2 and, thus, increasing P_AO_2. The alveolar gas equation can generally be used to quantify the degree of hypoxemia attributable to V/Q inequality versus shunt, however, reabsorption atelectasis of partially obstructed low V/Q units can convert these areas to an intrapulmonary shunt and introduce inaccuracy into the calculation.

The development of an A-a gradient can be lessened by effective hypoxic pulmonary vasoconstriction (HPV) in which pulmonary vessels constrict in response to the presence of regional alveolar hypoxia. HPV is strongest and can create the greatest diversion of blood flow when the hypoxic region of lung is small [22]. HPV is stimulated by a low P_AO_2 [23] with its site of action primarily at the small pulmonary arteries and veins [24]. A low mixed venous saturation can significantly limit the effectiveness of regional HPV, as a decrease in the P_AO_2 due to the lower SvO_2 may decrease perfusion to well ventilated lung regions and result in inappropriate shunting of blood to more poorly ventilated

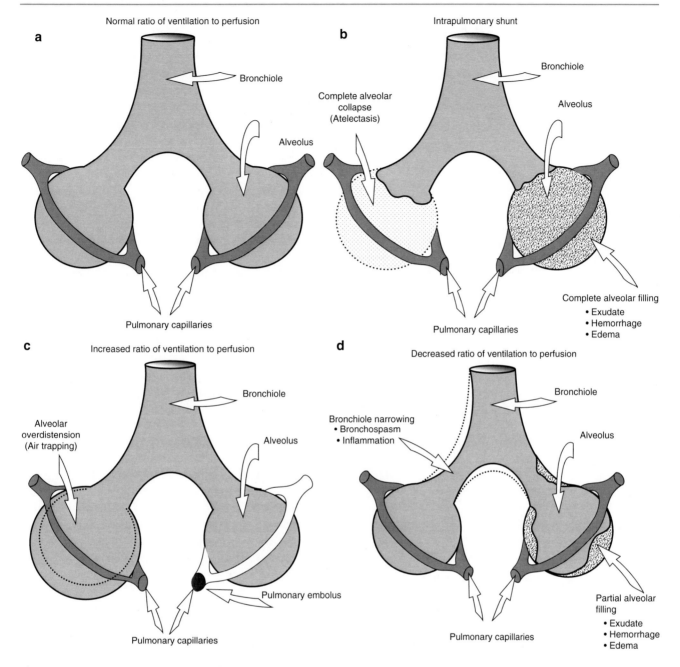

Fig. 31.5 Ventilation-perfusion inequality. (**a**) Normal. (**b**) Intrapulmonary shunt. (**c**) Increased ventilation-perfusion ratio. (**d**) Decreased ventilation-perfusion ratio (Courtesy of Neil W. Kooy, MD)

segments [25]. The effectiveness of HPV can be generally restored by augmenting cardiac output, and subsequently increasing the mixed venous saturation.

Shunting

Shunting results from deoxygenated blood entering the arterial system without first passing through ventilated regions of lung. Two types of shunt exist: (i) anatomic or fixed shunts

and (ii) intrapulmonary or true shunts. Anatomic shunts occur when systemic venous blood enters the left ventricle without having entered the pulmonary circulation. In a normal, healthy child, about 2–5 % of the total cardiac output represents a "normal" anatomic shunt (i.e., venous blood from the bronchial veins, the besian veins, anterior cardiac veins, and pleural veins directly enter the left-sided circulation). Anatomic shunts also include intracardiac shunts associated with congenital heart lesions. Conversely, intrapulmonary shunting (true shunts) can occur via either extra-alveolar

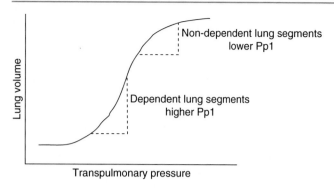

Fig. 31.6 Differential ventilation of dependent vs. non-dependent lung regions. During spontaneous ventilation, a greater proportion of inhaled gas is directed to the dependent regions of the lung. Gravitational forces create a less negative subatmospheric intrapleural pressure (Ppl) at the base compared to the apex of the lung. Alveolar pressure remains the same, so the transmural distending pressure (PA-Ppl) is reduced in the dependent lung segments

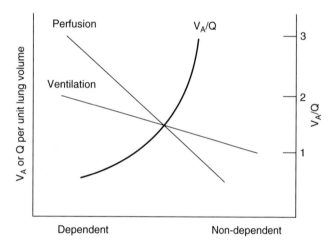

Fig. 31.7 Differential distribution of ventilation (V_A), perfusion (Q), and ventilation-perfusion ratio in the lung. The dependent lung regions preferentially receive better ventilation and perfusion compared to the non-dependent lung regions. However, the perfusion gradient is much steeper than the ventilation gradient, such that the ventilation-perfusion ratio is higher in the non-dependent (*apex*) regions compared to the dependent (*base*) regions (Adapted from West [44]. With permission from John Wiley & Sons, Inc.)

arteriovenous connections or, more typically, via capillaries perfusing alveoli that receive no ventilation. The degree of desaturation will be determined by the relative proportion of shunted versus unshunted blood. This shunted blood, or venous admixture, can be calculated as the amount of blood that would need to mix with arterial blood to account for the A-a gradient.

Measurement of the shunt fraction can be made when a patient is breathing 100 % oxygen. While this will not define the anatomic pathway of the shunt, it can be used as a useful marker to follow the efficacy of gas exchange.

$$Q_S / Q_T = (c_c - c_a)/(c_c - c_v)$$

Q_S is equal to shunt flow, Q_T is equal to total pulmonary blood flow, and c_c, c_a, and c_v represent the end capillaries, arteries and mixed venous O_2 content, respectively. The O_2 content can be calculated from pO_2 and hemoglobin saturation; arterial and mixed venous pO_2 are measured directly, while end capillary pO_2 is assumed to be equal to alveolar pO_2 calculated by the alveolar gas equation. Normally, there is less than 5 % shunt representing the admixture from the bronchial veins which supply the lungs. Supplemental O_2 will have minimal effect on the degree of hypoxemia secondary to shunting, because the red blood cells passing through the lungs are already near maximally saturated (approximately 97 %), and the supplemental O_2 never reaches the blood that bypasses non-ventilated regions of the lung.

Diffusion Impairment

Similar to V/Q inequality, alterations in diffusion capacity typically will present as hypoxemia, due to CO_2 diffusing more readily than O_2 through tissues. Diffusion impairment results in inequality of PO_2 between the alveolar gas and capillary blood gas. This can occur secondary to a thickening of the blood-gas barrier or decreased alveolar capillary volume due to lung injury or destruction. In practice, however, it is difficult to determine the degree to which hypoxemia is due to diffusion impairment rather than to V/Q inequality as the two often occur together. The rate of diffusion as determined by Fick's Law (below) is dependent on the thickness and area of the alveolar membrane and the difference in partial pressure of gas between the alveolus and the blood:

$$\text{Fick's Law of Diffusion}: V_{gas} = A * D * (P1 - P2)/T$$

where V_{gas} is the volume of air diffusing through the alveolar-capillary membrane per time, A is the surface area available for diffusion, D is the diffusion coefficient, T is the thickness of the alveolar-capillary membrane (or diffusion distance), and (P1-P2) is the partial pressure difference between the alveolus and the blood. Therefore, hypoxemia will ensue in disease processes where the alveolar membrane is thickened or the area is reduced (e.g., severe lung fibrosis), where transit time through the alveolar capillaries is increased (e.g., hyperdynamic circulation), or where the P_AO_2 is decreased because of low V/Q matching, low FiO_2, or low P_AO_2 secondary to high altitude. While limitation to diffusion is rarely thought to be the primary cause of hypoxemia, even in the case of pulmonary edema or fibrosis, it can significantly worsen hypoxemia due to V/Q mismatch or shunt. Supplemental

O_2 will increase the gradient between the alveolus and the capillary blood and, therefore, improve hypoxemia secondary to impairments in diffusion.

Evaluation of Respiratory Failure

The development of respiratory failure is often preceded by a period of increased work of breathing to compensate for worsening gas exchange. While the clinical signs of impending respiratory failure can be fairly nonspecific, recognizing these signs can provide an opportunity to anticipate and intervene before true respiratory failure develops. Tachypnea is typically the first manifestation of respiratory distress, particularly in infants, and is an attempt to minimize the work load of the muscles. While tachypnea is a sensitive sign of failure of gas exchange and the ventilatory pump, it is not specific and can be present in a number of other conditions. However, when combined with other signs of increased work of breathing or abnormal breathing patterns, it may signify impending respiratory failure. These signs include the presence of nasal flaring and the use of accessory muscles, especially the sternocleidomastoids. The presence of paradoxical abdominal movements may also indicate weakness or fatigue of the diaphragm. A prolonged expiratory phase and prominent use of abdominal muscles can indicate severe expiratory flow limitations as seen with asthma or airway obstruction. Expiratory grunting, caused by premature closure of the glottis during active exhalation, is an attempt to maintain or increase functional residual capacity and lessen atelectasis. Finally, cyanosis, while a major sign of hypoxemia, can be a late finding. The development of cyanosis requires at least 5 g /dL of deoxygenated hemoglobin. Therefore, a greater degree of desaturation is required for the development of cyanosis in an anemic patient. While clinical judgment is of primary importance in assessing the patient for impending respiratory failure, arterial blood gas measurements can also provide significant information in the diagnosis of respiratory failure and in monitoring the response to therapy.

Oxygenation

The most sensitive measure of the failure of gas exchange is the A-a gradient. This difference between the P_AO_2 and the P_aO_2 can help interpret the decrease in arterial oxygen tension. The P_AO_2 is calculated using the alveolar gas equation:

$$P_AO_2 = F_iO_2 \left(P_{atm} - P_{H2O} \right) - \left(P_aCO_2 / RQ \right)$$

The A-a gradient is then calculated by subtracting the measured P_aO_2 from the calculated P_AO_2. The normal A-a gradient in the supine position will increase with age [26] and can be calculated by

$$\text{Normal A} - \text{a gradient} = 2.5 + \left[0.21 * \text{age} \left(\text{years} \right) \right]$$

The presence of a decreased PaO_2 with an increased A-a gradient suggests the presence of V/Q mismatch, right to left shunt, and/or diffusion abnormality. Conversely, a decreased PaO_2 with a normal A-a gradient suggests hypoventilation as the etiology for the hypoxemia.

Carbon Dioxide Retention

Normal $PaCO_2$ is between 37 and 42 mmHg and is directly proportional to the amount of CO_2 produced and inversely proportional to that eliminated. To appropriately manage ventilatory failure, it is necessary to determine whether the CO_2 retention (respiratory acidosis) is acute or chronic. In the acute setting, pH will change by approximately 0.08 for every 10 mmHg change in pCO_2 from 40. As the renal tubules will conserve HCO_3^- during persistent acidosis, the chronicity of respiratory acidosis will be evident by the metabolic compensation, such that pH may only change by as little as 0.03 for every 10 mmHg chronic change in PCO_2 from 40. The presence of chronic respiratory failure with superimposed acute decompensation will present with an intermediate change in pH. A more severe lowering in pH suggests a combined metabolic acidosis. Conversely, patients may compensate for metabolic acidosis by decreasing their $PaCO_2$ [10].

Treatment of Respiratory Failure

Resuscitation of a patient with impending respiratory failure should initially include the administration of supplemental oxygen and an evaluation for airway patency. The airway should be cleared of secretions or mechanical obstruction and the head maintained in a neutral sniffing position. The use of an artificial oral or nasal airway can also be helpful to maintain patency of the airway. If, despite these interventions, the patient manifests severe hypoxemia, increasing hypercarbia with the development of significant acidosis, or develops the need for airway protection, mechanical ventilation is indicated. The need for mechanical ventilation must also be based on the clinical scenario, the rate of clinical deterioration, and the patient's response to therapy. The decision should be weighed keeping in mind the risks and benefits of tracheal intubation and mechanical ventilation [27]. Similarly, the presence of preexisting respiratory disease may result in an inability to compensate and the need for earlier tracheal intubation.

Mechanical ventilation provides a means of supporting the respiratory system rather than a therapeutic modality. As such, the primary goal of mechanical ventilation is to assure adequate oxygen delivery by adequately maintaining alveolar ventilation, maximizing V/Q matching, and optimizing patient work of breathing [28]. An additional important objective is to avoid the development of ventilator induced lung injury (VILI). VILI can be caused by several mechanisms, including oxygen toxicity, lung overdistension (i.e., volutrauma), excessive airway pressures (i.e., barotrauma), and *shear* injury to the alveoli (i.e., atelectrauma) caused by repeatedly opening collapsed lung regions; each of which serve to further exacerbate inflammation [29–31]. The attempt to achieve these two goals of treatment have led to the development of lung protective ventilation strategies [3, 32, 33], with goals of achieving adequate levels of oxygenation using a FiO_2 less than approximately 0.60, low peak inspiratory pressures, and small tidal volumes.

The profound hypoxemia seen in acute respiratory distress syndrome (ARDS) and other disorders manifested by V/Q mismatch and intrapulmonary shunting can be, at least partially, alleviated by re-recruiting and stabilizing nonventilated alveoli. Positive-end expiratory pressure (PEEP) can stabilize alveoli and decrease both V/Q mismatch and shunt, as well as prevent alveolar shear injury. However, high levels of PEEP may overdistend recruited alveoli and interfere with cardiac output by impeding systemic venous return [34].

The recognition that excessive distending pressure can cause significant ventilator induced injury, or volutrauma, has led to a decrease in set tidal volumes from the previously accepted use of tidal volumes of 10–15 mL/kg to generally less than 10 mL/kg in most populations and approximately 6 mL/kg in those patients with acute lung injury / ARDS [35, 36]. Acute lung injury is typically a heterogeneous process, and the use of larger tidal volumes results in overdistension of more compliant lung units and, therefore, greater injury to previously healthier lung. Use of lower tidal volumes result in significantly less overdistension and resultant volutrauma [36]. The low tidal volume study published by the ARDS Network in 2000 demonstrated a significant reduction in mortality in adults with acute lung injury ventilated with lower tidal volumes (6 mL/kg) when plateau pressures were limited to 30 cmH_2O or less [36].

The pressure-volume curve can be used to more effectively guide the application of PEEP and peak inspiratory pressure (PIP). The addition of PEEP can be used to improve compliance of the respiratory system above the lower inflection point on the pressure volume curve (Fig. 31.8). It should be noted that the lower inflection point on a dynamic pressure-volume loop will often overestimate the required PEEP because of the confounding variable of inspiratory flow. PIP can then be set to maintain inspiratory pressure below the upper inflection point. Beyond the upper inflection

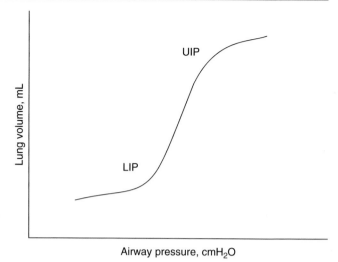

Fig. 31.8 Lung pressure-volume curve in a child with acute respiratory failure (*UIP* upper inflection point, *LIP* lower inflection point)

point, compliance again worsens as there is minimal increase in tidal volume for the increased pressure. The attempt to maintain tidal volumes of approximately 6 ml/kg and peak inspiratory pressures less than 30 cmH_2O may precipitate the development of hypercarbia and subsequent respiratory acidosis. This state of *permissive hypercapnia*, in which the $PaCO_2$ may be in excess of 60–80 Torr with pH less than 7.30, is well tolerated by most patients, and attenuates the inflammatory response, resulting in further lung protection [29, 37–39].

In summary, mechanical ventilation for respiratory failure should optimize alveolar ventilation, maximize V/Q matching, and improve patient work of breathing while reducing the risk of developing ventilator induced lung injury. This can typically be achieved by maintaining the FiO_2 less than 0.60, using an optimal level of PEEP to recruit and stabilize alveoli without causing overdistension or hemodynamic compromise, and setting low tidal volumes while maintaining the peak inspiratory pressure less than 30 cmH_2O. Inability to achieve these parameters using conventional mechanical ventilation, suggests the potential need for other modalities of support and alternative management strategies, which may include high-frequency oscillatory ventilation, high-frequency jet ventilation, and/or extracorporeal membrane oxygenation as discussed elsewhere in this textbook [40–43].

References

1. Farias JA, et al. Mechanical ventilation in pediatric intensive care units during the season for acute lower respiratory infection. A multicenter study. Pediatr Crit Care Med. 2012;13:158–64.
2. Hoyert DL, et al. Deaths: preliminary data for 2003. Natl Vital Stat Rep. 2005;53(15):1–48.

3. Dahlem P, van Aalderen WM, Bos AP. Pediatric acute lung injury. Paediatr Respir Rev. 2007;8(4):348–62.

4. Rogers MC, Nichols DG. Textbook of pediatric intensive care. 3rd ed. Baltimore: Williams & Wilkins; 1996. xviii, 1710 p.

5. Cote CJ, Todres ID, et al. A practice of anesthesia for infants and children. 3rd ed. Philadelphia: W.B. Saunders Company; 2001.

6. Leung AK, Kellner JD, Johnson DW. Viral croup: a current perspective. J Pediatr Health Care. 2004;18(6):297–301.

7. Roussos C, Macklem PT. The respiratory muscles. N Engl J Med. 1982;307(13):786–97.

8. Tobin MJ. Respiratory muscles in disease. Clin Chest Med. 1988;9(2):263–86.

9. Roussos C, Koutsoukou A. Respiratory failure. Eur Respir J Suppl. 2003;47:3s–14.

10. Tobin MJ. Principles and practice of mechanical ventilation. New York: McGraw-Hill, Inc; 1994. xv, 1300 p.

11. Taussig LM, Landau LI. Pediatric respiratory medicine. St. Louis: Mosby; 1999. xxiv, 1296 p.

12. Sieck GC, Fournier M. Diaphragm motor unit recruitment during ventilatory and nonventilatory behaviors. J Appl Physiol. 1989; 66(6):2539–45.

13. Robertson Jr CH, Foster GH, Johnson Jr RL. The relationship of respiratory failure to the oxygen consumption of, lactate production by, and distribution of blood flow among respiratory muscles during increasing inspiratory resistance. J Clin Invest. 1977;59(1): 31–42.

14. Rochester DF, Bettini G. Diaphragmatic blood flow and energy expenditure in the dog. Effects of inspiratory airflow resistance and hypercapnia. J Clin Invest. 1976;57(3):661–72.

15. Aubier M, et al. Respiratory muscle contribution to lactic acidosis in low cardiac output. Am Rev Respir Dis. 1982;126(4):648–52.

16. Sieck GC, Lewis MI, Blanco CE. Effects of undernutrition on diaphragm fiber size, SDH activity, and fatigue resistance. J Appl Physiol. 1989;66(5):2196–205.

17. Laghi F, Tobin MJ. Disorders of the respiratory muscles. Am J Respir Crit Care Med. 2003;168(1):10–48.

18. Braun NM, Arora NS, Rochester DF. Respiratory muscle and pulmonary function in polymyositis and other proximal myopathies. Thorax. 1983;38(8):616–23.

19. Mehta S. Neuromuscular disease causing acute respiratory failure. Respir Care. 2006;51(9):1016–21; discussion 1021–3.

20. West JB. Respiratory physiology: the essentials. 6th ed. Philadelphia: Lippincott Williams & Wilkins; 2000. p. 171.

21. Mansell A, Bryan C, Levison H. Airway closure in children. J Appl Physiol. 1972;33(6):711–4.

22. Marshall BE, et al. Hypoxic pulmonary vasoconstriction in dogs: effects of lung segment size and oxygen tension. J Appl Physiol. 1981;51(6):1543–51.

23. Scarpelli EM. Pulmonary physiology: fetus, newborn, child, and adolescent. 2nd ed. Philadelphia: Lea & Febiger; 1990. xi, 500 p.

24. Voelkel NF. Mechanisms of hypoxic pulmonary vasoconstriction. Am Rev Respir Dis. 1986;133(6):1186–95.

25. Benumof JL, et al. Interaction of PVO2 with PAO2 on hypoxic pulmonary vasoconstriction. J Appl Physiol. 1981;51(4):871–4.

26. Bates DV, Christie RV, Macklem PT. Respiratory function in disease; an introduction to the integrated study of the lung [by] David V. Bates, Peter T. Macklem [and] Ronald V. Christie. 2nd ed. Philadelphia: W.B. Saunders; 1971. xxi, 584 p.

27. Flori HR, et al. Pediatric acute lung injury: prospective evaluation of risk factors associated with mortality. Am J Respir Crit Care Med. 2005;171(9):995–1001.

28. Mesiano G, Davis GM. Ventilatory strategies in the neonatal and paediatric intensive care units. Paediatr Respir Rev. 2008;9(4):281–8; quiz 288–9.

29. Peltekova V, et al. Hypercapnic acidosis in ventilator-induced lung injury. Intensive Care Med. 2010;36(5):869–78.

30. Rimensberger PC. Mechanical ventilation in paediatric intensive care. Ann Fr Anesth Reanim. 2009;28(7–8):682–4.

31. Rotta AT, Steinhorn DM. Conventional mechanical ventilation in pediatrics. J Pediatr (Rio J). 2007;83(2 Suppl):S100–8.

32. Prodhan P, Noviski N. Pediatric acute hypoxemic respiratory failure: management of oxygenation. J Intensive Care Med. 2004; 19(3):140–53.

33. Turner DA, Arnold JH. Insights in pediatric ventilation: timing of intubation, ventilatory strategies, and weaning. Curr Opin Crit Care. 2007;13(1):57–63.

34. Cheifetz IM, et al. Increasing tidal volumes and pulmonary overdistention adversely affect pulmonary vascular mechanics and cardiac output in a pediatric swine model. Crit Care Med. 1998;26(4):710–6.

35. Gajic O, et al. Ventilator-associated lung injury in patients without acute lung injury at the onset of mechanical ventilation. Crit Care Med. 2004;32(9):1817–24.

36. Ventilation with lower tidal volumes as compared with traditional tidal volumes for acute lung injury and the acute respiratory distress syndrome. The Acute Respiratory Distress Syndrome Network. N Engl J Med. 2000;342(18):1301–8.

37. Bidani A, et al. Permissive hypercapnia in acute respiratory failure. JAMA. 1994;272(12):957–62.

38. Laffey JG, et al. Permissive hypercapnia–role in protective lung ventilatory strategies. Intensive Care Med. 2004;30(3):347–56.

39. Rotta AT, Steinhorn DM. Is permissive hypercapnia a beneficial strategy for pediatric acute lung injury? Respir Care Clin N Am. 2006;12(3):371–87.

40. Randolph AG. Management of acute lung injury and acute respiratory distress syndrome in children. Crit Care Med. 2009;37(8): 2448–54.

41. Wunsch H, Mapstone J, Takala J. High-frequency ventilation versus conventional ventilation for the treatment of acute lung injury and acute respiratory distress syndrome: a systematic review and cochrane analysis. Anesth Analg. 2005;100(6):1765–72.

42. Hansell DR. Extracorporeal membrane oxygenation for perinatal and pediatric patients. Respir Care. 2003;48(4):352–62; discussion 363–6.

43. Zabrocki LA, et al. Extracorporeal membrane oxygenation for pediatric respiratory failure: survival and predictors of mortality. Crit Care Med. 2011;39(2):364–70.

44. West JB. Ventilation/blood flow and gas exchange. 3rd ed. Oxford: Blackwell; 1977. p. 33–52.

The Multiply Injured Child

32

Gad Bar-Joseph, Amir Hadash, Anat Ilivitzki,
and Hany Bahouth

Abstract

Multiple trauma (MT) is an injury to more than one body system or at least two serious injuries to one body system. In the developed world, trauma is the leading cause of death and acquired disability in the 1–45 years age groups with staggering burden of medical and societal costs. Moreover, more than 95 % of pediatric injury deaths occur in the developing world, where the magnitude of trauma toll is increasing with the trends of expanding urbanization and motorization.

MT is a "systemic" disease, and is best approached according to the "two-hits hypothesis": The initial injury causes organ and tissue damage (first hits), that activate the neuroendocrine and metabolic stress response and the systemic inflammatory response (SIRS), causing 'second hits' such as respiratory distress syndrome, reperfusion injury, compartment syndromes and infections. Exogenous 'second hits' include surgical interventions, hypothermia, massive transfusions, inadequate or delayed surgical or intensive care interventions and line infections. Thus, MT increases the probability of secondary damage – especially to the brain. MT complicates the clinical course and the patient's management, makes clinical decision making far more complicated and requires different priority setting.

Management issues discussed in this chapter include pertinent aspects of pre-hospital, emergency room and intensive care evaluation and treatment, imaging of the multiply injured child, the pivotal role of the intensivist in the ICU care, approach to the bleeding patient with hypothermia and acidosis ("Triad of Death"), the damage control paradigm, and management of the multiply injured child with abdominal and chest trauma.

Keywords

Multiple trauma • Polytrauma • Children • Triad of death • Damage control surgery • Abdominal trauma • Chest trauma

G. Bar-Joseph, MD (✉)
Department of Pediatrics,
Bruce Rappaprot Faculty of Medicine,
Technion, Israel Institute of Technology,
Haifa, Israel

Pediatric Intensive Care, Meyer Children's Hospital,
Rambam Medical Center, Haifa, Israel
e-mail: g_barjoseph@rambam.health.gov.il

A. Hadash, MD
Pediatric Intensive Care, Meyer Children's Hospital,
Rambam Medical Center, Haifa, Israel
e-mail: a_hadash@rambam.health.gov.il

A. Ilivitzki, MD
Bruce Rappaprot Faculty of Medicine,
Technion, Israel Institute of Technology, Haifa, Israel

Department of Diagnostic Imaging, Pediatric Radiology,
Rambam Medical Center, Haifa, Israel
e-mail: a_ilivitzki@rambam.health.gov.il

H. Bahouth, MD
Bruce Rappaprot Faculty of Medicine, Technion Institute
of Technology, Trauma and Emergency Surgery, Haifa, Israel

Department of General Surgery, Rambam Medical Center, Haifa, Israel
e-mail: h_bahouth@rambam.health.gov.il

D.S. Wheeler et al. (eds.), *Pediatric Critical Care Medicine*,
DOI 10.1007/978-1-4471-6362-6_32, © Springer-Verlag London 2014

Introduction

Trauma is defined as a body injury or wound produced by physical force or energy, whether mechanical, chemical, thermal or electrical. It can be caused by accident (unintentional) or by violence (intentional) – including, in children, child abuse. Definition of Multiple trauma (MT) or Polytrauma is rather controversial [1]. Still, MT may be defined as injury to more than one body system or at least two serious injuries to one body system – such as multiple lower extremity fractures [1].

More children and young adults die from trauma than from all other diseases combined [2]. Moreover, the magnitude of this so called "neglected disease", in terms of acute morbidity and chronic disability, societal costs of direct medical and rehabilitation expenses, lost productivity by care providers and loss of years of potential productive life, let alone the immeasurable psychological burden, is staggering.

According to the trimodal model of the temporal course of trauma-related deaths, very early (immediate) deaths occur within minutes of the event and are practically unavoidable. The second, highest mortality peak occurs within the first 24 h, often within the first "platinum half hour" or the "golden hour", and these patients may benefit from aggressive, efficient and organized emergency medical services (EMSs) and hospital emergency departments (EDs) [3]. The third mortality peak occurs beyond the first 24 h as a consequence of the combination of the primary injury, secondary damage and the pathophysiologic processes initiated by them. These children usually die in the pediatric intensive care unit (PICU), and will be the focus of this chapter.

Trauma Related Mortality and Morbidity

In the developed world, trauma continues to be the leading cause of death and acquired disability among children (beyond their first year of life) and adults up to the age of 45 [2, 4, 5]. In the US, more children and adolescents die from injuries (including suicide) than from all other diseases combined [2]. Back in 1966, a special report by the American National Academy of Sciences defined trauma as the "neglected disease of modern society" [6]. Since then, significant advances in prevention, pre-hospital care and transport systems, emergency and hospital care – including intensive care – and subsequent rehabilitation, have resulted in substantial reductions in mortality, residual morbidity and disability. According to the Center for Disease Control (CDC) data, between 1981 and 1998, mortality rates due to unintentional trauma decreased by about 41 % in the 1–19 years age groups [5]. Between 1981 and 2007 crude mortality due to unintentional trauma decreased in the 0–14 years age groups by 43.2 % [5].

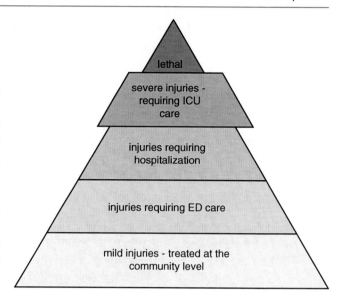

Fig. 32.1 Pyramid of injuries with added level for severe injuries requiring admission to an ICU

These numbers, however, grossly under-represent the true world-wide magnitude of trauma related toll: According to a recent World Health Organization (WHO) report [7, 8], more than 95 % of injury deaths occur in children and adolescents in the developing world, accounting for nearly one million deaths annually. Despite a full order of magnitude lower vehicle ownership rates, 95 % of road traffic crash deaths of children and adolescents occur in the low- and middle-income countries [7]. The magnitude of road traffic injuries is expected to further increase with the trends of increasing urbanization and motorization in the developing world: India and China alone are expected to see by 2020 an increase in the number of road-traffic deaths by 147 and 97 %, respectively [7].

Parallel to continuous decreases in the magnitude of other "traditional" causes of death among the young age groups, the relative importance of trauma as a worldwide health problem is therefore increasing. Based on the WHO database, Viner et al. analyzed global mortality trends for people aged 1–24 years across the past 50 years in low-, middle- and high-income countries [9]. Mortality in children aged 1–9 years declined by 80–93 % in this 50 years period, largely due to steep declines in mortality from communicable diseases. However, improvements in mortality in young people aged 15–24 years were only half those seen in children, largely due to static or rising injury-related deaths. In the UK, mortality in the 15–24 years age group has exceeded that of children aged 1–4 years since the 1970s due to increasing mortality from transport injuries, suicide and homicide [10].

Most statistics relate to trauma associated mortality, as it is the most convenient parameter to record. However, mortality represents only the tip of the "pyramid of injuries" (Fig. 32.1) that stratifies injuries according to severity and the level of medical attention they require. The basis of the pyramid consists of mild injuries treated at the community level; above it hypotension and hypoxia [35, 44, 45]. The Immediate stress response following injury is characterized by activation of the sympathetic nervous system and by increased pituitary hormone secretion that affect hormone secretion from target organs. These result in a massive release of catecholamines, glucagon, glucocorticoids (cortisol) and mineralocorticoids (aldosterone), anti-diuretic hormone, endorphins, growth hormone, TSH and prolactin. These increased hormone levels can be detected in the serum within minutes after the injury [35].

These concerted responses aim at achieving cardiovascular homeostasis, retention of salt and water to maintain fluid volume and at mobilizing substrates to provide energy sources. The combined effects of the stress response include vasoconstriction, redistribution of blood volume, increased cardiac output, increased oxygen consumption, increased minute ventilation, and increased catabolic rate with gluconeogenesis and glycogenolysis. During this initial phase, the injured patient is therefore relatively oliguric, catabolic and hyperglycemic [35, 45, 46].

Following initial stabilization, increased energy expenditure and catabolism are the hallmarks of the further adjustment of the body to injury. Catabolic metabolism includes fat, muscle and serum protein breakdown with enhanced amino acids mobilization towards the circulation. These amino acids are used by the liver to produce glucose for energy in the gluconeogenesis pathway.

Elevated levels of the stress hormones – cathecholamines, cortisol and glucagon – not only stimulate gluconeogenesis but also inhibit insulin secretion by the pancreas and cause insulin resistance, resulting in hyperglycemia. Early hyperglycemia was shown to be an independent predictor of mortality in both adult [47] and pediatric [27] trauma patients. It should be stressed that glucose stores are limited in young children and neonates, and once they are exhausted, dangerous hypoglycemia may occur.

During this phase, liver metabolic processes are shifted toward production of acute-phase proteins, resulting in a marked rise in the circulatory levels of C-reactive protein, fibrinogen, haptoglobin, alpha-1 antitrypsin and more. Concomitantly, production of nutrient transporters such as albumin is markedly decreased [48, 49]. Decreased production, increased breakdown by the catabolic processes and enhanced vascular permeability are the major causes of the marked hypoalbuminemia, typically seen early following severe multiple injury [50]. Admission serum albumin was predictive of outcome in critically ill adult trauma patients [51].

This phase of increased energy expenditure and enhanced catabolism peaks after 5–10 days and can last for 2 weeks. This adaptive mechanism, generating amino acids for wound healing and glucose for energy usage, is a very pronounced, short term compensatory mechanism in children. In the long run, if the metabolic and nutritional needs are not met by appropriate caloric support, these compensatory mechanisms become insufficient as they exhaust the body proteins stores. Progressive loss of muscle mass leads, among others, to respiratory compromise and cardiac dysfunction. Therefore, early and appropriate nutrition – either enteral or parenteral – is crucial. Following abatement of the catabolic phase, the final recovery anabolic phase gradually takes place, aiming at wound healing, buildup of new tissues and renewal of energy stores [35, 46].

The Systemic Inflammatory Response to Trauma

The delayed responses to trauma aim at clearance and repair of damaged tissues and incite a complex inflammatory response, which basically involves a twofold dysregulation of the immune system (Fig. 32.3). Initially, hyperinflammation dominates – clinically expressed as the systemic inflammatory response syndrome (SIRS). Subsequently the compensatory anti-inflammatory response syndrome (CARS) sets in, resulting in immune suppression and predisposing the patient to sepsis [35, 52]. If severe enough, these processes can result in multi-organ dysfunction syndrome (MODS), multiple organ failure (MOF) and death.

The innate immune system, the first line of defense against infection, recognizes pathogen-associated molecular patterns through pathogen recognition receptors (PRRs). PRRs also recognize products of tissue damage, known as 'alarmins' [53, 54]. These are intracellular components that, when released into the extracellular space, signal danger to surrounding tissue. Of the PRRs, the most extensively studied are the toll-like receptors (TLR) [54, 55]. PRRs are located on or in cells that act as sentinels of infection and tissue damage and initiate the complex inflammatory response – both locally and systematically, remote from the site of injury [53–55].

Binding of 'alarmins' to the PRRs induces production of proinflammatory cytokines like TNF-α, IL-6, IL-8, IL-10, chemokines and type I interferon [55, 56]. The degree of cytokine production correlates with the severity of injury and with outcome [57–59]. This binding also initiates the priming of neutrophils for increased release of toxic oxidants and enzymes, resulting – among others – in endothelial damage – again predisposing the patient to subsequent SIRS and MODS [57, 60–62].

MT further activates the complement system, the coagulation cascades, platelet activating factors and the arachidonic acid pathway producing various prostanoids [35, 52, 63]. These basically distinct systems are interconnected and usually exert mutual positive feedbacks, so that the activation of one system augments the activity of other systems.

are injuries requiring ED care, then injuries requiring hospitalization and the tip consists of lethal injuries. Clearly, a new level should be added to this traditional pyramid, namely severe injuries requiring admission to an ICU, as these obviously differ in every aspect from injuries occupying the "admission to hospital" level. In general, the available epidemiological data relate to the overall magnitude of injuries. No 'PICU specific' epidemiological and clinical data are available.

Age Distribution

Road accidents are the most frequent cause of mortality among children older than 1 year, and falls from height are the most frequent cause of injuries requiring hospitalization [11]. There are no major differences in the overall incidence of childhood injuries by age, though in the developed world the incidence increases with age, with the highest incidence in the teen-age group [12–14]. Overall age distributions by specific mechanisms of injury show distinct patterns: Injuries due to falls occur predominantly in the 1–4 years age group [12, 15, 16], pedestrian and bicyclists injuries peak in the 6–14 years age group [12, 13] and car occupant and sport and leisure-associated injuries peak in the 15–19 years age group [12, 13].

Injury Patterns and Mechanisms of Injury

The effects of injury on a child are related to the amount of delivered kinetic energy ($1/2$ mV^2, where m = mass, V = relative velocity). With increased body surface area to volume ratio, the delivered kinetic energy is compacted to a smaller volume and multiple organ involvement is common. Hence, injured small children are at high risk for mortality and morbidity because of their small body size and because of their limited physiologic reserves. Moreover, EMS and ED teams are relatively less trained in their acute care – especially in airway management and in obtaining vascular access. Therefore, a small body weight, especially <10 kg, receives a distinct unfavorable grade in the Pediatric Trauma Score (PTS) [17].

Similar mechanisms of trauma result in different injuries in adults and children. Because of their relatively large and heavy heads, falling children tend to land on their heads – accounting for the very high incidence of traumatic brain injury (TBI) among children admitted to hospital and PICU following falls. Among 188 children admitted to our PICU following falls from height, 92 % suffered TBI, 20 % had facial injuries, 18 % chest injuries and only ten had skeletal injuries.

The increased elasticity of the immature bones results in fewer fractures but in more soft tissue injuries. Thoracic trauma is generally associated with a high transmitted kinetic energy and therefore with high mortality rates [18, 19]. In children it results in injuries to the mediastinum and lungs but only rarely in rib fractures due to their elasticity.

The clinician taking care of the severely injured child should pay careful attention to the injury mechanism, as this determines to a great extent the "quality" and "quantity" of the resultant injuries. Unfortunately, information regarding the actual circumstances or mechanism of injury is often unknown or inaccurate – especially in the early management phase. For example, the relative speed in motor vehicle crashes determines crash severity and influences injury severity [20], yet it is unknown to the clinician taking care of the injured child in the ED or later in the ICU. As a "rule of thumb", an automobile crash in which other occupants have suffered lethal injuries carries high risk for very severe injuries to other occupants as it usually involves very high impact energy. Children who are thrown out of a crashed vehicle often suffer very severe injuries because of the absorbed energy as their body impacts with a solid surface. As mentioned, rib fractures in children are a "red flag" as they often signify severe mechanism of trauma.

Several distinct injury patterns are associated with specific injury mechanisms. Pedestrian – motor vehicle crash often results in the Waddell's triad of injuries to the lower extremities and/or pelvis, torso and head [21] – although this association has been questioned [22]. Unrestrained car occupants often suffer head, face and neck injuries as their head hits the dashboard or the windshield. Restrained children – especially when using lap belt – may present with the "seatbelt syndrome", consisting of intraabdominal injuries (gastric or bowel contusions or ruptures and/or injuries to solid organs) and of Chance fractures of the lumbar or cervical vertebra [23, 24]. With the widespread use of helmets, resulting in reduced incidence of TBI, the major severe injuries among bicyclists has become abdominal trauma – including deep organs such as pancreas or duodenum, as a result of impact by the handlebar [25].

Incidence of Multiple Trauma and Trauma Scoring

Multiple injuries – as opposed to a single injury – have far reaching clinical implications: Their presence impacts on the patient's physiologic status, on the intensity and complexity of his management, on his chances of survival and of residual disability and on the decision making processes. MT require a coordinated teamwork of multiple subspecialties (a major factor in the development of dedicated trauma centers), longer ICU and hospital stays and therefore much higher resource utilization and costs.

TBI is the most frequent type of severe injury and the major cause of mortality and residual disability. Injuries to more than one organ system were diagnosed in 52.5–67 % of children with severe TBI [26, 27]. In fact, when whole-body computed tomography was utilized, MT was diagnosed in even 79 % of severe TBI cases [27]. The most frequently associated injuries were lung contusion and pleural effusion (62 %); bones fractures – mainly in the upper limbs, femoral shafts or pelvic ring (32 %); facial fractures and lacerations (29 %); abdominal solid organ lesions (20 %) and spinal cord injuries (5 %) [27].

Injury scoring systems are discussed elsewhere in this textbook. Basically, injury severity scores attempt to quantify the complexity of multiple injuries, and were shown to correlate with all of the above mentioned outcome variables. They are used mainly for epidemiological and research purposes, and, with the exception of the Revised Trauma Score (RTS) that is used for triage purposes, are of limited usefulness for clinical decision making or patient's management. In fact, it has been shown in both adults [28] and children [29], that the single worst injury actually predicts mortality more accurately than the complex cumulative scores. Furthermore, it seems that simpler, more readily available variables are as reliable as the combined scoring systems in predicting severity of trauma: For example, in severely injured children, with or without severe TBI, admission base deficit reflected injury severity and predicted mortality [30–32]. Base deficit less than −8 mEq/L should alert the clinician to the presence of potentially lethal injuries or uncompensated shock [31]. Recently, Borgman et al. [33] have proposed a simple pediatric trauma mortality prediction score developed in military hospitals in Iraq and Afghanistan and validated in civilian patients. This BIG score takes into account only three, early available variables (base deficit, international normalized ratio – INR – and the Glasgow Coma Scale score) and showed a higher sensitivity compared to other commonly used pediatric trauma scores.

Pathophysiology of Major Trauma and Mechanisms of Secondary Damage

TBI and hemorrhagic shock are responsible for the great majority of immediate and early traumatic deaths [34]. Late mortality and the complex clinical course that dominates the care of the multiply injured child in the PICU are caused mostly by secondary TBI and by the systemic inflammatory effects of the host defense responses [3].

The "two-hits hypothesis" states that this complex cascade of host defense responses is stimulated by both primary (first hits) and secondary (second hits) insults [35, 36]. The initial trauma causes primary organ and tissue damage (trauma load, first hits), and it activates the systemic inflammatory response (SIRS) that is then involved in causing secondary complications (second hits) such as respiratory distress syndrome, repeated cardiovascular instability, ischemia and reperfusion injury, metabolic acidosis, compartment syndromes and infections. Other "second hits" are exogenous, including surgical interventions with severe tissue damage, hypothermia or blood loss, massive transfusions, inadequate or delayed surgical or intensive care interventions and line infections (interventional Load) [35]. These second hits often further stimulate the SIRS in a vicious cycle pattern.

The pathophysiologic consequences of major injury can be grossly categorized into a) impaired oxygen delivery due to hypoxemia or shock, resulting in cellular hypoxia, dysfunction and cell death; b) the cascades of biochemical processes following reperfusion after "successful" resuscitation and c) the multiple mechanisms aiming at restoration of homeostasis, clearance of necrotic cells and repair of damaged tissues that are needed to ensure survival and recovery.

All of these processes are intertwined, and although they are discussed separately for didactic purposes, their combined effect creates an extremely complicated pathophysiologic picture. Even after successful resuscitation that ensures immediate survival, the effects of these complex processes turn major trauma into a systemic disease, cause secondary damage and multisystem organ failure that often dominate the clinical picture and impact heavily on the ICU course, residual disability and survival.

Hypoperfusion, Hypoxemia and Tissue Hypoxia

Oxygen delivery to the tissues (VO_2) is the product of arterial blood oxygen content (CaO_2) multiplied by cardiac output (CO); CaO_2 depends mostly on the hemoglobin concentration and oxygen saturation (O_2 Sat), that depends on PaO_2 and the affinity of hemoglobin for oxygen:

$$VO_2\left(ml\,O_2/minute\right) = CaO_2\left(ml\,O_2/dL\right) \times CO/100$$
$$= \left[Hb\right]\left(gr/dL\right) \times 1.36 \times O_2Sat/100 \times CO\left(ml/minute\right)/100$$

Multiple injuries – rather than injury to a single organ – frequently expose the trauma victim to profound compromise of each or several of these physiologic variables. Unfortunately, we still can not routinely monitor cellular PO_2 and therefore do not have direct measures of cellular hypoxia.

When trauma causes significant bleeding, both hemoglobin concentration and blood volume decrease. Decreased circulating blood volume decreases cardiac preload and stroke volume, resulting in hemorrhagic shock and tissue ischemia. Direct injury to the heart or chest can cause, among others, hemopericardium with cardiac tamponade or tension pneumothorax – both reduce cardiac output precipitously by interfering with blood return to the heart and cause traumatic cardiogenic shock.

PaO_2 and O_2 Sat can be critically reduced by multiple mechanisms. In the setting of trauma, the most frequent are central hypoventilation and inability to maintain patent airway as a result of TBI. Facial injuries, aspiration, chest trauma with lung contusion, rib fractures or tension pneumothorax, abdominal distention due to intra-abdominal bleeding and cervical spine injury make up only a partial list of other pathologies causing hypoxemia. Finally, the use of analgesic and sedative drugs during resuscitation and failure to secure patent airway and provide effective ventilation and

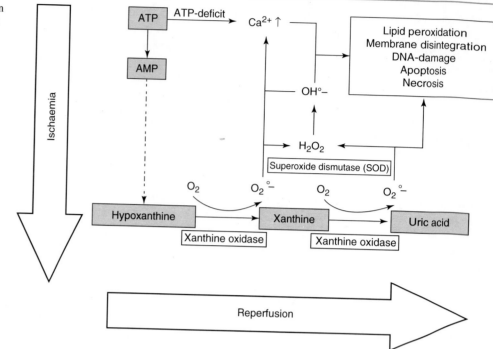

Fig. 32.2 Ischemia – reperfusion injury (Reprinted from Keel and Trentz [35]. With permission from Elsevier)

oxygenation are a rather frequent cause of hypoventilation and hypoxemia in the injured child.

The injured brain is extremely sensitive to secondary insults, and hypotension and hypoxemia in the early stages following TBI were identified as the most deleterious factors contributing to secondary brain damage in both adults [37, 38] and children [39–41].

Ducrocq et al. [26] have analyzed a large cohort of children with severe TBI treated at the scene by the SAMU emergency teams in Paris, and found that hypotension at hospital's arrival was an independent predictor of death and poor neurological outcome. Zebrack et al. [42] found that untreated hypotension – but not untreated hypoxemia – during the early care of children with TBI, was associated with much higher odds for death and residual disability when compared with treated hypotension. In both studies the untreated hypoxemic groups were too small to draw any conclusions, and it may be a grave mistake to conclude that hypoxemia should not be corrected promptly.

Reperfusion Injury

Systemic hypoxemia and hypoperfusion (shock), local hypoperfusion due to contusions, lacerations, vascular injuries or compartment syndromes lead to cellular hypoxia and energy depletion [35] (see Fig. 32.2). Hypoxia leads to decreased production and increased consumption of adenosine triphosphate (ATP), that is degraded to ADP and AMP, which are further degraded to hypoxantine [35, 43]. Cellular energy depletion result in intracellular accumulation of Na^+ and Ca^{++} that may lead to structural cell damage and death.

Following effective resuscitation and organ reperfusion, hypoxantine is degraded to xantine and finally to uric acid, with the generation of superoxide anions (O_2^-) that are further reduced to hydrogen peroxide (H_2O_2) and hydroxyl ions (OH^-) by superoxide dismutase [35, 43]. These free oxygen radicals enhance disturbances in intracellular Ca^{++} homeostasis and induce lipid peroxidation, membrane disintegration and DNA damage, resulting in cell apoptosis and necrosis [35] (Fig. 32.2).

Pathophysiologic Responses to Major Trauma

Regardless of the specific mechanism and organ injured, MT trauma is a systemic disease, involving complex, predictable systemic changes. This systemic reaction encompasses a wide range of responses, including activation of the sympathetic nervous system, neuro-endocrinological "stress response" and complex immunological-hematological effects [35, 44, 45]. Following injury, these measures aim at restoration of homeostasis, clearance of necrotic cells and repair of damaged tissues to ensure survival and recovery.

Neuroendocrine and Metabolic Stress Response

The metabolic neuroendocrine response to stress, including multiple injuries, can be triggered by pain, stress, fear and other stimuli that occur in trauma and is augmented by tissue damage, hemorrhage, decreased intravascular volume,

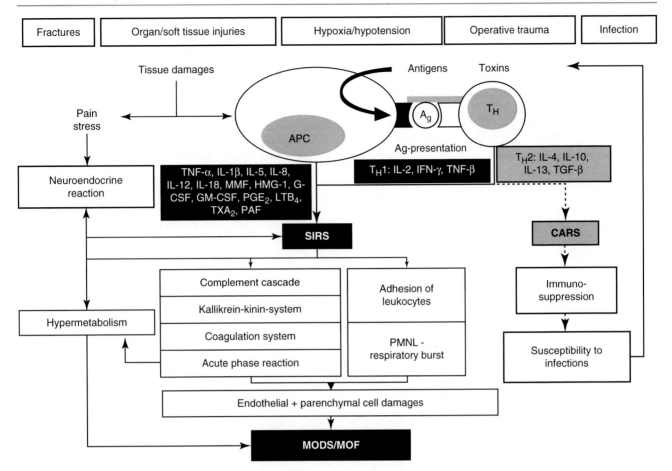

Fig. 32.3 Host defence response after trauma. *APC* antigen presenting cells, *TH* T-helper cells, *SIRS* systemic inflammatory response syndrome, *CARS* compensatory anti-inflammatory response syndrome, *PMNL* polimorphonuclear leukocytes, *MODS* multiorgan dysfunction syndrome, *MOF* multiple organ failure (Reprinted from Keel and Trentz [35] With permission from Elsevier)

The immune response to trauma has been modeled by Bone et al. to consist of the pro-inflammatory SIRS arm followed by a compensatory anti-inflammatory response arm (CARS), aiming at deactivation of the "hyperactive" immune system and restoration of homeostasis [64] (Fig. 32.3). The resultant immune suppression predisposes the trauma patient to local infection and to sepsis, which are associated with late mortality. More recently, it has been hypothesized that following trauma, these two divergent response arms are in fact concurrent, and that their timing and relative magnitude have a profound impact on patient outcome [65, 66].

The activation of all of these basically protective mechanisms may result in multiple, variable, often unpredictable, potentially deleterious physiologic responses, including increased microvascular permeability and edema, vasodilation and decreased cardiac output that may progress to irreversible shock, vasoconstriction that can cause thrombosis and local ischemia, pulmonary vasoconstriction, coagulopathies including DIC, intense catabolic state causing hypoalbuminemia, hyperglycemia and insulin-resistance, direct endothelial damage, acidosis, fever and more. These

processes are augmented by hemorrhage, shock and hypoxia and also by antecedent therapeutic measures like fluid resuscitation and the administration of vasopressors. These intense responses may evolve into dysfunctions and failure of various body systems such as the respiratory, cardiovascular, gastrointestinal, hepatic, renal, coagulation and immune systems, that often dominate the clinical course following MT, require complex therapeutic measures and are associated with prolonged ICU stay, high ICU costs, worsened outcome and increased risk of mortality.

Multi-Organ Dysfunction Syndrome (MODS) and Multiple Organ Failure (MOF) Following Trauma in Children

With the advancement of life-support care of major trauma, resulting in impressive decreases in early mortality, multiple organ failure has emerged as a major pathway to delayed death in intensive care units [67]. It has been further recognized that regardless of age, organ dysfunction represents a continuum of physiologic derangements rather than a dichotomous state of "normal" vs. "failure"- hence the more appropriate terminology of multi-organ dysfunction syndrome (MODS) rather than multi-organ failure (MOF) [67].

Calkins et al. [68] reported no MODS in 334 children admitted to the PICU with isolated brain injury. Only 3 % of multiply injured children developed MOF – defined as moderate to severe MODS – with a low (17 %) mortality. Compared with adults, seriously injured children had a four- to eightfold lower incidence of MODS and of MOF related mortality [52, 68, 69]. It is unclear whether this low rate of MOF is due to a different inflammatory response, as speculated by Calkins [68], or whether it is due to other factors, including comorbidities [70]. Wood et al., suggested that differences in the innate immune response of children may go beyond simple intensity of responsiveness and that children have a fundamentally unique inflammatory system with a relatively protective response to traumatic injury [52].

Clinical Implications of Multiple Trauma

The presence of MT, especially if associated with severe TBI, has several important clinical implications: First, it increases the probability of secondary damage – especially to the brain. Second, it complicates the clinical course, impacts on patient's management, worsens the outcome of each single injury and is associated with a higher case-fatality rate. This basically obvious fact is quantified by the various injury severity scoring systems (ISS, NISS etc.). Lastly, MT requires different priority setting and makes clinical decision taking in the PICU far more complicated.

Pre-hospital Care of the Multiply Injured Child

The crucial importance of prompt and effective resuscitation of the multiply injured child at the scene, during transport and in the emergency department (ED) cannot be overemphasized. The paradigm of preventing early hypoxemia and hypotension to prevent secondary brain damage has become a firm cornerstone of all adult and pediatric guidelines for the care of severe injuries [41, 71, 72]. Efficient emergency medical services (EMS's) and well trained medical and paramedical teams, capable of rapidly providing professional primary treatment at the scene, followed by safe and expedite evacuation – preferably to a designated trauma center – have reduced the frequency of critical complications and were repeatedly shown to improve the outcome of severely traumatized patients [42, 73–76].

Discussion of basic and advanced life support is provided in specific chapters in this textbook. The following paragraphs discuss aspects that are specific to the multiply injured child.

Pre-hospital Airway Management

Inadequate airway management in the field and on the way to hospital is the major cause of secondary damage. While endotracheal intubation (ETI) is considered a "gold standard" in the hospital setting, it was not shown to provide unequivocal outcome benefit over bag-valve mask (BVM) ventilation in the field. Retrospective studies comparing pre-hospital ETI and BVM in both adult and pediatric trauma and in urban and rural settings reached contradicting results: Some studies found better survival with ETI [76–79], while others found no benefit [80] or even worse outcome [81–85]. Gauche et al. conducted a large, prospective trial on children requiring airway intervention in the pre-hospital setting in the Los Angeles County [86]. The results indicated no difference in survival or neurologic outcome between paramedic ETI versus BVM ventilation. It should be noted that ETI skills were added to the paramedic scope of practice for the purpose of this study, resulting in paucity of practical experience, poor ETI success rate (57 %) and relatively high complications rate. Moreover, the mean transport time to the nearby ED was only 6 min. These results, therefore, may be relevant to trauma occurring in a densely populated, inner-city environment with abundance of medical facilities but not to trauma occurring in different circumstances, such as rural environments.

Importantly, most of the studies reported high rates of ETI failures and complications, and in many of them ETI's were performed without adequate sedation [83, 85–89] – both factors contributing to adverse outcome. Hence, the lack of a proven outcome benefit of pre-hospital ETI possibly stems from deficient operator's skills combined with the difficult nature of performing ETI in the field [90, 91].

Active gag and cough reflexes are maintained even in the comatose patient with severe TBI, and when ETI with inadequate sedation is attempted, he often becomes combative. This may result in laryngospasm, vomiting, coughing, aspiration, hypoxemia, aggravated cervical spine damage, elevated intracranial pressure, hypertension and enhanced bleeding – all contributing to intubation failure and potentially to secondary damage [85, 88, 92, 93]. Experienced emergency teams using sedation protocols that included neuromuscular blockage reported high ETI success rates and very low complication rates [77, 94, 95].

Rapid sequence intubation (RSI) with muscle paralysis is the recommended approach to ETI in emergency situations. Etomidate and midazolam are the most commonly used sedatives, while opiates and thiopental are hardly ever used in the pre-hospital setting. Midazolam, opiates and thiopental may decrease blood pressure – more so in the unstable trauma patient, and a significant number of children respond paradoxically to benzodiazepines and become more agitated and combative [96].

Ketamine is a safe and effective sedative-hypnotic and may be optimal for short interventions in emergency situations, including RSI [97–101]. Within its therapeutic range it does not depress spontaneous ventilation nor lowers blood pressure. Its use in trauma situations and especially in patients with TBI was very limited due to its alleged effect of ICP elevation [100, 102, 103]. This notion has been recently refuted in a prospective controlled trial demonstrating that ketamine was in fact effective in decreasing elevated ICP and in preventing untoward ICP elevations during distressing activities in ventilated children [98]. It is currently used successfully and extensively not only in the ED but also by civilian and military emergency services [104–106].

Emergency Department Management of the Multiply Injured Child

The complicated, very demanding rapid sequence of actions undertaken in the admitting ED is organized in a standardized scheme, aiming at detecting and treating immediate life-endangering conditions (primary survey) and subsequently at diagnosing all other injuries (secondary survey) and constructing the treatment plan. This standardized approach is crucial in face of the wide variability of major trauma, the very short time frame available to prevent secondary damage, loss of organs or death (the "platinum half hour" or the "golden hour") and the dramatic nature of caring for a severely injured child in the ED. Without a systematic approach and a concerted teamwork under one team leader overseeing the entire scene, the intricate situation may become chaotic, more subtle injuries may be missed and wrong decisions may be taken – leading to potentially catastrophic results.

Role of the PICU Physician

The role of the pediatric intensivist in the pre-PICU management of the severely injured child varies according to local organizational structures and policies. Pediatric intensivists often lead ground or air medical transport teams. In the ED, the trauma team leader is most frequently a surgeon or an emergency physician, and the pediatric intensivist is often responsible for airway management, ventilation or intravenous line placement. Subsequently, again according to local policies and the patient's condition, the pediatric intensivist may be in charge of attending the ventilated child through imaging and during transport to the operating room or PICU.

Primary Survey, Resuscitation and Initial Stabilization

The primary survey follows the Airway, Breathing, Circulation, Disability and Exposure sequence (ABCDE), though in reality the evaluation of the neurological status (part of "Disability") is performed as a first step concomitant with airway evaluation. Treatment of life threatening conditions often takes place concurrent with the primary survey.

Airway

Airway compromise, the most urgent medical problem in the severely injured child, is caused first and foremost by altered sensorium. In the comatose child the relatively large tongue, the floppy epiglottis, secretions, blood or foreign body in the oral cavity and loss of effective coughing are the main mechanisms of upper airway obstruction. In the neurologically intact child, maxillo-facial trauma, facial burns or direct laryngeal injury can obstruct the airway. All ETI's in the ED should be performed under the same RSI approach outlined above.

Clear cut indications for securing the airway through ETI in the ED include clinical signs of upper airway obstruction, inability to cough or clear secretions and inadequate respiratory effort or a GCS ≤8 [41]. Of note: children with GCS ≤8 may temporarily be able to maintain airway and ventilate effectively, and this should not be mistakenly interpreted as if they do not need ETI, as their sensorium should be expected to deteriorate further. When this happens, they may be out of the closely observed surrounding of the trauma bay, on intra- or inter-hospital transport or in the imaging department, under far less favorable conditions for emergency ETI.

There are some "relative" indications for ETI in the ED: The multiply injured child with no major TBI is typically painful, frightened and combative. To reduce pain and anxiety and to enable effective, thorough evaluation and rapid initiation of treatment, he will require generous doses of analgesics and sedatives. Uncompensated shock presents another relative indication for early assisted ventilation. The injured child will be much safer and his management much smoother if he will undergo "semi-elective" ETI in the ED. Similarly, if the child is planned for surgery under general anesthesia, or even imaging procedures that require heavy sedation, ETI should not be postponed. The disadvantage of this approach is the loss of the ability to clinically monitor the child, but in reality most management decisions are made on the basis of the initial evaluation in the pre-hospital phase or upon ED admission and according to imaging findings.

Breathing and Mechanical Ventilation

Once the airway is secured, adequacy of breathing should be evaluated clinically, by oxygen saturation and by blood gases analysis. In the injured child, ventilation may be compromised mainly due to decreased central ventilatory drive or to thoracic injury. Very frequently, however, hypoventilation or apnea are iatrogenic, caused by sedative-anesthetic medications, and obviously by muscle relaxants, used during RSI.

Every intubated child must be mechanically ventilated. No child, certainly not the injured child, should ever be expected to breathe effectively through a narrow pipe that typically reduces the diameter of the trachea by half and therefore increase resistance to airflow by 16.

The injured child should initially be ventilated with $FiO_2 = 1.0$. Although there is insufficient evidence to recommend any specific FiO_2, it is reasonable to titrate it to maintain $SatO_2 > 94$ % [107]. In many ventilators available in ambulances and in the ED, FiO_2 is not adjustable, but can be set to FiO_2 of 0.4 or 1.0. As long as there is no clear cut evidence that short-term hyperoxemia is detrimental, it seems safer to avoid hypoxemia and use the higher FiO_2.

Circulation

Shock in the multiply injured child is primarily hemorrhagic. The classical assessment of end-organ perfusion may be of limited value in this situation: CNS function is often depressed due to TBI or the use of sedatives, tachycardia may also result from pain and anxiety, skin temperature and capillary refill are affected by exposure to environmental temperature and urinary output is not indicative during the primary survey. The more "reliable" signs of shock include tachycardia in the sedated or comatose child, thready or absent pulses and hypotension.

Shock is conveniently categorized into compensated and uncompensated: In compensated shock blood pressure is maintained above the lower limit (5th percentile) of age-adjusted values. In uncompensated shock, blood pressure drops below these values, sensorium is usually markedly depressed and peripheral pulses are not palpable. It should be stressed that hypotension is a relatively late sign, developing following loss of at least 30 % of blood volume. The response to resuscitation measures and fluid boluses is extremely helpful in the evaluation of the hemodynamic status.

Uncontrolled hemorrhage occurs usually in hidden body cavities and compartments – the abdominal cavity, retroperitoneum, pleural space and thighs. Scalp lacerations can cause fatal hemorrhage and may be easily missed as the child is lying supine, covered with a blanket and the blood accumulates posteriorly, under his back on the stretcher – hence the utmost importance of examining the child's "back". Less frequent causes of shock in the traumatized child are tension pneumothorax and pericardial tamponade, and more rarely spinal cord or severe traumatic brain injuries ('neurogenic' shock).

Vascular Access

Vascular access may be challenging in the injured child and should be obtained as early as possible, preferably in the pre-hospital phase before shock develops. Two large bore peripheral catheters should be inserted, at least one of them in an upper extremity, ensuring effective fluid resuscitation in case of intra-abdominal injury.

Intraosseous (IO) needle is an excellent alternative whenever peripheral line insertion fails, especially in infants and young children and during shock [107, 108]. Several IO insertion devices are currently marketed: The traditional Jamshidi needle is available in 15G and 18G diameters. We prefer the larger, 15G needle for all ages beyond the neonatal period as the smaller 18G needles tend to bend during insertion. Significant force should be applied for successful insertion and care should be given to correct placement and fixation to avoid needle displacement.

Other mechanical IO insertion devices are available for use in children. The Bone Injection Gun (BIG) is a spring-loaded single-use device that "shoots" the needle into the bone, and is available in pediatric and adult sizes. The EZ-IO is a hand-held drill with detachable IO needle. Although clinical data in pediatric patients are very limited, these mechanical devices seem to be easier for use and to have a higher insertion success rates compared with the Jamshidi needle [109]. Tested on turkey bone model, the EZ-IO had a higher insertion success rate compared to BIG and was the preferred device by the users [110].

In the ED setup, central venous catheters are used infrequently. They may be indicated when no other vascular access can be established or when a very large bore catheter is needed for massive blood and coagulation factors transfusion. The pediatric intensivist is relatively more trained in central line placement and may undertake this task.

Fluid Resuscitation

After over 30 years of controversy, the issue of colloids versus crystalloids is still debated. A recent comprehensive meta-analysis of 56 randomized controlled clinical trials that compared colloids and crystalloids in patients requiring volume replacement, concluded that there is no evidence that resuscitation with colloids reduces the risk of death compared to resuscitation with crystalloids in patients with trauma, burns or following surgery [111].

Clinical trials of fluid resuscitation in children with trauma were not published. Rather small size randomized trials in children with septic shock or dengue shock syndrome found no clinical benefit of colloids over isotonic crystalloid resuscitation [112–114].

Another unsettled issue is that of hypertonic (7.5 % saline or 7.5 % saline + 6 % dextran 70) vs. isotonic (normal saline or lactated Ringer's) solutions. Potential benefits of hypertonic solutions include restoration of intravascular volume and tissue perfusion with smaller fluid volumes, and attenuation of the inflammatory response and secondary ischemia-reperfusion injury. Thus, they may reduce the development of MOF and ARDS, and prevent brain edema and intracranial hypertension in patients with both TBI and shock [115–118].

Though earlier clinical trials demonstrated some overall survival benefit for patients resuscitated with hypertonic solutions [119], two recent large multicenter clinical trials failed to demonstrate any advantage of hypertonic solutions over normal saline in adult patients with either traumatic shock [120] or severe TBI [121].

Hydroxyethyl starch (HES), an artificial colloid, has been used extensively in adults. Recent controlled clinical trials documented increased incidence of acute kidney injury and acute renal failure requiring dialysis in adult ICU patients [122] and in adults with severe sepsis [123], assigned to fluid resuscitation with HES as compared with those receiving normal saline or Ringer's acetate.

A recent meta-analysis [124] concluded that the use of HES – compared with other resuscitation solutions – in critically ill patients requiring acute volume resuscitation, was associated with a significant increased risk of mortality and acute kidney injury. The authors concluded that the use of HES for acute volume resuscitation is not warranted due to serious safety concerns.

Blood and Coagulation Factors Transfusion

If signs of shock persist after three fluid boluses (60 ml/Kg), red blood cells (RBC's) transfusion should be initiated at 15 ml/Kg or one adult unit. Although the great majority of children stabilize after the initial fluid resuscitation and a single RBC's transfusion, bleeding in the mutiply injured child may be massive and coagulaties may develop due to dilution or consumption of platelets and coagulation factors and due to hypothermia. Recent evidence in adult trauma patients indicates that earlier and increased plasma and platelet to RBC's ratio improve outcome following massive transfusion [125–127]. This has led to the development of massive transfusion protocols that include empiric early transfusion of RBC's, FFP, platelets and cryoprecipitate in balanced ratios for adults [128, 129] and children [130–132] (see Fig. 32.4). A recent study in children [131] showed that the introduction of massive transfusion protocol to a pediatric trauma center resulted in earlier FFP transfusion but was of a far too small scale to detect any potential effects on outcome.

Imaging of the Multiply Injured Child

Patients who are referred to a Trauma Center usually have undergone imaging studies in the referring hospital. It is very helpful to obtain the original images as they serve as 'reference point' and help avoiding repetition of examinations and radiation exposure.

Chest x-ray is the first and usually the only x-ray needed in the ED. Multiply injured patients and those with suspected isolated abdominal trauma should undergo focused abdominal sonography for trauma (FAST) scan in the ED, preferably by a radiologist. To detect free fluid – that will usually be due to internal bleeding – FAST is directed to four locations: the hepato renal fossa (Morison's pouch), subxyphoid view (pericardium), perisplenic space and the pelvis [133].

Ultrasound is a sensitive tool for diagnosing small amounts of intra-peritoneal fluid (200 ml), but is an operator dependent examination. In adults, FAST was shown to have a high sensitivity (73–88 %), very high specificity (98–100 %) and accuracy of 96–98 % [134]. In a recent prospective study sensitivities and specificities of FAST scans for blunt and penetrating trauma were even higher – 93.1 and 100 %, and 90.0 and 100 %, respectively [135]. In the pediatric population, FAST has not gained the same enthusiasm by clinicians, as the indices were lower (sensitivity around 75 %). These examinations, however, were performed by surgeons: When performed by a radiologist, FAST was shown to have sensitivity of 92.5 %, specificity of 97.2 % and accuracy of 95.5 % [136].

In children with less severe trauma, FAST may be used alongside the clinical assessment as a discriminative tool, and can safely exclude the need for computed tomography (CT) scan [137]. The multiply injured child will usually proceed to CT regardless of the FAST findings, which are mainly used for initial assessment of unstable patients who may require immediate surgery.

Multiply injured children should have a 'whole body' CT scan, including a non- contrast head and neck scan, CT angiography (CTA) of the chest, and arterial and venous phase scans of the abdomen and pelvis with no enteral contrast media. With reconstructions in the coronal and sagittal planes, CT scans allow excellent characterization of multiple injuries and CTA has virtually supplanted interventional angiography. Reconstruction images of bone fractures waive the need for additional x-rays of the bony trunk.

CT provides a quick overview of the extent of injuries and additional studies may be required as judged by the radiologist and the case manager. As with all pediatric CT, efforts should be made to minimize radiation dose through technical settings [138, 139]: Effective radiation dose from radiologic studies in pediatric trauma patients admitted to trauma centers was calculated as 14.9 mSv [140] and 12 mSv [141]. CT accounted for 97.5 % of total effective dose [140]. However, when weighing immediate benefits versus potential radiation 'costs' to the multiply injured child, whole body CT scan is 'logically' justified.

In the acute setting Magnetic Resonance Imaging (MRI) is used mainly in cases of complicated cervical injuries. Compared to CT, MRI has superior contrast resolution with higher sensitivity for soft tissue injuries, and is the imaging modality of choice in assessing soft tissue injuries, spinal cord injury, and intervertebral discs and ligaments.

Fig. 32.4 Rambam Medical Center's pediatric massive transfusion protocol (Courtesy of E. Dann MD, Rambam Medical Center, Haifa, Israel)

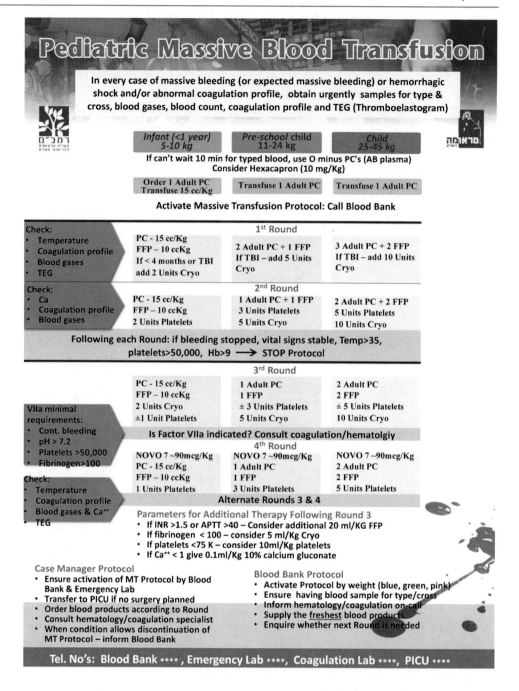

Management of the Multiply Injured Child in the Intensive Care Unit

The child with multiple, severe injuries, represents a difficult and complex management case. Although the involved surgeon will perform necessary surgeries and will make decisions regarding management of the specific organ system under his 'jurisdiction', it is the intensivist's responsibility to overview the entire clinical picture and to be deeply involved in the decision making processes and in leading all clinical activities. In the PICU, the intensivist should assume the role of "case manager": He is at the patient's bedside 24/7, and is

basically the only person able to integrate the complexity of the patient's clinical problems, physiologic parameters, laboratory and imaging results and the various consultants' opinions and recommendations. We have adopted this approach for many years and time and time again realize that its cardinal value cannot be overemphasized.

As the pediatric intensivist oversees the entire clinical picture, one of his crucial roles is to set priorities: He should determine what are the most critical, life or organ endangering problems and prevent or postpone the performance of interventions with potential to cause secondary damage. For example, as the child with low intracranial compliance is exquisitely sensitive to any external stimulus, it is worthwhile to minimize interventions and delay those considered postponable if they can potentially increase ICP. In general, activities in- and outside the PICU (imaging, surgeries) should be coordinated to minimize patient's risk, pain and discomfort, to avoid excessive use of analgesics and sedatives, and to reduce both nursing and medical staff workload.

Multiply injured children may present some of the most difficult to manage clinical problems, such as MOD and MSOF. One of the more complicated, life-endangering conditions, encountered early in the clinical course, is that of the bleeding patient with hypothermia and acidosis – the so called "Triad of Death". These patients may be admitted to the PICU following surgery or for stabilization prior to surgery.

Triad of Death

Injured patients presenting with hypothermia, acidosis and coagulopathy have been identified at very high risk of death, hence the term 'triad of death'. The triad can develop rapidly in the exsanguinating trauma patient, and is the result of the primary trauma and the secondary systemic response. Once established, it forms a vicious circle that may be impossible to overcome [45, 142–144].

Hypothermia is both a marker of profound injury and is by itself deleterious, promoting this vicious cycle in the bleeding patient. Hypothermia can occur in the field and subsequently in the various hospital environments, due to exposure and heat loss, transfusion of cold fluids and impaired thermogenesis (use of muscle relaxants, for example). It develops more rapidly in infants and children due to their small body mass and large surface area to volume ratio. Hypothermia induces multiple adverse effects: It causes cardiac dysfunction (arrhythmias, decreased contractility) and increased inotropic requirement. It shifts the oxyhaemoglobin dissociation curve to the left and impairs oxygen delivery, thereby aggravating tissue hypoxia in the trauma patient with a preexisting 'oxygen debt'. Hypothermia suppresses enzymatic activity, induces endotheliopathy and increases fluid leak, and promotes platelet dysfunction and coagulopathy [45, 145–149].

Although metabolic acidosis has been considered not harmful per se in this setting, but rather a marker of tissue hypoxia [45, 150], recent studies indicate that low pH by itself severely impairs thrombin generation and accelerates fibrinogen degradation [151]. Tissue hypoxia may be due to direct tissue damage, hypotension or impairment of the microcirculation by hypovolemia, disseminated coagulation, intravascular sludging and endothelial damage. Tissue hypoxia leads to anaerobic metabolism and lactic acid production that may be aggravated by abundant glucose supply and by hepatic function impairment. In pediatric trauma, the probability of mortality increases precipitously in children with a base deficit less than -8 mEq/L [31].

Coagulopathy after major trauma is a multifactorial, global failure of the coagulation system to sustain adequate hemostasis [146]. Derangements in coagulation are detectable already in the hyperacute phase following severe trauma, driven by the combination of tissue trauma and systemic hypoperfusion, and are characterized by global anticoagulation and hyperfibrinolysis [146, 152]. Subsequently, coagulopathy proceeds due to continued blood loss, hemodilution and consumption of platelets and clotting factors, and is exacerbated by hypothermia and acidemia [147, 153].

Studies analyzing the effects of the 'triad of death' on mortality in pediatric trauma patients are lacking. Mortality in adult trauma patients presenting with this triad approximates 50 % [143, 154]. Hypothermia contributes to mortality over and above the mortality associated with multiple severe injuries, independent of hypotension, fluid requirements, age, or duration of surgery [143, 145, 148]. Coagulopathy on presentation has been associated with a fourfold increase in overall mortality [152].

The presence of all three conditions not only adds to mortality, but they further potentiate each other, forming a "vicious cycle resulting in death" [155]. Continuing attempts to stop hemorrhage and repair the injury in the hypoperfused patient result in deepening hypothermia and coagulopathy. SIRS is evolving, further lowers blood pressure, worsens tissue acidosis and enhances capillary leak. The intravascular hypovolemia requires further transfusion and crystalloids volume infusion, resulting in dilution of coagulation factors and enhanced SIRS. The patient is now "oozing" extensively and the vicious cycle spirals down, often resulting in the patient's death in the OR.

Even if the bleeding can be eventually stopped, the patient will arrive at the ICU with massive fluid overload and ongoing capillary leak and is at high risk of developing MODS, MOF and abdominal compartment syndrome. If he also has a significant TBI, the previously incurred hypoperfusion and generalized edema will negatively impact on the brain's ability to recover and on the development of cerebral edema.

The recognition of the poor outcome of these multiply injured, bleeding patients, had led in the early 1990s to a paradigm shift – to the 'damage control surgery' and subsequently to the 'damage control resuscitation' paradigms.

Damage Control in the Unstable Injured Child

"Damage control (DC) surgery" was coined in 1993 by Rotondo et al. [156], though the concept of 'staged laparotomy' has been pioneered by several groups since the mid-1970s [155]. The 'traditional' approach up to this time has been adopted from the elective surgery paradigm, calling for definitive repair of all injuries with abdominal wall closure in a

Table 32.1 The three stages of damage control surgery

1. Theatrer – damage control surgery
Rapid haemostasis
Control contamination
Temporary abdominal closure
2. Intensive care – resuscitation
Re-warming
Correct shock – optimize oxygen delivery
Correct coagulopathy
Correct acidosis
Detect abdominal compartment syndrome
3. Theatre – second look laparotomy
Definitive repair
Abdominal closure
Primary
Prosthetic

Reprinted from Hamill [150]. With permission from Elsevier

single operative session. The paradigm shift to staged laparotomy was driven by the recognition of the 'triad of death' and the realization of the disastrous results of continuing attempts to perform definitive repair of massive injuries in these unstable patients. The focus has been directed to the injured patient's physiology rather than to the completeness of anatomy.

The accepted indications for damage control surgery include hypothermia (temperature <35°), acidosis (pH <7.2 or base deficit >8 mEq/L), clinical coagulopathy or massive transfusion (whole blood volume replacement or – in adults – ≥10 units of pRBC's), hemodynamic instability or profound hypoperfusion and prohibitive operative time needed for definitive repair (>90 min).

Although DC surgery was conceptualized for hepatic and other major abdominal trauma, it was later adopted by other specialties, especially orthopedic [157] and vascular surgery. DC in children follows the same principles as in adults [45, 150, 158] (Table 32.1).

The first stage is targeted at rapid damage control. It includes surgery to control hemorrhage in the abdominal cavity, chest, neck or extremities, and at alleviating contamination, such as fecal spillage from damaged bowel. This is achieved by packing of organs or spaces to control nonsurgical bleeding and by resection of damaged bowel without performing anastomoses or stomas. Because of the high probability of developing abdominal compartment syndrome (ACS), the abdomen is often closed temporarily with loose retention sutures or left open, covered with a prosthetic material. Fractures are immobilized, not definitively reduced.

The second stage is resuscitation and stabilization in the ICU. It includes re-warming of hypothermic patients, correcting coagulopathy and acidosis and restoring adequate cardiovascular state. Resuscitation in this setting calls for several specific considerations. The patient should remain mechanically ventilated to ensure adequate oxygenation, sedation and

pain control. He is at a significant danger of developing ARDS and is planned for repeated surgery in a few days; hence attempts at weaning are unadvisable. Hemodynamic resuscitation should be guided by few crucial endpoints – there is no need to 'normalize' all values. Blood pressure should be targeted to values sufficient to achieve urinary output of 1 ml/Kg/h and lactate clearance (to correct acidosis) and to maintain minimal cerebral perfusion pressure in case of coexisting TBI. Normal – and certainly elevated – blood pressure should be avoided in light of the bleeding tendency.

Fluid resuscitation should be judicious as the child is already fluid overloaded and is at a high risk of developing brain edema, respiratory insufficiency and ACS. Blood products, needed for correcting the coagulopathy, are excellent volume expanders. When appropriate, we prefer the use of judicious dosages of cathecholamines rather than 'fill the patient up' with crystalloids. Central venous pressure monitoring is of limited value and should serve as an adjunct guide – not as a targeted endpoint. If the hemodynamic status cannot be stabilized, cardiac echocardiography is indicated to exclude myocardial contusion and to provide useful information regarding myocardial function and volume status. High index of suspicion towards the possibility of ACS is mandatory, even if the abdomen was left partly or entirely open, as discussed elsewhere in this Textbook.

The third stage, reoperation, should be undertaken after the patient's condition has stabilized. This 'second look' aims at searching for missed injuries, definitive repair and, if possible, formal closure of the abdominal wall. In the adult patient population with massive injuries and the catastrophic 'triad of death', the DC approach has reduced mortality to around 50 % [159]. Data regarding outcome of DC surgery in children is minimal, probably because the numbers are much smaller. Stylianos et al. [160] reported on DC in 22 children aged 6 days to 20 years, 13 of whom were trauma patients and 90 % had the 'triad of death': packing controlled hemorrhage in 95 % and survival rate was 82 %. Porras-Ramirez [161] reported on four pediatric MT patients – three of them with multiple penetrating abdominal injuries – managed with DC surgery. Yin et al. [162] compared 32 children who have undergone DC surgery with 17 children who have undergone conventional surgery for serious abdominal diseases. Recovery rates were 84.4 % in the DC group compared to 52.9 % in the conventional group.

Blunt Abdominal Trauma in the Multiply Injured Child

The spleen and the liver are the most frequently injured organs in blunt abdominal injury, each accounting for a third of abdominal injuries. In the hemodynamically stable child, non-operative management has become standard practice. Should these patients be taken care of in the PICU? Guidelines based on a retrospective review of 832 children with isolated liver or spleen injury proposed no ICU admission for isolated injuries with CT grades I, II, and III, and only one ICU day observation for grade IV injury [163]. A follow-up study, however, found that in 19 % of the cases admitted to 'committed' pediatric surgical centers, actual practice deviated from these recommendations – assumingly towards a more cautious approach towards ICU admission [164]. Jim et al. [165] concluded that nonoperative management of splenic injury must include close monitoring, because 16 % required delayed operation. For high grade liver or spleen injuries it seems justified to prefer the safer approach over the "limitation of resource utilization" approach.

Until the late 1990s, the non-operative approach was limited to isolated liver or spleen injuries. The approach to these injuries in multiply injured children, especially those with associated TBI, remained controversial as their clinical evaluation is unreliable. Based on analysis of children with combined spleen and/or liver and head injuries, registered in the National Pediatric Trauma Registry, Keller et al. [166] found that when stratified for type of injury and severity, both mortality and abdominal and neurologic morbidity were improved in children managed non-operatively. Similarly, Coburn et al. [167] concluded that non-operative management of splenic and hepatic injury in multiply injured pediatric patients, including those with head injury and injury remote from the abdomen that requires surgical intervention, is successful and is not associated with a prohibitive morbidity.

In our PICU we routinely apply the non-operative approach to children with combined abdominal and brain trauma, as long as they are hemodynamically stable. Obviously, clinical evaluation of the abdomen is impaired in comatose or heavily sedated patients, but they can be reliably monitored through hemodynamic parameters (all must have an arterial line) and hematocrit, abdominal girth measurement and abdominal ultrasound when needed. For high grade liver or spleen lacerations, elective mechanical ventilation with complete rest under sedation and minimal handling for at least 24–48 h is indicated.

ICP monitoring should always be applied in patients with MT involving severe TBI. In a child with "borderline" severe TBI (GCS 8–9), one may consider clinical follow up with early cessation of sedatives and early extubation. However, if this child has a significant abdominal or chest trauma and requires mechanical ventilation and sedation, ICP monitoring is indicated as no other follow up is available.

Thoracic Injury in the Multiply Injured Child

Thoracic injury is common among multiply injured children and is an important marker of the severity of injury. Pedestrian and car occupant injuries are the major cause of blunt chest trauma, while penetrating injuries are caused mainly by gunshot or stab wounds. Direct blunt trauma to the chest results in lung contusions or lacerations, rib fractures, pneumo- and/or hemothorax, major vascular disruption or myocardial contusion [18, 45, 168–170].

Severe thoracic injury (AIS ≥3) was detected in 38 % of multiply injured children in the German trauma registry [171]. In two French studies of severe TBI, the most frequently associated injury was chest trauma [26, 27]. Several other studies reported far lower incidence of chest trauma among hospitalized pediatric trauma patients [18, 172–174].

Lung contusions are detected very frequently with advanced CT technology, though their clinical significance is incompletely understood [175, 176]. While lung contusions occupying >20 % of total lung volume were shown to be highly predictive of the need for assisted ventilation in adults [175], similarly large lung contusions did not carry the same morbidity in children [176].

In children, chest trauma as a single injury only rarely results in death [19, 168, 172]. On the other hand, mortality rates in multiply injured children with chest trauma are very high [18, 19, 169, 170, 172, 173, 177].

Peclet et al. [18] analyzed thoracic injuries in children admitted to a level 1 pediatric trauma center. Although thoracic injury was detected in only 4.4 % of this patient population, it was strongly associated with severity of injury: 71 % of the children with thoracic injury were admitted to the PICU, and MT was present in 81.7 % of the children with thoracic injury. Mortality rates were 20 times higher for children with thoracic injury compared to those with no thoracic injury. Mortality was 28.6 % for children with injuries to the chest and another body region, compared to 5.3 % for children with thoracic injury alone. Multiple rib fractures and contusions to several pulmonary lobes were strongly correlated with the risk of death [18].

Chest injuries in multiple trauma victims resulted in a mortality of 19 % in children and 9 % in adults (P<0.05) [19]. Mortality was highest in combined head, chest and abdominal trauma: 25 % percent in children and 28 % in adults. For comparison, mortality of multiply injured children with TBI but with no chest injury was only 3 % [19].

Injuries to head, abdomen and chest were associated with the highest overall mortality in the study by Meier et al. [169]. Thoracic injury was associated with the highest odds ratios for death compared to all other injured regions.

The grave consequences of thoracic injury as part of a MT, relate to several factors. First and foremost, thoracic injuries are caused by high energy impacts absorbed by relatively small bodies. In children, bony thoracic structures are more elastic, and if an impacting force is of sufficient energy to result in rib fracture, major intrathoracic injury and trauma to other regions can be expected [18, 19, 169, 170]. Moreover, chest injuries contribute to the unfavorable outcome in multiply injured children as they may interfere with pulmonary gas exchange and cause hypoxemia and secondary brain damage. Children with chest injury had significantly greater physiological derangement compared to those with no chest injury, reflected by their lower Trauma Scores [18]. Thus, a significant, treatable chest injury, such as pnemo/hemothorax represents true emergency in the initial care of the multiply injured child.

References

1. Butcher N, Balogh ZJ. The definition of polytrauma: the need for international consensus. Injury. 2009;40 Suppl 4:S12–22.
2. Hoyert DL, Xu J. Deaths: preliminary data for 2011. Natl Vital Stat Rep. 2012;61:6.
3. Acosta JA, Yang JC, Winchell RJ, et al. Lethal injuries and time to death in a level I trauma center. J Am Coll Surg. 1998;186:528–33.
4. Allshouse MJ, Rouse T, Eichelberger MR. Childhood injury: a current perspective. Pediatr Emerg Care. 1993;9:159–64.
5. Center for Disease Control and Prevention. WISQARS. Web-Based Injury Statistics Query and Reporting System www.cdc.gov/ncipc/wisqars. Accessed 22 Aug 2011.
6. Accidental death and disability: the neglected disease of modern society. In: National Research Council NAoS. Committee on trauma and committee on shock DoMS. Washington: National Academy of Sciences; 1966.
7. Peden M OK, Ozanne-Smith J, et al. *World Report on Child Injury Prevention.* Geneva, Switzerland: World Health Organization; 2008.
8. Rivara FP. The global problem of injuries to children and adolescents. Pediatrics. 2009;123:168–9.
9. Viner RM, Coffey C, Mathers C, et al. 50-year mortality trends in children and young people: a study of 50 low-income, middle-income, and high-income countries. Lancet. 2011;377:1162–74.
10. Viner RM, Barker M. Young people's health: the need for action. BMJ. 2005;330:901–3.
11. Rivara FP, Grossman DC, Cummings P. Injury prevention. First of two parts. N Engl J Med. 1997;337:543–8.
12. Gallagher SS, Finison K, Guyer B, et al. The incidence of injuries among 87,000 Massachusetts children and adolescents: results of the 1980–81 Statewide Childhood Injury Prevention Program Surveillance System. Am J Public Health. 1984;74:1340–7.
13. Agran PF, Winn D, Anderson C, et al. Rates of pediatric and adolescent injuries by year of age. Pediatrics. 2001;108:E45.
14. Danseco ER, Miller TR, Spicer RS. Incidence and costs of 1987–1994 childhood injuries: demographic breakdowns. Pediatrics. 2000;105:E27.
15. Bar-Joseph N B-JG, Tamir, A, Rennert G. Comparison of major pediatric trauma due to falls from height and due to road accidents. Paper presented at: 12th Annual Congress of the European Society of Pediatric and Neonatal Intensive Care 2001; Luebeck.
16. Hyder AA, Sugerman D, Ameratunga S, et al. Falls among children in the developing world: a gap in child health burden estimations? Acta Paediatr. 2007;96:1394–8.
17. Tepas 3rd JJ, Mollitt DL, Talbert JL, et al. The pediatric trauma score as a predictor of injury severity in the injured child. J Pediatr Surg. 1987;22:14–8.
18. Peclet MH, Newman KD, Eichelberger MR, et al. Thoracic trauma in children: an indicator of increased mortality. J Pediatr Surg. 1990;25:961–5; discussion 965–6.
19. Sharma OP, Oswanski MF, Stringfellow KC, et al. Pediatric blunt trauma: a retrospective analysis in a level I trauma center. Am Surg. 2006;72:538–43.
20. Ehrlich PF, Brown JK, Sochor MR, et al. Factors influencing pediatric injury severity score and Glasgow Coma Scale in pediatric automobile crashes: results from the Crash Injury Research Engineering Network. J Pediatr Surg. 2006;41:1854–8.
21. Waddell JP, Drucker WR. Occult injuries in pedestrian accidents. J Trauma. 1971;11:844–52.
22. Orsborn R, Haley K, Hammond S, et al. Pediatric pedestrian versus motor vehicle patterns of injury: debunking the myth. Air Med J. 1999;18:107–10.
23. Le TV, Baaj AA, Deukmedjian A, et al. Chance fractures in the pediatric population. J Neurosurg Pediatr. 2011;8:189–97.
24. Santschi M, Lemoine C, Cyr C. The spectrum of seat belt syndrome among Canadian children: results of a two-year population surveillance study. Paediatr Child Health. 2008;13:279–83.
25. Abu-Kishk I, Vaiman M, Rosenfeld-Yehoshua N, et al. Riding a bicycle: do we need more than a helmet? Pediatr Int. 2010;52:644–7.
26. Ducrocq SC, Meyer PG, Orliaguet GA, et al. Epidemiology and early predictive factors of mortality and outcome in children with traumatic severe brain injury: experience of a French pediatric trauma center. Pediatr Crit Care Med. 2006;7:461–7.
27. Tude Melo JR, Di Rocco F, Blanot S, et al. Mortality in children with severe head trauma: predictive factors and proposal for a new predictive scale. Neurosurgery. 2010;67:1542–7.
28. Kilgo PD, Osler TM, Meredith W. The worst injury predicts mortality outcome the best: rethinking the role of multiple injuries in trauma outcome scoring. J Trauma. 2003;55:599–606; discussion 606–7.
29. Tepas 3rd JJ, Leaphart CL, Celso BG, et al. Risk stratification simplified: the worst injury predicts mortality for the injured children. J Trauma. 2008;65:1258–61; discussion 1261–3.
30. Jung J, Eo E, Ahn K, et al. Initial base deficit as predictors for mortality and transfusion requirement in the severe pediatric trauma except brain injury. Pediatr Emerg Care. 2009;25:579–81.
31. Kincaid EH, Chang MC, Letton RW, et al. Admission base deficit in pediatric trauma: a study using the National Trauma Data Bank. J Trauma. 2001;51:332–5.
32. Peterson DL, Schinco MA, Kerwin AJ, et al. Evaluation of initial base deficit as a prognosticator of outcome in the pediatric trauma population. Am Surg. 2004;70:326–8.
33. Borgman MA, Maegele M, Wade CE, et al. Pediatric trauma BIG score: predicting mortality in children after military and civilian trauma. Pediatrics. 2011;127:e892–7.
34. Esposito TJ, Sanddal ND, Hansen JD, et al. Analysis of preventable trauma deaths and inappropriate trauma care in a rural state. J Trauma. 1995;39:955–62.
35. Keel M, Trentz O. Pathophysiology of polytrauma. Injury. 2005;36:691–709.
36. Rotstein OD. Modeling the two-hit hypothesis for evaluating strategies to prevent organ injury after shock/resuscitation. J Trauma. 2003;54:S203–6.
37. Chesnut RM, Marshall LF, Klauber MR, et al. The role of secondary brain injury in determining outcome from severe head injury. J Trauma. 1993;34:216–22.
38. Chi JH, Knudson MM, Vassar MJ, et al. Prehospital hypoxia affects outcome in patients with traumatic brain injury: a prospective multicenter study. J Trauma. 2006;61:1134–41.
39. Pigula FA, Wald SL, Shackford SR, et al. The effect of hypotension and hypoxia on children with severe head injuries. J Pediatr Surg. 1993;28:310–4; discussion 315–6.
40. Chiaretti A, Piastra M, Pulitano S, et al. Prognostic factors and outcome of children with severe head injury: an 8-year experience. Childs Nerv Syst. 2002;18:129–36.
41. Kochanek PM, Carney N, Adelson PD, et al. Guidelines for the acute medical management of severe traumatic brain injury in infants, children, and adolescents–second edition. Pediatr Crit Care Med. 2012;13 Suppl 1:S1–82.

42. Zebrack M, Dandoy C, Hansen K, et al. Early resuscitation of children with moderate-to-severe traumatic brain injury. Pediatrics. 2009;124:56–64.

43. Tsukamoto T, Chanthaphavong RS, Pape HC. Current theories on the pathophysiology of multiple organ failure after trauma. Injury. 2010;41:21–6.

44. Desborough JP. The stress response to trauma and surgery. Br J Anaesth. 2000;85:109–17.

45. Wetzel RC, Burns RC. Multiple trauma in children: critical care overview. Crit Care Med. 2002;30:S468–77.

46. Hill AG, Hill GL. Metabolic response to severe injury. Br J Surg. 1998;85:884–90.

47. Laird AM, Miller PR, Kilgo PD, et al. Relationship of early hyperglycemia to mortality in trauma patients. J Trauma. 2004;56:1058–62.

48. Durward A, Mayer A, Skellett S, et al. Hypoalbuminaemia in critically ill children: incidence, prognosis, and influence on the anion gap. Arch Dis Child. 2003;88:419–22.

49. Horowitz IN, Tai K. Hypoalbuminemia in critically ill children. Arch Pediatr Adolesc Med. 2007;161:1048–52.

50. Safavi M, Honarmand A. The impact of admission hyperglycemia or hypoalbuminemia on need ventilator, time ventilated, mortality, and morbidity in critically ill trauma patients. Ulus Travma Acil Cerrahi Derg. 2009;15:120–9.

51. Sung J, Bochicchio GV, Joshi M, et al. Admission serum albumin is predictive of outcome in critically ill trauma patients. Am Surg. 2004;70:1099–102.

52. Wood JH, Partrick DA, Johnston Jr RB. The inflammatory response to injury in children. Curr Opin Pediatr. 2010;22:315–20.

53. Oppenheim JJ, Yang D. Alarmins: chemotactic activators of immune responses. Curr Opin Immunol. 2005;17:359–65.

54. Prince JM, Levy RM, Yang R, et al. Toll-like receptor-4 signaling mediates hepatic injury and systemic inflammation in hemorrhagic shock. J Am Coll Surg. 2006;202:407–17.

55. Kumar P, Shen Q, Pivetti CD, et al. Molecular mechanisms of endothelial hyperpermeability: implications in inflammation. Expert Rev Mol Med. 2009;11:e19.

56. Majetschak M, Borgermann J, Waydhas C, et al. Whole blood tumor necrosis factor-alpha production and its relation to systemic concentrations of interleukin 4, interleukin 10, and transforming growth factor-beta1 in multiply injured blunt trauma victims. Crit Care Med. 2000;28:1847–53.

57. Napolitano LM, Ferrer T, McCarter Jr RJ, et al. Systemic inflammatory response syndrome score at admission independently predicts mortality and length of stay in trauma patients. J Trauma. 2000;49:647–52; discussion 652–3.

58. Sakamoto Y, Mashiko K, Matsumoto H, et al. Systemic inflammatory response syndrome score at admission predicts injury severity, organ damage and serum neutrophil elastase production in trauma patients. J Nippon Med Sch. 2010;77:138–44.

59. Stensballe J, Christiansen M, Tonnesen E, et al. The early IL-6 and IL-10 response in trauma is correlated with injury severity and mortality. Acta Anaesthesiol Scand. 2009;53:515–21.

60. Bhatia R, Dent C, Topley N, et al. Neutrophil priming for elastase release in adult blunt trauma patients. J Trauma. 2006;60:590–6.

61. Ramaiah SK, Jaeschke H. Role of neutrophils in the pathogenesis of acute inflammatory liver injury. Toxicol Pathol. 2007;35:757–66.

62. Zallen G, Moore EE, Johnson JL, et al. Circulating postinjury neutrophils are primed for the release of proinflammatory cytokines. J Trauma. 1999;46:42–8.

63. Harris BH, Gelfand JA. The immune response to trauma. Semin Pediatr Surg. 1995;4:77–82.

64. Bone RC. Sir Isaac Newton, sepsis, SIRS, and CARS. Crit Care Med. 1996;24:1125–8.

65. Kasten KR, Goetzman HS, Reid MR, et al. Divergent adaptive and innate immunological responses are observed in humans following blunt trauma. BMC Immunol. 2010;11:4.

66. Ward NS, Casserly B, Ayala A. The compensatory anti-inflammatory response syndrome (CARS) in critically ill patients. Clin Chest Med. 2008;29:617–25, viii.

67. American College of Chest Physicians/Society of Critical Care Medicine Consensus Conference: definitions for sepsis and organ failure and guidelines for the use of innovative therapies in sepsis. Crit Care Med. 1992;20:864–74.

68. Calkins CM, Bensard DD, Moore EE, et al. The injured child is resistant to multiple organ failure: a different inflammatory response? J Trauma. 2002;53:1058–63.

69. Proulx F, Joyal JS, Mariscalco MM, et al. The pediatric multiple organ dysfunction syndrome. Pediatr Crit Care Med. 2009;10:12–22.

70. Thomas NJ, Lucking SE, Dillon PW, et al. Is the injured child different or just treated differently with respect to the development of multiple organ dysfunction syndrome? J Trauma. 2003;55:181–2; author reply 183–4.

71. Badjatia N, Carney N, Crocco TJ, et al. Guidelines for prehospital management of traumatic brain injury 2nd edition. Prehosp Emerg Care. 2008;12 Suppl 1:S1–52.

72. Bratton SL, Chestnut RM, Ghajar J, et al. Guidelines for the management of severe traumatic brain injury. I. Blood pressure and oxygenation. J Neurotrauma. 2007;24 Suppl 1:S7–13.

73. Celso B, Tepas J, Langland-Orban B, et al. A systematic review and meta-analysis comparing outcome of severely injured patients treated in trauma centers following the establishment of trauma systems. J Trauma. 2006;60:371–8; discussion 378.

74. Chiaretti A, De Benedictis R, Della Corte F, et al. The impact of initial management on the outcome of children with severe head injury. Childs Nerv Syst. 2002;18:54–60.

75. Harris T, Davenport R, Hurst T, et al. Improving outcome in severe trauma: trauma systems and initial management: intubation, ventilation and resuscitation. Postgrad Med J. 2012;88:588–94.

76. Klemen P, Grmec S. Effect of pre-hospital advanced life support with rapid sequence intubation on outcome of severe traumatic brain injury. Acta Anaesthesiol Scand. 2006;50:1250–4.

77. Regel G, Stalp M, Lehmann U, et al. Prehospital care, importance of early intervention on outcome. Acta Anaesthesiol Scand Suppl. 1997;110:71–6.

78. Winchell RJ, Hoyt DB. Endotracheal intubation in the field improves survival in patients with severe head injury. Trauma Research and Education Foundation of San Diego. Arch Surg. 1997;132:592–7.

79. Berlot G, La Fata C, Bacer B, et al. Influence of prehospital treatment on the outcome of patients with severe blunt traumatic brain injury: a single-centre study. Eur J Emerg Med. 2009;16:312–7.

80. Cooper A, DiScala C, Foltin G, et al. Prehospital endotracheal intubation for severe head injury in children: a reappraisal. Semin Pediatr Surg. 2001;10:3–6.

81. DiRusso SM, Sullivan T, Risucci D, et al. Intubation of pediatric trauma patients in the field: predictor of negative outcome despite risk stratification. J Trauma. 2005;59:84–90; discussion 90–1.

82. Eckstein M, Chan L, Schneir A, et al. Effect of prehospital advanced life support on outcomes of major trauma patients. J Trauma. 2000;48:643–8.

83. Lockey D, Davies G, Coats T. Survival of trauma patients who have prehospital tracheal intubation without anaesthesia or muscle relaxants: observational study. BMJ. 2001;323:141.

84. Stockinger ZT, McSwain Jr NE. Prehospital endotracheal intubation for trauma does not improve survival over bag-valve-mask ventilation. J Trauma. 2004;56:531–6.

85. Wang HE, Peitzman AB, Cassidy LD, et al. Out-of-hospital endotracheal intubation and outcome after traumatic brain injury. Ann Emerg Med. 2004;44:439–50.

86. Gausche M, Lewis RJ, Stratton SJ, et al. Effect of out-of-hospital pediatric endotracheal intubation on survival and neurological outcome: a controlled clinical trial. JAMA. 2000;283:783–90.

87. Davis DP, Ochs M, Hoyt DB, et al. Paramedic-administered neuromuscular blockade improves prehospital intubation success in severely head-injured patients. J Trauma. 2003;55:713–9.

88. Ehrlich PF, Seidman PS, Atallah O, et al. Endotracheal intubations in rural pediatric trauma patients. J Pediatr Surg. 2004;39:1376–80.

89. Orf J, Thomas SH, Ahmed W, et al. Appropriateness of endotracheal tube size and insertion depth in children undergoing air medical transport. Pediatr Emerg Care. 2000;16:321–7.

90. Boswell WC, McElveen N, Sharp M, et al. Analysis of prehospital pediatric and adult intubation. Air Med J. 1995;14:125–7; discussion 127–8.

91. Bochicchio GV, Ilahi O, Joshi M, et al. Endotracheal intubation in the field does not improve outcome in trauma patients who present without an acutely lethal traumatic brain injury. J Trauma. 2003; 54:307–11.

92. Karch SB, Lewis T, Young S, et al. Field intubation of trauma patients: complications, indications, and outcomes. Am J Emerg Med. 1996;14:617–9.

93. Murray JA, Demetriades D, Berne TV, et al. Prehospital intubation in patients with severe head injury. J Trauma. 2000;49:1065–70.

94. Garner A, Rashford S, Lee A, et al. Addition of physicians to paramedic helicopter services decreases blunt trauma mortality. Aust N Z J Surg. 1999;69:697–701.

95. Harrison TH, Thomas SH, Wedel SK. Success rates of pediatric intubation by a non-physician-staffed critical care transport service. Pediatr Emerg Care. 2004;20:101–7.

96. Golparvar M, Saghaei M, Sajedi P, et al. Paradoxical reaction following intravenous midazolam premedication in pediatric patients – a randomized placebo controlled trial of ketamine for rapid tranquilization. Paediatr Anaesth. 2004;14:924–30.

97. Aroni F, Iacovidou N, Dontas I, et al. Pharmacological aspects and potential new clinical applications of ketamine: reevaluation of an old drug. J Clin Pharmacol. 2009;49:957–64.

98. Bar-Joseph G, Guilburd Y, Tamir A, et al. Effectiveness of ketamine in decreasing intracranial pressure in children with intracranial hypertension. J Neurosurg Pediatr. 2009;4:40–6.

99. Sehdev RS, Symmons DA, Kindl K. Ketamine for rapid sequence induction in patients with head injury in the emergency department. Emerg Med Australas. 2006;18:37–44.

100. Filanovsky Y, Miller P, Kao J. Myth: ketamine should not be used as an induction agent for intubation in patients with head injury. CJEM. 2010;12:154–7.

101. Jamora C, Iravani M. Unique clinical situations in pediatric patients where ketamine may be the anesthetic agent of choice. Am J Ther. 2010;17:511–5.

102. Dershwitz M, Rosow C. Pharmacology of intravenous anesthetics. In: Longbecker DE, Brown D, Newman MF, Zapol WM, editors. Anesthesiology. New York: McGraw-Hill; 2008. p. 849–68.

103. Heard CMB, Fletcher JE. Sedation and analgesia. In: Fuhrman BP, Zimmerman JJ, editors. Pediatric critical care. 3rd ed. Philadelphia: Mosby, Elsevier; 2006. p. 1748–79.

104. Bredmose PP, Grier G, Davies GE, et al. Pre-hospital use of ketamine in paediatric trauma. Acta Anaesthesiol Scand. 2009;53: 543–5.

105. Melamed E, Oron Y, Ben-Avraham R, et al. The combative multi-trauma patient: a protocol for prehospital management. Eur J Emerg Med. 2007;14:265–8.

106. Svenson JE, Abernathy MK. Ketamine for prehospital use: new look at an old drug. Am J Emerg Med. 2007;25:977–80.

107. Kleinman ME, Chameides L, Schexnayder SM, et al. Part 14: pediatric advanced life support: 2010 American Heart Association Guidelines for Cardiopulmonary Resuscitation and Emergency Cardiovascular Care. Circulation. 2010;122:S876–908.

108. Fiorito BA, Mirza F, Doran TM, et al. Intraosseous access in the setting of pediatric critical care transport. Pediatr Crit Care Med. 2005;6:50–3.

109. Weiser G, Hoffmann Y, Galbraith R, et al. Current advances in intraosseous infusion – a systematic review. Resuscitation. 2012;83: 20–6.

110. Shavit I, Hoffmann Y, Galbraith R, et al. Comparison of two mechanical intraosseous infusion devices: a pilot, randomized crossover trial. Resuscitation. 2009;80:1029–33.

111. Perel P, Roberts I. Colloids versus crystalloids for fluid resuscitation in critically ill patients. Cochrane Database Syst Rev. 2013;2:CD000567.

112. Dung NM, Day NP, Tam DT, et al. Fluid replacement in dengue shock syndrome: a randomized, double-blind comparison of four intravenous-fluid regimens. Clin Infect Dis. 1999;29:787–94.

113. Upadhyay M, Singhi S, Murlidharan J, et al. Randomized evaluation of fluid resuscitation with crystalloid (saline) and colloid (polymer from degraded gelatin in saline) in pediatric septic shock. Indian Pediatr. 2005;42:223–31.

114. Wills BA, Nguyen MD, Ha TL, et al. Comparison of three fluid solutions for resuscitation in dengue shock syndrome. N Engl J Med. 2005;353:877–89.

115. Angle N, Hoyt DB, Coimbra R, et al. Hypertonic saline resuscitation diminishes lung injury by suppressing neutrophil activation after hemorrhagic shock. Shock. 1998;9:164–70.

116. Deitch EA, Shi HP, Feketeova E, et al. Hypertonic saline resuscitation limits neutrophil activation after trauma-hemorrhagic shock. Shock. 2003;19:328–33.

117. Ducey JP, Mozingo DW, Lamiell JM, et al. A comparison of the cerebral and cardiovascular effects of complete resuscitation with isotonic and hypertonic saline, hetastarch, and whole blood following hemorrhage. J Trauma. 1989;29:1510–8.

118. Traverso LW, Bellamy RF, Hollenbach SJ, et al. Hypertonic sodium chloride solutions: effect on hemodynamics and survival after hemorrhage in swine. J Trauma. 1987;27:32–9.

119. Wade CE, Kramer GC, Grady JJ, et al. Efficacy of hypertonic 7.5 % saline and 6 % dextran-70 in treating trauma: a meta-analysis of controlled clinical studies. Surgery. 1997;122:609–16.

120. Bulger EM, May S, Kerby JD, et al. Out-of-hospital hypertonic resuscitation after traumatic hypovolemic shock: a randomized, placebo controlled trial. Ann Surg. 2011;253:431–41.

121. Bulger EM, May S, Brasel KJ, et al. Out-of-hospital hypertonic resuscitation following severe traumatic brain injury: a randomized controlled trial. JAMA. 2010;304:1455–64.

122. Myburgh JA, Finfer S, Bellomo R, et al. Hydroxyethyl starch or saline for fluid resuscitation in intensive care. N Engl J Med. 2012;367:1901–11.

123. Perner A, Haase N, Guttormsen AB, et al. Hydroxyethyl starch 130/0.42 versus Ringer's acetate in severe sepsis. N Engl J Med. 2012;367:124–34.

124. Zarychanski R, Abou-Setta AM, Turgeon AF, et al. Association of hydroxyethyl starch administration with mortality and acute kidney injury in critically ill patients requiring volume resuscitation: a systematic review and meta-analysis. JAMA. 2013;309: 678–88.

125. Holcomb JB, Wade CE, Michalek JE, et al. Increased plasma and platelet to red blood cell ratios improves outcome in 466 massively transfused civilian trauma patients. Ann Surg. 2008;248: 447–58.

126. Shaz BH, Dente CJ, Nicholas J, et al. Increased number of coagulation products in relationship to red blood cell products transfused improves mortality in trauma patients. Transfusion. 2010;50: 493–500.

127. Peiniger S, Nienaber U, Lefering R, et al. Balanced massive transfusion ratios in multiple injury patients with traumatic brain injury. Crit Care. 2011;15:R68.

128. Cotton BA, Au BK, Nunez TC, et al. Predefined massive transfusion protocols are associated with a reduction in organ failure and postinjury complications. J Trauma. 2009;66:41–8; discussion 48–9.

129. Dente CJ, Shaz BH, Nicholas JM, et al. Improvements in early mortality and coagulopathy are sustained better in patients with blunt trauma after institution of a massive transfusion protocol in a civilian level I trauma center. J Trauma. 2009;66:1616–24.

130. Dehmer JJ, Adamson WT. Massive transfusion and blood product use in the pediatric trauma patient. Semin Pediatr Surg. 2010;19:286–91.

131. Hendrickson JE, Shaz BH, Pereira G, et al. Implementation of a pediatric trauma massive transfusion protocol: one institution's experience. Transfusion. 2012;52:1228–36.

132. Paterson NA. Validation of a theoretically derived model for the management of massive blood loss in pediatric patients – a case report. Paediatr Anaesth. 2009;19:535–40.

133. McKenney KL, Nunez Jr DB, McKenney MG, et al. Sonography as the primary screening technique for blunt abdominal trauma: experience with 899 patients. AJR Am J Roentgenol. 1998;170:979–85.

134. Rothlin MA, Naf R, Amgwerd M, et al. Ultrasound in blunt abdominal and thoracic trauma. J Trauma. 1993;34:488–95.

135. Smith ZA, Wood D. Emergency focussed assessment with sonography in trauma (FAST) and haemodynamic stability. Emerg Med J. 2013.

136. Soudack M, Epelman M, Maor R, et al. Experience with focused abdominal sonography for trauma (FAST) in 313 pediatric patients. J Clin Ultrasound. 2004;32:53–61.

137. Patel JC, Tepas 3rd JJ. The efficacy of focused abdominal sonography for trauma (FAST) as a screening tool in the assessment of injured children. J Pediatr Surg. 1999;34:44–7; discussion 52–4.

138. Hartin Jr CW, Jordan JM, Gemme S, et al. Computed tomography scanning in pediatric trauma: opportunities for performance improvement and radiation safety. J Surg Res. 2013;180:226–31.

139. Sodickson A. Strategies for reducing radiation exposure in multidetector row CT. Radiol Clin North Am. 2012;50:1–14.

140. Kim PK, Zhu X, Houseknecht E, et al. Effective radiation dose from radiologic studies in pediatric trauma patients. World J Surg. 2005;29:1557–62.

141. Kharbanda AB, Flood A, Blumberg K, et al. Analysis of radiation exposure among pediatric trauma patients at national trauma centers. J Trauma Acute Care Surg. 2013;74:907–11.

142. Danks RR. Triangle of death. How hypothermia acidosis & coagulopathy can adversely impact trauma patients. JEMS. 2002;27 (61–66):68–70.

143. Mitra B, Cameron PA, Parr MJ, et al. Recombinant factor VIIa in trauma patients with the 'triad of death'. Injury. 2012;43:1409–14.

144. Murphy P, Colwell C, Pineda G. Understand the trauma triad of death: know its components to help protect patients. EMS World. 2012;41:44–51.

145. Rutherford EJ, Fusco MA, Nunn CR, et al. Hypothermia in critically ill trauma patients. Injury. 1998;29:605–8.

146. Davenport R. Pathogenesis of acute traumatic coagulopathy. Transfusion. 2013;53 Suppl 1:23S–7.

147. Moffatt SE. Hypothermia in trauma. Emerg Med J. 2012.

148. Shafi S, Elliott AC, Gentilello L. Is hypothermia simply a marker of shock and injury severity or an independent risk factor for mortality in trauma patients? Analysis of a large national trauma registry. J Trauma. 2005;59:1081–5.

149. Soreide K. Clinical and translational aspects of hypothermia in major trauma patients: from pathophysiology to prevention, prognosis and potential preservation. Injury. 2014;45:647–54. pii: S0020-1383(13)00009-0.

150. Hamill J. Damage control surgery in children. Injury. 2004;35(7):708–12.

151. Martini WZ. Coagulopathy by hypothermia and acidosis: mechanisms of thrombin generation and fibrinogen availability. J Trauma. 2009;67:202–8; discussion 208–9.

152. Brohi K, Cohen MJ, Ganter MT, et al. Acute coagulopathy of trauma: hypoperfusion induces systemic anticoagulation and hyperfibrinolysis. J Trauma. 2008;64:1211–7; discussion 1217.

153. Hess JR, Brohi K, Dutton RP, et al. The coagulopathy of trauma: a review of mechanisms. J Trauma. 2008;65:748–54.

154. Sharp KW, Locicero RJ. Abdominal packing for surgically uncontrollable hemorrhage. Ann Surg. 1992;215:467–74; discussion 474–5.

155. Moore EE, Thomas G. Orr memorial lecture. Staged laparotomy for the hypothermia, acidosis, and coagulopathy syndrome. Am J Surg. 1996;172:405–10.

156. Rotondo MF, Schwab CW, McGonigal MD, et al. 'Damage control': an approach for improved survival in exsanguinating penetrating abdominal injury. J Trauma. 1993;35:375–82; discussion 382–3.

157. Giannoudis PV, Giannoudi M, Stavlas P. Damage control orthopaedics: lessons learned. Injury. 2009;40 Suppl 4:S47–52.

158. Mooney JF. The use of 'damage control orthopedics' techniques in children with segmental open femur fractures. J Pediatr Orthop B. 2012;21:400–3.

159. Shapiro MB, Jenkins DH, Schwab CW, et al. Damage control: collective review. J Trauma. 2000;49:969–78.

160. Stylianos S. Abdominal packing for severe hemorrhage. J Pediatr Surg. 1998;33:339–42.

161. Porras-Ramirez G. Damage control surgery in pediatric trauma. Rev Mex Cir Pediatr. 2008;15:30–4.

162. Yin Q, Zhou XY, Xiao YL, et al. Application of damage control surgery in serious pediatric abdominal surgery. Zhongguo Dang Dai Er Ke Za Zhi. 2009;11:729–32.

163. Stylianos S. Evidence-based guidelines for resource utilization in children with isolated spleen or liver injury. The APSA Trauma Committee. J Pediatr Surg. 2000;35:164–7; discussion 167–9.

164. Stylianos S. Compliance with evidence-based guidelines in children with isolated spleen or liver injury: a prospective study. J Pediatr Surg. 2002;37:453–6.

165. Jim J, Leonardi MJ, Cryer HG, et al. Management of high-grade splenic injury in children. Am Surg. 2008;74:988–92.

166. Keller MS, Sartorelli KH, Vane DW. Associated head injury should not prevent nonoperative management of spleen or liver injury in children. J Trauma. 1996;41:471–5.

167. Coburn MC, Pfeifer J, DeLuca FG. Nonoperative management of splenic and hepatic trauma in the multiply injured pediatric and adolescent patient. Arch Surg. 1995;130:332–8.

168. Ceran S, Sunam GS, Aribas OK, et al. Chest trauma in children. Eur J Cardiothorac Surg. 2002;21:57–9.

169. Meier R, Krettek C, Grimme K, et al. The multiply injured child. Clin Orthop Relat Res. 2005;432:127–31.

170. Tovar JA, Vazquez JJ. Management of chest trauma in children. Paediatr Respir Rev. 2013;14:86–91.

171. Buschmann C, Kuhne CA, Losch C, et al. Major trauma with multiple injuries in German children: a retrospective review. J Pediatr Orthop. 2008;28:1–5.

172. Cooper A, Barlow B, DiScala C, et al. Mortality and truncal injury: the pediatric perspective. J Pediatr Surg. 1994;29:33–8.

173. Inan M, Ayvaz S, Sut N, et al. Blunt chest trauma in childhood. ANZ J Surg. 2007;77:682–5.

174. Black TL, Snyder CL, Miller JP, et al. Significance of chest trauma in children. South Med J. 1996;89:494–6.

175. Hamrick MC, Duhn RD, Ochsner MG. Critical evaluation of pulmonary contusion in the early post-traumatic period: risk of assisted ventilation. Am Surg. 2009;75:1054–8.

176. Hamrick MC, Duhn RD, Carney DE, et al. Pulmonary contusion in the pediatric population. Am Surg. 2010;76:721–4.

177. Ismail MF, al-Refaie RI. Chest trauma in children, single center experience. Arch Bronconeumol. 2012;48:362–6.

Coma and Altered Mental Status

Alexis Topjian and Nicholas S. Abend

Abstract

Coma is a neurologic state that is described as loss of wakefulness and decreased awareness of one's surroundings. It is caused by multiple etiologies and is a medical emergency that must be rapidly evaluated and treated. Treatable causes (meningitis and intracranial hypertension) and emergently required interventions (neurosurgical procedures) should be addressed after evaluation of airway, breathing, and circulation. Further investigation into etiology should be performed systematically, taking into account age, history and physical exam findings. Thorough neurologic examination, laboratory evaluation and imaging can help derive the etiology of coma. Patients may fully recover, remain in a minimally conscious state or persistent vegetative state, or progress to brain death. Recovery is dependent on the underlying coma etiology. Prognostication of outcome can be performed using multimodal neurologic monitoring modalities including repeated neurologic examination, evoked potentials, electroencephalography, neuroimaging, and natural history of disease. Clinician experience, prognostics data, and familial values together can impact the long term outcomes of the patients.

Keywords

Coma • Herniation • Hypoxic ischemia • Traumatic brain injury prognosis • Vegetative state • Neurologic examination

Introduction

Coma is a neurologic state that can result from a wide variety of etiologies including both primary neurologic and systemic conditions. Evaluation of the comatose child starts with immediate assessment of airway, breathing, and circulation. History and physical examination should be rapid and thorough. Diagnosis and treatment should be tiered to initially target life threatening etiologies that are reversible and treatable. Determination of the etiology of the underlying cause will direct management. In this chapter we will (1) define coma and other states of altered consciousness, (2) review the pathophysiology underlying coma, (3) discuss the differential diagnosis of coma, (4) outline an approach to the evaluation and management of the comatose child, (5) review specifics of herniation syndromes and management, and (6) discuss prognosis.

A. Topjian, MD, MSCE (✉)
Department of Anesthesia and Critical Care,
The Children's Hospital of Philadelphia,
3401 Civic Center Boulevard, Philadelphia, PA 19104, USA
e-mail: topjian@email.chop.edu

N.S. Abend, MD
Department of Neurology and Pediatrics, The Children's Hospital of Philadelphia, 3501 Civic Center Blvd, CTRB 10016, Philadelphia, PA 19104, USA
e-mail: abend@email.chop.edu

Epidemiology

The incidence of non-traumatic coma is 30/100,000 children per year [1] and the incidence of traumatic coma in children is 140/100,000 [2], with the most severe cases comprising 5.6/100,000 [3]. Non-traumatic coma is more common in

D.S. Wheeler et al. (eds.), *Pediatric Critical Care Medicine*,
DOI 10.1007/978-1-4471-6362-6_33, © Springer-Verlag London 2014

younger children and has a 46 % 12 month mortality rate [1]. Mortality is highly dependent on the etiology for coma, and ranges from 3 % to 84 %. Traumatic brain injury is often responsible for coma. Approximately 27 % of patients with traumatic brain injury had an initial Glasgow Coma Score of less than nine [3].

Consciousness and Coma and Altered Mental Status Definitions

Normal consciousness is a state of wakefulness and awareness of self and surroundings. *Coma* is a state of altered consciousness, with loss of both wakefulness (arousal, vigilance) and awareness of the self and environment. Coma is characterized by closed eyes and inability to be aroused to respond appropriately to stimuli [4]. Sleep-wake cycles are absent. Coma is a temporary state and evolves towards normal consciousness, a minimally conscious state, a vegetative state, or brain death.

Between normal consciousness and coma is a spectrum of states of decreasing consciousness. Decreased consciousness states are lethargy, obtundation, and stupor. *Lethargy* is a state of reduced wakefulness where subjects are sleepy but can be easily roused. *Obtundation* is characterized by sleepiness that persists even with stimulation. *Stupor* is a state of unresponsiveness with little or no spontaneous movement. Stupor resembles deep sleep, but differs from coma because vigorous stimulation induces temporary arousal. *Delirium* is an acute state characterized by decreased awareness of the environment, with changes in level of consciousness, impaired attention, and a waxing and waning course.

If a patient does not improve from coma toward a normal state, they may evolve into a vegetative state or minimally conscious state. A patient in the *persistent vegetative state* is awake but unaware and has sleep-wake cycles, but has no detectable cerebral cortical function. The eyes may be open, but there is no visual fixation or pursuit. Generally this state is not diagnosed until 1 month after the coma onset. A patient in a *minimally conscious state* has severely altered consciousness with minimal, but definite evidence of self or environmental awareness, such as following simple commands or making simple non-reflexive gestures. Recent use of functional neuroimaging has initiated controversy as to whether patients who are presumed to be in a persistent vegetative state based on clinical exam may actually be in a minimally conscious state [5]. *Akinetic mutism* is a condition of extreme slowing or absence of bodily movement with loss of speech. Wakefulness and awareness are preserved but cognition is slowed. This is caused by extensive injury to the bilateral inferior frontal lobes, paramedian mesencephalic reticular formation, or the posterior diencephalon. The *locked-in syndrome* is a state of preserved consciousness and cognition with complete paralysis of the voluntary motor

system. Cortical function is intact and electroencephalogram (EEG) patterns are normal. Vertical eye movements may be preserved, allowing for some communication. The locked-in state may result from lesions of the corticospinal and corticobulbar pathways at or below the pons, posterior circulation infarcts, or severe peripheral nervous system disease such as Guillain-Barre syndrome, botulism, and critical illness polyneuropathy. Finally, coma must also be distinguished from brain death. The determination of brain death (irreversible cessation of neurologic function) is based on the absence of neurologic function with a known etiology, including absence of all brain activity, including brainstem function [6]. The diagnosis of brain death is discussed in detail in another chapter of this textbook.

Anatomy of the Brain in Relation to Coma

The reticular activating system constitutes the central core of the brainstem and extends from the caudal medulla to the thalamus and the basal forebrain. The reticular activating system transmits sensory input from the periphery through the brainstem to the cerebral cortices. The reticular activating system activates the cortex, participates in feedback control and is responsible for regulating arousal. Bilateral cortical injury or brainstem injury impacting the reticular activating system connections results in coma.

Causes of Coma

The causes of coma are broad and are listed in Table 33.1. Non-traumatic coma may be due to primary brain dysfunction, such as seizures or encephalitis, or secondary impact on

Table 33.1 Causes of coma

Trauma
Parenchymal injury
Intracranial hemorrhage
Epidural hematoma
Subdural hematoma
Subarachnoid hemorrhage
Intracerebral hematoma
Diffuse axonal injury
Accidental vs non-accidental
Concussion
Non-traumatic causes
Hypoxic ischemic encephalopathy
Shock
Cardiopulmonary arrest
Near drowning
Carbon monoxide poisoning
Stroke

Table 33.1 (continued)

Toxins

    Medications: narcotics, sedatives, antiepileptics, antidepressants, analgesics, aspirin

    Environmental toxins: organophosphates, heavy metals, cyanide, mushroom poisoning

    Illicit substances: alcohol, heroine, amphetamines, cocaine

Systemic metabolic disorders

    Substrate deficiencies

        Hypoglycemia

        Cofactors: thiamine, niacin, pyridoxine, B12

    Electrolyte and acid-base imbalance: sodium, magnesium, calcium

    Diabetic ketoacidosis

    Thyroid/adrenal/other endocrine disorders

    Uremic coma

    Hepatic coma

    Reye syndrome

    Inborn errors of metabolism

        Urea cycle disorders

        Amino acidopathies

        Organic acidopathies

        Mitochondrial disorders

    Sepsis

Infections/postinfectious/inflammatory

    Meningitis and encephalitis: bacterial, viral, rickettsial, fungal

    Acute demyelinating diseases

        Acute disseminated encephalomyelitis (ADEM)

        Multiple sclerosis

Inflammatory/autoimmune

    Sarcoidosis

    Sjogren's disease

    Lupus cerebritis

Mass lesions

    Neoplasms

    Abscess, granuloma

    Hydrocephalus

Paroxysmal neurologic disorders

    Seizures/status epilepticus

    Acute confusional migraine

Vascular

    Intracranial hemorrhage – SAH/SDH/ epidural hematomas

    Arterial infarcts

    Venous sinus thromboses with venous infarcts

    Vasculitis

the brain due to global derangements. Causes of coma may be multifactorial such as meningitis leading to an epidural empyema and elevated intracranial pressure, sinus venous thrombosis, and status epilepticus. In a population-based study, 278 of over 600,000 children between the ages of 1 month and 16 years had 345 episodes of coma [1]. Infection was the most common cause of non-traumatic coma, accounting for 38 % of cases. Intoxication, epilepsy, and complications of congenital abnormalities each accounted for 8–10 %

of cases, while accidents and metabolic causes were each responsible for 6 % of cases. Incidence of non-traumatic coma also varies with age, with the highest incidence age group being less than 1 year of age. Traumatic brain injury results in an annual hospitalization rates of 129 per 100,000 of adolescents and 80 per 100,000 for children younger than years of age [7]. Major causes of traumatic brain injury requiring care in the ICU are inflicted trauma less <1 year of age (30 per 100,000 children annually) and non-inflicted trauma in toddlers (10 per 100,000 children annually). Inflicted trauma is more common than non-inflicted trauma for children under 1 year of age.

Evaluation of the Comatose Child

The evaluation of the comatose child must be performed rapidly and thoroughly to identify and manage the immediate life threatening causes of coma. Interventions to stabilize, diagnose, and then treat the comatose patient should follow a tiered approach. Initially, one must address airway, breathing, and circulation and then move on to rapidly correctable derangements. Diagnosis and management should happen concurrently. An algorithm for initial evaluation of coma is outlined in Table 33.2 and discussed below. The Pediatric Accident and Emergency Research Group of the Royal College of Paediatrics and Child Health and the British Association for Emergency Medicine have published related guidelines, including a management algorithm (www.nottingham.ac.uk/paediatric-guideline) [8].

History

A detailed history may not always be available on initial evaluation of the comatose child, but historical information must be gathered as quickly as possible, as it may be crucial in identifying the cause of coma. The history must include a detailed description of events leading to coma, with particular attention to timing of events, potential exposures, and accompanying symptoms. Preceding somnolence suggests a metabolic or toxic or infectious cause, such as toxin ingestion, liver failure, or encephalitis; sudden onset of coma without trauma suggests spontaneous intracranial hemorrhage, seizure, or cardiac arrhythmia resulting in hypoxic-ischemic encephalopathy. Previous fever with or without neck stiffness may suggest meningitis or encephalitis, but may also be a symptom of autoimmune processes such as acute disseminated encephalomyelitis or lupus cerebritis. Acute onset of headache may be due to spontaneous intracranial hemorrhage from arteriovenous malformation rupture, aneurysm rupture, or unwitnessed trauma. Chronic headache may suggest hydrocephalus, an expanding mass lesion such

Table 33.2 Initial evaluation of coma

Airway, breathing, and circulation assessment and stabilization.
Ensure adequate ventilation and oxygenation
Blood pressure management depends on considerations regarding underlying coma etiology. If hypertensive encephalopathy or intracranial hemorrhage then lower blood pressure. If perfusion dependent state such as some strokes or elevated intracranial pressure then reducing blood pressure may reduce cerebral perfusion
Draw blood for glucose, electrolytes, ammonia, arterial blood gas, liver and renal function tests, complete blood count, and toxicology screen
Neurological assessment
GCS score
Evidence of gag reflex and pupillary exam
Assess for evidence of raised intracranial pressure and herniation
Assess for abnormalities suggesting focal neurologic disease
Assess for history or signs of seizures
Administer glucose intravenously if hypoglycemic
If there is concern for infection with fever of neck rigidity and LP must be delayed broad spectrum infection coverage to treat bacterial and viral meningitis (e.g., Vancomycin/cefotaxime (ampicillin if less than 1 month to treat listeria) and acyclovir for potential HSV)
Give specific antidotes if toxic exposures are known
For opiate overdose administer naloxone
Identify and treat critical elevations in intracranial pressure
Neutral head position, elevated head by 20°, sedation
Hyperosmolar therapy with mannitol 0.5–1 g/K or hypertonic saline
Hyperventilation as temporary measure
Secure the airway
Consider intracranial monitoring
Consider neurosurgical intervention
Head CT
Treat seizures with IV anticonvulsants. Consider prophylactic anticonvulsants
Investigate source of fever and use antipyretics and/or cooling devices to reduce cerebral metabolic demands
Detailed history and examination

Consider: lumbar puncture, EEG or extended long term EEG monitoring, MRI, metabolic testing (amino acids, organic acids, acylcarnitine profile), autoimmune testing (ANA panel, antithyroid antibodies), thyroid testing (TSH, T3, T4)

as tumor, or indolent infection. Questions about possible toxic ingestions should include a survey of medications and poisons kept in the places the child has recently been.

The child's past medical history may be valuable. A history of multiple episodes of coma, developmental delay, or other prior neurologic abnormalities suggest inborn errors of metabolism, but may also indicate the presence of epilepsy with ongoing non-convulsive seizures or a post-ictal state. Toxic ingestions or inflicted childhood neurotrauma are also suggested by multiple episodes of coma. Recent weight changes or other constitutional abnormalities suggest endocrine dysfunction. Previous history of immunosuppression or HIV may suggest atypical CNS infections. A history of uncontrolled hypertension may suggest Posterior Reversible Encephalopathy Syndrome (PRES). Previously existing cardiac disease raises the possibility of dysrhythmia or cardiac failure leading to hypoxic ischemic encephalopathy. Travel history may explain exposure to infections prevalent in certain areas, such as Lyme Disease in the northeastern Unites States. Exposure to kittens in a patient with axillary or inguinal lymphadenopathy may be a clue to infection with *Bartonella henselae*, which causes cat scratch encephalopathy.

Eliciting a history of trauma, whether accidental or inflicted, is crucial. Understanding the mechanism of injury can direct further investigation. Intracranial lesions such as epidural hematomas may result in delayed loss of consciousness and require emergent intervention. Base of the skull fractures may compromise blood flow in the carotid artery or result in dissection of the artery as it enters the skull or travels in the petrous canal. In children under 2 years of age or in non-verbal children with developmental delay or intellectual disability, it is critical to have a high index of suspicion for non-accidental trauma. A broad approach to physical exam and diagnostic testing can often uncover the source of coma in these situations.

Physical Examination

The general examination should start with assessment and continuous monitoring of the vital signs. *Hyperthermia* suggests infection, autoimmune processes, heat stroke and anticholinergic ingestion. *Hypothermia* may also be due to sepsis as well as hypothyroidism, adrenal insufficiency, chronic malnutrition, or environmental exposure. *Hypotension* may be due to sepsis, cardiac dysfunction (which may cause or be due to neurologic injury), toxic ingestion, or adrenal insufficiency, and may lead to poor cerebral perfusion thereby causing or worsening brain injury. If not quickly normalized, diffuse or watershed hypoxic-ischemic injury may occur. *Hypertension* can be a physiologic response to increased intracranial pressure that functions to maintain cerebral perfusion pressure. Hypertension with bradycardia and a change in breathing pattern (Cushing's triad) is an ominous sign of elevated intracranial pressure and suggests impending herniation. In this situation, acutely lowering blood pressure may worsen neurologic injury by reducing cerebral perfusion. However, hypertension may be caused by toxin ingestion such as cocaine, thyrotoxicosis or renal disease, and may produce hypertensive encephalopathy (posterior reversible leukoencephalopathy) in which case management focuses on reducing blood pressure. Differentiating reactive/compensatory hypertension from a hypertensive encephalopathy may be difficult. While treating hypotension is critical to maintain cerebral perfusion, treating hypertension without understanding its cause can result in secondary neurologic injury and potential systemic injury. *Tachycardia* should raise concerns of pain, seizures, toxic ingestions, sepsis, and cardiogenic shock. *Bradycardia* is concerning for a patient who may be in a pre-arrest state from hypoxia or hypotension, hypothermia, toxic ingestion, chronic malnutrition, or intracranial hypertension.

Abnormalities in respiratory rate and pattern of breathing may indicate a systemic hypermetabolic state such as fever, intrinsic lung pathology, acid-base derangement, toxin ingestion or nervous system dysfunction. Cheyne-Stokes respiration describes a rhythmic and cycling pattern of accelerating hyperpnea followed by a fall in amplitude of breathing, decelerating rate of breathing, and apnea. It is a nonspecific pattern observed with extensive bihemispheric cerebral dysfunction, diencephalic (thalamic and hypothalamic) dysfunction, or cardiac failure. Pontine or midbrain tegmental lesions may result in central neurogenic hyperventilation. Apneustic breathing is characterized by a pause at the end of inspiration, and reflects damage to respiratory centers at the mid or lower pontine levels, at or below the level of the trigeminal motor nucleus. Apneusis occurs with basilar artery occlusion (leading to pontine infarction), hypoglycemia, anoxia, or meningitis. Ataxic breathing is completely irregular in rate and tidal volume, and occurs with damage to the reticular formation of the dorsomedial medulla [4]. Kussmaul respirations are large tidal volume, deep sighing breaths that are usually in response to severe acidosis usually seen in diabetic ketoacidosis or renal failure. Often the patient's arterial partial pressure of carbon dioxide will be low in the attempts to compensate for severe systemic acidosis.

A complete general examination may yield other important findings. Meningeal signs include involuntary hip flexion with passive flexion of the neck (Brudzinski's sign) and resistance to knee extension with hips flexed (Kernig's sign). Skin examination provides information about trauma (bruises, lacerations), systemic disease (jaundice in liver failure, uremic frost, hyperpigmentation in adrenal insufficiency), and infection (superficial lacerations in cat scratch fever, erythema migrans in Lyme disease, petechiae and purpura in meningococcemia). Organomegaly raises suspicion of metabolic, hematologic, and hepatic diseases. Cardiac murmurs or a gallop, hepatomegaly, jugular venous distention, or pitting edema should raise concerns of cardiogenic shock and systemic hypoperfusion.

Neurologic Examination

While coma or altered mental status is the presenting symptom in patients, specific findings on the neurologic exam can be highly useful for determining the cause of coma as well directing further management. The neurologic examination is directed toward localizing brain dysfunction, identifying coma etiology, and determining early indicators of prognosis. As therapies are instituted for specific disease processes, continuous reassessment of the neurologic exam can help determine therapeutic impact.

Glasgow Coma Score (GCS)

Initial rapid assessment of neurologic status can be summarized in part by the Glasgow Coma Score (GCS). This score allows objective description of a patient's degree of impairment and allow the patient's state to be tracked over time and conveyed quickly to other caregivers. The GCS which was initially developed to evaluate adults with head injury [9]. Pediatric adaptations to the GCS, more developmentally appropriate for infants and children, include the Pediatric Coma Scale, the Children's Coma Scale, and the Glasgow Coma Scale-Modified for Children (Table 33.3) [10–12]. The GCS and the pediatric adaptations categorize the patient based on measures of verbal response, eye opening, and movement. Combined with other modalities, the initial GCS score may have limited prognostic value (described below). While the GCS allows efficient standardized communication of a child's state, more detailed description of the child's clinical findings is often more useful for relaying detailed information and detecting changes over time.

Response to Stimuli

Evaluation of responsiveness must include vigorous auditory and sensory stimulation inducing nail-bed pressure, pinching, and sternal rubbing. Responsiveness must be evaluated in terms of lack of verbal, motor, and cranial nerve responses.

Table 33.3 Glasgow coma scale and modification for children

Sign	Glasgow comas scale	Modification for children	Score
Eye opening	Spontaneous	Spontaneous	4
	To command	To sound	3
	To pain	To pain	2
	None	None	1
Verbal response	Oriented	Age appropriate verbalization, orients to sound, fixes and follows, social smile	5
	Confused	Cries, but consolable	4
	Disoriented – inappropriate words	Irritable, uncooperative, aware of environment – irritable, persistent cries, inconsistently consolable	3
	Incomprehensible sounds	Inconsolable crying, unaware of environment or parents, restless, agitated	2
	None	None	1
Motor response	Obeys commands	Obeys commands, spontaneous movement	6
	Localizes pain	Localizes pain	5
	Withdraws	Withdraws	4
	Abnormal flexion to pain	Abnormal flexion to pain	3
	Abnormal extension	Abnormal extension	2
	None	None	1
Best total score			15

In a comatose child, much of the examination that requires patient cooperation (such as mental status and sensory testing) cannot be performed. Thus, the exam primarily assesses function and responsiveness of the brainstem and motor systems.

A comatose child may be flaccid, or may display an abnormal posture. *Decorticate posturing* describes flexion of the arms and extension of the legs, while *decerebrate posturing* describes extension and internal rotation of the arms and legs. Traditionally, decorticate posturing has been considered to relate to dysfunction primarily in the supratentorial compartment, while decerebrate posturing has been considered to relate to brainstem dysfunction. Plum and Posner [4] describe the following guidelines to interpreting abnormal postures:

1. Flexor arm responses with or without extensor responses in the legs typically reflect less severe supratentorial damage
2. Extensor responses in the arm and leg correlate with more severe supratentorial dysfunction
3. Arm extension with leg flexion suggests pontine damage
4. Diffuse flaccidity correlates with brainstem damage below the pontomedullary level.

Cranial Nerve Examination

Examination of the cranial nerves allows investigation of both the brainstem and the cortical control of cranial nerve pathways.

Fundoscopic Examination

Fundoscopic examination evaluates the retina and optic nerves. Papilledema may be seen with increased intracranial pressure but may take hours or days to develop, so its absence does not confirm normal intracranial pressure [13]. Retinal hemorrhages may be seen in inflicted childhood neurotrauma and flame shaped hemorrhages and cotton-wool spots are seen in hypertensive encephalopathy. To obtain a reliable fundoscopic exam it is almost always necessary to dilate the pupils, which can last for up to 24 h. As will be discussed below, the pupillary exam not only contributes to the diagnosis of coma but is one of the few rapid and reliable repeated neurologic assessments. Therefore, careful thought regarding whether the pupillary exam can be forgone is needed.

Pupillary Exam

Pupillary exam should be one of the first neurologic exams performed in the comatose patient. Abnormalities in pupillary response or asymmetry in conjunction with history may require immediate life saving intervention. Asymmetric pupils are either caused by oculomotor nerve (cranial nerve III) disruption or impairment of sympathetic fibers (Horner's syndrome). Because the oculomotor nerve innervates the pupil constrictors, oculomotor nerve impairment results in an abnormally dilated pupil with an absent pupillary light reflex. Oculomotor nerve palsy also results in ptosis and ophthalmoparesis and may be a sign of uncal herniation. Horner's syndrome describes disruption of the sympathetic innervation to the face, characterized by mild ptosis over an abnormally small pupil (meiosis). In traumatic coma, Horner's syndrome may suggest dissection of the carotid artery, along which the sympathetic fibers travel, or an injury to the lower brachial plexus (C8-T1). Anisocoria (asymmetric pupils) is an important physical finding, and differentiating whether a pupil is abnormally large or abnormally small is crucial to identifying underlying pathology. When pupils are more asymmetric in bright light, the pathology lies within the larger pupil and is likely the result of oculomotor nerve palsy. Investigations to rule out uncal herniation or an aneurysm of the posterior communicating artery should follow. As uncal herniation is a potentially treatable emergency, pupillary asymmetry and lack of pupillary reactivity require immediate assessment and treatment. Fixed and dilated pupils are concerning for herniation progressing to brain death, recent hypoxic ischemic injury, or anticholinergic administration, and thus require immediate attention.

When pupils are more asymmetric in darkness, the pathology lies with the smaller pupil. Investigation of the carotid artery, the low cervical-high thoracic spinal cord, or brachial plexus roots should follow to find causes of the Horner's syndrome. If subjects have received sympathomimetic or anticholinergic sprays or drops, it is possible that local effects have impacted one pupil leading to the asymmetry.

Eye Position and Motility

Abnormalities of eye position and motility may be signs of cortical, midbrain, or pontine dysfunction. Conjugate lateral eye deviation is caused by destructive lesions of the ipsilateral cortex or pons, or focal seizures in the contralateral hemisphere. Rarely thalamic lesions may cause "wrong-way eyes," in which the eyes deviate away from the side of the destructive lesion [14]. Tonic down gaze suggests dorsal midbrain compression.

Dysconjugate gaze suggests extraocular muscle weakness or, more commonly, abnormalities of the third, fourth, or sixth cranial nerves or nuclei. Unilateral or bilateral abducens nerve (cranial nerve VI) palsies are commonly seen in increased intracranial pressure, presumably because the nerve is stretched. An eye with an oculomotor nerve (cranial nerve III) palsy is ptotic, depressed and abducted, and has a dilated pupil. As discussed below, oculomotor nerve palsy in a comatose patient suggests uncal herniation with midbrain compression, and thus requires urgent intervention. Trochlear nerve (cranial nerve IV) palsy causes hypertropia in the affected eye.

Roving eye movements are seen in comatose patients with intact brainstem function. Their disappearance may signal the onset of brainstem dysfunction. Periodic alternating gaze (ping-pong gaze) describes conjugate horizontal eye movements back and forth with a pause at each end. It may be seen with extensive bilateral hemispheric, basal ganglia, or thalamic-midbrain damage with an intact pons, and is thought to result from disconnection of cortical influences on oculovestibular reflex generators. It has also been reported in reversible coma from monoamine oxidase and tricyclic antidepressant toxicity.

Oculocephalic and Oculovestibular Reflexes

Oculocephalic and oculovestibular reflexes are useful for assessing the integrity of the midbrain and pons in a coma-
tose patient. To test oculocephalic reflexes ("Dolls eye" reflex), the examiner holds the patient's eyelids open and quickly moves the head to one side. In a comatose patient with an intact brainstem, the eyes will move in the direction opposite the head motion. For example, if the head is moved to the right, the eyes will move conjugately to the left. After several seconds, the eyes may return to a neutral position. The head should be tested in both horizontal and vertical directions. Oculocephalic reflexes should not be tested if the patient has sustained cervical spine trauma or if the spine has not been cleared.

The oculovestibular reflex, commonly referred to as cold calorics, tests the function above the pontomedullary junction. The child must have an open external auditory canal with an intact tympanic membrane (including the absence of pressure equalization tubes), so visual inspection of the canal is an important first step. With the head elevated at 30°, up to 120 mL of ice water is introduced in the ear canal with a small catheter. A conscious patient would experience nystagmus with slow deviation of the eyes toward the irrigated ear and a fast corrective movement away from the ear. In a comatose patient, the fast correction mediated by the cortex is not seen. Instead, the eyes will deviate slowly toward the irrigated ear and remain fixed there. If the brainstem vestibular nuclei (located at the pontomedullary junction) are impaired, no movement will be seen. In brain death, where there is no brainstem function, no eye movement is seen with both ears tested. Five minutes should be allowed before the second ear is tested to allow return of temperature equilibrium between the two ears.

Gag Reflex

The gag reflex is elicited when the soft palate is stimulated and produces elevation of the soft palate. The afferent and efferent signals are carried by the glossopharyngeal and vagus nerves respectively, with processing in the medulla. Absence of the gag reflex should be assessed during the initial airway assessment of the comatose patient. Absence of a gag reflex should raise the concern for the need for tracheal intubation for airway protection, even if the patient is spontaneously breathing with adequate oxygenation and ventilation.

Other Brainstem Reflexes

The remaining brainstem reflexes provide information about the integrity of lower regions of the brainstem. The *corneal reflex* is tested by tactile stimulation of the cornea, which should elicit bilateral eyelid closure. The afferent signal is carried by the trigeminal nerve (cranial nerve V), and the efferent pathway is carried by the facial nerve (cranial nerve VII). Completion of the reflex loop requires intact trigeminal and facial nerve nuclei in the mid and lower pons. The *cough reflex*, which may be seen with stimulation of the carina when a patient is intubated or undergoes suctioning, is mediated by medullary cough centers; sensory and motor signals are carried by the glossopharyngeal (cranial nerve IX) and vagus (cranial nerve X) nerves. Narcotics may suppress cough reflex, an important consideration for accurate assessment of brainstem function [15].

Diagnostic Testing

Diagnostic testing should occur simultaneously with the history and physical examination. Initial blood sampling should include serum glucose, sodium, calcium and magnesium levels as hypoglycemia and electrolyte abnormalities can produce altered mental status, coma, and seizures. Hypoglycemia (capillary glucose <2.6 mmol/L) can cause direct brain injury and must be treated emergently and aggressively with intravenous dextrose. Other initial tests should include a chemistry panel to evaluate for acidosis and renal function, a hepatic function panel to evaluate for signs of elevated bilirubin or hepatitis, a complete blood count to evaluate for signs of infection, anemia or thrombocytopenia, an ammonia level for metabolic dysfunction, and a blood gas to assess for adequate ventilation and metabolic derangements. If fever is present then a blood culture should also be obtained. A lumbar puncture to evaluate for the presence of meningoencephalitis (specifically cell count, gram stain and culture, protein and glucose and herpes PCR) should be performed. However, if the patient is not stable for lumbar puncture or cerebrospinal fluid cannot be obtained, then antibiotic and/or antiviral administration should not be delayed. A serum toxicology screen to evaluate for serum levels of ethanol, tricyclic antidepressants, acetaminophen and salicylates should be performed and urine test for narcotics, benzodiazepines, cocaine, and barbiturates.

After initial laboratory assessment, other laboratory tests are based upon the clinical context and may yield information about the metabolic state of the patient. These include serum or cerebrospinal fluid lactate, pyruvate, organic acids, amino acids, and acylcarnitine profile. If the cause of coma remains unknown, additional studies may be directed at uncommon causes of coma in pediatrics such as Hashimoto's encephalitis (thyroid function tests and thyroid autoantibodies), cerebral vasculitis (ESR, ANA panel, and possibly angiography) or paraneoplastic disorders.

After initial resuscitation, a CT scan of the brain should be performed in all children to evaluate for the presence of intracranial hemorrhage, space occupying lesions (such as tumor or abscess), cerebral edema, focal hypodensities (such as acute disseminated encephalitis, herpes simplex encephalitis, infarct), or hydrocephalus. If the patient is febrile, prior to performing a lumbar puncture, a CT scan

should be evaluate for intracranial hypertension, however, antibiotics should not be delayed for imaging. If there is clinical or radiological evidence for intracranial hypertension, then lumbar puncture should be deferred and treatment should be initiated for possible infections (bacterial and viral) until the clinician deems it safe to perform and lumbar puncture. Importantly, a normal CT scan does not rule out elevated intracranial pressure, sinus venous thrombosis, early ischemic stroke, hypertensive encephalopathy, or demyelinating processes. Once the patient has been stabilized and the etiology of coma remains unclear, a brain MRI may be performed for diagnostic and prognostic purposes.

An electroencephalogram (EEG) may detect useful background changes and may identify subclinical seizures. A prolonged EEG may be required to detect subclinical seizures. If there is clinical evidence of seizures then benzopdiazepines or other anticonvulsants should be administered while awaiting the EEG.

Associated Problems

Intracranial Hypertension

Depending on etiology of coma, patients may develop intracranial hypertension. The Monro- Kelli doctrine states that the skull is a fixed space with three compartments: blood, cerebral spinal fluid and brain parenchyma. Increases in one compartment will lead to a compensatory decrease in the other compartments. When there is a chronic increase in one compartment, then other compartments may gradually accommodate the increase. For example, if a tumor expands, some CSF reduction (reduced ventricle size) may occur, keeping intracranial pressure normal. However, when there is an acute change, such as an epidural hematoma or cerebral abscess, the ability of other compartments to compensate may be overwhelmed, producing an elevation in intracranial pressure. This may produce herniation which if not emergently treated can lead to brain death. Additionally, this may further compromise cerebral perfusion, resulting in further hypoxic-ischemic injury and swelling, and thus further elevations in intracranial pressure.

Numerous processes can result in elevated intracranial pressure. Hydrocephalus in an acute setting is generally the result of a blockage in cerebrospinal fluid flow, leading to its accumulation and resultant elevated intracranial pressure. Blockage can occur due to structural lesions, such as intraventricular hemorrhage or tumor or abscess blocking a usual flow path. Intracranial blood due to hemorrhage can be epidural, subdural, subarachnoid, intraparenchymal or intraventricular. Finally, cerebral edema may be vasogenic, cytotoxic or osmolar in origin. Vasogenic edema is due to a breakdown in the blood brain barrier allowing intravascular proteins into the parenchymal space. This can be sewn following traumatic brain injury or with parenchymal tumors or abscesses. Cytotoxic edema is due to cellular derangements as a consequence of homeostatic processes to control excitotoxicity or acidosis with sodium and water accumulation leading to cellular necrosis. Osmolar edema can occur with electrolyte derangements and fluid influx to the brain such as in hyperosmolar coma.

In the event that these processes produce continuing elevation in intracranial pressure, herniation occurs. There are multiple types of herniation, but most involve compression or distortion of the reticular activating system producing worsening altered mental status, compression of the brainstem producing new cranial nerve deficits and vital sign changes, and compression of arteries further reducing cerebral perfusion. Initial management of critically elevated intracranial pressure includes evaluation of airway breathing and circulation and determining whether the airway should be secured. Initial hyperventilation should be instituted to acutely decrease cerebral blood flow. Further reduction in pCO2 may be necessary to achieve rapid but temporary reductions in cerebral blood flow and thus intracranial pressure, but excessive or prolonged hyperventilation may compromise cerebral perfusion resulting in further hypoxic ischemic brain injury. The head of the bed should be elevated to 30° to aid in venous drainage. Maintaining a neutral neck position may also improve venous drainage. Hyperosmolar therapy can be instituted to decrease cerebral edema. Mannitol will remove water from the brain parenchyma and lead to a large urinary osmotic dieresis and 3 % hypertonic saline will act as a volume expander while removing fluid from the brain parenchyma. Depending on the cause of intracranial hypertension these may only be temporizing solutions. Tracheal intubation should be considered to decrease the metabolic demand of the brain, control ventilation and oxygenation and allow for administration of medications. Barbiturate coma or hypothermia may reduce cellular energy requirements and may thus help protect the brain during periods of hypoxia and ischemia. Similarly, providing adequate sedation and paralysis may further reduce energy demand and prevent spikes in intracranial pressure. Surgical intervention for placement of a ventriculostomy is warranted it here is severe hydrocephalus. Surgical evacuation of hematomas and abscesses can reduce intracranial pressure. At times a decompressive craniectomy will allow brain contents to herniate outward, thereby reducing intracranial pressure. Herniation syndromes are summarized in Table 33.4. While neuroimaging will demonstrate the exact nature of the herniation, waiting and transport for neuroimaging may be detrimental and medical interventions should be implemented.

Table 33.4 Herniation syndromes

Herniation syndrome	Location	Signs
Central herniation	Increased pressure in both cerebral hemispheres causing downward displacement of the diencephalon through the tentorium, causing brainstem compression	**Diencephalic stage**: withdraws to noxious stimuli, increased rigidity or decorticate posturing; small reactive pupils with preserved oculocephalic and oculovestibular reflexes; yawns, sighs, or Cheyne-Stokes breathing
		Midbrain-upper pons stage: decerebrate posturing or no movement; midposition pupils which may become irregular and unreactive; abnormal or absent oculocephalic and oculovestibular reflexes; hyperventilation
		Lower pons-medullary stage: no spontaneous motor activity but lower extremities may withdraw to plantar stimulation; mid-position fixed pupils; absent oculocephalic and oculvestibular reflexes; ataxic respirations
		Medullary stage: generalized flaccidity; absence pupillary reflexes and ocular movements; slow irregular respirations, death
Uncal herniation	Uncus of the temporal lobe is displaced medially over the free edge of the tentorium	Ipsilateral third nerve palsy (ptosis, pupil fixed and dilated, eye deviated down and out)
		Ipsilateral hemiparesis from compression of the contralateral cerebral peduncle (Kernohan's notch)
		Other signs of brainstem dysfunction from ischemia secondary to compression of posterior cerebral artery
Subfalcine (Cingulate) herniation	Increased pressure in one cerebral hemisphere leads to herniation of cingulated gyrus underneath falx cerebri	Compression of anterior cerebral artery leads to paraparesis
Tonsillar herniation	Increased pressure in the posterior fossa leads to brainstem compression	Loss of consciousness from compression of reticular activating system
		Focal lower cranial nerve dysfunction
		Respiratory and cardiovascular function can be significantly affected early with relative preservation of upper brain stem function such as pupillary light reflexes and vertical eye movements

Seizures

Subclinical seizures in critically ill patients may be an under-recognized phenomenon, so the index of suspicion in a comatose child should be high. Recent studies of critically ill children demonstrate a high occurrence of subclinical seizures and status epilepticus [16–19]. Studies in adults have demonstrated that non-convulsive seizure duration and time to detection predict outcome in patients with NCSE. When NCSE was diagnosed within 30 min of onset mortality was 36 %, whereas when diagnosis was delayed for over 24 h, mortality increase to 75 %. When NCSE lasted less than 10 h, 60 % of patients returned home. However, when NCSE lasted more than 20 h none of the patients returned home and 85 % died [20].

Outcome Prediction

General Considerations

Coma is a non-specific behavioral state that can be the consequence of multiple processes, and therefore outcomes are closely related to the underlying etiology. Wong [1] reported that in 283 episodes of pediatric coma (defined as GCS <12 for at least 6 h) mortality at about 1 year ranged from 3 % to 84 % depending on etiology. Children less than a year of age were more likely to die, however, this was closely associated with etiology of coma. Accidents (smoke inhalation, strangulation, burns, drowning) and infections had higher mortality rates (60–85 %) than causes such as metabolic changes (diabetic ketoacidosis, inborn errors of metabolism), epilepsy, and intoxication (3–26 %). Morbidity, defined by severity of neurologic impairment, was more common in older children, but was not associated with specific etiology of coma.

Traumatic brain injury outcome is associated with the initial severity of brain injury. The overall US pediatric mortality for children <15 years is 11.8/100,000. Age impacts outcome, in part tied to etiology of trauma. Children <4 years old have a higher mortality than children between 5 and 9 years and 10 and 14 years (5.3 vs 2.6 vs 3.9/100,000) [21]. Younger children may have more severe long term brain injury when compared to older children [7]. Young children with non-accidental traumatic brain injury have worse outcomes than children with accidental traumatic brain injury (see the chapter on inflicted trauma later in this textbook).

Prognosticating outcome is important to help guide future management and prepare families' expectations. An overly negative prediction may lead to withdrawal of treatment in a child with a potentially salvageable quality of life. Alternatively, providing an overly positive prediction in a child who has a high probability of never regaining con-sciousness may lead to survival past the acute stage with return of spontaneous breathing and resultant prolonged persistent vegetative state, a condition that the child or family may not have wanted. Therefore, reliable and accurate prognostic evaluations are important to guide families' and practitioners' decision making.

Many studies provide little information regarding the exact definitions of terms such as "good" or "poor" outcome or "mild", "moderate", or "severe" neurological disability. Further, neurologic disability is not equivalent to quality of life, which depends on individual's and family's personal set of values. As Shewmon [22] described, the terms "poor/unfavorable" and "good/favorable" which are used as the outcome measures in most studies of coma prognosis are not descriptive of neuro-developmental state, but convey judgment regarding quality of life. For some, a good outcome requires the child to be fully interactive and self-sufficient, while for others a good outcome is a child who lives in any state. Furthermore, a family's perception may change over time as they live with the disabled child. Therefore, data on prognosis cannot be used in isolation to make judgments regarding quality of life, since so many factors (i.e., psychological traits related to resilience, social support) beyond neurological disability are intertwined.

Data suggests that improvement may continue for several years after injury, so determining when to measure outcome is complicated. In children with severe traumatic brain injury, the percent of children who were independent in all areas of function increased from 37 % at discharge from the hospital to 65 % at a median follow-up of 24 months [23]. While most children who are survive to discharge after a cardiac arrest are alive at 1 year, detailed long term neurologic outcomes for this survivors in a small study does not show long term neurologic improvement [24]. Many studies have evaluated prognostic tools based on hospital discharge thereby, leaving clinicians without important data regarding long term recovery. While data regarding prognosis are useful and needed, the goal may be to distinguish between a persistent vegetative state and some degree of consciousness (even with severe disability) as opposed to distinguishing between different levels of disability.

Scoring Tools

Multiple tools have been developed to repeatedly assess a patient's function and progress. These tools assess neurologic examination, daily function, and overall quality of life. The Pediatric Cerebral Performance Category (PCPC) and Pediatric Cerebral Outcome Category (POPC) are validated tools which evaluate patient neurologic outcome at ICU discharge and up to 6 months following discharge. They have been validated against more robust measures [25–27]. The

Glasgow Outcome Score is a five point scale initially used to assess outcomes for patients who have suffered traumatic brain injury [28]. These gross measures are used mainly for research purposes and can be followed over time. Tools for more granular assessment of outcome following pediatric brain injury take into account communication, daily living, social, and motor domains of adaptive behavior. The Vineland Adaptive Behavioral Score is validated from birth to 18 years of age and can be administered to a care provider [29]. The Bayley Development Score can assess outcomes in children from 0 to 3 years of age whereas other scores such as the Wee-Fim can measure disabilities in older children. Other tools can evaluate executive processing, memory and learning and may be helpful to evaluate long term functional impact. Quality of life tools can evaluate the impact of residual injury on both patients and families. Measuring these outcomes can assess the impact of injury on patients and families.

Adjunct Tools

While prognosis from coma is dependent upon etiology, certain adjunctive tools can be helpful to determine outcomes. Helpful factors include neurologic examination, neurophysiologic studies such as EEG and evoked potential testing, and neuroimaging. The reliability and validity of these tools is closely linked to patient population in which they were studied and therefore may not be generalizable to the heterogeneous comatose population.

Neurologic Exam
Specific neurologic exam findings can guide outcome prediction, especially in the acute period. While no specific early physical exam finding is 100 % predictive of outcome, certain findings in conjunction with other modalities can guide the practitioner. Following adult cardiac arrest, poor outcome is predicted by the absence of pupillary responses and absent corneal reflexes within days 1–3 after CPR, as well as absent or extensor motor responses after 3 days [30]. Several small pediatric cardiac arrest studies draw similar conclusions [31–33]. In children with coma due to multiple etiologies, the absence of motor response to pain on day three after injury had PPV for unfavorable outcome of 100 % [34].

Neurophysiology
Electrophysiological measures such as electroencephalography (EEG) and somatosensory evoked potentials may be helpful in predicting outcome early on in coma. The EEG is a good indicator of thalamocortical function, but the utility of a single EEG is limited by the lack of specificity of findings. EEG patterns may evolve over time and combined with

clinical findings may help prognosticate outcome. Specific background patterns such as low amplitude, discontinuity, lack of reactivity and electrocerebral silence are associated with poor outcome in comatose children [31, 35, 36]. The sensitivity and specificity of these findings are less robust as the cause of coma becomes more heterogeneous and therefore clinicians should evaluate the multiple factors contributing to a patient's state.

Somatosensory evoked potentials measure the cortical response to a peripherally provided sensory stimulus. Absent or delayed waves between the stimulus and recording electrode suggest anatomic disruption in the conduction pathways. Evoked potentials are not affected by sedative administration or environmental electrical noise, but, intracranial lesions may alter the evoked potential signal. In children with coma due to multiple etiologies abnormal sensory evoked potentials (SEPs) predicted unfavorable outcome with sensitivity of 75 % and specificity of 92 % [33]. On initial testing, abnormal SEPs have a PPV for unfavorable outcome of 98 % when absent bilaterally and PPV for favorable outcome of 91 % when present [34]. In children who were comatose from cardiac arrest 24 h after resuscitation, the finding of bilateral absent N20 waves on the SEP had 100 % PPV for unfavorable outcome, with 63 % sensitivity [31]. While N20 SEPs are highly sensitive for poor outcome, the presence of N20 SEP's is not sensitive for favorable outcome. Visual evoked potentials (VEP) use a flickering light to activate the visual system and have mixed results. Small series of patient suggest that absence of VEP may predict death, but presence of VEPs may not predict good outcome [37, 38].

Neuroimaging
Neuroimaging may be helpful for prognosis following certain disease conditions. Following hypoxic ischemic injury and cardiac arrest, magnetic resonance imaging (MRI), especially diffusion weighted imaging (DWI), can characterize the location and severity of injury. Injury to the basal ganglia and watershed regions are highly sensitive for poor outcome [39, 40]. Following adult traumatic brain injury MRI findings of diffuse axonal injury, thalamic injury and ischemic injury are associated with more severe outcomes [41]. DAI is associated with poor outcome when located in the brain stem [42]. In children, lesions in the pons or caudal medulla were associated with 100 % mortality [43].

Newer MR imaging techniques have been useful in predicting outcome after TBI. Susceptibility weighted MR imaging detects hemorrhagic diffuse axonal injury particularly well, and in children with TBI the lesion volume using this technique accounted for 32 % of the variance in cognitive performance [44]. MRS determines metabolic ratios in specific brain regions and may allow the clinician to determine the impact of ongoing metabolic injury.

Conclusion

Coma refers to an abnormality in consciousness in which both wakefulness and awareness are disturbed. There are many etiologies for coma including those that primarily neurologic or those that secondarily affect the brain. Coma is a medical emergency. The history, physical examination, laboratory analysis, imaging, and electrophysiological evaluation may disclose the etiology of coma, allowing specific treatment. A tiered evaluation should rapidly take place to identify and treat reversible causes and to prevent secondary injury. Prognosis of outcome from coma is dependent on etiology and thus prognostic information should not be provided for the family until the etiology is determined. The combined expertise of intensivists and neurologists, while taking into account the views of a patient's family, can help guide the long term care and outcomes of these children.

References

1. Wong CP, et al. Incidence, aetiology, and outcome of non-traumatic coma: a population based study. Arch Dis Child. 2001;84(3):193–9.
2. Michaud LJ, et al. Predictors of survival and severity of disability after severe brain injury in children. Neurosurgery. 1992;31(2):254–64.
3. Parslow RC, et al. Epidemiology of traumatic brain injury in children receiving intensive care in the UK. Arch Dis Child. 2005; 90(11):1182–7.
4. Plum F, Posner JB. The diagnosis of stupor and coma. 3rd ed. Philadelphia: Oxford University Press; 1980.
5. Bernat JL. Current controversies in states of chronic unconsciousness. Neurology. 2010;75(18 Suppl 1):S33–8.
6. Nakagawa TA, et al. Clinical report-guidelines for the determination of brain death in infants and children: an update of the 1987 task force recommendations. Pediatrics. 2011;128:e720–40.
7. Keenan HT, Bratton SL. Epidemiology and outcomes of pediatric traumatic brain injury. Dev Neurosci. 2006;28(4–5):256–63.
8. The management of a child (aged 0–18 years) with a decreased conscious level. The Paediatric Accident and Emergency Research Group. 2006. http://www.nottingham.ac.uk/paediatric-guideline/. Accessed Nov 2006.
9. Teasdale G, Jennett B. Assessment of coma and impaired consciousness. A practical scale. Lancet. 1974;2(7872):81–4.
10. Reilly PL, et al. Assessing the conscious level in infants and young children: a paediatric version of the Glasgow Coma Scale. Childs Nerv Syst. 1988;4(1):30–3.
11. Raimondi AJ, Hirschauer J. Head injury in the infant and toddler. Coma scoring and outcome scale. Childs Brain. 1984;11(1):12–35.
12. Hahn YS, et al. Head injuries in children under 36 months of age. Demography and outcome. Childs Nerv Syst. 1988;4(1):34–40.
13. Allen ED, et al. The clinical and radiological evaluation of primary brain tumors in children, part I: clinical evaluation. J Natl Med Assoc. 1993;85(6):445–51.
14. Messe SR, Cucchiara BL. Wrong-way eyes with thalamic hemorrhage. Neurology. 2003;60(9):1524.
15. O'Connell F. Central pathways for cough in man–unanswered questions. Pulm Pharmacol Ther. 2002;15(3):295–301.

16. Hosain SA, Solomon GE, Kobylarz EJ. Electroencephalographic patterns in unresponsive pediatric patients. Pediatr Neurol. 2005;32(3):162–5.
17. Alehan FK, Morton LD, Pellock JM. Utility of electroencephalography in the pediatric emergency department. J Child Neurol. 2001;16(7):484–7.
18. Jette N, et al. Time to first seizure in pediatric patients with nonconvulsive seizures on continuous EEG monitoring. In: annual meeting of the American Epilepsy Society. New Orleans; 2004.
19. Abend NS, et al. Non-convulsive seizures are common in critically ill children. Neurology. 2011;76(12):1071–7.
20. Young GB, Jordan KG, Doig GS. An assessment of nonconvulsive seizures in the intensive care unit using continuous EEG monitoring: an investigation of variables associated with mortality. Neurology. 1996;47(1):83–9.
21. Coronado VG, et al. Surveillance for traumatic brain injury-related deaths–United States, 1997–2007. MMWR Surveill Summ. 2011;60(5):1–32.
22. Shewmon DA. Coma prognosis in children. Part II: clinical application. J Clin Neurophysiol. 2000;17(5):467–72.
23. Thakker JC, et al. Survival and functional outcome of children requiring endotracheal intubation during therapy for severe traumatic brain injury. Crit Care Med. 1997;25(8):1396–401.
24. Rodriguez-Nunez A, et al. Effectiveness and long-term outcome of cardiopulmonary resuscitation in paediatric intensive care units in Spain. Resuscitation. 2006;71(3):301–9.
25. Fiser DH. Assessing the outcome of pediatric intensive care. J Pediatr. 1992;121(1):68–74.
26. Fiser DH, et al. Relationship of pediatric overall performance category and pediatric cerebral performance category scores at pediatric intensive care unit discharge with outcome measures collected at hospital discharge and 1- and 6-month follow-up assessments. Crit Care Med. 2000;28(7):2616–20.
27. Fiser DH, Tilford JM, Roberson PK. Relationship of illness severity and length of stay to functional outcomes in the pediatric intensive care unit: a multi-institutional study. Crit Care Med. 2000;28(4):1173–9.
28. Jennett B, Bond M. Assessment of outcome after severe brain damage. Lancet. 1975;1(7905):480–4.
29. Sparrow S, Cicchetti D, Balla D. Vineland adaptive behavioral scales. 2nd ed. Circle Pines: American Guidance Service; 2005.
30. Wijdicks EF, et al. Practice parameter: prediction of outcome in comatose survivors after cardiopulmonary resuscitation (an evidence-based review): report of the quality standards subcommittee of the American Academy of Neurology. Neurology. 2006;67(2):203–10.
31. Mandel R, et al. Prediction of outcome after hypoxic-ischemic encephalopathy: a prospective clinical and electrophysiologic study. J Pediatr. 2002;141(1):45–50.
32. Bratton SL, Jardine DS, Morray JP. Serial neurologic examinations after near drowning and outcome. Arch Pediatr Adolesc Med. 1994;148(2):167–70.
33. Carter BG, Butt W. A prospective study of outcome predictors after severe brain injury in children. Intensive Care Med. 2005;31(6):840–5.
34. Beca J, et al. Somatosensory evoked potentials for prediction of outcome in acute severe brain injury. J Pediatr. 1995;126(1):44–9.
35. Tasker RC, et al. Monitoring in non-traumatic coma. Part II: electroencephalography. Arch Dis Child. 1988;63(8):895–9.
36. Ramachandrannair R, et al. Reactive EEG patterns in pediatric coma. Pediatr Neurol. 2005;33(5):345–9.
37. Taylor MJ, Farrell EJ. Comparison of the prognostic utility of VEPs and SEPs in comatose children. Pediatr Neurol. 1989;5(3):145–50.

38. Mewasingh LD, et al. Predictive value of electrophysiology in children with hypoxic coma. Pediatr Neurol. 2003;28(3):178–83.
39. Christophe C, et al. Value of MR imaging of the brain in children with hypoxic coma. AJNR Am J Neuroradiol. 2002;23(4):716–23.
40. Dubowitz DJ, et al. MR of hypoxic encephalopathy in children after near drowning: correlation with quantitative proton MR spectroscopy and clinical outcome. AJNR Am J Neuroradiol. 1998;19(9):1617–27.
41. Adams JH, et al. Neuropathological findings in disabled survivors of a head injury. J Neurotrauma. 2011;28(5):701–9.
42. Skandsen T, et al. Prognostic value of magnetic resonance imaging in moderate and severe head injury: a prospective study of early MRI findings and one-year outcome. J Neurotrauma. 2011;28(5):691–9.
43. Woischneck D, et al. Prognosis of brain stem lesion in children with head injury. Childs Nerv Syst. 2003;19(3):174–8.
44. Babikian T, et al. Susceptibility weighted imaging: neuropsychologic outcome and pediatric head injury. Pediatr Neurol. 2005;33(3):184–94.

Cecilia D. Thompson, Michael T. Bigham,
and John S. Giuliano Jr.

Abstract

Pediatric medicine has become increasingly complex and strategies supporting regionalization have gained popularity. Regionalization has placed a new focus on pediatric interfacility transport, allowing a broader group of patients to receive specialized care at tertiary and quaternary medical centers. Pediatric transport medicine was officially recognized by the American Academy of Pediatrics (AAP) in 1986, and achieved Section status in 1990. More recently, the AAP Section of Transport Medicine (AAP-SOTM) published a consensus statement focused on the establishment of dedicated medical directors and team members, transport team accreditation, and clinical research to further improve pediatric transport. Since its recognition, it has been transformed from a concept, to an area of active development.

Keywords

Pediatric • Transport medicine • EMTALA • Aeromedical • Transport modes • Altitude physiology

Introduction

Pediatric medicine has become increasingly complex and strategies supporting regionalization have gained popularity [1–4]. Regionalization has placed a new focus on pediatric interfacility transport, allowing a broader group of patients to receive specialized care at tertiary and quaternary medical centers [5]. Pediatric transport medicine was officially recognized by the American Academy of Pediatrics (AAP) in 1986, and achieved Section status in 1990. More recently, the AAP Section of Transport Medicine (AAP-SOTM) published a consensus statement focused on the establishment of dedicated medical directors and team members, transport team accreditation, and clinical research to further improve pediatric transport [6]. Since its recognition, it has been transformed from a concept, to an area of active development.

C.D. Thompson, MD
Division of Critical Care Medicine, Mount Sinai Kravis
Children's Hospital, New York, NY, USA
e-mail: cecilia.thompson@mssm.edu

M.T. Bigham, MD
Department of Pediatrics, Division of Critical Care Medicine,
Akron Children's Hospital, Akron, OH, USA
e-mail: mbigham@chmca.org

J.S. Giuliano Jr., MD (✉)
Department of Pediatrics, Yale University School of Medicine,
333 Cedar Street, 305 LLCI, New Haven, CT 06520, USA
e-mail: john.giuliano@yale.edu

Historical Perspective

The medical transport of patients was developed by military forces in response to the mass casualties of warfare [7]. Napoleon was the first to develop triage and used a structured ambulance corps, outfitted with a dedicated surgeon and horse drawn carriages [8]. This method continued with little advancement until World War I when the Serbian Army, followed by the French and United States, first used airplanes to evacuate the wounded [7]. However, it was not until World

D.S. Wheeler et al. (eds.), *Pediatric Critical Care Medicine*,
DOI 10.1007/978-1-4471-6362-6_34, © Springer-Verlag London 2014

War II when aeromedical evacuation gained widespread acceptance [9]. During the Korean War, helicopters were used successfully to evacuate the wounded from front lines [7, 9]. The success of rotor-wing medical evacuation was further expanded during the Vietnam conflict [7, 8]. With the implementation of a well-designed triage system and the use of helicopters for medical transport, the military was able to significantly reduce the amount of time between injury and definitive care which improved mortality [7].

With the success of Armed Forces aeromedical evacuation, civilian medical transport systems were developed in the mid 1960s. The National Research Council of the National Academy of Sciences published *Accidental Death and Disability: The Neglected Disease of Modern Society* which highlighted the need for improved first aid, triage skills and medical transportation in the civilian medical sector [10]. This report suggested that helicopters could improve civilian transport by delivering patients quickly to hospitals [10]. This concept gained popularity when Dr. R.A. Cowley, a trauma specialist, coined the term "golden hour," which referred to providing advanced care to critically ill and injured individuals within the first hour after injury [11]. Under Dr. Cowley, the first specialized aeromedical transport team for civilians in the United States was established to support the Maryland Shock Trauma Unit. Despite a report by the Department of Transportation in 1972 suggesting that using helicopters for civilian medical transport was not economically feasible, rotor-wing based civilian programs (federal, state, and local) increased in the 1970s and 1980s [12, 13]. As of 2010, there were a total of 309 air ambulance programs reported in the United States [14]. With the availability and advancements in medical transport, especially aeromedical transport, the support for the regionalization of medicine became more widespread.

Driving the continued momentum toward regionalization of care was the growing evidence of improved outcomes for patients receiving care at higher-volume, tertiary centers. In 1970, Dr. Usher described a 50 % reduction in the infant mortality rate of critically ill newborns cared for in regional centers compared with community hospitals [15]. These findings were reproduced and supported in multiple studies comparing high volume regional neonatal intensive care units with lower volume community hospitals [16–21]. In 1991 Pollack et al first suggested regionalization would improve pediatric critical care outcomes as well [22]. This was supported by a large, multicenter study that confirmed high volume regional pediatric intensive care units had better outcomes [23].

The Transport Team

Most pediatricians believe that critically ill or injured infants and children should receive the same level of care during transport that they will receive at the accepting facility within the constraints of the transport environment. This can only be accomplished by a transport program with a well-organized, specialty-trained, critical care transport team.

Medical Director

The medical director of the program is a physician with acute care and transport expertise. The medical director is responsible and accountable for supervising and evaluating the quality of medical care provided by the transport team personnel. In concert with the transport coordinator, this person ensures competency and currency of all medical personnel working with the service [24]. There is no specific sub-specialty training in pediatrics for transport medicine, although, fellowships in neonatology, pediatric critical care, and emergency medicine generally offer training in this area. A pediatric transport consensus statement described medical director responsibilities to include: (1) team development and supervision (including team selection, periodic review, and development of a mission statement), (2) training and education, (3) establishment of standards, protocols, and guidelines, (4) compliance with local and national standards, (5) team accreditation, (6) acting as a liaison to the hospital administration and to the community, (7) quality assurance and improvement, (8) selection of equipment and medications, (9) financial planning and revenue generation, (10) research coordination, (11) development of transport agreements with referring hospitals, (12) introduction of new technologies and treatments, and (13) community outreach [6].

Transport Coordinator

The transport coordinator's (or manager's) role may be undertaken by the medical director, or by a separate individual who acts as a liaison between the director and the transport team personnel. This individual should have intimate knowledge of the day-to-day operations of the transport team.

Transport Team Personnel

Pediatric and neonatal critical care transport teams are composed of personnel who are specifically trained to provide advanced critical care to neonates, infants, and children. Team composition can vary widely among programs based on availability of professionals at the facility, anticipated patient condition, and financial support for the program. Teams may include: specialty-trained attending physicians, transport physicians, physicians-in-training, advanced practitioners, critical care, emergency, or neonatal nurses, respiratory therapists, EMT-paramedics, or EMTs [25]. Teams may be hospital unit based or dedicated specialty-trained personnel that are capable of caring for the full spectrum of pediatric ages and maladies. Expertise in the management of pediatric respiratory and neurologic conditions is of paramount importance, as these represent the first and second most common problems encountered, respectively [26]. Although team compositions may change depending on patient acuity, all critical care transport teams must have personnel that are capable of establishing and maintaining the airway of a child, establishing vascular access, performing advanced pediatric assessment skills, resuscitation, and dosing and administering medications commonly used in a critical care setting [26].

The necessity for a physician to be a member of the transport team is not well established. Historically, physicians staffing transport teams were resident physicians or fellows. Because of the increasingly complex work hour restrictions, physicians-in-training are less available to participate in a primary role at most transport programs. Recent studies have supported the use of specialty trained nurses and respiratory therapists to lead transport teams without direct physician accompaniment [27–31]. Adams et al found that specialty trained respiratory care practitioners had a 92 % success rate in intubation compared to a 77 % success rate among resident physicians on pediatric interfacility transports [29]. King et al similarly found high intubation success rates among transport-team trained nurses and also found that nurse led teams had a faster response time and overall transport time, compared to resident physician led teams [28].

Smith and Hackel suggested that transport team personnel should be selected based on particular skills that may be required during a transport [32]. Data collected at the first telephone contact with the referring facility would permit "tailored" staffing specific to the needs of that patient. However, numerous studies have demonstrated the difficulty of predicting this need. For example, pre-transport Pediatric Risk of Mortality (PRISM) scores underestimated the requirements for intensive care, as well as the need for major interventions during interhospital transport [33]. Using a pre- and post-assessment survey that took into account vital signs, diagnoses and current therapies and interventions, McCloskey and Johnston found that in 25 % of transports studied, a physician was likely sent unnecessarily [34].

Training and Education

Currently, there are no standard curriculums or published guidelines regarding team training, though one transport accreditation agency suggests a minimum of 3 years of acute care experience prior to transport hire [24]. There are no recommendations for EMTs or respiratory therapists at this time. Along with certification and training through courses such as Pediatric Advanced Life Support (PALS) and Neonatal Resuscitation Program (NRP), team members should receive instruction in basic diagnostic skills and technical procedures while in the transport environment. Methods for teaching these skills may include formal lectures, clinical practice, and simulation, with ongoing continuing education. Training should also include a thorough understanding of transport team protocols. The development and frequent review of protocols designed for specific situations should be established and approved by the transport medical director. In most situations, the protocols are not designed to stand alone but rather to augment the online medical control.

Equipment

Along with established protocols to guide clinical care during emergency situations, each transport team must be appropriately equipped with medications, supplies and equipment necessary for the resuscitation and stabilization of critically ill or injured children. State regulations govern the minimum standards for stocking clinical and safety equipment, though most critical care teams exceed these standards [35–37]. The supply of medications, intravenous fluids, and oxygen should be sufficient to last the entire transport plus additional time and the transport team should not rely on the referring institution for these critical supplies. When transporting patients using oxygen cylinders, the supply can be determined using the following formula:

$$\text{Minutes of oxygen flow} = \text{Cylinder pressure} \times \text{Cylinder Factor} / \text{Flow of oxygen (liters/minute)}$$

where the cylinder factor of a size D, E, and H tank is 0.16, 0.28, and 3.15, respectively. Equipment should also be lightweight, portable, rugged, easy to clean, meet all hospital, local, state, federal and Federal Aviation Administration (FAA) requirements, and have been tested in the transport environment [25]. To ensure the safety of patients and personnel while en route, transport team members should be trained in the appropriate way to secure patients, equipment, and themselves.

Communications Center

The communications center serves as the central contact between the referring hospital and transport team. The design of the communications center serves to streamline access to transport services through the notification and mobilization of the transport team. The American Academy of Pediatrics (AAP) published guidelines state that a fully

Table 34.1 Modes of transportation

Ground	Rotor wing (helicopter)	Fixed wing
Advantages	Advantages	Advantages
Availability	Rapid transit time	Rapid transit time over extremely long distances
Relative cost	Ability to reach inaccessible or remote areas	Able to fly above or around inclement weather
Space available for staff, patient and medical equipment		Cabin size larger than helicopter
		Cabin pressurized
Disadvantages	Disadvantages	Disadvantages
Not ideal for long distance transports	Adequate, unobstructed landing space required (field, helipad, etc.)	Airport required
Limitations of road and traffic conditions	Limitations of weather conditions	Multiple patient transfers of patient required
	Multiple transfers of patient may be required	
	Limited range because of fuel capacity (compared with fixed wing)	Noise and vibration interfere with monitoring of patient
	Limited cabin space	Environmental stresses of altitude
	Lack of cabin pressurization	High maintenance costs
	Ambient air has less moisture	Expensive
	Hypothermia if isolette not used for infants	
	Noise and vibration interfere with monitoring of patient	
	High maintenance costs	
	Expensive	
	Safety(?)	

implemented centralized communications center should include the following essential features: (1) operations 24 hours a day, 7 days a week, (2) trained communication specialists, (3) administrative transport policies and procedures in place, (4) information about local and regional emergency care resources, and (5) communication technology and equipment, including the ability to record all transport-related contacts [25].

Mode of Transport

Determining the appropriate mode of transport is influenced by several key factors: (1) the acuity and stability of a patient's condition and the need for unavailable local services at the referring facility, (2) vehicle availability, (3) weather, (4) distance, (5) geography, (6) transport time, and (7) transport "logistics" [25]. Critical care transport includes surface (ground) and air (fixed and rotor wing) ambulances. Potential advantages and disadvantages of each mode of transport are listed in Table 34.1 [38]. Any vehicle selected should provide adequate space, power sources compatible with transport equipment, sufficient oxygen, safety equipment, and climate control.

Aeromedical Transport Considerations

Altitude Physiology

Aeromedical transport allows for the rapid collection and delivery of sick and injured patients, but also carries a number of potential risks not encountered when traveling by ground. Changes in altitude can have a significant impact on patient's or team members' cardiorespiratory status, as well as the functionality of transport equipment. Dalton's Law states that the pressure of a gas is equal to the sum of the partial pressure of the individual gases in that mixture:

$$P_{atm} = PN_2 + PO_2 + etc.$$

where P_{atm} is the partial pressure of the atmosphere, PN_2 is the partial pressure of nitrogen and PO_2 is the partial pressure of oxygen. Therefore at higher altitudes, atmospheric pressure is lower than at sea level. This translates into lower partial pressures of individual gasses. Conversely, the fractional content of gasses remains fixed. For example, oxygen comprises 21 % of the Earth's atmosphere until about 70,000 ft above sea level. The PO_2 at any given altitude can be calculated as follows:

$$P_{atm} (sea\ level) = 760\ mmHg$$

$$PO_2 = 760 \ mmHg \times 0.21 = 160 \ mmHg$$

Alveolar PO_2 (PAO_2) can then be calculated using the alveolar gas equation:

$$PAO_2 = FiO_2 \left(P_{atm} - P_{H2O} \right) - PaCO_2 / RQ$$

where FiO_2 is the fractional inspired oxygen, P_{H2O} is the partial pressure of water, $PaCO_2$ is the arterial partial pressure of carbon dioxide and RQ is the respiratory quotient. Assuming no significant intrapulmonary shunt, PAO_2 will closely approximate the arterial PO_2 (PaO_2), with a normal alveolar to arterial gradient less than 10 mmHg. Fixed wing aircraft can adjust cabin pressures to reduce the effects of altitude but most large aircraft pressurize their cabins to about 7,000–8,000 ft instead of sea level to conserve fuel. When an aircraft cabin is pressurized to an altitude of 8,000 ft, the atmospheric pressure will be much lower than sea level despite a constant FiO_2 of 0.21. This will lead to a decrease in the partial pressure of oxygen in the air, as well as in the alveoli. In turn, the decrease in PAO2 may lead to lower PaO_2 and increased pulmonary vascular resistance secondary to hypoxic pulmonary vasoconstriction, unless supplemental FiO_2 is administered. This clinical consequence is variable and will depend upon the patient's physiologic stability.

The effects of pressure changes on gas volume are best described by Boyle's law. This law states that the product of the pressure (P_1) and volume (V_1) of a gas is constant, given constant temperature.

$$P_1 V_1 = P_2 V_2$$

Clinically, if the pressure of a gas decreases, as occurs with increased altitude, the volume of the gas will increase. Therefore, the volume of a gas in any enclosed space (i.e., bowel, endotracheal tube cuff, pneumothorax) will increase with increasing altitude. Transport personnel must address these issues prior to ascending in an aircraft by evacuating pneumothoraces, placing chest tubes to suction, deflating or instilling saline into cuffs of an endotracheal tubes or laryngeal mask airways (LMA), or by placing nasogastric tubes to continuous suction in order to decompress the bowel in children with bowel obstructions [39–41].

Finally, Henry's law states that the amount of gas dissolved in a liquid is determined by the partial pressure and the solubility of the gas. With significant changes in barometric pressure, gasses will emerge from solution. The most well known example of this is when nitrogen bubbles form in the blood of deep sea divers who surface too quickly, otherwise known as "the bends." Although theoretically important, clinical changes are rare, except in patients who have recently been scuba diving or when people are exposed to altitudes exceeding 25,000 ft.

Safety in Transport

Unfortunately, with the increase in both ground and air transport programs, there has also been an increase in transport related accidents. Between 2003 and 2008 the number of air ambulance accidents rose to historic levels and has fluctuated between 11 and 15 accidents per year, with multiple fatalities reported in 2008 [13]. While aeromedical accidents may end in fatalities more frequently, ground ambulance accidents are more prevalent and can result in a wide range of injuries. Data sources regarding ground ambulance crashes involving pediatric occupants in the U.S. are limited. However, it is estimated that up to 1,000 ambulance crashes involve pediatric patients each year [42].

Currently, there are no standardized approaches to restraining infants and children in ambulances. Responding to a study that identified 35 states which did not require children or infants to be restrained while being transported in an ambulance [43], the National Highway Traffic Safety Administration (NHTSA) and the U.S. Department of Health and Human Services' Health Resources and Services Administration (HRSA) Emergency Medical Services for Children program (EMS-C) published *The Dos and Don'ts of Transporting Children in an Ambulance* [44]. Unfortunately, a follow-up study in 2006 demonstrated continued unsafe practices among EMS providers and found that nearly 30 % of providers surveyed could not identify the correct method of transport for a stable 2-year-old. Additionally 40 % could not identify the correct method of securing a child seat in the back of the ambulance, despite the majority reporting some training in child-restraint use and "a lot" or "very much" knowledge about securing a critically ill child for transport [45]. In the same study specialized pediatric transport providers were more likely to report safe pediatric restraint practices than were community EMS providers [45].

Safety concerns are not isolated to patient and personnel restraints within the transport vehicle. Environmental factors, specifically weather and traffic conditions, sleep deprivation, and poor team communication can also affect the safety environment during a transport. Although weather conditions exert greater effects on aircraft, ground transport vehicles are also affected by icy roads, snow and heavy rain. Since using lights and sirens only decreases transport time by minutes and significantly increases the risk posed to transport personnel and patients, protocols should be in place to dictate when ground crews are allowed to use these and should be strictly limited to situations requiring time-sensitive interventions [46, 47]. Personnel alertness, related to lack of sleep or disruptions in circadian rhythm also affect transport safety and patient care. Attention should be provided to ensure that transport teams have adequate rest between shifts and that all drivers and pilots adhere strictly to regulations governing shift work hours. Finally, emphasis should be placed on team training by teaching concepts used to strengthen communication between team members in order to help improve safety and prevent errors [48, 49].

Medicolegal Issues

Interfacility transport is regulated by laws that protect patients who present to facilities for emergency care services (ECS). In 1986, Congress enacted the Consolidated Omnibus Budget Reconciliation Act (COBRA) to ensure public access to ECS regardless of a patient's ability to pay. One part of the COBRA legislation was the Emergency Medical Treatment and Labor Act (EMTALA). This act additionally required medical screening exams, as well as stabilizing treatments to be performed at the presenting hospital to the best of that hospital's ability prior to transfer to a more suitable institution [50]. EMTALA also prevented the transfer of a patient from one institution to another solely based on their ability to pay. In 2010, EMTALA was extended to cover admitted patients that required further stabilizing care beyond the scope of the original institution [51].

Additionally under EMTALA, the patient is protected as soon as a patient-physician relationship is established [50]. However, the specific time when a relationship is established during interhospital transport is controversial especially since most accepting physicians initially act as consultants without physically meeting or examining the transferring patient. Medical control liability was examined in the case of *Sterling v. Johns Hopkins Hospital*, which found that a patient-physician relationship was not established between an accepting physician and a patient during interfacility transport. In this case, a severely pre-eclamptic pregnant woman was referred to a tertiary care center for further management. There was a disagreement between the referring and accepting physician as to the appropriate mode of transportation. In the end, the accepting physician's recommendation for ground transport was chosen and the patient died en route after developing an intraventricular hemorrhage. The courts ruled that a patient-physician relationship had not been established by the accepting hospital and the mode of transportation was ultimately decided by the referring physician [52, 53]. Similar cases have been ruled differently making this distinction challenging. For further information on EMTALA and the medicolegal aspects of transport, the interested reader is referred to the following references [25, 50–53].

Clinical Care Stabilization of the Critically Ill or Injured Child for Transport

Only 10 % of EMS calls involve children, with only a small proportion for true emergencies [54]. Because paramedics rarely respond to pediatric emergencies, non-specialized teams may be uncomfortable with and be under-prepared to provide appropriate care for critically ill infants and children. A survey in 1990 found that paramedics were not only less likely to assess vital signs in children less than 2 years of age, but were also less confident in their ability to interpret their vital signs [55]. Because of this, the emphasis in paramedic training for infants and children focuses on patient assessment and recognition of specific clinical states. It also encourages rapid delivery to the closest medical center (i.e., "scoop and run") rather than field intervention [56]. Therefore, stabilization frequently occurs at community hospitals without pediatric/neonatal intensive care units or pediatric/neonatal specialty staff. This necessitates interhospital transfer once initial stabilization has occurred. Depending on the mode of transport selected, pediatric patients may require multiple transfers. Each transfer carries with it increased risk for clinical deterioration from a recurrence or progression of the original problem or from new complications while en route [57].

Accepting the risk of transporting a critically ill or injured child in need of pediatric/neonatal intensive care is often justifiable since children cared for in PICUs have better outcomes than children cared for in adult intensive care units [22, 58]. Previous reports have shown conflicting results regarding adverse outcomes related solely to interhospital transport [59, 60]. These studies however, did not use similarly trained teams for transport, making comparative conclusions difficult. A recent study found improved survival rates and fewer unplanned events during transport when specialized pediatric transport teams were used when compared to nonspecialized teams and controlling for severity of illness [56]. The investigators found that children transported by nonspecialized teams had more than two times greater odds of death than children transported by a specialized team [56]. Besides advanced training, specialized teams often approach the transport of a critically ill or injured child differently. As discussed previously, nonspecialized teams are often driven by the "golden hour" concept that suggests a rapid transport to a tertiary hospital saves lives [11, 56, 61]. Conversely, specialized pediatric transport teams are trained to begin treatment and perform stabilizing procedures upon first encounter at the referring hospital. Although this often prolongs on-scene times at the referring hospital and delays arrival to the tertiary care center, it may explain in part why specialized teams have better results [57, 61–63].

Airway and Respiratory Care

Respiratory interventions are required during approximately 50 % of pediatric interhospital transports [64] and those requiring intubation are at risk for tracheal intubation adverse events (TIAEs) [64, 65]. As was discussed earlier in this chapter, all team members should be comfortable with airway management techniques and at least one member of the transport team should be proficient in pediatric tracheal intubation. Critical care transport teams frequently begin positive pressure ventilation to treat diseases of lower and upper airways [60, 66]. Most specialized pediatric transport teams may have the capabilities to provide non-invasive positive pressure ventilation (NIPPV) using bi-level positive airway pressure (BiPAP), continuous positive airway pressure (CPAP) or high flow nasal cannula.

When preparing for an interhospital transport, a conservative approach to the child's airway is most appropriate favoring intubation for securing an unstable airway. Auscultation, end-tidal carbon dioxide measurement, and chest radiography should confirm proper placement of the endotracheal tube prior to departure from the referring facility. The endotracheal tube should be properly secured and an appropriate amount of sedation and, if necessary, muscle relaxants should be administered to prevent accidental extubation while en route. LMAs should not be considered first line therapy because of potential dislodgement during transport but have been successfully used when endotracheal intubation attempts were unsuccessful [67]. If bag-mask-valve ventilation as opposed to mechanical ventilation is elected, care should be taken to provide consistent minute ventilation using continuous end-tidal CO_2 monitoring, as studies have found wide variation in pCO_2 with this form of ventilation [68, 69].

Sepsis

Since early goal-directed therapy has been shown to improve outcomes in pediatric septic shock, transport personnel should initiate resuscitative measures and antibiotic therapy at the referring hospital instead of waiting for arrival at the tertiary care center [61, 70]. Critical care specialty transport teams offer this benefit. The interested reader can find a complete overview of sepsis management further in this text.

Vascular Access

Critically ill infants and children should have stable vascular access to accommodate resuscitation during transport. Peripheral intravenous access is acceptable if it can be placed quickly. According to PALS guidelines, central venous access during an emergency is no longer necessary prior to vasoactive medication administration [71]. Intraosseous access is an acceptable alternative when peripheral access is unable to be obtained quickly and has been found to be stable and effective in the transport environment [72].

Family Centered Care and Interfacility Transport

The AAP has recognized that family centered care, not only creates a stronger alliance between families and medical staff, but also improves communication and health outcomes while decreasing anxiety among the child and their loved ones [73]. Although family centered care is becoming standard practice in many emergency departments and intensive care units, its inclusion during interfacility transport has not been standardized [74]. Historically, concerns by transport personnel regarding parental accompaniment during transport have included: dealing with belligerent and difficult parents, difficulty controlling a child in the presence of a parent, lack of space in the vehicle, and anxiety about providing medical care or performing procedures in front of family members [74–76]. Recent data, discounted many of these concerns showing that the majority of transport staff found parental accompaniment to be non- or minimally stressful, while 98 % found little to no difficulty in performing medical procedures with parents present [76]. Additionally, the majority of parents questioned favored accompanying their children during interfacility transport [75]. It should be noted that parental accompaniment during interfacility transport is only allowable if the safety of the parent, child, and team can be assured. Thus, parental accompaniment should be deferred in situations where the family member has demonstrated hostility, belligerence, or is under the influence. Parent riders must also wear appropriate restraints and children should never be transported in a parent's lap or arms.

Unique Transport Situations

Scene Flights

Aeromedical transport from the scene of injury or illness to a tertiary care center can be a valuable transport mode in cases requiring time-sensitive specialized medical care. That said, several studies have demonstrated that scene flights are not cost effective and may not be medically necessary [77–81]. Additionally, it has been established that pediatric patients are more successfully endotracheally intubated with fewer complications when this procedure occurs at a hospital rather than in the field [82, 83].

Organ Procurement

The success of solid organ transplant depends, not only on the cooperation of multiple agencies, programs and personnel, but also on time to harvest and time to transplant following harvest. It is often necessary for a transplant team to travel to harvest an organ and then to transport the organ back to the transplant center in a timely fashion. Transport teams may be requested to facilitate the transport of medical personnel or of the organs themselves because they can be assembled quickly. The personnel used for organ procurement deviates greatly from the specialty trained critical care transport team. Guidelines for the transport of organs can be found on the Organ Procurement and Transplantation Network (OPTN), a section of the U.S. Department of Health and Human Services at http://optn.transplant.hrsa.gov.

Extracorporeal Membrane Oxygenation (ECMO)

ECMO is provided at approximately 115 centers in the United States, with a recent increase in cases secondary to the H1N1 influenza pandemic [84]. Patients may either be referred to an institution for ECMO evaluation or may be transported on ECMO using a specialized team. Several single center studies have demonstrated that patients can be safely transported while on ECMO [85–89]. Indications for transport ECMO include the inability to wean from cardiopulmonary bypass, extracorporeal cardiopulmonary resuscitation, and the need to move a patient on ECMO for specialized services such as organ transplant [85]. If ECMO transport is offered, specialized team personnel including perfusionists, surgeons, specialty care nursing staff, and a more spacious transport environment are required to safely and effectively manage the patient en route. Recently, smaller, portable ECMO circuits have been developed which may improve ECMO transport and increase its availability in the future [90, 91].

Burns

Although adult burn units are commonly found at major medical centers, specialized care for pediatric burn patients is concentrated among a small number of facilities. Interfacility transport from not only community hospitals, but also tertiary care centers to pediatric burn centers is not uncommon. The American Burn Association has published patient referral guidelines which can be found at www.ameriburn.org. Referring physicians often inaccurately estimate burn severity which accounts for the overuse of transport, especially aeromedical modes in cases of burn injury [92–94]. Protocolized burn management is needed to delineate when it is appropriate to utilize aeromedical transport to minimize costs and "over triage."

Quality Improvement in Transport

Monitoring and evaluation of transport programs are essential in order to continue to provide high quality patient care. Quality Improvement (QI) activities are often under the direction of the Transport Medical Director and are executed by a multidisciplinary QI committee. Currently there are no established national standards for transport benchmarking. Candidate quality metrics suitable for benchmarking may include resource utilization, patient/family/referral satisfaction, response times, incidence of unplanned adverse events, airway management outcomes, protocol compliance, pain control, use of sedation and neuromuscular blockade, timeliness of initiation of goal-directed therapy, and accuracy of documentation and billing [6, 25]. The development of a national database of quality metrics would be invaluable for the development of national standards in transport medicine.

Future of Pediatric Transport

In 2002, the AAP-SOTM recognized that research in pediatric transport medicine was necessary for the growth and improvement of the field [6]. Committee members stated that an organized national transport research network should be established to investigate important clinical questions and to develop a centralized interactive secure database [6]. However, the subsequent decade has produced few meaningful studies focused on pediatric interfacility transport. With the mounting national interest in quality care following the Institute of Medicine (IOM's) "Crossing the Quality Chasm" report, the future of cooperation around benchmarking, quality improvement, and clinical research is bright.

References

1. Chang RK, Klitzner TS. Resources, use, and regionalization of pediatric cardiac services. Curr Opin Cardiol. 2003;18(2):98–101.
2. Staebler S. Regionalized systems of perinatal care: health policy considerations. Adv Neonatal Care. 2011;11(1):37–42.
3. Feudtner C, Silveira MJ, Shabbout M, Hoskins RE. Distance from home when death occurs: a population-based study of Washington State, 1989–2002. Pediatrics. 2006;117(5):e932–9.
4. Saugstad OD. Reducing global neonatal mortality is possible. Neonatology. 2011;99(4):250–7.
5. Council of the Society of Critical Care Medicine. Consensus report for regionalization of services for critically ill or injured children. Crit Care Med. 2000;28(1):236.
6. Woodward GA, Insoft RM, Pearson-Shaver AL, Jaimovich D, Orr RA, Chambliss R, et al. The state of pediatric interfacility transport: consensus of the second national pediatric and neonatal interfacility transport medicine leadership conference. Pediatr Emerg Care. 2002;18(1):38–43.
7. Meier DR, Samper ER. Evolution of civil aeromedical helicopter aviation. South Med J. 1989;82(7):885–91.
8. Dorland P, Nanney J. Dust off: army aeromedical evacuation in Vietnam. Washington, DC: US Army Center of Military History; 1982. p. 4–8.
9. Carter G, Couch R, O'Brien DJ. The evolution of air transport systems: a pictorial review. J Emerg Med. 1988;6(6):499–504.
10. National Academy of Sciences NRC. Accidental death and disability, the neglected disease of modern society. Washington, DC: US Government Printing Office; 1966.
11. Cowley RA, Hudson F, Scanlan E, Gill W, Lally RJ, Long W, et al. An economical and proved helicopter program for transporting the emergency critically ill and injured patient in Maryland. J Trauma. 1973;13(12):1029–38.

12. Thomas F. The development of the nation's oldest operating civilian hospital-sponsored aeromedical helicopter service. Aviat Space Environ Med. 1988;59(6):567–70.

13. Potential strategies to address air ambulance safety concerns: hearing before the subcommittee on aviation, Committee on Transportation and Infrastructure, House of Representatives 2009.

14. Flanigan M, Blatt A. Atlas and Database of Air Medical Services (ADAMS). 2010. http://www.adamsairmed.org. Accessed 19 July 2012.

15. Usher R. Changing mortality rates with perinatal intensive care and regionalization. Semin Perinatol. 1977;1(3):309–19.

16. Holmstrom ST, Phibbs CS. Regionalization and mortality in neonatal intensive care. Pediatr Clin North Am. 2009;56(3):617–30. Table of Contents.

17. Paneth N, Kiely JL, Wallenstein S, Marcus M, Pakter J, Susser M. Newborn intensive care and neonatal mortality in low-birth-weight infants: a population study. N Engl J Med. 1982;307(3):149–55.

18. Phibbs CS, Bronstein JM, Buxton E, Phibbs RH. The effects of patient volume and level of care at the hospital of birth on neonatal mortality. JAMA. 1996;276(13):1054–9.

19. Verloove-Vanhorick SP, Verwey RA, Ebeling MC, Brand R, Ruys JH. Mortality in very preterm and very low birth weight infants according to place of birth and level of care: results of a national collaborative survey of preterm and very low birth weight infants in The Netherlands. Pediatrics. 1988;81(3):404–11.

20. Phibbs CS, Baker LC, Caughey AB, Danielsen B, Schmitt SK, Phibbs RH. Level and volume of neonatal intensive care and mortality in very-low-birth-weight infants. N Engl J Med. 2007;356(21):2165–75.

21. Chung JH, Phibbs CS, Boscardin WJ, Kominski GF, Ortega AN, Needleman J. The effect of neonatal intensive care level and hospital volume on mortality of very low birth weight infants. Med Care. 2010;48(7):635–44.

22. Pollack MM, Alexander SR, Clarke N, Ruttimann UE, Tesselaar HM, Bachulis AC. Improved outcomes from tertiary center pediatric intensive care: a statewide comparison of tertiary and nontertiary care facilities. Crit Care Med. 1991;19(2):150–9.

23. Tilford JM, Simpson PM, Green JW, Lensing S, Fiser DH. Volume-outcome relationships in pediatric intensive care units. Pediatrics. 2000;106(2 Pt 1):289–94.

24. 8th Edition Accreditation Standards of the Commission on Accreditation of Medical Transport System. 117 Chestnut Lane, Anderson: Commission on Accreditation of Medical Transport System (CAMTS); 2009. 8th edn. http://www.camts.org/04_8th_Edition_1_.pdf. Accessed 19 July 2012.

25. Woodward G, Insoft R, Kleinman M, Alexander N. Guidelines for air and ground transport of neonatal and pediatric patients. 3rd ed. Elk Grove Village: American Academy of Pediatrics; 2007.

26. Ajizian SJ, Nakagawa TA. Interfacility transport of the critically ill pediatric patient. Chest. 2007;132(4):1361–7.

27. King BR, Foster RL, Woodward GA, McCans K. Procedures performed by pediatric transport nurses: how "advanced" is the practice? Pediatr Emerg Care. 2001;17(6):410–3.

28. King BR, King TM, Foster RL, McCans KM. Pediatric and neonatal transport teams with and without a physician: a comparison of outcomes and interventions. Pediatr Emerg Care. 2007;23(2):77–82.

29. Adams K, Scott R, Perkin RM, Langga L. Comparison of intubation skills between interfacility transport team members. Pediatr Emerg Care. 2000;16(1):5–8.

30. Leslie A, Stephenson T. Neonatal transfers by advanced neonatal nurse practitioners and paediatric registrars. Arch Dis Child Fetal Neonatal Ed. 2003;88(6):F509–12.

31. Harrison TH, Thomas SH, Wedel SK. Success rates of pediatric intubation by a non-physician-staffed critical care transport service. Pediatr Emerg Care. 2004;20(2):101–7.

32. Smith DF, Hackel A. Selection criteria for pediatric critical care transport teams. Crit Care Med. 1983;11(1):10–2.

33. Orr RA, Venkataraman ST, Cinoman MI, Hogue BL, Singleton CA, McCloskey KA. Pretransport Pediatric Risk of Mortality (PRISM) score underestimates the requirement for intensive care or major interventions during interhospital transport. Crit Care Med. 1994;22(1):101–7.

34. McCloskey KA, Johnston C. Critical care interhospital transports: predictability of the need for a pediatrician. Pediatr Emerg Care. 1990;6(2):89–92.

35. New Jersey State First Aid Council 2009 Standards Committee Ambulance Equipment Checklist. 2009. http://www.njsfac.org/forms/2009standards_checklist.pdf. Accessed 19 July 2012.

36. State of Vermont Ambulance Equipment Standards Emergency Medical Services Rules 5.9–5.91. 2003. http://healthvermont.gov/hc/ems/documents/AMBINSPFORMREV2006pg2.pdf. Accessed 19 July 2012.

37. Ohio Medical Transportation Board Ohio Administrative Code Chapter 4766-2 Ambulance. 2009. http://omtb.ohio.gov/omt-blancerule.pdf. Accessed 19 July 2012.

38. Wheeler DS, Poss BW. Pediatric Transport Medicine. In: Wheeler DS, Wong HR, Shanley TP, editors. Pediatric critical care medicine basic science and clinical evidence. 1st ed. London: Springer; 2007. p. 313.

39. Henning J, Sharley P, Young R. Pressures within air-filled tracheal cuffs at altitude–an in vivo study. Anaesthesia. 2004;59(3):252–4.

40. Mann C, Parkinson N, Bleetman A. Endotracheal tube and laryngeal mask airway cuff volume changes with altitude: a rule of thumb for aeromedical transport. Emerg Med J. 2007;24(3):165–7.

41. Smith RP, McArdle BH. Pressure in the cuffs of tracheal tubes at altitude. Anaesthesia. 2002;57(4):374–8.

42. Transportation Do, Administration NHTS. Public meeting on draft recommendations for safely transporting children in specific situations in emergency ground ambulances. 2010. http://edocket.access.gpo.gov/2010/pdf/2010-17513.pdf. Accessed 19 July 2012.

43. Seidel JS, Greenlaw J. Use of restraints in ambulances: a state survey. Pediatr Emerg Care. 1998;14(3):221–3.

44. Administration TNHTS, Transportation USDo. Recommendations of the safe transport of children in ground ambulances. 2010. http://www.nasemso.org/documents/EMS_Child_Transport_Working_Group_July_Final_Draft_7-2-20105.pdf. Accessed 19 July 2012.

45. Johnson TD, Lindholm D, Dowd MD. Child and provider restraints in ambulances: knowledge, opinions, and behaviors of emergency medical services providers. Acad Emerg Med. 2006;13(8):886–92.

46. Hunt RC, Brown LH, Cabinum ES, Whitley TW, Prasad NH, Owens CF, et al. Is ambulance transport time with lights and siren faster than that without? Ann Emerg Med. 1995;25(4):507–11.

47. Marques-Baptista A, Ohman-Strickland P, Baldino KT, Prasto M, Merlin MA. Utilization of warning lights and siren based on hospital time-critical interventions. Prehosp Disaster Med. 2010;25(4):335–9.

48. Sherwood G, Thomas E, Bennett DS, Lewis P. A teamwork model to promote patient safety in critical care. Crit Care Nurs Clin North Am. 2002;14(4):333–40.

49. Seamster T, Boehm-Davis D, Holt R, Schultz K. Developing Advanced Crew Resource Management (ACRM) training: a training manual. Federal Aviation Administration Office of the Chief Scientific and Technical Advisor for Human Factors AAR-100; 1 Aug 1998.

50. Federal Register Volume 77, Number 22, by Department of Health and Human Services Centers for Medicaid and Medicare Services. Published Feb 2012. http://www.cms.gov/EMTALA. Accessed 19 Jul 2012.

51. Federal Register 75 FR 246. In: Services DoHaH, Services CfMaM, editors; 23 Dec 2010.

52. Cartwright-Smith L, Rosenbaum S, Belli K, Singh Weik T. Legal issues in interfacility transfer. Washington, DC: The George Washington University; 2010.

53. Edwin Sterling, Personal Representative of the Estate of Laverne Sterling et al. v. Johns Hopkins Hospital. No. 398, Sept. Term, 2001. Court of Special Appeals of Maryland. July 1, 2002 Thieme, Raymond G. Jr: Court of Special Appeals of Maryland; 2002.

54. Seidel JS, Hornbein M, Yoshiyama K, Kuznets D, Finklestein JZ, St Geme JW. Emergency medical services and the pediatric patient: are the needs being met? Pediatrics. 1984;73(6):769–72.

55. Gausche M, Henderson DP, Seidel JS. Vital signs as part of the prehospital assessment of the pediatric patient: a survey of paramedics. Ann Emerg Med. 1990;19(2):173–8.

56. Orr RA, Felmet KA, Han Y, McCloskey KA, Dragotta MA, Bills DM, et al. Pediatric specialized transport teams are associated with improved outcomes. Pediatrics. 2009;124(1):40–8.

57. Wallen E, Venkataraman ST, Grosso MJ, Kiene K, Orr RA. Intrahospital transport of critically ill pediatric patients. Crit Care Med. 1995;23(9):1588–95.

58. Thompson DR, Clemmer TP, Applefeld JJ, Crippen DW, Jastremski MS, Lucas CE, et al. Regionalization of critical care medicine: task force report of the American College of Critical Care Medicine. Crit Care Med. 1994;22(8):1306–13.

59. Black RE, Mayer T, Walker ML, Christison EL, Johnson DG, Matlak ME, et al. Special report. Air transport of pediatric emergency cases. N Engl J Med. 1982;307(23):1465–8.

60. Kanter RK, Boeing NM, Hannan WP, Kanter DL. Excess morbidity associated with interhospital transport. Pediatrics. 1992;90(6):893–8.

61. Stroud MH, Prodhan P, Moss MM, Anand KJ. Redefining the golden hour in pediatric transport. Pediatr Crit Care Med. 2008;9(4):435–7.

62. Borrows EL, Lutman DH, Montgomery MA, Petros AJ, Ramnarayan P. Effect of patient- and team-related factors on stabilization time during pediatric intensive care transport. Pediatr Crit Care Med. 2010;11(4):451–6.

63. Chen P, Macnab AJ, Sun C. Effect of transport team interventions on stabilization time in neonatal and pediatric interfacility transports. Air Med J. 2005;24(6):244–7.

64. Fuller J, Frewen T, Lee R. Acute airway management in the critically ill child requiring transport. Can J Anaesth. 1991;38(2):252–4.

65. Nishisaki A, Marwaha N, Kasinathan V, Brust P, Brown CA, Berg RA, et al. Airway management in pediatric patients at referring hospitals compared to a receiving tertiary pediatric ICU. Resuscitation. 2011;82(4):386–90.

66. Beyer AJ, Land G, Zaritsky A. Nonphysician transport of intubated pediatric patients: a system evaluation. Crit Care Med. 1992;20(7):961–6.

67. Trevisanuto D, Verghese C, Doglioni N, Ferrarese P, Zanardo V. Laryngeal mask airway for the interhospital transport of neonates. Pediatrics. 2005;115(1):e109–11.

68. Dockery WK, Futterman C, Keller SR, Sheridan MJ, Akl BF. A comparison of manual and mechanical ventilation during pediatric transport. Crit Care Med. 1999;27(4):802–6.

69. Hurst JM, Davis K, Branson RD, Johannigman JA. Comparison of blood gases during transport using two methods of ventilatory support. J Trauma. 1989;29(12):1637–40.

70. Hicks P, Cooper DJ, Committee TAaNZICSABaCTGE. The surviving sepsis campaign: international guidelines for management of severe sepsis and septic shock: 2008. Crit Care Resusc. 2008;10(1):8.

71. Kleinman ME, Chameides L, Schexnayder SM, Samson RA, Hazinski MF, Atkins DL, et al. Part 14: pediatric advanced life support: 2010 American Heart Association Guidelines for cardiopulmonary resuscitation and emergency cardiovascular care. Circulation. 2010;122(18 Suppl 3):S876–908.

72. Fiorito BA, Mirza F, Doran TM, Oberle AN, Cruz EC, Wendtland CL, et al. Intraosseous access in the setting of pediatric critical care transport. Pediatr Crit Care Med. 2005;6(1):50–3.

73. Pediatrics CoHCAAo. Family-centered care and the pediatrician's role. Pediatrics. 2003;112(3 Pt 1):691–7.

74. Woodward GA, Fleegler EW. Should parents accompany pediatric interfacility ground ambulance transports? Results of a national survey of pediatric transport team managers. Pediatr Emerg Care. 2001;17(1):22–7.

75. Woodward GA, Fleegler EW. Should parents accompany pediatric interfacility ground ambulance transports? The parent's perspective. Pediatr Emerg Care. 2000;16(6):383–90.

76. Davies J, Tibby SM, Murdoch IA. Should parents accompany critically ill children during inter-hospital transport? Arch Dis Child. 2005;90(12):1270–3.

77. Cocanour CS, Fischer RP, Ursic CM. Are scene flights for penetrating trauma justified? J Trauma. 1997;43(1):83–6. discussion 6–8.

78. Jones JB, Leicht M, Dula DJ. A 10-year experience in the use of air medical transport for medical scene calls. Air Med J. 1998;17(1):7–11. discussion -2.

79. Falcone RE, Johnson R, Janczak R. Is air medical scene response for illness appropriate? Air Med J. 1993;12(6):191. 3–5.

80. Moront ML, Gotschall CS, Eichelberger MR. Helicopter transport of injured children: system effectiveness and triage criteria. J Pediatr Surg. 1996;31(8):1183–6. discussion 7–8.

81. Bledsoe BE, Wesley AK, Eckstein M, Dunn TM, O'Keefe MF. Helicopter scene transport of trauma patients with nonlife-threatening injuries: a meta-analysis. J Trauma. 2006;60(6):1257–65. discussion 65–6.

82. Ehrlich PF, Seidman PS, Atallah O, Haque A, Helmkamp J. Endotracheal intubations in rural pediatric trauma patients. J Pediatr Surg. 2004;39(9):1376–80.

83. DiRusso SM, Sullivan T, Risucci D, Nealon P, Slim M. Intubation of pediatric trauma patients in the field: predictor of negative outcome despite risk stratification. J Trauma. 2005;59(1):84–90. discussion -1.

84. Extracorporeal Life Support Organization. 2011. Ann Arbor. http://www.elso.med.umich.edu/. Accessed 19 July 2012.

85. Coppola CP, Tyree M, Larry K, Coppola CP, Tyree M, Larry K, DiGeronimo R. A 22-year experience in global transport extracorporeal membrane oxygenation. J Pediatr Surg. 2008;43(1):46–52. discussion.

86. Clement KC, Fiser RT, Fiser WP, Chipman CW, Taylor BJ, Heulitt MJ, et al. Single-institution experience with interhospital extracorporeal membrane oxygenation transport: a descriptive study. Pediatr Crit Care Med. 2010;11(4):509–13.

87. Forrest P, Ratchford J, Burns B, Herkes R, Jackson A, Plunkett B, et al. Retrieval of critically ill adults using extracorporeal membrane oxygenation: an Australian experience. Intensive Care Med. 2011;37(5):824–30.

88. Burns BJ, Habig K, Reid C, Kernick P, Wilkinson C, Tall G, et al. Logistics and safety of extracorporeal membrane oxygenation in medical retrieval. Prehosp Emerg Care. 2011;15(2):246–53.

89. Foley DS, Pranikoff T, Younger JG, Swaniker F, Hemmila MR, Remenapp RA, et al. A review of 100 patients transported on extracorporeal life support. ASAIO J. 2002;48(6):612–9.

90. Müller T, Philipp A, Lubnow M, Weingart C, Pfeifer M, Riegger GA, et al. First application of a new portable, miniaturized system for extracorporeal membrane oxygenation. Perfusion. 2011;26(4):284.

91. Philipp A, Arlt M, Amann M, Lunz D, Müller T, Hilker M, et al. First experience with the ultra compact mobile extracorporeal membrane oxygenation system Cardiohelp in interhospital transport. Interact Cardiovasc Thorac Surg. 2011;12:978–81.

92. Saffle JR, Edelman L, Morris SE. Regional air transport of burn patients: a case for telemedicine? J Trauma. 2004;57(1):57–64. discussion.

93. Slater H, O'Mara MS, Goldfarb IW. Helicopter transportation of burn patients. Burns. 2002;28(1):70–2.

94. Chipp E, Warner RM, McGill DJ, Moiemen NS. Air ambulance transfer of adult patients to a UK regional burns centre: who needs to fly? Burns. 2010;36(8):1201–7.

Multiple Organ Dysfunction Syndrome

François Proulx, Stéphane Leteurtre,
Jean Sébastien Joyal, and Philippe Jouvet

Abstract

Multiple organ dysfunction syndrome (MODS) occurs after a life-threatening primary insult, including severe infection, hypoxic-ischemic injury, or other serious injuries. It represents a continuum of physiological abnormalities rather than a distinct state (present or absent). Young age and chronic health conditions are the most important risk factors for the development of MODS. Increasing number of dysfunctional organs is correlated with mortality, greater use of resources, and prolonged stay in pediatric intensive care units. Severe insults converge towards a common systemic response resulting in organ dysfunctions, yet the underlying mechanism remains ill-defined. Acute illnesses may trigger severe inflammatory response resulting in cytokine liberation, activation of coagulation, development of shock and capillary leak. Most experimental therapies to date have focused on attenuating the initial inflammatory response with little benefits in humans. As the initial inflammatory storm subsides, relative immune suppression becomes a major contributor to the disease process. Consequently, MODS patients are highly vulnerable to nosocomial infections. Metabolic demands and neuroendocrine responses also follow a similar seesaw pattern of over-activation followed by a state of relative suppression. Therefore, MODS may emerge from the cumulative suppression of metabolic, neuroendocrine, and immune functions resembling a state of dormancy, hypothesized to be an evolutionary protective cellular mechanism in response to overwhelming injuries. Diagnosis of MODS should encourage physicians to uncover the underlying etiology that may require a specific therapy. The symptomatic management of organ dysfunctions must be carefully assessed in the context of systemic interactions with other failing organs. Although long term outcome data of critically ill children with MODS is limited, 60 % of survivors are reported to have a normal quality of life with minimal health problems.

Keywords

Systemic inflammatory response syndrome • Sepsis • Multiple organ dysfunction syndrome • Cytokines • Immunoparalysis

F. Proulx, MD (✉) • J.S. Joyal, MD, PhD
P. Jouvet, MD, PhD
Department of Pediatrics, Sainte-Justine,
3175 Chemin Côte Sainte Catherine,
Montreal, Québec H3T 1C5, Canada
e-mail: fproulx_01@yahoo.ca; js.joyal@gmail.com;
philippe.jouvet@umontreal.ca

S. Leteurtre, MD, PhD
Department of Pediatrics, Jeanne de Flandre,
Avenue Eugène Avinée, Lille, France
e-mail: stephane.leteurtre@chru-lille.fr

Introduction

Progressive organ dysfunctions were first reported 50 years ago in the surgical literature. In 1963, adult patients with severe peritonitis were found to develop a state of high output shock and respiratory failure requiring mechanical ventilation. Biochemical and mechanical factors were presumed to explain the severe deterioration in these patients [1].

D.S. Wheeler et al. (eds.), *Pediatric Critical Care Medicine*,
DOI 10.1007/978-1-4471-6362-6_35, © Springer-Verlag London 2014

Table 35.1 Definitions of systemic inflammatory response syndrome (SIRS), infection, sepsis, severe sepsis, and septic shock

SIRS[a]

The presence of at least two of the following four criteria, one of which must be abnormal temperature or leukocyte count:

Core[b] temperature of >38.5 °C or <36 °C

Tachycardia, defined as a mean heart rate >2 SD above normal for age in the absence of external stimulus, chronic drugs, or painful stimuli; or otherwise unexplained persistent elevation over a 0.5–4-h time period OR for children <1 year old: bradycardia, defined as a mean heart rate <10th percentile for age in the absence of external vagal stimulus, β-blocker drugs, or congenital heart disease; or otherwise unexplained persistent depression over a 0.5-h time period

Mean respiratory rate >2 SD above normal for age or mechanical ventilation for an acute process not related to underlying neuromuscular disease or the receipt of general anesthesia

Leukocyte count elevated or depressed for age (not secondary to chemotherapy-induced leukopenia) or >10 % immature neutrophils

Infection

A suspected or proven (by positive culture, tissue stain, or polymerase chain reaction test) infection caused by any pathogen OR a clinical syndrome associated with a high probability of infection. Evidence of infection includes positive findings on clinical exam, imaging, or laboratory tests (e.g., white blood cells in a normally sterile body fluid, perforated viscus, chest radiograph consistent with pneumonia, petechial or purpuric rash, or purpura fulminans)

Sepsis

SIRS in the presence of or as a result of suspected or proven infection

Severe sepsis

Sepsis plus one of the following: cardiovascular organ dysfunction or acute respiratory distress syndrome or two or more other organ dysfunctions. Organ dysfunctions are defined in Table 35.3

Septic shock

Sepsis and cardiovascular organ dysfunction as defined in Table 35.3

Adapted from Goldstein et al. [10]. With permission from Wolter Kluwers Health
[a]See Table 35.2 for age-specific ranges for physiologic and laboratory variables
[b]Core temperature must be measured by rectal, bladder, oral, or central catheter probe

Table 35.2 Age-specific vital signs and laboratory variables [10, 13]

Age group	Heart rate, beats/min		Respiratory rate, (breaths/min)	Leukocyte count, (10⁹/L)	Hypotension (mmHg)
	Tachycardia (beat/min)	Bradycardia (beat/min)			
0 days to 1 week	>180	<100	>50	>34	<59
1 week to 1 month	>180	<100	>40	>19.5 or <5	<79
1 month to 1 year	>180	<90	>34	>17.5 or <5	<75
2–5 years	>140	NA	>22	>15.5 or <6	<74
6–12 years	>130	NA	>18	>13.5 or <4.5	<83
13 to <18 year	>110	NA	>14	>11 or <4.5	<90

Lower values for heart rate, leukocyte count, and systolic blood pressure are for the 5th and upper values for heart rate, respiration rate, or leukocyte count for the 95th percentile
NA not applicable

A sequential pattern of organ failures was identified during the 1970s among patients with ruptured aortic aneurysms [2]. Improvement in the medical management of shock states began to change disease progression and more reports of multiple organ failures in shock survivors emerged [3, 4]. Several studies uncovered a relationship between an increasing number of failing organs and mortality [5] or the length of stay in the intensive care unit (ICU) [5]. Multiple organ dysfunctions were found to occur with or without any identifiable infectious source [6], changing in severity over time, and being potentially reversible. Faced with this new entity, adult diagnostic criteria for the systemic inflammatory response syndrome (SIRS) [7], sepsis, and organ dysfunctions were proposed in 1992 [6] and were revisited in 2003 [8]. These definitions helped to distinguish the insult (infection, trauma, etc.), from the host response (SIRS) and the subsequent number of organ dysfunctions, while emphasizing

the pathophysiological continuum culminating in these organ dysfunctions [9].

Definition of Pediatric Multiple Organ Dysfunction Syndrome (MODS)

Diagnostic criteria currently used to define the infectious insults, the host response (SIRS), and the number of organ dysfunction in children were established in 2002 [10] and are summarized here. *Systemic inflammatory response syndrome* [7] refers to any combination of two or more symptoms including fever or hypothermia; tachycardia or bradycardia in infants (<12 months of age); tachypnea or hypocapnia; leukocytosis or leukopenia (Tables 35.1 and 35.2) [6]. The host response is called "*sepsis*" when these symptoms are suspected to be triggered by an infection.

Multiple organ failure in critically ill children is defined as the simultaneous dysfunction of at least two organ systems [11, 12]. Criteria for organ failures (Table 35.3) were established according to severity of illness scoring systems used in critically ill children [10, 13]. The aim of using a common definition for MODS is to provide a reproducible assessment of organ dysfunction that allows for tracking of changes in organ function. However, the reproducibility and relative strength of these criteria has not been evaluated. MODS can be classified as primary or secondary, depending on the timing of organ dysfunctions. *Primary MODS* develops rapidly after pediatric ICU (PICU) admission [14–16] and is generally the consequence of a well-defined insult. In one study, the maximal number of organ failures was noted within 72 h in the majority of patients [14]. *Secondary MODS* corresponds to children who develop evidence of organ damages after the first week of PICU admission and/or develop a sequential pattern of organ dysfunction [17].

Pediatric MODS Scoring Systems

Two scores were developed to quantify the severity of MODS and follow its evolution over time: *(1)* Leteurtre et al. developed and validated the PELOD score [18, 19], which is derived from six independent physiological variables (Table 35.4) [18]; *(2)* Graciano et al. developed the Pediatric-MODS score, which relies exclusively on laboratory values (lactic acid, PaO_2/FiO_2 ratio, bilirubin, fibrinogen, blood urea nitrogen) and therefore does not take into consideration the neurological function [20]. This may be a serious limitation of the Pediatric-MODS score, since 80 % of the variability in PELOD scores is attributable to cardiovascular and neurologic dysfunctions [18]. Although both scores have good discriminative values and are useful tools to describe the severity of MODS in critically ill children, the calibration of the PELOD score has been recently criticized [21, 22]. Since mortality is low (around 5 %) and incidence of MODS higher (from 6 % to 57 %) in critically ill children (Table 35.5), the PELOD score has been used as a surrogate outcome measure in pediatric clinical trials for risk adjustment [23] or secondary outcome [24]. Daily PELOD scores of critically ill children effectively identified survivors from non survivors [25]. Fifty percent of 115 deaths were associated with an increase in the score from day 1 to day 2 and from day 2 to day 4 [25].

Epidemiology

Pediatric mortality is closely correlated with the number of organ dysfunctions [11, 12]. Conversely, the number of children who die in the PICU without reaching criteria for MODS is low [12, 15, 18]. MODS may stem from pediatric

Table 35.3 Organ dysfunction criteria (2002)

Cardiovascular dysfunction

Despite administration of isotonic intravenous fluid bolus ≥40 mL/kg in 1 h

  Decrease in BP (hypotension) <5th percentile for age or systolic BP <2 SD below normal for age[a]

    OR

  Need for vasoactive drug to maintain BP in normal range (dopamine >5 µg/kg/min or dobutamine, epinephrine, or norepinephrine at any dose)

    OR

  Two of the following

Unexplained metabolic acidosis: base deficit >5.0 mEq/L

Increased arterial lactate >2 times upper limit of normal

Oliguria: urine output <0.5 mL/kg/h

Prolonged capillary refill: >5 s

Core to peripheral temperature gap >3 °C

Respiratory[b]

  PaO_2/FIO_2 <300 in absence of cyanotic heart disease or preexisting lung disease

    OR

  $PaCO_2$ >65 Torr or 20 mmHg over baseline $PaCO_2$

    OR

  Proven need[c] or >50 % FIO_2 to maintain saturation ≥92 %

    OR

  Need for nonelective invasive or noninvasive mechanical ventilation[d]

Neurologic

  Glasgow coma score ≤11

    OR

  Acute change in mental status with a decrease in Glasgow Coma Score ≥3 points from abnormal baseline

Hematologic

  Platelet count <80,000/mm³ or a decline of 50 % in platelet count from highest value recorded over the past 3 days (for chronic hematology/oncology patients)

    OR

  International normalized ratio >2

Renal

  Serum creatinine ≥2 times upper limit of normal for age or 2-fold increase in baseline creatinine

Hepatic

  Total bilirubin ≥4 mg/dL (not applicable for newborn)

    OR

  ALT 2 times upper limit of normal for age

Adapted from Goldstein et al. [10]. With permission from Wolter Kluwers Health

BP blood pressure, *ALT* alanine transaminase

[a]See Table 35.1

[b]Acute respiratory distress syndrome must include a PaO_2/FIO_2 ratio ≤200 mmHg, bilateral infiltrates, acute onset, and no evidence of left heart failure. Acute lung injury is defined identically except the PaO_2/FIO_2 ratio must be ≤300 mmHg

[c]Proven need assumes oxygen requirement was tested by decreasing flow with subsequent increase in flow if required

[d]In postoperative patients, this requirement can be met if the patient has developed an acute inflammatory or infectious process in the lungs that prevents him or her from being extubated

Table 35.4 The pediatric logistic organ dysfunction score

Organ dysfunction and variable	Scoring system			
	0	1	10	20
Neurological[a]				
Glasgow coma score	12–15	7–11	4–6	3
	and		**or**	
Pupillary reactions	Both reactive	NA	Both fixed	NA
Cardiovascular[b]				
Heart rate (beats/min)				
<12 years	≤195	NA	>195	NA
≥12 years	≤150	NA	>150	NA
	and		**or**	
Systolic blood pressure (mmHg)				
<1 month	>65	NA	35–65	<35
1 month–1 year[c]	>75	NA	35–75	<35
1–12 years[c]	>85	NA	45–85	<45
≥12 years	>95	NA	55–95	<55
Renal				
Creatinine (μmol/L)				
<7 days	<140	NA	≥140	NA
7 days–1 year[c]	<55	NA	≥55	NA
1–12 years[c]	<100	NA	≥100	NA
≥12 years	<140	NA	≥140	NA
Respiratory[d]				
PaO_2 (kPa)/FIO_2 ratio	>9·3	NA	≤9·3	NA
	and		**or**	
$PaCO_2$ (kPa)	≤11·7	NA	>11·7	NA
	and			
Mechanical ventilation[d]	No Ventilation	Ventilation	NA	NA
Haematological				
White blood cell count (×10^9/L)	≥4·5	1·5–4·4	<1·5	NA
	and	**or**		
Platelets (×10^9/L)	≥35	<35	NA	NA
Hepatic				
Aspartate transaminase (IU/L)	<950	≥950	NA	NA
	and	**or**		
Prothrombin time[e] (or INR)	>60 (<1·40)	≤60 (≥1·40)	NA	NA

Adapted from Leteurtre et al. [18]. With permission from Elsevier
PaO₂ arterial oxygen pressure, *FIO₂* fraction of inspired oxygen, *PaCO₂* arterial carbon dioxide pressure, *INR* international normalised ratio
[a]Glasgow coma score: use lowest value. If patient is sedated, record estimated Glasgow coma score before sedation. Assess patient only with known or suspected acute central nervous system disease. Pupillary reactions: non-reactive pupils must be >3 mm. Do not assess after iatrogenic pupillary dilatation
[b]Heart rate and systolic blood pressure: do not assess during crying or iatrogenic agitation.
[c]Strictly less than
[d]PaO₂: use arterial measurement only
[e]Percentage of activity. PaO₂/FIO₂ ratio, which cannot be assessed in patients with intracardiac shunts, is considered as normal in children with cyanotic heart disease. PaCO₂ may be measured from arterial, capillary, or venous samples. Mechanical ventilation: the use of mask ventilation is not counted as mechanical ventilation

Table 35.5 Epidemiology of pediatric MODS

	Patients	Incidence[a]	Mortality[b]
General pediatric ICU population			
Wilkinson et al. [12]	831	27 %	26 %
Proulx et al. [170]	777	11 %	51 %
Tan et al. [171]	283	6 %	56 %
Leteurtre et al. [19]	594	45 %	19 %
Tantalean et al. [15]	276	57 %	42 %
Leteurtre et al. [18]	1,806	53 %	12 %
Khilnani et al. [172]	1,722	17 %	26 %
Typpo et al. [33]	44,693	19 %	10 %
Sepsis			
Wilkinson et al. [11]	726	24 %	47 %
Proulx et al. [173]	1,058	18 %	36 %
Goh et al. [16]	495	17 %	57 %
Kutko et al. [48]	80	73 %	19 %
Leclerc et al. [35]	593	45 %	19 %
Congenital heart diseases			
Seghaye et al. [38]	460	4 %	56 %
Trauma			
Calkins et al. [43]	534	3 %	17 %
Liver or bone marrow transplantation			
Feickert et al. [45]	114	27 %	72 %
Keenan et al. [174]	121	55 %	94 %
Lamas et al.[c] [175]	49	90 %	69 %

Adapted from Proulx et al. [176]. With permission from Wolter Kluwers Health
MODS Multiple organ dysfunction syndrome, *ICU* Intensive care unit; Incidence[a] and mortality rate[b] of MODS; [c]MODS was defined as 3 organ dysfunctions

conditions, including sepsis, congenital heart diseases, trauma, and liver or bone marrow transplantations [26]. The incidence and mortality rate of MODS varies between studies in part due to disparities in case-definition and case-mix (see Table 35.5).

Risk factors for MODS in adults include delayed or inadequate resuscitation, persistent infectious or inflammatory focus, advancing age, malnutrition, or cancer [27]. In children, MODS most frequently affects *children under 1 year of age* [28]. The incidence and mortality of MODS is higher in neonates compared to older children [29] and a distinct pattern of organ dysfunctions was noted in the neonatal population [30, 31]. Indeed, important developmental changes occur during the first year of life that govern the maturation of renal, hepatic, gastrointestinal, and central nervous systems, which may predispose infants to MODS [32].

The presence of *comorbid conditions* increases the incidence of MODS and mortality. While one fourth of children with MODS were reported to have chronic condition in the mid-80s [12], now almost two thirds of pediatric ICU patients have an underlying chronic condition [33]. Not surprisingly, the incidence of MODS is twofold greater among children with a comorbid condition, which independently increases the risk of death [33].

Table 35.6 Etiologies of multiple organ dysfunction in children

Severe hypoxia or cardiorespiratory arrest [170]
Shock states: septic[a], cardiogenic[b], hemorrhagic
Severe dehydration[c]
Multiple trauma [44]
Burns [104]
Inhalation pneumonia
Acute liver failure [177–179]
Acute pancreatitis
Intestinal ischemia[d]
Acute leukemia[e]
Solid organ[f] or bone marrow transplantation[g]
Familial or secondary hemophagocytic lymphohystiocytosis[h] [180, 181]
Thrombotic microangiopathy[i]
Sickle cell [182]
Vasculitis [183]
Inborn errors of metabolism[j] [179, 184]
Malignant hyperthermia [185]
Toxic ingestion
Snake bite

[a]Including purpura fulminans, toxic shock syndrome, severe pneumonia, bacterial meningitis, viral meningoencephalitis
[b]Myocarditis, left heart obstructive lesions, prolonged cardiopulmonary bypass, univentricular physiology
[c]May occur in neonates or children with encephalopathy
[d]Intestinal volvulus, intussusception, perforation, necrotizing enterocolitis
[e]Promyelocytic leukemia
[f]May occur with vascular thrombosis, massive bleeding, occult intestinal perforation, post transplant lymphoproliferative disease
[g]Veno-occlusive disease, graft versus host disease
[h]Secondary hemophagocytosis may also occur during MODS itself [186]
[i]Post diarrheal or atypical hemolytic uremic syndrome, thrombotic thrombocytopenic purpura
[j]Urea cycle defect, congenital lactic acidosis, organic acidemia

Etiology

The initial life-threatening insult leading to MODS also influences mortality. A diagnosis of MODS compels the physician to identify the underlying cause since several diseases with multi-systemic manifestations may require a specific therapy. An overview of common and less usual causes of pediatric MODS are presented in Table 35.6.

Sepsis

Pediatric MODS in sepsis is associated with a poor prognosis compared to non-infectious SIRS [34]. Moreover, severity of organ failures and mortality rates are closely correlated with the severity of the infectious process [15, 16, 35, 36]. A detailed discussion of sepsis is found later in this textbook.

Congenital Heart Diseases

Children with congenital heart diseases sometimes develop organ dysfunction both before and after cardiac surgery requiring cardiopulmonary bypass. Pre-operative imbalances of the pulmonary and systemic circulations may lead to organ dysfunctions. This is the case of children with hypoplastic left heart syndrome and pulmonary overcirculation associated with poor systemic perfusion. Afterload reduction has been reported to improve hepatic, renal, and gastrointestinal functions pre-operatively in these patients [37]. MODS may also occur after cardiac surgery as a consequence of cardiopulmonary bypass and the surgical correction itself. Cardiovascular instability, endothelial damage, platelet and immune activations from cardiopulmonary bypass predispose to MODS [38]. Persistent renal failure, in the context of cardiac surgery has been associated with poor outcome [39, 40]. The surgical repair may sometimes exacerbate organ damage in the presence of low cardiac output syndrome, residual lesions, or a delayed adaptation to the postoperative physiology [37, 41]. Children with congenital heart diseases may be prone to "classical" adult-type MODS characterized by the development of immune paralysis, and susceptibility to a second-hit phenomenon [42]. For example, in the first week after surgery, Ben-Abraham et al. found that 80 % of mortality was due to MODS; thereafter, sepsis was believed to be the main cause of death [42].

Multiple Trauma

Multiple trauma is a cause of MODS in children, albeit less frequent than in adults. In a series of 334 children admitted to the PICU with isolated head injury, not a single patient developed MODS [43]. Only 3 % of children with multiple traumatic injuries acquired MODS 2 days after their admission to the PICU [43]. However, multiple trauma associated with abdominal compartment syndrome and MODS has a worse prognosis, with a reported mortality rate of 20 % in children [44]. Overall, the mortality from multiple trauma is threefold lower in children compared to adults [43], possibly because children have different mechanisms of injury, fewer comorbid conditions, and a different physiological response to traumatic injury.

Solid Organ or Bone Marrow Transplantations

MODS is a major determinant of early mortality after pediatric orthotopic liver transplantation due to vascular thrombosis, sepsis, or as a result of pre-transplant organ dysfunctions [45]. The extent of damage to the engrafted liver is a major contributor to organ dysfunction. In this regard, hepatic vascular thrombosis may lead to severe hemorrhagic shock and acute renal failure. This may then lead to polymicrobial sepsis due to intestinal perforation and malnutrition. Severe rejection is rare early after liver transplantation. Conversely, patients with rejections are less likely to develop MODS in the postoperative phase [45]. Long term survival depends on the underlying disease, the presence of MODS in the post-operative phase, or late sepsis [45]. The development of chronic graft failure or lymphoproliferative disease are also major determinants of outcome [45], the latter being associated with a 50 % mortality rate [46].

In bone marrow transplantation, pre-transplant conditioning leads to potentially reversible cytotoxicity including pancytopenia, capillary leak syndrome, acute graft versus host disease, and hepatic veno-occlusive disease. If important, this toxicity may create MODS. In one large prospective study, MODS was the only variable that had a negative impact on the outcome [47]. An increased mortality rate has been noted in children who developed septic shock and MODS after bone marrow transplantation, but not among those suffering from neoplasic disorders who did not have transplantation [48]. In the former group, pulmonary or neurological dysfunctions were important determinants of patient survival [49]. Respiratory insufficiency may be secondary to opportunistic infections, bronchiolitis obliterans, pulmonary edema, or toxicity. Combined neurological and renal dysfunctions may occur with cyclosporine or tacrolimus toxicity and the related bone marrow transplant thrombotic microangiopathy.

Pathogenesis

Evolutionary Ties Between Sepsis and Tissue Injury

Despite similar host responses to severe sepsis and post-traumatic SIRS suggestive of a unifying cause, the molecular mechanism has been poorly understood. Due to lower blood pressure and relative splanchnic hypoperfusion in severe trauma, the possibility of bacterial translocation from the gut was initially suggested. However, this hypothesis was later refuted. More recent evidence posits activation of the innate immune system through highly conserved molecules known as the pathogen-associated molecular patterns (PAMPs), expressed by a variety of pathogens. Similarly, host molecules released following tissue injury called damage-associated molecular patterns (DAMPs) also initiate the innate immune response through shared signalling pathways with PAMPs, even in the absence of microbial pathogens [50]. Recent evidence reveals that DAMPs, including the high mobility group protein (HMGB1) produced by nucleated cells, are released in the blood of injured patients and their levels correlate with the development of organ failures.

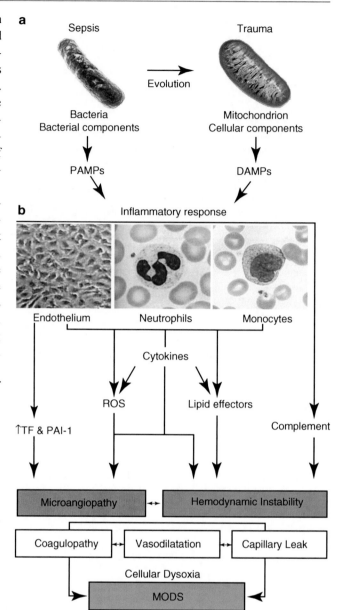

Fig. 35.1 Sepsis, tissue injury and the inflammatory response. (Panel **a**) Release of molecules called pathogen-associated molecular patterns (*PAMPs*) from bacteria and damage-associated molecular patterns (*DAMPs*) from tissue necrosis and mitochondrial fragments trigger the inflammatory response. (Panel **b**) Activation of innate immunity and the complement cascade leads to the release of cytokines, reactive oxygen species (*ROS*) and highly reactive lipid mediators. Hemodynamic instability is the outcome of changes in myocardial contractility, vasodilatation and capillary leak. The endothelium begins to express tissue factor (*TF*) launching the coagulation cascade, while plasminogen activator inhibitor-1 (*PAI-1*) decreases fibrinolysis; this results in microangiopathy and DIC. Together, cellular dysoxia culminate in organ dysfunctions (Adapted from Cohen [187]. With permission from Nature Publishing Group)

Mitochondria provide a plausible explanation for the common infectious and tissue injury triggers of the innate immune response (Fig. 35.1a). Mitochondrial and bacterial DNA share similar structural motifs as an evolutionary consequence of the bacterial origin of these organelles [51].

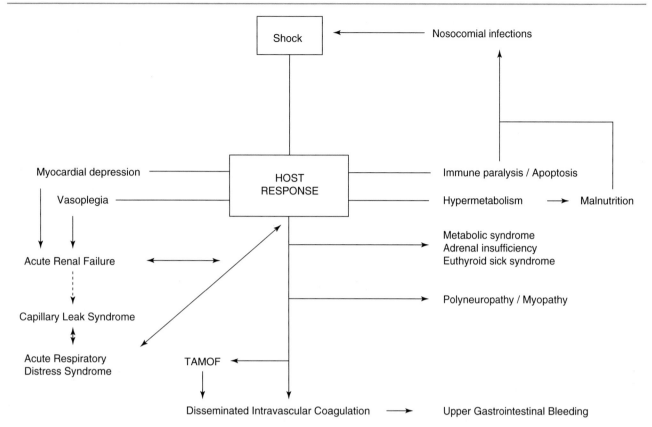

Fig. 35.2 Overview of the pathophysiology of multiple organ dysfunction syndrome. The host response to injury or infection is central to the development of multiple organ dysfunction syndrome (*MODS*). Shock states are characterized by abnormal microcirculatory blood flow, with variable degree of peripheral vasoplegia and myocardial depression that may cause acute renal failure. The latter may aggravate capillary leak syndrome. Renal failure itself may result in worse lung injury or other organ failure. Inflammatory processes, including the cytokine and chemokine response, lead to endothelial cell activation, which is clinically recognized as disseminated intravascular coagulation, capillary leak as well as acute respiratory distress syndrome. Hypermetabolism, also called "septic autocannibalism", may result in a state of severe malnutrition which is associated with secondary immunoparalysis. Overall, impaired mechanisms of tissue repair may lead to the development of nosocomial infections, usually 7–10 days later. The biological significance of other clinical conditions highlighted above remains to be clarified (*TAMOF* Thrombocytopenia associated multiple organ failure)

Zhang et al. therefore postulated that mitochondrial components spilled by necrotic tissue after severe trauma (DAMPs) could mimic PAMPs and activate host response [52]. Administration of mitochondrial DAMPs in rats induced acute lung injury. Severe trauma in humans caused a rapid release of mitochondrial DNA and mitochondrial DAMPs such as formyl peptides, which attracted neutrophils and initiated the immune response through pattern-recognition receptors (PRRs), such as toll-like receptor 4 (TLR-4). Conserved molecular motifs between bacteria and mitochondria may therefore provide an explanation for a shared immune response to injury and infections [52].

Inflammation and Immune System

Sepsis and MODS were traditionally believed to result from over-activation of the immune system and the ensuing inflammatory cascade (Fig. 35.1b). Overwhelming stimulation of innate immune cells expressing PRRs rapidly initiate host defence after tissue damage or microbial infection [53]. TLRs are a subfamily of PRRs crucial to the initiation of the inflammatory response. TLR4-mediated recognition of lipopolysaccharide and DAMPs (such as mitochondrial DNA), rapidly initiates host response and facilitate crosstalk with the complement system [53]. Activated neutrophils and macrophages produce cytokines, chemokines, and complement-activation products, resulting in a markedly imbalanced cytokine response (or 'cytokine storm'). This pro-inflammatory environment triggers the liberation of powerful secondary lipid mediators and reactive oxygen species that further amplify the inflammatory storm, leading to host tissue damage. Children who died from meningococcal sepsis presented higher concentrations of several pro-inflammatory cytokines, as well as increased serum levels of anti-inflammatory mediators (IL-10, soluble TNF receptors) [54, 55]. Hereditary markers of innate immunity influence the outcome of sepsis [56, 57]. However, if most patients die during the initial phase of sepsis and MODS, several succumb later during the second phase characterized by protracted immune suppression (Fig. 35.2).

Adaptive Immunity and Immune Suppression

In contrast to the innate immune system, adaptive immunity develops over several days and provides a more specific line of defence against pathogens. T cells orchestrate the inflammatory response, particularly CD4+ T helper 1 (T_H1) and 2 (T_H2) cells, with distinct cytokine profiles. During sepsis, adaptive immunity shifts from a T_H1 cell mediated inflammatory response (interferon-γL-2 and IL-12), to a T_H2-cell response (IL-4, IL-5, IL-10 and IL-13), which can contribute to immunosuppresion.

Multiple cellular mechanisms underlie the immune suppression in sepsis. Increased levels of apoptosis in lymphocytes and dendritic cells contribute to immune suppression [58]. Moreover, apoptotic cells intensify the process of 'immune paralysis' in remaining immune cells characterized by shut-down of cytokine response and signalling capacity [59, 60], albeit not a generalized phenomenon [61]. In contrast to circulating immune cells, those derived from tissues appear to remain fully responsive, thereby indicating compartmentalization of inflammatory processes [61]. Intracellular reprogramming may be responsible for the hyporeactivity of circulating leukocytes and may represent a physiological adaptation with protective effects. This observation is reminiscent of the phenomenon of endotoxin tolerance well described in sepsis models [62–64].

Autopsies of pediatric and adult patients that died of sepsis and MODS revealed significant lymphoid depletion. An absolute lymphocyte count of less than 1,000 for more than 7 days was only observed in children with MODS [65]. Lymphopenia and lymphoid depletion predispose to anergy, a state of non-responsiveness to antigens. Together, this immune reprogramming (or 'immunoparesis') referred to as the compensatory anti-inflammatory response syndrome (CARS), is an adaptive mechanism to restrain the initial aggressive inflammatory burst. However, relative immune suppression also predisposes critically ill patients to viral reactivation [66], nosocomial infections and death [65].

Coagulation and Fibrinolysis

The sepsis triad refers to the activation of coagulation and inhibition of fibrinolysis triggered by inflammation [67] (see again Fig. 35.1b). The extent of pro-thrombotic and anti-fibrinolytic plasma activation is correlated with the severity of pediatric MODS and mortality [68–75]. Tissue factor (TF) is pivotal to the initiation of the coagulation cascade. In sepsis, inflammation results in the expression of TF on endothelial cells, the activation of coagulation and ensuing disseminated intravascular coagulation (DIC). Tissue factor

binds and activates factor VII, X and V, thereby increasing thrombin activation, fibrin deposition, and microthrombi formation [76]. Inflammation also elevates the levels of plasminogen-activator inhibitor 1 (PAI-1) and thrombin-activatable fibrinolysis inhibitor (TAFI) which impair fibrin removal [77]. The general consumption of factors that regulate thrombin formation, such as antithrombin III, protein C and tissue-factor pathway inhibitor (TFPI) further exacerbates DIC [78].

Thrombocytopenia-associated multiple organ failure (TAMOF) is a clinical entity associated with sepsis. It comprises a spectrum of similar conditions including disseminated intravascular coagulation (DIC) and secondary thrombotic microangiopathy (TMA) [79]. Autopsies of children with TAMOF revealed a predominance of von Willebrand factor-rich (vWF) thrombi in the microvasculature of their brain, lung and kidney [80]. Recent evidence also suggests that as many as 30 % of children with severe sepsis have moderately decreased (20 % activity) ADAMTS-13 protease activity [81], which may increase the risk of thrombosis and organ dysfunction in this population.

Capillary Leak Syndrome

MODS has been associated with abnormal systemic vascular permeability resulting in the development of the capillary leak syndrome [82, 83]. In meningococcemia, the amount of circulating endotoxin and complement activation determines the severity of capillary leakage [84]. Susceptibility to the development of edema after cardiopulmonary bypass [85, 86] or bone marrow transplantation [87] is also related to activation of the complement system. More importantly, a positive fluid balance is associated with prolonged mechanical ventilation and increased mortality [88, 89]. PICU survivors had less fluid overload and were more likely to attain their target dry weight during continuous renal replacement therapy [90–92]. However, it is unclear whether endothelial dysfunction and the ensuing edema is simply an epiphenomena or contributes to the disease process. Recent work explored the role of adherens junctions that binds endothelial cells together to prevent vascular leak. Slit proteins and its receptor Robo4 are important to neuronal and vascular development. London and colleagues recently demonstrated that Slit and Robo4 proteins can stabilize VE-cadherin on endothelial adherens junction thereby decreasing vascular permeability [93]. In three different mouse model of infection, intravenous injection of Slit prevented vascular leakage and reduced mortality [93]. The role of the microvascular barrier in severe infections is now considered a therapeutic target [94]. Although confirmation in human is required, this may suggest a critical role of the endothelium and the capillary leak syndrome in sepsis.

Neuroendocrine Response

The initial phase of MODS results in a massive release of stress hormones, including adrenocorticotropic hormone (ACTH) and cortisol, catecholamines, vasopressin, glucagon, and growth hormone [95]. These hormones help supply the increased demand by maintaining circulation and the liberation of energy substrate, namely glucose, fatty acids and amino acids. Insulin resistance is a common manifestation of this overwhelming neuroendocrine response, although the mechanism remains ill-defined [95]. Intracellular metabolism, energy expenditure and tissue oxygen consumption doubles during that initial period. Concurrently, less vital systems are shut down and anabolism is halted.

In the second phase of MODS, the hormonal response recedes. Vasopressin levels are often insufficient, the adrenals become less responsive to ACTH, and sick euthyroid syndrome begins to appear [95]. Suppression of the hypothalamus-pituitary-adrenal axis is presumed to be a consequence of hypoperfusion, cytokine, and nitric oxide signalling in situ [96]. The transition between the first and second phase of the hormonal response may result from the abnormal pulsatile secretion of growth hormone, thyrotropin, and prolactin [95]. The later endocrine changes may also in part be the consequence of inhibitory feedbacks from the initial burst of hormonal activation. As such, high cortisol levels prevent the secretion of growth hormone, and together with prolactin repress the secretion of gonadotropins. Cortisol may also modulate thyroid metabolism by promoting the generation of metabolically inactive reverse T3, contributing to the development of the sick euthyroid syndrome.

In children, non-survivors from meningococcal sepsis had variable aldosterone levels [97, 98], lower serum cortisol, and severely decreased cortisol to ACTH ratio, indicating a state of adrenal insufficiency [97, 99, 100]. They also had acquired sick euthyroid syndrome (decreased total T_3 and T_4, increased reverse T_3, normal free T_4 and TSH) [96, 101, 102]. In newborns, dopamine curbs the secretion of growth hormone, thyrotropin and prolactin, which could aggravate partial hypopituitarism and sick euthyroid syndrome [103].

Hyper and Hypometabolism

At the onset of severe infections or thermal injury, a decreased metabolic rate with hypothermia and stimulation of the neuroendocrine response has been referred to as the ebb phase [104]. Hypermetabolism has then been noted during the flow phase, usually about 24 h after injury [105]. Normal metabolic requirements were noted in children with SIRS or sepsis without any organ dysfunction [106]. Briassoulis et al. noted a predominance of a hypermetabolic pattern which declined within 1 week of an acute stress [107]. In adults, hypermetabolism occurs as a result of an increased oxidation of glucose and fatty acids [108], as well as an increased rate of neoglucogenesis through the use of lactate, glycerol or amino acids (alanine, glutamine, serine, glycine).

Humoral factors released by the wound have been shown to trigger skeletal muscle proteolysis. TNF-α, also known as "cachectin", plays a major role along with IL-1 in the development of "septic autocannibalism" [108]. Decreased lipoprotein lipase activity induced by TNF-α leads to increased serum levels of triglycerides, cholesterol and hyperglycemia, a clinical condition known as the "metabolic syndrome". Glucose-lactate metabolism between skeletal muscle and liver is known as the Cori cycle. Under hypoxic conditions of tissue injury or infection, glucose is transformed into lactate which is further converted within liver into glucose, before returning to the injured area. This process resulted in a net loss of 4 mol of adenosine triphosphate per cycle which may explain in part the drainage of energetic reserve. In the most severely ill patients, muscle protein breakdown with consumption of branched amino acids and increased nitrogen urinary losses, may lead to muscular cachexia, atrophy of intestinal epithelium, abnormal wound healing and secondary immune dysfunction.

Cellular Dysoxia

Compromised oxygen delivery in shock is a major determinant of organ failures. Inducible nitric oxide synthase (iNOS) triggered by the inflammatory response liberates large concentrations of nitric oxide (NO), far exceeding the regional production [109]. This may lead to abnormal regional vascular blood flow and would contribute to inadequate oxygen delivery [109]. The severity of arterial hypotension in pediatric sepsis is correlated with serum concentrations of nitrites and nitrates [74]. Neuroendocrine and inflammatory factors can exacerbate hypoperfusion as discussed. Although organ failure is classically believed to result from hypoxia and cellular damage, histological inspection of dysfunctional organs is often normal [110]. This would suggest a functional rather than a structural deficit.

Cytopathic dysoxia is therefore potentially important to the pathogenesis of MODS. Mitochondrial respiration generally increases in the acute phase of critical illness, but tends to fall with prolonged inflammation [111]. The presence of glucocorticoids and thyroid receptors on mitochondria

[112] suggests the integration of neurohormonal demands with corresponding energy supply at the cellular level. However, NO and cytokines have been shown to inhibit enzymes of the mitochondrial respiratory chain, which curtails energy production [113]. Markers of oxidative and nitrosative stress also correlate with decreased mitochondrial respiratory chain activity (mainly Complex I) [114]. Despite reduced ATP production from cytopathic dysoxia, ATP levels are largely maintained in surviving septic patients, thereby implying a state of diminished cellular energy consumption [115]. Based on these observations, Singer et al. have argued that multiorgan failure is a survival mechanism instating a dormant state analogous to hibernation that may increase the chances of survival when faced with a potentially overwhelming insult [116].

Organ Dysfunctions in Critically Ill Children

Cardiovascular Dysfunction and Septic Shock

Hemodynamic profiles noted in critically ill children with septic shock are more unpredictable than initially recognized [117–119]. Indeed, only 20 % of children with fluid refractory septic shock presented the classical picture of high cardiac index and low systemic vascular resistance [120]. Nearly 60 % of patients showed low cardiac index with high systemic vascular resistance, and both parameters might even be decreased [120]. During shock, sympathetic stimulation preferentially directs blood flow toward the brain and myocardium, diverting it from the splanchnic circulation (the so-called "dive reflex"). This may lead to increased serum lactate concentrations [121, 122]. In contrast to adults, most studies performed in critically ill children did not find the gastric pH to be predictive of developing MODS or death [121, 123–126]. However, decreased intestinal pH in very low birth weight infants was associated with a higher risk of developing necrotizing enterocolitis [127].

Acute Lung Injury (ALI) and Acute Respiratory Distress Syndrome (ARDS)

Pulmonary congestion with protein-rich pulmonary edema is a cardinal feature of the acute respiratory distress syndrome (ARDS) [26, 128], which has been associated with a 20 % mortality rate in children [129]. This can be due to a direct pulmonary insult such as infection (so-called "direct ARDS") or secondary to systemic inflammation (so-called "indirect ARDS"). Abnormally increased vascular pulmonary permeability has been associated with platelet activation, neutrophils and macrophage infiltration [128], as well as with fibrin exudate resulting in hyaline membrane formation [128].

During the early phase of pulmonary injury, a restrictive pattern is noted with a decrease in respiratory system compliance and forced vital capacity [130]. The natural course of ARDS has been characterized by inadequate gas exchanges requiring more aggressive mechanical ventilation. This leads to the production of inflammatory mediators that would further increase pulmonary capillary permeability and generates deleterious mechanical forces that leads to further damage of the alveolar-capillary membrane [131].

Gut Mucosal Barrier Dysfunction

Gut injury and inflammation have been proposed as the "motor of MODS" [132]. The mechanism was thought to be related to intestinal bacteria and/or endotoxin translocating to the systemic circulation via the portal vein. However, neither clinical studies nor animal studies demonstrated bacterial translocation via the portal vein [133]. Instead it appears that mesenteric lymph translocates factors which activate neutrophils and injure endothelial cells [133]. In neonates, the development of necrotizing enterocolitis resulted in increased plasma endotoxin levels [134]. Endotoxemia was more severe at the onset of illness among infants with necrotizing enterocolitis and play a critical role in the development of MODS [134]. Theorically, measures to improve gut epithelial barrier may improve or prevent MODS.

MODS is a significant risk factor to develop upper gastrointestinal bleeding [135–137]. Clinically significant upper gastrointestinal bleeding occurs in 2 % of PICU admissions [137]. It is most frequently observed among mechanically ventilated patients with a PRISM score higher than 10, and with evidence of systemic coagulopathy [137].

Neuromuscular Syndromes

Neuromuscular syndromes, including critical illness polyneuropathy, pure motor polyneuropathy, thick-filament myopathy, and necrotizing myopathy have been described [138–141]. Prolonged weakness has been identified in 2 % of critically ill children studied prospectively, of whom 63 % had MODS and 57 % had transplantation [142]. SIRS has been proposed as a common underlying pathogenic process, which may have been potentiated by the use of corticosteroids or neuromuscular blocking agents [138]. Patients showed flaccid quadriplegia with the inability to wean from ventilatory support [138]. In most severe cases, deep tendon reflexes were abolished. Electrophysiological abnormalities usually showed a pattern of axonal polyneuropathy or abnormalities of neuromuscular transmission [138]. Recovery in strength most frequently occurred over a period of weeks to months.

Outcome of Pediatric MODS

Development of MODS is associated with greater resource use and an increased length of stay in the PICU [28]. A normal quality of life with minimal health problems is reported in 60 % of children with MODS, while 32 % indicated a fair quality of life with ongoing health, emotional, social, physical or cognitive problems that required some intervention or hospitalization; 2 % had a poor quality of life [143]. The return of organ function in children who developed MODS has not been examined in a systematic manner. There are few small case series in children with ARDS or those with MODS after cardiac surgery [144, 145]. In one study, 78 % of children who left the hospital after acute renal failure in the ICU survived beyond 24 months [146].

Treatment of Pediatric MODS

The care of children with MODS is best performed by a multidisciplinary team that carefully balances multiple therapeutic modalities. These modalities include general supportive care and organ specific therapeutics. The patient clinical condition should be reassessed periodically as for the need to perform complementary exams or invasive procedures in order to distinguish between possible, probable or definitive diagnosis.

General Supportive Care

Control of the infectious focus is of major importance. *Antibiotic therapy* should be started early with appropriate resection of infected or necrotic tissue. However, the prolonged use of large spectrum antibiotic therapy should be avoided when cultures are negative, and the risk-benefit of invasive catheters must be re-evaluated periodically. The use of recombinant human activated protein C reduced mortality and improved organ dysfunction among adults with severe sepsis [147]. However, in the RESOLVE trial, a pediatric trial in which children with sepsis-induced cardiovascular and respiratory failure were randomly assigned to receive placebo or recombinant human activated protein, there was no difference between treatment groups in either organ failure resolution or mortality [148]. While overall bleeding events were not different between groups, there was an increased incidence of central nervous system bleeding in the treated group among children younger than 2 months. Based upon follow-up trials in adults showing no benefit, the manufacturer removed activated protein C from the market and it is no longer available for clinical use [149]. Results of the CORTICUS trial in adults suggest that although shock reversal may occur more rapidly with corticsteroids, overall survival is not improved, apparently due to an increased rate of infections [150]. In the case of a transplanted patient with active systemic infection, *immunosuppressive therapy should be minimized.* Lymphopenia may occur with the prolonged use of dopamine or steroids, and prolonged lymphopenia has been associated with secondary infection and MODS [65].

A large-scale multicenter clinical trial in PICU patients who were hemodynamically stable, the TRIPICU study, showed that a *restrictive transfusion strategy* based on an hemoglobin transfusion threshold of 70 g/L, was not inferior to a liberal approach (threshold: 95 g/L) with regard to the number of patients with "new or progressive MODS or death" [151]. The incidence rate of "new and/or progressive MODS" in the TRIPICU study was 12 %, while the death rate was, as expected, only 4 %.

Critically ill children should receive *appropriate sedation and analgesia.* Vet et al. have recently shown that increased disease severity resulted in lower clearance of midazolam (decreased cytochrome 3A activity), without decreasing midazolam dose requirements [152]. Several drugs used in critical care have a narrow therapeutic index. Caution should be applied when using nephrotoxic or hepatotoxic drugs, with a special emphasis on timely drug dosages, metabolic clearance and drug interaction. Iatrogenic complications may typically occur due to difficult vascular catheterization, or overactive cardio-respiratory support usually based on a blind treatment of numbers.

While inadequate oxygen delivery to tissues results in organ dysfunction initially, MODS itself may well occur as a result of mitochondrial dysfunction [153]. As children with septic shock have better outcomes than adults, it is suggestive that their mitochondrial functions are relatively preserved compared to that of adults. This is a new area of research as therapies are being developed to affect mitochondrial function in sepsis [154]. There is some evidence that *blood glucose control* can improve mitochondrial dysfunction in patients with sepsis [155]. What remains unclear at this point is whether therapy aimed at reversing the metabolic response is helpful in critically ill patients [156]. In medical or surgical adult ICUs, tight glycemic control with intensive insulin therapy has been reported to decrease morbidity or mortality; other studies suggested no benefit or potential harm due to hypoglycemia [157–159].

Organ Therapeutic Management

In this section, only some specificities of organ dysfunction management are reported. For more details in the management, readers should refer to the appropriate and relevant chapters later in this textbook.

Hemodynamic Management

Early goal-directed therapy has been shown to decrease mortality and the severity of MODS in adults with sepsis [160]. Guidelines developed in 2002 proposed a time-dependent flow diagram in the hemodynamic support of children with sepsis [161].

Lung Protective Ventilation

There is no clear data in children. Expert opinions recommend to keep positive inspiratory pressures below 30 cmH$_2$O and consider small tidal volume ventilation (physiologic tidal volumes in a normal subject are in the range of 6–8 ml/kg). The other therapies such as endotracheal surfactant, high-frequency oscillatory ventilation, prone positioning, bronchodilators or corticosteroids for lung inflammation and fibrosis need further research before they can be recommended in clinical practice [162].

Renal Failure Management

Renal replacement therapy can be continuous or intermittent according to team experience and patient tolerance. High dialysis dose did not demonstrate any benefits in adults [163, 164] and no data are available in children. Although, fluid overload is a risk factor of death in adults [165, 166] and children [90, 167, 168], no data are available on the impact of negative fluid balance on critically ill children outcome [169]. Such aggressive ultrafiltration needs to be balanced with the risk of hypovolemia.

Nutritional Support

Nutritional support may allow sufficient protein-calorie intake. Early enteric feeding has been proposed to prevent intestinal disuse with secondary mucosal atrophy, decreasing the susceptibility to bacterial translocation and systemic inflammation. Indeed, the capacity to tolerate enteral feedings, as for the mobilization of third space and peripheral edema, usually represent a trend for clinical improvement.

Withdrawal of Curative Care

Despite the willingness to provide as good as possible intensive care to children with MODS, several patients simply persistently fail to improve or spontaneously further deteriorate, presenting several complications, that may ultimately be viewed as an inexorable pathway to death. Therefore, the issue of medical futility and palliative care is frequently encountered in children with MODS. The pro's and con's of not escalating the level of care, the withdrawal of cardiopulmonary resuscitation (CPR), or discontinuing some of the therapeutic modalities, are usually evaluated by the members of the multidisciplinary team. With the aim of reaching a consensus between the medical team and family, honest clinical information should be provided at least daily to the family, including when standard of medical care fails to lead to recovery.

References

1. Burke J, Pontoppidan H, Welch C. High output respiratory failure: an important cause of death ascribed to peritonitis or ileus. Ann Surg. 1963;158(4):581–95.
2. Tilney NL, Bailey GL, Morgan AP. Sequential system failure after rupture of abdominal aortic aneurysms: an unsolved problem in postoperative care. Ann Surg. 1973;178(2):117–22.
3. Pinsky M. The definition and history of multiple-system organ failure. In: Charbonneau P, Société de Réanimation de Langue Française, editors. Syndrome de défaillance multiviscérale. Paris: Expansion scientifique français; 1991. p. 3–7.
4. Fry D, Pearlstein L, Fulton R, Polk H. Multiple system organ failure: the role of uncontrolled infection. Arch Surg. 1980;115(2): 136–40.
5. Knauss W, Wagner D. Multiple organ failure: epidemiology and prognosis. Crit Care Clin. 1989;5(2):221–32.
6. American College of Chest Physicians, Society of Critical Care Medicine. American College of Chest Physicians/society of critical care medicine consensus conference: definitions for sepsis and organ failure and guidelines for the use of innovative therapies in sepsis. Crit Care Med. 1992;20(6):864–74.
7. Rangel-Frausto MS, Pittet D, Costigan M, Hwang T, Davis CS, Wenzel RP. The natural history of the systemic inflammatory response syndrome (SIRS). A prospective study. JAMA. 1995;273: 117–23.
8. Levy M, Fink M, Marshall J, Abraham E, Angus D, Cook D, et al. 2001 SCCM/ESICM/ACCP/ATS/SIS international sepsis definitions conference. Crit Care Med. 2003;31(4):1250–6.
9. Montgomery VL, Strotman JM, Ross MP. Impact of multiple organ system dysfunction and nosocomial infections on survival of children treated with extracorporeal membrane oxygenation after heart surgery. Crit Care Med. 2000;28(2):526–31.
10. Goldstein B, Giroir B, Randolph A. International pediatric sepsis consensus conference: definitions for sepsis and organ dysfunction in pediatrics. Pediatr Crit Care Med. 2005;6(1):2–8.
11. Wilkinson JD, Pollack MM, Glass NL, Kanter RK, Katz RW, Steinhart CM. Mortality associated with multiple organ system failure and sepsis in pediatric intensive care unit. J Pediatr. 1987;111(3): 324–8.
12. Wilkinson JD, Pollack MM, Ruttimann UE, Glass NL, Yeh TS. Outcome of pediatric patients with multiple organ system failure. Crit Care Med. 1986;14(4):271–4.
13. Gebara BM. Values for systolic blood pressure. Pediatr Crit Care Med. 2005;6(4):500. [Comment Letter]; author reply 500-1.
14. Proulx F, Grunberg F. Suicide in hospitalized patients. Sante Ment Que. 1994;19(2):131–43.
15. Tantalean JA, Leon RJ, Santos AA, Sanchez E. Multiple organ dysfunction syndrome in children. Pediatr Crit Care Med. 2003;4(2): 181–5.
16. Goh A, Lum L. Sepsis, severe sepsis and septic shock in paediatric multiple organ dysfunction syndrome. J Paediatr Child Health. 1999;35(5):488–92.
17. Proulx F, Lacroix J, Farrell CA, Lambert M. Blood lactate and gastric intramucosal pH during severe sepsis. Crit Care Med. 1996;24(6):1092.
18. Leteurtre S, Martinot A, Duhamel A, Proulx F, Grandbastien B, Cotting J, et al. Validation of the paediatric logistic organ dysfunction (PELOD) score: prospective, observational, multicentre study. Lancet. 2003;362(9379):192–7.
19. Leteurtre S, Martinot A, Duhamel A, Gauvin F, Grandbastien B, Nam TV, et al. Development of a pediatric multiple organ dysfunction score: use of two strategies. Med Decis Making. 1999;19(4): 399–410.
20. Graciano AL, Balko JA, Rahn DS, Ahmad N, Giroir BP. The Pediatric Multiple Organ Dysfunction Score (P-MODS):

development and validation of an objective scale to measure the severity of multiple organ dysfunction in critically ill children. Crit Care Med. 2005;33(7):1484–91.

21. Tibby SM. Does PELOD measure organ dysfunction…and is organ function a valid surrogate for death? Intensive Care Med. 2010;36(1):4–7.

22. Garcia PC, Eulmesekian P, Branco RG, Perez A, Sffogia A, Olivero L, et al. External validation of the paediatric logistic organ dysfunction score. Intensive Care Med. 2010;36(1):116–22.

23. Vlasselaers D, Milants I, Desmet L, Wouters PJ, Vanhorebeek I, van den Heuvel I, et al. Intensive insulin therapy for patients in paediatric intensive care: a prospective, randomised controlled study. Lancet. 2009;373(9663):547–56. Randomized Controlled Trial Research Support, Non-U.S. Gov't.

24. Lacroix J, Hebert PC, Hutchison JS, Hume HA, Tucci M, Ducruet T, et al. Transfusion strategies for patients in pediatric intensive care units. N Engl J Med. 2007;356(16):1609–19.

25. Leteurtre S, Duhamel A, Grandbastien B, Proulx F, Cotting J, Gottesman R, et al. Daily estimation of the severity of multiple organ dysfunction syndrome in critically ill children. CMAJ. 2010;182(11):1181–7.

26. Berkowitz FE, Vallabh P, Altman DI, Diamantes F, Van Wyk HJ, Stroucken JM. Jarisch-Herxheimer reaction in meningococcal meningitis. Am J Dis Child. 1983;137(6):599.

27. Baue AE. Multiple, progressive, or sequential systems failure. A syndrome of the 1970s. Arch Surg. 1975;110(7):779–81.

28. Johnston J, Yi M, Britto M, Mrus J. Importance of organ dysfunction in determining hospital outcomes in children. J Pediatr. 2004;144(5):595–601.

29. Bestati N, Leteurtre S, Duhamel A, Proulx F, Grandbastien B, Lacroix J, et al. Differences in organ dysfunctions between neonates and older children: a prospective, observational, multicenter study. Crit Care. 2010;14(6):R202.

30. Avanoglu A, Ergun O, Bakirtas F, Erdener A. Characteristics of multisystem organ failure in neonates. Eur J Pediatr Surg. 1997;7(5):263–6.

31. Shah P, Riphagen S, Beyene J, Perlman M. Multiorgan dysfunction in infants with post-asphyxial hypoxic-ischaemic encephalopathy. Arch Dis Child Fetal Neonatal Ed. 2004;89(2):F152–5.

32. Kearns G, Abdel-Rahman S, Alander S, Blowey D, Leeder J, RE K. Developmental pharmacology: drug disposition, action, and therapy in infants and children. N Engl J Med. 2003;349(12):1157–67.

33. Typpo K, Petersen N, Hallman D, Markovitz B, Mariscalco M. Impact of premorbid conditions on multiple organ dysfunction syndrome in the PICU. Crit Care Med. 2007;35(12):A10.

34. Carvalho PR, Feldens L, Seitz EE, Rocha TS, Soledade MA, Trotta EA. Prevalence of systemic inflammatory syndromes at a tertiary pediatric intensive care unit. J Pediatr (Rio J). 2005;81(2):143–8.

35. Leclerc F, Leteurtre S, Duhamel A, Grandbastien B, Proulx F, Martinot A, et al. Cumulative influence of organ dysfunctions and septic state on mortality of critically ill children. Am J Respir Crit Care Med. 2005;171(4):348–53.

36. Aneja RK, Carcillo JA. Differences between adult and pediatric septic shock. Minerva Anestesiol. 2011;77(10):986–92.

37. Stieh J, Fischer G, Scheewe J, Uebing A, Dutschke P, Jung O, et al. Impact of preoperative treatment strategies on the early perioperative outcome in neonates with hypoplastic left heart syndrome. J Thorac Cardiovasc Surg. 2006;131(5):1122–9. e2.

38. Seghaye MC, Engelhardt W, Grabitz RG, Faymonville ME, Hornchen H, Messmer BJ, et al. Multiple system organ failure after open heart surgery in infants and children. Thorac Cardiovasc Surg. 1993;41(1):49–53.

39. Baslaim G, Bashore J, Al-Malki F, Jamjoom A. Can the outcome of pediatric extracorporeal membrane oxygenation after cardiac surgery be predicted? Ann Thorac Cardiovasc Surg. 2006;12(1):21–7.

40. Aharon AS, Drinkwater Jr DC, Churchwell KB, Quisling SV, Reddy VS, Taylor M, et al. Extracorporeal membrane oxygenation in children after repair of congenital cardiac lesions. Ann Thorac Surg. 2001;72(6):2095–101. discussion 101–2.

41. Shime N, Ashida H, Hiramatsu N, Kageyama K, Katoh Y, Hashimoto S, et al. Arterial ketone body ratio for the assessment of the severity of illness in pediatric patients following cardiac surgery. J Crit Care. 2001;16:102–7.

42. Ben-Abraham R, Efrati O, Mishali D, Yulia F, Vardi A, Barzilay Z, et al. Predictors for mortality after prolonged mechanical ventilation after cardiac surgery in children. J Crit Care. 2002;17(4):235–9.

43. Calkins CM, Bensard DD, Moore EE, McIntyre RC, Silliman CC, Biffl W, et al. The injured child is resistant to multiple organ failure: a different inflammatory response? J Trauma. 2002;53(6):1058–63.

44. Steinau G, Kaussen T, Bolten B, Schachtrupp A, Neumann UP, Conze J, et al. Abdominal compartment syndrome in childhood: diagnostics, therapy and survival rate. Pediatr Surg Int. 2011;27(4):399–405.

45. Feickert HJ, Schepers AK, Rodeck B, Geerlings H, Hoyer PF. Incidence, impact on survival, and risk factors for multi-organ system failure in children following liver transplantation. Pediatr Transplant. 2001;5(4):266–73.

46. Pinho-Apezzato ML, Tannuri U, Tannuri AC, Mello ES, Lima F, Gibelli NE, et al. Multiple clinical presentations of lymphoproliferative disorders in pediatric liver transplant recipients: a single-center experience. Transplant Proc. 2010;42(5):1763–8.

47. Diaz M, Vicent M, Prudencio M, Rodriguez F, Marin C, Serrano A, et al. Predicting factors for admission to an intensive care unit and clinical outcome in pediatric patients receiving hematopoietic stem cell transplantation. Haematologica. 2002;87(3):292–8.

48. Kutko M, Calarco M, Flaherty M, Helmrich R, Ushay H, Pon S, et al. Mortality rates in pediatric septic shock with and without multiple organ system failure. Pediatr Crit Care Med. 2003;4(3):333–7.

49. Rossi R, Shemie SD, Calderwood S. Prognosis of pediatric bone marrow transplant recipients requiring mechanical ventilation. Crit Care Med. 1999;27(6):1181–6.

50. Mollen KP, Anand RJ, Tsung A, Prince JM, Levy RM, Billiar TR. Emerging paradigm: toll-like receptor 4-sentinel for the detection of tissue damage. Shock. 2006;26(5):430–7.

51. Gray MW, Burger G, Lang BF. The origin and early evolution of mitochondria. Genome Biol. 2001;2(6):Reviews1018.

52. Zhang Q, Raoof M, Chen Y, Sumi Y, Sursal T, Junger W, et al. Circulating mitochondrial DAMPs cause inflammatory responses to injury. Nature. 2010;464(7285):104–7.

53. Bianchi ME, Manfredi AA. High-mobility group box 1 (HMGB1) protein at the crossroads between innate and adaptive immunity. Immunol Rev. 2007;220:35–46.

54. Hazelzet JA, van der Voort E, Lindemans J, ter Heerdt PG, Neijens HJ. Relation between cytokines and routine laboratory data in children with septic shock and purpura. Intensive Care Med. 1994;20(5):371–4.

55. Kornelisse RF, Hazelzet JA, Savelkoul HF, Hop WC, Suur MH, Borsboom AN, et al. The relationship between plasminogen activator inhibitor-1 and proinflammatory and counterinflammatory mediators in children with meningococcal septic shock. J Infect Dis. 1996;173(5):1148–56.

56. Viktorov VV, Viktorova TV, Mironov PI, Khustnutdinova EK. Significance of hereditary factors in multiple organ dysfunction syndrome in children with infections. Anesteziol Reanimatol. 2000;1:32–4.

57. Mariscalco MM. Infection and the host response. In: Fuhrman BP, Zimmerman JJ, editors. Pediatric critical care. 3rd ed. Philadelphia: Mosby; 2006. p. 1299–319.

58. Hotchkiss RS, McConnell KW, Bullok K, Davis CG, Chang KC, Schwulst SJ, et al. TAT-BH4 and TAT-Bcl-xL peptides protect against sepsis-induced lymphocyte apoptosis in vivo. J Immunol. 2006;176(9):5471–7.

59. Singh-Naz N, Sprague BM, Patel KM, Pollack MM. Risk factors for nosocomial infection in critically ill children: a prospective cohort study. Crit Care Med. 1996;24(5):875–8.

60. Hall MW, Knatz NL, Vetterly C, Tomarello S, Wewers MD, Volk HD, et al. Immunoparalysis and nosocomial infection in children with multiple organ dysfunction syndrome. Intensive Care Med. 2011;37(3):525–32.

61. Cavaillon J, Adib-Conquy M, Cloez-Tayarani I, Fitting C. Immunodepression in sepsis and SIRS assessed by ex vivo cytokine production is not a generalized phenomenon: a review. J Endotoxin Res. 2001;7(2):85–93.

62. Adib-Conquy M, Moine P, Asehnoune K, Edouard A, Espevik T, Miyake K, et al. Toll-like receptor-mediated tumor necrosis factor and interleukin-10 production differ during systemic inflammation. Am J Respir Crit Care Med. 2003;168(2):158–64.

63. Adib-Conquy M, Adrie C, Moine P, Asehnoune K, Fitting C, Pinsky MR, et al. NF-kappaB expression in mononuclear cells of patients with sepsis resembles that observed in lipopolysaccharide tolerance. Am J Respir Crit Care Med. 2000;162(5):1877–83.

64. Cavaillon J, Fitting C, Adib-Conquy M. Mechanisms of immuno-dysregulation in sepsis. Contrib Nephrol. 2004;144:76–93.

65. Felmet KA, Hall MW, Clark RS, Jaffe R, Carcillo JA. Prolonged lymphopenia, lymphoid depletion, and hypoprolactinemia in children with nosocomial sepsis and multiple organ failure. J Immunol. 2005;174(6):3765–72.

66. Limaye AP, Kirby KA, Rubenfeld GD, Leisenring WM, Bulger EM, Neff MJ, et al. Cytomegalovirus reactivation in critically ill immunocompetent patients. JAMA. 2008;300(4):413–22. Research Support, N.I.H., Extramural Research Support, Non-U.S. Gov't.

67. Short M. Linking the sepsis triad of inflammation, coagulation and suppressed fibrinolysis to infants. Adv Neonat Care. 2004;4(5):258–73.

68. Doughty L, Carcillo JA, Kaplan S, Janosky J. The compensatory anti-inflammatory cytokine interleukin 10 response in pediatric sepsis-induced multiple organ failure. Chest. 1998;113(6):1625–31.

69. Doughty L, Carcillo JA, Kaplan S, Janosky J. Plasma nitrite and nitrate concentrations and multiple organ failure in pediatric sepsis. Crit Care Med. 1998;26(1):157–62.

70. Doughty LA, Kaplan SS, Carcillo JA. Inflammatory cytokine and nitric oxide responses in pediatric sepsis and organ failure. Crit Care Med. 1996;24(7):1137–43.

71. Hatherill M, Tibby SM, Turner C, Ratnavel N, Murdoch IA. Procalcitonin and cytokine levels: relationship to organ failure and mortality in pediatric septic shock. Crit Care Med. 2000;28(7):2591–4.

72. Whalen MJ, Doughty LA, Carlos TM, Wisniewski SR, Kochanek PM, Carcillo JA. Intercellular adhesion molecule-1 and vascular cell adhesion molecule-1 are increased in the plasma of children with sepsis-induced multiple organ failure. Crit Care Med. 2000;28(7):2600–7.

73. Han YY, Doughty LA, Kofos D, Sasser H, Carcillo JA. Procalcitonin is persistently increased among children with poor outcome from bacterial sepsis. Pediatr Crit Care Med. 2003;4(1):21–5.

74. Wong HR, Carcillo JA, Burckart G, Shah N, Janosky JE. Increased serum nitrite and nitrate concentrations in children with the sepsis syndrome. Crit Care Med. 1995;23(5):835–42.

75. Green J, Doughty L, Kaplan SS, Sasser H, Carcillo JA. The tissue factor and plasminogen activator inhibitor type-1 response in pediatric sepsis-induced multiple organ failure. Thromb Haemost. 2002;87(2):218–23.

76. Anisimova IN, Shvets OL, Guliaev DV, Tsinzerling VA, Belebez'ev GI. Morphologic aspects of hemostasis disturbances in meningococcemia in children. Arkh Patol. 1993;55(5):16–22.

77. Zeerleder S, Schroeder V, Hack CE, Kohler HP, Wuillemin WA. TAFI and PAI-1 levels in human sepsis. Thromb Res. 2006;118(2):205–12.

78. Levi M, de Jonge E, van der Poll T. New treatment strategies for disseminated intravascular coagulation based on current understanding of the pathophysiology. Ann Med. 2004;36(1):41–9.

79. Nguyen TC, Carcillo JA. Bench-to-bedside review: thrombocytopenia-associated multiple organ failure–a newly appreciated syndrome in the critically ill. Crit Care. 2006;10(6):235.

80. Nguyen T, Hall M, Han Y, Fiedor M, Hasset A, Lopez-Plaza I, et al. Microvascular thrombosis in pediatric multiple organ failure: is it a therapeutic target? Pediatr Crit Care Med. 2001;2(3):187–96.

81. Nguyen TC, Liu A, Liu L, Ball C, Choi H, May WS, et al. Acquired ADAMTS-13 deficiency in pediatric patients with severe sepsis. Haematologica. 2007;92(1):121–4.

82. Foley K, Keegan M, Campbell I, Murby B, Hancox D, Pollard B. Use of single-frequency bioimpedance at 50 kHz to estimate total body water in patients with multiple organ failure and fluid overload. Crit Care Med. 1999;27(8):1472–7.

83. Shime N, Ashida H, Chihara E, Kageyama K, Katoh Y, Yamagishi M, et al. Bioelectrical impedance analysis for assessment of severity of illness in pediatric patients after heart surgery. Crit Care Med. 2002;30(3):518–20.

84. Hazelzet JA, de Groot R, van Mierlo G, Joosten KF, van der Voort E, Eerenberg A, et al. Complement activation in relation to capillary leakage in children with septic shock and purpura. Infect Immun. 1998;66(11):5350–6.

85. Zhang S, Wang S, Li Q, Yao S, Zeng B, Ziegelstein RC, et al. Capillary leak syndrome in children with C4A-deficiency undergoing cardiac surgery with cardiopulmonary bypass: a double-blind, randomised controlled study. Lancet. 2005;366(9485):556–62.

86. Zhang S, Wang S, Yao S. Evidence for development of capillary leak syndrome associated with cardiopulmonary bypass in pediatric patients with the homozygous C4A null phenotype. Anesthesiology. 2004;100(6):1387–93.

87. Nurnberger W, Heying R, Burdach S, Gobel U. C1 esterase inhibitor concentrate for capillary leakage syndrome following bone marrow transplantation. Ann Hematol. 1997;75(3):95–101.

88. Naran N, Sagy M, Bock KR. Continuous renal replacement therapy results in respiratory and hemodynamic beneficial effects in pediatric patients with severe systemic inflammatory response syndrome and multiorgan system dysfunction. Pediatr Crit Care Med. 2010;11(6):737–40.

89. Flori HR, Church G, Liu KD, Gildengorin G, Matthay MA. Positive fluid balance is associated with higher mortality and prolonged mechanical ventilation in pediatric patients with acute lung injury. Crit Care Res Pract. 2011;2011:854142.

90. Goldstein SL, Currier H, Graf C, Cosio CC, Brewer ED, Sachdeva R. Outcome in children receiving continuous venovenous hemofiltration. Pediatrics. 2001;107(6):1309–12.

91. Goldstein SL, Somers MJ, Baum MA, Symons JM, Brophy PD, Blowey D, et al. Pediatric patients with multi-organ dysfunction syndrome receiving continuous renal replacement therapy. Kidney Int. 2005;67(2):653–8.

92. Michael M, Kuehnle I, Goldstein S. Fluid overload and acute renal failure in pediatric stem cell transplant patients. Pediatr Nephrol. 2004;19(1):91–5.

93. London NR, Zhu W, Bozza FA, Smith MCP, Greif DM, Sorensen LK, et al. Targeting Robo4-dependent Slit signaling to survive the cytokine storm in sepsis and influenza. Sci Transl Med. 2010;2(23):23ra19.

94. Ye X, Ding J, Zhou X, Chen G, Liu SF. Divergent roles of endothelial NF-kappaB in multiple organ injury and bacterial clearance in mouse models of sepsis. J Exp Med. 2008;205(6):1303–15.

95. Van den Berghe G, de Zegher F, Bouillon R. Acute and prolonged critical illness as different neuroendocrine paradigms. J Clin Endocrinol Metab. 1998;83(2):1827–34.

96. Joosten KF, de Kleijn ED, Westerterp M, de Hoog M, Eijck FC, Hop WCJ, et al. Endocrine and metabolic responses in children with meningococcal sepsis: striking differences between survivors and nonsurvivors. J Clin Endocrinol Metab. 2000;85(10):3746–53.

97. den Brinker M, Joosten KF, Liem O, de Jong FH, Hop WC, Hazelzet JA, et al. Adrenal insufficiency in meningococcal sepsis: bioavailable cortisol levels and impact of interleukin-6 levels and intubation with etomidate on adrenal function and mortality. J Clin Endocrinol Metab. 2005;90(9):5110–7.

98. Lichtarowicz-Krynska E, Cole T, Camacho-Hubner C, Britto J, Levin M, Klein N, et al. Circulating aldosterone levels are unexpectedly low in children with acute meningococcal disease. J Endocrinol Metab. 2004;89(3):1410–4.

99. Riordan F, Thomson A, Ratcliffe J, Sills J, Diver M, Hart C. Admission cortisol and adrenocorticotrophic hormone levels in children with meningococcal disease; evidence for adrenal insufficiency? Crit Care Med. 1999;27(10):2257–61.

100. De Kleijn ED, Joosten KF, Van Rijn B, Westerterp M, De Groot R, Hokken-Koelega AC, et al. Low serum cortisol in combination with high adrenocorticotrophic hormone concentrations are associated with poor outcome in children with severe meningococcal disease. Pediatr Infect Dis J. 2002;21(4):330–6.

101. den Brinker M, Joosten KF, Visser TJ, Hop WC, de Rijke YB, Hazelzet JA, et al. Euthyroid sick syndrome in meningococcal sepsis: the impact of peripheral thyroid hormone metabolism and binding proteins. J Clin Endocrinol Metab. 2005;90(10):5613–20.

102. den Brinker M, Dumas B, Visser TJ, Hop WC, Hazelzet JA, Festen DA, et al. Thyroid function and outcome in children who survived meningococcal septic shock. Intensive Care Med. 2005;31(7):970–6.

103. Van den Berghe G, de Zegher F, Lauwers P. Dopamine suppresses pituitary function in infants and children. Crit Care Med. 1994;22(11):1747–53.

104. Herndon DN, Gore D, Cole M, Desai MH, Linares H, Abston S, et al. Determinants of mortality in pediatric patients with greater than 70% full-thickness total body surface area thermal injury treated by early total excision and grafting. J Trauma. 1987;27(2):208–12.

105. Frayn K. Hormonal control of metabolism in trauma and sepsis. Clin Endocrinol. 1986;24(5):577–99.

106. Turi RA, Petros AJ, Eaton S, Fasoli L, Powis M, Basu R, et al. Energy metabolism of infants and children with systemic inflammatory response syndrome and sepsis. Ann Surg. 2001;233(4):581–7.

107. Briassoulis G, Venkataraman S, Thompson A. Cytokines and metabolic patterns in pediatric patients with critical illness. Clin Dev Immunol. 2010;2010:354047.

108. Cerra FB. Hypermetabolism-organ failure syndrome: a metabolic response to injury. Crit Care Clin. 1989;5(2):289–302.

109. Schwartz D, Mendonca M, Schwartz I, Xia Y, Satriano J, Wilson CB, et al. Inhibition of constitutive nitric oxide synthase (NOS) by nitric oxide generated by inducible NOS after lipopolysaccharide administration provokes renal dysfunction in rats. J Clin Invest. 1997;100(2):439–48.

110. Hotchkiss RS, Swanson PE, Freeman BD, Tinsley KW, Cobb JP, Matuschak GM, et al. Apoptotic cell death in patients with sepsis, shock, and multiple organ dysfunction. Crit Care Med. 1999;27:1230–51.

111. Singer M, Brealey D. Mitochondrial dysfunction in sepsis. Biochem Soc Symp. 1999;66:149–66.

112. Scheller K, Seibel P, Sekeris CE. Glucocorticoid and thyroid hormone receptors in mitochondria of animal cells. Int Rev Cytol. 2003;222:1–61.

113. Borutaite V, Budriunaite A, Brown GC. Reversal of nitric oxide-, peroxynitrite- and S-nitrosothiol-induced inhibition of mitochondrial respiration or complex I activity by light and thiols. Biochim Biophys Acta. 2000;1459(2–3):405–12.

114. Clementi E, Brown GC, Feelisch M, Moncada S. Persistent inhibition of cell respiration by nitric oxide: crucial role of S-nitrosylation of mitochondrial complex I and protective action of glutathione. Proc Natl Acad Sci U S A. 1998;95(13):7631–6.

115. Brealey D, Brand M, Hargreaves I, Heales S, Land J, Smolenski R, et al. Association between mitochondrial dysfunction and severity and outcome of septic shock. Lancet. 2002;360(9328):219–23.

116. Singer M. Multiorgan failure is an adaptive, endocrine-mediated, metabolic response to overwhelming systemic inflammation. Lancet. 2004;364:S45–7.

117. Pollack MM, Fields AI, Ruttimann UE. Sequential cardiopulmonary variables of infants and children in septic shock. Crit Care Med. 1984;12(7):554–9.

118. Pollack MM, Fields AI, Ruttimann UE. Distributions of cardiopulmonary variables in pediatric survivors and nonsurvivors of septic shock. Crit Care Med. 1985;13(6):454–9.

119. Mercier JC, Beaufils F, Hartmann JF, Azema D. Hemodynamic patterns of meningococcal shock in children. Crit Care Med. 1988;16(1):27–33.

120. Roth BL, Suba EA, Carcillo JA, Litten RZ. Alterations in hepatic and aortic phospholipase-C coupled receptors and signal transduction in rat intraperitoneal sepsis. Prog Clin Biol Res. 1989;286:41–59.

121. Duke TD, Butt W, South M. Predictors of mortality and multiple organ failure in children with sepsis. Intensive Care Med. 1997;23(6):684–92.

122. Siegel LB, Dalton HJ, Hertzog JH, Hopkins RA, Hannan RL, Hauser GJ. Initial postoperative serum lactate levels predict survival in children after open heart surgery. Intensive Care Med. 1996;22(1):1418–23.

123. Casado-Flores J, Mora E, Perez-Corral F, Martinez-Azagra A, Garcia-Teresa MA, Ruiz-Lopez MJ. Prognostic value of gastric intramucosal pH in critically ill children. Crit Care Med. 1998;26(6):1123–7.

124. Dugas MA, Proulx F, de Jaeger A, Lacroix J, Lambert M. Markers of tissue hypoperfusion in pediatric septic shock. Intensive Care Med. 2000;26(1):75–83.

125. Calvo RC, Ruza TF, Delgado Dominguez MA, Lopez-Herce CJ, Dorao Martinez-Romillo P. Effectiveness of hemodynamic treatment guided by gastric intramucosal pH monitoring. An Esp Pediatr. 2000;52(4):339–45.

126. de Souza RL, de Carvalho WB. Preliminary study about the utility of gastric tonometry during the weaning from mechanical ventilation. Rev Assoc Med Bras. 2002;48(1):66–72.

127. Campbell ME, Costeloe KL. Measuring intramucosal pH in very low birth weight infants. Pediatr Res. 2001;50(3):398–404.

128. Matthay M, Zimmerman G. Acute lung injury and the acute respiratory distress syndrome: four decades of inquiry into pathogenesis and rational management. Am J Respir Cell Mol Biol. 2005;33(4):319–27.

129. Flori HR, Glidden DV, Rutherford GW, Matthay MA. Pediatric acute lung injury: prospective evaluation of risk factors associated with mortality. Am J Respir Crit Care Med. 2005;171(9):995–1001.

130. Newth C, Stretton M, Deakers T, Hammer J. Assessment of pulmonary function in the early phase of ARDS in pediatric patients. Pediatr Pulmonol. 1997;23(3):169–75.

131. Fishel RS, Are C, Barbul A. Vessel injury and capillary leak. Crit Care Med. 2003;31(8 Suppl):S502–11.

132. Fink MP, Delude RL. Epithelial barrier dysfunction: a unifying theme to explain the pathogenesis of multiple organ dysfunction at the cellular level. Crit Care Clin. 2005;21(2):177–96.

133. Senthil M, Brown M, Xu DZ, Lu Q, Feketeova E, Deitch EA. Gut-lymph hypothesis of systemic inflammatory response syndrome/multiple-organ dysfunction syndrome: validating studies in a porcine model. J Trauma. 2006;60(5):958–65. discussion 65–7.

134. Sharma R, Tepas 3rd JJ, Hudak ML, Mollitt DL, Wludyka PS, Teng RJ, et al. Neonatal gut barrier and multiple organ failure: role of endotoxin and proinflammatory cytokines in sepsis and necrotizing enterocolitis. J Pediatr Surg. 2007;42(3):454–61.

135. Lacroix J, Nadeau D, Laberge S, Gauthier M, Lapierre G, Farrell CA. Frequency of upper gastrointestinal bleeding in a pediatric intensive care unit. Crit Care Med. 1992;20(1):35–42.

136. Gauvin F, Dugas MA, Chaibou M, Morneau S, Lebel D, Lacroix J. The impact of clinically significant upper gastrointestinal bleeding acquired in a pediatric intensive care unit. Pediatr Crit Care Med. 2001;2(4):294–8.

137. Chaibou M, Tucci M, Dugas MA, Farrell CA, Proulx F, Lacroix J. Clinically significant upper gastrointestinal bleeding acquired in a pediatric intensive care unit: a prospective study. Pediatrics. 1998;102(4 Pt 1):933–8.

138. Jordan I, Cambra FJ, Alcover E, Colomer J, Campistol J, Caritg J, et al. Neuromuscular pathology in a critical pediatric patient. Rev Neurol. 1999;29(5):432–5.

139. Sheth RD, Bolton CF. Neuromuscular complications of sepsis in children. J Child Neurol. 1995;10(5):346–52.

140. Petersen B, Schneider C, Strassburg HM, Schrod L. Critical illness neuropathy in pediatric intensive care patients. Pediatr Neurol. 1999;21(4):749–53.

141. Ohto T, Iwasaki N, Ohkoshi N, Aoki T, Ichinohe M, Tanaka R, et al. A pediatric case of critical illness polyneuropathy: clinical and pathological findings. Brain Dev. 2005;27(7):535–8.

142. Banwell BL, Mildner RJ, Hassall AC, Becker LE, Vajsar J, Shemie SD. Muscle weakness in critically ill children. Neurology. 2003;61(12):1779–82.

143. Morrison AL, Gillis J, O'Connell AJ, Schell DN, Dossetor DR, Mellis C. Quality of life of survivors of pediatric intensive care. Pediatr Crit Care Med. 2002;3(1):1–5.

144. Fanconi S, Kraemer R, Weber J, Tschaeppeler H, Pfenninger J. Long-term sequelae in children surviving adult respiratory distress syndrome. J Pediatr. 1985;106(2):218–22.

145. Ben-Abraham R, Weinbroum AA, Roizin H, Efrati O, Augarten A, Harel R, et al. Long-term assessment of pulmonary function tests in pediatric survivors of acute respiratory distress syndrome. Med Sci Monit. 2002;8(3):CR153–7.

146. Askenazi DJ, Feig DI, Graham NM, Hui-Stickle S, Goldstein SL. 3–5 year longitudinal follow-up of pediatric patients after acute renal failure. Kidney Int. 2006;69(1):184–9.

147. Bernard GR, Vincent JL, Laterre PF, LaRosa SP, Dhainaut JF, Lopez-Rodriguez A, et al. Efficacy and safety of recombinant human activated protein C for severe sepsis. N Engl J Med. 2001;344(10):699–709.

148. Nadel S, Goldstein B, Williams MD, Dalton H, Peters M, Macias WL, et al. Drotrecogin alfa (activated) in children with severe sepsis: a multicentre phase III randomised controlled trial. Lancet. 2007;369(9564):836–43.

149. Wheeler DS. An after action report of drotrecogin alpha (activated) and lessons for the future. Pediatr Crit Care Med. 2012;13:692–4.

150. Sprung CL, Annane D, Keh D, Moreno R, Singer M, Freivogel K, et al. Hydrocortisone therapy for patients with septic shock. N Engl J Med. 2008;358(2):111–24.

151. Bailey D, Phan V, Litalien C, Ducruet T, Merouani A, Lacroix J, et al. Risk factors of acute renal failure in critically ill children: a prospective descriptive epidemiological study. Pediatr Crit Care Med. 2007;8(1):29–35.

152. Vet NJ, de Hoog M, Tibboel D, de Wildt SN. The effect of inflammation on drug metabolism: a focus on pediatrics. Drug Discov Today. 2011;16(9–10):435–42.

153. Singer M. Mitochondrial function in sepsis: acute phase versus multiple organ failure. Crit Care Med. 2007;35(9):S441–8.

154. Piel DA, Gruber PJ, Weinheimer CJ, Courtois MR, Robertson CM, Coopersmith CM, et al. Mitochondrial resuscitation with exogenous cytochrome c in the septic heart. Crit Care Med. 2007;35(9):2120–7.

155. Vanhorebeek I, Langouche L, Van den Berghe G. Glycemic and nonglycemic effects of insulin: how do they contribute to a better outcome of critical illness? Curr Opin Crit Care. 2005;11(4):304–11.

156. Verbruggen SC, Joosten KF, Castillo L, van Goudoever JB. Insulin therapy in the pediatric intensive care unit. Clin Nutr. 2007;26(6):677–90.

157. Van den Berghe G, Wilmer A, Hermans G, Meersseman W, Wouters PJ, Milants I, et al. Intensive insulin therapy in the medical ICU. N Engl J Med. 2006;354(5):449–61.

158. van den Berghe G, Wouters P, Weekers F, Verwaest C, Bruyninckx F, Schetz M, et al. Intensive insulin therapy in the critically ill patients. N Engl J Med. 2001;345(19):1359–67.

159. Brunkhorst FM, Reinhart K. Sepsis therapy: present guidelines and their application. Chirurg. 2008;79(4):306–14.

160. Rivers E, Nguyen B, Havstad S, Ressler J, Muzzin A, Knoblich B, et al. Early goal-directed therapy in the treatment of severe sepsis and septic shock. N Engl J Med. 2001;345(19):1368–77.

161. Carcillo JA, Fields AI. Clinical practice parameters for hemodynamic support of pediatric and neonatal patients in septic shock. Crit Care Med. 2002;30(6):1365–78.

162. Randolph AG. Management of acute lung injury and acute respiratory distress syndrome in children. Crit Care Med. 2009;37(8):2448–54. Review.

163. Palevsky PM, Zhang JH, O'Connor TZ, Chertow GM, Crowley ST, Choudhury D, et al. Intensity of renal support in critically ill patients with acute kidney injury. N Engl J Med. 2008;359(1):7–20. Multicenter Study Randomized Controlled Trial Research Support, N.I.H., Extramural Research Support, U.S. Gov't, Non-P.H.S.

164. Bellomo R, Cass A, Cole L, Finfer S, Gallagher M, Lo S, et al. Intensity of continuous renal-replacement therapy in critically ill patients. N Engl J Med. 2009;361(17):1627–38. Multicenter Study Randomized Controlled Trial Research Support, Non-U.S. Gov't.

165. Payen D, de Pont AC, Sakr Y, Spies C, Reinhart K, Vincent JL. A positive fluid balance is associated with a worse outcome in patients with acute renal failure. Crit Care. 2008;12(3):R74. Multicenter Study Research Support, Non-U.S. Gov't.

166. Bouchard J, Soroko SB, Chertow GM, Himmelfarb J, Ikizler TA, Paganini EP, et al. Fluid accumulation, survival and recovery of kidney function in critically ill patients with acute kidney injury. Kidney Int. 2009;76(4):422–7. Multicenter Study Research Support, N.I.H., Extramural Research Support, Non-U.S. Gov't.

167. Foland JA, Fortenberry JD, Warshaw BL, Pettignano R, Merritt RK, Heard ML, et al. Fluid overload before continuous hemofiltration and survival in critically ill children: a retrospective analysis. Crit Care Med. 2004;32(8):1771–6.

168. Sutherland SM, Zappitelli M, Alexander SR, Chua AN, Brophy PD, Bunchman TE, et al. Fluid overload and mortality in children receiving continuous renal replacement therapy: the prospective pediatric continuous renal replacement therapy registry. Am J Kidney Dis. 2010;55(2):316–25. Multicenter Study Research Support, Non-U.S. Gov't.

169. Claure-Del Granado R, Mehta RL. Assessing and delivering dialysis dose in acute kidney injury. Semin Dial. 2011;24(2):157–63. Research Support, Non-U.S. Gov't Review.

170. Proulx F, Gauthier M, Nadeau D, Lacroix J, Farrell CA. Timing and predictors of death in pediatric patients with multiple organ system failure. Crit Care Med. 1994;22(6):1025–31.

171. Tan G, Tan T, Goh D, HK Y. Risk factors for predicting mortality in a paediatric intensive care unit. Ann Acad Med Singapore. 1998;27(6):813–8.

172. Khilnani P, Sarma D, Zimmerman J. Epidemiology and peculiarities of pediatric multiple organ dysfunction syndrome in New Delhi, India. Intensive Care Med. 2006;32:1856–62.

173. Proulx F, Fayon M, Farrell CA, Lacroix J, Gauthier M. Epidemiology of sepsis and multiple organ dysfunction syndrome in children. Chest. 1996;109(4):1033–7.

174. Keenan HT, Bratton SL, Martin LD, Crawford SW, Weiss NS. Outcome of children who require mechanical ventilatory support after bone marrow transplantation. Crit Care Med. 2000;28(3): 830–5.

175. Lamas A, Otheo E, Ros P, Vazquez JL, Maldonado MS, Munoz A, et al. Prognosis of child recipients of hematopoietic stem cell transplantation requiring intensive care. Intensive Care Med. 2003;29(1):91–6.

176. Proulx F, Joyal JS, Mariscalco MM, Leteurtre S, Leclerc F, Lacroix J. The pediatric multiple organ dysfunction syndrome. Pediatr Crit Care Med. 2009;10(1):12–22.

177. Mack CL, Ferrario M, Abecassis M, Whitington PF, Superina RA, Alonso EM. Living donor liver transplantation for children with liver failure and concurrent multiple organ system failure. Liver Transpl. 2001;7(10):890–5.

178. Kamat P, Kunde S, Vos M, Vats A, Heffron T, Romero R, et al. Invasive intracranial pressure monitoring is a useful adjunct in the management of severe hepatic encephalopathy associated with pediatric acute liver failure. Pediatr Crit Care Med. 2012;13(1): e33–8.

179. Ozanne B, Nelson J, Cousineau J, Lambert M, Phan V, Mitchell G, et al. Threshold for toxicity from hyperammonemia in critically ill children. J Hepatol. 2012;56(1):123–8.

180. Karapinar B, Yilmaz D, Balkan C, Akin M, Ay Y, Kvakli K. An unusual cause of multiple organ dysfunction syndrome in the pediatric intensive care unit: hemophagocytic lymphohistiocytosis. Pediatr Crit Care Med. 2009;10(3):285–90.

181. Castillo L, Carcillo J. Secondary hemophagocytic lymphohistiocytosis and severe sepsis/systemic inflammatory response syndrome/multiorgan dysfunction syndrome/macrophage activation syndrome share common intermediate phenotypes on a spectrum of inflammation. Pediatr Crit Care Med. 2009;10(3):387–92. Research Support, N.I.H., Extramural.

182. Chehal A, Taher A, Shamseddine A. Sicklemia with multi-organ failure syndrome and thrombotic thrombocytopenic purpura. Hemoglobin. 2002;26(4):345–51.

183. Brenner JL, Jadavji T, Pinto A, Trevenen C, Patton D. Severe Kawasaki disease in infants: two fatal cases. Can J Cardiol. 2000;16:1017–23.

184. Liet JM, Pelletier V, Robinson BH, Laryea MD, Wendel U, Morneau S, et al. The effect of short term dimethylglycine treatment on oxygen consumption in cytochrome oxidase deficiency: a double-blind randomized crossover trial. J Pediatr. 2003;142:62–6.

185. Brossier T, Gwinner N, Fontaine P, Girard C. Anesthetic malignant hyperthermia and multiple organ dysfunction syndrome. Ann Fr Anesth Reanim. 2001;20:647–50.

186. Gauvin F, Toledano B, Champagne J, Lacroix J. Reactive hemophagocytic syndrome presenting as a component of multiple organ dysfunction syndrome. Crit Care Med. 2000;28: 3341–5.

187. Cohen J. The immunopathogenesis of sepsis. Nature. 2002; 420(6917):885–91.

Withdrawal of Life Support

36

Ajit A. Sarnaik and Kathleen L. Meert

Abstract

Decisions regarding the limitation or withdrawal of life-sustaining therapies for critically ill children are intellectually and emotionally difficult. A working knowledge of the basic principles of biomedical ethics and their compassionate application are needed to guide the decision-making process. Health professionals and families must work together to achieve that which is in the best interest of the child. Optimal care during limitation or withdrawal of life support places a strong emphasis on palliation, which includes assessing the impact of each device, medication, and procedure on the comfort of the child. Additionally, the physical and emotional environment of the PICU can influence patients' and families' level of comfort at the time of death. Parents and families suffer greatly after the loss of a child. Follow-up of parents and families after a child's death is an important part of end-of-life care.

Keywords

Withdrawal of support • Ethics • Organ donation • Pediatrics

Introduction

Many of the treatment modalities available for supporting children with life-threatening illnesses are technologically complex and invasive, and consume considerable resources. Although intended to promote recovery and restore health, such treatment modalities can at times increase suffering and prolong the dying process if used indiscriminately in children who will ultimately succumb to their illness. To avoid unnecessary suffering, decisions to limit or withdraw support are often made [1]. In an analysis of more than 900 deaths in 35 U.S. PICUs occurring among children who did not meet brain death criteria, 85 % occurred after limitation or withdrawal of support [2]. Decisions regarding the forgoing of life-sustaining therapies for an individual child are intellectually and emotionally difficult. Thus, it is important for pediatric intensivists to have a working knowledge of the principles of biomedical ethics, and to be facile with the compassionate application of these principles in end-of-life care for children.

Ethical Framework

The teachings of Hippocrates instruct physicians to "refuse to treat those who are overmastered by their diseases, realizing that in such cases that medicine is powerless." Situations of medical futility include those in which treatment of a progressive or irreversible illness merely delays death, or leads to survival with excessive physical or mental impairment or unbearable suffering [3]. Thus, physicians are under no moral, legal, or ethical obligation to offer medically futile therapy. It is also widely accepted that competent persons have the right to refuse life-sustaining treatment. In order to avoid the dangers of medical futility on one end, and respect the sanctity of life on the other, physicians may apply the

A.A. Sarnaik, MD • K.L. Meert, MD (✉)
Department of Pediatrics,
Children's Hospital of Michigan,
3901 Beaubien Ave, Detroit, MI, USA
e-mail: asarnai@med.wayne.edu; kmeert@med.wayne.edu

principles of biomedical ethics as proposed by Beauchamp and Childress, which are autonomy, beneficence, nonmaleficence, and justice [4]. Although these ethical principles do not carry equal weight in the end-of-life care of an individual child, none can stand alone, and should thus be applied together to guide the decision-making process. Whether the best interest of a child is served by a life-sustaining treatment depends on the degree of suffering inflicted, potential future benefit, the level of support required to sustain life, and the views of the child, parents and professional caregivers [3].

Autonomy

The ethical principle of *autonomy*, or *respect for persons*, provides adults with decision-making power over what is done to their own bodies, and includes the right to refuse life-sustaining therapies. In the case of incapacitated adults, the ethical principle of *substituted judgment* is invoked. This is based on the premise that incapacitated adults are likely to have had prior expressed wishes concerning their end-of-life care, and that individuals close to them know what these wishes are. It is then the responsibility of the surrogate decision-maker to make the choice that the incapacitated patient would have wanted. Advanced directives preserve an individual's autonomy should he or she become incapacitated at some time in the future. Most children for whom decisions regarding the use of life support are being made have not reached the requisite developmental or cognitive level to meaningfully participate in such decision-making. However, there is evidence to suggest that children are often not consulted even when they are capable of contributing to the decision-making process regarding their own care [5]. American Academy of Pediatrics guidelines emphasize that physicians and parents should give great weight to the expressed views of children [6].

Beneficence and Nonmaleficence

The ethical principle of *beneficence* obliges physicians to base decisions about potential treatments on the benefits they are likely to provide the child. The accompanying ethical principle of *nonmaleficence* requires physicians to avoid or minimize potential harm to the child as a result of treatment. These two principles help physicians and family members create the *best interest standard* in the context of life-sustaining therapies, as with all medical decisions. Potential harms in continuing life-sustaining therapies may include exposure to invasive procedures, undesirable side effects, or a prolongation of an underlying illness that is accompanied with tremendous suffering. Potential benefits may include increased duration of life or other consequences of therapy

perceived as beneficial by parents, physicians or the patient. In applying the best interest standard, physicians and families are often faced with assessing what the child's quality of life would likely be if life-sustaining therapies were continued. However, quality of life is difficult to assess and perceptions of what constitutes quality may differ among individuals. Some may perceive adequate quality of life in the face of severe cognitive disability and technology dependence. For others, adequate quality of life may depend on the capacity for interpersonal relationships or perception of surroundings.

Justice

In the context of end-of-life care, *justice* considerations focus on the high cost to society of life-sustaining therapy provided to few, compared to the low-cost basic care being denied to many. In addition, life-sustaining therapy can be associated with harm and marginal benefit, whereas basic, preventative care would likely provide tremendous benefit to those who do not have access. Although justice is an important consideration, it should not be a major determinant of end-of-life decisions for an individual patient.

Family Centered Care and Conflict

Availability, honest communication, and sensitivity on the part of the medical team are extremely important in optimal interactions with families. Physicians and other healthcare providers should be willing and able to conduct family meetings on a regular basis that are ideally multi-disciplinary, thereby involving the child's primary physician, consultants, nurses, social work, and spiritual care where appropriate. The purpose of these meetings is to impart information, explore parents' concerns, and answer questions [7]. Adequate information is essential to good decision-making [6, 8–10]. However, it is not enough to simply enumerate facts and options, only to leave the entire burden of decision-making on the parents [3]. Physicians should make an independent assessment of what is in the child's best interest and provide guidance, which may range from sharing experience and perspective to making recommendations on a course of action [6]. General pediatricians and sub-specialists who have longstanding relationships with the child and family can be extremely helpful in discussions with families regarding the withholding or withdrawal of life support from a critically ill child. Among the many physicians and services that frequently contribute to the child's care, parents should know the identity of the attending physician ultimately responsible. Physicians from different specialties and backgrounds may however have different views. As such, they should discuss their views and ideally reach consensus among themselves before making recommendations to parents. Disagreements among physicians, real or perceived, regarding the forgoing of life support places undue stress on parents and leads to mistrust [11].

Conflicts between physicians and parents regarding what is in the child's best interest are common. Families may advocate continuing what physicians may deem futile care due to unrealistic expectations or overly optimistic hope of recovery. On the opposite end of the spectrum, parents may be unduly pessimistic or underestimate the potential for quality of life for a disabled child [3]. The physician should start with an honest and compassionate recommendation, which can emphasize to parents the shared nature of the decision-making and help relieve any doubt or guilt the parents may feel. Good communication and allowing more time can resolve most of these disagreements. If the conflict is not resolved, physicians are not obligated to provide treatments that in their judgment will not benefit the patient [12]. Hospitals should have mechanisms to address unresolved conflicts between physicians, patients and families. For example, one role of institutional ethics committees is to provide a forum for open discussion of medical, moral and legal issues involving decisions to forgo life support in a particular case [13]. However, ethics committees do not have the authority to force a decision one way or the other. Studies suggest that ethics committee consultations are useful in resolving conflicts regarding end-of-life decisions, and reduce the use of nonbeneficial treatments in intensive care units [14, 15]. When physician-parent consensus cannot be reached, it may be possible to transfer the child's care to another physician or institution that is willing to comply with the parents' wishes, if such is available [6, 16].

Providing Care During Withdrawal of Life Support

The term "forgo" in the context of life-sustaining therapy refers to withholding and withdrawing treatment, which are deemed by most to be morally and legally equivalent [6, 17]. In the intensive care setting, a decision to withhold life support usually refers to establishing with the family that support will not be escalated, and cardiopulmonary resuscitation will not be performed. A decision to withdraw life support usually refers to discontinuing one or more treatment modalities (e.g. mechanical ventilation) with the expectation that death will occur as a result. Such decisions must be accompanied by a careful evaluation of the child's palliative care needs [18, 19]. The focus of palliative care is on relief of the child's symptoms rather than cure of the underlying disease. Experts agree that certain elements of palliative care are appropriate for most critically ill children and should be applied regardless of whether or not their illness is likely to be terminal [18, 19]. However, a child's palliative care needs are almost certain to change once a decision to withdraw life support has been made. It is important to recognize that such patients continue to require considerable care in relation to their physical, emotional, social and spiritual needs.

Compassionate withdrawal of life support requires clinicians to assess each monitoring device or treatment modality applied to the patient with respect to the patient and family's goals [20]. For example, the goals for a dying child may include alleviation of pain, an opportunity to be held, and avoidance of a prolonged death. Blood tests, radiographs and vital sign monitoring may be more burdensome to the child than beneficial and therefore best discontinued. Two methods for withdrawing mechanical ventilator support from critically ill patients have been described, *terminal extubation* and *terminal weaning* [21–23]. Terminal extubation involves removal of the endotracheal tube from a ventilator dependent patient. Proponents of terminal extubation argue that it is direct and minimizes patient discomfort by shortening the dying process. Terminal weaning involves a rapid decrease (i.e. occurring over a few hours or less) in FiO_2, and ventilator rate and pressures to minimal settings, followed by extubation. Proponents of terminal weaning argue that it minimizes dyspnea and aspiration. Either method is acceptable depending on the patient's comfort level [21, 24]. In the case of brain death, extubation should be performed rather than weaning since the patient is already dead and patient comfort is no longer a concern.

Opiates and benzodiazepines are routinely used for treating pain, anxiety and dyspnea in dying children [9, 24, 25]. Meperidine is not recommended since its active metabolite, normeperidine, produces central nervous system excitation that can manifest as anxiety, tremors and seizures [9]. Clinicians should apply the concept of anticipatory dosing when administering sedatives and analgesics. For example, terminal extubation is likely to produce an abrupt change in the patient's ability to ventilate. Since dyspnea can be anticipated, sedatives and analgesics should be administered prior to extubation in order to prevent symptoms of air hunger [23]. Many critically ill children have been receiving opiates and benzodiazepines prior to a decision to forgo life support and may have developed some degree of tolerance. Dosages of such agents should be rapidly titrated to achieve adequate symptom control. Physicians recognize that increasing dosages of sedatives and analgesics may, in addition to controlling pain and suffering, hasten death. Increasing dosages of sedatives and analgesics may be administered to dying patients as long as the intent is to treat pain and suffering, and not to cause the patient's death. It has been suggested that intent be documented in the medical record [9]. For example, when medications are prescribed on an "as needed" basis, the order should explicitly state what the medication is to be given for (i.e. pain). The doctrine of *double effect*, which in this context the "good effect" is patient comfort, and the "bad effect" is hastening of the patient's death, renders this practice morally and ethically acceptable and minimizes discomfort at end-of-life [26, 27] The four conditions that must be met to satisfy this doctrine include the following [28]:

1. The act must be morally good or at least indifferent
2. The intention must cause the good effect, and there is no way to achieve the good effect without the occurrence of the bad effect
3. The bad effect must not be the means of producing the good effect
4. The good effect must be sufficiently desirable to compensate for the occurrence of the bad effect

The practices of euthanasia, in which the medical caregiver administers a lethal medication, and physician-assisted suicide, in which the patient delivers a lethal medication, are not supported by major professional organizations such as the American Medical Association, the American Academy of Pediatrics, and the American Thoracic Society [18, 29, 30]. However, there is some support for these practices, as euthanasia is legal in Belgium and the Netherlands, [31] and physician-assisted suicide is legal in the state of Oregon as well as in Switzerland. In those practices, the bad effect (causing the patient's death) is the means of producing the good effect (relief of suffering), thereby violating condition #3 above in the doctrine of double effect. Similarly, neuromuscular blocking agents have no role in treating patients' pain or suffering since they merely hasten death, but have no analgesic or sedating properties. Neuromuscular blockade also masks patients' symptoms thereby preventing their adequate assessment and treatment. Neuromuscular blocking agents should be discontinued and their effect worn off prior to withdrawing life support. In rare situations where neuromuscular blocking agents have been used for a long duration, clearance of the drug may be delayed and pharmacologic reversal incomplete. Physicians will have to weigh the degree of suffering caused by withdrawing life support from a patient without full neuromuscular function versus continuing treatment that has become unduly burdensome. The practice of *terminal sedation*, the use of high dose barbiturates and even propofol to sedate the patient to the point of unconsciousness at time of death, has been defended by some [9]. However, we do not advocate this approach since the distinction between alleviating suffering and euthanasia becomes obscure, and the doctrine of double effect may be violated [30, 32].

Other factors such as noise, lighting, privacy and the emotional attitudes of staff can influence patients and families' level of comfort at the time of death [11, 33–35]. Staff must be cognizant of how their words and body language can be perceived by families as kind and empathetic, or as uncaring and detached. Staff must demonstrate a caring presence without interfering with family privacy and togetherness. For patients in whom death appears imminent on withdrawal of life support, care is usually best provided in the ICU in order to provide continuity. Patients who are likely to survive for more than a few days are best taken care of on a general ward where a more intimate and less stressful environment can be created. Some parents may request that their child be taken home to die. With appropriate home care resources and support, death at home may be the most compassionate and respectful way to die [36, 37].

One of the most important needs of parents is maintaining relationship with their child at the time of the death [34, 35]. Parents should be given the option of being with their child when life support is withdrawn and during the death. Parents may want to hold their dying infant or toddler, or lie in bed with a child that is older. Most parents prefer unrestricted visiting but may need help from staff in directing and supporting other family members. Staff can help parents create memories of their child's last days that bring comfort in the future. For example, mementos such as a lock of hair, handprint, picture, blanket, favorite toy or article of clothing serve as symbols of the child's life and are especially meaningful to parents. Parents should be allowed the opportunity for religious rituals and family customs at the time of death. These practices help to maintain the parent-child relationship and build lasting memories.

Providing Care Around the Time of Death

Sensitivity and discernment are required to determine the most appropriate time to discuss the options of organ donation and autopsy with parents. Parents and families should be allowed to stay with their child's body as long as they wish after the child's death. Federal regulations require that institutions receiving Medicaid or Medicare have a trained, designated person approach families of deceased patients for organ donation [38]. The designated person is most often a representative of the local organ procurement agency. The representative will usually come to the hospital to discuss organ donation with the family and make the request. Research has shown that factors enhancing families' consent rate for organ donation include decoupling informing the parents of the death from the request for organs, participation of an organ procurement worker in the request, and making the request in a quiet, private place [39]. Many parents find comfort in the altruistic act of donating their child's organs. Even in situations where the organ procurement agency decides that the child is not an eligible donor, the child's lack of eligibility should be explained to the parents who may otherwise wonder in the future why they were not asked to donate [11]. In the past few decades, recovery of vital organs has generally been from brain dead donors. However, many hospitals have recently adopted protocols to recover organs from non-brain dead donors after the declaration of cardiac death, which usually occurs in the context of withdrawal of life support. This practice, known as donation after cardiac death (DCD), has drawn some ethical concerns which include, among others, potential violation of the Dead Donor Rule stating that the a donor must be irreversibly dead prior to the donation of vital organs [40–44]. However, the Institute of Medicine, Society of Critical Care Medicine, and more recently the American Academy of Pediatrics have endorsed DCD as a means to recover organs for transplantation [45–47].

Physicians also need to explain and request permission for autopsy from parents. Depending on the location and circumstances of the death, autopsy may not be an option but rather required by law. In some jurisdictions when the law requires an autopsy, the parent may be allowed to identify the child's body at the hospital thereby avoiding a distressing trip to the county morgue. If organ donation is possible and the law requires an autopsy, the medical examiner's office should be contacted in order to request their permission for organ donation and coordinate plans.

Follow-up of parents and families after the child's death is an important part of end-of-life care. Parents suffer greatly after the loss of a child, and adverse health outcomes are common, especially among parents whose child dies in the ICU [48, 49]. Sympathy cards, letters, and telephone calls from staff are deeply appreciated by most parents [50]. Formal memorial services and bereavement support for families are powerful means of helping families adjust to their loss. Meeting with the child's physician at some point after the death may help parents make sense of their experiences [51, 52]. Physicians can use these meetings to review the course of the child's illness, discuss the cause of death and autopsy findings, answer questions, inquire about family coping, and provide referrals. Most parents perceive these activities as a willingness on the part of the hospital and staff to provide ongoing emotional and informational support.

References

1. Devictor D, Latour JM, Tissieres P. Forgoing life-sustaining or death-prolonging therapy in the pediatric ICU. Pediatr Clin North Am. 2008;55(3):791–804. xiii.
2. Lee KJ, Tieves K, Scanlon MC. Alterations in end-of-life support in the pediatric intensive care unit. Pediatrics. 2010;126(4):e859–64.
3. Wellesley H, Jenkins IA. Withholding and withdrawing life-sustaining treatment in children. Paediatr Anaesth. 2009;19(10):972–8.
4. Beauchamp TL, Childress J. Principles of biomedical ethics. 5th ed. New York: Oxford; 2001.
5. McCallum DE, Byrne P, Bruera E. How children die in hospital. J Pain Symptom Manage. 2000;20(6):417–23.
6. American Academy of Pediatrics Committee on Bioethics: guidelines on foregoing life-sustaining medical treatment. Pediatrics. 1994;93 3:532–6.
7. Michelson KN, Emanuel L, Carter A, Brinkman P, Clayman ML, Frader J. Pediatric intensive care unit family conferences: one mode of communication for discussing end-of-life care decisions. Pediatr Crit Care Med. 2011;12(6):e336–43.
8. Kurz R. Decision making in extreme situations involving children: withholding or withdrawal of life supporting treatment in paediatric care. Statement of the ethics working group of the Confederation of the European Specialists of Paediatrics (CESP). Eur J Pediatr. 2001;160(4):214–6.
9. Truog RD, Cist AF, Brackett SE, et al. Recommendations for end-of-life care in the intensive care unit: the ethics Committee of the Society of Critical Care Medicine. Crit Care Med. 2001;29(12):2332–48.
10. Bell EF. Noninitiation or withdrawal of intensive care for high-risk newborns. Pediatrics. 2007;119(2):401–3.
11. Meert KL, Thurston CS, Sarnaik AP. End-of-life decision-making and satisfaction with care: parental perspectives. Pediatr Crit Care Med. 2000;1(2):179–85.
12. Guidelines for the appropriate use of do-not-resuscitate orders. Council on Ethical and Judicial Affairs, American Medical Association. JAMA. 1991;265 14:1868–71.
13. Institutional ethics committees. Committee on bioethics. Pediatrics. 2001;107(1):205–9.
14. Schneiderman LJ, Gilmer T, Teetzel HD, et al. Effect of ethics consultations on nonbeneficial life-sustaining treatments in the intensive care setting: a randomized controlled trial. JAMA. 2003;290(9):1166–72.
15. Yen BM, Schneiderman LJ. Impact of pediatric ethics consultations on patients, families, social workers, and physicians. J Perinatol. 1999;19(5):373–8.
16. Texas Health & Safety Code – Section 166.052. Statements explaining patient's right to transfer.
17. Rachels J. Active and passive euthanasia. N Engl J Med. 1975;292(2):78–80.
18. American Academy of Pediatrics. Committee on Bioethics and Committee on Hospital Care. Palliative care for children. Pediatrics. 2000;106(2 Pt 1):351–7.
19. Field MJ, Behrman RE. When children die: improving palliative and end-of-life care for children and their families. Washington, DC: National Academy Press; 2003.
20. Brody H, Campbell ML, Faber-Langendoen K, Ogle KS. Withdrawing intensive life-sustaining treatment – recommendations for compassionate clinical management. N Engl J Med. 1997;336(9):652–7.
21. Faber-Langendoen K. The clinical management of dying patients receiving mechanical ventilation. A survey of physician practice. Chest. 1994;106(3):880–8.
22. Gilligan T, Raffin TA. Withdrawing life support: extubation and prolonged terminal weans are inappropriate. Crit Care Med. 1996;24(2):352–3.
23. Billings JA. Humane terminal extubation reconsidered: the role for pre-emptive analgesia and sedation. Crit Care Med. 2012;40(2):625–30.
24. Burns JP, Mitchell C, Outwater KM, et al. End-of-life care in the pediatric intensive care unit after the forgoing of life-sustaining treatment. Crit Care Med. 2000;28(8):3060–6.
25. Zernikow B, Michel E, Craig F, Anderson BJ. Pediatric palliative care: use of opioids for the management of pain. Paediatr Drugs. 2009;11(2):129–51.
26. Quill TE, Dresser R, Brock DW. The rule of double effect–a critique of its role in end-of-life decision making. N Engl J Med. 1997;337(24):1768–71.
27. Sulmasy DP, Pellegrino ED. The rule of double effect: clearing up the double talk. Arch Intern Med. 1999;159(6):545–50.

28. Doctrine of double effect. Stanford Encyclopedia of Philosophy. 2004. http://plato.stanford.edu/entries/double-effect. Accessed 18 Jul 2011.

29. Council on Ethical and Judicial Affairs, American Medical Association. Decisions near the end of life. JAMA. 1992;267(16): 2229–33.

30. Lanken PN, Terry PB, Delisser HM, et al. An official American Thoracic Society clinical policy statement: palliative care for patients with respiratory diseases and critical illnesses. Am J Respir Crit Care Med. 2008;177(8):912–27.

31. Manthous CA. Why not physician-assisted death? Crit Care Med. 2009;37(4):1206–9.

32. Rady MY, Verheijde JL. Continuous deep sedation until death: palliation or physician-assisted death? Am J Hosp Palliat Care. 2009;27(3):205–14.

33. Meert KL, Briller SH, Schim SM, Thurston CS. Exploring parents' environmental needs at the time of a child's death in the pediatric intensive care unit. Pediatr Crit Care Med. 2008;9(6): 623–8.

34. Meert KL, Briller SH, Schim SM, Thurston C, Kabel A. Examining the needs of bereaved parents in the pediatric intensive care unit: a qualitative study. Death Stud. 2009;33(8):712–40.

35. Meert KL, Thurston CS, Briller SH. The spiritual needs of parents at the time of their child's death in the pediatric intensive care unit and during bereavement: a qualitative study. Pediatr Crit Care Med. 2005;6(4):420–7.

36. Needle JS. Home extubation by a pediatric critical care team: providing a compassionate death outside the pediatric intensive care unit. Pediatr Crit Care Med. 2009;11(3):401–3.

37. Sarnaik AP. A student, a nun, and a professor. Pediatr Crit Care Med. 2000;1(2):176–8.

38. Federal register final rule: hospital conditions for participation for organ donation. 42 CFR Part 482,2000.

39. Gortmaker SL, Beasley CL, Sheehy E, et al. Improving the request process to increase family consent for organ donation. J Transpl Coord. 1998;8(4):210–7.

40. Robertson JA. The dead donor rule. Hastings Cent Rep. 1999;29(6): 6–14.

41. Carcillo JA, Orr R, Bell M, et al. A call for full public disclosure and moratorium on donation after cardiac death in children. Pediatr Crit Care Med. 2010;11(5):641–3. author reply 643-645.

42. Rady MY, Verheijde JL, McGregor J. Organ donation after cardiac death: are we willing to abandon the dead-donor rule? Pediatr Crit Care Med. 2007;8(5):507. author reply 507-509.

43. Veatch RM. Donating hearts after cardiac death–reversing the irreversible. N Engl J Med. 2008;359(7):672–3.

44. Hornby K, Hornby L, Shemie SD. A systematic review of autoresuscitation after cardiac arrest. Crit Care Med. 2010;38(5):1246–53.

45. Policy statement--pediatric organ donation and transplantation. Pediatrics. 2010;125 4:822–8.

46. Herdman R, Beauchamp TL, Potts JT. The Institute of Medicine's report on non-heart-beating organ transplantation. Kennedy Inst Ethics J. 1998;8(1):83–90.

47. A position paper by the Ethics Committee, American College of Critical Care Medicine, Society of Critical Care Medicine. Recommendations for nonheartbeating organ donation. Crit Care Med. 2001;29(9):1826–31.

48. Meert KL, Donaldson AE, Newth CJ, et al. Complicated grief and associated risk factors among parents following a child's death in the pediatric intensive care unit. Arch Pediatr Adolesc Med. 2010;164(11):1045–51.

49. Hendrickson KC. Morbidity, mortality, and parental grief: a review of the literature on the relationship between the death of a child and the subsequent health of parents. Palliat Support Care. 2009;7(1): 109–19.

50. Macdonald ME, Liben S, Carnevale FA, et al. Parental perspectives on hospital staff members' acts of kindness and commemoration after a child's death. Pediatrics. 2005;116(4):884–90.

51. Meert KL, Eggly S, Pollack M, et al. Parents' perspectives regarding a physician-parent conference after their child's death in the pediatric intensive care unit. J Pediatr. 2007;151(1):50–5. 55 e51-52.

52. Eggly S, Meert KL, Berger J, et al. A framework for conducting follow-up meetings with parents after a child's death in the pediatric intensive care unit. Pediatr Crit Care Med. 2010;12(2): 147–52.

Sam D. Shemie and Sonny Dhanani

Abstract

The concept of brain death was influenced by two major advances in health care in the 1960s: the development of intensive care units with artificial airways and mechanical ventilators that treated irreversible apnea, thus interrupting the natural evolution from brain failure to cardiocirculatory death, and, to address ethical concerns associated with organ donation arising from the then-new discipline of transplant surgery. Brain death is defined as the irreversible loss of the capacity for consciousness combined with the irreversible loss of all brainstem functions, including the capacity to breathe. For patients who die as a result of severe brain injury, standard end-of-life care should include offering the option of organ and tissue donation for eligible patients. All patients who are suspected of being brain dead should have an assessment to document this fact, to diagnose death, and establish donor eligibility. This chapter reviews the history of brain death, pathophysiology, and diagnostic criteria for declaration including minimum clinical criteria and ancillary testing. Current variability and practice controversies are discussed.

Keywords

Brain death • Brainstem death • Organ donation • End of life care • Death declaration • Brainstem reflexes • Apnea testing • Confounding factors • Ancillary testing

History of the Brain Death Concept

The concept of brain death was influenced by two major advances in health care in the 1960s: (1) the development of intensive care units with artificial airways and mechanical ventilators that treated irreversible apnea, thus interrupting the natural evolution from brain failure to cardiocirculatory death, and, (2) to address ethical concerns associated with organ donation arising from the then-new discipline of transplant surgery. Prior to the introduction of mechanical ventilators in the mid twentieth century and the evolution of resuscitative measures, a non-brain or circulation formulation was used to determine death. Historical records indicate that Rabbi Moses Maimonides was the first to suggest that the brain was of primary importance in sustaining life when he noted that decapitated individuals would invariably die. The clinical appearance of brain death was first described in seminal work by the French in 1959 and termed "coma dépassé" [1] meaning "a state beyond coma", which described 23 cases in which loss of consciousness, brain stem reflexes, and spontaneous respiration was associated with absent encephalographic activity. In 1968, the Ad Hoc Committee of the Harvard Medical School, lead by neurologists Schwab and Adams, undertook to define irreversible coma and brain death [2]. They established a new, neurologically based definition of death defined as "*unresponsiveness and lack of receptivity, the absence of movement*

S.D. Shemie, PhD
Department of Critical Care, Montreal Children's Hospital,
2300 Tupper Street room C-806, Montreal, QC, Canada
e-mail: sam.shemie@mcgill.ca

S. Dhanani, Bsc (Pharm), MD, FRCPC (✉)
Pediatric Critical Care, Children's Hospital of Eastern Ontario,
Ottawa, ON, Canada
e-mail: sdhanani@cheo.on.ca

D.S. Wheeler et al. (eds.), *Pediatric Critical Care Medicine*,
DOI 10.1007/978-1-4471-6362-6_37, © Springer-Verlag London 2014

and breathing, the absence of brain-stem reflexes and coma whose cause had been identified". Also recommended was an isoelectric EEG with repetition of all tests after a period of at least 24 h.

In the 1970s Mohandas and Chou emphasized the importance of irreversible loss of brainstem function in brain death [3], the importance of which was then the focus of a published statement by the Conference of Medical Royal Colleges and Their Faculties in the United Kingdom (UK) in 1976 [4]. Subsequently championed by Pallis and Harley, the brainstem formulation of brain death was formally adopted in the UK in 1995 [5]. In the United States, the Uniform Determination of Death Act [6] codifies the whole-brain formulation in stating "an individual who has sustained irreversible cessation of all functions of the entire brain, including the brainstem, is dead." This formulation is the one most commonly applied worldwide and forms the foundation for legal codification in many Western nations.

Brain death declaration has been used to initiate withdrawal of mechanical support discussions and is a prerequisite to organ donation. Its concept has been internationally accepted as a medical and legal definition of death in many countries with advanced health care systems. Despite the widespread acceptance of the criteria, there are limitations in the levels of evidence to support many of the procedures and substantial variability of clinical practice internationally and within nations [7, 8]. This chapter will focus on the medical aspects of the diagnosis to guide PICU practitioners in the field.

The Neurological Determination of Death: Concept, Terminology and Clinical Relevance

Whole-Brain Versus Brainstem Death

Brain death is defined as the irreversible loss of the capacity for consciousness combined with the irreversible loss of all brainstem functions, including the capacity to breathe. It is important to understand that the clinical evaluation documents the complete loss of brainstem function, but it does not distinguish between brainstem death, as may be seen in massive brainstem infarction, or whole brain death that involves the cerebrum and brainstem. The *whole-brain formulation* accepted in the USA is characterized by irreversible loss of function of both the cerebral hemispheres and the brainstem. An intact brainstem is integral to the preservation of most regulatory and homeostatic mechanisms, while the reticular formation, thalamus, and cerebral hemispheres all play roles

in the preservation of consciousness. Global disruption of these structures forms the basis for whole-brain death.

Clinical evaluation of these structures in the context of brainstem death is essentially identical to that used for the evaluation of whole-brain death. The *brainstem formulation* accepted in the UK requires irreversible cessation of brainstem functioning and is based on the fact that the reticular formation forms the basis of consciousness and that the brainstem nuclei preserve regulatory and homeostatic mechanisms. Destruction of the brainstem and reticular formation should result in unconsciousness [9]. US experts have argued against using the brainstem formulation because of the possibility of a "super locked-in syndrome" in which awareness might be retained in the absence of all other signs of brainstem activity [10, 11].

Brain Death Versus Brain Arrest

Brain death is a term and a concept that remains a source of misunderstanding for many practitioners, casual observers, and the public. There is ongoing animated discourse in bioethical, religious, socio-anthropological and philosophical circles [12, 13]. International variability in criteria or definitions may fuel this debate and lay doubt to the credibility of the diagnosis. It may be difficult to comprehend 'death' in an individual whose vital functions – heart beat, the warmth of circulation, and tidal movement of the lungs – are maintained by support technology. Persistence of some neuroregulatory function may be observed with variable preservation of anterior pituitary function [14] and theoretical argument occurs as to the possibility of functioning nests of neurons [15]. While brain death may be discussed, perceived or argued as death of the brain, from an ICU-based physiological perspective, it is better understood as irreversible brain arrest or complete brain failure. It is the maximum clinical expression of irreversible neurological failure [16].

The event of a cardiac arrest, if irreversible, leads to death that is subsequently determined by cardiocirculatory criteria based on the absence of heartbeat and circulation. Once brain arrest occurs and is irreversible, death is subsequently determined by neurological criteria. This neurological determination of death is the *process and procedure* to determine death. It should never be confused with other forms of severe brain injury, such as persistent vegetative state, cortical death or anencephaly. Brain injury in these conditions may be catastrophic and irreversible, but it is not complete as clinical signs of residual brainstem function persist [17].

The concept of brain death has been criticized as a social construct created for utilitarian purposes to permit transplantation [13, 18, 19]. However, traditional cardiopulmonary definitions of death (asystole, circulatory arrest, and apnea) are no longer sufficient in the face of advancing technology that may support and/or replace complete and irreversible loss of heart and/or lung function. Every solid organ can be supported by ICU-based technology or replaced by transplantation *except* the brain. If the heart is completely and irreversibly arrested, death has not occurred if the circulation is being supported by a machine such as extracorporeal membrane oxygenation (ECMO) or other forms of artificial heart technology, as long as neurological function is salvageable [20]. Cardiorespiratory function can be sustained in any form or severity brain failure. Although it was once considered that brain death invariably leads to hemodynamic stability and cardiac arrest [21, 22], it is now clear that aggressive cardiorespiratory support, hormonal therapy, and nursing care can maintain somatic functions indefinitely [23–25]. These continued advances in technology and transplantation have made brain- based determination of death more relevant and valid but also more complex today than in its origin.

End-of-Life Care and the Obligations of the PICU

For patients who die as a result of severe brain injury, standard end-of-life care should include offering the option of organ and tissue donation for eligible patients. Routine provision of the opportunity to donate has become law in a number of jurisdictions, reflecting strong societal support for organ donation. Although the benefits of organ donation have been traditionally linked to the needs of transplant recipients, it is increasingly apparent that families desire the opportunity as a fundamental part of, rather than distinct from, end-of-life care. Families of children who die in the PICU may offer organs despite being ineligible and in follow-up, of those who were not asked to donate, 37 % wanted the opportunity to be presented [26, 27].

All patients who are suspected of being brain dead should have an assessment to document this fact, to diagnose death and establish donor eligibility [28]. Diagnosis of brain death should be made to support the family's wishes and in a timely fashion. Brain death is the exclusive domain of ICU practice and the determination of death should be made as per accepted medical standards in the local jurisdiction. Families should be supported through the declaration and the death process. Correspondingly, the PICU, in collaboration with regional organ donation/procurement services, should be responsible for ensuring that the opportunity for donation occurs [29].

Demographics and Etiology

The most common etiologies of brain injury leading to brain death in children are traumatic brain injury and hypoxic-ischemic encephalopathy after cardiac arrest, followed up relatively rarely by cerebrovascular accidents and CNS tumors. The demographics have changed over time in adults, where cerebrovascular accidents now exceed traumatic brain injury as the primary cause leading to brain death [30, 31]. Acute neurosurgical lesions account for the majority of cases and include traumatic brain injury, intracranial hemorrhage related to vascular malformations or tumors, and acute hydrocephalus. Other causes in children include infection (meningitis, encephalitis), metabolic encephalopathies (hepatic failure, diabetic ketoacidosis, inborn errors of metabolism, hyponatremia) and vasculitis [29].

The true incidence of brain death is not known, as there is currently no mechanism for mandatory reporting. This is problematic, as countries report their organ donor rates as "per million population", which does not account for the wide variation of motor vehicle, cerebrovascular fatality rates, and medical/surgical resources between countries and within geographic regions of each country. Indirect estimates suggest the incidence of brain death is progressively decreasing [32]. Successful public health policy is reducing the incidence of traumatic brain injury, early field interventions and advances in neuroprotective therapy decreases mortality, and earlier neuroprognostication leads to recommendations to withdraw to life sustaining therapy prior to brain death occurring. Table 37.1 lists the demographics of brain death in children from a large single center experience [29]. Of all deaths in the PICU, 16–38 % are brain death (Fig. 37.1), dependent on the geographic location and type of unit, disease severity, end-of-life practices and the application of the diagnostic criteria.

Pathophysiology

Regardless of the primary etiology of brain injury, tissue edema or mass effect leads to the final common pathway characterized by increasing intracranial pressure, which progressively impairs cerebral blood flow. As pressure rises inside the rigid intracranial vault, it may do so heterogeneously throughout the brain or selectively within compartments. Pressure-related ischemia ensues leading to further neuronal/glial injury, abnormal vascular autoregulation, and edema [33]. This contributes to a continued rise in ICP until intracerebral pressure exceeds arterial inflow pressure and cerebral circulatory arrest occurs. In response to rising intracranial pressure, the brain herniates through paths of least resistance

(Fig. 37.2), most commonly seen as downward descent of the brainstem and cerebellum through the foramen magnum (Fig. 37.3a, b). Cellular disruption and herniation triggers an inflammatory cascade that affects cardiorespiratory function, and hormonal regulation [34]. This cascade affects pituitary and hypothalamic function resulting in catecholamine, thyroid, and vasopressin abnormalities [22, 35–37].

The duration of time from injury to brain death may vary, depending on mechanism and severity of initial injury and the response to neuroprotective therapies. Acute and massive rises in ICP as seen with explosive brain death [38], as may be seen with sudden intracranial hemorrhage, may present immediately with herniation. Slower rises in ICP, in response to acute injury and gradual cerebral edema e.g. hypoxia-ischemia, make take many days.

Table 37.1 Demographics of pediatric brain death (Hospital for Sick Children, Toronto, from January 1990 to December 1997)

Etiology	n=199 (%)
Acute neurosurgical lesions	91 (46 %)
Hypoxic-ischemic encephalopathy	66 (33 %)
Infection	24 (12 %)
Miscellaneous	18 (9 %)
Age	Mean 5.80 +/- 5.2 years
	Median 4.15 years

Adapted from Tsai et al. [29]. With permission from Wolter Kluwers Health

1. Acute Neurosurgical Lesions (*ANL*)- includes head trauma from motor vehicle accident, intracranial bleed from arterio-venous malformations, non-accidental injury, intracranial tumour in isolation and acute hydrocephalus
2. Hypoxic-Ischemic Encephalopathy (*HIE*) including post-cardiac arrest or respiratory arrest patients, near SIDS, near drowning, asphyxia and hypovolemic shock
3. Infection including meningitis, encephalitis and generalized sepsis
4. Miscellaneous diagnoses such as metabolic encephalopathy from liver disease, diabetic ketoacidosis, inborn errors of metabolism, hyponatremia and vasculitis

Minimum Clinical Criteria

Brainstem Reflexes

Brain death is fundamentally a detailed clinical examination that documents the *complete and irreversible loss of consciousness and absence of brainstem function including the capacity to breathe.* The following criteria in the clinical assessment for brain death determination are not uniform but still remarkably similar throughout the world, most based on initial American Academy of Pediatric guidelines in 1987 (Table 37.2) [39–43].

Etiology and Coma

The fundamental principle of organ donation continues to reflect adherence to the 'dead donor rule' [44]. As a result, an absolute prerequisite is the absence of clinical neurological function with a known, proximate cause that is irreversible. There must be definite clinical and/or neuroimaging evidence of an acute central nervous system (CNS) event that is consistent with the irreversible loss of neurological function. Coma of unclear mechanism or etiology precludes the diagnosis.

Absent Motor Response

Deep unresponsive coma implies a Glasgow Coma Score (GCS) of 3 and specifically an absence of centrally mediated response to pain. This should be tested with deep central stimulation at the sternum or clavicles bilaterally. Any motor response in the cranial nerve distribution, CNS-mediated motor response to pain in any distribution, seizures, decorticate and/or decerebrate responses is not compatible with the diagnosis. Spinal reflexes, or motor responses confined to spinal distribution, may persist. A proportion of patients may continue to display some reflex spinal activity, which can confuse the bedside staff or the inexperienced clinician and

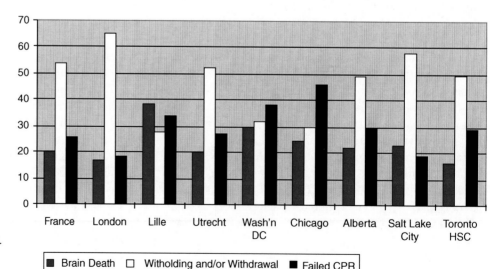

Fig. 37.1 Modes of death in PICU: comparison of literature rates of different modes of death for children admitted to the paediatric intensive care units (Adapted from Martinot et al. [28]. With permission from John Wiley & Sons, Inc.)

be disturbing to family members. They should be anticipated and explanations should be provided to families. Observed spinal reflex activity may range from subtle twitches to the more complex "Lazarus sign" and may be seen in 13–39 % of cases [45–47]. Persistence of these reflexes is compatible with brain death [48]. If disagreement arises as to their interpretation, an ancillary test should be performed.

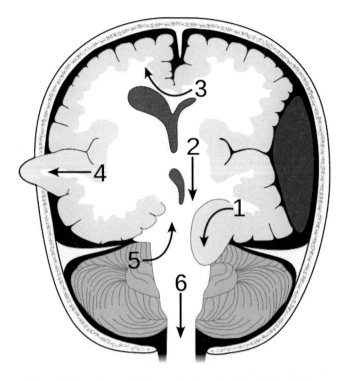

Fig. 37.2 Sites of potential herniation in response to intracranial pressure. (1) Supratentorial herniation (**a**) uncal, (**b**) central (transtentorial), (**c**) cingulate (subfalcine), (**d**) transcalvarial. (2) Infratentorial herniation (**e**) upward (upward cerebellar or upward transtentorial), (**f**) tonsillar (downward cerebellar) (Reprinted from Wikipedia Commons. File: brain herniation types-2.svg. http://commons.wikimedia.org/wiki/File:Brain_herniation_types-2.svg with permission from the Creative Commons License)

Absent Brainstem Reflexes

Brainstem reflexes should be tested by localizing specific cranial nerves. Any response excludes brain death. A suction catheter should be inserted into the endotracheal tube to stimulate the trachea. A Yankauer suction or tongue depressor should be inserted into the back of the pharynx to observe for a gag response. Corneal responses should be evaluated by absence of blink response by opening the eye to expose the cornea and lightly touching the cornea with tissue. The pupils should be tested with a specific ophthalmoscope for direct and indirect response to light and should be dilated >4 mm and non-reactive. Interpretation should be cautious when topical ocular instillations or systemic atropine has been used. The oculo-cephalic, or so-called "dolls eyes" reflex is a less potent stimulus to the vestibular system, contraindicated when cervical spine injury is suspected and is generally not required. This should be performed by briskly moving the head side to side, observing for movement of the pupils. The pupils should remain mid-positioned. Ashwal recommends that the oculo-cephalic reflex be evaluated and documented in neonates and infants in whom the oculo-vestibular reflex may be more difficult to determine [49]. In newborns, the suck reflex may be included [40]. The oculo-vestibular reflex or so-called 'caloric test' should be performed with the head at 30°, irrigating the canals with 50 ml of ice water via a catheter into the ear canal. Both eyes should be observed for 5 min with any eye deviation from the midline excluding brain death. Auditory canal should be patent and trauma to the tympanic membrane should be ruled out first [41, 50].

Apnea Testing

Determination of persistent apnea is required as a fundamental part of the clinical criteria and is based on the absence of any sign of respiratory effort (mediated by the medullary

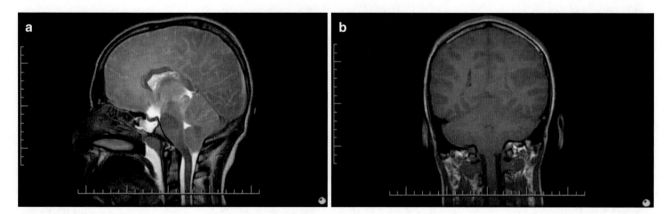

Fig. 37.3 Sagittal T2 (**a**) and coronal T1 (**b**) series MRI after brain death, demonstrating downward herniation of brain stem and cerebellum through the foramen magnum

Table 37.2 Clinical criteria for brain death

1. Established etiology
Capable of causing brain death in the absence of reversible conditions capable of mimicking brain death
2. Deep unresponsive coma
3. Absent motor responses, excluding spinal reflex or mycolonus
4. Absent brainstem reflexes
Gag and cough response
Corneal responses
Pupillary responses to light with pupils at mid size or greater
Oculo-cephalic and oculo-vestibular responses
5. Absent respiratory effort based on the apnea test
6. Absent confounding factors

Based on Refs. [40, 43]

Table 37.3 Confounding factors in the diagnosis of brain death

1. Unresuscitated shock or hypotension
2. Hypothermia
3. Severe metabolic disorders capable of causing a potentially reversible coma
4. Peripheral nerve, muscle dysfunction or neuromuscular blockade potentially accounting for unresponsiveness e.g. Guillain-Barre syndrome
5. Clinically significant drug intoxications (e.g., alcohol, barbiturates, sedatives, hypnotics)
6. The acute post resuscitation phase after cardiac arrest

Based on Refs. [40, 43]

respiratory center) in response to acute hypercarbic stimulation. In less technically advanced centers, apnea determined by ventilator disconnection may be sufficient [18]. However, most guidelines require documentation of apneic threshold as determined by arterial blood gas analysis. Most require a starting pH of 7.40 with normalized $PaCO_2$. American [51] and Canadian [40] guidelines recommend an apneic threshold $PaCO_2 \geq 60$ mmHg and increase of 20 mmHg above baseline [43]. Some guidelines also require documentation of an acidemic pH < 7.28 [40].

Optimal performance of the apnea test requires a period of preoxygenation followed by 100 % oxygen delivered via to the trachea (e.g. insufflation via endotracheal catheter inserted into distal trachea) upon disconnection from mechanical ventilation. Oxygen flow can be maintained at 4–5 L/min to support oxygenation. High flow rates could cause CO_2 washout and delay arterial $PaCO_2$ rise. Alternatively, endotracheal CPAP can be provided to minimize any potential respiratory instability [52]. To correctly interpret an apnea test, the certifying physician must continuously observe the patient for respiratory effort throughout the performance of the test. The rate of rise of $PaCO_2$ during the apnea test is non-linear, depends on body temperature (metabolic rate) and basal $PaCO_2$ [53] and often requires up to 10–20 min off the ventilator. It is estimated that approximately 3–6 mmHg/min rise of $PaCO_2$ occurs after disconnection from the ventilator. Serial arterial blood gases should be drawn to monitor the rise of $PaCO_2$ and determine the end of testing once thresholds are reached [42]. Optimally, the ventilator should be disconnected during testing to prevent autotriggering and being confused for respiratory effort [54].

There are risks of hypoxemia, hemodynamic instability, arrhythmia or cardiac arrest during the apnea test, occurring in up to 21 % [55, 56]. This may be anticipated with coexisting respiratory dysfunction, myocardial injury or hemodyamic instability and reduced by preoxygenation. The blood pressure should be supported throughout the apnea test. In those with high risk of apnea test complications, the time off the ventilator can be minimized by reducing the ventilator rate prior to the test, lung recruitment and CPAP prior to disconnecting the ventilator, and maintaining CPAP [57] or administering exogenous CO_2 during testing [41, 58]. Maintaining tidal volume and PEEP during the test has been shown to maintain stability [52].

The recommended apneic thresholds are based on substantial and long term clinical experience, but are somewhat empirical. Higher hypercarbic breathing thresholds beyond those recommended has been reported in an isolated pediatric case report [59]. Caution must be exercised in considering the validity of the apnea test if in the physician's judgment there is a history suggestive of chronic respiratory insufficiency and responsiveness to only supra-normal levels of carbon dioxide, or if the patient is dependent on hypoxic drive. The apnea test should be performed with the goal of minimizing further hypoxic injury, minimal compromise of perfusion to end-organs, and minimizing risk of further injury to potentially recoverable brain tissue in case death of the brain stem has not actually occurred [43]. For these reasons, the apnea test should only be performed if other brainstem functions appear to be irreversibly absent [60]. Though standard of practice, the apnea test continues to create some controversy [61, 62]. Inability to perform or complete the apnea test for technical or stability reasons mandates ancillary testing [41].

Confounding Factors

The confounding factors listed in Table 37.3 preclude the clinical diagnosis of brain death. It is well recognized that hypothermia (core temperature < 32.2 °C) induces hyporeflexia and that at temperatures < 28 °C areflexia may ensue [63]. Despite this fact, level of consciousness and core temperature may be poorly correlated [64] and the effect of brain injury on temperature is unclear. Hypothermia is now being used more often as therapy for acute brain injury post-trauma or after cardiac arrest and practice may impact timing of declaration [65, 66]. Many guidelines include specific core temperature thresholds for clinical determination of brain death but recommended thresholds are wide, ranging from 32.2 °C to 36.5 °C [40] [43].

Severe metabolic abnormalities including hyperglycemia or hypoglycemia, electrolyte imbalances, inborn errors of metabolism, and liver or renal dysfunction may play a role in the patient's clinical presentation. Reversible coma with hypernatremia >160 has been documented. Hypokalemia below 2 mmol/L as well as hypophosphatemia and hypomagnesemia can present with flaccid paralysis or encephalopathy [67–69]. Specifically, abnormal thyroxine, ammonia, and urea levels can be implicated in potentially reversible coma [41]. It is important to distinguish metabolic abnormalities that play a role in the presentation, e.g. acute hyponatremia and resultant cerebral edema, from those that may arise during the ICU treatment phase but do not necessarily contribute to brain arrest (e.g. hypernatremia from diabetes insipidous). If the primary etiology does not fully explain the clinical picture, and if in the treating physician's judgment the metabolic abnormality may play a role, it should be corrected or an ancillary test should be performed.

Brain death determination in the presence of recognized therapeutic or self-administered drug intoxication requires attentiveness to the pharmacokinetic profile of the identified agent [30]. Common therapeutic agents such as narcotics, benzodiazepines, and anaesthetic agents such as propofol should be stopped prior to testing with appropriate time for drug clearance. Muscle relaxant effect should be ruled out with train-of-four stimulation if needed. Elimination of these drugs may be slower in brain injured patients and may confound clinical brainstem testing thus imitating brain death [70–72]. Where the identity of a suspected ingestion is unknown, drug screening should be considered and time should be allotted for metabolism and elimination of the drug. Alternatively, ancillary testing to confirm cerebral circulatory arrest is recommended. Importantly, therapeutic levels and/or therapeutic dosing of anticonvulsants, sedatives and analgesics do *not* preclude the diagnosis.

It is important to distinguish barbiturate intoxication as the primary etiology of coma, where cerebral blood flow persists, versus high dose barbiturates used for the treatment of refractory intracranial hypertension. The EEG is of limited use to distinguish these situations. Existing evidence suggests that for patients who fulfill minimum clinical criteria under the circumstances of high dose barbiturate therapy utilized for refractory intracranial hypertension to achieve deep coma or electrocerebral silence, death can be confirmed by the demonstration of absent intracerebral blood flow [43, 73].

Neurological assessments may be unreliable in the acute post-resuscitation phase after cardiorespiratory arrest especially after therapeutic hypothermia [66, 73, 74]. Case reports have been identified where initial clinical exam after therapeutic hypothermia was consistent with brain death but were subsequently reevaluated [72, 75]. Some studies report more reliable neurologic exam after 3 days post therapeutic hypothermia [76]. In cases of acute hypoxic-ischemic brain injury, most guidelines recommend that clinical evaluation should be delayed for at least 24 h subsequent to the cardiorespiratory arrest or an ancillary test should be performed [77–79]. Further caution and delay is advised after the use of therapeutic hypothermia, although evidence for the duration of this time delay is yet to be clearly established [43].

Physician Expertise

The level of expertise and specialty of declaring physicians vary by country and region, most often including intensivist, neurologist and/or neurosurgeon [39]. Some guidelines recommend attending staff level to augment the rigor of the determination [40] but this is not uniform throughout the world. Regardless of specialty, the physician should be experienced in the ICU-based management of severe brain injury and neurological evaluation. Appropriate training supplemented by substantial clinical experience may be more important than the specialization of the attending physician. Most guidelines explicitly exclude those physicians involved in organ transplantation from brain death determination processes [40, 42].

Subsequent Clinical Examinations and Time Intervals

The presumed purpose of a second examination is to assure independent confirmation and/or confirm irreversibility over time. Most clinical guidelines require two clinical examinations within a predetermined time interval depending upon the etiology of brain injury, ranging from 2 to 24 h. However, some advocate for single brain death examination citing that the second exam may be associated with delays leading to increased cost and loss of viable organs [80, 81]. Most commonly, it is recommended that a 24-h observation period between examinations be observed in hypoxic-ischemic brain injury. Guidelines, however, tend to be less specific regarding appropriate interval times in all other clinical circumstances.

Interval waiting times have progressively diminished since the earliest guidelines of the Ad Hoc Committee of the Harvard Medical School. Some guidelines such as those developed by the Australia and New Zealand Intensive Care Society [82] mandate that two different physicians determine brain death when organ transplantation is being considered; most do not. More commonly a single physician may perform both clinical examinations. Canadian guidelines [40] mandate two physician examinations in accordance with

Table 37.4 Age adjustments

>37 weeks CGA–1 month	1 month–1 year	Over 1 year
48 h after birth	Suggest 24 h after primary anoxic injury	Suggest 24 h after primary anoxic injury
24 h between exams	12 h between exams	12 h between exams
Exam includes suck, and oculocephalic reflex		

Based on Refs. [40, 43]

existing legislation, but have eliminated the requirement for any predefined time interval between examinations for all age groups outside of the newborn period, regardless of the mechanism of brain injury.

Age Related Adjustments

Guidelines specific to infants and children are lacking do to limited experience, emerging evidence, and concerns about the ability to reliably confirm irreversibility, especially under 2 months of age (Table 37.4). Some conclude that it is difficult to confirm brain death in this group [41]; however, recommendations for the purposes of organ donation do exist in many jurisdictions [32]. It is widely accepted that adult criteria may be applied in children, although the age limits are inconsistent amongst guidelines. There is little or no scientific basis for published age-related adjustments and disagreement on whether clinical examination alone is sufficient in children below 1 year. The interval times between examinations and requirements for ancillary testing in the newborn and infant period are inconsistent [43].

Farrell et al [83] indicate that the clinical history, physical examination and an apnea test are sufficient in diagnosing pediatric brain death, where adult guidelines may be used in infants > 7 days of age. Nakagowa et al. recently published an update of 1987 American Academy of Pediatrics guidelines where review of the literature has suggested that declaration can be suitable for infants >37 weeks gestation and older providing the clinicians are aware of the limitations of clinical exam and ancillary tests in this age group [43, 84] Similarly, Canadian guidelines emphasize that brain death in term newborns, infants and children remains a clinical diagnosis and ancillary testing by cerebral blood flow imaging should be reserved for cases where the minimum clinical criteria cannot be completed or confounding factors exist [40].

Legal Time of Death

The medical literature and daily practice is often unclear on the issue of timing of legal death in the case of brain dead patients because two examinations for brain death are required in most jurisdictions. Following the first determination of brain death, Pallis states that the patient becomes a "ventilated cadaver" [5]. It is acknowledged that, in experienced hands, the second examination for brain death is invariably consistent with the first and that an apnea test need not be repeated during the second evaluation [39]. In some jurisdictions, two examinations are mandated for postmortem donation, but only one for the diagnosis of death without donation [40]. While regional legal statutes should be clarified, it is most reasonable to conclude that the declaration of death should be legally established at the completion of the first brain death examination [40]. However, recent American guidelines state that death is certified on the second examination [43].

Ancillary Testing

Brain death is fundamentally a clinical examination and where all the minimum clinical criteria have been met, there is no need to consider ancillary diagnostic testing (excluding age adjustments) [51]. However, the indications for ancillary testing vary by jurisdiction and age [40, 41, 43]. A number of international guidelines still mandate ancillary diagnostic testing to establish brain death [39]. These advocate for increased reliance on routine ancillary blood flow tests to corroborate clinical exam in cases of unknown confounding factors [72, 85]. In general, the following indications should apply:

1. the inability to complete any part of the minimum clinical criteria e.g. spinal cord injury that precludes motor testing, or respiratory instability that precludes apnea testing, ocular trauma that precludes eye examination etc.
2. the presence of confounding conditions that cannot be resolved.
3. the uncertainty or disagreement amongst certifying physicians.
4. the need to help families understand brain death

In most jurisdictions the use of ancillary testing is limited, provided that a well-established etiology for brainstem death is identified and that conditions known to mimic absent brainstem function are excluded. There are currently no techniques available to directly evaluate flow or function of the brainstem in isolation.

Electroencephalography (EEG)

The EEG is readily available in most tertiary medical centers worldwide, has a long historical experience in practice, and is the most common ancillary test recommended. It was a component of the first guidelines for brain death [2] and remains strongly recommended in the United States [42, 43, 86, 87]. It can be performed at the bedside but has significant limitations. The EEG detects cortical electrical activity but is unable to detect deep cerebral or brainstem function and thus it may be isoelectric in the presence of viable neurons and blood flow in the brain stem and elsewhere [88]. Some patients may remain indefinitely in a vegetative state with a flat EEG, but are clearly not brain dead [89, 90]. The high sensitivity requirement for recording may result in detection of electric interference from many of the devices that are commonplace in the ICU setting. The EEG is also significantly affected by hypothermia, drug administration and metabolic disturbances. These factors, resulting in false positives or false negatives, diminish its clinical utility [91]. While it is still required in many jurisdictions, the relevance of the EEG for brain death is under question and a number of recent guidelines recommend testing of intracerebral blood flow as the ancillary test of choice especially in infants [43, 92, 93].

Tests of Intracerebral Blood Flow

Tests that show absent blood flow to the brain are generally accepted as establishing whole brain death with certainty, as it is accepted that the brain without a blood supply for an extended period of time is completely and irreversibly arrested. They provide evidence of global brain death; i.e. both the cerebral hemispheres and posterior fossa structures can be assessed. Because these tests have been used to define brain death, there are no reliable studies to assess their validity *before* clinical brain death has occurred [92]. The tests are not confounded by drugs, metabolic disorders or hypothermia. Blood pressure stability should be ensured as damaged brain may have lost autoregulation and blood flow will vary with changes in perfusion pressure. Rarely, perfusion tests give "false negative" results, in which some perfusion of arterial or venous intracranial structures is found in the presence of clinically and pathologically confirmed brain death [93, 94]. This occurs principally in those conditions in which intracranial pressure is lowered through some decompressive mechanism, e.g., decompressive craniectomies, skull fractures, ventricular shunts or infants with pliable skulls. While a number techniques are in evolution, the two generally recommended diagnostic tests capable of identifying complete cerebral circulatory arrest are cerebral angiography and Tc-99 m hexamethylpropylene-amine oxime (Tc-HMPAO) radionuclide angiograph [93].

4-Vessel Cerebral Angiography

Visualizing both the anterior and posterior cerebral circulation is the traditional "gold standard" among ancillary testing for brain death [95]. Cerebral-circulatory arrest occurs when intracranial pressure exceeds arterial inflow pressure. External carotid circulation should be evident, and filling of the superior sinus may be present. The absence of any intracranial filling of internal carotid or vertebral arteries should be demonstrated [96]. Angiography requires technical expertise and is performed in the radiology department, necessitating transport. Arterial puncture and catheter-related complications have been described. Radiocontrast can produce idiosyncratic reactions and renal dysfunction.

Nuclear Medicine Imaging Techniques

Radionuclide angiography for brain death confirmation has been widely accepted for a number of years and is easy to perform [97]. Radiopharmaceuticals, such as Tc-99 m hexamethylpropylene-amine oxime (Tc-99 m HMPAO) and ethyl cysteinate dimer (ECD), have been studied extensively in the last decade with enhanced detection of intracerebral, posterior fossa and brainstem blood flow [92]. They are lipid soluble, crossing the blood-brain barrier and penetrate into the brain parenchyma in proportion to regional blood flow. They are detected with single photon emission computed tomography (SPECT) and provide information on both arterial cerebral blood flow and uptake of tracer within perfused brain tissue. Their ability to show the presence or absence of brain perfusion rather than just intracranial circulation makes them close to the ideal test [98, 99]. The lack of signal from the intracranial compartment and the normal uptake in other parts of the head produce the "empty light bulb" (Fig. 37.4) and "hot nose" signs [100]. Access to radionucleotides is time consuming and requires specific technical expertise. As well, traditional gamma cameras used for this technique are immobile necessitating patient transfer for study. Newer technologies are portable, allowing for studies to be performed at the bedside where available [101, 102].

Transcranial Doppler Ultrasonography

Using a pulse doppler instrument, the intracranial arteries are isolated bilaterally, including the vertebral or basilar arteries. Brain-dead patients display either absent or reversed diastolic flow or small systolic spikes [103]. The non-invasiveness and portability of this technique are advantageous, but the technology requires substantial clinical expertise for proper application and is not widely available. Up to 20 % may fail Doppler scanning because of inappropriate visualization [104]. Use of this technique is being studied and is thought to be a possible future sensitive alternative to angiography [105, 106]. At present; however, its use alone is still limited [107].

Fig. 37.4 Nuclear medicine based cerebral blood flow scan (^{99m}Tc-labelled hexamethylpropyleneaminoxime (*HMPAO*)) demonstrating the absence of intracerebral blood flow in a child after brain death. Intact scalp and facial blood flow support the image of the 'empty light bulb' (Reprinted from Bonetti et al. [101]. With permission from Springer Science+Business Media)

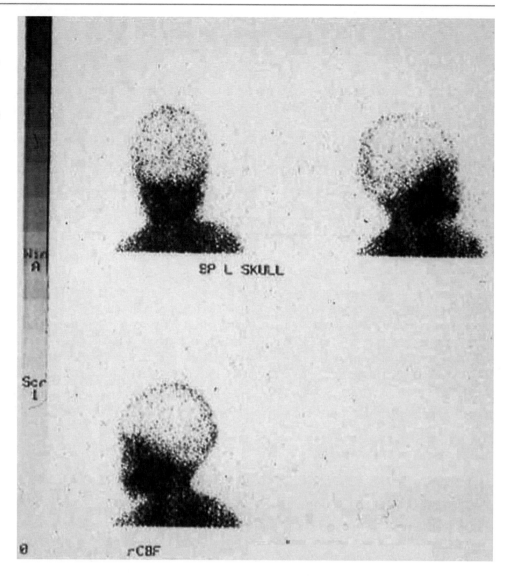

Magnetic Resonance Angiography with Magnetic Resonance Imaging (MRA with MRI)

Loss of intracranial perfusion with MRA is the most definitive aspect of MRI perfusion. In addition, there is loss of intracranial flow, transtentorial and tonsillar herniation, variable gray-white differentiation and relative contrast enhancement of the nose and scalp, similar to that found with nuclear medicine tests [108]. MRA for diagnosis of brain death has been shown to have high sensitivity but most studies lack inclusion of non-brain dead patients to assess precision of false positives [42]. The addition of diffusion weighted images may increase the sensitivity, specificity, and the positive predictive values thus allowing for an increase role [109]. Widespread experience in its use for confirming brain death is still lacking [92].

Computed Tomographic Angiography (CTA)

CTA is a recent addition to CT technology, which follows the intravenously injected contrast into the arterial circulation. The test provides adequate resolution for purposes of assessing whether intracranial perfusion is present or not. Similar to MRA, widespread experience in its use for this indication is growing and holds future promise. As a rapid, non-invasive, and widely available technique, its use is more accepted. Studies show high sensitivity and specificity for detecting cerebral circulatory arrest that accompanies clinical brain death [110]. However, CTA has not yet been well validated against the gold standard angiography and interpretation can be difficult leading to false [111] positives of blood flow [94, 112].

Other Tests of Interest

At this time, there are no other convincing contenders for ancillary testing. Somatosensory **evoked potentials** and brainstem auditory evoked responses have been studied in brain death but are limited in suitability [112, 113]. Each test activates a discrete sensory pathway and thus examines specific and anatomically limited tracts through the brainstem. They do not test the functional integrity of other CNS structures and are not sufficient stand-alone tests for brain death [104]. **Bispectral index** monitoring is a continuous, simple method to correlate cerebral blood flow. Studies have only shown that this method might be useful to alert the clinician to the possibility of progression to brain death but not to confirm it [114]. The **Atropine test**, whereby the expected rise in heart rate is absent, allows too limited an assessment of medullary function to be very useful [115]. Its anticholinergic action is meant to abolish any residual vagal tone mediated by the dorsal motor vagal nucleus in the medulla.

Variability and Practice Controversies

Numerous investigators have described consistency in concept, but significant variability in diagnostic criteria in Canadian [116], American [117, 118] international [39] and pediatric studies [8, 119, 120]. While the brainstem criteria are quite uniform, inconsistencies are evident in observation time, apnea testing, examination intervals, provisions for anoxic brain death, pediatric age adjusted criteria, confirmatory laboratory testing, required expertise of physicians and legal standards. Although various publications have been used as reference documents [2, 40, 84], hospitals or regions may make individual adjustments to existing guidelines, thus exaggerating the inconsistencies between different hospitals in the same country [118]. Hopefully newer consensus statements have addressed ambiguities in earlier documents [42, 43]. With the addition of newer resuscitation techniques such as hypothermia and extracorporeal life support, the timing and techniques needed for brain death confirmation might need adaptation [20, 72, 75]. In addition, there are concerns incomplete brain death documentation in medical charts [121] that may reflect a problem of documentation or a more concerning, a lapse in performing the full clinical examination. These inconsistencies risk damaging the credibility of the determination and there is a strong need for standardization of brain death criteria within countries and internationally [122, 123]. Checklist-based documentation should be ensured to minimize variability, an example of which is shown in Fig. 37.5 [42, 43, 111, 124].

Brain Death Examination for Infants and Children
Two physicians must perform independent examinations separated by specified intervals.

Age of Patient	Timing of first exam	Inter-exam. interval
Term newborn 37 weeks gestational age and up to 30 days old	☐ First exam may be performed 24 hours after birth OR following cardiopulmonary resuscitation or other severe brain injury	☐ At least 24 hours ☐ Interval shortened because ancillary study (section 4) is consistent with brain death
31 days to 18 years old	☐ First exam may be performed 24 hours following cardiopulmonary resuscitation or other severe brain injury	☐ At least 12 hours OR ☐ Interval shortened because ancillary study (section 4) is consistent with brain death

Section 1. PREREQUISITES for brain death examination and apnea test
A. IRREVERSIBLE AND IDENTIFIABLE Cause of Coma (Please check)
☐ Traumatic brain injury ☐ Anoxic brain injury ☐ Known metabolic disorder ☐ Other (Specify)
_____

B. Correction of contributing factors that can interfere with the neurologic examination	Examination One		Examination Two	
a. Core Body Temp is over 95° F (35° C)	☐ Yes	☐ No	☐ Yes	☐ No
b. Systolic blood pressure or MAP in acceptable range (Systolic BP not less than 2 standard deviations below age appropriate norm) based on age	☐ Yes	☐ No	☐ Yes	☐ No
c. Sedative/analgesic drug effect excluded as a contributing factor	☐ Yes	☐ No	☐ Yes	☐ No
d. Metabolic intoxication excluded as a contributing factor	☐ Yes	☐ No	☐ Yes	☐ No
e. Neuromuscular blockade excluded as a contributing factor	☐ Yes	☐ No	☐ Yes	☐ No

☐If ALL prerequisites are marked YES, then proceed to section 2, OR
☐_____confounding variable was present. Ancillary study was therefore performed to document brain death. (Section 4).

Section 2. Physical Examination (Please check) NOTE: SPINAL CORD REFLEXES ARE ACCEPTABLE	Examination One Date/ time: _____		Examination Two Date/ Time: _____	
a. Flaccid tone, patient unresponsive to deep painful stimuli	☐ Yes	☐ No	☐ Yes	☐ No
b. Pupils are midposition or fully dilated and light reflexes are absent	☐ Yes	☐ No	☐ Yes	☐ No
c. Corneal, cough, gag reflexes are absent	☐ Yes	☐ No	☐ Yes	☐ No
Sucking and rooting reflexes are absent (in neonates and infants)	☐ Yes	☐ No	☐ Yes	☐ No
d. Oculovestibular reflexes are absent	☐ Yes	☐ No	☐ Yes	☐ No
e. Spontaneous respiratory effort while on mechanical ventilation is absent	☐ Yes	☐ No	☐ Yes	☐ No

☐The _____ (specify) element of the exam could not be performed because_____.
Ancillary study (EEG or radionuclide CBF) was therefore performed to document brain death. (Section 4).

Section 3. APNEA Test	Examination One Date/ Time _____	Examination Two Date/ Time _____
No spontaneous respiratory efforts were observed despite final PaCO$_2$ ≥ 60 mm Hg and a ≥ 20 mm Hg increase above baseline. (Examination One) No spontaneous respiratory efforts were observed despite final PaCO$_2$ ≥ 60 mm Hg and a ≥ 20 mm Hg increase above baseline. (Examination Two)	Pretest PaCO$_2$: _____ Apnea duration: _____min Posttest PaCO$_2$: _____	Pretest PaCO$_2$: _____ Apnea duration: _____min Posttest PaCO$_2$: _____

Apnea test is contraindicated or could not be performed to completion because_____.
Ancillary study (EEG or radionuclide CBF) was therefore performed to document brain death. (Section 4).

Section 4. ANCILLARY testing is required when (1) any components of the examination or apnea testing cannot be completed; (2) if there is uncertainty about the results of the neurologic examination; or (3) if a medication effect may be present. **Ancillary testing can be performed to reduce the inter-examination period however a second neurologic examination is required. Components of the neurologic examination that can be performed safely should be completed in close proximity to the ancillary test**	Date/Time: _____
☐ Electroencephalogram (EEG) report documents electrocerebral silence OR	☐ Yes ☐ No
☐ Cerebral Blood Flow(CBF) study report documents no cerebral perfusion	☐ Yes ☐ No

Section 5. Signatures
Examiner One
I certify that my examination is consistent with cessation of function of the brain and brainstem. Confirmatory exam to follow.

_____   _____
(Printed Name)   (Signature)

_____   _____   _____   _____
(Specialty)   (Pager #/License #)   (Date mm/dd/yyyy)   (Time)

Examiner Two
☐I certify that my examination☐ and/or ancillary test report ☐confirms unchanged and irreversible cessation of function of the brain and brainstem. The patient is declared brain dead at this time.
Date/Time of death: _____

_____   _____
(Printed Name)   (Signature)

_____   _____   _____   _____
(Specialty)   (Pager #/License #)   (Date mm/dd/yyyy)   (Time)

Fig. 37.5 Sample brain death declaration checklist (Reprinted from Nakagawa et al. [43]. With permission from Wolter Kluwers Health)

References

1. Mollaret P, Goulon M. Le coma dépassé. Rev Neurol (Paris). 1959;101:3–15.
2. A definition of irreversible coma: report of the Ad Hoc Committee of the Harvard Medical School to examine the definition of brain death. JAMA. 1968;205:337–40.
3. Mohandas A, Chou SN. Brain death-A clinical and pathological study. J Neurosurg. 1971;35:211–8.
4. Diagnosis of brain death: statement issued by the honorary secretary of the conference of Medical Royal Colleges and their faculties in the United Kingdom on 11 October 1976. BMJ. 1976;2:1187–8.
5. Pallis C, Harley DH. ABC of brainstem death. 2nd ed. London: BMJ Publishing Group; 1996.
6. Uniform Determination of Death Act, 12 Uniform Laws Annotated (U.L.A.) 589 (West 1993 and West Supp.1997).
7. Wijdicks EF. Brain death worldwide: accepted fact but no global consensus in diagnostic criteria. Neurology. 2002;58:20–5.
8. Mathur M, Peterson L, Stadtler M, et al. Variability in pediatric brain death determination and documentation in Southern California. Pediatrics. 2008;121:998–3.
9. Parvizi J, Damasio AR. Neuroanatomical correlates of brainstem coma. Brain. 2003;126(Pt 7):1524–36.
10. Bernat JL. The concept and practice of brain death. Prog Brain Res. 2005;150:369–79.
11. Bernat JL. Philosophical and ethical aspects of brain death. In: Wijdicks EFM, editor. Brain death. Philadelphia: Lippincott Williams & Wilkins; 2000. p. 171–87.
12. Lock M. Twice dead: organ transplants and the reinvention of death. Berkley/Los Angeles: University of California Press; 2002.
13. Souter M, Van Norman G. Ethical controversies at end of life after traumatic brain injury: defining death and organ donation. Crit Care Med. 2010;38(9 Suppl):S502–9.
14. Howlett TA, Keogh AM, Perry L, Touzel R, Rees LH. Anterior and posterior pituitary function in brain-stem-dead donors. Transplantation. 1989;47:828–34.
15. Bernat JL, Culver CM, Gert B. On the definition and criterion of death. Ann Intern Med. 1981;94:389–94.
16. The President's Council on Bioethics: controversies in the determination of death: a white paper by the President's Council on Bioethics 2008. http://bioethics.georgetown.edu/pcbe/reports/death/index.html. Accessed 27 Aug 2012.
17. Bernat JL. Contemporary controversies in the definition of death. Prog Brain Res. 2009;177:21–31.
18. Taylor RM. Reexamining the definition and criteria of death. Semin Neurol. 1997;17(3):265–70.
19. Truog RD, Miller FG. The dead donor rule and organ transplantation. Engl J Med. 2008;359:674–5.
20. Muralidharan R, Mateen FJ, Shinohara RT, Schears GJ, Wijdicks EF. The challenges with brain death determination in adult patients on extracorporeal membrane oxygenation. Neurocrit Care. 2011;14(3):423–6.
21. Lagiewska B, Pacholczyk M, Szostek M, Walaszewski J, Rowinski W. Hemodynamic and metabolic disturbances observed in brain dead organ donors. Transplant Proc. 1996;28:165–6.
22. Salim A, Martin M, Brown C, et al. Complications of brain death: frequency and impact on organ retrieval. Am Surg. 2006;72(5):377–81.
23. Powner DJ, Bernstein IM. Extended somatic support for pregnant women after brain death. Crit Care Med. 2003;31(4):1241–9.
24. Salim A, Velmahos GC, Brown C, et al. Aggressive organ donor management significantly increases the number of organs available for transplantation. J Trauma. 2005;58(5):991–4.
25. Wood KE, Becker BN, McCartney JG, et al. Care of the potential organ donor. N Engl J Med. 2004;351(26):2730–9.
26. Cloutier R, Baran D, Morin JE, Dandavino R, Marleau D, Naud A, Gagnon R, Billard M. Brain death diagnoses and evaluation of the number of potential organ donors in Quebec hospitals. Can J Anaesth. 2006;53(7):716–21.
27. Meert KL, Thurston CS, Sarnaik AP. End-of-life decision-making and satisfaction with care: parental perspectives. Pediatr Crit Care Med. 2000;1(2):179–85.
28. Martinot A, Grandbastien B, Leteurtre S, Duhamel A, Leclerc F. No resuscitation orders and withdrawal of therapy in French paediatric intensive care units. Groupe Francophone de Reanimation et d'Urgences Pediatriques. Acta Paediatr. 1998;87(7):769–73.
29. Tsai E, Shemie SD, Hebert D, Furst S, Cox PN. Organ donation in children. The role of the pediatric intensive care unit. Ped Crit Care Med. 2000;1:156–60.
30. Badovinac K, Greig PD, Ross H, Doig CJ, Shemie SD. Organ utilization among deceased donors in Canada, 1993–2002. Can J Anaesth. 2006;53(8):838–44.
31. U.S. Department of Health & Human Services. Organ procurement and transplant network. http://optn.transplant.hrsa.gov/latestData/rptData.asp. Accessed 14 Aug 2011.
32. Shemie SD, Doig C, Belitsky P. Advancing towards a modern death: the path from severe brain injury to neurological determination of death. CMAJ. 2003;168(8):993–5.
33. Philip S, Udomphorn Y, Kirkham FJ, Vavilala MS. Cerebrovascular pathophysiology in pediatric traumatic brain injury. J Trauma. 2009;67(2 Suppl):S128–34.
34. Venkateswaran RV, Dronavalli V, Lambert PA, et al. The proinflammatory environment in potential heart and lung donors: prevalence and impact of donor management and hormonal therapy. Transplantation. 2009;88(4):582–8.
35. Katz K, Lawler J, Wax J, et al. Vasopressin pressor effects in critically ill children during evaluation for brain death and organ recovery. Resuscitation. 2000;47(1):33–40.
36. Dimopoulou I, Tsagarakis S, Anthi A, et al. High prevalence of decreased cortisol reserve in brain-dead potential organ donors. Crit Care Med. 2003;31(4):1113–7.
37. Pérez López S, Otero Hernández J, Vázquez Moreno N, et al. Brain death effects on catecholamine levels and subsequent cardiac damage assessed in organ donors. J Heart Lung Transplant. 2009;28(8):815–20.
38. Shivalkar B, Van Loon J, Wieland W, Tjandra-Maga TB, Borgers M, Plets C, Flameng. Variable effects of explosive or gradual increase of intracranial pressure on myocardial structure and function. Circulation. 1993;87(1):230–9.
39. Wijdicks EFM. Brain death worldwide – accepted fact but no global consensus in diagnostic criteria. Neurology. 2002;58:20–5.
40. Shemie SD, Doig C, Dickens B, Byrne P, et al. Severe brain injury to neurological determination of death: Canadian Council for Donation and Transplantation forum recommendations. CMAJ. 2006;174(6):S1–13.
41. A code of practice for the diagnosis and confirmation of death. London: Academy of Medical Royal Colleges; 2008.
42. Wijdicks EF, Varelas PN, Gronseth GS, Greer DM, American Academy of Neurology. Evidence-based guideline update: determining brain death in adults: report of the Quality Standards Subcommittee of the American Academy of Neurology. Neurology. 2010;74(23):1911–8.
43. Nakagawa TA, Ashwal S, Mathur M, Mysore MR, Bruce D, Conway Jr EE, Duthie SE, Hamrick S, Harrison R, Kline AM, Lebovitz DJ, Madden MA, Montgomery VL, Perlman JM, Rollins N, Shemie SD, Vohra A, Williams-Phillips JA, Society of Critical Care Medicine, The Section on Critical Care and Section on Neurology of the American Academy of Pediatrics, The Child Neurology Society. Guidelines for the determination of brain death in infants and children: an update of the 1987 task force recommendations. Crit Care Med. 2011;39(9):2139–55.

44. Robertson JA. The dead donor rule. Hastings Cent Rep. 1999;29:6–14.

45. Saposnik G, Bueri JA, Maurino J, Saizar R, Garretto NS. Spontaneous and reflex movements in brain death. Neurology. 2000;54(1):221–3.

46. Dosemeci L, Cengiz M, Yilmaz M, Ramazanoglu A. Frequency of spinal reflex movements in brain-dead patients. Transplant Proc. 2004;36(1):17.

47. Jain S, DeGeorgia M. Brain death-associated reflexes and automatisms. Neurocrit Care. 2005;3(2):122–6.

48. Saposnik G, Basile VS, Young GB. Movements in brain death: a systematic review. Can J Neurol Sci. 2009;36(2):154–60.

49. Ashwal S. Clinical diagnosis and confirmatory testing of brain death in children. In: Wijdicks EFM, editor. Brain death. Philadelphia: Lippincott Williams & Wilkins; 2000.

50. Swartz M, editor. Textbook of physical diagnosis. 6th ed. Philadelphia: WB Saunders; 2010.

51. The Quality Standards Subcommittee of the American Academy of Neurology. Practice parameters for determining brain death in adults (summary statement). Neurology. 1995;45:1012–24.

52. Mascia L, Pasero D, Slutsky AS, Arguis MJ, Berardino M, Grasso S, Munari M, Boifava S, Cornara G, Della Corte F, Vivaldi N, Malacarne P, Del Gaudio P, Livigni S, Zavala E, Filippini C, Martin EL, Donadio PP, Mastromauro I, Ranieri VM. Effect of a lung protective strategy for organ donors on eligibility and availability of lungs for transplantation: a randomized controlled trial. JAMA. 2010;304(23):2620–7.

53. Dominguez-Roldan JM, Barrera-Chacon JM, Murillo-Cabezas F, Santamaria-Mifsut JL, Rivera-Fernandez V. Clinical factors influencing the increment of blood carbon dioxide during the apnea test for the diagnosis of brain death. Transplant Proc. 1999;31(6):2599–600.

54. Dodd-Sullivan R, Quirin J, Newhart J. Ventilator autotriggering: a caution in brain death diagnosis. Prog Transplant. 2011;21(2):152–5.

55. Goudreau JL, Wijdicks EF, Emery SF. Complications during apnea testing in the determination of brain death: predisposing factors. Neurology. 2000;55(7):1045–8.

56. Wu XL, Fang Q, Li L, Qiu YQ, Luo BY. Complications associated with the apnea test in the determination of the brain death. Chin Med J (Engl). 2008;121(13):1169–72.

57. Lévesque S, Lessard MR, Nicole PC, Langevin S, LeBlanc F, Lauzier F, Brochu JG. Efficacy of a T-piece system and a continuous positive airway pressure system for apnea testing in the diagnosis of brain death. Crit Care Med. 2006;34(8):2213–6.

58. Sharpe MD, Young GB, Harris C. The apnea test for brain death determination: an alternative approach. Neurocrit Care. 2004;1(3):363–6.

59. Vardis R, Pollack MM. Increased apnea threshold in a pediatric patient with suspected brain death. Crit Care Med. 1998;26(11):1917–9.

60. Yee AH, Mandrekar J, Rabinstein AA, Wijdicks EF. Predictors of apnea test failure during brain death determination. Neurocrit Care. 2010;12(3):352–5.

61. Joffe AR, Anton NR, Duff JP. The apnea test: rationale, confounders, and criticism. J Child Neurol. 2010;25(11):1435–43.

62. Tibballs J. A critique of the apneic oxygenation test for the diagnosis of "brain death". Pediatr Crit Care Med. 2010;11(4):475–8.

63. Danzl DR, Pozos RD. Accidental hypothermia. N Engl J Med. 1994;331:1756–60.

64. Wijdicks EFM. Brain death. Philadelphia: Lippincott Williams & Wilkins; 2000.

65. Hutchison JS, Ward RE, Lacroix J, Hébert PC, Barnes MA, Bohn DJ, Dirks PB, Doucette S, Fergusson D, Gottesman R, Joffe AR, Kirpalani HM, Meyer PG, Morris KP, Moher D, Singh RN, Skippen PW, Hypothermia Pediatric Head Injury Trial Investigators, Canadian Critical Care Trials Group. Hypothermia therapy after traumatic brain injury in children. N Engl J Med. 2008;358(23):2447–56.

66. Doherty DR, Parshuram CS, Gaboury I, Hoskote A, Lacroix J, Tucci M, Joffe A, Choong K, Farrell R, Bohn DJ, Hutchison JS, Canadian Critical Care Trials Group. Hypothermia therapy after pediatric cardiac arrest. Circulation. 2009;119(11):1492–500. Epub 2009.

67. Polderman KH, Bloemers FW, Peerdeman SM, Girbes AR. Hypomagnesemia and hypophosphatemia at admission in patients with severe head injury. Crit Care Med. 2000;28(6):2022–5.

68. Mégarbane B, Guerrier G, Blancher A, Meas T, Guillausseau PJ, Baud FJ. A possible hypophosphatemia-induced, life-threatening encephalopathy in diabetic ketoacidosis: a case report. Am J Med Sci. 2007;333(6):384–6.

69. Pothiwala P, Levine SN. Analytic review: thyrotoxic periodic paralysis: a review. J Intensive Care Med. 2010;25(2):71–7.

70. Meinitzer A, Zink M, März W, Baumgartner A, Halwachs-Baumann G. Midazolam and its metabolites in brain death diagnosis. Int J Clin Pharmacol Ther. 2005;43(11):517–26.

71. Auinger K, Müller V, Rudiger A, Maggiorini M. Valproic acid intoxication imitating brain death. Am J Emerg Med. 2009;27(9):e5–6. 1177.

72. Joffe AR, Kolski H, Duff J, deCaen AR. A 10-month-old infant with reversible findings of brain death. Pediatr Neurol. 2009;41(5):378–82.

73. López-Navidad A, Caballero F, Domingo P, et al. Early diagnosis of brain death in patients treated with central nervous system depressant drugs. Transplantation. 2000;70:131–5.

74. Booth CM, Boone RH, Tomlinson G, Detsky AS. Is this patient dead, vegetative, or severely neurologically impaired? Assessing outcome for comatose survivors of cardiac arrest. JAMA. 2004;291(7):870–9.

75. Bisschops LL, van Alfen N, van der Hoeven JG, Hoedemaekers CW. Predictive value of neurologic prognostic indicators in hypothermia after cardiac arrest. Ann Neurol. 2011;70(1):176.

76. Webb AC, Samuels OB. Reversible brain death after cardiopulmonary arrest and induced hypothermia. Crit Care Med. 2011;39(6):1538–42.

77. Fugate JE, Wijdicks EF, Mandrekar J, Claassen DO, Manno EM, White RD, Bell MR, Rabinstein AA. Predictors of neurologic outcome in hypothermia after cardiac arrest. Ann Neurol. 2010;68(6):907–14.

78. Safar PJ, Kochanek PM. Therapeutic hypothermia after cardiac arrest. N Engl J Med. 2002;346(8):612–3.

79. Young GB. Clinical practice. Neurologic prognosis after cardiac arrest. N Engl J Med. 2009;361(6):605–11.

80. Shemie SD, Langevin S, Farrell C. Therapeutic hypothermia after cardiac arrest: another confounding factor in brain-death testing. Pediatr Neurol. 2010;42(4):304. author reply 304–5.

81. Lustbader D, O'Hara D, Wijdicks EF, MacLean L, Tajik W, Ying A, Berg E, Goldstein M. Second brain death examination may negatively affect organ donation. Neurology. 2011;76(2):119–24. Epub 2010 Dec 15.

82. Varelas PN, Rehman M, Abdelhak T, Patel A, Rai V, Barber A, Sommer S, Corry JJ, Venkatasubba Rao CP. Single brain death examination is equivalent to dual brain death examinations. Neurocrit Care. 2011;15:547–53.

83. Pearson IY. Australia and New Zealand intensive care society statement and guidelines on brain death and model policy on organ donation. Aneasth Intensive Care. 1995;23:104–8.

84. Farrell MM, Levin DL. Brain death in the pediatric patient: historical, sociological, medical, religious, cultural, legal and ethical considerations. Crit Care Med. 1993;21:1951–65.

85. American Academy of Pediatrics Task Force on Brain Death in Children. Guidelines for the determination of brain death in children. Pediatrics. 1987;80:298–300.

86. Roberts DJ, MacCulloch KA, Versnick EJ, Hall RI. Should ancillary brain blood flow analyses play a larger role in the neurological determination of death? Can J Anaesth. 2010;57(10):927–35. Epub 2010 Aug 13.

87. Banasiak KJ, Lister G. Brain death in children. Curr Opin Pediatr. 2003;15(3):288–93.

88. American Electroencephalographic Society. Guideline three: minimum technical standards for EEG recording in suspected cerebral death. J Clin Neurophysiol. 1994;11:10–3.

89. Brierley JB, Graham DI, Adams JH, Simpson JA. Neocortical death after cardiac arrest: a clinical, neurophysiological and neuropathological report of two cases. Lancet. 1971;2:560–5.

90. Blend MJ, Oavel DG, Highes JR, et al. Normal radionuclide angiogram in a child with electrocerebral silence. Neuropediatrics. 1986;17:168–70.

91. Rimmelé T, Malhière S, Ben Cheikh A, Boselli E, Bret M, Ber CE, Petit P, Allaouchiche B. The electroencephalogram is not an adequate test to confirm the diagnosis of brain death. Can J Anaesth. 2007;54(8):652–6.

92. Young GB, Shemie SD, Doig C, Teitelbaum J. A brief review: the role of ancillary tests in the neurological determination of death. Can J Anaesth. 2006;53(6):620–7.

93. Shemie SD, Lee D, Sharpe M, Tampieri D, Young B, Canadian Critical Care Society. Brain blood flow in the neurological determination of death: Canadian expert report. Can J Neurol Sci. 2008;35(2):140–5.

94. Heran MK, Heran NS, Shemie SD. A review of ancillary tests in evaluating brain death. Can J Neurol Sci. 2008;35(4):409–19.

95. Flowers WM, Patel BR. Persistence of cerebral blood flow after brain death. South Med J. 2000;93:364–70.

96. Greer DM, Strozyk D, Schwamm LH. False positive CT angiography in brain death. Neurocrit Care. 2009;11(2):272–5.

97. Wilkening M, Lowvier N, D'Athis P, Freysz M. Validity of cerebral angiography via the venous route in the diagnosis of brain death. Bull Acad Natl Med. 1995;179:41–8.

98. Savard M, Turgeon AF, Gariépy JL, Trottier F, Langevin S. Selective 4 vessels angiography in brain death: a retrospective study. Can J Neurol Sci. 2010;37(4):492–7.

99. Wieler H, Marohl K, Kaiser KP, Klawki P, Frossler H. Tc-99 m HMPAO cerebral scitigraphy. A reliable, noninvasive method for determination of brain death. Clin Nucl Med. 1993;18:104–9.

100. Spieth ME, Ansari AN, Kawada TK, Kimura RL, Siegel ME. Direct comparison of Tc-99 m DPTA and TC-99 m HMPAO for evaluating brain death. Clin Nucl Med. 1994;19:867–72.

101. Donohoe KJ, Frey KA, Gerbaudo VH, Mariani G, Nagel JS, Shulkin B. Procedure guideline for brain death scintigraphy. J Nucl Med. 2003;44(5):846–51. PubMed.

102. Bonetti MG, Ciritella P, Valle V, Perrone E. 99mTc HM-PAO brain perfusion SPECT in brain death. Neuroradiology. 1995;37:365–9.

103. Okuyaz C, Gücüyener K, Karabacak NI, Aydin K, Serdaroğlu A, Cingi E. Tc-99 m-HMPAO SPECT in the diagnosis of brain death in children. Pediatr Int. 2004;46(6):711–4.

104. Munari M, Zucchetta P, Carollo C, Gallo F, De Nardin M, Marzola MC, Ferretti S, Facco E. Confirmatory tests in the diagnosis of brain death: comparison between SPECT and contrast angiography. Crit Care Med. 2005;33(9):2068–73.

105. Ducrocq X, Braun M, Debouverie M, et al. Brain death and transcranial Doppler: experience in 130 cases of brain dead patients. J Neurol Sci. 1998;160:41–6.

106. Young GB, Lee D. A critique of ancillary tests for brain death. Neurocrit Care. 2004;1(4):499–508. Review.

107. Poularas J, Karakitsos D, Kouraklis G, Kostakis A, De Groot E, Kalogeromitros A, Bilalis D, Boletis J, Karabinis A. Comparison between transcranial color Doppler ultrasonography and angiography in the confirmation of brain death. Transplant Proc. 2006;38(5):1213–7.

108. Sharma D. Early TCD monitoring in brain death: what may be relevant? Neurol Sci. 2011;32(4):749–50. author reply 751–2.

109. Monteiro LM, Bollen CW, van Huffelen AC, Ackerstaff RG, Jansen NJ, van Vught AJ. Transcranial Doppler ultrasonography to confirm brain death: a meta-analysis. Intensive Care Med. 2006;32(12):1937–44.

110. Karantanas AH, Hadjigeorgiou GM, Paterakis K, Sfiras D, Komnos A. Contribution of MRI and MR angiography in early diagnosis of brain death. Eur Radiol. 2002;12(11):2710–6.

111. Selcuk H, Albayram S, Tureci E, Hasiloglu ZI, Kizilkilic O, Cagil E, Kocer N, Islak C. Diffusion-weighted imaging findings in brain death. Neuroradiology. 2011.

111. Escudero D, Otero J, Marqués L, Parra D, Gonzalo JA, Albaiceta GM, Cofiño L, Blanco A, Vega P, Murias E, Meilan A, Roger RL, Taboada F. Diagnosing brain death by CT perfusion and multislice CT angiography. Neurocrit Care. 2009;11(2):261–71.

112. Combes JC, Chomel A, Ricolfi F, d'Athis P, Freysz M. Reliability of computedtomographic angiography in the diagnosis of brain death. Transplant Proc. 2007;39(1):16–20.

113. Facco E, Munari M, et al. Role of short latency evoked potentials in the diagnosis of brain death. Clin Neurophysiol. 2002;113:1855–66.

114. Machado C. An early approach to brain death diagnosis using multimodality evoked potentials and eletroretinography. Minerva Anestesiol. 1994;60:573–7.

115. Misis M, Raxach JG, Molto HP, Vega SM, Rico PS. Bispectral index monitoring for early detection of brain death. Transplant Proc. 2008;40(5):1279–81.

116. Hüttemann E, Schelenz C, Sakka SG, Reinhart K. Atropine test and circulatory arrest in the fossa posterior assessed by transcranial Doppler. Intensive Care Med. 2000;26:422–5.

117. Shemie SD. Varibility in brain death practices. Crit Care Med. 2004;32(12):2564–5.

118. Powner DJ, Hernandez M, Rives TE. Variability among hospital policies for determining brain death in adults. Crit Care Med. 2004;31(6):1284–8.

119. Greer DM, Varelas PN, Haque S, Wijdicks EF. Variability of brain death determination guidelines in leading US neurologic institutions. Neurology. 2008;70(4):284–9. Epub 2007 Dec 12.

120. Mejia RE, Pollack MM. Variability in brain death determination practices in children. JAMA. 1995;274(7):550–3.

121. Chang MY, McBride LA, Ferguson MA. Variability in brain death declaration practices in pediatric head trauma patients. Pediatr Neurosurg. 2003;39(1):7–9.

122. Wang MY, Wallace P, Gruen JP. Brain death documentation: analysis and issues. Neurosurgery. 2002;51(3):731–5.

123. Busl KM, Greer DM. Pitfalls in the diagnosis of brain death. Neurocrit Care. 2009;11(2):276–87. Epub 2009 May 15.

124. Stockwell JA, Pham N, Fortenberry JD. Impact of a computerized note template/checklist on documented adherence to institutional criteria for determination of neurologic death in a pediatric intensive care unit. Pediatr Crit Care Med. 2011; 12(3):271–6.

The Physiology of Brain Death and Organ Donor Management

38

Sam D. Shemie and Sonny Dhanani

Abstract

Brain death is associated with complex physiologic changes that may impact the management of the potential organ donor. Medical management is critical to actualizing the individual or family's intent to donate and maximizing the benefit of that intent. This interval of care in the PICU begins with brain death and consent to donation and culminates with surgical organ procurement. During this phase, risks for hemodynamic instability and compromise of end organ function are high. The brain dead organ donor is in a distinct and challenging pathophysiologic condition that culminates in multifactorial shock. The potential benefits of aggressive medical management of the organ donor may include increased number of donors providing transplantable organs and increased number of organs transplanted per donor. This may improve graft function, graft survival, and patient survival in those transplanted. In this chapter, pathophysiologic changes occurring after brain death are reviewed. General and organ specific donor management strategies and logistic considerations are discussed. There is a significant opportunity for enhancing donor multi-organ function and improving organ utilization with appropriate PICU management.

Keywords

Brain death • Brainstem death • Organ donation • Donor management • Organ yield

Introduction

Successful medical management of the organ donor is critical to actualizing the individual or family's intent to donate and maximizing the benefit of that intent. This interval of care in the PICU begins with brain death and consent to donation and culminates with surgical organ procurement. It generally ranges from 12 to 48 h or longer and is related to the

S.D. Shemie, MD, FRCPC
Department of Critical Care,
Montreal Children's Hospital, Montreal, QC, Canada
e-mail: sam.shemie@mcgill.ca

S. Dhanani, Bsc (Pharm), MD, FRCPC (✉)
Pediatric Critical Care,
Children's Hospital of Eastern Ontario, Ottawa, ON, Canada
e-mail: sdhanani@cheo.on.ca

time required for repeated brain death declarations, consent discussions with the family, procurement logistics of donor/organ evaluation, and donor/recipient matching. During this phase, risks for hemodynamic instability and compromise of end organ function are high (Table 38.1). There is a significant opportunity for enhancing donor multi-organ function and improving organ utilization with appropriate medical management [1].

The brain dead organ donor is in a distinct and challenging pathophysiological condition that culminates in a state of multifactorial shock. The current level of evidence supporting practices in pediatric donor management is limited by the inherent lack of prospective trial data, and based largely on adult human and animal studies; however, donor management practice is of increasing importance [2–5]. PICU care should be tailored by principles similar to the management of any patient with multifactorial shock. It is important to treat the donor as one would treat the transplant recipient.

D.S. Wheeler et al. (eds.), *Pediatric Critical Care Medicine*,
DOI 10.1007/978-1-4471-6362-6_38, © Springer-Verlag London 2014

This can be accomplished by understanding the physiology of brain death coupled with aggressive and attentive PICU management.

Figure 38.1 shows the Canadian experience of organ utilization across all age groups, comparable to international rates [6–8]. Utilization rates vary from region to region and transplant center to transplant center. Rates for heart and lung utilization have the greatest capacity for quantitative improvement. For the purposes of most international reports, a "donor" is one who has provided at least one organ that has been transplanted (Table 38.2). Initial interventions to increase transplantation focused on identification, referral, and consent of the donor, recent pursuit of organ yield has

gained importance [9]. Pediatric investigators have reported rates of 3.6 organs per donor (of eight possible organs), but 22 % of consented pediatric donors failed to provide *any* transplantable organs primarily due to hemodynamic instability during the phase of PICU donor care [10].

The goal of PICU based donor management is to improve the utilization of organs from consented donors to transplant recipients. The potential benefits of aggressive medical management of the organ donor may include increased number of donors providing transplantable organs and increased number of organs transplanted per donor. This may improve graft function, graft survival and patient survival in those transplanted [11].

Table 38.1 Incidence of pathophysiologic changes occurring after brain stem death requiring intensive care management of the potential organ donor

Hypotension	81 %
Diabetes insipidus	65 %
Disseminated intravascular coagulation	28 %
Cardiac arrhythmias	25 %
Pulmonary edema	18 %
Metabolic acidosis	11 %

[Based on data from ref. 298]

Table 38.2 Organ-specific donation numbers for pediatric deceased brain dead donors in United States, UNOS

	2010	2009
All donors	841	916
Kidney	792	854
Liver	739	794
Heart	477	480
Pancreas	321	365
Lung	212	204
Intestine	100	138

[Based on data from Ref. 299]

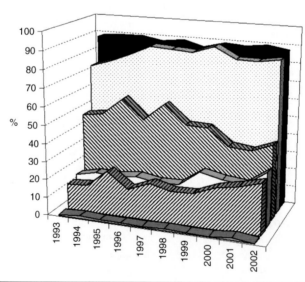

	1993	1994	1995	1996	1997	1998	1999	2000	2001	2002
▣ Intestine/Multivisceral	0.7	1.5	0.7	0.7	0.7	1.0	0.5	0.4	1.7	0.2
▨ Lungs	14.3	15.0	24.2	15.5	20.7	17.8	18.2	22.7	25.0	28.3
▢ Pancrease	16.1	18.6	17.9	19.3	17.7	17.8	26.2	23.6	22.4	30.6
▨ Heart	47.9	49.6	59.2	48.7	58.3	47.8	47.4	38.6	37.6	42.2
▢ Liver	73.6	77.4	82.3	87.4	86.5	85.8	89.5	83.7	83.1	85.0
■ Kidneys	88.4	89.3	89.4	87.2	88.7	85.5	88.6	87.5	88.7	87.0

Fig. 38.1 Organ-specific utilization rates for deceased donors, Canada, 1993–2002 (Reprinted from Badovinac et al. [6]. With permission from Springer Science + Business Media.)

The Physiology of Brain Death

The deterioration of cardiovascular and pulmonary function associated with intracranial hypertension will vary with the rapidity of rise of intracranial pressure (ICP) [12], time after herniation, and presence of coexisting forms of myocardial injury e.g., traumatic myocardial contusion, ischemia after cardiac arrest, shock, or hypoxemia [13, 14]. In the face of markedly elevated ICP, mean arterial pressure (MAP) rises in an effort to maintain cerebral perfusion pressure. As ICP rises further, cerebral herniation into the brainstem ensues, and brainstem ischemia is initiated in an orderly, rostral-caudal fashion. Initial apnea, bradycardia, hypotension and drop in cardiac output are mediated by vagal (parasympathetic) activation resulting from midbrain ischemia. Brainstem ischemia then progresses toward the pons, where sympathetic stimulation is superimposed on the initial vagal response, resulting in bradycardia and hypertension (the classic Cushing's reflex) [15]. During this period, the ECG may be characterized by sinus bradycardia, junctional escape beats, and even complete heart block [16]. Further extension into the medulla oblongata occurs, at which point the vagal cardiomotor nucleus becomes ischemic, preventing tonic vagal stimuli. This results in unopposed sympathetic stimulation which may last for minutes to hours and manifests as arterial hypertension with elevated cardiac output with the potential for tachyarrhythmias [16]. This period of unopposed sympathetic stimulation is often termed the "autonomic" or "sympathetic storm" during which time cardiotoxicity occurs and severe vasoconstriction may compromise end organ perfusion [17, 18]. Subsequent changes occur in oxygen consumption and delivery [19]. Herniation triggers an inflammatory cascade that affects cardiorespiratory function, and hormonal regulation [20]. This cascade affects pituitary and hypothalamic function resulting in catecholamine, thyroid, and vasopressin abnormalities [21–24].

Neurogenic Myocardial Dysfunction

The sympathetic storm is responsible for potentially reversible myocardial injury and has been best studied in subarachnoid hemorrhage [25], where is called "neurogenically stunned myocardium" [26, 27]. Endogenous catecholamine-related increases in peripheral resistance may result in a sudden increase in myocardial work and oxygen consumption leading to myocardial ischemia or infarction and subsequent elevation of cardiac troponin I and T [15, 28]. Patients dying of acute intracranial events show scattered foci of transmural myocardial injury that are not seen in patients dying of noncerebral causes [29]. Myocardial necrosis after subarachnoid hemorrhage is a neurally mediated process that is dependent on the severity of neurological injury [30]. Brain dead

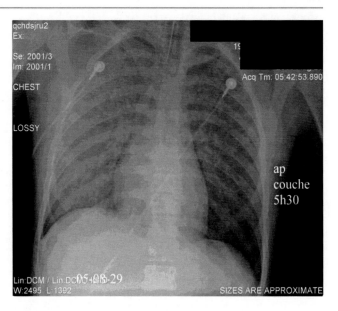

Fig. 38.2 Chest x-ray showing neurogenic pulmonary edema in an adolescent with acute intracranial hypertension

cardiac donors with elevations in cardiac troponin I have been shown to have diffuse subendocardial myocytolysis and coagulative necrosis and a high incidence of graft failure after transplantation [31]. The magnitude of the rise of epinephrine after brain death and the extent of myocardial damage have also been shown to depend on the rate of rise in ICP in a canine model [12, 32]. Dogs given a sudden rise in ICP demonstrated a higher epinephrine surge and poorly functioning donor hearts. Surgical sympathectomy [33] or pharmacologic sympathetic blockade in humans [34] and animals [35, 36] effectively prevents the ICP-related catecholamine cardiotoxicity and the electrophysiologic, biochemical and pathologic changes characteristic of neurogenic injury in the heart. While the ICP-related sympathetic storm is characterized by myocardial injury and high systemic vascular resistance, it is soon followed by period of sympathetic depletion and a low SVR state. Brain dead patients become functionally decapitated and the sympathetic system is anatomically interrupted, similar to high spinal cord injuries [37].

Neurogenic Pulmonary Edema

This unopposed sympathetic stimulation mediates the myocardial injury and is also likely responsible for the neurogenic pulmonary edema often seen in the management of patients with acute elevations of ICP (Fig. 38.2) [38]. Practitioners should be aware of this fulminant presentation of sudden onset respiratory failure with large volume, frothy tracheal secretions. In primate models of acute intracranial hypertension, acute heart failure ensues with reversal of flow in the pulmonary circulation due to massive rises in left atrial pressure [33]. Rupture of pulmonary capillaries can occur from this retrograde increase in vascular hydrostatic pressure [39]. This hydrostatic pulmonary edema is responsive to high PEEP and is generally reversible with time [40, 41].

Inflammatory State

Brain death is also associated with the up-regulation and induction of the inflammatory response in all somatic organs [42], triggering a cascade of mediators that may affect graft function [43]. Transient focal cerebral ischemia upregulates the transcriptional levels of TNF-α, IL-6, and other markers [44, 45]. Rapid rises of ICP causes immune activation in peripheral organs resulting in enhanced immunogenicity [32]. In animal models, brain death has a detrimental effect on hepatic dysfunction related to immune activation and appears to be independent of hemodynamic instability [46] and magnified by longer ischemic times [47]. In comparison to living related kidney donors, kidneys from brain dead donors have significantly higher levels of pro-inflammatory mediators on biopsy (endothelial E-selectin and proximal tubular expression of HLA-DR antigens, intracellular adhesion molecule-1, and vascular cell adhesion molecule-1) [48, 49]. Delayed renal graft function and acute rejection in the recipient is correlated to higher indices of free radical mediated injury in the donor [50, 51]. Evidence that neurogenic pulmonary edema may be alleviated with glucocorticoids also suggests that an inflammatory component exists in this process [52, 53]. Recent animal work suggests that this inflammation is triggered by the acute hemodynamic effects of ICP-related neurogenic myocardial dysfunction, resulting in hydrostatic pressure based neurogenic pulmonary edema and rupture of the alveolar-capillary membrane [39, 54].

Brain death is an important risk factor itself and influences graft outcomes, mediated by postischemic reperfusion injury and other nonantigen-dependent inflammatory pathways [55, 56]. Deleterious processes such as inflammation and fibrosis occur in donor organs [57] potentiating graft immunogenicity and increases host alloresponsiveness organs, developing and contributing to reduced graft survival [58]. These findings may used to introduce specific cytoprotective interventions in the brain dead donor to reduce the immunogenicity or the pro-inflammatory status of the graft and better maintain or increase organ viability. Anti-inflammatory therapies may be beneficial on eventual graft status [45].

Donor Management: General

Cardiovascular Performance and Monitoring

The etiology of low cardiac output in brain dead patients is complex and time dependent. It may be characterized by low preload due to vascular volume depletion, contractile myocardial dysfunction, and variable SVR states ranging from extreme vasoconstriction from ICP-related sympathetic storm to vasodilation from sympathetic arrest. Resuscitation of the cardiopulmonary system benefits the function of all end organs in the brain dead donor. The variety of changes in volume status, cardiac inotropy, and peripheral vascular resistance that occur after brain death are similar to those in any pediatric critically ill patient with shock of diverse etiology. Intensivists should titrate cardiovascular therapy to clinical, biochemical and hemodynamic endpoints that ensure restoration of intravascular volume status, and appropriate support of the myocardium and vascular system to ensure optimal cardiac output for organ perfusion. Optimization with aggressive intensive care can optimize transplantation [59].

Evaluation of cardiocirculatory status is a global assessment of multiple variables. Traditional and vigilant hemodynamic assessments should be provided, based on physical findings, vital signs, central venous pressure, urine output, central or mixed venous oximetry and serial lactate measurements. Escalation of support should be accompanied by escalation of hemodynamic monitoring.

Echocardiographic parameters have also been demonstrated to be beneficial in predicting successful cardiac transplant outcomes [60, 61]. Echocardiographic systolic myocardial dysfunction is present in 42 % of adult brain death and associated with ventricular arrhythmias [60]. Diffuse wall motion abnormalities are a risk factor for 30-day heart transplant mortality [62]. Evaluation of left ventricular end diastolic diameter, ventricular wall thickness, and coronary flow are felt to influence transplantation [63]. Single echocardiographic evaluations may have limitations in detecting the reversible myocardial dysfunction often seen after brain injury [26]. Recent studies advocate pharmacologic stress evaluation for organ suitability [64]. The utility of serial echocardiograms to evaluate improvement in myocardial dysfunction in the brain dead donor and to better predict cardiac allograft survival has been reported in adults [65] and is evolving into routine practice. Studies show that serial echocardiogram lacked specificity but was particularly useful in showing improvements following aggressive donor management [66].

Right-sided pressures may underestimate left-sided pressures after brain death and may increase risk for elevated left-sided filling pressures and pulmonary edema [67]. Expert consensus supports pulmonary arterial catheterization (PAC) and cardiac output monitoring in adults, particularly if the donors are hemodynamically unstable or initial ejection fraction is less than 40–45 % [68, 69]. PAC and goal-directed hemodynamic therapy of initially unacceptable donors, in conjunction with hormonal therapy may improve the rate of organ procurement without compromising transplant outcomes [70]. A significant increase in heart recovery was seen with the use of PAC in adult studies [71]. The Transplantation Committee of the American College of Cardiology has recommended titrating volume infusions and dopamine to thermodilution indices [72]. Justifications for PAC are not limited to the precise titration of hemodynamic support but are also required for the evaluation of suitability for heart and lung transplantation. As the use of PAC in PICU care is limited, serial echocardiography at q6-12 hourly intervals has been recommended [69].

Newer non-invasive methods of monitoring cardiac output are becoming more common because of their ease of use and safety, but are still not well validated for use in donor management, especially in children [73, 74]. Though management of the donor is similar to other shock states, monitoring of central venous saturations has not been recommended because of the lack of normal values in the donor patient [75]. Monitoring of other biochemical markers such as acidosis, lactates, and electrolytes is essential [76].

Hemodynamic Targets and Supports

Following the sympathetic storm, a subsequent reduction in catecholamines and sympathetic hormones result in a normotensive or hypotensive phase. This stage is characterized by impaired cardiac inotropy and chronotropy, impaired vascular tone and a reduced cardiac output. Clinical deterioration (progressive hypotension, hypoxia, anuria ± cardiac arrest) during the interval from brain death to procurement is common without aggressive intervention [77]. Cardiovascular support should be based on rational physiology and should be preceded by volume resuscitation to normovolemia.

Preload

Significant volume depletion is anticipated in brain-injured patients after brain death due to fluid restriction, diuretics, hyperosmolar therapy, third space losses, hemorrhage and/or diabetes insipidus. In addition, a low SVR state may result in relative hypovolemia. In a Canadian study of 77 pediatric organ donors [2], 53 % suffered sustained hypotension and 35 % deteriorated to cardiac arrest. This was more common in patients treated with inotropic agents in the presence of a low central venous pressure and in those without anti-diuretic hormone replacement, emphasizing the importance adequate restoration of intravascular volume. Organ transplantation may be less favourable in preload dependent donors, possibly related to higher inflammatory response [78].

The optimal volume status of the brain dead patient is controversial and transplant-organ specific. Disparity exists between lung and kidney interests ("dry lungs" versus "wet kidneys"). In a study of crystalloid fluid management in 26 brain dead donors, a significant increase in the alveolar-arterial oxygen gradient was seen in those who achieved a central venous pressure (CVP) of 8–10 compared to those whose CVP was maintained at 4–6 mmHg [67]. Some authors advocate maintaining a CVP of 10–12 mmHg to volume replete those patients in whom only abdominal organs are to be procured, a CVP < 8 mmHg for potential

lung donors and a CVP of 8–10 mmHg if both thoracic and abdominal organs are to be harvested [79]. This approach is impractical since all organs should initially be considered potentially transplantable. Effectively, euvolemia is the reasonable goal and the assessment of volume status should be based on experienced clinical evaluation [80–82].

Contractility

The preferred choice of contractility agents in PICU practice varies according to individual center. Traditionally, dopamine or dobutamine has been used as the initial inotrope of choice in the brain dead patient. However, no randomized trials exist comparing the hemodynamic effects of dopamine to other inotropes or vasopressors and their influence on graft survival. β-agonist therapy should be used with caution in potential heart donors given concerns about myocardial adenosine triphosphate (ATP) depletion and desensitization of β-receptors [83]. If the heart is being considered for donation, dopamine or its equivalent should not be escalated beyond 10 μg/kg/min due to risks of increases oxygen demand [69]. High dose dopamine has been related to poor graft survival for hearts but favourable for other organs such kidneys [84, 85]. Use of epinephrine alone or as an adjunct may be appropriate in these cases.

Systemic Vascular Resistance

The functional sympathectomy associated with brain death results in low SVR that often requires the use of vasoconstricting agents. The concern over the use of alpha-agonists such as norepinephrine or phenylephrine has arisen because of the fear of inducing central and peripheral vasoconstriction and subsequent ischemia in coronary and vascular beds supplying potentially transplantable organs. However, in studies of other causes of shock states with low SVR (septic patients), norepinephrine, as compared to dopamine, was demonstrated to increase mean perfusion pressures without adverse effects to renal and splanchnic blood flow [86–88]. Early use of vasoconstrictor agents alone or in adjunction with inotropes is suggested [69].

Vasopressin and Catecholamine Sparing in Brain Death

Arginine vasopressin (AVP) is a unique agent because it can be used for a variety of applications in donor management, e.g. hemodynamic vasopressor support, diabetes insipidus therapy, and hormonal therapy. Brain death and hypotension are often associated with vasopressin deficiency [89]. Low-dose AVP infusions have been shown to improve hemodynamic stability and spare catecholamine use [89, 90]. Prolonged hemodynamic stability can be maintained after brain death with low-dose AVP (1–2 units/h), permitting a significant decrease in epinephrine and extended preservation of renal function [91]. In a rigorous, randomized study of volume-resuscitated brain dead organ donors supported with dopamine, 0.30 mU/kg/min infusion of AVP significantly increased MAP and SVR and spared dopamine use compared to further fluid loading [92]. Pediatric donors given AVP (41 ± 69 mU/kg/h) respond by increasing MAP and weaning alpha-agonists (norepinephrine, epinephrine, phenylephrine) without significant differences in the quality of kidneys, livers and hearts recovered [21, 93]. Similar catecholamine-sparing effects of AVP have been demonstrated in septic shock patients with low SVR [94, 95].

Optimal dosing of AVP in relation to its effects on organ procurement and graft survival are unclear. Concern has been expressed regarding risks of splanchnic ischemia in vasodilatory shock [96, 97]. Practitioners should be cautioned regarding the multiple and confusing dosing units used throughout the literature. Although it is suggested that doses of AVP exceeding 0.04 U/min (approx. 40 mU/kg/h) may be associated with excessive vasoconstriction in sepsis [94] brain dead donors respond to AVP infusions of 0.04–0.1 U/min (40–100 mU/kg/h) [89] without histologic evidence of cardiac damage [98]. Recent evidence shows that systemic and SMA flow may be compromised with AVP versus dopamine [99]. Available literature suggests that the use of AVP at doses up to 0.04 U/min in adults (2.4 U/h) and 0.0003–0.0007 U/kg/min (0.3–0.7 mU/kg/min) in children can be recommended to support the MAP and spare catecholamines [69].

Oxygenation and Ventilation Strategies

Many potential donors have various etiologies of donor-related lung injury and dysfunction that may include neurogenic pulmonary edema, aspiration, atelectasis, pulmonary contusion, bronchopulmonary infection, alveolar-capillary inflammation, and diffuse alveolar damage [59]. Pulse oximetry, serial arterial blood gas monitoring, endotracheal tube suctioning, and serial chest x-rays are considered standard in donors [100]. Mechanical ventilation should be tailored to the following empirical recommendations: fraction of inspired oxygen (FiO_2) titrated to keep oxygen saturation ≥ 95 %, partial pressure of arterial oxygen (PaO_2) ≥ 80 mmHg, pH 7.35–7.45, $PaCO_2$ 35–45 mmHg, positive end expiratory pressure (PEEP) of 5 cm H_2O [69, 101, 102]. A prospective, randomized control trial in potential adult donors, ARDS-type lung protective strategies with tidal volumes of 6–8 mL/kg and 8–10 cmH2O PEEP significantly increased lung utilization for transplantation [103].

Metabolic and Endocrine

Glycemia and Nutrition

Hyperglycemia is common in brain dead donors [77]. It may be secondary to insulin resistance as pancreatic function appears to be preserved [104], which may be aggravated by corticosteroid therapy and dextrose-based fluid replacements used for diabetes insipidus. Insulin is variably and inconsistently considered as part of hormonal resuscitation cocktails. The hypothesis that tight glycemic control in the brain dead donor improves graft survival has not been tested, but has been recommended by expert consensus [68, 69]. Hyperglycemia has been shown to be an independent risk factor for poor outcome after severe brain injury in children [105] and adults [106].

Dextrose infusions and nutrition are generally withheld in the acute PICU management after brain injury [107], a practice supported by animal models [108]. Malnutrition or depletion of cellular glycogen stores may be common during the phase of care leading to brain death [109]. The influence of donor nutrition on graft survival has been studied in several animal studies but not formally in humans. In a rabbit and porcine model, improved liver transplant survival was shown from donors receiving enteral nutrition versus fasting donors [110]. A significant improvement in hepatic sinusoidal lining cell viability has been demonstrated in rats with liver grafts from donors receiving enteral feeding and intraperitoneal glucose prior to liver procurement. Glycogen appears to protect the hepatic graft upon rewarming in rats [111].

The importance of nutritional support in the human multi-organ donor, however, is not clear but is of increased interest [112]. Studies of donor-specific predictors of graft function following liver transplantation suggested a length of stay in the ICU of greater than 3 days as a risk factor [113]. A contributing factor to this association may be the effect of starvation on the liver with depletion of glycogen stores. In a controlled prospective randomized study of 32 patients it was shown that an intraportal infusion of insulin (1 IU/kg/h) and glucose reglycogenates the liver, increases glycogen utilization during cold and rewarming periods, and improves transaminase levels [114]. However, the only human series of liver transplants that included donor nutritional status failed to identify an independent effect of donor nutrition on postoperative liver graft function [115]. As a general approach, intravenous dextrose infusions should be given routinely and routine enteral or parenteral feeding should be initiated or continued as tolerated [116].

Diabetes Insipidus and Hypernatremia

Dysfunction of the posterior pituitary in brain dead donors is common; anterior pituitary function is often preserved [117]. Histologic observations of the pituitary gland demonstrate various degrees of edema, hemorrhage, and tissue necrosis depending on the mechanism and site of traumatic or ischemic brain injury [118, 119]. This is likely to be a result of compromised blood supply to the cell bodies arising in the deep supraventricular and paraventricular nuclei of the hypothalamus, whose neurons supply the posterior pituitary and regulate AVP secretion. Anterior pituitary function is often preserved, implying that some blood supply via the hypophyseal arteries, which arise extradurally, is reaching the median eminence of the hypothalamus [117]. Undetectable levels of antidiuretic hormone (ADH) have been noted in 75 % of brain dead donors, and diabetes insipidus is present in up to 87 % [29, 30, 54, 55]. Diabetes insipidus may commonly appear prior to the diagnosis of brain death [118] and is associated with hemodynamic instability and the compromise of transplantable organ function [2, 23, 77].

Hypernatremia is frequently encountered, resulting from the preceding hyperosmolar therapy for initial brain injury or poorly controlled diabetes insipidus. Donor hypernatremia > 155 mmol/L at procurement has been shown to be independently associated with hepatic and renal dysfunction or graft loss after transplantation [115, 120–122], although new evidence may show that these concerns may be less significant [123]. A prospective study demonstrated the benefit of correcting donor sodium (Na) $\leq$ 155 mmol/L with equivalent graft success compared to donors who were never hypernatremic [124]. The mechanism of hepatic and kidney injury related to hypernatremia is unclear but may be related polyuria and dehydration and to the accumulation of idiogenic osmoles resulting in intracellular swelling after transplantation into the normonatremic recipient.

Ideal serum sodium (Na) target range is $\geq$130 $\leq$150 mmol/L [25]. A reasonable urine output target range is 0.5–3 ml/kg/h after brain death. Diabetes insipidus can be defined as a urine output > 4 ml/kg/h associated with rising serum Na $\geq$145 mmol/L and serum osmolarity $\geq$300 mosM and decreasing urine osmolarity $\leq$ 200 mosM [69].

DDAVP (analog 1-desamino-8-D-arginine vasopressin, or desmopressin) is commonly used for the treatment of diabetes insipidus in brain death without adverse effect on early or late graft function after renal transplantation [125]. It is highly selective for the vasopressin V_2 receptor subtype found in the renal collecting duct and thus has a relatively pure antidiuretic effect with no significant vasopressor activity [126]. DDAVP has multiple potential routes of administration (iv, im, sc, intranasal, ETT) and corresponding variability of dose recommendations. In brain death, it is preferable to rely on the i.v. route with a recommended dosing range is 0.5–10 µg iv every 6–8 h [127]. Given its lack of vasopressor action, it can be safely titrated to the effect of ablating polyuria and normalizing serum sodium. Improved organ yield is associated with DDAVP use in donor management [11, 128].

Many authors have advocated the use of AVP for the treatment of diabetes insipidus in organ donors to modulate both diabetes insipidus and support cardiovascular system [68, 69, 74, 93, 129, 130]. In pediatric case series, doses of vasopressin between 0.25 and 2.7 mU/kg/h have been used to successfully treat hypothalamic diabetes insipidus [131–134]. Doses between 0.5 and 15 U/h of AVP have been advocated in adults, though there are concerns about high doses causing coronary, renal and splanchnic vasoconstriction, potentially jeopardizing cardiac, renal, pancreatic and

hepatic function [99, 127]. The safety and efficacy of a combination of DDAVP (for its antidiuretic effect) with AVP as a vasopressor on cardiovascular and laboratory endpoints has been described [21, 92, 135]. Many protocols recommend separate dosing regimens for diabetes insipidus and support for perfusion. The upper limit of AVP recommended by the Transplantation Committee of the American College of Cardiology is 0.8–1.0 U/h (13–17 mU/kg/h) to treat diabetes insipidus [72].

Thyroid Hormone

Thyroid hormone increases cardiac output by improving both contractility and chronotropy, as well as by decreasing systemic vascular resistance [136]. The use of thyroid hormone therapy in brain dead donors is largely based on experimental animal models and human case series. Investigators describe variable levels of thyroid hormones after brain death and varying and conflicting effects of thyroid hormone administration. Thyroid-stimulating hormone (TSH), T_4 and T_3 levels were below normal in a majority of 22 brain dead donors [137]. Other studies have shown that these patients are suffering from "sick euthyroid syndrome" rather than TSH deficiency and do not require thyroid supplementation [54]. In the baboon model, T_3 levels become depleted after brain death and the resulting transition to anaerobic metabolism is reversed with T_3 replacement [138]. The positive effects on myocardial gene expression have been demonstrated [139].

In a comparative study in brain dead patients, T_3, cortisol and insulin promoted aerobic metabolism, reduced the need for inotropic support and improved the rate of cardiac graft procurement [140, 141]. Other investigators were unable to demonstrate any improvement in echocardiographic function or organ retrieval rates with a similar hormone regimen [142]. Serum free T_3 concentrations in organ donors may not correlate with hemodynamic stability [118] but replacement of thyroid hormone (T3) has shown to reduce need for vasopressor support and may improve the likelihood of heart transplantations [143–146]. There is equipoise for routine use since many other studies did not show improvement in cardiac and hemodynamic status [147, 148].

T_4 infusion rather than T3 does not reduce vasopressor requirements or especially in pediatric donors [21] but this may be related to impaired peripheral conversion to T_3. While there are numerous theoretical advantages of parenteral T_3 over T_4 (stability for iv infusion, does not require peripheral tissue conversion), it is extremely expensive in comparison to intravenous T_4 and may not be commercially available in many countries. In those UNOS patients receiving hormone therapy, T_4 was used in 93 % and T_3 in 6.9 % of cases, with insufficient numbers to discriminate any benefit of T_3 over T_4 [Rosendale, Kauffman, personal communication]. Most studies for thyroid replacement in the context of the organ donor are of low quality with poor study design, thus limiting objective analysis [149].

Corticosteroids

Several publications have advocated the use of high-dose methylprednisolone in an effort to diminish inflammation thought to be present in donor lungs [102, 130, 150] and other organs. The initial evidence for this was largely based on a single retrospective analysis of 118 consecutive lung donors administered a non-uniform protocol of methylprednisolone (mean 14.5 mg/kg) compared with 38 donors not receiving methylprednisolone and demonstrating a significant improvement in donor oxygenation and lung procurement rate [151]. A recent analysis of the California Donor Network database demonstrated an independent effect of methylprednisolone on the successful procurement of lungs from the donor [152]. The UNOS database showed that heart graft survival benefit was also found in those donors receiving corticosteroids alone [150]. Recent studies do reveal a highly proinflammatory environment in donors but do not actually show benefit from methyprednisolone replacement [20]. Although the optimal dose and time effect (if any) of corticosteroids in brain dead donors are uncertain, guidelines recommend methylprednisolone 15 mg/kg q24h [69].

Combined Hormonal Therapy

Despite conflicting literature regarding use of hormones individually, there is strong evidence supporting the use of combined hormonal therapy in organ donors, defined as vasopressin, thyroid hormone, and methylprednisolone (insulin is inconsistently included in this strategy). The United Network for Organ Sharing (UNOS) database shows a 46 % reduced odds of post-transplant death within 30 days and a 48 % reduced odds of early cardiac graft dysfunction with the use of combined hormonal therapy in a large retrospective cohort [150]. Benefit was also found in those donors receiving corticosteroids alone or in combination with T_3/T_4 which is supported by independent studies [153, 154]. Recovery of organs was most beneficial to heart and lung transplantation [155]. Analysis of UNOS data suggests a substantial benefit from hormone therapy with minimal risk. A multivariate logistic regression analysis of 18,726 brain dead donors showed significant increases in kidney, liver and heart utilization from donors receiving three-drug hormonal therapy. Significant improvements in 1-year kidney graft survival and heart transplant patient survival were also demonstrated [147, 148, 150]. More recently, however, in a prospective randomized study T3 and methylprednisolone did not add to the effect on cardiac index shown by vasopressin and aggressive cardiovascular support [156]. Despite this recent finding, current expert consensus still strongly recommends the use of combined hormonal therapy for any donor with hemodynamic instability or reduced ejection fraction on echocardiography [68, 69].

Transfusion Thresholds

There are no rigorous studies that assess the role of red blood cell transfusions for short-term organ preservation during organ donor maintenance specifically. Prospective studies for transfusion thresholds suggest outcomes are similar with hemoglobin level at 7 g/dL in critically ill children [157]. However, consensus conferences recommend maintaining a hemoglobin level ≥ 10 g/dL or a hematocrit greater than 30 % [127, 130]. Large platelet transfusion requirements during liver transplant surgery are independently associated with more severe hepatic dysfunction after transplantation, but this is likely more indicative of a more technically complicated procedure and sicker recipient [115]. There is no literature identified to guide platelet or plasma factor replacement in the donor. Invasive procedures associated with bleeding risk may require correction of thrombocytopenia and coagulation status. Blood drawing for donor serology and tissue typing should occur prior to transfusions to minimize the risk of false results related to hemodilution. In regions where blood is routinely leukocyte depleted, and the risk of transmission of cytomegalovirus (CMV) is negligible and it may not be necessary to give CMV-negative blood to CMV-negative donors [69].

Invasive Bacterial Infections

Isolated cases of transmission of solid organ infection from donor to recipient may have significant consequences including graft infection, sepsis, and poor initial graft function [158–163]. While approximately 5 % of all donors will be bacteremic at the time of procurement, the routine use of broad spectrum antibiotics (vancomycin and ceftazidime/cefotaxime) in the recipient has been shown to prevent transmission of bacterial infection in organ recipients [164, 165]. Importantly, donor infections do not show differences in acute mortality or graft survival. The current expansion of potential marginal donors has increased the risk of infection. One study quoted bacteremia rates in the donor up to 21 % [166]. Donors with ICU stays greater than 3 days, rescue CPR, and inotropic agents are at increased risk [167]. Though rates of infections in donors may be up, organs obtained from donors with positive cultures continue to be transplanted safely, likely due to vigilant screening and polymicrobial therapy given to recipients [168, 169]. Other authors have described the successful transplantation of organs from donors declared brain dead from meningitis caused by *Neisseria meningitides*, *Streptococcus pneumoniae* and *Escherichia coli* without transmission to the recipient [170]. The finding of positive cultures does not preclude donation but may delay procurement until 24–48 h of treatment has been established. Prophylactic antibiotic therapy in the organ donor is generally not recommended.

Viral infections in the donor can affect recipients especially with post transplant immunosuppression. However, many chronic infections such as hepatitis B and C virus no longer preclude donation. Knowledge of potential risks is essential but often manageable in the appropriate recipient [171, 172].

Initial baseline blood, urine and endotracheal cultures should be obtained for all donors and repeated daily. PCR screens for common chronic viral infection are common. Positive blood cultures or presumed infections are not contraindications to organ donation but antibiotic therapy should be initiated early in cases of proven or presumed infection. Duration of therapy depends on the virulence of the organism and should be determined in consultation with the transplant team and infectious disease services.

Donor Management: Organ Specific

Heart

Wait list mortality among US children listed for heart transplant has decreased by two-thirds over the last 20 years [173]. Mostly this is related to extended donor and recipient criteria including ABO incompatible transplantation [174, 175]. This has not compromised clinical outcomes after transplantation [176]. Reasons for this are multifactorial but include improved donor management [177].

The majority of studies linking donor variables to heart transplant outcomes are in adults and related to known risk factors such as coronary artery disease, left ventricular hypertrophy, older age, diabetes mellitus, and chronic hypertension [62, 130, 178, 179]. While these variables may be indications for coronary angiography in the adult donor, they generally are not relevant to the pediatric population. Extrapolation from adult studies would suggest that myocardial dysfunction in the pediatric donor, as manifest by greater inotropic support [62, 180], pacemaker support [181], and reduced ejection fraction and/or wall motion abnormalities by echocardiography [62, 130] are important factors. Interestingly, donor CPR has not shown to be a negative factor for heart transplant survival [182, 183].

Potential heart donors should undergo routine screening by electrocardiogram (ECG) and 2D echocardiography. In children, initial echocardiography for heart donor evaluation should be performed only after hemodynamic resuscitation and repeat echocardiography should be considered after ≥6 h [69]. Intensive donor management has been show to improve function on serial echocardiography and may improve transplantability in up to 50 % [66, 184, 185]. Some advocate that the majority of echographic abnormalities in donor hearts resolve in the transplant recipient prior to discharge [186]. Reduced function should not preclude consideration

for transplantation based on a single evaluation. Ejection fractions < 40–45 % do not necessarily translate into high transplant risk, as they may be related to related to inadequate cardiovascular resuscitation or neurogenic myocardial dysfunction that is reversible with time (see earlier sections). Adult data has shown significant improvements in echocardiographic function with time and conventional support [65], with up to 78 % of potential donors demonstrating clinically significant improvements [63, 184].

Serological markers such as donor troponin I and T have been linked to early cardiac graft failure [31, 187, 188] and should also be measured. However, these markers do not necessarily relate to graft dysfunction in recipients [189]. Though Tri-iodothyronine and methylprednisolone therapy is recommended, a recent study of 80 cardiac donors did not show acute improvement to cardiovascular function or donor yield [156].

Pulmonary artery catheterization (PAC) data has been linked to favorable transplant outcomes [70]. Reduced ejection fraction or hemodynamic instability has been recommended as an indication for PAC in adults to allow for both precision of hemodynamic support and evaluation of suitability for heart and lung transplantation especially in marginal donors [68, 190]. PAC use in pediatrics is still limited.

Lungs

Though lower yield than other organs donated, lung transplantation in pediatrics has increased with better techniques and improved management [191–193]. A relatively scarce donor pool has limited wider application for lung transplantation [194]. This has led to relaxation of donor criteria, specific donor management protocols that preserve lung function, and development of ex-vivo perfusion techniques to recondition suboptimal lungs, all of which have optimized transplantation [195, 196]. Outcomes for pediatric lung recipients are similar to adults but young children often do better due to a decreased incidence of rejection. Adolescent outcomes are poor mainly due to bronchiliolitis obliterans [197].

The 'ideal' lung donor has been previously defined but significant advances have been made in donor and recipient management allowing for increased use of marginal or 'extended criteria' donors [198–200]. There is some evidence that organs transplanted using extended donor criteria may have higher rates of early graft rejection [201, 202]. The quality of the lung donor and the subsequent recipient outcomes are related to the possibility of this primary graft dysfunction which is a result of multifactorial hemodynamic, metabolic, and inflammatory insults resulting from the brain dead donor [203]. Primary pulmonary allograft failure has pathological features of acute lung injury (ALI) and occurs in 12–50 % of transplanted patients [204–206]. This is often associated with inadequate lung preservation, ischemia-reperfusion injury and cellular rejection [207]. Despite this, many centers have adopted extended criteria in order to increase the number of potential donors [208, 209].

Traditional oxygenation criteria used as a threshold in the acceptance of donor lungs include a donor $PaO_2 > 300$ mmHg on FiO_2 of 100 % and PEEP of 5 cm H_2O (P/F ratio > 300) [210]. However, recent and evolving efforts have improved the current criteria for donor selection [191, 211]. Physiological, microbiological and histological evaluation of rejected lungs from the California transplant registry show 41 % of rejected lungs were judged suitable for transplantation based on pulmonary edema, intact alveolar fluid clearance, and histology [212]. In a case series of 15 brain dead adults, lung grafts that did not meet the usual criteria for transplantation were found to have higher dynamic and static elastance measurements than donor lungs that met standard transplantation criteria [213]. The outcomes of 49 marginal donors (i.e., failing to meet one or more of the ideal criteria) showed no significant difference in duration of post-transplant mechanical ventilation or P/F ratio compared to ideal donors [211]. Investigators have also challenged donor PaO_2 criteria by arguing that physiological donor factors influence peripheral arterial PaO_2 independent of isolated individual lung function [214]. Despite poor global oxygenation, parenchymal abnormalities isolated to one lung may not preclude procurement of the contralateral lung [215].

The cause of brain death does not correlate with lung transplant outcomes, but there is improved outcomes with longer time interval before retrieval suggesting longer and specific donor management may reduce lung injury over time [101, 216]. Pulse oximetry, serial arterial blood gas monitoring, endotracheal tube suctioning, rotational positioning, chest x-ray, bronchoscopy and bronchoalveolar lavage are considered standard in the lung specific care of donor [100]. Mechanical ventilation should be tailored to the general targets (see previous section) [103]. Similar to the management of lung injury in general, alveolar recruitment and pressure limited ventilation strategies should be used in potential donors [59]. New strategies for the improvement of lung function in the donor such as airway pressure release ventilation have been utilized [217]. Excessive fluid administration deteriorates alveolar-arterial oxygenation gradients in potential donors [67] and may be an indication for diuresis. Steroid administration may also reduce progressive lung water accumulation [101]. Prolonged ventilation in the supine position results in loss of alveolar expansion and microatelectasis. In an experimental rat model, donor lungs develop microatelectasis despite PEEP and a relatively short ventilatory period before organ procurement [218]. Prevention of alveolar collapse enhances post mortem preservation of pulmonary grafts in a rabbit model [219]. Recruitment maneuvers in the form of high sustained PEEP for short durations may be a useful adjunct to prevent alveolar stress and collapse [220]. Lung

donors failing traditional oxygenation criteria (P/F < 300) respond to aggressive bronchial toilet using bronchoscopy, physiotherapy, increasing tidal volume and increasing PEEP with improvements in P/F ratio > 300. Lungs were subsequently transplanted without differences in ICU length of stay or 30-day mortality compared to recipients of ideal donors [221]. Hemodynamic and reperfusion injury seem to play a significant role in donor lung injury [222]. The early use of norepinephrine or vasopressin may reduce lung injury [223].

Recent guidelines suggest that there should be no predefined lower limit for the P/F ratio that precludes consideration for transplantation. Timing of evaluation, temporal changes, response to alveolar recruitment and recipient status should be considered [69]. In cases of unilateral lung injury, pulmonary venous partial pressure of oxygen during intraoperative assessment is required to reliably evaluate contralateral lung function.

Bronchoscopy and Bronchopulmonary Infections

The consensus of expert opinion supports the use of bronchoscopy for the purposes of examining the tracheobronchial tree for abnormalities and collecting microbiological specimens [68, 129, 211]. Pathological studies of lungs rejected for donation have indicated that bronchopneumonia, diffuse alveolar damage, and diffuse lung consolidation are the three most common reasons for being deemed unsuitable [214]. Between 76 % and 97 % of bronchoalveolar lavages (BAL) will grow at least one organism [224, 225]. The most commonly identified organisms included *Staphylococcus aureus* and *Enterobacter*, and in 43 % of transplants, similar organisms were isolated from recipient bronchoscopy. Pulmonary infection in the graft recipient results in significantly lower survival compared with recipients who do not develop early graft infection [226]. Recipients with donor BAL cultures positive for either gram positive or gram negative bacteria had longer mean mechanical ventilation times and inferior 6-month to 4-year survival than those with negative bacterial BAL cultures [227]. Trauma donors (versus intracerebral hemorrhage) may be at higher risk for aspiration and for intubation under less sterile field conditions and were generally ventilated longer [228]. The etiology of donor death is not associated with lung transplant mortality [204] but may influence the type of organisms found on BAL and subsequent graft infection risk. The high rates of positive bacterial and fungal BAL results suggest the need for more aggressive critical care management and antibiotic therapy [229].

Liver

Liver transplantation from deceased donors has become accepted as standard of care for many children with liver failure. Advances in donor and recipient management has optimized graft survival with 80–90 % 5 year survival rates

[230]. Whole liver transplants are still more successful with less morbidity and mortality than split liver grafts [231, 232]. Potential liver donors should be assessed by the following: aspartate aminotransferase (AST), alanine aminotransferase (ALT), bilirubin (direct and indirect where available), INR (or prothrombin time [PT]) (repeat q6h), serum electrolytes, creatinine, urea, Hepatitis B surface antigen (HBsAG), hepatitis B antibody (HBcAb), hepatitis C virus antibody positive (HCV Ab). There is no indication for routine liver imaging. The use of donor characteristics (donor risk index) and recipient matching using bicochemical models in end stage liver disease (MELD) are becoming more useful in predicting liver transplant outcomes [233–235].

There is variation in organ quality and recipient outcomes; larger volume centers tend to use higher risk organs but also have higher disease severity resulting in worse outcomes [236]. Predictors of early graft dysfunction or failure for whole or split liver transplantation include donor history of cardiac arrest, older donor age in adult transplantation (>40 years), [113, 237, 238], very young age in pediatric transplantation [113], reduced size livers, moderate to severe steatosis on liver biopsy, prolonged cold ischemia time (>6 h) [121, 239, 240] and donor hypernatremia (Na > 155 mmol/L). Donor hypernatremia is independently associated with death or retransplantation at 30 days [121] but this risk reverses with the correction of hypernatremia [124].

Although liver allograft dysfunction has been reported to be associated with prolonged ICU stay [113, 241], this was supported by univariate analysis but did not hold true by multivariate analysis [241]. In a cohort of 323 orthotopic liver transplants (OLT), longer donor hospitalization was not found to be associated with primary liver graft dysfunction [239]. Large platelet transfusion requirements during surgery are independently associated with more severe hepatic dysfunction after transplantation [115], although this may be indicative of a more technically complicated procedure, sicker recipient, or poor quality graft with subsequently greater sequestration of platelets within the donor liver [242]. As with other organs, the mechanisms of brain death itself impact the donor liver [243]. With the use of marginal livers for transplantation, studies are identifying more factors that may impact graft survival such as the liver's gross appearance, the donor P/F ratio, and the donor hemoglobin [244].

The sinusoidal lining cells (SLC) of the liver are particularly vulnerable to the effects of preservation-reperfusion injury, the extent of which depends on the duration of cold ischemia rather than reperfusion. Cold preservation causes the SLC to become edematous and detach into the sinusoidal lumen [245]. While some authors recommend routine donor liver biopsies in all liver donors in an effort to decrease the rate of early graft dysfunction or failure [246, 247], the use of a biopsy in the decision making of liver suitability has generally been restricted to evaluating the amount of steatosis or in the presence of active hepatitis C in the appropriate risk groups.

Kidney

Donor age ≥ 40 or ≤10 years were thought to be independently associated with risk for graft failure [248, 249]. Now, recipients of kidneys from young donors < 5 years old have equivalent patient and graft survival [250]. En bloc kidneys from pediatric donors now show comparable outcomes with living kidney donation [251]. Older kidneys have a higher incidence of renovascular or parenchymal injury [249]. Adult donor characteristics that are independently associated with graft failure risk include creatinine > 133 μmol/L, history of hypertension independent of duration and cerebrovascular accident (CVA) as the cause of donor death [248]. During the past few years, there has been a renewed interest in the use of expanded criteria donors for kidney transplantation to increase number of donations with improving outcomes [252]. However, these kidneys have worse long-term survival and are only recommended for older recipients [253, 254].

A normal creatinine clearance (>80 ml/min/1.73 m^2), as estimated by the Schwartz formula [255], defines the optimal function threshold for transplantation. However, an abnormal serum creatinine or calculated creatinine clearance in a donor does not necessarily preclude use of the kidneys [256]. Urinalysis is essential to rule out kidney abnormalities and serum creatinine and serum urea (blood urea nitrogen) measurements should be obtained q6h. Ultrasound with Doppler flow of renal vessels is often requested if creatinine levels are abnormal. If contrast angiography is performed (e.g. cerebral, coronary) N-acetylcysteine with hydration should be administered both before and after the angiographic procedure in order reduce the risk of contrast nephropathy [257] in potential donors, particularly in those with reduced renal function.

Delayed graft function predicts the development of adverse events such as decreased graft survival, decreased recipient survival and increased allograft nephropathy [258]. Most studies do not link a specific cause of brain death as a predictor of graft function in children [259]. The brain death process itself can affect acute rejection in renal transplantation [260, 261]. Greater sympathetic activity during the process produces endothelial damage, complement activation, and a proinflammatory state increases organ immunogenicity, then promoting rejection after transplant [262, 263]. Targeting this inflammatory state may improve outcomes of recipients [264, 265].

Other donor risk factors predicting kidney allograft dysfunction include hemodynamics, age, last creatinine level prior to donation, and cold ischemic time [266]. Donor hemodynamic instability is correlated with post-transplant acute tubular necrosis in adults [77, 267, 268] and children [2]. Reduced graft survival or acute tubular necrosis may occur in organs retrieved from donors receiving high-dose dopamine (>10 μg/kg/min) but these effects may be limited to donors who are hypotensive at the time of organ retrieval

[268]. Hemodynamic resuscitation may improve outcome as donor use of dopamine and/or noradrenaline is independently associated with a lower risk of acute rejection [269], lower rate of delayed graft function [84, 270], and reduces the need for recipient dialysis [271]. In adults, donor hypertension is also a risk factor for inferior outcomes [272]. It is suggested that the time taken to optimize donor cardiovascular status may reduce renal ischemic injury and optimize donor yield [273, 274].

In an analysis of the Collaborative Transplant Study database of kidney transplants, cold ischemic preservation time > 12 h resulted in progressively worsening recipient graft survival, particularly once the cold ischemia time (CIT) was ≥48 h [275]. Other analyses have suggested that CIT is predictive of poorer graft survival [248] or function [267] if it was >24 h. Preservation incorporating pulsatile perfusion, rather than cold storage, may reduce the incidence of delayed graft function [276, 277].

Intestine

Small bowel transplantation has been become an increasingly feasible option for short bowel syndrome and liver failure [278]. Long term survival following intestinal transplant is above 60 %, but the incidence of morbidity and mortality is still significant [279, 280]. Because of this, many feel that intestinal transplantation as an option is still premature and remains unique to specialized centres only [281, 282]. For the brain dead donor, non-absorbable antibiotics for selective bowel decontamination are sometimes used for liver and intestine transplantation to prevent postoperative infections. Results are best if given >3 days prior to transplantation [283]. A meta-analysis showed an 84 % relative risk reduction in the incidence of gram negative infection following liver transplantation; however, the risk of antimicrobial resistance should be considered [284]. More recent studies have not duplicated these results. At this time, selective bowel decontamination is not routinely administered [285].

Logistics of Organ Donation

Donor Management Protocols and Education

One of the main reasons for insufficient organ procurement has been low organ yield due to poor multiorgan failure management in the potential donor [82]. Evidence has shown that multidisciplinary donor management protocols can improve donation outcomes [286, 287]. When these strategies are used, there are a significantly improved number of organs transplanted per donor [3, 4]. This is mostly

attributed to the improvement in basic cardiovascular and respiratory monitoring and treatment [288–290]. Improved multimodal strategies aimed at preserving organ function specifically may increase numbers of potential donors, especially with the increasing use of "marginal" donors [81]. These protocols need to be supported with appropriate medical and nursing education [291–293] and influencing attitudinal changes for the role of donor [294]. Policies for organ donation and management should be developed with aim to change the culture at the bedside and with hospital administration [295, 296].

Optimal Time of Organ Procurement

In general, after brain death has been declared and consent to organ donation has been granted, all efforts are made to complete logistics and initiate procurement as quickly as possible. Expediting the interval from brain death to surgical procurement may allow grieving families to leave the hospital sooner and reduce ICU length of stay. This approach may also have been influenced by the misperception that brain dead patients are irretrievably unstable [77].

As a concept fundamental to ICU multiorgan support, resuscitation of the cardiopulmonary system benefits all end organs. Neurogenic myocardial injury related to primary brain injury is largely reversible with time and treatment [30, 65, 184]. Australian investigators advocate a delay in organ procurement until marginal donor lungs have been optimized with aggressive bronchial toilet using bronchoscopy, physiotherapy, increasing tidal volume and increasing (PEEP) [152, 221]. In a large cohort study of 1,106 renal transplant recipients, longer duration of brain death (time from declaration of brain death to onset of cold ischemia) was associated with improved initial graft function and graft survival, suggesting that the time taken to optimize donor cardiovascular status may reduce ischemic injury [273]. Despite early reports to the contrary [113], liver allograft dysfunction is not associated with prolonged ICU stay by multivariate analysis [239, 241]. A period of time may be needed to determine the trend of elevated AST or ALT, as generally accepted upper limits may be exceeded if the levels are falling rapidly (e.g., following a hypotensive episode with resuscitation).

Temporal changes in multi-organ function after brain death demand flexibility in identifying the optimal time of procurement. Recent consensus guidelines stress the importance of taking the necessary time in the ICU to optimize multi-organ function for the purposes of improving organ utilization and transplant outcomes [69]. Reversible organ dysfunction can be improved with resuscitation and re-evaluation and may include:

- Myocardial/cardiovascular dysfunction
- Oxygenation impairment related to potentially reversible lung injury
- Invasive bacterial infections
- Hypernatremia
- The need to evaluate temporal trends in aspartate aminotransferase (AST) and alanine aminotransferase (ALT)
- The need to evaluate temporal trends in creatinine
- Any other potentially treatable situation.

This treatment period may be extended 24–48 or longer and should be accompanied by frequent re-evaluation to demonstrate improvement in organ function toward defined targets. Extending the interval of donor care in the ICU to optimize transplant outcomes should be factored into donation consent discussions and should be consistent with the wishes of the family or surrogate decision maker. Adequate PICU resource allocation should be anticipated.

Decisions Regarding Transplantability

End-of-life care in the ICU includes all efforts to actualize the opportunity and expressed intent to donate organs. Given the management of brain death and the organ donor is the exclusive domain of ICU practice, it is incumbent on critical care practitioners to assume leadership in this regard, in collaboration with organ procurement agencies and transplant programs. Table 38.3 provides an example of standing orders for pediatric donors to help guide practice [69].

It is important for ICU staff to know that individual programs may have different function thresholds for accepting organs, dependent on program experience and urgency of recipient need. Although the non-utilization of organs is most commonly related to organ dysfunction, it is also related to donor characteristics and/or flaws in the processes of transplant evaluation and decision making. A four-center Canadian review of heart and lung utilization identified deficits in the consent to individual organs, the offering of organs, and the utilization of offered organs unrelated to organ dysfunction [297]. Consent should be requested for all organs regardless of baseline function and all organs should be offered. Ideally, final decisions about transplantability should rest with the individual transplant programs represented by the organ-specific transplant doctors.

Management of marginal organs should include resuscitation and reevaluation to allow for potential organ rescue and utilization. Transplant programs should be accountable to the donor family and ICU donation efforts for the non-utilization of organs, to ensure that all useable organs are used. This evolving collaboration to establish best donor management practices in the ICU must be linked to ensuring optimal organ utilization, which in turn, must be linked to transplant graft and patient outcomes.

Table 38.3 Standing orders for organ donor management: pediatrics

Standard monitoring
1. Urine catheter to straight drainage, strict intake and output
2. Nasogastric tube to straight drainage
3. Vital signs q1h
4. Pulse oximetry, 3-lead electrocardiogram (EKG)
5. Central venous pressure (CVP) monitoring
6. Arterial line pressure monitoring

Laboratory investigations
1. Arterial blood gas (ABG), electrolytes, glucose q4h and PRN
2. CBC q8h
3. Blood urea nitrogen (BUN), creatinine q6h
4. Urine analysis
5. AST, ALT, bilirubin (total and direct), international normalized ratio (INR) (or prothrombin time [PT]), partial thromboplastin time (PTT) q6h

Hemodynamic monitoring and therapy
General targets: age-related norms for pulse and blood pressure (BP)
1. Fluid resuscitation to maintain normovolemia, CVP 6–10 mmHg
2. Age-related treatment thresholds for arterial hypertension:

Newborns–3 months	>90/60
>3 m–1 year	>110/70
>1 year–12 year	>130/80
>12 year–18 year	>140/90

    a. Wean inotropes and vasopressors, and, if necessary
    b. Start
       Nitroprusside 0.5–5.0 µg/kg/min, or
       Esmolol 100–500 µg/kg bolus followed by 100–300 µg/kg/min
3. Serum lactate q2–4h
4. Central venous oximetry q2–4h; titrate therapy to central $SVO_2 \geq 60\%$

Agents for hemodynamic support
1. Dopamine 1–10 µg/kg/min
2. Vasopressin 0.0003–0.0007 U/kg/min (0.3–0.7 mU/kg/min) to a maximum dose of 2.4 U/h
3. Norepinephrine, epinephrine, phenylephrine (caution with doses > 0.2 µg/kg/min)

Glycemia and nutrition
1. Routine intravenous (iv) dextrose infusions
2. Continue enteral feeding as tolerated
3. Continue parenteral nutrition if already initiated
4. Initiate and titrate insulin infusion to maintain serum glucose 6–10 mmol/L

Fluid and electrolytes
Targets:
    1. Urine output 0.5–3 ml/kg/h
    2. Serum sodium (Na) $\geq 130 \leq 150$ mM
    3. Normal ranges for potassium, calcium, magnesium, phosphate

Diabetes insipidus
Defined as:
    1. Urine output > 4 ml/kg/h, associated with:
       a. Rising serum Na ≥ 145 mmol/L and/or
       b. Rising serum osmolarity ≥ 300 mosM and/or
       c. Decreasing urine osmolarity ≤ 200 mosM

(continued)

Table 38.3 (continued)

Diabetes insipidus therapy

1. Titrate therapy to urine output ≤ 3 ml/kg/h

   a. iv vasopressin infusion 0.0003–0.0007 U/kg/min (0.3–0.7 mU/kg/min) to a maximum dose of 2.4 U/h, and/or

   b. Intermittent 1-desamino-D-arginine vasopression (DDAVP) 0.25–10 µg iv q6h

Combined hormonal therapy

Defined as:

1. Tetra-iodothyronine (T_4) 20 µg iv bolus followed by 10 µg/h iv infusion (or 50–100 µg iv bolus followed by 25–50 µg iv bolus q12h)

2. Vasopressin 0.0003–0.0007 U/kg/min (0.3–0.7 mU/kg/min) to a maximum dose of 2.4 U/h

3. Methylprednisolone 15 mg/kg (≤1 g) iv q24h

Indications:

1. 2D echocardiographic ejection fraction ≤ 40 %, or

2. Hemodynamic instability (includes shock unresponsive to restoration of normovolemia and requiring vasoactive support [dopamine >10 µg/min or any other vasopressor agent])

3. Consideration should be given to its use in all donors

Hematology

1. Hemoglobin (Hgb) optimal ≥ 100 g/L for unstable donors, lowest acceptable ≥ 70 g/L

2. Platelets, INR, PTT no predefined targets, transfuse in cases of clinically relevant bleeding

3. No special transfusion requirements

Microbiology (baseline, Q24h and PRN)

1. Daily blood cultures

2. Daily urine cultures

3. Daily endotracheal tube (ETT) cultures

4. Antibiotics for presumed or proven infection

Heart Specific

1. 12-lead EKG

2. Troponin I or T, q12h

3. 2D echocardiography

   a. Should only be performed after fluid and hemodynamic resuscitation

   b. If 2D echo ejection fraction ≤ 40 % then repeat echocardiography at q6–12 h intervals

Lung specific

1. Chest x-ray q24h and PRN

2. Bronchoscopy and bronchial wash gram stain and culture

3. Routine ETT suctioning, rotation to lateral position q2h

4. Mechanical ventilation targets:

   a. Tidal volume (Vt) 8–10 ml/kg, positive end expiratory pressure (PEEP) 5 cm H_2O, peak inspiratory pressure (PIP) ≤ 30 cm H_2O

   b. pH 7.35–7.45, partial pressure of arterial carbon dioxide ($PaCO_2$) 35–45 mmHg, partial pressure of arterial oxygen (PaO_2) ≥ 80 mmHg, oxygen (O_2) sat ≥ 95 %

5. Recruitment maneuvers for oxygenation impairment may include:

   a. Periodic increases in PEEP up to 15 cm H_2O

   b. Sustained inflations (PIP @ 30 cm H_2O × 30–60 s)

   c. Diuresis to normovolemia

[Based on data from ref. 69]

References

1. Smith M. Physiologic changes during brain stem death–lessons for management of the organ donor. J Heart Lung Transplant. 2004;23(9 Suppl):S217–22.

2. Finfer S, Bohn D, Colpitts D, Cox P, Fleming F, Barker G. Intensive care management of paediatric organ donors and its effect on post-transplant organ function. Intensive Care Med. 1996;22(12):1424–32.

3. Hagan ME, McClean D, Falcone CA, Arrington J, Matthews D, Summe C. Attaining specific donor management goals increases number of organs transplanted per donor: a quality improvement project. Prog Transplant. 2009;19(3):227–31.

4. Franklin GA, Santos AP, Smith JW, Galbraith S, Harbrecht BG, Garrison RN. Optimization of donor management goals yields increased organ use. Am Surg. 2010;76(6):587–94.

5. Malinoski DJ, Daly MC, Patel MS, Oley-Graybill C, Foster 3rd CE, Salim A. Achieving donor management goals before deceased donor procurement is associated with more organs transplanted per donor. J Trauma. 2011;71(4):990–5. discussion 996.

6. Badovinac K, Greig P, Ross H, Doig C, Shemie SD. Organ utilization among deceased donors in Canada, 1993-2002. Can J Anaesth. 2006;53(8):838–44.

7. Punch JD, Hayes DH, LaPorte FB, McBride V, Seely MS. Organ donation and utilization in the United States, 1996-2005. Am J Transplant. 2007;7(5 Pt 2):1327–38.

8. Klein AS, Messersmith EE, Ratner LE, Kochik R, Baliga PK, Ojo AO. Organ donation and utilization in the United States, 1999-2008. Am J Transplant. 2010;10(4 Pt 2):973–86.

9. Messersmith EE, Arrington C, Alexander C, Orlowski JP, Wolfe R. Development of donor yield models. Am J Transplant. 2011;11(10):2075–84.

10. Tsai E, Shemie SD, Hebert D, Furst S, Cox PN. Organ donation in children. The role of the pediatric intensive care unit. Pediatr Crit Care Med. 2000;1:156–60.

11. Selck FW, Deb P, Grossman EB. Deceased organ donor characteristics and clinical interventions associated with organ yield. Am J Transplant. 2008;8(5):965–74.

12. Shivalkar B, Van Loon J, Wieland W, Tjandra-Maga TB, Borgers M, Plets C, Fleming W. Variable effects of explosive or gradual increase of intracranial pressure on myocardial structure and function. Circulation. 1993;87(1):230–9.

13. Powner DJ, Bernstein IM. Extended somatic support for pregnant women after brain death. Crit Care Med. 2003;31(4):1241–9.

14. Wood KE, Becker BN, McCartney JG, et al. Care of the potential organ donor. N Engl J Med. 2004;351(26):2730–9.

15. Philip S, Udomphorn Y, Kirkham FJ, Vavilala MS. Cerebrovascular pathophysiology in pediatric traumatic brain injury. J Trauma. 2009;67(2 Suppl):S128–34.

16. Novitzky D. Detrimental effects of brain death on the potential organ donor. Transplant Proc. 1997;29:3770–2.

17. Novitzky D, Wicomb WN, Cooper DKC, Rose AG, Fraser RC, Barnard CW. Electrocardiographic, hemodynamic and endocrine changes occurring during experimental brain death in the chacma baboon. Heart Transplant. 1984;4:63–9.

18. Ferrera R, Hadour G, Tamion F, Henry JP, Mulder P, Richard V, Thuillez C, Ovize M, Derumeaux G. Brain death provokes very acute alteration in myocardial morphology detected by echocardiography: preventive effect of beta-blockers. Transpl Int. 2011;24(3):300–6.

19. Li J, Konstantinov IE, Cai S, Shimizu M, Redington AN. Systemic and myocardial oxygen transport responses to brain death in pigs. Transplant Proc. 2007;39(1):21–6.

20. Venkateswaran RV, Dronavalli V, Lambert PA, et al. The proinflammatory environment in potential heart and lung donors: prevalence and impact of donor management and hormonal therapy. Transplantation. 2009;88(4):582–8.

21. Katz K, Lawler J, Wax J, et al. Vasopressin pressor effects in critically ill children during evaluation for brain death and organ recovery. Resuscitation. 2000;47(1):33–40.

22. Dimopoulou I, Tsagarakis S, Anthi A, et al. High prevalence of decreased cortisol reserve in brain-dead potential organ donors. Crit Care Med. 2003;31(4):1113–7.

23. Salim A, Martin M, Brown C, et al. Complications of brain death: frequency and impact on organ retrieval. Am Surg. 2006;72(5):377–81.

24. Pérez López S, Otero Hernández J, Vázquez Moreno N, et al. Brain death effects on catecholamine levels and subsequent cardiac damage assessed in organ donors. J Heart Lung Transplant. 2009;28(8):815–20.

25. Mayer SA, Fink ME, Raps EC, et al. Cardiac injury associated with neurologic pulmonary edema following subarachnoid hemorrhage. Neurology. 1994;44:815–20.

26. Kono T, Morita H, Kuroiwa T, Onaka H, Takatsuka H, Fujiwara A. Left ventricular wall motion abnormalities in patients with subarachnoid hemorrhage: neurogenic stunned myocardium. J Am Coll Cardiol. 1994;24:636–40.

27. Temes RE, Tessitore E, Schmidt JM, Naidech AM, Fernandez A, Ostapkovich ND, Frontera JA, Wartenberg KE, Di Tullio MR, Badjatia N, Connolly ES, Mayer SA, Parra A. Left ventricular dysfunction and cerebral infarction from vasospasmafter subarachnoid hemorrhage. Neurocrit Care. 2010;13(3):359–65.

28. Macmillan CSA, Grant IS, Andrews PJD. Pulmonary and cardiac sequelae of subarachnoid haemorrhage: time for active management? Intensive Care Med. 2002;28:1012–23.

29. Kolin A, Norris JW. Myocardial damage from acute cerebral lesions. Stroke. 1984;15:990–3.

30. Tung P, Kopelnik A, Banki N, Ong K, Ko N, Lawton MT, Gress D, Drew B, Foster E, Parmley W, Zaroff J. Predictors of neurocardiogenic injury after subarachnoid hemorrhage. Stroke. 2004;35(2):548–51. Epub 2004 Jan 22.

31. Grant J, Canter CE, Spray TL, Landt YS, Jeffrey E, Ladenson JH, Jaffe AS. Elevated donor cardiac troponin I: a marker of acute graft failure in infant heart recipients. Circulation. 1994;90(6):2618–21.

32. Takada M, Nadeau KC, Hancock WW, Mackenzie HS, Shaw GD, Waaga AM, Chandraker A, Sayegh MH, Tilney NL. Effects of explosive brain death on cytokine activation of peripheral organs in the rat. Transplantation. 1998;65:1533–42.

33. Novitzky D, Wicomb WN, Rose AG, Cooper DK, Reichart B. Pathophysiology of pulmonary edema following experimental brain death in the chacma baboon. Ann Thorac Surg. 1987;43(3):288–94.

34. Cruickshank JM, Meil-Dwyer G, Degaute JP, Kuurne T, Kytta J, Carruthers ME, Patel S. Reduction of stress/catecholamine-induced cardiac necrosis by beta 1 selective blockade. Lancet. 1987;2:585–9.

35. Siaghy EM, Halejcio-Delophont P, Mertes PM, et al. Protective effects of labetalol on myocardial contractile function in brain-dead pigs. Transplant Proc. 1998;30:2842–3.

36. Hall SR, Wang L, Milne B, Ford S, Hong M. Intrathecal lidocaine prevents cardiovascular collapse and neurogenic pulmonary edema in a rat model of acute intracranial hypertension. Anesth Analg. 2002;94(4):948–53.

37. Baguley IJ. Autonomic complications following central nervous system injury. Semin Neurol. 2008;28(5):716–25. Epub 2008 Dec 29. Review.

38. Sedý J, Zicha J, Kunes J, Jendelová P, Syková E. Mechanisms of neurogenicpulmonary edema development. Physiol Res. 2008; 57(4):499–506. Epub 2007 Nov 30.

39. Avlonitis VS, Wigfield CH, Kirby JA, Dark JH. The hemodynamic mechanisms of lung injury and systemic inflammatory response following brain death in the transplant donor. Am J Transplant. 2005;5(4 Pt 1):684–93.

40. Fontes RB, Aguiar PH, Zanetti MV, Andrade F, Mandel M, Teixeira MJ. Acute neurogenic pulmonary edema: case reports and literature review. J Neurosurg Anesthesiol. 2003;15(2):144–50.

41. Bruder N, Rabinstein A, The Participants in the International Multidisciplinary Consensus Conference on the Critical Care Management of Subarachnoid Hemorrhage. Cardiovascular and pulmonary complications of aneurysmal subarachnoid hemorrhage. Neurocrit Care. 2011;15(2):257–69.

42. Pratschke J, Wilhelm MJ, Kusaka M, Hancock WW, Tilney NL. Activation of proinflammatory genes in somatic organs as a consequence of brain death. Transplant Proc. 1999;31:1003–5.

43. Barklin A. Systemic inflammation in the brain-dead organ donor. Acta Anaesthesiol Scand. 2009;53(4):425–35. Epub 2009 Feb 18. Review.

44. Amado JA, Lopez-Espadas F, Vazquez-Barquero A, Salas E, Riancho JA, Lopez-Cordovilla JJ, et al. Blood levels of cytokines in brain-dead patients: relationship with circulating hormones and acute phase reactants. Metabolism. 1995;44:812–6.

45. Kuecuek O, Mantouvalou L, Klemz R, Kotsch K, Volk HD, Jonas S, Wesslau C, Tullius S, Neuhaus P, Pratschke J. Significant reduction of proinflammatory cytokines by treatment of the brain-dead donor. Transplant Proc. 2005;37(1):387–8.

46. van der Hoeven JA, Ter Horst GJ, Molema G, de Vos P, Girbes AR, Postema F, Freund RL, Wiersema J, van Schilfgaarde R, Ploeg RJ. Effects of brain death and hemodynamic status on function and immunologic activation of the potential donor liver in the rat. Ann Surg. 2000;232:804–13.

47. van der Hoeven JA, Lindell S, van Schilfgaarde R, Molema G, Ter Horst GJ, Southard JH, Ploeg RJ. Donor brain death reduces survival after transplantation in rat livers preserved for 20 hr. Transplantation. 2001;72:1632–6.

48. Koo DDH, Welsh KI, McLaren AJ, Roake JA, Morris PJ, Fuggle SV. Cadaver versus living donor kidneys: impact of donor factors on antigen induction before transplantation. Kidney Int. 1999;56:1551–9.

49. Nijboer WN, Schuurs TA, van der Hoeven JA, Fekken S, Wiersema-Buist J, Leuvenink HG, Hofker S, Homan van der Heide JJ, van Son WJ, Ploeg RJ. Effect of brain death on gene expression and tissue activation in human donor kidneys. Transplantation. 2004;78(7):978–86.

50. Kosieradzki M, Kuczynska J, Piwowarska J, Wegrowicz-Rebandel I, Kwiatkowski A, Lisik W, et al. Prognostic significance of free radical mediated injury occurring in the kidney donor. Transplantation. 2003;75(8):1221–7.

51. Nijboer WN, Schuurs TA, van der Hoeven JA, Leuvenink HG, van der Heide JJ, van Goor H, Ploeg RJ. Effects of brain death on stress and inflammatory response in the human donor kidney. Transplant Proc. 2005;37(1):367–9.

52. Minnear FL, Connell RS. Prevention of aconitine-induced neurogenic pulmonary oedema with hypovolemia or methylprednisolone. J Trauma. 1982;22:121–8.

53. Edmonds HLJ, Cannon HCJ, Garretson HD, Dahlquist G. Effects of aerosolized methylprednisolone on experimental neurogenic pulmonary injury. Neurosurgery. 1986;19:36–40.

54. Zweers N, Petersen AH, van der Hoeven JA, de Haan A, Ploeg RJ, de Leij LF, Prop J. Donor brain death aggravates chronic rejection after lung transplantation in rats. Transplantation. 2004;78(9):1251–8.

55. Land WG. The role of postischemic reperfusion injury and other nonantigen-dependent inflammatory pathways in transplantation. Transplantation. 2005;79(5):505–14.

56. van der Hoeven JA, Molema G, Ter Horst GJ, Freund RL, Wiersema J, van Schilfgaarde R, Leuvenink HG, Ploeg RJ. Relationship between duration of brain death and hemodynamic (in)stability on progressive dysfunction and increased immunologic activation of donor kidneys. Kidney Int. 2003;64(5):1874–82.

57. Schuurs TA, Gerbens F, van der Hoeven JA, Ottens PJ, Kooi KA, Leuvenink HG, Hofstra RM, Ploeg RJ. Distinct transcriptional changes in donor kidneys upon brain death induction in rats: insights in the processes of brain death. Am J Transplant. 2004;4(12):1972–81.

58. Pratschke J, Neuhaus P, Tullius SG. What can be learned from brain-death models? Transpl Int. 2005;18(1):15–21.

59. Powner DJ, Hewitt MJ, Levine RL. Interventions during donor care before lung transplantation. Prog Transplant. 2005;15(2):141–8. Review.

60. Dujardin KS, McCully RB, Wijdicks EF, Tazelaar HD, Seward JB, McGregor CG, Olson LJ. Myocardial dysfunction associated with brain death: clinical, echocardiographic, and pathologic features. J Heart Lung Transplant. 2001;20:350–7.

61. Yokoyama Y, Cooper DKC, Sasaki H, Snow TR, Akutsu T, Zuhdi N. Donor-heart evaluation by monitoring the left ventricular pressure-volume relationship: clinical observations. J Heart Lung Transplant. 1992;11:685–92.

62. Young JB, Naftel DC, Bourge RC, Kirklin JK, Clemson BS, Porter CB, Rodeheffer RJ. Matching the heart donor and heart transplant recipient. Clues for successful expansion of the donor pool: a multivariable, multi-institutional report. J Heart Lung Transplant. 1994;13:353–65.

63. Hashimoto S, Kato TS, Komamura K, Hanatani A, Niwaya K, Funatsu T, Kobayashi J, Sumita Y, Tanaka N, Hashimura K, Asakura M, Kanzaki H, Kitakaze M. Utility of echocardiographic evaluation of donor hearts upon the organ procurement for heart transplantation. J Cardiol. 2011;57(2):215–22. Epub 2011 Jan 14.

64. Fine NM, Pellikka PA. Pharmacologic stress echocardiography for the assessment of organ suitability for heart transplantation: casting a broader net in search of donors. J Am Soc Echocardiogr. 2011;24(4):363–6.

65. Babcock WD, Menza RL, Zaroff JG. Increased donor heart utilization using serial echocardiography during donor management. J Heart Lung Transplant. 2003;22(1S):74.

66. Venkateswaran RV, Townend JN, Wilson IC, Mascaro JG, Bonser RS, Steeds RP. Echocardiography in the potential heart donor. Transplantation. 2010;89(7):894–901.

67. Pennefather S, Bullock RE, Dark JH. The effect of fluid therapy on alveolar arterial oxygen gradient in brain-dead organ donors. Transplantation. 1993;56(6):1418–22.

68. Rosengard BR, Feng S, Alfrey EJ, Zaroff JG, Emond JC, Henry ML, Garrity ER, Roberts JP, Wynn JJ, Metzger RA, Freeman RB, Port FK, Merion RM, Love RB, Busuttil RW, Delmonico FL. Report of the crystal city meeting to maximize the use of organs recovered from the cadaver donor. Am J Transplant. 2002;2:701–11.

69. Shemie SD, Ross H, Pagliarello J, Baker AJ, Greig PD, Brand T, Cockfield S, Keshavjee S, Nickerson P, Rao V, Guest C, Young K, Doig C, Pediatric Recommendations Group. Organ donor management in Canada: recommendations of the forum on Medical Management to Optimize Donor Organ Potential. CMAJ. 2006;174(6):S13–32.

70. Wheeldon DR, Potter CDO, Oduro A, Wallwork J, Large SR. Transforming the "unacceptable" donor: outcomes from the adoption of a standardized donor management technique. J Heart Lung Transplant. 1995;14:734–42.

71. Hadjizacharia P, Salim A, Brown C, Inaba K, Chan LS, Mascarenhas A, Margulies DR. Does the use of pulmonary artery catheters increase the number of organs available for transplantation? Clin Transplant. 2010;24(1):62–6. Epub 2009 Feb 14.

72. Hunt SA, Baldwin J, Baumgartner W, Bricker JT, Costanzo MR, Miller L, Mudge G, O'Connell JB. Cardiovascular management

of a potential heart donor: a statement from the Transplantation Committee of the American College of Cardiology. Crit Care Med. 1996;24:1599–601.

73. Powner DJ, Hergenroeder GW. Measurement of cardiac output during adult donor care. Prog Transplant. 2011;21(2):144–50. quiz 151.

74. Su BC, Yu HP, Yang MW, Lin CC, Kao MC, Chang CH, Lee WC. Reliability of a new ultrasonic cardiac output monitor in recipients of living donor liver transplantation. Liver Transpl. 2008;14(7):1029–37.

75. Powner DJ, Doshi PB. Central venous oxygen saturation monitoring: role in adult donor care? Prog Transplant. 2010;20(4):401–5.

76. Huang J, Trinkaus K, Huddleston CB, Mendeloff EN, Spray TL, Canter CE. Risk factors for primary graft failure after pediatric cardiac transplantation: importance of recipient and donor characteristics. J Heart Lung Transplant. 2004;23(6):716–22.

77. Lagiewska B, Pacholczyk M, Szostek M, Walaszewski J, Rowinski W. Hemodynamic and metabolic disturbances observed in brain dead organ donors. Transplant Proc. 1996;28:165–6.

78. Murugan R, Venkataraman R, Wahed AS, Elder M, Carter M, Madden NJ, Kellum JA, HIDonOR Study Investigators. Preload responsiveness is associated with increased interleukin-6 and lower organ yield from brain-dead donors. Crit Care Med. 2009;37(8):2387–93.

79. Tuttle-Newhall JE, Collins BH, Kuo PC, Schroeder R. Organ donation and treatment of multi-organ donor. Curr Probl Surg. 2003;40(5):266–310.

80. Kutsogiannis DJ, Pagliarello G, Doig C, Ross H, Shemie SD. Medical management to optimize donor organ potential: review of the literature. Can J Anaesth. 2006;53(8):820–30.

81. Mascia L, Mastromauro I, Viberti S, Vincenzi M, Zanello M. Management to optimize organ procurement in brain dead donors. Minerva Anestesiol. 2009;75(3):125–33.

82. Dictus C, Vienenkoetter B, Esmaeilzadeh M, Unterberg A, Ahmadi R. Critical care management of potential organ donors: our current standard. Clin Transplant. 2009;23 Suppl 21:2–9.

83. D'Amico TA, Meyers CH, Koutlas TC, Peterseim DS, Sabiston DC, Van Trigt P, et al. Desensitization of myocardial β-adrenergic receptors and deterioration of left ventricular function after brain death. J Thorac Cardiovasc Surg. 1995;110:746–51.

84. Schnuelle P, Yard BA, Braun C, Dominguez-Fernandez E, Schaub M, Birck R, Sturm J, Post S, van der Woude FJ. Impact of donor dopamine on immediate graft function after kidney transplantation. Am J Transplant. 2004;4(3):419–26.

85. Santise G, D'Ancona G, Falletta C, Pirone F, Sciacca S, Turrisi M, Biondo D, Pilato M. Donor pharmacological hemodynamic support is associated with primary graft failure in human heart transplantation. Interact Cardiovasc Thorac Surg. 2009;9(3):476–9. Epub 2009 Jun 29.

86. Marik PE, Mohedin M. The contrasting effects of dopamine and norepinephrine on systemic and splanchnic oxygen utilization in hyperdynamic sepsis. JAMA. 1994;272:1354–7.

87. Martin C, Papazian L, Perrin G, Saux P, Gouin F. Norepinephrine or dopamine for the treatment of hyperdynamic septic shock? Chest. 1993;103:1826–31.

88. De Backer D, Creteur J, Silva E, Vincent JL. Effects of dopamine, norepinephrine, and epinephrine on the splanchnic circulation in septic shock: which is best? Crit Care Med. 2003;31(6):1659–67.

89. Chen JM, Cullinane S, Spanier TB, Artrip JH, John R, Edwards NM, Oz MC, Landry DW. Vasopressin deficiency and pressor hypersensitivity in hemodynamically unstable organ donors. Circulation. 1999;100(suppl II):II-246.

90. Kinoshita Y, Yahata K, Yoshioka T, Onishi S, Sugimoto T. Long-term renal preservation after brain death maintained with vasopressin and epinephrine. Transplant Int. 1990;3:15–8.

91. Yoshioka T, Sugimoto H, Uenishi M. Prolonged haemodynamic maintenance by the combined administration of vasopressin and epinephrine in brain death: a clinical study. Neurosurgery. 1986;18:565–7.

92. Pennefather SH, Bullock RE, Mantle D, Dark JH. Use of low dose arginine vasopressin to support brain-dead organ donors. Transplantation. 1995;59(1):58–62.

93. Nakagawa K, Tang JF. Physiologic response of human brain death and the use of vasopressin for successful organ transplantation. J Clin Anesth. 2011;23(2):145–8.

94. Holmes CL, Patel BM, Russell JA, Walley KR. Physiology of vasopressin relevant to management of septic shock. Chest. 2001;120:989–1002.

95. Brierley J, Carcillo JA, Choong K, Cornell T, Decaen A, Deymann A, Doctor A, Davis A, Duff J, Dugas MA, Duncan A, Evans B, Feldman J, Felmet K, Fisher G, Frankel L, Jeffries H, Greenwald B, Gutierrez J, Hall M, Han YY, Hanson J, Hazelzet J, Hernan L, Kiff J, Kissoon N, Kon A, Irazuzta J, Lin J, Lorts A, Mariscalco M, Mehta R, Nadel S, Nguyen T, Nicholson C, Peters M, Okhuysen-Cawley R, Poulton T, Relves M, Rodriguez A, Rozenfeld R, Schnitzler E, Shanley T, Kache S, Skippen P, Torres A, von Dessauer B, Weingarten J, Yeh T, Zaritsky A, Stojadinovic B, Zimmerman J, Zuckerberg A. Clinical practice parameters for hemodynamic support of pediatric and neonatal septic shock: 2007 update from the American College of Critical Care Medicine. Crit Care Med. 2009;37(2):666–88.

96. Guzman JA, Rosado AE, Kruse JA. Vasopressin vs norepinephrine in endotoxic shock: systemic, renal, and splanchnic hemodynamic and oxygen transport effects. J Appl Physiol. 2003; 95(2):803–9.

97. Dunser MW, Mayr AJ, Ulmer H, Knotzer H, Sumann G, Pajk W, Friesenecker B, Hasibeder WR. Arginine vasopressin in advanced vasodilatory shock: a prospective, randomized, controlled study. Circulation. 2003;107(18):2313–9. Epub 2003 May 5.

98. Kinoshita Y, Okamoto K, Yahata K, Yoshioka T, Sugimoto T, Kawaguchi N, Onishi S. Clinical and pathological changes of the heart in brain death maintained with vasopressin and epinephrine. Pathol Res Pract. 1990;186:173–9.

99. Martikainen TJ, Kurola J, Kärjä V, Parviainen I, Ruokonen E. Vasopressor agents after experimental brain death: effects of dopamine and vasopressin on vitality of the small gut. Transplant Proc. 2010;42(7):2449–56.

100. Mascia L, Bosma K, Pasero D, Galli T, Cortese G, Donadio P, Bosco R. Ventilatory and hemodynamic management of potential organ donors: an observational survey. Crit Care Med. 2006; 34(2):321–7.

101. Venkateswaran RV, Patchell VB, Wilson IC, Mascaro JG, Thompson RD, Quinn DW, Stockley RA, Coote JH, Bonser RS. Early donor management increases the retrieval rate of lungs for transplantation. Ann Thorac Surg. 2008;85(1):278–86.

102. Mallory Jr GB, Schecter MG, Elidemir O. Management of the pediatric organ donor to optimize lung donation. Pediatr Pulmonol. 2009;44(6):536–46. Review.

103. Mascia L, Pasero D, Slutsky AS, Arguis MJ, Berardino M, Grasso S, Munari M, Boifava S, Cornara G, Della Corte F, Vivaldi N, Malacarne P, Del Gaudio P, Livigni S, Zavala E, Filippini C, Martin EL, Donadio PP, Mastromauro I, Ranieri VM. Effect of a lung protective strategy for organ donors on eligibility and availability of lungs for transplantation: a randomized controlled trial. JAMA. 2010;304(23):2620–7.

104. Masson F, Thicoipe M, Gin H, De Mascarel A, Angibeau RM, Favarel-Garrigues JF, Erny P. The endocrine pancreas in brain-dead donors. Transplantation. 1993;56(2):363–7.

105. Cochran A, Scaife ER, Hansen KW, Downey EC. Hyperglycemia and outcomes from pediatric traumatic brain injury. J Trauma. 2003;55(6):1035–8.

106. Rovlias A, Kotsou S. The influence of hyperglycemia on neurological outcome in patients with severe head injury. Neurosurgery. 2000;46(2):335–42. discussion 342–3.

107. Kelly DF. Neurosurgical postoperative care. Neurosurg Clin North Am. 1994;5:789–810.

108. Cherian L, Goodman JC, Robertson CS. Effect of glucose administration on contusion volume after moderate cortical impact injury in rats. J Neurotrauma. 1998;15(12):1059–66.

109. Singer P, Cohen J, Cynober L. Effect of nutritional state of brain-dead organ donor on transplantation. Nutrition. 2001;17(11–12):948–52.

110. Boudjema K, Lindell SL, Southard JH, Belzer FO. The effects of fasting on the quality of liver preservation by simple cold storage. Transplantation. 1990;50:943–8.

111. Wakiyama S, Yanaga K, Soejima Y, Nishizaki T, Sugimachi K. Significance of donor nutritional status for rewarming injury of the hepatic graft in rats. Eur Surg Res. 1997;29(5):339–45.

112. Singer P, Shapiro H, Cohen J. Brain death and organ damage: the modulating effects of nutrition. Transplantation. 2005;80(10):1363–8.

113. Greig PD, Forster J, Superina RA, Strasberg SM, Mohamed M, Blendis LM, Taylor BR, Levy GA, Langer B. Donor-specific factors predict graft function following liver transplantation. Transplant Proc. 1990;22:2072–3.

114. Cywes R, Greig PD, Morgan GR, Sanabria JR, Clavien PA, Harvey PR, Strasberg SM. Rapid donor liver nutritional enhancement in a large animal model. Hepatology. 1992;16:1271–9.

115. Gonzalez FX, Rimola A, Grande L, Antolin M, Garcia-Valdecasas JC, Fuster J, Lacy AM, Cugat E, Visa J, Rodes J. Predictive factors of early postoperative graft function in human liver transplantation. Hepatology. 1994;20:565–73.

116. Shah VR. Aggressive management of multiorgan donor. Transplant Proc. 2008;40(4):1087–90.

117. Howlett TA, Keogh AM, Perry L, Touzel R, Rees LH. Anterior and posterior pituitary function in brain-stem-dead donors. Transplantation. 1989;47:828–34.

118. Gramm H, Meinhold H, Bickel U, Zimmermann J, Von Hammerstein B, Keller F, Dennhardt R, Voigt K. Acute endocrine failure after brain death. Transplantation. 1992;54(5):851–7.

119. Agha A, Phillips J, Thompson CJ. Hypopituitarism following traumatic brain injury (TBI). Br J Neurosurg. 2007;21(2):210–6.

120. Avolio AW, Agnes S, Magalini SC, Foco M, Castagneto M. Importance of donor blood chemistry data (AST, serum sodium) in predicting liver transplant outcome. Transplant Proc. 1991;23:2451–2.

121. Figueras J, Busquets J, Grande L, Jaurrieta E, Perez-Ferreiroa J, Mir J, Margarit C, Lopez P, Vazquez J, Casanova D, Bernardos A, De-Vicente E, Parrilla P, Ramon JM, Bou R. The deleterious effect of donor high plasma sodium and extended preservation in liver transplantation. A multivariate analysis. Transplantation. 1996;61:410–3.

122. Kazemeyni SM, Esfahani F. Influence of hypernatremia and polyuria of brain-dead donors before organ procurement on kidney allograft function. Urol J. 2008;5(3):173–7.

123. Mangus RS, Fridell JA, Vianna RM, Milgrom ML, Chestovich P, Vandenboom C, Tector AJ. Severe hypernatremia in deceased liver donors does not impact early transplant outcome. Transplantation. 2010;90(4):438–43.

124. Totsuka E, Dodson F, Urakami A, Moras N, Ishii T, Lee MC, Gutierrez J, Gerardo M, Molmenti E, Fung JJ. Influence of high donor serum sodium levels on early postoperative graft function in human liver transplantation: effect of correction of donor hypernatremia. Liver Transpl Surg. 1999;5:421–8.

125. Ourahma S, Guesde R, Leblanc I, Riou B, Goarin JP, Bitker MO, Coriat P. Administration of desmopressin in brain-dead donors does not modify renal function in kidney recipients. Transplant Proc. 1998;30:2844.

126. Richardson DW, Robinson AG. Desmopressin. Ann Intern Med. 1985;103:228–39.

127. Van Bakel AB. The cardiac transplant donor: identification, assessment, and management. Heart Transplant Symp. 1997; 314(3):152–63.

128. Blasi-Ibanez A, Hirose R, Feiner J, Freise C, Stock PG, Roberts JP, Niemann CU. Predictors associated with terminal renal function in deceased organ donors in the intensive care unit. Anesthesiology. 2009;110(2):333–41.

129. Rosendale JD, Chabalewski FL, McBride MA, Garrity ER, Rosengard BR, Delmonico FL, Kauffman HM. Increased transplanted organs from the use of a standardized donor management protocol. Am J Transplant. 2002;2:761–8.

130. Zaroff JG, Rosengard BR, Armstrong WF, Babcock WD, D'Alessandro A, Dec GW, Edwards NM, Higgins RS, Jeevanandum V, Kauffman M, Kirklin JK, Large SR, Marelli D, Peterson TS, Ring WS, Robbins RC, Russell SD, Taylor DO, Van Bakel A, Wallwork J, Young JB. Consensus conference report maximizing use of organs recovered from the cadaver donor: cardiac recommendations. Circulation. 2002;106:836–41.

131. Lee YJ, Shen EY, Huang FY, Kao HA, Shyur SD. Continuous infusion of vasopressin in comatose children with neurogenic diabetes insipidus. J Pediatr Endocrinol Metab. 1995;8:257–62.

132. Lee YJ, Yang D, Shyur SD, Chiu NC. Neurogenic diabetes insipidus in a child with fatal Coxsackie virus B1 encephalitis. J Pediatr Endocrinol Metab. 1995;8:301–4.

133. Lugo N, Silver P, Nimkoff L, Caronia C, Sagy M. Diagnosis and management algorithm of acute onset of central diabetes insipidus in critically ill children. J Pediatr Endocrinol Metab. 1997;10:633–9.

134. Ralston C, Butt W. Continuous vasopressin replacement in diabetes insipidus. Arch Dis Child. 1990;65:896–7.

135. Meyer S, Gortner L, McGuire W, Baghai A, Gottschling S. Vasopressin incatecholamine-refractory shock in children. Anaesthesia. 2008;63(3):228–34. Epub 2007 Dec 13.

136. Klein I, Ojamaak K. Thyroid hormone and the cardiovascular system. NEJM. 2001;344(7):501.

137. Sazontseva IE, Kozlov IA, Moisuc YG, Ermolenko AE, Afonin VV, Illnitskiy VV. Hormonal response to brain death. Transplant Proc. 1991;23(5):2467.

138. Novitzky D, Cooper DKC, Morrell D, Isaacs S. Change from aerobic to anaerobic metabolism after brain death, and reversal following triiodothyronine therapy. Transplantation. 1988;45(1):32–6.

139. James SR, Ranasinghe AM, Venkateswaran R, McCabe CJ, Franklyn JA, Bonser RS. The effects of acute triiodothyronine therapy on myocardial gene expression in brain stem dead cardiac donors. J Clin Endocrinol Metab. 2010;95(3):1338–43.

140. Novitzky D, Cooper DKC, Reichart B. Hemodynamic and metabolic responses to hormonal therapy in brain-dead potential organ donors. Transplantation. 1987;43(2):852–4.

141. Novitzky D, Cooper DKC, Chaffin JS, Greer AE, Debault LE, Zuhdi N. Improved cardiac allograft function following triiodothyronine therapy to both donor and recipient. Transplantation. 1990;49(2):311–6.

142. Roels L, Pirenne J, Delooz H, Lauwers P, Vandermeersch E. Effect of triiodothyronine replacement therapy on maintenance characteristics and organ availability in hemodynamically unstable donors. Transplant Proc. 2000;32:1564–6.

143. Zuppa AF, Nadkarni V, Davis L, Adamson PC, Helfaer MA, Elliott MR, Abrams J, Durbin D. The effect of a thyroid hormone infusion on vasopressor support incritically ill children with cessation of neurologic function. Crit Care Med. 2004;32(11):2318–22.

144. Ranasinghe AM, Quinn DW, Pagano D, Edwards N, Faroqui M, Graham TR, Keogh BE, Mascaro J, Riddington DW, Rooney SJ, Townend JN, Wilson IC, Bonser RS. Glucose-insulin-potassium and tri-iodothyronine individually improve hemodynamic performance and are associated with reduced troponin I release after on-pumpcoronary artery bypass grafting. Circulation. 2006;114(1 Suppl):I245–50.

145. Cooper DK, Novitzky D, Wicomb WN, Basker M, Rosendale JD, Myron Kauffman H. A review of studies relating to thyroid hormone therapy in brain-dead organ donors. Front Biosci. 2009;14:3750–70. Review.

146. Pérez-Blanco A, Caturla-Such J, Cánovas-Robles J, Sanchez-Payá J. Efficiency of triiodothyronine treatment on organ donor hemodynamic management and adeninenucleotide concentration. Intensive Care Med. 2005;31(7):943–8.

147. Novitzky D, Cooper DK, Rosendale JD, Kauffman HM. Hormonal therapy of the brain-dead organ donor: experimental and clinical studies. Transplantation. 2006;82(11):1396–401. Review.

148. Rosendale JD, Kauffman HM, McBride MA, Skjei TC, Zaroff JG, Garrity ER, Delmonico FL, Rosengard BR. Hormonal resuscitation associated with more transplanted organs with no sacrifice in survival. Transplantation. 2004;78(Sup 2):17.

149. Powner DJ. Treatment goals during care of adult donors that can influence outcomes of heart transplantation. Prog Transplant. 2005;15(3):226–32.

150. Rosendale JD, Kauffman HM, McBride MA, Chabalewski FL, Zaroff JG, Garrity ER, Delmonico FL, Rosengard BR. Hormonal resuscitation yields more transplanted hearts, with improved early function. Transplantation. 2003;75(8):1336–41.

151. Follette DM, Rudich SM, Babcock WD. Improved oxygenation and increased lung donor recovery with high-dose steroid administration after brain death. J Heart Lung Transplant. 1998;17(4):423–9.

152. McElhinney DB, Khan JH, Babcock WD, Hall TS. Thoracic organ donor characteristics associated with successful lung procurement. Clin Transplant. 2001;15:68–71.

153. Abdelnour T, Rieke S. Relationship of hormonal resuscitation therapy and central venous pressure on increasing organs for transplant. J Heart Lung Transplant. 2009;28(5):480–5.

154. Nicolas-Robin A, Barouk JD, Amour J, Coriat P, Riou B, Langeron O. Hydrocortisone supplementation enhances hemodynamic stability in brain-dead patients. Anesthesiology. 2010;112(5):1204–10.

155. Nath DS, Ilias Basha H, Liu MH, Moazami N, Ewald GA. Increased recovery of thoracic organs after hormonal resuscitation therapy. J Heart Lung Transplant. 2010;29(5):594–6. Epub 2010 Mar 6.

156. Venkateswaran RV, Steeds RP, Quinn DW, Nightingale P, Wilson IC, Mascaro JG, Thompson RD, Townend JN, Bonser RS. The haemodynamic effects of adjunctive hormone therapy in potential heart donors: a prospective randomized double-blind factorially designed controlled trial. Eur Heart J. 2009;30(14):1771–80.

157. Lacroix J, Hébert PC, Hutchison JS, Hume HA, Tucci M, Ducruet T, Gauvin F, Collet JP, Toledano BJ, Robillard P, Joffe A, Biarent D, Meert K, Peters MJ, TRIPICU Investigators, Canadian Critical Care Trials Group, Pediatric Acute Lung Injury and Sepsis Investigators Network. Transfusion strategies for patients in pediatric intensive care units. N Engl J Med. 2007;356(16):1609–19.

158. Ciancio G, Burke G, Roth D, Zucker K, Tzakis A, Miller J. The significance of infections in donor organs. Transpl Immunol. 1996;12:3–11. Abstract.

159. Doig RL, Boyd PJ, Eykyn S. Staphylococcus aureus transmitted in transplanted kidneys. Lancet. 1975;2:243–5.

160. Gottesdiener KM. Transplanted infections: donor-to-host transmission with the allograft. Ann Intern Med. 1989;110:1001–16.

161. Nery JR, Weppler D, Ketchum P, Olson L, Fragulidis GP, Khan MF, Webb MG, Miller J, Tzakis AG. Donor infection and primary nonfunction in liver transplantation. Transplant Proc. 1997;29:481–3.

162. Weber TR, Freier DT, Turcotte JG. Transplantation of infected kidneys: clinical and experimental results. Transplantation. 1979;27:63–5.

163. Powner DJ, Allison TA. Bacterial infection during adult donor care. Prog Transplant. 2007;17(4):266–74. Review.

164. Freeman RB, Giatras I, Falagas ME, Supran S, O'Connor K, Bradley J, Snydman DR, Delmonico FL. Outcome of

transplantation of organs procured from bacteremic donors. Transplantation. 1999;68:1107–11.

165. Lumbreras C, Sanz F, Gonzalez A, Perez G, Ramos MJ, Aguado JM, Lizasoain M, Andres A, Moreno E, Gomez MA, Noriega AR. Clinical significance of donor-unrecognized bacteremia in the outcome of solid-organ transplant recipients. Clin Infect Dis. 2001;33:722–6.

166. Cerutti E, Stratta C, Romagnoli R, Serra R, Lepore M, Fop F, Mascia L, Lupo F, Franchello A, Panio A, Salizzoni M. Bacterial- and fungal-positive cultures in organ donors: clinical impact in liver transplantation. Liver Transpl. 2006;12(8):1253–9.

167. Wu TJ, Lee CF, Chou HS, Yu MC, Lee WC. Suspect the donor with potential infection in the adult deceased donor liver transplantation. Transplant Proc. 2008;40(8):2486–8.

168. Ruiz I, Gavaldà J, Monforte V, Len O, Román A, Bravo C, Ferrer A, Tenorio L, Román F, Maestre J, Molina I, Morell F, Pahissa A. Donor-to-host transmission of bacterial and fungal infections in lung transplantation. Am J Transplant. 2006;6(1):178–82.

169. Mattner F, Kola A, Fischer S, Becker T, Haverich A, Simon A, Suerbaum S, Gastmeier P, Weissbrodt H, Strüber M. Impact of bacterial and fungal donor organ contamination in lung, heart-lung, heart and liver transplantation. Infection. 2008;36(3):207–12. Epub 2008 May 9.

170. Lopez-Navidad A, Domingo P, Caballero F, Gonzalez C, Santiago C. Successful transplantation of organs retrieved from donors with bacterial meningitis. Transplantation. 1997;64:365–8.

171. Natov SN, Pereira BJ. Transmission of viral hepatitis by kidney transplantation: donor evaluation and transplant policies (Part 1: hepatitis B virus). Transpl Infect Dis. 2002;4(3):117–23.

172. Huskey J, Wiseman AC. Chronic viral hepatitis in kidney transplantation. Nat Rev Nephrol. 2011;7(3):156–65. Epub 2011 Feb 1. Review.

173. Singh TP, Almond CS, Piercey G, Gauvreau K. Trends in wait-list mortality in children listed for heart transplantation in the United States: era effect across racial/ethnic groups. Am J Transplant. 2011;11(12):2692–9.

174. Dipchand A, Cecere R, Delgado D, Dore A, Giannetti N, Haddad H, Howlett J, Leblanc MH, Leduc L, Marelli A, Perron J, Poirier N, Ross H. Canadian Consensus on cardiac transplantation in pediatric and adult congenital heart disease patients 2004: executive summary. Can J Cardiol. 2005;21(13):1145–7.

175. West LJ, Karamlou T, Dipchand AI, Pollock-BarZiv SM, Coles JG, McCrindle BW. Impact on outcomes after listing and transplantation, of a strategy to accept ABO blood group-incompatible donor hearts for neonates and infants. J Thorac Cardiovasc Surg. 2006;131(2):455–61.

176. Forni A, Luciani GB, Chiominto B, Pizzuti M, Mazzucco A, Faggian G. Results with expanded donor acceptance criteria in heart transplantation. Transplant Proc. 2011;43(4):953–9.

177. Tjang YS, Stenlund H, Tenderich G, Hornik L, Körfer R. Pediatric heart transplantation: current clinical review. J Card Surg. 2008;23(1):87–91.

178. McGiffin DC, Savunen T, Kirklin JK, Naftel DC, Bourge RC, Paine TD, White-Williams C, Sisto T, Early L. A multivariable analysis of pretransplantation risk factors for disease development and morbid events. J Thorac Cardiovasc Surg. 1995;109:1081–9.

179. Hong KN, Iribarne A, Worku B, Takayama H, Gelijns AC, Naka Y, Jeevanandam V, Russo MJ. Who is the high-risk recipient? Predicting mortality after heart transplant using pretransplant donor and recipient risk factors. Ann Thorac Surg. 2011;92(2):520–7. Epub 2011 Jun 17.

180. Sweeney MS, Lammermeier DE, Frazier OH, Burnett CM, Haupt HM, Duncan JM. Extension of donor criteria in cardiac transplantation: surgical risk versus supply-side economics. Ann Thorac Surg. 1990;50:7–11.

181. Michaelides A, Koen W. Effect of donor selection on the early outcome of heart transplant recipients. Prog Transplant. 2005;15(1):24–6.

182. Matsumoto CS, Kaufman SS, Girlanda R, Little CM, Rekhtman Y, Raofi V, Laurin JM, Shetty K, Fennelly EM, Johnson LB, Fishbein TM. Utilization of donors who have suffered cardiopulmonary arrest and resuscitation in intestinal transplantation. Transplantation. 2008;86(7):941–6.

183. L'ecuyer T, Sloan K, Tang L. Impact of donor cardiopulmonary resuscitation on pediatric heart transplant outcome. Pediatr Transplant. 2011;15(7):742–5.

184. Zaroff JG, Solinger LL, Babcock WD. Temporal changes in donor left ventricular function: results of serial echocardiography. J Heart Lung Transplant. 2003;22(4):383–8.

185. Paul JJ, Tani LY, Shaddy RE, Minich LL. Spectrum of left ventricular dysfunction in potential pediatric heart transplant donors. J Heart Lung Transplant. 2003;22(5):548–52.

186. Sopko N, Shea KJ, Ludrosky K, Smedira N, Hoercher K, Taylor DO, Starling RC, Gonzalez-Stawinski GV. Survival is not compromised in donor hearts with echocardiographic abnormalities. J Surg Res. 2007;143(1):141–4.

187. Potapov E, Ivanitskaia E, Loebe M, Mumlckel M, Mumller C, Sodian R, Meyer R, Hetzer R. Value of cardiac troponin I and T for selection of heart donors and as predictors of early graft failure. Transplantation. 2001;71(10):1394–400.

188. Venkateswaran RV, Ganesh JS, Thekkudan J, Steeds R, Wilson IC, Mascaro J, Thompson R, Bonser RS. Donor cardiac troponin-I: a biochemical surrogate of heart function. Eur J Cardiothorac Surg. 2009;36(2):286–92. discussion 292. Epub 2009 Apr 25.

189. Boccheciampe N, Audibert G, Rangeard O, Charpentier C, Perrier JF, Lalot JM, Voltz C, Strub P, Loos-Ayav C, Meistelman C, Mertes PM, Longrois D. Serum troponin Ic values in organ donors are related to donor myocardial dysfunction but not to graft dysfunction or rejection in the recipients. Int J Cardiol. 2009;133(1):80–6. Epub 2008 Feb 5.

190. Stoica SC, Satchithananda DK, Charman S, Sharples L, King R, Rozario C, Dunning J, Tsui SS, Wallwork J, Large SR. Swan-Ganz catheter assessment of donor hearts: outcome of organs with borderline hemodynamics. J Heart Lung Transplant. 2002;21(6):615–22.

191. Solomon M, Grasemann H, Keshavjee S. Pediatric lung transplantation. Pediatr Clin North Am. 2010;57(2):375–91.

192. LaRosa C, Baluarte HJ, Meyers KE. Outcomes in pediatric solid-organ transplantation. Pediatr Transplant. 2011;15(2):128–41.

193. Zafar F, Heinle JS, Schecter MG, Rossano JW, Mallory Jr GB, Elidemir O, Morales DL. Two decades of pediatric lung transplant in the United States: have we improved? J Thorac Cardiovasc Surg. 2011;141(3):828–32.

194. Yusen RD, Shearon TH, Qian Y, Kotloff R, Barr ML, Sweet S, Dyke DB, Murray S. Lung transplantation in the United States, 1999-2008. Am J Transplant. 2010;10(4 Pt 2):1047–68.

195. Cypel M, Yeung JC, Keshavjee S. Novel approaches to expanding the lung donor pool: donation after cardiac death and ex vivo conditioning. Clin Chest Med. 2011;32(2):233–44.

196. Kotloff RM, Thabut G. Lung transplantation. Am J Respir Crit Care Med. 2011;184(2):159–71.

197. Sweet SC. Pediatric lung transplantation. Proc Am Thorac Soc. 2009;6(1):122–7.

198. Orens JB, Boehler A, de Perrot M, Estenne M, Glanville AR, Keshavjee S, Kotloff R, Morton J, Studer SM, Van Raemdonck D, Waddel T, Snell GI, Pulmonary Council, International Society for Heart and Lung Transplantation. A review of lung transplant donor acceptability criteria. J Heart Lung Transplant. 2003;22:1183–200.

199. Snell GI, Westall GP. Selection and management of the lung donor. Clin Chest Med. 2011;32(2):223–32. Epub 2011 Mar 22.

200. Van Raemdonck D, Neyrinck A, Verleden GM, Dupont L, Coosemans W, Decaluwé H, Decker G, De Leyn P, Nafteux P, Lerut T. Lung donor selection and management. Proc Am Thorac Soc. 2009;6(1):28–38.

201. Botha P. Extended donor criteria in lung transplantation. Curr Opin Organ Transplant. 2009;14(2):206–10.

202. Mangi AA, Mason DP, Nowicki ER, Batizy LH, Murthy SC, Pidwell DJ, Avery RK, McCurry KR, Pettersson GB, Blackstone EH. Predictors of acute rejection after lung transplantation. Ann Thorac Surg. 2011;91(6):1754–62. Epub 2011 May 4.

203. Naik PM, Angel LF. Special issues in the management and selection of the donor for lung transplantation. Semin Immunopathol. 2011;33(2):201–10.

204. Christie JD, Kotloff RM, Pochettino A, Arcasoy SM, Rosengard BR, Landis JR, Kimmel SE. Clinical risk factors for primary graft failure following lung transplantation. Chest. 2003;124(4):1232–41.

205. Christie JD, Bavaria JE, Palevski HI, Litzky L, Blumenthal NP, Kaiser LR, Kotloff RM. Primary graft failure following lung transplantation. Chest. 1998;114:51–60.

206. Thabut G, Vinatier I, Stern J-B, Leseche G, Loirat P, Fournier M, Mal H. Primary graft failure following lung transplantation. Predictive factors of mortality. Chest. 2002;121:1876–82.

207. Jahania MS, Mullett TW, Sanchez JA, Narayan P, Lasley RD, Mentzer RM. Acute allograft failure in thoracic organ transplantation. J Card Surg. 2000;15:122–8.

208. Aigner C, Winkler G, Jaksch P, Seebacher G, Lang G, Taghavi S, Wisser W, Klepetko W. Extended donor criteria for lung transplantation–a clinical reality. Eur J Cardiothorac Surg. 2005;27(5):757–61.

209. Moretti MP, Betto C, Gambacorta M, Vesconi S, Scalamogna M, Benazzi E, Ravini M. Lung procurement for transplantation: new criteria for lung donor selection. Transplant Proc. 2010;42(4):1053–5.

210. Davis RD, Pasque MK. Pulmonary transplantation. Ann Surg. 1995;221(1):14–28.

211. Sundaresan S, Semenkovich J, Ochoa L, Richardson G, Trulock EP, Cooper JD, Patterson GA. Successful outcome of lung transplantation is not compromised by the use of marginal donor lungs. J Thorac Cardiovasc Surg. 1995;109:1075–80.

212. Ware R, Fang X, Wang Y, Sakuma T, Hall TS, Matthay MA. Lung edema clearance: 20 years of progress selected contribution: mechanisms that may stimulate the resolution of alveolar edema in the transplanted human lung. J Appl Physiol. 2002;93:1869–74.

213. Labrousse L, Sztark F, Kays C, Thicoipe M, Lassie P, Couraud L, Marthan R. Improvement of brain-dead lung assessment based on the mechanical properties of the respiratory system. Transplant Proc. 1996;28(1):354.

214. Aziz T, El-Gamel A, Saad RAG, Migliore M, Campbell CS, Yonan NA. Pulmonary vein gas analysis for assessing donor lung function. Ann Thorac Surg. 2002;73:1559–605.

215. Puskas JD, Winton TL, Miller JD, Scavuzzo M, Patterson GA. Unilateral donor lung function does not preclude successful contralateral single lung transplantation. J Thorac Cardiovasc Surg. 1992;103:1015–7.

216. Wauters S, Verleden GM, Belmans A, Coosemans W, De Leyn P, Nafteux P, Lerut T, Van Raemdonck D. Donor cause of brain death and related time intervals: does it affect outcome after lung transplantation? Eur J Cardiothorac Surg. 2011;39(4):e68–76.

217. Hanna K, Seder CW, Weinberger JB, Sills PA, Hagan M, Janczyk RJ. Airway pressure release ventilation and successful lung donation. Arch Surg. 2011;146(3):325–8.

218. Taskar V, John J, Evander E, Wollmer P, Robertson B, Johnson B. Healthy lungs tolerate repetitive collapse and reopening during short periods of mechanical ventilation. Acta Anaesthesiol Scand. 1995;39:370–6.

219. Van Raemdonck DEM, Jannis NCP, De Leyn PRJ, Flameng WJ, Lerut TE. Alveolar expansion itself but not continuous oxygen supply enhances postmortem preservation of pulmonary grafts. Eur J Cardiothorac Surg. 1998;13:431–41.

220. Moran I, Zavala E, Fernandez R, Blanch L, Mancebo J. Recruitment manoeuvres in acute lung injury/acute respiratory distress syndrome. Eur Respir J Suppl. 2003;42:37s–42.

221. Gabbay E, Williams TJ, Griffiths AP, Macfarlane LM, Kotsimbos TC, Esmore DS, Snell GI. Maximizing the utilization of donor organs offered for lung transplantation. Am J Respir Crit Care Med. 1999;160:265–71.

222. Avlonitis VS, Wigfield CH, Golledge HD, Kirby JA, Dark JH. Early hemodynamic injury during donor brain death determines the severity of primary graft dysfunction after lung transplantation. Am J Transplant. 2007;7(1):83–90.

223. Rostron AJ, Avlonitis VS, Cork DM, Grenade DS, Kirby JA, Dark JH. Hemodynamic resuscitation with arginine vasopressin reduces lung injury after brain death in the transplant donor. Transplantation. 2008;85(4):597–606.

224. Dowling RD, Zenati M, Yousem SA, Pasculle AW, Kormos RL, Armitage JA, Griffith BP, Hardesty RL. Donor-transmitted pneumonia in experimental lung allogafts. Successful prevention with donor antibiotic therapy. J Thorac Cardiovasc Surg. 1992;103:767–72.

225. Low DE, Kaiser LR, Haydock DA, Trulock E, Cooper JD. The donor lung: infectious and pathologic factors affecting outcome in lung transplantation. J Thorac Cardiovasc Surg. 1995;109:1263–4.

226. Zenati M, Dowling RD, Dummer JS, Paradis IL, Arena VC, Armitage JM, Kormos RL, Hardesty RL, Griffith BP. Influence of the donor lung on development of early infections in lung transplant recipients. J Heart Transplant. 1990;9:502–9.

227. Avlonitis VS, Krause A, Luzzi L, Powell H, Phillips J, Corris PA, et al. Bacterial colonization of the donor lower airways is a predictor of poor outcome in lung transplantation. Eur J Cardiothorac Surg. 2003;24:601–7.

228. Waller DA, Thompson AM, Wrightson WN, Gould FK, Corris PA, Hilton CJ, Forty J, Dark JH. Does the mode of donor death influence the early outcome of lung transplantation? A review of lung transplantation from donors involved in major trauma. J Heart Lung Transplant. 1995;14(2):318–21.

229. Shafaghi S, Dezfuli AA, Makki SS, Marjani M, Mobarhan M, Ghandchi G, Khoddami-Vishteh HR, Ghorbani F, Najafizadeh K. Microbial pattern of bronchoalveolar lavage in brain dead donors. Transplant Proc. 2011;43(2):422–3.

230. Tiao GM, Alonso MH, Ryckman FC. Pediatric liver transplantation. Semin Pediatr Surg. 2006;15(3):218–27.

231. Hong JC, Yersiz H, Farmer DG, et al. Longterm outcomes for whole and segmental liver grafts in adult and pediatric liver transplant recipients: a ten year outcome comparative analysis of 2,988 cases. J Am Coll Surg. 2009;208(5):682–9.

232. Vagefi PA, Parekh J, Ascher NL, Roberts JP, Freise CE. Outcomes with split liver transplantation in 106 recipients: the University of California, San Francisco, experience from 1993 to 2010. Arch Surg. 2011;146(9):1052–9.

233. Feng S, Goodrich NP, Bragg-Gresham JL, Dykstra DM, Punch JD, DebRoy MA, Greenstein SM, Merion RM. Characteristics associated with liver graft failure: the concept of a donor risk index. Am J Transplant. 2006;6(4):783–90.

234. Bonney GK, Aldersley MA, Asthana S, Toogood GJ, Pollard SG, Lodge JP, Prasad KR. Donor risk index and MELD interactions in predicting long-term graft survival: a single-centre experience. Transplantation. 2009;87(12):1858–63.

235. Avolio AW, Cillo U, Salizzoni M, De Carlis L, Colledan M, Gerunda GE, Mazzaferro V, Tisone G, Romagnoli R, Caccamo L, Rossi M, Vitale A, Cucchetti A, Lupo L, Gruttadauria S, Nicolotti N, Burra P, Gasbarrini A, Agnes S, On behalf of the

Donor-to-Recipient Italian Liver Transplant (D2R-ILTx) Study Group. Balancing donor and recipient risk factors in liver transplantation: the value of D-MELD with particular reference to HCV recipients. Am J Transplant. 2011;11(12):2724–36.

236. Volk ML, Reichert HA, Lok AS, Hayward RA. Variation in organ quality between liver transplant centers. Am J Transplant. 2011;11(5):958–64.

237. Alexander JW, Vaughn WK, Carey MA. The use of marginal donors for organ transplantation: the older and younger donors. Transplant Proc. 1991;23:905–9.

238. Lee KW, Cameron AM, Maley WR, Segev DL, Montgomery RA. Factors affecting graft survival after adult/child split-liver transplantation: analysis of the UNOS/OPTN data base. Am J Transplant. 2008;8(6):1186–96.

239. Ploeg RJ, D'Alessandro AM, Knechtle SJ, Stegall MD, Pirsch JD, Hoffmann RM, Sasaki T, Sollinger HW, Belzer FO, Kalayoglu M. Risk factors for primary dysfunction after liver transplantation—a multivariate analysis. Transplantation. 1993;55:807–13.

240. Porte RJ, Ploeg RJ, Hansen B, van Bockel JH, Thorogood J, Persijn GG, Terpstra OT. Long-term graft survival after liver transplantation in the UW era: late effects of cold ischemia and primary dysfunction. European Multicentre Study Group. Transpl Int. 1998;11 Suppl 1:S164–7.

241. Brokelman W, Stel AL, Ploeg RJ. Risk factors for primary dysfunction after liver transplantation in the University of Wisconsin solution era. Transplant Proc. 1999;31:2087–90.

242. Alper I, Ulukaya S. Anesthetic management in pediatric liver transplantation: a comparison of deceased or live donor liver transplantations. J Anesth. 2010;24(3):399–406.

243. Zhang SJ, Wang T. The influence of brain death on donor liver and the potential mechanisms of protective intervention. Front Med. 2011;5(1):8–14.

244. Nafidi O, Marleau D, Roy A, Bilodeau M. Identification of new donor variables associated with graft survival in a single-center liver transplant cohort. Liver Transpl. 2010;16(12):1393–9.

245. Clavien PA, Harvey PR, Strasberg SM. Preservation and reperfusion injuries in liver allografts. An overview and synthesis of current studies. Transplantation. 1992;53:957–78.

246. Busuttil RW, Tanaka K. The utility of marginal donors in liver transplantation. Liver Transpl. 2003;9:651–63.

247. Strasberg SM, Howard TK, Molmenti EP, Hertl M. Selecting the donor liver: risk factors for poor function after orthotopic liver transplantation. Hepatology. 1994;20:829–38.

248. Port FK, Bragg-Gresham JL, Metzger RA, Dykstra DM, Gillespie BW, Young EW, Delmonico FL, Wynn JJ, Merion RM, Wolfe RA, Held PJ. Donor characteristics associated with reduced graft survival: an approach to expanding the pool of kidney donors. Transplantation. 2002;74:1281–6.

249. Wigmore SJ, Seeney FM, Pleass HC, Praseedom RK, Forsythe JL. Kidney damage during organ retrieval: data from UK National Transplant Database. Kidney Advisory Group. Lancet. 1999; 354:1143–6.

250. Moudgil A, Martz K, Stablein DM, Puliyanda DP. Good outcome of kidney transplants in recipients of young donors: a NAPRTCS data analysis. Pediatr Transplant. 2011;15(2):167–71.

251. Sharma A, Fisher RA, Cotterell AH, King AL, Maluf DG, Posner MP. En bloc kidney transplantation from pediatric donors: comparable outcomes with living donor kidney transplantation. Transplantation. 2011;92(5):564–9.

252. Kim JM, Kim SJ, Joh JW, Kwon CH, Song S, Shin M, Kim BN, Lee SK. Is it safe to use a kidney from an expanded criteria donor? Transplant Proc. 2011;43(6):2359–62.

253. Merion RM, Ashby VB, Wolfe RA, Distant DA, Hulbert-Shearon TE, Metzger RA, Ojo AO, Port FK. Deceased-donor characteristics and the survival benefit of kidney transplantation. JAMA. 2005;294(21):2726–33.

254. Pascual J, Zamora J, Pirsch JD. A systematic review of kidney transplantation from expanded criteria donors. Am J Kidney Dis. 2008;52(3):553–86. Review.

255. Schwartz GJ, Brion LP, Spitzer A. The use of plasma creatinine concentration for estimating glomerular filtration rate in infants, children, and adolescents. Pediatr Clin North Am. 1987;34(3):571–90.

256. Lee S, Shin M, Kim E, Kim J, Moon J, Jung G, Choi G, Kwon C, Joh J, Lee S, Kim S. Donor characteristics associated with reduced survival of transplanted kidney grafts in Korea. Transplant Proc. 2010;42(3):778–81.

257. Birck R, Krzossok S, Markowetz F, Schnulle P, van der Woude FJ, Braun C. Acetylcysteine for prevention of contrast nephropathy: meta-analysis. Lancet. 2003;362:598–603.

258. Melk A, Gourishankar S, Halloran P. Long-term effects of nonimmune tissue injury in renal transplantation. Curr Opin Organ Transplant. 2002;7:171–7.

259. Marconi L, Moreira P, Parada B, Bastos C, Roseiro A, Mota A. Donor cause of brain death in renal transplantation: a predictive factor for graft function? Transplant Proc. 2011;43(1):74–6.

260. Morariu AM, Schuurs TA, Leuvenink HG, van Oeveren W, Rakhorst G, Ploeg RJ. Early events in kidney donation: progression of endothelial activation, oxidative stress and tubular injury after brain death. Am J Transplant. 2008;8(5):933–41.

261. Westendorp WH, Leuvenink HG, Ploeg RJ. Brain death induced renal injury. Curr Opin Organ Transplant. 2011;16(2):151–6.

262. Sánchez-Fructuoso A, Naranjo Garcia P, Calvo Romero N, Ridao N, Naranjo Gómez P, Conesa J, Barrientos A. Effect of the brain-death process on acute rejection in renal transplantation. Transplant Proc. 2007;39(7):2214–6.

263. de Vries DK, Lindeman JH, Ringers J, Reinders ME, Rabelink TJ, Schaapherder AF. Donor brain death predisposes human kidney grafts to a proinflammatory reaction after transplantation. Am J Transplant. 2011;11(5):1064–70.

264. Nijboer WN, Ottens PJ, van Dijk A, van Goor H, Ploeg RJ, Leuvenink HG. Donor pretreatment with carbamylated erythropoietin in a brain death model reduces inflammation more effectively than erythropoietin while preserving renal function. Crit Care Med. 2010;38(4):1155–61.

265. Damman J, Hoeger S, Boneschansker L, Theruvath A, Waldherr R, Leuvenink HG, Ploeg RJ, Yard BA, Seelen MA. Targeting complement activation in brain-dead donors improves renal function after transplantation. Transpl Immunol. 2011;24(4):233–7. Epub 2011 Apr 1.

266. Jung GO, Yoon MR, Kim SJ, Sin MJ, Kim EY, Moon JI, Kim JM, Choi GS, Kwon CH, Cho JW, Lee SK. The risk factors of delayed graft function and comparison of clinical outcomes after deceased donor kidney transplantation: single-center study. Transplant Proc. 2010;42(3):705–9.

267. Troppmann C, Gillingham KJ, Benedetti E, Almond S, Gruessner RWG, Najarian JS, Matas AJ. Delayed graft function, acute rejection, and outcome after cadaver renal transplantation. Transplantation. 1995;59(7):962–8.

268. Walaszewski J, Rowinski W, Pacholczyk M, Lagiewska B, Cajzner S, Chmura A, et al. Multiple risk factor analysis of delayed graft function (ATN) after cadaveric transplantation: positive effect of lidocaine donor pretreatment. Transplant Proc. 1991;23:2475–6.

269. Schnuelle P, Lorenz D, Mueller A, Trede M, Van Der Woude FJ. Donor catecholamine use reduces acute allograft rejection and improves graft survival after cadaveric renal transplantation. Kidney Int. 1999;56:738–46.

270. Domínguez J, Lira F, Troncoso P, Aravena C, Ortiz M, Gonzalez R. Factors that predict duration of delayed graft function in cadaveric kidney transplantation. Transplant Proc. 2009;41(6):2668–9.

271. Schnuelle P, Gottmann U, Hoeger S, Boesebeck D, Lauchart W, Weiss C, Fischereder M, Jauch KW, Heemann U, Zeier M,

Hugo C, Pisarski P, Krämer BK, Lopau K, Rahmel A, Benck U, Birck R, Yard BA. Effects of donor pretreatment with dopamine on graft function after kidney transplantation: a randomized controlled trial. JAMA. 2009;302(10):1067–75.

272. Singh RP, Farney AC, Rogers J, Gautreaux M, Reeves-Daniel A, Hartmann E, Doares W, Iskandar S, Adams P, Stratta RJ. Hypertension in standard criteria deceased donors is associated with inferior outcomes following kidney transplantation. Clin Transplant. 2011;25(4):E437–46.

273. Kunzendorf U, Hohenstein B, Oberbarnscheid M, Muller E, Renders L, Schott GE, Offermann G. Duration of donor brain death and its influence on kidney graft function. Am J Transplant. 2002;2:282–94.

274. Nijboer WN, Moers C, Leuvenink HG, Ploeg RJ. How important is the duration of the brain death period for the outcome in kidney transplantation? Transpl Int. 2011;24(1):14–20.

275. Opelz G. Cadaver kidney graft outcome in relation to ischemia time and HLA match. Collaborative Transplant Study. Transplant Proc. 1998;30:4294–6.

276. Wight JP, Chilcott JB, Holmes MW, Brewer N. Pulsatile machine perfusion vs. cold storage of kidneys for transplantation: a rapid and systemic review. Clin Transplant. 2003;17:293–307.

277. Ojo AO, Hanson JA, Meier-Kriesche H, Okechukwu CN, Wolfe RA, Leichtman AB, Agodoa LY, Kaplan B, Port FK. Survival in recipients of marginal cadaveric donor kidneys compared with other recipients and wait-listed transplant candidates. J Am Soc Nephrol. 2001;12:589–97.

278. Berg CL, Steffick DE, Edwards EB, Heimbach JK, Magee JC, Washburn WK, Mazariegos GV. Liver and intestine transplantation in the United States 1998-2007. Am J Transplant. 2009; 9(4 Pt 2):907–31.

279. Kaufman SS, Atkinson JB, Bianchi A, Goulet OJ, Grant D, Langnas AN, McDiarmid SV, Mittal N, Reyes J, Tzakis AG, American Society of Transplantation. Indications for pediatric intestinal transplantation: a position paper of the American Society of Transplantation. Pediatr Transplant. 2001;5(2):80–7.

280. Gupte GL, Beath SV, Protheroe S, Murphy MS, Davies P, Sharif K, McKiernan PJ, de Ville de Goyet J, Booth IW, Kelly DA. Improved outcome of referrals for intestinal transplantation in the UK. Arch Dis Child. 2007;92(2):147–52.

281. Goulet O, Sauvat F. Short bowel syndrome and intestinal transplantation in children. Curr Opin Clin Nutr Metab Care. 2006;9(3):304–13.

282. Sudan D. Long-term outcomes and quality of life after intestine transplantation. Curr Opin Organ Transplant. 2010;15(3):357–60.

283. Arnow PM, Carandang GC, Zabner R, Irwin ME. Randomized controlled trial of selective bowel decontamination for prevention of infections following liver transplantation. Clin Infect Dis. 1996;22(6):997–1003.

284. Safdar N, Said A, Lucey MR. The role of selective digestive decontamination for reducing infection in patients undergoing liver transplantation: a systematic review and meta-analysis. Liver Transpl. 2004;10(7):817–27.

285. Hellinger WC, Yao JD, Alvarez S, Blair JE, Cawley JJ, Paya CV, O'Brien PC, Spivey JR, Dickson RC, Harnois DM, Douglas DD, Hughes CB, Nguyen JH, Mulligan DC, Steers JL. A randomized, prospective, double-blinded evaluation of selective bowel decontamination in liver transplantation. Transplantation. 2002;73(12):1904–9.

286. Arbour R. Clinical management of the organ donor. AACN Clin Issues. 2005;16(4):551–80.

287. Kong AP, Barrios C, Salim A, Willis L, Cinat ME, Dolich MO, Lekawa ME, Malinoski DJ. A multidisciplinary organ donor council and performance improvement initiative can improve donation outcomes. Am Surg. 2010;76(10):1059–62.

288. Salim A, Martin M, Brown C, Rhee P, Demetriades D, Belzberg H. The effect of a protocol of aggressive donor management: implications for the national organ donor shortage. J Trauma. 2006;61(2):429–33.

289. DuBose J, Salim A. Aggressive organ donor management protocol. J Intensive Care Med. 2008;23(6):367–75.

290. Kirschbaum CE, Hudson S. Increasing organ yield through a lung management protocol. Prog Transplant. 2010;20(1):28–32.

291. Bardell T, Hunter DJ, Kent WD, Jain MK. Do medical students have the knowledge needed to maximize organ donation rates? Can J Surg. 2003;46(6):453–7.

292. Cohen J, Ami SB, Ashkenazi T, Singer P. Attitude of health care professionals to brain death: influence on the organ donation process. Clin Transplant. 2008;22(2):211–5.

293. Bener A, El-Shoubaki H, Al-Maslamani Y. Do we need to maximize the knowledge and attitude level of physicians and nurses toward organ donation and transplant? Exp Clin Transplant. 2008;6(4):249–53.

294. Hobeika MJ, Simon R, Malik R, Pachter HL, Frangos S, Bholat O, Teperman S, Teperman L. U.S. surgeon and medical student attitudes toward organ donation. J Trauma. 2009;67(2):372–5.

295. Griffiths J, Verble M, Falvey S, Bell S, Logan L, Morgan K, Wellington F. Culture change initiatives in the procurement of organs in the United Kingdom. Transplant Proc. 2009; 41(5):1459–62.

296. Committee on Hospital Care, Section on Surgery, and Section on Critical Care. Policy statement- -pediatric organ donation and transplantation. Pediatrics. 2010;125(4):822–8.

297. Hornby K, Ross H, Keshavjee S, Rao V, Shemie SD. Factors contributing to non-utilization of heart and lungs after consent for donation: a Canadian multicentre study. Can J Anaesth. in press, 2006.

298. Scheinkestel CD, Tuxen DV, Cooper DJ, Butt W. Medical management of the (potential) organ donor. Anaesth Intensive Care. 1995;23(1):51–9.

299. U.S. Department of Health & Human Services. Organ procurement and transplantation network. Donors : donation year (2009–2010) by donor type, age type, organ. Based on OPTN data as of October 7, 2011. http://optn.transplant.hrsa.gov. Accessed 10 Aug 2012.

Part IV

Monitoring the Critically Ill or Injured Child

Shane M. Tibby

Derek S. Wheeler and Peter C. Rimensberger

Abstract

Vital functions such as respiration have to be continuously monitored in a critically ill or injured child. The two main components of respiratory function that can be monitored at the bedside are gas exchange and mechanical behavior of the respiratory system. The goals of respiratory monitoring are twofold. First, respiratory monitoring should help the clinician to be able to recognize acute respiratory failure and to quantify its severity and progression. Second, respiratory monitoring should provide the necessary therapeutic endpoints for management of acute respiratory failure and lung disease in the pediatric intensive care unit (PICU). This chapter will review the various techniques available for respiratory monitoring and discuss how multimodal respiratory monitoring might help to improve ventilator settings during non-invasive or invasive mechanical ventilation.

Keywords

Respiratory failure • Respiratory monitoring • Respiratory mechanics • End-tidal CO_2 • Capnography • Respiratory graphics

Introduction

The lungs are highly unique in that they are internal organs, yet at the same time they are constantly exposed to the external environment. For example, with each breath, the lungs are exposed to pollens, viruses, bacteria, smoke and other pollutants, and all of the other substances in the environment. At the same time, at any one point in time the lungs receive approximately half of the cardiac output and all of the potential internal toxins (proinflammatory cytokines, drugs, etc). As such, there is a vast array of diseases that affect the human respiratory tract. Dr. George A. Gregory, one of the founding fathers of pediatric critical care medicine, once stated that acute respiratory failure accounts for approximately 50 % of all admissions to the pediatric intensive care unit (PICU) [1]. More recent studies continue to support Dr. Gregory's claim – acute respiratory failure and the need for respiratory support remains one of the most common reasons children are admitted to the PICU [2–5]. In this context, monitoring the function of the respiratory system assumes critical importance. The two main components of respiratory function that can be monitored at the bedside are gas exchange and mechanical behavior of the respiratory system. The goals of respiratory monitoring are twofold. First, respiratory monitoring should help the clinician to be able to recognize acute respiratory failure and to quantify its severity and progression. Second, respiratory monitoring should provide the necessary therapeutic endpoints for management of acute respiratory failure and lung disease in the PICU. This chapter will review the various techniques available for respiratory monitoring and discuss how multimodal respiratory

D.S. Wheeler, MD, MMM (✉)
Division of Critical Care Medicine, Cincinnati Children's Hospital Medical Center, University of Cincinnati College of Medicine, 3333 Burnet Avenue, Cincinnati, OH 45229-3039, USA
e-mail: derek.wheeler@cchmc.org

P.C. Rimensberger, MD
Department of Pediatrics, Service of Neonatology and Pediatric Intensive Care, University Hospital of Geneva, 6, Rue Willy-Donzé, Geneva CH-1211, Switzerland
e-mail: peter.rimensberger@hcuge.ch

monitoring might help to improve ventilator settings during non-invasive or invasive mechanical ventilation. Importantly, in the interest of space limitations, we will not discuss physical examination of the respiratory system and imaging techniques (i.e. chest radiograph, ultrasound, CT, etc.). Even with all of the dramatic advances in technology pertaining to monitoring of the respiratory system, the physical examination continues to remain a vital aspect of the evaluation and management of the critically ill and/or injured child. The importance of the physical examination can't be overemphasized. Indeed, tachypnea, nasal flaring, retractions, and accessory muscle use are the earliest and usually most sensitive signs of impending respiratory failure in the PICU.

Monitoring Gas Exchange

Gas exchange consists of two mutually independent processes – oxygenation and ventilation (i.e. CO_2 elimination). Hypoxemia is generally defined as a PaO_2 ≤60 mmHg and most often occurs due to ventilation-perfusion mismatching, the presence of either fixed or physiologic shunts, global hypoventilation, impairment of diffusion, and low ambient oxygen (as would occur at altitude with a lower than normal PAO_2 due to a low atmospheric pressure, or lowered FIO_2, as in the setting of manipulating pulmonary vascular resistance and Qp/Qs ratio in critically ill infants with single ventricle physiology). Conversely, hypercarbia (an elevated $PaCO_2$) is usually due to low alveolar minute ventilation (recall that $PaCO_2$ is inversely proportional to minute ventilation).

Monitoring Oxygenation

Arterial Blood Gas Monitoring

There are multiple methods for monitoring the systemic arterial oxygen saturation (SaO_2). Invasive methods include arterial blood gas (ABG) monitoring, while the most common non-invasive method is pulse oximetry. The primary purpose of monitoring SaO_2 is to assure adequate oxygen delivery. Importantly, oxygen delivery is dependent upon cardiac output (CO) (L/min) and arterial oxygen content (CaO_2) (mL/dL). CaO_2 in turn is dependent upon the hemoglobin concentration (Hb, mg/dL), SaO_2, and PaO_2 (mm Hg), which comprises a very small proportion of the total arterial oxygen content.

$$DO_2 = CO \times CaO_2 = CO \times \left[\begin{array}{c} (1.34 \times Hb \times SaO_2) \\ + (0.003 \times PaO_2) \end{array} \right] \quad (39.1)$$

The Hb and PaO_2 can be easily measured in the clinical laboratory or with a point-of-care (POC) test, while the oxygen saturation can be obtained via pulse oximetry (see below). The measurement of cardiac output is more difficult,

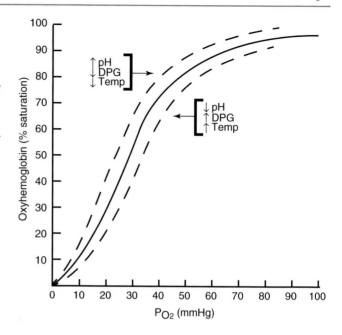

Fig. 39.1 Oxygen-hemoglobin dissociation curve

though there are now several non-invasive methods of monitoring cardiac output in critically ill children currently used in the PICU setting (please see Chap. 40).

While the partial pressure of oxygen dissolved in plasma (PaO_2) is only a small part of the total arterial oxygen content, the relationship between PaO_2 and the amount of oxygen bound to hemoglobin (Hb) is described by the sigmoid shaped oxyhemoglobin dissociation curve. The most important factors that influence the shape and position of the dissociation curve are temperature, pH, 2,3 diphosphoglycerate (2,3-DPG) levels in the blood, and the type of hemoglobin (Fig. 39.1). There are a couple of rules of thumb – first, assuming normal physiologic conditions, the oxygen saturation at a PaO_2 of 50 mmHg should be around 80 %, while the oxygen saturation at a PaO_2 of 60 mmHg should be around 90 %. The P50 is defined as the PaO_2 at which the hemoglobin is 50 % saturated (which is approximately 25 mmHg in most cases). A rightward shift of the oxyhemoglobin dissociation curve implies an increase in the P50 and is due to a lower affinity of hemoglobin for oxygen (oxygen is released to the tissues). Conversely, a leftward shift of the oxyhemoglobin dissociation curve implies a decrease in the P50 and is due to a higher affinity of hemoglobin for oxygen (oxygen is more tightly bound). The factors that affect the standard oxyhemoglobin dissociation curve are listed in Table 39.1 and shown in Fig. 39.1. Factors that shift the curve to the right are theoretically advantageous to the patient since this means that more oxygen can be released from hemoglobin to the tissues (i.e. reduced affinity of oxygen for hemoglobin). Inversely, factors that shift the curve to the left (e.g. in the case of anemia) will be less advantageous for oxygen delivery to the tissue.

Table 39.1 Factors that affect the standard oxyhemoglobin dissociation curve

	Left shift (↓P50, high affinity for O_2)	Right shift (↑P50, low affinity for O_2)
Temperature	Decrease	Increase
2, 3-DPG	Decrease	Increase
CO_2	Decrease	Increase
pH (Bohr effect)	Increase (alkalosis)	Decrease (acidosis)
Type of Hb	Fetal hemoglobin	Adult hemoglobin

Given that dissolved oxygen comprises such a small (and insignificant) portion of the total arterial oxygen content, one could certainly question the utility of measuring PaO_2 in the clinical setting. The information provided by an isolated PaO_2 measurement is not very helpful. Knowing where on the oxyhemoglobin dissociation curve an individual patient's oxygenation status is at a particular moment in time could potentially be of use – for example, if the patient is on the steep portion of the oxyhemoglobin dissociation curve, small changes in PaO_2 will be associated with large changes in oxygen saturation. For similar reasons, if avoiding toxic levels of oxygen is the concern, PaO_2 is much better than the oxygen saturation. On the flat portion of the oxyhemoglobin dissociation curve, oxygen saturation remains at or near 100 % despite marked changes in PaO_2. Regardless, a single measurement of PaO_2 only provides information at a specific point in time – serial PaO_2 measurements would be of significantly greater utility.

There are several clinically relevant measures of oxygenation that require knowledge of the PaO_2 (Table 39.2). The 'gold standard' for assessing oxygenation is the venous admixture, or shunt fraction (Qs/Qt), which quantifies the extent of venous blood that bypasses oxygenation in the pulmonary capillaries.

$$Qs/Qt = \left(CcO_2 - CaO_2 \right) / \left(CcO_2 - CvO_2 \right) \quad (39.2)$$

where Qs/Qt is the intra-pulmonary shunt fraction, CcO_2 is the capillary oxygen content, CaO_2 is the arterial oxygen content, and CvO_2 is the mixed venous oxygen content (Fig. 39.2). The derivation of the shunt fraction is an important concept that is provided in the Table 39.3.

$$CcO_2 = \left(Hb \times 1.34 \times 1.0 \right) + \left(0.003 \times PaO_2 \right) \quad (39.3)$$

$$CvO_2 = \left(Hb \times 1.34 \times SvO_2 \right) + \left(0.003 \times PvO_2 \right) \quad (39.4)$$

Under normal conditions, approximately 2–5 % of the cardiac output bypasses the pulmonary capillaries (includes venous blood from the bronchial veins, the thebesian veins, and the pleural veins – this is the normal anatomic shunt, often called the physiologic shunt). Note that calculation of the shunt fraction requires invasive hemodynamic monitoring, e.g. Swan-Ganz or

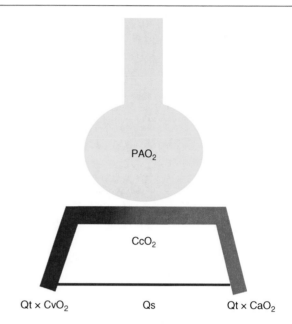

Fig. 39.2 Single compartment model of the lung and pulmonary circulation. PAO_2 is the partial pressure of oxygen in the alveolus. Qt is the total cardiac output, while Qs is that portion of the cardiac output that passes through the pulmonary circulation without becoming oxygenated. CcO_2, CvO_2, and CaO_2 refer to the oxygen content of the pulmonary capillaries (fully saturated blood with oxygen saturation of 100 %), mixed venous blood, and arterial blood. The model is useful for deriving the Qs/Qt shunt equation (venous admixture)

Pulmonary Artery (PA) catheter. The shunt fraction can be estimated using the ISO shunt diagram (Fig. 39.3), which assumes normal ranges of Hb, $PaCO_2$, and cardiac output. However, the shunt fraction most accurately reflects intrapulmonary shunt when the patient is breathing 100 % oxygen. When the FIO_2 is less than 1.0, the shunt fraction will include true shunt (venous blood completely bypasses the pulmonary capillaries, i.e. V/Q is zero), as well as areas of low V/Q and diffusion impairment [7]. In essence, this is the basis for the oxygen challenge test for neonates with suspected cyanotic congenital heart disease (increasing the FIO_2 to 1.0 should increase PaO_2 in patients with lung disease, but not anatomic shunts). Therefore, as shown in multiple studies and computer models, there is a lot of variation in the shunt fraction in critically ill patients with lung disease (especially when the FIO_2 is <1.0) [8–11]. This particular limitation and the need for invasive hemodynamic monitoring make the shunt fraction relatively impractical for assessing oxygenation status in the PICU setting.

There are several so-called tension-based measures of oxygenation (i.e., measures based on the partial pressure of oxygen in either the alveolus or the arterial blood) [7]. The major advantage of these measures is that they do not require a PA catheter. For example, the $P(A-a)O_2$ gradient reflects the ability of the lungs to transfer oxygen from the inspired air to the alveolar capillaries. The normal $P(A-a)O_2$ gradient is about 5 mmHg and generally increases with age:

Table 39.2 Clinically useful measures of oxygenation status

Measure	Normal values	Formula
PaO_2	80–100 mmHg	–
PAO_2	100–673 mmHg (FIO_2 0.21–1.0)	$^a FIO_2\left(P_{atm} - P_{H_2O}\right) - PaCO_2/RQ$
PaO_2/FIO_2 ratio	380–475	PaO_2/FIO_2
PaO_2/PAO_2	0.8–1.0	PaO_2/PAO_2
Oxygenation index (OI)	<5	$(MAP \times FIO_2)/PaO_2$
A-a gradient	5–10 mmHg (FIO_2 0.21)	$PAO_2 - PaO_2$
	30–60 mmHg (FIO_2 1.0)	
Respiratory index		$(PAO_2 - PaO_2)/PaO_2$
Arterial oxygen content (CaO_2)	20 vol%	$[SaO_2 \times Hb \times 1.34] + 0.003 \times PaO_2$
Mixed venous O_2 content (CvO_2)	15 vol%	
Shunt fraction (Qs/Qt)	2–5 %	$\dfrac{\left(CcO_2 - CaO_2\right)}{\left(CcO_2 - CvO_2\right)}$

^{a}Note: The actual Alveolar Gas Equation [6] states that $PAO_2 = FIO_2\left(P_{atm} - P_{H_2O}\right) - \dfrac{\left(PaCO_2\left(1 - FIO_2\left[1 - RQ\right]\right)\right)}{RQ}$

where $P_{atm} = 760$ mmHg at sea level, $P_{H_2O} = 47$ mmHg at 37 °C, and RQ (respiratory quotient, VCO_2/VO_2) = 0.8 on a mixed carbohydrate-protein-fat diet. However, if FIO_2 is small (≤ 0.6), then $FIO_2[1-RQ] \approx 0$, so the alveolar-gas equation can be further simplified to
$PAO_2 = FIO_2\left(P_{atm} - P_{H_2O}\right) - PaCO_2/RQ$

Table 39.3 Derivation of the shunt equation

The major assumption of the shunt equation is that all there are only two types of alveolar-capillary units – those with well-matched ventilation and perfusion and those with a ventilation/perfusion ratio of zero. The shunt equation combines anatomic shunt, physiologic shunt, and shunt-like regions of the lung (extremely low V/Q ratios) into one group

1. The blood entering the lungs will have an "oxygen flux" determined by the mixed venous oxygen content (CvO_2) multiplied by the cardiac output (Qt)
2. The blood leaving the lungs will have an "oxygen flux" given by the arterial oxygen content (CaO_2) multiplied by the cardiac output (Qt)
3. The total cardiac output consists of that portion that bypasses the lungs (Qs) and that portion which flowed through the pulmonary capillaries to become oxygenated (Qc): $Qt = Qs + Qc$
4. The above equation can be solved for Qc by re-arranging: $Qc = Qt - Qs$
5. Using the above two equations, the overall "oxygen flux" in the system can then be derived:
$\left(Qt \times CaO_2\right) = \left(Qs \times CvO_2\right) + \left[\left(Qt - Qs\right) \times CcO_2\right]$
6. Now we multiply out the brackets: $Qt \times CaO_2 = Qs \times CvO_2 + Qt \times CcO_2 - Qs \times CcO_2$
7. Now we re-arrange to get the Qs and Qt terms on the same side of the equation: $Qs \times CcO_2 - Qs \times CvO_2 = Qt \times CcO_2 - Qt \times CaO_2$
8. Factor out the Q terms: $Qs\left(CcO_2 - CvO_2\right) = Qt\left(CcO_2 - CaO_2\right)$
9. Now solve for Qs/Qt by dividing by Qt and ($CcO_2 - CvO_2$): $Qs/Qt = \left(CcO_2 - CaO_2\right)/\left(CcO_2 - CvO_2\right)$

$$P\left(A-a\right)O_2 \text{ gradient} = \left(Age/4\right) + 4 \qquad (39.5)$$

Changes in lung function (e.g., V/Q mismatch, shunt, diffusion defects) will cause the PaO_2 to decrease in relation to the PAO_2, resulting in an increase in the $P(A-a)O_2$ gradient. However, this measure is somewhat dependent upon the FIO_2 and is therefore not very accurate when the FIO_2 is high (as would be the case in a critically ill patient with acute lung injury or ARDS) [7, 10, 12]. The respiratory index (ratio of $P(A-a)O_2$ to PaO_2) was proposed to address this particular

issue. The ratio of PaO_2 to PAO_2 has also been proposed as a measure of oxygenation. Unfortunately, both the respiratory index and the ratio of PaO_2 to PAO_2 are subject to the same limitations as the other tension-based measures (poor validity and accuracy at low V/Q ratio and/or high FIO_2) [7, 10, 13–15]. The PaO_2/FIO_2 ratio, which may be calculated without the cumbersome PAO_2 formula, is still used in the definition of acute lung injury (ALI) and acute respiratory distress syndrome (ARDS). With the new Berlin criteria for ALI/ARDS, a P/F ratio <300 is used in the definition of ALI, while a P/F

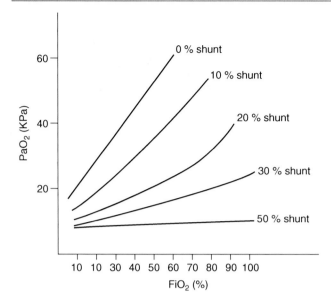

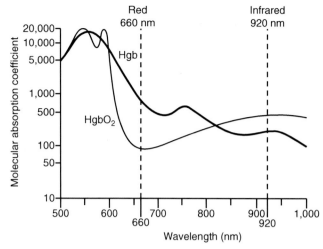

Fig. 39.4 Absorption spectra for O₂Hb and HHb. See text for details

Fig. 39.3 ISO shunt diagram. Note that as the venous admixture (% shunt fraction) increases, increasing the FIO₂ has less of an effect on PaO₂. Under these conditions, reducing the shunt fraction is the key to improving gas exchange

ratio <200 is used in the definition of ARDS [16–18]. The main criticism of the P/F ratio is that it does not take into account the "effort" (i.e. the degree of ventilatory requirements and FIO₂) required to generate a certain PaO₂. Hence, the oxygenation index (OI) has become commonly used in the critical care setting. An OI >40 was historically used (and still is in many centers) as a threshold criteria for initiating extracorporeal membrane oxygenation (ECMO) [19]. Both the OI [19–22] and P/F ratio [21–23] appear to correlate with outcome in critically ill children with acute respiratory failure. One important thing to bear in mind is that obtaining PaO₂ measurements (especially serial measurements) will require arterial access, with all its attendant risks (infection, bleeding, nerve damage, etc.). Notably, the risk of catheter-related infection appears to be as high in arterial catheters as it is with central venous catheters [24, 25].

Pulse Oximetry

Importantly, many (if not all) blood gas instruments do not actually measure oxygen saturation (SaO₂), but instead calculate (or estimate) the SaO₂ based on assumptions about the shape of the oxyhemoglobin dissociation curve. Unfortunately, calculated oxygen saturation levels are usually unreliable (as there are several conditions that are common in the PICU that impact the normal oxyhemoglobin dissociation curve), particularly in the case when true oxygen saturation levels are <90 % [26]. As such, continuous measurement of oxygen saturation by pulse oximetry (SpO₂) has become an essential first-line monitoring tool in the PICU. SpO₂ has even been called the "fifth vital sign"

[27, 28]. Interestingly, in the early days of this technology, pulse oximetry was subjected to a randomized, controlled clinical trial involving over 20,000 adult surgical patients. While pulse oximetry significantly improved the early detection of hypoxemia in the operating room and post-anesthesia recovery unit (PACU), there was not an overall reduction in the rate of postoperative complications [29]. More recently, a prospective observational trial showed that continuous pulse oximetry on a postsurgical ward did not reduce the need for ICU transfer or hospital mortality [30]. There have been no clinical trials on the effects of pulse oximetry on outcome in the PICU population [31] – there will probably never be such a trial! Pulse oximetry has essentially become the standard of care in most ICUs in the developed world, virtually with no evidence basis aside from anecdote and decades of experience [32]. However, the utility of this technology and the impact that it has had on the management of critically ill children in the PICU is without question.

Unfortunately, despite its widespread use, many health care providers do not fully understand the principles behind pulse oximetry or appreciate the limitations of this technology [33–37]. Pulse oximetry is based upon the principles of spectral analysis (i.e., the quantification of different components in a solution by their unique light absorption characteristics) [38]. Two principles are important for understanding how pulse oximetry works in the clinical setting. First, Beer's Law states that the intensity of transmitted light decreases exponentially as the concentration of the substance increases. Second, Lambert's Law states that the intensity of transmitted light decreases exponentially as the distance through which the substance travels increases. The pulse oximeter probe is composed of two light emitting diodes and a photodetector. The diodes emit light at two different wavelengths – 660 nm (red) and 940 nm (infrared). Oxyhemoglobin (O₂Hb) and deoxyhemoglobin (HHb) absorb light differently at these two wavelengths (Fig. 39.4). O₂Hb absorbs greater

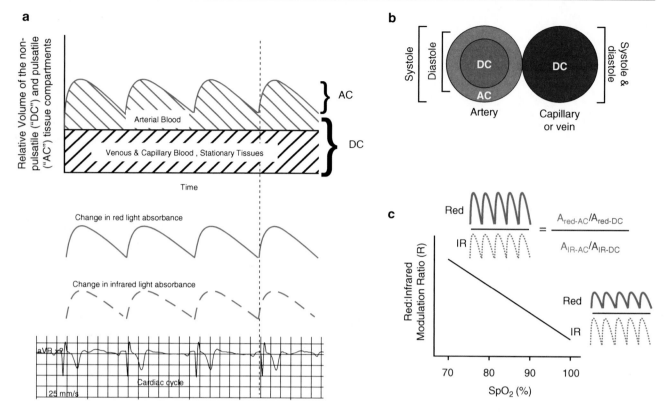

Fig. 39.5 Schematic diagram of light absorbance by a pulse oximeter. (**a**) In a patient with normal cardiac function, the onset of systole (as denoted by the onset of the QRS complex on the ECG tracing) results in an increase in the arterial blood volume. The relative amounts of red and near-infrared light that is absorbed in the arterial compartment also fluctuates with the cardiac cycle. The increase in arterial blood volume during systole is often referred to as "Alternating Current" or AC, while the fixed component of the volume of blood in the veins, capillaries, and tissues is often referred to as the "Direct Current" or DC. (**b**) Cross-sectional diagram of an artery and vein showing the relative increase and decrease in arterial blood volume during systole and diastole, respectively. Note that the volume in the vein remains fixed and does not fluctuate. (**c**) A calibration curve of the Red:IR Modulation Ratio ("R") in relation to the SpO_2 is shown. Increased R corresponds to increased absorption of red light, which is associated with increased HHb (i.e. lower SpO_2). Conversely, decreased R corresponds to increased absorption of near-infrared light, which is associated with increased O_2Hb (i.e. higher SpO_2) (Reprinted from Chan et al. [40]. With permission from Elsevier)

amounts of near-infrared light and lower amounts of red light (this is why oxygenated blood appears bright red – O_2Hb scatters more red light). Conversely, HHb absorbs greater amounts of red light and lower amounts of near-infrared light (and therefore appears less red). These absorption characteristics are fortuitous, in that red and near-infrared light penetrates tissues well, while blue, green, yellow, and far-infrared light are significantly absorbed [39]. The light that is transmitted by the pulse oximeter probe can therefore be detected by a photodiode on the opposite arm of the probe. Using the Beer-Lambert Law, the relative proportion of O_2Hb and Hb can then be determined.

The ability of pulse oximetry to measure the oxygen saturation of arterial blood (as opposed to venous blood, capillary blood, tissue, etc.) is based upon the pulsatile nature of blood flow. During an arterial pulsation, the amount of red and near-infrared light that is absorbed changes with the cardiac cycle. The volume of blood passing through the arteries increases transiently during systole, while the volume of blood in the veins, capillaries, and tissues remains

relatively constant. By measuring these changes literally hundreds of times per second, the photodiode is able to distinguish a variable, pulsatile component (analogous to an alternating current signal, AC) versus a nonpulsatile, fixed component (analogous to a direct current, DC) (Fig. 39.5). The ratio of the red signal (AC_{660nm}/DC_{660nm}) to the near-infrared signal (AC_{940nm}/DC_{940nm}) can then be used to determine the relative proportion of HHb to O_2Hb, which is called R [40].

$$R = AC_{660nm} / DC_{660nm} \div AC_{940nm} / DC_{940nm} \quad (39.6)$$

Importantly, there is no physiologic relationship between R and SpO_2. Rather, both R and oxygen saturation (measured using co-oximetry – see below) were measured in healthy volunteers breathing subambient concentrations of O_2 in order to change their oxygen saturation from 70 to 100 %. A calibration curve was then constructed, which the microprocessor in the pulse oximeter uses to determine SpO_2 [39, 41–43] For this reason, SpO_2 is less accurate at oxygen saturations less than 70 % [44–49].

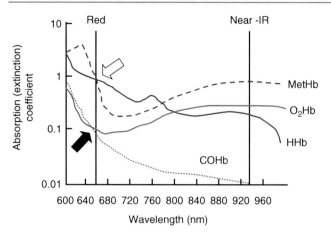

Fig. 39.6 Absorption spectra for O_2Hb, HHb, COHb, and MetHb (available on standard co-oximetry) (Reprinted from Chan et al. [40]. With permission from Elsevier). Note that the absorption of red light by COHb and O_2Hb are very similar (*black arrow*). In addition, the red light absorption of MetHb and HHb are also very similar (*white arrow*).

Importantly, pulse oximeters, which employ two light-emitting diodes measure *functional oxygen saturation*, which is the percentage of O_2Hb relative to the sum of O_2Hb and HHb.

$$\text{Functional SaO}_2 = O_2Hb / O_2Hb + HHb \quad (39.7)$$

Conversely, co-oximeters employ between four to six light-emitting diodes (and hence measure absorption at four to six different wavelengths) and measure *fractional oxygen saturation*, that is the percentage of O_2Hb relative to the sum of O_2Hb, HHb, carboxyhemoglobin (CO-Hb), and methemoglobin (met-Hb) (Fig. 39.6).

$$\text{Fractional SaO}_2 = O_2Hb / \left(\begin{array}{c} O_2Hb + HHb + CO \\ -Hb + met - Hb \end{array} \right) \quad (39.8)$$

Therefore, in presence of pathologic hemoglobins (dyshemoglobinemias), functional oxygen saturation will be spuriously high (discussed further below).

Proper site selection for the pulse oximeter probe is essential for appropriate reading and interpretation. Tissue beds with a high vascular density are particularly important – these include the finger, toe, nose, ear lobe, or forehead. The ear lobe or forehead location may be preferable in critically ill children with poor peripheral perfusion (due to vasoconstriction and hypotension) or in hypothermic patients [40, 50, 51]. In addition, it is also important to remember that in the presence of an anatomic right-to-left shunt (e.g. ductal-dependent, cyanotic congenital heart disease), any placement at a post-ductal location cannot reflect real oxygenation of the upper limb and brain and might lead to inappropriate clinical decisions (in this case, many providers choose to monitor both pre- and post-ductal oxygen saturation).

There are several issues that can impact the reliability of pulse oximetry readings (Table 39.4) [38]. As alluded to above, poor probe positioning, movement artifact, and/

Table 39.4 Common causes of falsely high or low SpO_2 readings

Conditions associated with falsely high or normal SpO_2 readings
Carbon monoxide poisoning
Sickle cell anemia vasoocclusive crises
Methemoglobinemia[a]
Sulfhemoglobinemia[a]
Sepsis/septic shock[a]
Poor probe positioning[a]
Conditions associated with falsely low SpO_2 readings
Hypotension
Shock
Vasoconstriction
Hypothermia
Fingernail polish
Excessive movement artifact
Severe anemia
Poor probe positioning
Congenital dyshemoglobinemias

[a]These conditions may also cause a falsely low SpO_2 reading (see text for details)

or poor peripheral perfusion (due to shock, hypotension, hypothermia, or vasoconstriction secondary to endogenous or exogenous catecholamines) are usually associated with a falsely low SpO_2 or inability to read SpO_2 (intermittent drop-out). Poor probe positioning may also result in a falsely high SpO_2 – in this situation, the light emitted from the probe bypasses tissues completely and hits the photodetector (the R value approaches 1, as both transmitted red and near-infrared light is largely unabsorbed) [40]. Carbon monoxide (CO) poisoning will elicit a falsely elevated SpO_2 reading. Recall that CO has a much greater affinity for Hb (about 240x more) than oxygen, which results in the formation of carboxyhemoglobin (COHb). Both O_2Hb and COHb absorb red light in a similar fashion (which is not very well – again, this is why oxygenated blood appears red and why patients with CO poisoning are frequently described as having a "cherry red" appearance) and COHb doesn't absorb near-infrared light at all. The photodetector on a standard pulse oximeter therefore can't distinguish between COHb and O_2Hb – the net effect is a decreased absorption of red light, which results in a lower R than predicted (and hence a falsely normal or higher SpO_2 reading than the actual oxygen saturation). Note that the SpO_2 reading on the pulse oximeter is normal or higher than what would be predicted by the fractional SaO_2 (as measured by co-oximetry) (Fig. 39.7). There are conflicting reports on the accuracy of pulse oximetry in patients with sickle cell anemia vasoocclusive crises [40, 52–55]. However, in general the discrepancies in measurement are clinically insignificant, except in severe cases when the oxygen saturation is usually falsely elevated (due to greater concentration of COHb – due to hemolysis).

Excessive movement and venous pulsations (as occurs if the probe is placed too tightly around the fingertip or in the presence of a widened pulse pressure and "warm shock")

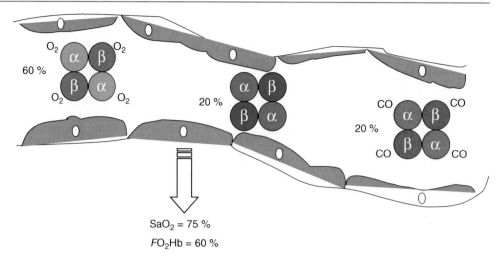

Fig. 39.7 Distinction between functional oxygen saturation (*SaO₂*) and fractional oxygen saturation (*FO₂Hb*). In this particular case, the arterial blood contains 60 % O₂Hb, 20 % HHb, and 20 % COHb. Using Eq. 39.7, the functional oxygen saturation is 60/(60 + 20), or 75 %. Using Eq. 39.8, the fractional oxygen saturation is 60/(60 + 20 + 20), or 60 % (Reprinted from Chan et al. [40]. With permission from Elsevier)

$SaO_2 = 75$ %

$FO_2Hb = 60$ %

falsely lower the SpO₂ reading. Intravenous dyes such as methylene blue (used in the treatment of methemoglobinemia) or iodocyanine green (used in certain diagnostic tests) also falsely lower the SpO₂ reading. Of note, the peak absorption of methylene blue occurs at 668 nm, which is close to the strong red light absorption by HHb – methylene blue therefore mimics HHb, which leads to a lower R than normal (and hence, lower SpO₂ reading) [56]. Congenital dyshemoglobinemias also falsely lower SpO₂, again due to a similar absorption spectrum with HHb [40]. Older studies raised concerns about particular shades of fingernail polish impacting SpO₂ readings, though the newer models of pulse oximeters have largely fixed this problem [40, 42, 43]. Finally, patients with severe anemia may also have a falsely lower SpO₂ reading (it is important to note that anemia reduces the overall oxygen content of the blood, but does not normally lower the oxygen saturation of the blood). The physics behind this phenomenon are complex to say the least – suffice it to say that the lower number of red blood cells in patients with severe anemia results in decreased light scatter [57]. Recall that the R versus SpO₂ curves were calibrated in otherwise healthy individuals with normal amounts of light scatter. Overall, the result is that the SpO₂ underestimates the true oxygen saturation in patients with severe anemia and hypoxemia, though this effect is limited in patients with severe anemia and normoxia [40, 58–60].

MetHb (formed when the iron in the heme moiety is oxidized from Fe^{2+} to Fe^{3+}) absorbs more near-infrared light than either O₂Hb or HHb, though it absorbs red light similar to HHb (this, in fact, is the reason that these patients appear quite cyanotic and the blood often appears a very dark blue). As further shown in Fig. 39.6, MetHb absorbs both red and near-infrared light equally well, which results in an R value that approaches 1. The net result is that patients with methemoglobinemia will have a SpO₂ of 80–85 % [38, 40, 42, 61]. Similarly, sulfhemoglobin (SulfHb), which is formed by the irreversible oxidation of iron in the heme moiety to Fe^{3+} (just like MetHb) with the incorporation of a sulfur atom into the porphyrin ring, can be a side effect of certain oxidizing drugs, such as aniline dyes, nitrates, metoclopramide, or dapsone. SulfHb does not carry oxygen, so these patients have markedly reduced oxygen transport. However, while MetHb shifts the oxyhemoglobin dissociation curve to the left (inhibiting oxygen unloading at the tissue level), SulfHb shifts the curve to the right (which facilitates oxygen unloading to the tissue). Similar to MetHb, SulfHb absorbs red light and near-infrared light equally well – these patients will have a SpO₂ of 80–85 % as well [40]. Finally, there are conflicting data on the accuracy of pulse oximetry in critically ill patients with severe sepsis and septic shock [40]. The discrepancy is small and probably clinically irrelevant, though the mechanisms are poorly understood. In the case of a "warm shock" state, venous pulsations may falsely lower SpO₂ readings [62–64]. Conversely, other studies suggest that the septic state falsely elevates SpO₂ (the mechanism is poorly understood) [65, 66]. Further studies in this population are warranted. For now, clinicians should be aware of these potential issues.

Monitoring Ventilation

The partial pressure of carbon dioxide (CO_2) in the arterial blood is inversely proportional to alveolar minute ventilation (i.e. increased minute ventilation = decreased $PaCO_2$). The efficiency of ventilation, i.e. the efficiency of CO_2 elimination, can therefore be measured directly using arterial blood gas analysis. Alternatively, CO_2 can be measured in expiratory gases either via the concentration of CO_2 reached at the end of expiration (partial pressure of CO_2 at end-tidal; $P_{et}CO_2$ or $EtCO_2$) or the amount of CO_2 expired per breath as measured by volumetric capnography (CO_2 elimination; VCO_2, the net volume of CO_2 eliminated per minute). Finally, ventilation can be monitored using transcutaneous $PtCO_2$ monitoring.

Table 39.5 Conditions associated with changes in $P_{et}CO_2$

		Increase $P_{et}CO_2$	Decrease $P_{et}CO_2$	Absent $P_{et}CO_2$
Rapid change		Increase in cardiac output (e.g. seizure)	Decreased cardiac output (e.g. cardiac arrest)	Esophageal intubation
			Pulmonary embolus	Inadvertent extubation
			Air embolus	Ventilator disconnect
			Tracheal tube obstruction	
			Large tracheal tube leak	
Slow change		Inadequate minute ventilation	Increased minute ventilation	
		Increased CO_2 production (e.g. fever)	Decreased CO_2 production (e.g. sedation, paralysis, hypothermia)	
		Equipment malfunction	Increased dead space ventilation	

Arterial Blood Gas Analysis

The *gold standard* of CO_2 determination remains the arterial blood gas (ABG). Routine blood gas analysis directly measures the pH and the PCO_2. Measurement of $PaCO_2$ requires obtaining an arterial blood specimen, via either intermittent sampling or an indwelling arterial catheter. However, measurement of PCO_2 in a free flowing capillary specimen (so-called capillary blood gas) is a reasonable approximation of $PaCO_2$ [67–71]. Venous blood samples drawn from free-flowing blood through a central line [71–75] or peripheral intravenous catheter [71, 75–79] may also reflect arterial pH and PCO_2 values reasonably well.

End-Tidal CO_2 Monitoring

Capnometry refers to the measurement of exhaled CO_2 (i.e. the measurement is displayed numerically), whereas capnography refers to the graphical display of the change in exhaled CO_2 over time (with each breath). Capnometry includes the colorimetric detection of CO_2 in exhaled air used by certain devices (usually disposable) to confirm proper tracheal tube placement (i.e. placement in the trachea versus the esophagus), which will not be discussed here (these devices are discussed in the Basic Airway Management chapter).

End-tidal CO_2 ($EtCO_2$) measurements by capnometry give the peak value of the PCO_2 at the end of expiration ($P_{et}CO_2$). There are several conditions which can be associated with changes in $P_{et}CO_2$ (Table 39.5) [80]. Under normal conditions, the $P_{et}CO_2$ is about 2–6 mmHg lower than the $PaCO_2$ value, as a result of physiologic ventilation-perfusion (V/Q) mismatching (i.e. physiologic shunt). In general, an increase in $P_{et}CO_2$ is almost always due to an increase in $PaCO_2$. Conversely, a decrease in $P_{et}CO_2$ doesn't necessarily correspond to a decrease in $PaCO_2$ (in fact, the $PaCO_2$ can be increased, decreased, or normal in this situation). The difference between $P_{et}CO_2$ and $PaCO_2$ can be significantly increased in critically ill patients with significant dead-space ventilation, cyanotic heart disease, decreased pulmonary blood-flow (classically in presence of an extra-pulmonary R-L shunt), and impaired cardiac output.

End-tidal CO_2 is almost universally monitored in critically ill children on mechanical ventilatory support in the PICU [80–82] to continuously monitor and evaluate respiratory rate and rhythm, quantify dead-space (see below), confirm proper tracheal tube placement to avoid inadvertent extubation, and monitor patient-ventilator asynchrony [80, 83, 84]. In addition, end-tidal CO_2 can be monitored in patients who are breathing spontaneously during procedural sedation to improve safety [85–89]. Almost all commercially available devices use infrared absorption to detect CO_2 – these devices therefore consist of an infrared light source, an exhalation gas collection chamber, and a photodiode (similar to pulse oximetry, discussed above). The end-tidal CO_2 monitor is connected to the end of the tracheal tube and quantifies the adsorption of infrared light as it passes through the exhaled gas to detect and quantify CO_2. Oxygen, helium, and nitrogen do not absorb infrared light and therefore do not interfere with CO_2 measurement. These monitors are generally classified into two types based upon the gas sampling method – mainstream or sidestream [80]. Mainstream analyzers are attached inline to the tracheal tube and directly sample exhaled gas, while sidestream analyzers continuously sample an aliquot of exhaled gas. Mainstream analyzers usually have a faster response time and do not remove any aliquots of exhaled gas from the circuit (which could influence exhaled tidal volume measurements). However, they are bulkier and tend to place tension on the tracheal tube. In addition, mainstream analyzers can't be used in non-intubated patients. Sidestream analyzers, on the other hand, have a slight delay in response time but are smaller, lighter, and able to be used in non-intubated patients [80, 85, 86, 90–92].

As stated above, an increase in the difference between $P_{et}CO_2$ and $PaCO_2$ usually is indicative of either an increase in dead-space or a decrease in cardiac output [93]. Recall that minute ventilation is the sum of alveolar ventilation and dead-space ventilation. The dead-space is that portion of the lung (including the conducting airways) that does not participate in gas exchange. All patients have some proportion of dead-space, known as the anatomic dead-space (conducting airways, which essentially includes that portion of the respiratory tract from the mouth to the bronchioles). However, there is also a portion of dead-space that is due to the regional ventilation-perfusion heterogeneity, known as the alveolar dead-space. Regions of the lung that are ventilated but not perfused comprise the alveolar dead-space (in contrast, regions of the lung that are perfused but not ventilated comprise the intra-pulmonary shunt). Physiologic dead-space is therefore the sum of the anatomic dead-space and alveolar dead-space. Increased physiologic dead-space has been shown to correlate with outcomes in both critically ill children [94] and adults [95–98] with ARDS. In addition, the dead-space (determined via the Bohr equation – below) can be used to set the optimal positive end-expiratory pressure (PEEP), which has been defined as the pressure level with the highest compliance in conjunction with the lowest calculated dead-space [99, 100]. Optimal PEEP during mechanical ventilation should theoretically decrease dead-space ventilation by recruiting alveoli to participate in gas exchange. Similarly, the $PaCO_2$–$P_{et}CO_2$ gradient is smallest at optimal recruitment [101, 102].

The measurement of end-tidal CO_2 can be used in the modified Bohr equation to calculate the dead-space ventilation (ratio of physiologic dead-space to tidal volume):

$$V_D / V_T = \left(PaCO_2 - PeCO_2 \right) / PaCO_2 \quad (39.9)$$

$$V_{D\text{-}Alv} / V_T = \left(PaCO_2 - P_{et}CO_2 \right) / PaCO_2 \quad (39.10)$$

where V_D is the physiologic dead-space, $V_{D\text{-}Alv}$ is the alveolar dead-space, V_T is tidal volume, $PaCO_2$ is the partial pressure of CO_2 in the arterial blood, $PeCO_2$ is the partial pressure of CO_2 in expired air, and $P_{et}CO_2$ is the end-tidal CO_2 concentration. A normal value is <0.3. Note that when using $PetCO_2$ instead of $PeCO_2$, the alveolar dead-space is being calculated (as end-tidal CO_2 reflects alveolar ventilation and not the anatomic dead-space – see below). The validity of dead-space calculations depends on the validity of the end-tidal CO_2 value, which should reflect true alveolar gas CO_2 concentration. Incomplete expiration, maldistribution of inspired gas, or acute hyperventilation will lead to an end-tidal CO_2 value that does not correspond to true alveolar gas CO_2 concentration, and hence an erroneous calculation of dead-space ventilation.

Classically, the shape of the CO_2-expiration curve is characterized by three distinct phases (Fig. 39.8). The initial phase I characterizes the beginning of expiration with the release of "dead-space" gases, i.e. CO_2 poor gas mixture from conducting airways (i.e. the anatomic dead-space). During the phase II, there is a rapid upswing caused by the increasing amounts of exhaled alveolar gas that contains CO_2 mixed with a reduced amount of dead-space gas. The alpha angle represents the transition from phase II to phase III.

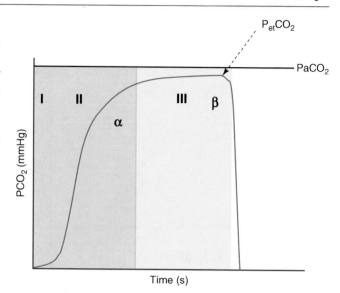

Fig. 39.8 The single-breath CO_2 curve (normal capnograph) consists of three phases. See text for detailed explanation

Finally, during phase III, more and more of the alveoli have emptied and the CO_2 concentration in the exhaled gas contains reaches a plateau that approaches (but does not reach) $PaCO_2$. The presence of a plateau phase at end-expiration is required for valid measures of $P_{et}CO_2$. In absence of such a plateau, $P_{et}CO_2$ values will be underestimated and the derived calculation of V_D/V_T will be erroneous. The beta angle represents the change to the inspiratory phase. When inspiration starts, the CO_2 level drops rapidly back to zero. The point at which phase III ends immediately prior to the start of the next inspiration is the true $P_{et}CO_2$ [80, 81, 103]. The length and shape of the three phases may provide some useful information (Fig. 39.9). For example, a prolonged phase I suggests the presence of increased anatomic dead-space or low expiratory flow conditions, a flattened slope of phase II indicates prolonged expiratory times and can be seen with important obstructive airway disease, and a upslope within phase III has been shown to correlate with the degree of obstructive airway disease [81, 83, 103].

Although the shape of the traditional capnography curve can theoretically give some information on the characteristics of the underlying lung disease, it is difficult to analyze in detail at the bedside. CO_2 elimination (VCO_2) measurements (i.e. the amount of CO_2 exhaled per breath), which corresponds to the area under the expiratory CO_2 curve, by volumetric capnography theoretically are a much better reflection of ventilation efficiency than a single point measure of the patient via traditional time-based end-tidal CO_2 monitoring. Volumetric capnography (also known as single breath carbon dioxide ($SBCO_2$) elimination) combines a CO_2 sensor and a pneumotachometer to measure the net CO_2 expired as a volume exhaled over time. The volumetric capnograph is very similar to the traditional time-based capnograph (Fig. 39.10).

Fig. 39.9 Capnography interpretation can be clinically useful. The normal capnograph is shown in the *shaded green* tracing. (**a**) Capnography from a patient with obstructive lung disease (e.g., status asthmaticus). Note the prolonged expiratory phase (phase II) and the lack of a plateau phase (phase III). The "ramping up" pattern is highly characteristic. (**b**) Capnograph from a patient whose tracheal tube has been dislodged into the right main bronchus (in this case, the capnograph reveals an abrupt change from this patient's previous baseline). (**c**) Capnograph from a patient with patient-ventilator asynchrony. The *bold arrows* indicate spontaneous breaths during intermittent mandatory ventilation. (**d**) Capnograph from a patient whose tracheal tube is malpositioned in the esophagus. There is no discernible CO_2

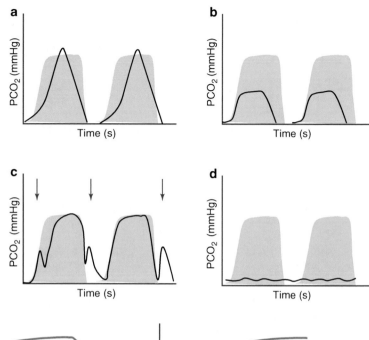

Fig. 39.10 Time-based and volume-based (volumetric) capnograms

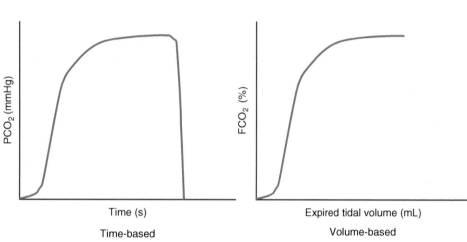

While volumetric capnography requires a different set of equipment, these devices are readily available in the clinical setting. During mechanical ventilation volumetric capnography can be used breath-to-breath to immediately determine the effect of any change in ventilator settings on CO_2 elimination [104, 105]. In addition, volumetric capnography can assess dead-space ventilation more accurately than time-based capnography [106–112].

Transcutaneous CO_2 (TcCO$_2$) Measurements

Whereas transcutaneous O_2 monitors correlate poorly with PaO_2 (and with pulse oximetry, these monitors are probably not necessary anyway) [113, 114], transcutaneous CO_2 (TcCO$_2$) monitors can reasonably approximate $PaCO_2$, particularly in certain settings [113, 115–120]. These monitors heat the skin from 41 to 43 °C to cause localized vasodilation and diffusion of CO_2 into the dermal and epidermal layers. CO_2 then diffuses across the membrane of the probe and into

the reservoir where the partial pressure of the gas is detected electrochemically. TcCO$_2$ monitoring provides continuous data and allows for trending of TcCO$_2$ levels over time – readings closely approximate $PaCO_2$ levels to within 6–10 mmHg [121]. TcCO$_2$ measurements can provide non-invasive monitoring of $PaCO_2$ when EtCO$_2$ and/or VCO$_2$ is not available or even not feasible, such as during high-frequency oscillatory ventilation [120, 122]. However, TcCO$_2$ monitoring does have some significant limitations. For example, the accuracy of these devices is complicated by drifting and the probes require frequent calibration to address this issue. Additionally, the accuracy of the probe is affected by skin temperature and tissue perfusion. The heated probe may locally increase the metabolic rate of the skin and yield a falsely elevated carbon dioxide level. Additionally, during states of hypoperfusion (as commonly occurs in critically ill children in the PICU), carbon dioxide levels increase in the tissue and the TcCO$_2$ may overestimate the true $PaCO_2$. Skin

Fig. 39.11 The six basic waveform shapes for ventilator graphics

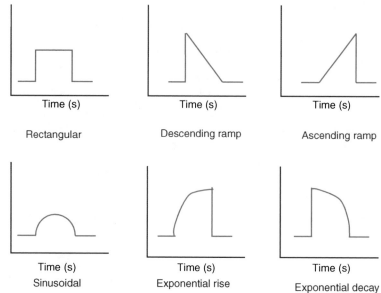

Rectangular

Descending ramp

Ascending ramp

Sinusoidal

Exponential rise

Exponential decay

thickness also limits the accuracy of the $TcCO_2$ and likely explains the decreasing accuracy of this modality in older children and adults [114]. Despite the theoretical advantages of $TcCO_2$ monitoring, it is not widely used in the PICU setting due to these limitations, as well as the comparatively slower response time and the need to frequently relocate the sensors to prevent skin burn.

Monitoring the Mechanics of the Respiratory System

Ventilator waveforms are graphic representations of the mechanics of the respiratory system. They are essential components of the respiratory monitoring armamentarium in the PICU. Proper interpretation of these waveforms is crucial to clinical decision making in the management of critically ill children on mechanical ventilation. There are three waveforms (also called scalars) of interest to the clinician in the PICU – pressure, volume, and flow, all of which are displayed versus time. In addition, pressure-volume (P-V) and flow-volume (F-V) loops also provide useful information.

Importantly, ventilator pressures are typically measured in cm H_2O and referenced to atmospheric pressure (i.e. baseline value is zero). Pressure and flow generated by the ventilator are measured by transducers in the ventilator itself, while volume is derived mathematically as the integral of the flow waveform over time. The total pressure applied to the respiratory system during mechanical ventilation is comprised of the sum of the pressures generated by the ventilator (Pvent) and the pressure generated by the respiratory musculature (Pmus). These pressures generate flow, which delivers volume to the respiratory system. In order to generate flow, these pressures must exceed that of

the elastic recoil pressure of the lungs and chest wall, the resistance to flow through the airways, and frictional forces of the tissues in the respiratory tract (which is usually considered negligible under most conditions), as summarized in the equation of motion:

$$Pvent + Pmus = Elastic\,recoil\,pressure \\ + Resistive\,pressure \qquad (39.11)$$

The elastic recoil pressure is the product of elastance (the inverse of compliance) and volume, while resistive pressure is the product of resistance and flow.

$$Pvent + Pmus = (Elastance \times Volume) \\ + (Resistance \times Flow) \qquad (39.12)$$

Again, as elastance (i.e. the tendency of the respiratory system to return to its original shape) is the inverse of compliance (i.e. the distensibility of the respiratory system), the equation can be re-written as:

$$Pvent + Pmus = (Volume\,/\,Compliance) \\ + (Resistance \times Flow) \qquad (39.13)$$

Note that the ventilator can control the left-side of the equation by controlling Pvent (i.e. pressure-control ventilation) or the right-side of the equation by controlling volume and flow (i.e. volume-control ventilation). The individual patient characteristics and disease condition determine the compliance and resistance.

There are six basic shapes to the various waveforms or scalars (pressure versus time, flow versus time, and volume versus time) (Fig. 39.11). By convention, time is plotted on the x-axis, while pressure, flow, or volume are plotted on the y-axis. In general, pressure waveforms are usually rectangu-

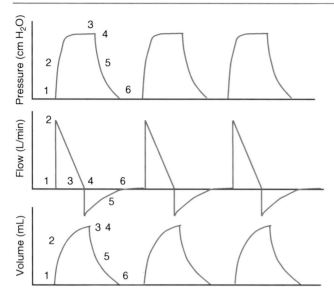

Fig. 39.12 Representative scalars for a patient in a pressure-control mode of mechanical ventilation. Each breath is divided into six phases: (*1*) Beginning of inspiration: as shown on the pressure-time scalar, the pressure-controlled inspiration starts at the baseline, in contrast to a spontaneous breath which starts with a negative deflection (decrease in pressure). (*2*) Inspiration: as shown on the flow-time scalar, there is a rapid increase to peak inspiratory flow, followed by a decelerating flow phase (which is characteristic of pressure-controlled ventilation). As shown on the pressure-time scalar, the peak inspiratory pressure is rapidly attained and held constant for the duration of the inspiratory phase. The shape of the pressure-time scalar changes according to the pre-set rise time (i.e. the time in which the ventilator achieves the target peak inspiratory pressure) and inspiratory time. The volume achieved may vary from breath to breath, and due to the decelerating flow pattern, there is a curvilinear upslope on the volume-time scalar. (*3*) End of inspiration: the inspiratory phase is terminated at the end of the inspiratory time (time-cycled) that is set by the clinician. At this point, the expiratory valve on the ventilator opens, leading to the start of the expiratory phase. The delivered tidal volume depends upon the patient's lung and chest wall compliance. Note that the flow reaches zero at or just before the end of the inspiratory time. (*4*) Beginning of expiration: expiration is largely passive – the shape of the expiratory phase on the three scalars are determined by the patient's airway resistance, resistance of the artificial airway (e.g., tracheal tube), and the elastic recoil pressure of the lung and chest wall. (*5*) Expiration (*6*) End of expiration: termination occurs at the end of the expiratory time set by the clinician (time-cycled). Pressure returns to the baseline (0 cm H_2O) or the level of PEEP set by the clinician

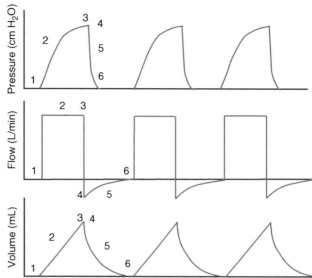

Fig. 39.13 Representative scalars for a patient in a volume-control mode of mechanical ventilation. Each breath is divided into six phases: (*1*) Beginning of inspiration: the initiation of inspiration depends upon the triggering mode (i.e. Control, Assist/Control, SIMV) and can be time-triggered (at a predetermined time set by the clinician) or patient-triggered (triggered by the patient's own respiratory effort). (*2*) Inspiration: the shape of the flow, volume, and pressure scalars depends upon the airway resistance, lung compliance, the set flow (rate and pattern), and the preset tidal volume being delivered. For example, as shown on the flow-time scalar, there is a rapid increase to peak inspiratory flow which is then held constant for the duration of the inspiratory phase (resulting in a rectangular waveform). As shown on the pressure-time scalar, the peak inspiratory pressure (*PIP*) is not reached until the end of inspiration (see below). Due to the constant flow pattern during inspiration, volume is delivered in fixed increments per unit time, which results in a straight-line, linear upslope to the pre-set tidal volume. (*3*) End of inspiration: the inspiratory phase is terminated at the end of the inspiratory time (time-cycled) that is set by the clinician. The PIP necessary to attain the preset tidal volume depends upon the patient's lung and chest wall compliance. An end-inspiratory hold will allow the pressures within the respiratory system to equilibrate, which occurs at the plateau pressure (not shown). At the end of the inspiratory phase, the expiratory valve on the ventilator opens, leading to the start of the expiratory phase. (*4*) Beginning of expiration: expiration is largely passive – the shape of the expiratory phase on the three scalars are determined by the patient's airway resistance, resistance of the artificial airway (e.g., tracheal tube), and the elastic recoil pressure of the lung and chest wall. (*5*) Expiration (*6*) End of expiration: termination occurs at the end of the expiratory time set by the clinician (time-cycled). Pressure returns to the baseline (0 cm H_2O) or the level of PEEP set by the clinician

lar or rising exponential, whereas volume waveforms are usually ascending ramp or sinusoidal. Flow waveforms can take several shapes. Pressure-time, volume-time, and flow-time scalars are generally displayed together by the ventilator graphics software, as shown in Fig. 39.12 (patient in pressure-control ventilation) and (Fig. 39.13), (patient in volume-control ventilation). Based upon the information provided in these scalars, each breath can be divided into distinct phases (as shown on the accompanying figures) – beginning of inspiration, inspiration, end of inspiration, beginning of expiration, expiration, and end of expiration. Each scalar is discussed in greater detail below.

Scalars

Flow-Time Scalars

The flow-time scalar can help distinguish between pressure-control versus volume-control ventilation. During pressure-control ventilation (Fig. 39.12), there are two components to the inspiratory flow waveform. There is an accelerating flow component at the beginning of inspiration (which almost immediately reaches peak inspiratory flow) followed by a

Fig. 39.14 Flow-time scalar showing what occurs when the inspiratory time is set at a level that is not appropriate for the patient. In the *top* graphic, the inspiratory time is too short for the patient, as flow does not return to baseline. Conversely, in the *bottom* graphic, the inspiratory time is too long for the patient. The area demarcated by the *blue circle* is called a "zero-flow state"

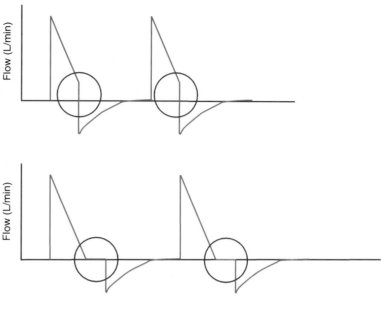

decelerating flow component (air entry slows as the lung approaches its capacity). The expiratory flow waveform similarly has an accelerating flow phase at the beginning of expiration (which almost immediately reaches peak expiratory flow), followed by a slower decelerating phase back to baseline. In contrast, during volume-control ventilation (Fig. 39.13), the flow waveform has a characteristic square or rectangular waveform, in which flow accelerates to a plateau and is held constant until the beginning of expiration, at which time expiratory flow rapidly decreases to baseline. The decelerating inspiratory flow waveform that is characteristic of pressure-control ventilation theoretically minimizes the pressure needed to deliver adequate tidal volumes (i.e. the same tidal volume can be delivered with a lower peak inspiratory pressure), thereby minimizing ventilator-induced lung injury (VILI), though there are several newer modes of volume-control ventilation with this feature (e.g. pressure-regulated volume control, PRVC mode of ventilation).

The flow-time scalar also provides information on whether the respiratory cycle time settings (inspiratory and expiratory time) are adequate according to the respiratory system's time constant. The time constant is the product of respiratory compliance (Crs) and resistance (Rrs).

$$T = Crs \times Rrs \qquad (39.14)$$

Recall that the inspiratory time (Ti) is defined as the time required for complete inspiration, which is determined according to the following equation:

$$Ti = V_T / Flow\ rate \qquad (39.15)$$

where V_T is the tidal volume (in mL) and the flow rate is expressed in mL/s. The cycle time (Tc) is the sum of the inspiratory time (Ti) and the expiratory time (Te) and depends upon the selected respiratory rate. In intubated patients, the

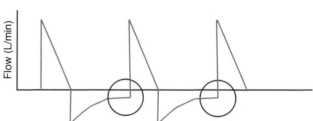

Fig. 39.15 Flow-time scalar showing air-trapping (i.e. rinsic PEEP or "auto-PEEP"). The expiratory flow doesn't return to baseline before the start of the next breath, which can occur in the presence of airway obstruction (e.g. asthma, bronchiolitis, etc.) or if the expiratory time is too short

resistance of the tracheal tube will have an effect on calculation of the time constant. The time constant describes the amount of time needed for complete filling or emptying of the respiratory system, which generally occurs within about five to six time constants. To calculate the time constant at the bedside in every patient and situation is cumbersome, whereas to simply search for a static (i.e. no-flow) condition on the flow-time curve at end-inspiration or end-expiration is more practical. A no-flow condition indicates that no further volume will be delivered to or exhaled by the patient, indicating pressure equilibrium between the respiratory system and airway opening. Searching at the bedside for an inspiratory time that allows for a very short no-flow condition at end-inspiration facilitates selection of the lowest airway pressures needed to deliver a desired tidal volume (Fig. 39.14). Similarly, searching for an expiratory time that allows for flow termination at end-expiration helps to avoid intrinsic PEEP, also called auto-PEEP (i.e. dynamic hyperinflation) (Fig. 39.15).

A "zig-zag" (or saw-tooth) pattern, which occurs most commonly during the expiratory phase of the flow-time scalar is classically observed as a result of flow variations due to

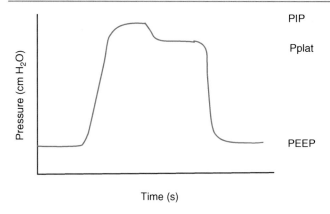

Fig. 39.16 Pressure-time scalar with inspiratory hold maneuver. See text for explanation

secretions in the airways. A sudden change in the expiratory flow shape will occur when the patient tries to inspire spontaneously when the expiratory valve is still open (i.e. the ventilator is still in expiratory phase). In this situation a drop in the airway pressure is observed simultaneously with a short and often modest increase in flow, which is indicative of inspiratory trigger failure (patient-ventilator asynchrony).

Pressure-Time Scalar

The pressure-time curve scalar can also help distinguish between pressure-control ventilation versus volume-control ventilation. During pressure-control ventilation, the pressure-time scalar classically shows a "rectangular-wave form" with a clear plateau phase (see again Fig. 39.12). The airway pressure rapidly rises (the rate of rise depends upon the rise time set by the clinician) to the peak inspiratory pressure and remains constant throughout the inspiratory phase. Conversely, during volume-control ventilation (i.e. constant flow pattern delivered by the ventilator), the pressure-time scalar takes the shape of a shark's fin. There is a rapid rise in pressure at the beginning of the inspiratory phase, as gas flow encounters the frictional resistance of the airways. Later during the inspiratory phase, there is a more gradual increase in airway pressure as the flow of gas confronts the opposing elastic forces of the lung and chest wall. Once the set tidal volume is reached, the expiratory valve opens and the airway pressure abruptly falls to baseline (the PEEP). The peak inspiratory pressure (PIP) necessary to attain this tidal volume will depend upon the patient's respiratory system compliance. Importantly, an inspiratory hold maneuver will reveal the pressure-time scalar at static (i.e. no flow conditions). In this case, the airway pressure falls to the plateau pressure (Pplat) (Fig. 39.16). Therefore the peak pressure (PIP) value gives an indication of the resistance of the respiratory system, while the Pplat is the actual pressure that reaches the alveoli. Importantly, static compliance is measured at static, or no-flow conditions, as opposed to dynamic compliance which is measured during periods of gas flow.

$$Cstat = V_T / \left(Pplat - PEEP \right) \qquad (39.16)$$

Dynamic compliance is always either less than or equal to the static lung compliance (as Pplat is always lower than PIP).

$$Cdyn = V_T / \left(PIP - PEEP \right) \qquad (39.17)$$

Note that during pressure-control ventilation, the PIP and Pplat are essentially the same. Spontaneous breaths during either volume-control or pressure-control ventilation are sinusoidal in shape and start with a negative deflection on the pressure-time scalar. Spontaneous breaths are therefore negative during inspiration and positive during expiration. If the patient is in a pressure support mode of ventilation, the spontaneous breaths are will trigger a ventilator-assisted breath, which is typically set to reach a lower peak inspiratory pressure than a normal ventilator breath.

Volume-Time Scalar

The volume-time scalar provides less information than either the flow-time or pressure-time scalars. During volume-control ventilation, volume is delivered in fixed increments per unit time (due to the rectangular flow pattern), such that there is a linear increase in volume to the tidal volume set by the clinician. Once the set tidal volume is attained, the expiratory valve opens and the volume decreases back to the baseline, resulting in a triangular or "mountain top" shape. Conversely, during pressure-control ventilation, there is a curvilinear increase in volume due to the decelerating flow pattern. The tidal volume that is reached depends entirely on the patient's respiratory system compliance. The volume-time scalar can easily detect the presence of a leak in either the ventilator circuit or around the tracheal tube. In the presence of a leak, the volume-time scalar does not return to zero at end-inspiration – a visible plateau phase above 0 cm H_2O is frequently observed. Most of the modern ventilators provide a numerical reading of both the inspired and expired tidal volume, as well as a percentage value for the measured leak. However, as previously mentioned, this reading is not as accurate due to the compressible volume in the ventilator circuit. Volumes measured at the tracheal tube are much more accurate [123].

Loops

Various loops can be displayed (i.e. flow-volume and pressure-volume). Loops display graphical information of the inspiratory and expiratory portions of a single breath, as opposed to time. Information can be derived from both the numerical values as well as the shapes of the waveforms themselves (as is the case with scalars described above).

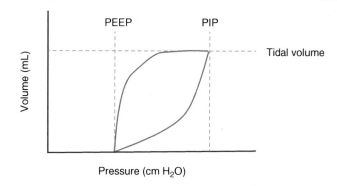

Fig. 39.17 Characteristic pressure-volume loop during positive pressure ventilation

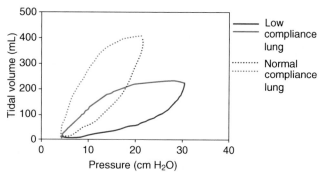

Fig. 39.18 Pressure-volume loops from a patient with poor lung compliance and a patient with normal lung compliance

Pressure-Volume (PV) Loops

The pressure-volume curve loop gained major interest over the last decade, certainly because of the recognition that mechanical ventilation needs to be applied in a gentle way to avoid ventilator-induced lung injury (VILI). Ventilator-induced overdistention (e.g. volutrauma and barotrauma) and under-recruitment (e.g., atelectrauma) are both recognized as potential putative mechanisms for VILI and lead to decreased respiratory system compliance, less efficient ventilation, and, in the patient who is spontaneously breathing, increased work of breathing. With the evidence that suggests that VILI can be limited by avoiding overdistention and the repetitive opening and collapsing of alveoli, analysis and careful monitoring of the shape of the inspiratory and expiratory limb of the dynamic PV loop gained major interest.

PV loops display the interaction between pressure (on the x-axis) and volume (on the y-axis), which can then be used to assess the patient's respiratory system compliance. During spontaneous ventilation, the PV loop moves in a clockwise direction (starting at the intersection of the x- and y-axes). The inspiratory portion is negative (i.e. to the left of the y-axis, as the pressure in the airways decreases below atmospheric pressure to generate flow), while the expiratory portion is positive (i.e. to the right of the y-axis, as airway pressure increases above atmospheric pressure in order to exhale). Conversely, during positive pressure mechanical ventilation, the PV loop moves in a counterclockwise direction an remains positive (to the right of the y-axis) for both the inspiratory and expiratory phases of the breath. The PV loop starts at PEEP and reaches its maximum pressure (PIP) before starting the expiratory phase. The maximal volume attained is of course the tidal volume that is delivered (Fig. 39.17).

In general, the PV loop of a patient with normal lung compliance has about a 45° angle (if a line was drawn from the peak pressure/volume to the baseline pressure/volume, bisecting the inspiratory and expiratory limbs). The shape of the PV loop provides a relative indication

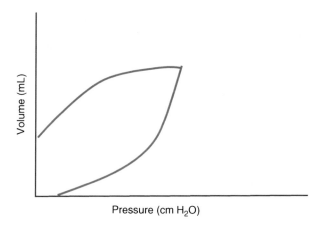

Fig. 39.19 Pressure-volume loop from a patient with a large leak around the tracheal tube. Note that the size of the leak can be determined by close examination of the y-axis. The point at which the expiratory limb intersects the y-axis is the volume of leaked air around the tracheal tube (this will also be shown numerically on the ventilator's inspiratory and expiratory tidal volumes)

of the patient's underlying lung compliance (recall that compliance is the change in volume for a given change in pressure, which is the slope of the PV loop referred to above). Figure 39.18 shows two PV loops from a patient with normal lung compliance and a patient with poor lung compliance.

An incomplete PV loops suggests the presence of an air-leak within the ventilator circuit, around the tracheal tube (most common), or in the respiratory tract (e.g., broncho-pleural fistula) (Fig. 39.19). A patient-triggered breath creates a "trigger tail" on the PV loop (Fig. 39.20). As discussed above, a spontaneous breath is shown as a clockwise movement with the inspiratory phase on the negative side. Therefore, a patient-triggered breath creates an initial clockwise movement, followed by the normal counterclockwise movement of the ventilator breath, as the patient triggers the ventilator. The size of the "trigger tail" provides a rough estimation of the patient's respiratory effort (i.e. the bigger the effort, the bigger the tail).

Recruitment/Derecruitment

Commonly the presence of a so called lower inflection point (point of maximal change in curvature) on the lower part of the inflation limb of the dynamic PV loop is interpreted as the point where lung opening (i.e. recruitment) starts (Fig. 39.21). Many authorities recommend setting PEEP slightly above the lower inflection point (LIP). However, this concept of optimizing PEEP by graphic analysis is of questionable value and may even be potentially harmful in certain situations. As discussed in the chapter on Mechanical Ventilation, there are several methods that have been proposed to set PEEP for optimal alveolar recruitment – none of these methods have been shown to be superior to any other.

Overdistention

Pulmonary overdistention occurs when the volume limit of some component of the lungs is approached. It will be manifest as a dramatic reduction in compliance at the terminal end of the breath, which is commonly referred to as "beaking" on the PV loop (Fig. 39.21). Overdistention should be avoided as it has several deleterious effects on the cardiovas-

cular and pulmonary system. First, overdistention puts the patient at risk for barotrauma and volutrauma. Second, overdistention can increase dead space and therefore render ventilation less efficient. Third, overdistention will result in a dramatic increase in pulmonary vascular resistance from compression of the pulmonary vessels by the overdistended alveoli (see chapter on Respiratory Physiology) and a resultant reduction in cardiac output. When terminal "beaking" is observed, the clinician should reduce the set PIP or V_T to reduce the risk of overdistention of some lung areas. Just as there is a LIP on the PV loop, there is an upper inflection point (UIP) which corresponds to the point at which maximal recruitment has been attained – beyond this point, further increases in pressure or tidal volume will result in lung overdistention (Fig. 39.21). For this reason, many authorities recommend setting the ventilator so that PIP's are below the UIP of the PV loop.

Flow-Volume (FV) Loops

The recognition and treatment of increased airway resistance (especially expiratory airway obstruction) is essential and the flow-volume (FV) loop is the most commonly used ventilator graphic to assess changes in respiratory system resistance. In contrast to the classical presentation of lung function measurements in the Pulmonary Function laboratory, typically, the inspiratory flow limb of the FV loop is shown above the x-axis (i.e. positive flow value), while the expiratory limb of the FV loop is shown below the x-axis (i.e. negative flow value) (Fig. 39.22). However, some ventilators display the FV loop in the opposite manner as well (consistent with the classic depiction on FV obtained obtained in the ambulatory setting in the Pulmonary Function laboratory). Limitation of the inspiratory flow (flattening of the inspiratory limb) is commonly observed in the presence of an extrathoracic airway obstruction (recall that extrathoracic airway obstruction is worse during inspiration – e.g.

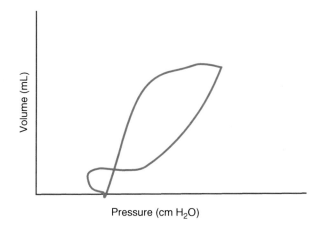

Fig. 39.20 Pressure-volume loop showing a "trigger tail." The "trigger tail" is due to the patient's spontaneous breath, triggering a ventilator breath

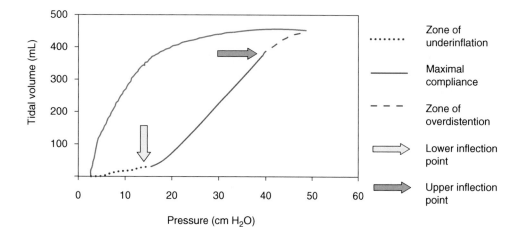

Fig. 39.21 Pressure-volume loop showing upper and lower inflection points

Fig. 39.22 Normal flow-volume loop. The inspiratory limb is on the positive side of the y-axis, while the expiratory limb is on the negative side of the y-axis (this arrangement can of course change, depending on the different ventilators that are used in the PICU)

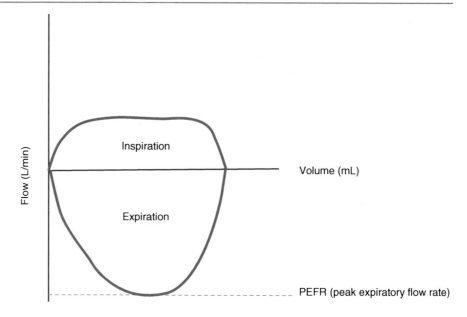

Fig. 39.23 Flow-volume loop of a patient with extrathoracic obstruction. The normal inspiratory limb of the FV loop is depicted as a *dotted line*. Recall that extrathoracic obstruction is worse during inspiration. Therefore, the inspiratory limb of the FV loop is flattened in appearance in a patient with extrathoracic obstruction (e.g. kinked or obstructed tracheal tube, croup, supraglottitis, bacterial tracheitis, etc)

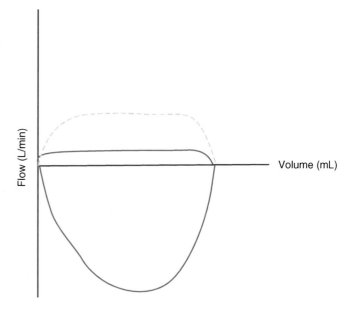

croup presents with inspiratory stridor) (Fig. 39.23), while limitation of the expiratory flow (flattening of the inspiratory limb) is commonly observed in the presence of intrathoracic airway obstruction (recall that intrathoracic airway obstruction is worse during expiration – e.g. asthma presents with expiratory wheeze) (Fig. 39.24).

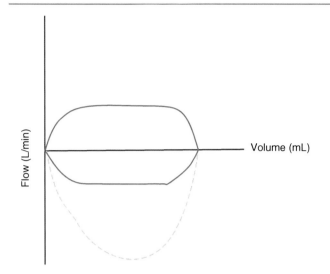

Fig. 39.24 Flow-volume loop of a patient with intrathoracic obstruction. The normal expiratory limb of the FV loop is depicted as a *dotted line*. Recall that intrathoracic obstruction is worse during expiration. Therefore, the expiratory limb of the FV loop is flattened in appearance in a patient with intrathoracic obstruction (e.g. asthma, bronchiolitis, etc)

Conclusion

Respiratory monitoring is an integral part in the overall care of the critically ill child in the PICU. In this chapter, we have focused primarily on the most commonly available respiratory monitoring techniques. There are certainly more advanced types of respiratory monitoring that are becoming more widely available. Regardless, an in-depth understanding of these most commonly used respiratory monitoring techniques is essential. The interested reader is referred to other reviews and chapters for a more in-depth discussion of the less commonly used, more advanced techniques, such as extravascular lung water measurement, esophageal pressure monitoring, electrical bioimpedance tomography (EIT), etc.

References

1. Gregory GA. Respiratory failure in the child. New York: Churchill Livingstone; 1981.
2. Farias JA, Frutos F, Esteban A, Flores JC, Retta A, Baltodano A, et al. What is the daily practice of mechanical ventilation in pediatric intensive care units? A multicenter study. Intensive Care Med. 2004;30:918–25.
3. Khemani RG, Markovitz BP, Curley MA. Characteristics of children intubated and mechanically ventilated in 16 PICUs. Chest. 2009;136:765–71.
4. Wolfler A, Calderoni E, Ottonello G, Conti G, Baroncini S, Santuz P, et al. Daily practice of mechanical ventilation in Italian pediatric intensive care units: a prospective survey. Pediatr Crit Care Med. 2011;12:141–6.
5. Farias JA, Fernandez A, Monteverde E, Flores JC, Baltodano A, Menchacha A, et al. Mechanical ventilation in pediatric intensive care units during the season for acute lower respiratory infection: a multicenter study. Pediatr Crit Care Med. 2012;13:158–64.
6. Curran-Everett D. A classic learning opportunity from Fenn, Rahn, and Otis (1946): the alveolar gas equation. Adv Physiol Educ. 2006;30:58–62.
7. Armstrong JAM, Guleria A, Girling K. Evaluation of gas exchange deficit in the critically ill. Contin Educ Anaesth Crit Care Pain. 2007;7:131–4.
8. Douglas ME, Downs JB, Dannemiller FJ, Hodges MR, Munson ES. Changes in pulmonary venous admixture with varying inspired oxygen. Anesth Analg. 1976;55:688–95.
9. Wandrup JH. Quantifying pulmonary oxygen transfer deficits in critically ill patients. Acta Anaesthesiol Scand Suppl. 1995;107:37–44.
10. Gowda MS, Klocke RA. Variability of indices of hypoxemia in adult respiratory distress syndrome. Crit Care Med. 1997;25:41–5.
11. Kathirgamanathan A, McCahon RA, Hardman JG. Indices of pulmonary oxygenation in pathological lung states: an investigation using high-fidelity, computational modelling. Br J Anaesth. 2009;103:291–7.
12. Cane RD, Shapiro BA, Templin R, Walther K. Unreliability of oxygen tension-based indices in reflecting intrapulmonary shunting in critically ill patients. Crit Care Med. 1988;16:1243–5.
13. Sganga G, Siegel JH, Coleman B, Giovannini I, Boldrini G, Pittiruti M. The physiologic meaning of the respiratory index in various types of critical illness. Circ Shock. 1985;17:179–93.
14. Gilbert R, Auchincloss JHJ, Kuppinger M, Thomas M. Stability of the arterial-alveolar oxygen partial pressure ratio. Effects of low ventilation/perfusion regions. Crit Care Med. 1979;7:267–72.
15. Aboab J, Louis B, Jonson B, Brochard L. Relation between PaO2/FIO2 ratio and FIO2: a mathematical description. Intensive Care Med. 2006;32:1494–7.
16. Bernard GR, Artigas A, Brigham KL, Carlet J, Falke K, Hudson L, et al. The American-European Consensus Conference on ARDS. Definitions, mechanisms, relevant outcomes, and clinical trial coordination. Am J Respir Crit Care Med. 1994;149:818–24.
17. Force ADT, Ranieri VM, Rubenfeld GD, Thompson BT, Ferguson ND, Caldwell E, et al. Acute respiratory distress syndrome: the Berlin definition. JAMA. 2012;307:2526–33.
18. Ferguson ND, Fan E, Camporota L, Antonelli M, Anzueto A, Beale R, et al. The Berlin definition of ARDS: an expanded rationale, justification, and supplementary material. Intensive Care Med. 2012;38:1573–82.
19. Pathan N, Ridout DA, Smith E, Goldman AP, Brown KL. Predictors of outcome for children requiring respiratory extra-corporeal life support: implications for inclusion and exclusion criteria. Intensive Care Med. 2008;34:2256–63.
20. Goldman AP, Tasker RC, Hosiasson S, Henrichsen T, Macrae DP. Early response to inhaled nitric oxide and its relationship to outcome in children with severe hypoxemic respiratory failure. Chest. 1997;112:752–8.
21. Flori HR, Glidden DV, Rutherford GW, Matthay MA. Pediatric acute lung injury: prospective evaluation of risk factors associated with mortality. Am J Respir Crit Care Med. 2005;171:995–1001.
22. Erickson S, Schibler A, Numa A, Nuthall G, Yung M, Pascoe E, et al. Acute lung injury in pediatric intensive care in Australia and New Zealand: a prospective, multicenter, observational study. Pediatr Crit Care Med. 2007;8:317–23.
23. Ben-Abraham R, Weinbroum AA, Augerten A, Toren A, Harel R, Vardi A, et al. Acute respiratory distress syndrome in children with malignancy – can we predict outcome? J Crit Care. 2001;16:54–8.
24. Wittekamp BH, Chalabi M, van Mook WN, Winkens B, Verbon A, Bermans DC. Catheter-related bloodstream infections: a prospective observational study of central venous and arterial catheters. Scand J Infect Dis. 2013;45(10):738–45.
25. Traore O, Liotier J, Souweine B. Prospective study of arterial and central venous catheter colonization and of arterial- and central venous catheter-related bacteremia in intensive care units. Crit Care Med. 2005;33:1276–80.

26. Salyer JW, Chatburn RL, Dolcini DM. Measured versus calculated oxygen saturation in a population of pediatric intensive care patients. Respir Care. 1989;34:342–8.

27. Neff T. Routine oximetry: a fifth vital sign? Chest. 1988;94:227.

28. Mower WR, Sachs C, Nicklin EL, Baraff LJ. Pulse oximetry as a fifth pediatric vital sign. Pediatrics. 1997;99:681–6.

29. Moller JT, Johannessen NW, Espersen K, Ravlo O, Pedersen PF, Rasmussen NH, et al. Randomized evaluation of pulse oximetry in 20,802 patients: II perioperative events and postoperative complications. Anesthesiology. 1993;78:445–53.

30. Ochroch EA, Russell MW, Hanson 3rd WC, Devine GA, Cucchiara AJ, Weiner MG, et al. The impact of continuous pulse oximetry monitoring on intensive care unit admissions from a postsurgical floor. Anesth Analg. 2006;102:868–75.

31. Salyer JW. Neonatal and pediatric pulse oximetry. Respir Care. 2003;48:386–96.

32. Cannesson M, Broccard A, Vallet B, Bendjelid K. Monitoring in the intensive care unit: its past, present, and future. Crit Care Res Pract. 2012;2012:452769.

33. Popovich DM, Richiuso N, Danek G. Pediatric health care providers' knowledge of pulse oximetry. Pediatr Nurs. 2004;30:14–20.

34. Stoneham MD, Saville GM, Wilson IH. Knowledge about pulse oximetry among medical and nursing staff. Lancet. 1994;344: 1339–42.

35. Rodriguez LR, Kotin N, Lowenthal D, Kattan M. A study of pediatric house staff's knowledge of pulse oximetry. Pediatrics. 1994; 93:810–3.

36. Davies G, Gibson AM, Swanney M, Murray D, Beckert L. Understanding of pulse oximetry among hospital staff. N Z Med J. 2003;116:U297.

37. Fouzas S, Politis P, Skylogianni E, Syriopoulou T, Priftis KN, Chatzimichael A, et al. Knowledge on pulse oximetry among pediatric health care professionals: a multicenter survey. Pediatrics. 2010;126:e657–62.

38. Fouzas S, Priftis KN, Anthracopoulos MB. Pulse oximetry in pediatric practice. Pediatrics. 2011;128:740–52.

39. Mannheimer P. The light-tissue interaction of pulse oximetry. Anesth Analg. 2007;105:S10–7.

40. Chan ED, Chan MM, Chan MM. Pulse oximetry: understanding its basic principles facilitates appreciation of its limitations. Respir Med. 2013;107:789–99.

41. Kelleher JF. Pulse oximetry. J Clin Monit. 1989;5:37–62.

42. Schnapp LM, Cohen NH. Pulse oximetry: uses and abuses. Chest. 1990;98:1244–50.

43. Sinex JE. Pulse oximetry: principles and limitations. Am J Emerg Med. 1999;17:59–67.

44. Faconi S. Reliability of pulse oximetry in hypoxic infants. J Pediatr. 1988;112:424–7.

45. Severinghaus JW, Naifeh KH, Koh SO. Errors in 14 pulse oximeters during profound hypoxemia. J Clin Monit. 1989;5:72–81.

46. Lebecque P, Shango P, Stijns M, Vliers A, Coates AL. Pulse oximetry versus measured arterial oxygen saturation: a comparison of the Nellcor N100 and Biox III. Pediatr Pulmonol. 1991;10:132–5.

47. Schmitt HJ, Schuetz WH, Proeschel PA, Jaklin C. Accuracy of pulse oximetry in children with cyanotic congenital heart disease. J Cardiothorac Vasc Anesth. 1993;7:61–5.

48. Trivedi NS, Ghouri AF, Lai E, Shah NK, Barker SJ. Pulse oximeter performance during desaturation and resaturation: a comparison of seven models. J Clin Anesth. 1997;9:184–8.

49. Carter BG, Carlin JB, Tibballs J, Mead H, Hochmann M, Osborne A. Accuracy of two pulse oximeters at low arterial hemoglobin-oxygen saturation. Crit Care Med. 1998;26:1128–33.

50. MacLeod DB, Cortinez LI, Keifer JC, Cameron D, Wright DR, White WD, et al. The desaturation response time of finger pulse oximeters during mild hypothermia. Anaesthesia. 2005;60: 65–71.

51. Berkenbosch JW, Tobias JD. Comparison of a new forehead reflectance pulse oximeter sensor with a conventional digit sensor in pediatric patients. Respir Care. 2006;51:726–31.

52. Comber JT, Lopez BL. Evaluation of pulse oximetry in sickle cell anemia patients presenting to the emergency department in acute vasoocclusive crisis. Am J Emerg Med. 1996;14:16–8.

53. Ortiz FO, Aldrich TK, Nagel RL, Benjamin LJ. Accuracy of pulse oximetry in sickle cell disease. Am J Respir Crit Care Med. 1999;159:447–51.

54. Fitzgerald RK, Johnson A. Pulse oximetry in sickle cell anemia. Crit Care Med. 2001;29:1803–6.

55. Ahmed S, Siddiqui AK, Sison CP, Shahid RK, Mattana J. Hemoglobin oxygen saturation discrepancy using various methods in patients with sickle cell vaso-occlusive painful crisis. Eur J Haematol. 2005;74:309–14.

56. Scheller MS, Unger RJ, Kelner MJ. Effects of intravenously administered dyes on pulse oximetry readings. Anesthesiology. 1986; 65:550–2.

57. Schmitt JM. Simple photon diffusion analysis of the effects of multiple scattering on pulse oximetry. IEEE Trans Biomed Eng. 1991; 38:1194–203.

58. Lee S, Tremper KK, Barker SJ. Effects of anemia on pulse oximetry and continuous mixed venous hemoglobin saturation monitoring in dogs. Anesthesiology. 1991;75:118–22.

59. Severinghaus JW, Koh SO. Effect of anemia on pulse oximeter accuracy at low saturation. J Clin Monit. 1990;6:85–8.

60. Jay GD, Hughes L, Renzi FP. Pulse oximetry is accurate in acute anemia from hemorrhage. Ann Emerg Med. 1994;24:32–5.

61. Tremper KK, Barker SJ. Pulse oximetry. Anesthesiology. 1989;70: 98–108.

62. Broome IJ, Mills GH, Spiers P, Reilly CS. An evaluation of the effect of vasodilation on oxygen saturations measured by pulse oximetry and venous blood gas analysis. Anaesthesia. 1993;48:415–6.

63. Secker C, Spiers P. Accuracy of pulse oximetry in patients with low systemic vascular resistance. Anaesthesia. 1997;52:127–30.

64. Hummler HD, Engelmann A, Pohlandt F, Hogel J, Franz AR. Decreased accuracy of pulse oximetry measurements during low perfusion caused by sepsis: is the perfusion index of any value? Intensive Care Med. 2006;32:1428–31.

65. Smatlak P, Knebel AR. Clinical evaluation of noninvasive monitoring of oxygen saturation in critically ill patients. Am J Crit Care. 1998;7:370–3.

66. Wilson BJ, Cowan HJ, Lord JA, Zuege DJ, Zygun DA. The accuracy of pulse oximetry in emergency department patients with severe sepsis and septic shock: a retrospective cohort study. BMC Emerg Med. 2010;10:9.

67. Courtney SE, Weber KR, Breakie LA, Malin SW, Bender CV, Guo SM, et al. Capillary blood gases in the neonate. A reassessment and review of ther literature. Am J Dis Child. 1990;144:168–72.

68. Harrison AM, Lynch JM, Dean JM, Witte MK. Comparison of simultaneously obtained arterial and capillary blood gases in pediatric intensive care unit patients. Crit Care Med. 1997;25:1904–8.

69. Escalante-Kanashiro R, Tantalean-Da-Fieno J. Capillary blood gases in a pediatric intensive care unit. Crit Care Med. 2000; 28:224–6.

70. Ueta I, Jacobs BR. Capillary and arterial blood gases in hemorrhagic shock: a comparative study. Pediatr Crit Care Med. 2002; 3:375–7.

71. Yildizdas D, Yapicioglu H, Yilmaz HL, Sertdemir Y. Correlation of simultaneously obtained capillary, venous, and arterial blood gases of patients in a paediatric intensive care unit. Arch Dis Child. 2004;89:176–80.

72. Fernandez EG, Green TP, Sweeney M. Low inferior vena caval catheters for hemodynamic and pulmonary function monitoring in pediatric critical care patients. Pediatr Crit Care Med. 2004;5: 14–8.

73. Malinoski DJ, Todd SR, Slone S, Mullins RJ, Schreiber MA. Correlation of central venous and arterial blood gas measurements in mechanically ventilated trauma patients. Arch Surg. 2005;140:1122–5.

74. Walkey AJ, Farber HW, O'Donnell C, Cabral H, Eagan JS, Philippides GJ. The accuracy of the central venous blood gas for acid-base monitoring. J Intensive Care Med. 2010;25:104–10.

75. Treger R, Pirouz S, Kamangar N, Corry D. Agreement between central venous and arterial blood gas measurements in the intensive care unit. Clin J Am Soc Nephrol. 2010;5:390–4.

76. Tobias JD, Meyer DJJ, Helikson MA. Monitoring of pH and PCO2 in children using the Paratrend 7 in a peripheral vein. Can J Anaesth. 1998;45:81–3.

77. Tobias JD, Connors D, Strauser L, Johnson T. Continuous pH and PCO2 monitoring during respiratory failure in children with Paratrend 7 inserted into the peripheral venous system. J Pediatr. 2000;136:623–7.

78. Kelly AM, McAlpine R, Kyle E. Venous pH can safely replace arterial pH in the initial evaluation of patients in the emergency department. Emerg Med J. 2001;18:340–2.

79. Kelly AM, Kyle E, McAlpine R. Venous pCO2 and pH can be used to screen for significant hypercarbia in emergency patients with acute respiratory distress. J Emerg Med. 2002;22:15–9.

80. Sullivan KJ, Kissoon N, Goodwin SR. End-tidal carbon dioxide monitoring in pediatric emergencies. Pediatr Emerg Care. 2005;21:327–32.

81. Thompson JE, Jaffe MB. Capnographic waveforms in the mechanically ventilated patients. Respir Care. 2005;50:100–9.

82. Hamel DS, Cheifetz IM. Do all mechanically ventilated pediatric patients require continuous capnography? Respir Care Clin N Am. 2006;12:501–13.

83. Carlton GC, Ray CJ, Miodownik S, Kopec I, Groeger JS. Capnography in mechanically ventilated patients. Crit Care Med. 1988;16:550–6.

84. Walsh BK, Crotwell DN, Restrepo RD. Capnograph/capnometry during mechanical ventilation: 2011. Respir Care. 2011;56:503–9.

85. Tobias JD, Flanagan JF, Wheeler TJ, Garrett JS, Burney C. Noninvasive monitoring of end-tidal CO2 via nasal cannulas in spontaneously breathing children during the perioperative period. Crit Care Med. 1994;22:1805–8.

86. Flanagan JF, Garrett JS, McDuffee A, Tobias JD. Noninvasive monitoring of end-tidal carbon dioxide tension via nasal cannulas in spontaneously breathing children with profound hypocarbia. Crit Care Med. 1995;23:1140–2.

87. Anderson JL, Junkins E, Pribble C, Guenther E. Capnography and depth of sedation during propofol sedation in children. Ann Emerg Med. 2007;49:9–13.

88. Krauss B, Hess DR. Capnography for procedural sedation and analgesia in the emergency department. Ann Emerg Med. 2007;50:172–81.

89. Deitch K, Miner J, Chudnofsky CR, Dominici P, Latta D. Does end tidal CO2 monitoring during emergency department procedural sedation and analgesia with propofol decrease the incidence of hypoxic events? A randomized, controlled trial. Ann Emerg Med. 2010;55:258–64.

90. Abramo TJ, Wiebe RA, Scott SM, Primm PA, McIntyre D, Mydler T. Noninvasive capnometry in a pediatric population with respiratory emergencies. Pediatr Emerg Care. 1996;12:252–4.

91. Abramo TJ, Wiebe RA, Scott S, Goto CS, McIntyre DD. Noninvasive capnometry monitoring for respiratory status during pediatric seizures. Crit Care Med. 1997;25:1242–6.

92. Abramo T, Cowan MR, Scott SM, Primm PA, Wiebe RA, Signs M. Comparison of pediatric end-tidal CO2 measured with nasal/oral cannula circuit and capillary PCO2. Am J Emerg Med. 1995;13:30–3.

93. McSwain SD, Hamel DS, Smith PB, Gentile MA, Srinivasan S, Meliones JN, et al. End-tidal and arterial carbon dioxide measurements correlate across all levels of physiologic dead space. Respir Care. 2010;55:288–93.

94. Coss-Bu JA, Walding DL, David YB, Jefferson LS. Dead space ventilation in critically ill children with lung injury. Chest. 2003;123:2050–6.

95. Nuckton TJ, Alonso JA, Kallet RH, Daniel BM, Pittet JF, Eisner MD, et al. Pulmonary dead-space fraction as a risk factor for death in the acute respiratory distress syndrome. N Engl J Med. 2002;346:1281–6.

96. Kallet RH, Alonso JA, Pittet JF, Matthay MA. Prognostic value of the pulmonary dead-space fraction during the first 6 days of acute respiratory distress syndrome. Respir Care. 2004;49:1008–14.

97. Lucangelo U, Bernabe F, Vatua S, Degrassi G, Villagra A, Fernandez RL, et al. Prognostic value of different dead space indices in mechanically ventilated patients with acute lung injury and ARDS. Chest. 2008;133:62–71.

98. Raurich JM, Vilar M, Colomar A, Ibanez J, Ayestaran I, Perez-Barcena J, et al. Prognostic value of the pulmonary dead-space fraction during the early and intermediate phases of acute respiratory distress syndrome. Respir Care. 2010;55:282–7.

99. Maisch S, Reissmann H, Feuellekrug B, Weismann D, Rutkowski T, Tusman G, et al. Compliance and dead space fraction indicate an optimal level of positive end-expiratory pressure after recruitment in anesthetized patients. Anesth Analg. 2008;106:175–81.

100. Fengmei G, Chen J, Songqiao L, Congshan Y, Yi Y. Dead space fraction changes during PEEP titration following lung recruitment in patients with ARDS. Respir Care. 2012;57:1578–85.

101. Blanch L, Fernandez R, Benito S, Mancebo J, Net A. Effect of PEEP on the arterial minus end-tidal carbon dioxide gradient. Chest. 1987;92:451–4.

102. Murray IP, Modell JH, Gallagher TJ, Banner MJ. Titration of PEEP by the arterial minus end-tidal carbon dioxide gradient. Chest. 1984;85:100–4.

103. Soubani AO. Noninvasive monitoring of oxygen and carbon dioxide. Am J Emerg Med. 2001;18:141–6.

104. Blanch L, Romero PV, Lucangelo U. Volumetric capnography in the mechanically ventilated patient. Minerva Anestesiol. 2006;72:577–85.

105. Cheifetz IM. Advances in monitoring and management of pediatric acute lung injury. Pediatr Clin North Am. 2013;60:621–39.

106. Riou Y, Leclerc F, Neve V, Dupuy L, Noizet O, Leteurtre S, et al. Reproducibility of the respiratory dead space measurements in mechanically ventilated children using the CO2SMO monitor. Intensive Care Med. 2004;30:1461–7.

107. Kallet RH, Daniel BM, Garcia O, Matthay MA. Accuracy of physiologic dead space measurements in patients with acute respiratory distress syndrome using volumetric capnography: comparison with the metabolic monitor method. Respir Care. 2005;50:462–7.

108. Almeida-Junior AA, da Silva MT, Almeida CC, Ribeiro JD. Relationship between physiologic deadspace/tidal volume ratio and gas exchange in infants with acute bronchiolitis on invasive mechanical ventilation. Pediatr Crit Care Med. 2007;8:372–7.

109. Tusman G, Sipmann FS, Borges JB, Hedenstierna G, Bohm SH. Validation of Bohr dead space measured by volumetric capnography. Intensive Care Med. 2011;37:870–4.

110. Tusman G, Sipmann FS, Bohm SH. Rationale of dead space measurement by volumetric capnography. Anesth Analg. 2012;114:866–74.

111. Sinha P, Soni N. Comparison of volumetric capnography and mixed expired gas methods to calculate physiological dead space in mechanically ventilated ICU patients. Intensive Care Med. 2012;38:1712–7.

112. Siobal MS, Ong H, Valdes J, Tang J. Calculation of physiologic dead space: comparison of ventilator volumetric capnography to

measurements by metabolic analyzer and volumetric CO2 monitor. Respir Care. 2013;58:1143–51.

113. Monaco F, Nickerson BG, McQuitty JC. Continuous transcutaneous oxygen and carbon dioxide monitoring in the pediatric ICU. Crit Care Med. 1982;10:765–6.

114. Hamilton PA, Whitehead MD, Reynolds EO. Underestimation of arterial oxygen tension by transcutaneous electrode with increasing age in infants. Arch Dis Child. 1985;60:1162–5.

115. Sivan Y, Eldadah MK, Cheah TE, Newth CJ. Estimation of arterial carbon dioxide by end-tidal and transcutaneous PCO2 measurement in ventilated children. Pediatr Pulmonol. 1992;12:153–7.

116. Palmisano BW, Severinghaus JW. Transcutaneous PCO2 and PO2: a multicenter study of accuracy. J Clin Monit. 1990;6:189–95.

117. Tobias JD, Wilson WRJ, Meyer DJ. Transcutaneous monitoring of carbon dioxide tension after cardiothoracic surgery in infants and children. Anesth Analg. 1999;88:531–4.

118. Tobias JD, Meyer DJ. Noninvasive monitoring of carbon dioxide during respiratory failure in toddlers and infants: end-tidal versus transcutaneous carbon dioxide. Anesthesiology. 1997;85:55–8.

119. Nosovitch MA, Johnson JO, Tobias JD. Noninvasive intraoperative monitoring of carbon dioxide in children: end-tidal versus transcutaneous techniques. Paediatr Anaesth. 2002;12:48–52.

120. Berkenbosch JW, Tobias JD. Transcutaneous carbon dioxide monitoring during high-frequency oscillatory ventilation in infants and children. Crit Care Med. 2002;30:1024–7.

121. Epstein MF, Cohen AR, Feldman HA, Raemer DB. Estimation of PaCO2 by two noninvasive methods in the critically ill newborn infant. J Pediatr. 1985;106:282–6.

122. Tobias JD. Transcutaneous carbon dioxide monitoring in infants and children. Paediatr Anaesth. 2009;19:434–44.

123. Cannon ML, Cornell J, Tripp-Hamel DS, Gentile MA, Hubble CL, Meliones JN, et al. Tidal volumes for ventilated infants should be determined with a pneumotachometer placed at the endotracheal tube. Am J Respir Crit Care Med. 2000;162:2109–12.

Hemodynamic Monitoring

Shane M. Tibby

Abstract

This chapter will cover key elements of hemodynamic monitoring, including pressure and flow measurements, constituents of cardiac output, markers of adequacy of flow and measures of regional perfusion. Emphasis will be on important physiological concepts, and how these relate to monitoring tools (for example, applications of the Fick principle). Newer modalities are introduced which were not included in the previous edition of the textbook, and include new methods for cardiac output measurement (transpulmonary ultrasound dilution, electrical velocimetry), Near Infrared Spectroscopy (NIRS), and Tissue Doppler Imaging.

Keywords

Hemodynamic monitoring • Cardiac output • Venous oxygen saturations • Perfusion

Introduction

Hemodynamic monitoring encompasses all pressure and flow measurements in relation to the cardiovascular system. The science of hemodynamics has its origins in the seventeenth and eighteenth centuries, from the pioneering work of William Harvey and the Reverend Stephen Hales. Hemodynamics incorporates monitoring within the wider consideration of the theoretical aspects of the forces responsible for the development and propagation of the pressure and flow pulses. Appreciation of hemodynamic monitoring requires an understanding of the structure of the heart and blood vessels, cardiovascular physiology, and fluid mechanics [1].

Vascular Pressure Measurement

Maintaining an adequate perfusion pressure is a vital adjunct to ensuring adequate oxygen delivery [2]. The two common invasive pressure measurements undertaken in the ICU are arterial and central venous pressures. Pressure measurement typically involves an in-dwelling catheter, fluid-filled non-compliant tubing, and a pressure chamber containing a diaphragm, which is connected to a pressure transducer. Pulsatile pressure transmitted from the blood vessel displaces the diaphragm; this movement is sensed by a transducer, which relays an electric signal to a visual monitor via a preamplifier. Blood sampling and zeroing to atmosphere are possible via a three-way tap within the tubing, and the system is kept patent via a continuous infusion of saline [1, 3].

The relationship between signal input and output is known as the transfer function. In a system measuring vascular pressures, the transfer function has two components – one relating to the steady state response, the other to the transient response [4]. The steady state response relates to the regular, periodic signals produced by an unchanging or minimally changing blood pressure and heart rate. Such a signal can be represented by Fourier analysis [5]. The transient response refers to how the system attempts to re-achieve a steady state when the input is rapidly altered, both in terms of frequency (heart rate) or amplitude (blood pressure). Two interacting components affect the transient response – the natural frequency of the system and the damping constant [6]. For each natural frequency there is a range of optimal dampening. If the system is overdamped, systolic pressure will be

S.M. Tibby, MBChB, MRCP, MSc (appl stat)
PICU Department, Evelina London Children's Hospital,
Westminster Bridge Road, London SE1 7EH, UK
e-mail: shane.tibby@gstt.nhs.uk

D.S. Wheeler et al. (eds.), *Pediatric Critical Care Medicine*,
DOI 10.1007/978-1-4471-6362-6_40, © Springer-Verlag London 2014

underestimated and diastolic pressure overestimated (however mean pressures will be relatively accurate). Conversely, an underdamped system will overestimate systolic pressure and give a distorted waveform overall [6]. Dampening can be estimated crudely at the bedside by (a) observation of the waveform and (b) a "fast-flush" test, where 1–2 mL of saline is flushed rapidly through the system at a pressure in excess of the systolic pressure and the ensuing signal observed. In an overdamped system, the pressure trace will be slow to return to the pulsatile waveform after the flush, and there will be no oscillation as it re-equilibrates with the blood pressure signal. The pressure trace in an underdamped system will return rapidly towards the blood pressure wave, but will show a series of rapid oscillations around the blood pressure as it re-equilibrates [6, 7]. The transient response can be optimized by utilizing tubing that is non-compliant and not of excessive length, monitoring for kinks in the tubing and the intravascular catheter, and avoiding small air bubbles and clots within the system [8, 9].

The arterial pressure pulse waveform is a function of a number of factors (in addition to dampening), including stroke volume, arterial compliance, arterial impedance, peripheral resistance, inertia, and wave reflection (see section "Arterial pulse contour analysis") [10, 11]. As these properties change along the arterial tree, so does the pulse pressure waveform. These changes are more marked in children than in adults [12]. This means that a centrally measured pressure will have a lower systolic pressure, higher diastolic pressure, and an approximately equal mean pressure to that from a peripherally measured site.

Cardiac Output

Cardiac output is the volume of blood ejected by the heart per minute. It is usually expressed relative to body surface area, which means that the normal range of 3.5–5.5 L/min/m^2 is applicable throughout the entire pediatric age range. Cardiac output is the net result of inter-relating factors affecting both myocardial systolic (heart rate, preload, contractility, and afterload) and diastolic function [13]. Measurement of cardiac output is uncommon in pediatrics, due to a variety of factors including perceived worth and technical difficulty [2]. However, the relevance of cardiac output monitoring in selected patients is underlined by the fact that: (a) the heart is one of the most common organs to fail during critical illness [14], (b) other failing organs and supportive therapies aimed at these organs can impact cardiac function (e.g. mechanical ventilation) [15], (c) it cannot be estimated clinically [16], and (d) low-flow states carry a higher mortality in certain diseases [17].

Traditionally cardiac output has been difficult to measure in small children. However, a variety of less invasive methods are now available. Nonetheless the decision to measure cardiac output represents a balance between the risks involved with the technique and the potential benefits gained from the additional hemodynamic information. The latter point requires a thorough understanding of both the modality used and the basic principles of cardiovascular physiology. If both of these criteria are not fulfilled there is potential for iatrogenic harm to the patient. Cardiac output monitoring is unnecessary in all ICU patients, but may be indicated for patients in the following categories: shock states, multiple organ failure, cardiopulmonary interactions during mechanical ventilation, congenital and acquired heart disease, assessment of selected new therapies and during clinical research which leads to a greater understanding of a disease process [18].

Common techniques for measurement of cardiac output can be categorized as utilizing indicator dilution, the Fick principle, Doppler ultrasound, impedance, pulse contour analysis, and other miscellaneous methods. In addition, these modalities can also be categorized as intermittent versus continuous, as well as invasive versus non- (or minimally invasive). When considering which modality to use for a particular patient, it is worth considering the eight desirable monitoring characteristics defined by Shephard: accuracy, reproducibility, rapid response time, operator independence, ease of application, no morbidity, continuous use, and cost effectiveness [19].

Indicator Dilution Techniques

Stewart published the first indicator dilution method for measurement of blood volume flow in 1897, based upon Hering's earlier work on blood velocity measurement [20]. Hamilton subsequently applied this principle to the measurement of cardiac output between 1928 and 1932 [21]. A number of dilution techniques are now available, however all follow the same principle, regardless of the indicator used (temperature, dye, charge) [22]. Blood flow can be calculated following a central venous injection of an indicator by measuring the change in indicator concentration over time at a point downstream of the injection. This can be expressed mathematically as:

$$\text{cardiac output} = \frac{\text{amount of indicator injected}}{\int_0^\infty \text{conc indicator}(t)dt}$$

The denominator refers to the integral of the indicator concentration with time. In other words, the area under the curve (AUC) for indicator concentration versus time measured between time of injection and infinity. Cardiac output is therefore inversely proportional to the AUC for the change in indicator concentration over time. Large AUC's therefore suggest low cardiac output, and vice versa. High flow situations produce small, peaked curves, while low flow situations

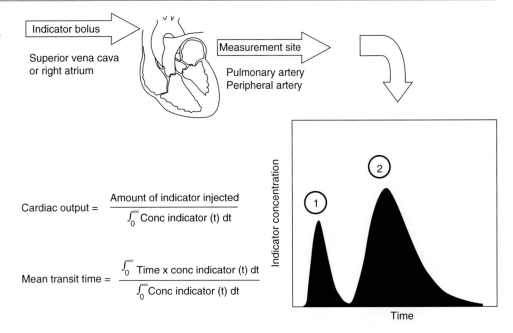

Fig. 40.1 Generalized schema for an indicator dilution method. *Curve 1* shows a typical curve seen with a high cardiac output; *curve 2*, occurring with a low cardiac output, is larger with an accentuated tail secondary to recirculation

Indicator bolus

Superior vena cava or right atrium

Measurement site

Pulmonary artery
Peripheral artery

$$\text{Cardiac output} = \frac{\text{Amount of indicator injected}}{\int_0^\infty \text{Conc indicator (t) dt}}$$

$$\text{Mean transit time} = \frac{\int_0^\infty \text{Time x conc indicator (t) dt}}{\int_0^\infty \text{Conc indicator (t) dt}}$$

produce curves which are larger, less peaked and with a longer tail (Fig. 40.1).

One problem inherent in dilution methods is that of recirculation. Recirculation refers to the phenomenon whereby the indicator within the initial portion of the concentration-time curve traverses the body and arrives back at the measurement site before the terminal portion of concentration-time curve has passed the measurement site. The net effect of this is a secondary (and sometimes tertiary) curve superimposed on the primary curve (Fig. 40.2). This may occur in states of low cardiac output. Calculation of cardiac output thus requires the "separation" of the primary curve from the composite. Several methods are available for doing this. The most widely used is that offered by Stewart and Hamilton, which assumes a monoexponential decay of the primary curve after a given time point [23]. Other methods include deconvolution [24], and fitting the declining part of the primary curve with lognormal, gamma and local density random walk probability distributions [25]. These methods are beyond the scope of this chapter. A possible source of extreme recirculation pertinent to pediatric practice is that which occurs in the presence of an anatomical shunt (either Left to Right shunts or Right to Left shunts), depending upon where the indicator is measured. In the presence of a large shunt, it may be impossible to identify the primary curve. Conversely, other authors have suggested methods for quantifying the shunt in relation to the appearance of the second peak [26–32].

Indicator dilution is accurate provided a series of conditions are met. These include rapid and even indicator injection, complete mixing of the indicator and blood, no loss of indicator between injection and measurement, no anatomical shunt, minimal valve regurgitation, and steady state flow [33].

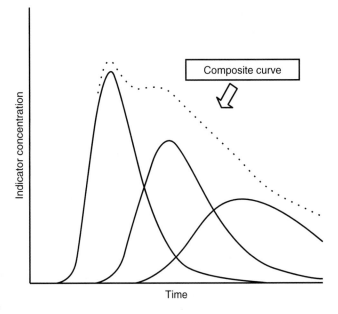

Composite curve

Fig. 40.2 Early recirculation, as in the case of an intracardiac shunt, may produce a composite curve with several peaks and a prolonged delay phase. Here the composite curve results from superposition of the primary, secondary and tertiary curves. Note the double peak, which may be seen with an anatomical shunt

Any of these conditions will impact the accuracy of measuring the change in indicator concentration over time.

Another useful property of indicator dilution curves is that they also allow for calculation of vascular volumes via the mean transit and exponential down slope times (see again, Fig. 40.1) [34]. Various vascular volumes have been used as measures of preload (see section "Transpulmonary thermodilution"). Indeed, other calculations relating to tissue volumes and liver function are also possible, depending on the indicator used.

Pulmonary Thermodilution (Swan-Ganz Catheters)

Pulmonary thermodilution utilizes temperature as the indicator and involves injection of a cooled solution into the right atrium (typically normal saline or 5 % dextrose), with temperature change sensed by thermistors at the injection site and in the pulmonary artery. This technique was first described in dogs by Fegler in 1954 [35], subsequently described in humans by Branthwaite and Bradley in 1968 [36], and introduced clinically with the development of the Swan-Ganz, or pulmonary artery catheter in 1970 [37]. Over the next 30 years this became the most widely used method for measurement of cardiac output in adults, although use in children remained limited, mainly due to technical constraints [18, 38–41]. Over the last 15 years the use of the pulmonary artery catheter has declined, considerably, possibly as a consequence of other, less-invasive methods becoming available, lack of benefit (and perhaps even harm) from several large studies, and also due to several authors questioning the value of cardiac output measurement, particularly via this technique [42–48]. This last point is supported by two large, trans-Atlantic surveys, which showed that many ICU clinicians lack the rudimentary skills for safe pulmonary artery catheter insertion and interpretation of readings [49, 50].

The Swan-Ganz catheter is typically inserted percutaneously through a sheath introducer (of a size larger than the catheter itself, e.g. 8.5 French introducer for a 7 French catheter) using the Seldinger technique. The left subclavian route is the preferred access point to encourage proper placement, although any of the major upper limb veins are appropriate. The femoral vein is an alternative site. The catheter is advanced until the tip lies within a branch pulmonary artery in a position suitable for measuring occlusion pressure (see below). A variety of sizes are available, including 7 French (suitable for older children), 5 French (10–18 kg) and 3 French (less than 10 kg) [51]. The larger catheters are typically four or five channel, including (a) a proximal lumen which sits in the right atrium for measurement of right atrial pressure and injection of the indicator, (b) a thermistor channel for measuring temperature of the injectate and blood within the pulmonary artery following injection, (c) an inflatable balloon to allow acquisition of occlusion pressure, (d) a distal lumen for measurement of pulmonary artery and occlusion pressures, and mixed venous blood sampling, (e) a fibreoptic line for continuous measurement of mixed venous oxygen saturation. Smaller catheters may contain fewer channels and are typically inserted under direct vision during cardiac surgery. Percutaneous insertion and placement is difficult in small children and carries complications [52, 53], including pneumothorax, hemothorax, catheter malposition, catheter

knotting, ventricular arrhythmias, balloon rupture, embolization, pulmonary artery occlusion, pulmonary infarction, and sepsis (central line infection) [53–55]. Interestingly, several studies have suggested that the subclavian route may be associated with a lower complication rate [55, 56].

Because of its long history of clinical use, pulmonary thermodilution is often regarded as the benchmark against which newer modalities are tested. However it must be stressed that pulmonary thermodilution is not a gold standard, and has many potential sources of inaccuracy [33, 57–59]. These include technical errors, variation in blood temperature within the pulmonary artery that is unrelated to indicator injection, and fluctuations in cardiac output. Perhaps the most common source of fluctuation in cardiac output pertinent to the ICU is that seen with mechanical ventilation. Positive pressure ventilation causes a transient drop in venous return and hence preload to the right ventricle, which produces a transient fall in right heart stroke volume. Because the time between injection and temperature sensing in the pulmonary artery is very short, the apparent cardiac output may vary, depending on when the measurement is taken in relation to the ventilatory cycle. To account for this, 3–4 measurements should be taken at systematic intervals throughout the ventilatory cycle and then averaged; this will produce an estimate within ±10 % of the true cardiac output in adults (provided all other sources of accuracy are dealt with) [60]. Stetz has concluded that there must be a minimal change of 12–15 % between serial averaged thermodilution measurements to represent a true change in cardiac output [61]. It is possible that this figure may be higher in children, however as thermodilution is thought to be less accurate and more variable [62].

In addition to measuring cardiac output, the pulmonary artery catheter can provide a measure of right ventricular function (ejection fraction), pulmonary artery occlusion pressure, pulmonary and right atrial pressures, and access to mixed venous oxygen saturations (via either direct intermittent measurement, or continuous oximetry). Right ventricular ejection fraction requires a thermistor with a rapid response time [63]. This reveals a characteristic series of temperature plateaus in the pulmonary artery after indicator injection into the right ventricle during diastole. These plateaus reflect intraventricular temperature during the previous heartbeat, and can be used to calculate ejection fraction via an algorithm, and hence end diastolic volume (since stroke volume is known from the thermodilution measurement and End Diastolic Volume = Stroke Volume/Ejection Fraction).

When the balloon near the tip of the pulmonary artery catheter is inflated so as to occlude upstream flow, a continuous column of non-flowing blood is then present between the catheter tip and the point of pulmonary venous convergence just behind the left atrium (J-1 point) [37, 64]. This is known as the occlusion pressure, and is thought to approximate left atrial pressure. Occlusion pressure is sometimes erroneously referred to as pulmonary capillary pressure, however the latter entity, as the name suggests refers to pressure within the pulmonary capillaries, which will be greater than the venous pressure by an amount influenced by both flow and pulmonary venous resistance (pulmonary vascular resistance has both an arterial and a venous component, which can be differentiated by a logarithmic plot of the pulmonary artery pressure decay after balloon occlusion) [65, 66]. Occlusion pressure is traditionally measured at end expiration. This is important because occlusion pressure will vary throughout the respiratory cycle, due to the influence of alveolar pressure. In situations where alveolar pressure greatly exceeds occlusion pressure, pulmonary vasculature distal to the catheter tip may collapse, and the pressure reading will reflect alveolar pressure rather than left atrial pressure. This may occur in West zones 1 and 2 of the lung, or in situations where high PEEP is used during mechanical ventilation [64]. This situation should be readily discernible from inspection of the pressure trace during occlusion, as large pressure swings will be seen in synchrony with the mechanical ventilator.

Occlusion pressure can be used in the calculation of pulmonary vascular resistance, and has been suggested as a measure of both left ventricular preload and performance. Unfortunately this is often not the case in clinical practice, for a variety of factors including technical problems, lack of user understanding, and difficulties in extrapolating a volume from a pressure reading [67, 68].

Transpulmonary Thermodilution

This principle is similar to pulmonary thermodilution, however here the temperature change is measured in a large artery, typically the femoral artery. Thus the journey from injection to measurement traverses the right atrium, right ventricle, pulmonary vascular bed, left atrium, left ventricle, and aorta [69]. At first glance this appears to violate one of the fundamental requirements of indicator measurement, i.e. no loss of indicator between injection and measurement. In fact it has been shown, that provided the injectate is cooled sufficiently (to less than 10 °C), the loss of heat is small and relatively constant and does not affect the accuracy of cardiac output measurement [70–73]. In addition, the loss of heat has been utilized to calculate extravascular lung water, which may be a marker of disease severity in certain states (e.g. Acute Respiratory Distress Syndrome) [74]. However, the utility of extravascular lung water measurement in pediatric practice is still largely unknown [75]. This may be partly due to errors in indexing this variable to body weight in young children [76]. Transpulmonary thermodilution, via a commercial system utilizes the theory of Newman to calculate a series of vascular volumes via the mean transit and exponential downslope times of the primary thermodilution curve [77]. These include intrathoracic blood volume and global end diastolic volume, which may be markers of preload, and cardiac function index (stroke volume divided by the global end diastolic volume in the heart), which may provide a measure of contractility. Application of these variables to pediatric practice is evolving. Concerns have been raised that global end diastolic volume is grossly overestimated by this method [78] and does not always bear a consistent relationship to stroke volume [79].

Transpulmonary thermodilution offers two main advantages over pulmonary thermodilution: (1) the need to access the pulmonary artery is obviated (all that is required is a central venous and arterial catheters) and (2) a commercially available device (PiCCO™, Pulsion Medical Systems, Munich, Germany) combines this modality with pulse contour analysis (calibration occurs via thermodilution), thereby representing an application of this technique to the provision of continuous cardiac output [80].

Transpulmonary Ultrasound Dilution

This new indicator dilution technique (CO-StatusTM–Transonic systems, Ithaca, NY, USA) utilizes an ultrasound beam which passes through an extracorporeal circuit attached to the arterial line. Measurement relies on the principle that ultrasound transit time will change when a small amount of saline is injected into the blood (via a central vein). Change is proportional to the volume of injectate and the cardiac output (typical ultrasound velocities through 0.9 % saline and blood are 1,533 and 1,580 m/s, respectively), thereby producing a typical dilution curve (Fig. 40.3) [81]. This technique has proven highly accurate in animal models and provides similar ancillary volumetric data to transpulmonary thermodilution (central blood volume, total end diastolic volume) [82]. Importantly, another potential advantage of both transpulmonary ultrasound and thermodilution techniques (in general) may be the ability to calculate cardiac output accurately in the presence of left to right shunts [83, 84].

Dye Dilution

Several dyes have been utilized as an indicator for calculation of cardiac output, though indocyanine green is the most commonly used. Injection is via a central vein, with measurement from a systemic artery traditionally utilizing a photometric technique. Three main limitations with this method have restricted its clinical application at the bedside. First, the concentration-time curve is measured using a densitometer, which requires calibration with samples of the patient's blood containing known concentrations of the dye, which can be time consuming. Second, measurement typically occurs extracorporeally, meaning that further blood must be withdrawn with each measurement. These two limitations have largely been overcome through the use of fiberoptic sensors utilizing the technique of pulse dye densitometry, a similar principle to pulse oximetry. Unfortunately the accuracy of this technique is questionable at low cardiac output, and also within certain patients [85, 86]. Third, because

Fig. 40.3 Typical concentration-time curve produced from transpulmonary ultrasound dilution

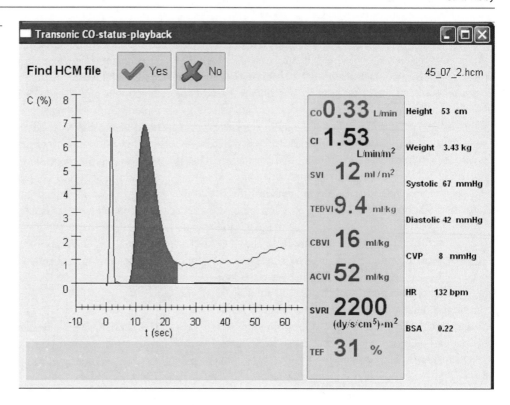

indocyanine green is removed by the liver, recirculation is guaranteed, which restricts the time between successive measurements. Obviously this is exacerbated in the face of significant hepatic impairment. For these reasons, use of dye dilution has been restricted chiefly to benchmarking newer modalities of cardiac output measurement.

Lithium Dilution

This innovation utilizes ionic concentration as the indicator [87, 88]. The ion used is lithium (injected as lithium chloride). Measurement occurs via a blood pump attached to the patient's arterial line, which transports the blood through a flow-through cell containing a lithium-selective electrode. The electrode contains a membrane which is selectively permeable to lithium ions, with change in voltage across the membrane being related to change in lithium ion concentration via the Nernst equation. Limitations are similar to dye dilution, in that blood sampling is required with every measurement, and rapid repeated measurements are not possible (however the time between injections is much less than that for the dye method). It is also thought that several drugs may interfere with readings, on the basis of their charge. Although this has proven accurate in pediatric patients [89], it is not currently licensed for patients less than 40 kg body weight.

The Fick Principle

Originally described in 1870, the Fick principle calculates flow by measuring the amount of indicator added (or removed)

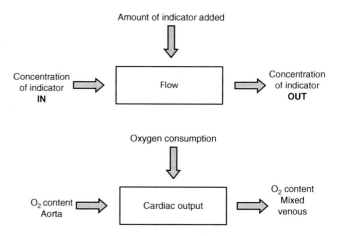

Fig. 40.4 Generalized representation of the Fick principle. It is assumed that the system is in steady state. Flow = amount of indicator added/change in indicator concentration; in the case of cardiac output this equation becomes: Cardiac output = oxygen consumption/change in oxygen content between aorta and mixed venous blood

from a system divided by the change in indicator concentration upstream and downstream of where the indicator is added (or removed) (Fig. 40.4) [90]. Calculation of systemic cardiac output may utilize one of two indicators: either O_2 (systemic oxygen consumption) or CO_2 (systemic carbon dioxide production), with upstream and downstream representing the systemic arterial and mixed venous sites, respectively. When these variables are measured directly, this is known as the direct Fick technique. Although accurate, the Fick principle has several sources of error and limitations, which will be elaborated on below. The following discussion refers primarily to the Fick calculation utilizing oxygen consumption, rather than carbon dioxide production.

Oxygen Consumption Measurement

The Fick principle for oxygen consumption measurement relies upon the assumption that oxygen consumption by the body is in equilibrium with oxygen uptake in the lung [91]. Traditionally the Douglas bag or spirometry have been used to measure oxygen uptake, however both are impractical in the ICU environment. Nowadays, portable metabolic monitors exist, which utilize a gas dilution principle to measure flow, a fast-response paramagnetic differential O_2 sensor to measure change in oxygen concentration, and an infrared CO_2 sensor [92, 93]. If flow and differential concentrations are known, content can be calculated via the Haldane transformation. Newer metabolic monitors are accurate within the pediatric range of oxygen consumption, CO_2 production, and gas flow, provided four conditions are met [93–96]:

1. There must be no loss of expired gas. This means that the technique is invalidated in the face of a pneumothorax with a chest drain, or if air leak occurs around the tracheal tube [97]. Several authors have suggested that the error may be acceptable in the absence of an audible leak [98], though this is controversial [99]. Others have claimed that the error may be acceptable if the measured leak is less than 5 % of expiratory tidal volume. However significant air leak is common [100] and may be difficult to quantify in an infant, given the inaccuracy of tidal volume measurement in most mechanical ventilators [101]. Thus a cuffed tube is recommended.
2. The partial pressure of water vapor within the system must be carefully controlled. Newer metabolic monitors use specialized tubing (e.g. Nafion) that equalizes the water vapor concentration of gas inside and outside the machine.
3. Conversion of gas volumes to standard conditions. Again, this occurs in all modern monitors.
4. Limitation of the fraction of inspired oxygen. When the FIO_2 is very high, for example in the face of significant lung disease, the difference between the fraction of inspired and expired oxygen may be very small. This creates an error in the denominator of the Haldane algorithm. Ideally the FIO_2 should be less than 0.60. At levels greater than 0.85 the error is likely to be large [102, 103].

A final source of error relates to oxygen consumption by the lung itself, which may occur with significant lung pathology. The numerator in the Fick equation is *systemic* oxygen consumption, however the metabolic monitor measures *total* oxygen consumption; that is, consumption by both the body and the lung. In health the majority of the pulmonary oxygen consumption occurs via the bronchial vessels, which can be regarded as being of systemic origin. However in disease states significant pulmonary oxygen consumption can occur

within the lung from the blood supplied by the pulmonary (right sided) circulation as well. This means that oxygen consumption as measured by the metabolic monitor will overestimate systemic oxygen consumption and hence cardiac output. An animal model using pneumococcal pneumonia has estimated this error to be of the order of 13–15 % [104]. A similar finding has been demonstrated in ventilated premature neonates at risk for chronic lung disease [105], though this is not seen in adults with pneumonia [106].

Arterial and Mixed Venous Oxygen Content

Oxygen content is a function of hemoglobin and dissolved oxygen and is calculated via the formula:

$$O_2 \text{ content } (ml\,O_2 \text{ per liter of blood}) = \left[1.34 \times Hgb\ (g\,/\,L) \times \%\,saturation\,/\,100\right] + \left[PaO_2\ (mmHg) \times 0.003\right].$$

Normally the contribution from dissolved O_2 is minimal and can be ignored without producing significant error. However this is not the case when the PaO_2 is very high (for example, a patient without significant lung disease who is receiving an $FIO_2 > 0.30$). Mixed venous sampling requires accessing the pulmonary artery, as blood taken from within the right atrium may inadvertently sample desaturated coronary sinus blood. Lastly, oxygen saturation must be measured via a co-oximeter, and not calculated from the blood gas PO_2 value.

Presence of Anatomical Shunt

The Fick equation can potentially allow for cardiac output estimation in the setting of an anatomical shunt [107]. This may be unrealistic at the bedside however, because shunting is often bi-directional and calculation may require blood sampling pre and post shunt. To understand these concepts it is necessary to apply the Fick equation to both the systemic (Qs) and pulmonary (Qp) blood flows.

The formulae are:

$$Qs = \frac{VO_2}{C_{aorta} - C_{mixed\ venous}} \quad Qp = \frac{VO_2}{C_{pulm\ vein} - C_{pulm\ artery}}$$

where "C" refers to the oxygen content in the respective sites. Thus in the absence of anatomical shunt Qs = Qp. This means that the formulae are essentially interchangeable, as mixed venous blood is sampled from the pulmonary artery and oxygen content in the pulmonary veins and systemic arteries are the same (ignoring the small R → L shunt that occurs from bronchial venous and thebesian drainage). However in the setting of L → R shunt (for example with a large ventricular septal defect), blood in the pulmonary artery is highly saturated, thus mixed venous sampling must occur proximal to the site of mixing. Options include right atrial sampling, or a weighted average of superior and inferior vena caval blood (weighting to reflect the assumed proportion of total venous return from each caval vessel, which is age dependent) [108]. In reality both methods may be inaccurate. Conversely in the setting of an R → L shunt, systemic arterial blood is less saturated than pulmonary venous, and so Qp can only be calculated if pulmonary venous blood is sampled. Lastly, these two formulae can be combined to provide a ratio of pulmonary to systemic blood flow; this is only ever undertaken in the cardiac cauterization laboratory because of the need to sample from multiple sites that are difficult to access.

$$Qp:Qs = \frac{C_{aorta} - C_{mixed\ venous}}{C_{pulm\ vein} - C_{pulm\ artery}}$$

Indirect Fick Principle

If the Fick principle is applied to CO_2 production, it may be possible to estimate the Fick parameters indirectly from the inspired and expired gases using a CO_2 re-breathe technique, whereby the patient rebreathes exhaled CO_2 for a short period of time whilst mechanically ventilated [109, 110]. Here the Fick equation relates to pulmonary capillary blood flow (in essence effective, or non-shunt blood flow) rather than total pulmonary blow. By measuring change in the parameters before and at the end of the CO_2 re-breathing period, pulmonary capillary blood flow is calculated from the following formula:

$$Q_{pcbf} = \frac{\Delta VCO_2}{\Delta C_{mixed\ venous} - \Delta C_{pulmonary\ end\ capillary}}$$

In this equation: (i) ΔVCO_2 is measured, (ii) it is assumed that a brief re-breathe period does not change mixed venous CO_2, hence ΔVCO_2 is zero, and (iii) $\Delta C_{pulmonary\ end\ capillary}$ is estimated from alveolar CO_2 content which is in turn estimated from end tidal PCO_2 via a correction factor. Intrapulmonary shunt flow is calculated from Nunn's iso-shunt diagrams [111] and added to pulmonary capillary blood flow, giving total pulmonary blood flow. As can be seen this technique relies on a series of assumptions, which may limit its validity in the ICU setting [112–114].

Doppler Ultrasound

Franklin applied the Doppler principle to measurement of blood flow in 1961 [115]. The principle states that the frequency shift of reflected ultrasound will be proportional to the velocity of the reflecting blood cells, and is related by the formula:

$$\text{Blood velocity} = \frac{\Delta frequency \times c}{2 \times f_t \times \cos\theta}$$

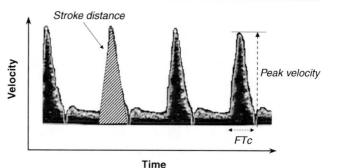

Hemodynamic state	Effect on Doppler parameter	
↓ Contractility	↓↑ FTc ±	↓ Peak velocity ++
↑ Afterload	↓ FTc ++	↓ Peak velocity +
Hypovolemia	↓ FTc ++	↓ Peak velocity ±

Fig. 40.5 Spectral representation of a Doppler velocity-time signal, showing effects of differing hemodynamic states. The area under the triangular waveform is stroke distance, which represents the distance a column of blood will travel down the descending aorta in one cardiac cycle. Peak velocity is affected predominantly by changes in contractility, and to a lesser extent by changes in preload and afterload. Corrected flow time (*FTc*) represents the systolic time corrected to a heart rate of 60 beats per minute. This parameter may be reduced in the face of diminished preload (e.g. hypovolemia) or an increased afterload. Both states can also decrease the peak velocity; they may be differentiated however on the basis of response to a fluid challenge

Where Δfrequency is the frequency shift between transmitted and reflected signal, c is the sound velocity in blood, f_t is the transmitting frequency, and θ is the angle of insonation (i.e. between the beam and blood flow).

Doppler ultrasound signals may be continuous or pulsed. Continuous signals react to all flow within their path, so that the point at which blood velocity is measured is unknown; this is known as range ambiguity. Pulsed signals allow for adjustment of the sampling depth and volume, but may be prone to errors in calculation of velocity, due to the relationship between the frequency (and hence wavelength) of the transmitted signal and the velocity being measured (this phenomenon is called aliasing). In essence, the chosen frequency represents a trade-off between velocity measurement and image resolution [116].

Doppler ultrasound can be applied to any pulsatile vessel, though measurement of cardiac output is typically performed in the aorta, either via the transthoracic or transesophageal approach (the latter allowing for continuous measurement) [117]. Spectral representation of the velocity-time signal characteristically shows a triangular shape, from which a variety of flow-related variables can be derived (Fig. 40.5) [118, 119]. The integral of velocity-time (area under the triangle) represents stroke distance, the distance that a column of blood will travel along the aorta in one cardiac cycle. Stroke distance is not stroke volume; conversion of the former to the latter requires multiplication by left heart outflow area. This can be achieved either via echocardiography [120] or a nomogram [119, 121, 122]. Both methods carry advantages and disadvantages.

Echocardiography, using either two-dimensional or M-Mode can be used to calculate outflow tract area at a variety of sites, including aortic valve annulus, aortic root and ascending aorta. Of these, measurement at the valve annulus in systole via two-dimensional mode appears to be the most accurate, producing a variation coefficient of approximately 6 % [123, 124]. Echocardiography in children can often be performed transthoracically, which is obviously less invasive than via the transesophageal route. In addition to providing a means of acquiring cardiac output, echocardiography, in the hands of a skilled operator also supplies a vast amount of functional and morphologic information, including indices of diastolic dysfunction, regional wall abnormalities, valve regurgitation, pericardial effusion, chamber dilatation, and cardiac chamber interdependence. The main disadvantage of echocardiography is the requirement for significant user expertise. Conversely, Doppler ultrasound requires little in the way of user training, and thus can be performed by any trained ICU practitioner [125]. Here left heart outflow area is estimated via a nomogram. Not surprisingly, the assumptions inherent in the nomogram produce an error in cardiac output unique to each patient, although changes in cardiac output are tracked accurately [121, 126]. Of the two modes, transesophageal Doppler has greater intra- and inter-user agreement [127], because the aorta lies approximately parallel to the esophagus, allowing the angle of insonation to be fixed at 45° and adjusted for. Unfortunately probe fixation is a significant problem in pediatrics. Both probe rotation and vertical movement can occur resulting in signal alteration. For this reason this modality cannot be considered as truly continuous. Transthoracic Doppler allows both the aortic and pulmonary outflow to be estimated via separate nomograms; however the angle of insonation is unknown and the coefficient of variation is generally higher than that for transesophageal Doppler [127]. More recently, a Doppler-based technique known as surface integration of velocity vectors, has been reported in animals with encouraging results [128]. This technique utilizes multi-planar Doppler sampling, which is reconstructed to a three-dimensional flow field [129]. Measurements take between 2 and 8 min to perform.

Doppler ultrasound typically utilizes a signal that is filtered to preferentially focus on blood flow (high frequency, low amplitude). However by altering the filter to detect low frequency, high amplitude signals, myocardial movement can be delineated (tissue Doppler). Although this does not calculate blood flow, it can provide a wealth of information about ventricular function, both systolic and diastolic, and also loading conditions of the heart [130, 131]. Speckle tracking is a two dimensional technique that tracks acoustic markers called speckles in grey scale throughout the cardiac cycle, followed by application of a post-processing algorithm to calculate cardiac deformation, known as strain

(change in length divided by original length). This can be calculated in three dimensions: longitudinal, radial and circumferential. Although strain can also be calculated using tissue Doppler, speckle tracking has the advantage that interrogation does not need to be parallel to the plane of contraction [132, 133]. Three dimensional echocardiography is a new development that allows multiplanar image reviews with structural reconstructions, providing exquisite detail of valvar and septal structures in particular [134]. It is likely that these applications will become increasingly important in the future, providing valuable information over and above a mere flow state (cardiac output).

Impedance/Conductance Methods

Impedance is the opposition to the flow of an alternating current, and can be defined using Ohm's law in the same manner as resistance for direct current:

$$\text{Impedance}(Z) = \frac{\text{potential difference}(V)}{\text{alternating current}(I)}$$

$$\text{Resistance}(R) = \frac{\text{potential difference}(V)}{\text{direct current}(I)}$$

Admittance is the reciprocal of impedance. Conductance is the reciprocal of resistance. Although described in relation to the cardiac cycle in 1953 [135], Kubicek was the first to apply this principle to the measurement of cardiac output in 1966 [136]. Here the chest is regarded as a conductor whose impedance is altered by the changes in blood volume and velocity that occur with each heartbeat; from this stroke volume is calculated. Impedance is measured via a series of voltage-sensing and current-transmitting electrodes. Alternating rather than direct current is used to achieve charge balancing and thus avoid any residual polarization at the interface between electrode and tissue, which would result in an increase in measured impedance [137]. The site of electrode placement defines the type of impedance measurement, from the non-invasive (thoracic bioimpedance, where electrodes are placed on the chest) to the highly invasive (intracardiac requiring electrode placement within the left ventricle).

Thoracic Impedance

A series of electrodes are placed at fixed intervals around the chest wall, and stroke volume calculated using the formula:

$$\text{stroke volume} = \frac{L^3 \times VET \times dZ/dt_{max}}{4.25 \times Z_0}$$

where L = thoracic segment length, VET = ventricular ejection time, dZ/dt_{max} = maximum rate of impedance change, and Zo = transthoracic baseline impedance. It is now known that the volume change sensed by thoracic bioimpedance is almost exclusively extracardiac, as the myocardium tends to shield the electrodes from the impedance changes occurring within the ventricle. Thus the change in impedance signal and hence stroke volume estimation comes predominantly from blood volume alterations within the systemic and pulmonary vessels inside the chest [138, 139]. Thoracic bioimpedance has not been widely adopted in the clinical setting. Indeed, several authors have expressed concern at the accuracy of this method in the ICU environment, particularly at states of low cardiac output, hypotension, and chest wall edema [140–143].

Electrical velocimetry is a recent refinement in the impedance algorithm, based upon the Bernstein–Osypka equation [144]. Standard ECG surface electrodes are placed side-to-side in a vertical direction to the patients' left middle and lower neck, and to the lower thorax at the left mid-axillary. Preliminary pediatric evaluation has proven to be promising when compared to Fick [145] and transthoracic echocardiography [146].

Intracardiac Impedance

Stroke volume is measured from catheters placed directly into the left ventricle. Accuracy is increased by utilizing multipolar catheters, which partition the ventricle into a series of cylindrical segments [147]. Several studies have reported a small but consistent underestimation of stroke volume, perhaps due to simultaneous conductance into surrounding tissues (atria, myocardium); this may be improved via a correction factor [148–150]. The invasiveness of this technique means that use in the ICU is effectively impossible, apart from when catheters are placed during cardiac surgery. Nonetheless, this technique can also provide valuable information concerning myocardial systolic function via either end-systolic elastance calculation or using preload recruitable stroke work [151–154]. The latter technique involves plotting the pressure-volume curves after manipulation of preload (typically reducing preload via progressive caval snaring). The area within the pressure-volume loop represents stroke work; when this is plotted against end diastolic volume, the slope of this relationship is termed preload recruitable stroke work, and is a load independent measure of contractility [153]. These techniques have provided insight into previously unsuspected degrees of cardiac dysfunction after relatively short periods on cardiopulmonary bypass [155].

Arterial Pulse Contour Analysis

Erlanger suggested a relationship between stroke volume and arterial pulse contour a century ago [156]. The advent of fast computer microprocessors has meant that a variety of pulse contour systems are now commercially available that estimate beat-to-beat changes in stroke volume. Interestingly, all utilize different techniques for pulse contour analysis, in part due to differing theories concerning both the relationship

between flow and pressure within the arterial system and the mechanism of pulse wave transmission along the arterial tree [1, 157–159]. In addition, the majority of commercial systems estimate only beat-to-beat *change* in cardiac output and therefore require initial calibration via an alternative method of cardiac output measurement.

An appreciation of several basic concepts and terminology is a pre-requisite for understanding pulse contour analysis, in essence how a volume change supplied from the left ventricle translates into a pressure change within the arterial system [1]. Both flow and pressure are primarily pulsatile events in the proximal arterial system and do not achieve non-pulsatile, or mean values until the level of the arterioles. Resistance to flow occurs in both the large and small arteries; in the vessels receiving pulsatile flow this is called impedance, while for those receiving non-pulsatile flow this is designated as resistance (also known as systemic peripheral resistance). The largest pressure drop occurs across the arterioles. In addition, arteries contain variable amounts of elastic tissue. In the largest vessels, such as the aorta, this means that they can expand to store volume (compliance) and contract in relation to the downstream load (elastic recoil). The relationship between stress (force applied to the arterial wall) and strain (reaction of the arterial wall to the stress applied) has traditionally been represented using a proportionality constant known as Young's modulus of elasticity. This in turn affects wave velocity via the formula:

$$\text{wave velocity} = \sqrt{\frac{E \times h}{2 \times \rho \times r}}$$

where, E = Young's modulus, h = vessel wall thickness, ρ = fluid density, and r = radius.

The phenomena of compliance and elastic recoil within the aorta partially explain the continuation of blood flow within small arteries after systole has terminated. In the aorta, compliance is non-linear (as is impedance), meaning that the pressure change for a given volume ejected by the heart will vary according to both the diastolic arterial pressure (and hence peripheral resistance) and stroke volume. This relationship, as well as the pressure wave reflected from the periphery back to the aorta, influences the shape of the arterial waveform (Fig. 40.6) [160]. Post mortem studies have shown that aortic compliance shows considerable interpatient variation [161, 162]. Although the shape of the aortic cross-sectional area versus pressure curve is relatively constant, it demonstrates differing intercepts between individuals, meaning that the error in estimating cross-sectional area (and hence compliance) can be as high as 30 % at maximal pressures (Fig. 40.7) [162–164]. Furthermore, compliance is also affected by a variety of factors, including age, disease and catecholamines. Lastly, pressure waves are also influenced by wave reflection back from the periphery to the proximal arteries.

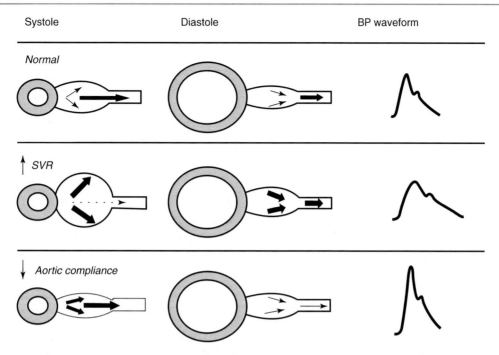

Fig. 40.6 Pulse pressure diagram. A simplified, 2-element Windkessel approach, utilizing aortic compliance and systemic vascular (peripheral) resistance is used to illustrate influences on the blood pressure waveform. The effects of aortic impedance and wave reflection are ignored. In the *top* diagram, the normal situation is shown, whereby a proportion of flow and pressure is channeled into the compliant aorta during systole. During diastole, the elastic recoil of the aorta causes a pressure and flow pulse to be transmitted into the distal arterial system. When systemic vascular resistance is increased (*middle*), more pressure and flow are transmitted to the aorta during systole, producing a greater flow and pressure in diastole. The net result is a narrower pulse pressure (lower systolic, higher diastolic). When aortic compliance is reduced (*lower* diagram), flow and pressure are greater in the distal arterial tree during systole, producing a characteristic spiky waveform

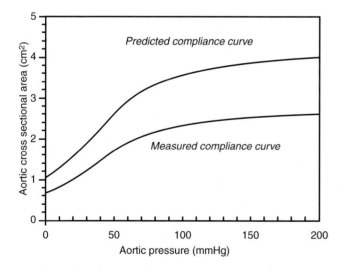

Fig. 40.7 "Typical" aortic compliance has been estimated in vitro from cadaveric studies, as following an arctangent relationship [161, 162]. In vivo, the shape of the aortic cross sectional area versus arterial pressure relationship (similar to compliance versus pressure) is relatively constant; however the intercept may vary between patients. The diagram shows this relationship in a 59-year-old patient, showing how aortic compliance may be overestimated using the in vitro formula (Reprinted de Vaal et al. [163]. With permission from Oxford University Press)

A variety of methods for continuous pulse contour analyses exist, all of which utilize a combination of calculations for aortic impedance, aortic compliance, total or systemic peripheral resistance, pressure wave reflection, and transfer function between large and small arteries (although not all components are included in every method) [1, 157–159, 163, 165–167]. Perhaps the best known of these is the modified Windkessel approach [168, 169]. This approach was first described by Otto Frank in 1899, who adopted the term Windkessel (German for "wind kettle") from Hales' eighteenth century description of the elastic arteries as being like a water pump [170]. The modified Windkessel approach describes the pressure response of the arterial system to an input of flow (stoke volume) as being a function of characteristic impedance of the proximal aorta, aortic compliance, and total systemic peripheral resistance. The latter two variables are described in parallel [168, 169]. The accuracy of this approach may be improved by either (a) ultrasonic measurement of aortic cross sectional area, which allows for a recalibration of the aortic compliance relationship for the individual patient (Modelflow™) [163] or (b) a more sophisticated analysis of the pressure waveform taking into account the shape as well as the area of the pressure wave (PiCCO™) [167]. An alternative method (LiDCO™plus) involves arterial pulse power analysis, and because it does not rely on waveform morphology, it is not strictly speaking a pulse contour method [157]. Questions remain over the accuracy of beat-to-beat methods of analysis when applied to pediatric patients; with animal work highlighting an inability to interpret correctly rapid changes in hemodynamic state (e.g. hemorrhage, cardiac consequences of vasoconstrictor initiation) [80, 171].

Other Methods

Several other methods exist for measurement of cardiac output. These include radionuclide techniques [172], magnetic resonance imaging [173, 174], and transluminal Doppler flow probes. All are as yet impractical for ICU use.

Measuring the Adequacy of Flow

Shock occurs when oxygen consumption is inadequate to meet the metabolic needs of the body [175]. This may occur for a variety of reasons, including inadequate global oxygen delivery, inadequate local oxygen delivery, excessive oxygen consumption, and inability of cells to consume oxygen (e.g. mitochondrial dysfunction) [175, 176]. The three components of oxygen delivery are cardiac output, hemoglobin concentration, and hemoglobin oxygen saturation [176], i.e. DO_2 = cardiac output × arterial oxygen content = cardiac output × [1.34 × Hgb (g/L) × %saturation/100]. This ignores the small contribution to content from dissolved oxygen. In many ways it is more important to decide whether flow is adequate to allow for required oxygen consumption, both on a global and a regional basis, than to merely derive an absolute value for flow [2]. Three global markers of adequacy are primarily used: mixed venous oxygen saturation, Near Infrared Spectroscopy (NIRS), and whole blood lactate.

Mixed Venous Oxygen Saturation

Mixed venous blood refers to the sum total of systemic venous return, i.e. that from the upper and lower body and the heart itself, which drain into the superior and inferior vena cavae and the coronary sinus, respectively. Provided there is no anatomical shunt, complete mixing occurs downstream of the right atrium, either in the right ventricle or pulmonary artery. It is customary to use the latter site for mixed venous sampling [177, 178].

When the oxygen delivery/consumption balance becomes perturbed, various compensatory mechanisms are triggered (these are described in detail in the chapter on shock) – one of these is an increase in oxygen extraction, resulting in a fall in mixed venous oxygen saturation. This is best understood by referring back to the Fick equation:

$$\text{Cardiac output} = \frac{VO_2}{C_{aorta} - C_{mixed\ venous}}$$

$$\approx \frac{VO_2}{O_2 sat_{aorta} - O_2 sat_{mixed\ venous}}$$

(VO_2, oxygen consumption; C, oxygen content; O_2 sat, oxygen saturation). Thus when cardiac output falls or oxygen

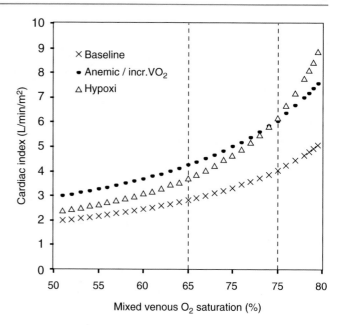

Fig. 40.8 Theoretical relationship between mixed venous oxygen saturation and cardiac index. The baseline relationship assumes typical values for hemoglobin of 120 g/L, oxygen consumption (VO_2) of 120 ml/min/m^2, and arterial oxygen saturation of 98 %. In situations of either increased VO_2 (220 ml/min/m^2) or anemia (80 g/L), the curve is shifted upwards. In all three situations, a fall in mixed venous saturation from 75 to 65 % represents a relative decrease in cardiac index of approximately 40 % (assuming all other variables remain constant). However in the case of mild baseline hypoxia (arterial oxygen saturation 90 %), the shape of the curve changes, such that the same drop in mixed venous saturation now represents a fall in cardiac index of 50 %

consumption rises (without a concomitant equivalent rise in cardiac output), the only way to balance this equation is for the denominator to increase. This can only be achieved by a fall in mixed venous oxygen saturation (i.e. an increase in oxygen extraction), as there is no mechanism for increasing arterial oxygen saturation acutely. It is important to appreciate that the relationship between cardiac output and mixed venous oxygen saturation is thus not linear and will vary according to the initial arterial oxygen saturation, oxygen consumption and hemoglobin concentration (Fig. 40.8).

The normal value for mixed venous oxygen saturation is approximately 73 % (range 65–75 %) [177–180]. As the oxygen delivery-supply ratio becomes perturbed, compensatory oxygen extraction will occur, and the mixed venous saturation will decrease. If this is inadequate, anaerobic metabolism will commence generating a subsequent lactic acidosis [176, 181]. The exact point at which oxygen extraction becomes inadequate or exhausted varies from patient to patient and is affected by chronicity. In the acute setting, lactic acidosis may occur when the mixed venous saturation falls below 50 %, however patients with long standing hypoxia (e.g. congenital cyanotic cardiac disease) or a chronically failing myocardium (e.g. cardiomyopathy) may exhibit mixed venous saturations below 50 % in the face of normal blood lactate levels [182]. Lastly it is important to appreciate that tissue hypoxia is not the only source of a raised blood lactate (see section "Blood lactate").

Hypoxia is common in pediatric practice (for example, in the setting of congenital heart disease) and may affect the mixed venous saturation [183]. Thus it may be preferable to monitor either the arteriovenous oxygen saturation difference or the oxygen extraction ratio. The latter is given by:

$$Oxygen\ Extraction\ Ratio = (SaO_2\ SvO_2)/SaO_2$$

Normal values are between 0.24 and 0.28 [2]. This equation is only valid if the contribution from dissolved oxygen is minimal. If this is not the case, then oxygen saturation should be substituted by oxygen content [107]. Other authors have suggested using the inverse of the oxygen extraction ratio, known as the oxygen excess factor, or omega (Ω) [184]:

$$Oxygen\ Excess\ Factor(W) = SaO_2/(SaO_2\ SvO_2)$$

The rationale for this is that Ω is mathematically equivalent to the ratio of oxygen delivery to oxygen consumption and is easier to assimilate clinically. It is also valid in states of hypoxia [185]. Normally this ratio is of the order of 4:1; it has also been shown that decompensation is more likely when Ω falls below 2:1 [186].

Unfortunately obtaining access to true mixed venous blood is difficult in pediatric practice. However placement of central venous catheters is common in critically ill patients and may represent an alternative to mixed venous blood [187]. Because of the wide variation in the oxygen saturation of venous blood draining organs below the diaphragm (Table 40.1), central venous blood should ideally be sampled from the superior vena cava, just before it enters the right atrium. However, the right atrium may also represent a suitable site. There is a theoretical risk that sampling from the right atrium may selectively sample desaturated blood from the coronary sinus. In reality, the probability of this is likely to be low [178, 187]. There are no large studies examining the relationship between central and mixed venous saturation in critically ill children, however in the immediate period after cardiac surgery, central venous values are, on average lower than mixed venous by between 7 and 17 % [189, 190]. Data from adult patients in shock of varying etiology suggest that, on average, the central venous saturation is 7 % higher than the mixed venous oxygen saturation [191, 192]. However, much larger differences (up to 20 %) are found within individual patients [193]. Reassuringly, when sequential sampling is performed, both sites trend in the same direction in the majority (90 %) of occasions [191]. The validity of central venous saturation as a monitoring tool has been shown in a large randomized controlled trial of adult patients in shock. In this study of early goal-directed resuscitation,

Table 40.1 Typical venous oxygen saturation values from organs and tissue beds [182, 187, 188]

Site	Saturation (%)
Brain	69
Heart	30–37
Liver	66
Gut	66
Kidney	92
Muscle	60–71
Skin	88

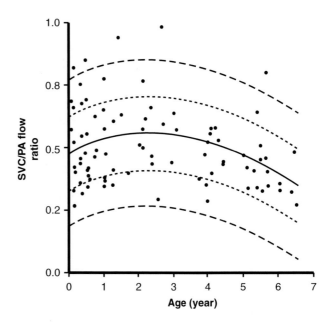

Fig. 40.9 Ratio of superior vena caval flow to total body venous return throughout childhood. Lines represent mean, one and two standard deviations (Reprinted from Salim et al. [197]. With permission from Wolter Kluwers Health)

mortality was decreased in the group in which normalization of central venous saturation was one of the end points (30.5 versus 46.5 %) [194]. A similar finding occurred in a pediatric study which utilized a similar protocol [195].

Application and interpretation of adult-derived values for central venous oxygen monitoring to children may be complicated by proportionate differences in superior vena caval flow between adults and children [196]. In adults, the superior vena cava carries approximately 35 % of the total body venous return. In childhood, this is age dependent, typically being 50 % in newborns, rising to a peak of 55 % by 2.5 years, and decreasing to adult values by age 6.5 years (Fig. 40.9). These represent average values in health however; there are major differences in these proportions within each age band, and whether the same relationship holds in disease states is unknown [196].

Finally, it is worth considering causes of an elevated mixed/central venous saturation in a critically ill patient. Broadly speaking this can be due to five causes: (1) a very high cardiac output, (2) functional arteriovenous shunting (typically occurring at the microcirculatory level), (3) impairment of cellular oxygen utilization, which includes mitochondrial dysfunction seen in sepsis, congenital defects of oxidative phosphorylation and with certain toxins, such as cyanide poisoning (4) organ death (5) extreme reductions in basal metabolic rate (e.g. during hypothermia).

Near Infrared Spectroscopy (NIRS)

This technology attempts to estimate tissue oxygenation beneath topically applied probes via transmitting and analyzing the absorbance of near-infrared light passing through the tissue adjacent to the probes (using the Beer-Lambert law). Different substances absorb light at preferential wavelengths. In the case of hemoglobin, this occurs in the near infrared range (650–850 nm). The oxygenation status of hemoglobin will further influence where in this spectrum preferential absorption occurs, with oxygenated hemoglobin absorbing more at 800–850 nm, and deoxygenated hemoglobin at 650–800 nm. Unlike pulse oximeters, which preferentially measure pulsatile signal (and hence arterial saturations), NIRS signals are returned from the entire vascular bed (arterial, capillary and venous). However, as most hemoglobin is located in the venous circulation, the NIRS signal represents a venous-weighted relative oxygen index of tissue beneath the probe. Thus NIRS does not directly measure tissue oxygenation per se [197, 198].

Typically NIRS is used cerebrally. However, there is growing interest in somatic application, with probe placement typically on the flank. A variety of monitors are now commercially available, each with a slightly different method of measurement and internal algorithm; with resultant inter-device variability [198, 199]. Of note, when used cerebrally, interference from superficial scalp vessels can increase the apparent NIRS saturation by 7–17 %, dependent upon the commercial device [200]. To date, the role of NIRS in critical illness has not been evaluated in a systematic fashion. Its most common use is in the setting of congenital heart disease [201], although there is growing interest in other disease states [198, 202].

Blood Lactate

As discussed above, lactic acidosis may result from tissue hypoxia [203]. However, it is important to appreciate that a rise in blood lactate may occur in the critically ill patient for reasons other than inadequate oxygen delivery [204]. In sepsis, muscles may generate lactate under aerobic conditions [205, 206]. This is probably due to catecholamine-induced stimulation of sarcolemmal Na^+–K^+–ATPase [207]. The energy supply for this enzyme is linked to the glycolytic and glycogenolytic pathways. Over stimulation produces pyruvate at a rate which outstrips the oxidative capacity of the mitochondria, resulting in lactate accumulation. Another mechanism for raised lactate is cytopathic hypoxia, or failure of the mitochondria to utilize delivered oxygen [208]. It is also becoming increasingly apparent that lactate serves as a currency for maintaining the redox potential both within and between cells; this is known as the lactate shuttle concept [209]. Nonetheless an elevated lactate, or more importantly an elevated lactate that does not fall has prognostic implications, and the cause should always be vigorously sought [210–213].

Regional Perfusion

Both mixed/central venous oxygen saturation and blood lactate are global markers. Delivery and consumption abnormalities can occur at the regional level. Unfortunately robust measures of regional perfusion at the bedside are lacking.

Tissue PCO_2 Monitoring Using Tonometry

Tonometry is a technique whereby a CO_2-permeable balloon is placed in proximity to a mucosal surface [214]. Hypoperfusion of the tissue bed in question causes tissue, and hence mucosal intracellular CO_2 accumulation. As CO_2 diffuses freely across cell membranes, it will equilibrate within the tonometer balloon. The difference between tonometric and arterial PCO_2 (PCO_2 gap) is thought to quantify the degree of hypoperfusion. This has been corroborated in several studies measuring splanchnic mucosal perfusion with other methods (microspheres, laser Doppler, flow probes) [215–217]. Gastric tonometry as a surrogate for splanchnic perfusion was the first application of this principle in the critical care setting. A vast number of studies utilizing this technique were published in the 1990s. Many of these studies appeared to show an adverse prognosis with the presence of an increased PCO_2 gap (particularly if this did not respond to resuscitation) [218–223]. Several suggested that early tonometric-guided therapy might improve outcome, however the results were by no means uniform. With hindsight, the results of many of the earlier studies have been questioned on the basis of methodological flaws [214]. These include the tonometer medium (air being more accurate than saline) [224, 225], use of buffers [224], gastric acid blockade [226], influence of feeding [227], inaccuracy in blood gas analyzers for measuring PCO_2 in saline [228], and use of calculated mucosal pH (using the Henderson-Hasselbalch equation and assuming mucosal and arterial bicarbonate to be equal) in preference to PCO_2. To date gastric tonometry has not been widely adopted as a routine monitoring tool in the intensive care unit. Recently sublingual tonometry has been suggested as a more accessible alternative, particularly during the early phases of resuscitation [229, 230].

Optical Monitoring Methods

A variety of optical methods for measuring tissue perfusion have recently become available, including Laser Doppler flowery [231], peripheral perfusion index [232, 233], and Orthogonal Polarization Spectral imaging [234]. Recently, NIRS (see above) has been adapted to estimate microvascular function and flow reserve, via a combination of placement on the thenar eminence, recurrent forearm cuff occlusion and measurement of the speed of signal decrement and return [235, 236].

Capillary Refill

Capillary refill figures prominently in the major resuscitation manuals and has been shown to be a marker of hypovolemia in the emergency room setting [237–239]. The significance of this variable in the ICU is less clear, perhaps due to the coexistence of confounding factors such as fever, hypothermia, and vasocative medication use [240]. In the ICU, capillary refill bears a weak relationship to stroke volume, with the optimal predictive value occurring with a capillary refill greater than 6 s (well above the traditional upper limit of 2 s) [240, 241]. It bears no relationship to systemic vascular resistance [240], however there are weak correlations with hemoglobin and central venous O_2 saturation (the latter being inverse) [242, 243]. Of note, it appears that senior, more experienced clinicians are more selective in their application of this marker, perhaps reflecting a better understanding of its utility and limitations [244].

Assessing the Components of Cardiac Output

If it appears that flow is inadequate, the next step is to attempt to isolate which component may be contributing – heart rate, preload, contractility, afterload, or diastolic function. One of the great problems is that all of these components are interdependent, thus an apparent deficiency in one parameter may be caused by abnormalities in one, or indeed several of the others. For example, the combination of a moderate sinus tachycardia (secondary to fever) coexistent with diastolic dysfunction may result in a functional preload deficit; the solution thus may not be to administer volume, but rather to slow the heart rate and give a lusitropic agent. It is also worth considering that many of the therapies aimed at increasing flow carry a cost. For example, increasing inotropy may also increase myocardial oxygen consumption, which may be undesirable in the setting

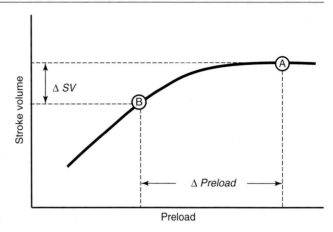

Fig. 40.10 Cyclical changes in stroke volume and pulse pressure induced by positive pressure ventilation can be used to predict a patient's response to fluid administration. However this can produce both false positive and false negative results. In position *A* the patient is optimally filled, and functioning at the top of the Starling curve. Ventilation with excessive tidal volumes produces a cyclical decrease in preload and hence stroke volume (to position *B*), suggesting that the patient may respond to volume administration. This is an example of a false positive result

of a failing myocardium. It may be preferable to decrease oxygen consumption (mechanical ventilation, increasing sedation, neuromuscular blockade, avoiding hyperthermia).

Heart Rate

Heart rate is the easiest component affecting cardiac function, but is often the most overlooked. Extreme tachycardia may compromise diastolic filling time, particularly if diastolic dysfunction coexists. Loss of atrio-ventricular synchrony will also compromise forward flow.

Preload Versus Volume Responsiveness

Preload relates to the variety of factors influencing the amount of ventricular fiber stretch at the end of diastole (and hence end diastolic volume) [245, 246]. Preload is both difficult to measure and interpret at the bedside. As a result, attention has recently focused towards the clinical question of identifying when a patient is likely to increase stroke volume in response to fluid administration [247]. In reality we may wish to address both issues simultaneously [248]. Failure of a patient to increase stroke volume following a fluid bolus when predicted to do so may occur for three reasons: (1) the prediction tool is inaccurate and the patient is already functioning at the top of the Starling curve (Fig. 40.10), (2) contractility is severely impaired, (3) the infusion volume is not sufficient to increase preload (this may be more common than we expect) [249]. In scenarios

(1) and (2), preload will increase, but they may be differentiated by a measure of contractility, while in scenario (3) preload will not increase [248].

Traditionally, the two commonly used measures of preload have been central venous pressure (right heart) and pulmonary artery occlusion pressure (left heart), however both perform poorly [68, 250]. This is because many factors affect the ability of a pressure measurement to act as a marker of volume status, including venous capacitance, cardiac chamber compliance, valve competence, pulmonary artery pressures, and the ability of the lung to function as a Starling resistor with positive pressure ventilation [64, 251]. Nonetheless it is reasonable to assume that a low central venous pressure may represent underfilling, and this parameter may be useful for trending [252].

Three volume-based measures, intrathoracic blood volume, global end diastolic volume and right ventricular end diastolic volume have been evaluated favorably in adult practice [68, 250, 253]. The former two are calculated from transpulmonary thermodilution, the latter from pulmonary thermodilution via a rapid response thermistor. Corrected flow time is a Doppler-derived measurement that has been used successfully in adults to guide intraoperative volume replacement [254–256], however it is also affected by afterload and contractility. Two echocardiographic indicators of preload have been suggested. The functional preload index requires specialized software and a series of calculations, thus limiting its clinical utility [257], while interpretation of mitral inflow velocity profiles is frequently difficult due to confounding variables [258].

In contrast to the static measures of preload, predictors of fluid responsiveness are dynamic. All relate to the cyclical fluctuations in right heart preload induced by positive pressure mechanical ventilation [247, 259]. These produce beat-to-beat variations in stroke volume, which are evident using any of the continuous measures of cardiac output described earlier. Fluid responsiveness can also be predicted from the arterial blood pressure trace [260]. Three measures have been suggested: pulse pressure variation, systolic pressure variation, and the downward portion of systolic pressure variation from baseline (delta down). All three show promise, however pulse pressure variation may be the most predictive, as it is theoretically more closely related to stroke volume (pulse pressure is influenced by stroke volume and arterial compliance, while systolic pressure is also influenced by diastolic pressure) [261]. The majority of studies suggest fluid responsiveness (an increase in stroke volume of greater than 10–15 %) is likely when the pulse pressure variation exceeds approximately 15 %.

One of the major difficulties in comparing any variability parameter based upon preload changes induced from positive pressure ventilation is the lack of standardization of the stimulus inducing the variation. Changes in preload are

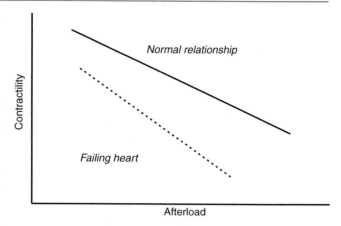

Fig. 40.11 Contractility versus afterload. A negative correlation exists between contractility and afterload [265]. When the heart is failing, this relationship may change in two ways: a decrease in intercept (*downward shift*), and the slope may become increasingly negative. Thus a failing heart may manifest both (**a**) a loss of contractility for a given afterload, and (**b**) a greater decline in contractility when afterload is increased

affected primarily by swings in pleural pressure, which are affected by tidal volume and transmural pressure gradient across the lung (which is in turn affected by factors such as pulmonary edema, consolidation). Thus there is potential for inducing both false positive readings due to excessive ventilation as well as false negative readings when low tidal volumes are used (Fig. 40.10) [262]. The latter situation may be avoided by using tidal volumes of at least 8 mL/kg [263]. Unfortunately, recent studies have highlighted that "real-world" utility of these predictive variables may be rather poor, as a consequence of numerous superimposing confounding factors that occur in the critically ill patient [264].

Contractility

Of all the parameters affecting cardiac output, contractility is perhaps the most difficult to measure at the bedside. The echocardiographic stress velocity index plots stress velocity (contractility) against end systolic wall stress (afterload) and has provided pathophysiological insight into several disease states [265–267]. This relationship changes in the failing heart in two ways: contractility is reduced for a given afterload, and the slope of the contractility-afterload relationship is steeper, meaning that afterload reduction may offer greater benefit (and conversely afterload increase greater harm, Fig. 40.11). Tissue Doppler is a relatively new modality which may provide information on diastolic function as well as contractility [130–133, 268, 269]. Cardiac function index, derived from transpulmonary thermodilution, is defined as stroke volume divided by global end diastolic volume, which is said to be a load independent measure of contractility. To date this has not been investigated in pediatric practice.

Stroke work index represents the area enclosed by the ventricular pressure-volume loop; however, this may be estimated at the bedside from stroke index and arterial pressure measurements. Although not a true measure of contractility, it allows some insight into cardiac reserve, namely how stoke index (volume) is adjusted in the face of changing afterload.

Afterload

Afterload is defined as the force opposing left ventricular fiber shortening during ventricular ejection, in other words left ventricular wall stress [270, 271]. Wall stress can be measured at various points throughout cardiac ejection, although it is thought that calculation at end systole provides the best measure of afterload [272]. Calculation of wall stress requires measurement of end systolic transmural ventricular pressure and echocardiographic measurement of left ventricular end systolic dimension and wall thickness. Here transmural pressure equals the difference between intra- and extraventricular (or intrathoracic) pressures. While intraventricular pressure can be estimated from the mean arterial pressure [273], accurate estimation of extraventricular/intrathoracic pressure is difficult and may involve measurement of esophageal or pleural pressures [274]. Using this approach it is easy to understand how factors that increase intrathoracic pressure, such as positive pressure ventilation, result in a reduction in afterload [15].

Systemic vascular resistance is commonly used as a surrogate measure of afterload in the clinical situation, predominantly because it is easier to measure than wall stress. It is important to appreciate that vascular resistance is not synonymous with afterload. Rather, it is one of several contributory factors. Systemic vascular resistance is analogous to Ohm's law, treating the heart as a "DC" (constant) rather than an "AC" (pulsatile) generator of flow, by measuring the ratio of mean pressure drop across the systemic vascular bed to the flow (see: section "Arterial pulse contour analysis")

$$SVR = \frac{79.9 \times (MAP - CVP)}{cardiac\ index}$$

(SVR, systemic vascular resistance; MAP, mean arterial pressure; CVP, central venous pressure. Units of measurement are dyn-s/cm^5/m^2)

Seen in this light, the limitations of this calculation are obvious. However, it provides the clinician with a single figure that may have prognostic value [275, 276]. The importance of minimizing afterload in the failing myocardium is well documented. However, the clinical dilemma is usually one of balancing afterload reduction against maintaining perfusion pressure (blood pressure). In reality this can only be optimized if cardiac output is measured.

Diastolic Function

The traditional definition of diastole covers the period from the end of aortic ejection (aortic valve closure) until the onset of ventricular tension occurring with the following beat [277]. Diastole is an energy-consuming process, which is influenced by both active and passive mechanisms. Active processes (relaxation) occur within the cardiomyocytes, while passive mechanisms (stiffness) involve external factors, including viscoelastic properties of the extracellular matrix, and changes in both diastolic load and afterload [278]. One of the primary active events concerns the regulation of cytosolic Ca^{2+} levels. Diastolic relaxation requires a drop in calcium concentration within the cytosol, thereby encouraging Ca^{2+} dissociation from troponin C and hence inhibition of actin-myosin cross-bridge activity [279]. Calcium concentration decrease in a variety of ways, the most important being re-uptake into the sarcoplasmic reticulum via a Ca^{2+}-ATPase pump (SERCA), which is in turn regulated by phospholamban. In its dephosphorylated form, phospholamban inhibits Ca^{2+} re-uptake [280]. However, when phosphorylated via a variety of agents, including β-adrenergic agents and phosphodiesterase inhibitors (e.g. milrinone), phospholamban increases Ca^{2+} uptake and hence diastolic relaxation (lusitropy) [281]. This same mechanism also improves systolic function by increasing the Ca^{2+} reservoir. Phosphodiesterase inhibitors appear to act via a second mechanism to increase lusitropy, namely a direct action on phosphodiesterase III located on the outer membrane of the sarcoplasmic reticulum [282].

The contribution of diastolic function to myocardial performance is now well established. Intracardiac pressure and volume measurements allow quantification of the active and passive components of diastolic function. Active relaxation can be estimated by (a) the time constant of isovolumic pressure decline (the time for ventricular pressure to fall by approximately two-thirds), (b) the isovolumic relaxation time, or (c) the maximum rate of pressure decay (−dP/dt) [278, 283]. Passive stiffness can be estimated by the diastolic slope of the pressure-volume curve. Unfortunately, the ability to measure diastolic function at the bedside is limited in pediatric practice. The most common technique is echocardiography. A variety of Doppler-derived parameters can be used to estimate (a) and (b) above, and also to examine patterns of mitral valve and pulmonary venous flow during left ventricular filling (including mitral E and A wave velocities). Unfortunately the majority of these measures are affected by many factors including age, heart rate, afterload, volume status and ventricular filling [278, 283, 284]. Recently, attention has focused towards tissue Doppler indices; however their utility as clinical monitoring tools is as yet relatively unexplored.

As a final note, the hemodynamic calculations discussed in this chapter are summarized in Table 40.2.

Table 40.2 Summary of hemodynamic variables [285, 286]

Parameter	Formula	Normal range	Units
Cardiac index	$CI = CO/\text{body surface area}$	3.5–5.5	$l/min/m^2$
Stroke index	$SI = CI/\text{heart rate}$	30–60	ml/m^2
Arterial oxygen content	$CaO_2 = (1.34 \times Hgb \times SaO_2) + (PaO_2 \times 0.003)$		ml/l
Oxygen delivery	$DO_2 = CI \times CaO_2$	570–670	$ml/min/m^2$
Fick principle	$CI = VO_2/(CaO_2 - CvO_2)$	160–180 (infant VO_2)	$ml/min/m^2$
		100–130 (child VO_2)	$ml/min/m^2$
Mixed venous oxygen saturation		65–75 %	
Oxygen extraction ratio[a]	$OER = (SaO_2 - SvO_2)/SaO_2$	0.24–0.28	
Oxygen excess factor[b]	$W = SaO_2/(SaO_2 - SvO_2)$	3.6–4.2	
Systemic vascular resistance index	$SVRI = 79.9 \times (MAP - CVP)/CI$	800–1,600	$dyn\text{-}s/cm^5/m^2$
Pulmonary vascular resistance index	$PVRI = 79.9 \times (MPAP - LAP)/CI$	80–240	$dyn\text{-}s/cm^5/m^2$
Left ventricular stroke work index	$LVSWI = SI \times MAP \times 0.0136$	50–62 (adult)	$g\text{-}m/m^2$

Abbreviations: *CO* cardiac output, *CI* cardiac index, *CVP* central venous pressure (mmHg), *CaO₂* arterial oxygen content, *CvO₂* mixed venous oxygen content, *DO₂* oxygen delivery, *Hgb* hemoglobin concentration (g/l), *LVSWI* left ventricular stroke work index, *MAP* mean systemic arterial pressure (mmHg), *MPAP* mean pulmonary arterial pressure, *LAP* left atrial pressure, *OER* oxygen extraction ratio, *PaO₂* partial pressure of dissolved oxygen, *SaO₂* arterial oxygen saturation, *SvO₂* mixed venous oxygen saturation, *SI* stroke index, *SVRI* systemic vascular resistance index, *PVRI* pulmonary vascular resistance index, *VO₂* oxygen consumption
[a]The equation is only valid if the contribution of dissolved oxygen is minimal
[b]The equations given for OER and Ω are only valid if the contribution from dissolved oxygen is minimal. If this is not the case, oxygen content (CaO_2, CvO_2) must be substituted for saturation (SaO_2, SvO_2).

References

1. Nichols WW, O'Rourke MF, Viachopoulos C, editors. McDonald's blood flow in arteries, 6th edition: theoretical, experimental and clinical principles. London: Hodder Arnold; 2011.
2. Tibby SM, Murdoch IA. Monitoring cardiac function in intensive care. Arch Dis Child. 2003;88:46–52.
3. Kaye W. Invasive monitoring techniques: arterial cannulation, bedside pulmonary artery catheterization, and arterial puncture. Heart Lung. 1983;12:395–427.
4. Fry DL. Physiologic recording by modern instruments with particular reference to pressure recording. Physiol Rev. 1960;40:753–88.
5. Patel DJ, Mason DT, Ross Jr J, Braunwald E. Harmonic analysis of pressure pulses obtained from the heart and great vessels of man. Am Heart J. 1965;69:785–94.
6. Gardner RM, Hollingsworth KW. Optimizing the electrocardiogram and pressure monitoring. Crit Care Med. 1986;14:651–8.
7. Kleinman B, Powell S, Kumar P, Gardner RM. The fast flush test measures the dynamic response of the entire blood pressure monitoring system. Anesthesiology. 1992;77:1215–20.
8. Gibbs NC, Gardner RM. Dynamics of invasive pressure monitoring systems: clinical and laboratory evaluation. Heart Lung. 1988;17:43–51.
9. Heimann PA, Murray WB. Medical construction and use of catheter-manometer systems. J Clin Monit. 1993;9:45–53.
10. O'Rourke MF. What is blood pressure? Am J Hypertens. 1990;3:803–10.
11. O'Rourke MF. What is the arterial pressure? Aust N Z J Med. 1988;18:649–50.
12. O'Rourke MF, Blazek JV, Morreels Jr CL, Krovetz LJ. Pressure wave transmission along the human aorta. Changes with age and in arterial degenerative disease. Circ Res. 1968;23:567–79.
13. Teitel DF. Cardiac physiology. In: Chang AC, Hanley FL, Wernovsky G, Wessel DL, editors. Pediatric cardiac intensive care. Philadelphia: Lippincott Williams & Wilkins; 1998. p. 25–9.
14. Proulx F, Gauthier M, Nadeau D, Lacroix J, Farrell CA. Timing and predictors of death in pediatric patients with multiple organ system failure. Crit Care Med. 1994;22:1025–31.
15. Shekerdemian L, Bohn D. Cardiovascular effects of mechanical ventilation. Arch Dis Child. 1999;80:475–80.
16. Tibby SM, Hatherill M, Marsh MJ, Murdoch IA. Clinicians' abilities to estimate cardiac index in ventilated children and infants. Arch Dis Child. 1997;77:516–8.
17. Mercier JC, Beaufils F, Hartmann JF, Azema D. Hemodynamic patterns of meningococcal shock in children. Crit Care Med. 1988;16:27–33.
18. Thompson AE. Pulmonary artery catheterization in children. New Horiz. 1997;5:244–50.
19. Shephard JN, Brecker SJ, Evans TW. Bedside assessment of myocardial performance in the critically ill. Intensive Care Med. 1994;20:513–21.
20. Stewart GN. Researches on the circulation time and on the influences which affect it. IV. The output of the heart. J Physiol. 1897;22:159–83.
21. Hamilton WF, Moore JW, Kinsman JM, et al. Studies on the circulation. IV. Further analysis of the injection method, and changes in hemodynamics under physiological and pathological conditions. Am J Physiol. 1932;99:534–42.
22. Zierler K. Indicator dilution methods for measuring blood flow, volume, and other properties of biological systems: a brief history and memoir. Ann Biomed Eng. 2000;28:836–48.
23. Millard RK. Indicator-dilution dispersion models and cardiac output computing methods. Am J Physiol. 1997;272:H2004–12.
24. Stephenson JL. Theory of measurement of blood flow by the dilution on an indicator. Bull Math Biophys. 1948;10:117–21.
25. Wise ME. Tracer dilution curves in cardiology and random walk and lognormal distributions. Acta Physiol Pharmacol Neerl. 1966;14:175–204.
26. Morady F, Brundage BH, Gelberg HJ. Rapid method for determination of shunt ratio using a thermodilution technique. Am Heart J. 1983;106:369–73.
27. Hedvall G. The applicability of the thermodilution method for determination of pulmonary blood flow and pulmonary vascular resistance in infants and children with ventricular septal defects. Scand J Clin Lab Invest. 1978;38:581–5.
28. Hedvall G, Kjellmer I, Olsson T. An experimental evaluation of the thermodilution method for determination of cardiac output and

of intracardiac right-to-left shunts. Scand J Clin Lab Invest. 1973;31:61–8.

29. Joji P, Werner O. Left-to-right shunt assessed by thermodilution during surgery for congenital heart disease. Scand J Thorac Cardiovasc Surg. 1987;21:203–6.

30. Saitoh M, Sudoh M, Haneda N, Watanabe K, Kajino Y, Mori C. Determination of left to right shunt by thermodilution in patients with ventricular septal defect. Jpn Circ J. 1989;53:1205–14.

31. Boehrer JD, Lange RA, Willard JE, Grayburn PA, Hillis LD. Advantages and limitations of methods to detect, localize, and quantitate intracardiac right-to-left and bidirectional shunting. Am Heart J. 1993;125:215–20.

32. Boehrer JD, Lange RA, Willard JE, Grayburn PA, Hillis LD. Advantages and limitations of methods to detect, localize, and quantitate intracardiac left-to-right shunting. Am Heart J. 1992;124:448–55.

33. Nishikawa T, Dohi S. Errors in the measurement of cardiac output by thermodilution. Can J Anaesth. 1993;40:142–53.

34. Zierler K. Equations for measuring blood flow by external monitoring of radioisotopes. Circ Res. 1965;16:309–21.

35. Fegler G. Measurement of cardiac output in anaesthetized animals by a thermodilution method. Q J Exp Physiol. 1954;39:153–64.

36. Branthwaite MA, Bradley RD. Measurement of cardiac output by thermal dilution in man. J Appl Physiol. 1968;24:434–8.

37. Swan HJ, Ganz W, Forrester J, Marcus H, Diamond G, Chonette D. Catheterization of the heart in man with use of a flow-directed balloon-tipped catheter. N Engl J Med. 1970;283:447–51.

38. Silove ED, Tynan MJ, Simcha AJ. Thermal dilution measurement of pulmonary and systemic blood flow in secundum atrial septal defect, and transposition of great arteries with intact interventricular septum. Br Heart J. 1972;34:1142–6.

39. Freed MD, Keane JF. Cardiac output measured by thermodilution in infants and children. J Pediatr. 1978;92:39–42.

40. Colgan FJ, Stewart S. An assessment of cardiac output by thermodilution in infants and children following cardiac surgery. Crit Care Med. 1977;5:220–5.

41. Pollack MM, Reed TP, Holbrook PR, Fields AI. Bedside pulmonary artery catheterization in pediatrics. J Pediatr. 1980;96:274–6.

42. Connors Jr AF, Speroff T, Dawson NV, et al. The effectiveness of right heart catheterization in the initial care of critically ill patients. SUPPORT Investigators. JAMA. 1996;276:889–97.

43. Takala J, Ruokonen E, Tenhunen JJ, Parviainen I, Jakob SM. Early non-invasive cardiac output monitoring in hemodynamically unstable intensive care patients: a multi-center randomized controlled trial. Crit Care. 2011;15:R148.

44. Sandham JD, Hull RD, Brant RF, et al.; Canadian Critical Care Clinical Trials Group. A randomized, controlled trial of the use of pulmonary-artery catheters in high-risk surgical patients. N Engl J Med. 2003;348:5–14.

45. Richard C, Warszawski J, Anguel N, et al.; French Pulmonary Artery Catheter Study Group Service. Early use of the pulmonary artery catheter and outcomes in patients with shock and acute respiratory distress syndrome: a randomized controlled trial. JAMA. 2003;290:2713–20.

46. Yu DT, Platt R, Lanken PN, et al.; AMCC Sepsis Project Working Group. Relationship of pulmonary artery catheter use to mortality and resource utilization in patients with severe sepsis. Crit Care Med. 2003;31:2734–41.

47. Binanay C, Califf RM, Hasselblad V, et al; ESCAPE Investigators and ESCAPE Study Coordinators. Evaluation study of congestive heart failure and pulmonary artery catheterization effectiveness: the ESCAPE trial. JAMA. 2005;294:1625–33.

48. Shah MR, Hasselblad V, Stevenson LW, Binanay C, O'Connor CM, Sopko G, Califf RM. Impact of the pulmonary artery catheter in critically ill patients: meta-analysis of randomized clinical trials. JAMA. 2005;294:1664–70.

49. Iberti TJ, Fischer EP, Leibowitz AB, et al. A multicenter study of physicians' knowledge of the pulmonary artery catheter. JAMA. 1990;264:2928–32.

50. Gnaegi A, Feihl F, Perret C. Intensive care physicians' insufficient knowledge of right-heart catheterization at the bedside: time to act? Crit Care Med. 1997;25:213–20.

51. Mori Y, Nakanishi T, Satoh M, Kondoh C, Momma K. Catheterization of the pulmonary artery using a 3 French catheter in patients with congenital heart disease. Cathet Cardiovasc Diagn. 1998;45:45–50.

52. Janik JE, Conlon SJ, Janik JS. Percutaneous central access in patients younger than 5 years: size does matter. J Pediatr Surg. 2004;39:1252–356.

53. Smith-Wright DL, Green TP, Lock JE, Egar MI, Fuhrman BP. Complications of vascular catheterization in critically ill children. Crit Care Med. 1984;12:1015–7.

54. Bagwell CE, Salzberg AM, Sonnino RE, Haynes JH. Potentially lethal complications of central venous catheter placement. J Pediatr Surg. 2000;35:709–13.

55. Johnson EM, Saltzman DA, Suh G, Dahms RA, Leonard AS. Complications and risks of central venous catheter placement in children. Surgery. 1998;124:911–6.

56. Finck C, Smith S, Jackson R, Wagner C. Percutaneous subclavian central venous catheterization in children younger than one year of age. Am Surg. 2002;68:401–4.

57. Jansen JRC. The thermodilution method for the clinical assessment of cardiac output. Intensive Care Med. 1995;21:691–7.

58. Levett JM, Replogle RL. Thermodilution cardiac output: a critical analysis and review of the literature. J Surg Res. 1979;27:392–404.

59. Moodie DS, Feldt RH, Kaye MP, et al. Measurement of cardiac output by thermodilution: development of accurate measurements at flows applicable to the pediatric patient. J Surg Res. 1978;25:305–11.

60. Jansen JRC, Schreuder JJ, Settels JJ, et al. An adequate strategy for the thermodilution technique in patients during mechanical ventilation. Intensive Care Med. 1990;16:422–5.

61. Stetz CW, Miller RG, Kelly GE, Raffin TA. Reliability of the thermodilution method in the determination of cardiac output in clinical practice. Am Rev Respir Dis. 1982;126:1001–4.

62. van Grondelle A, Ditchey RV, Groves BM, Wagner Jr WW, Reeves JT. Thermodilution method overestimates low cardiac output in humans. Am J Physiol. 1983;245:H690–2.

63. Nelson LD. The new pulmonary arterial catheters. Right ventricular ejection fraction and continuous cardiac output. Crit Care Clin. 1996;12:795–818.

64. O'Quin R, Marini JJ. Pulmonary artery occlusion pressure: clinical physiology, measurement, and interpretation. Am Rev Respir Dis. 1983;128:319–26.

65. Pinsky MR. Pulmonary artery occlusion pressure. Intensive Care Med. 2003;29:19–22.

66. Collee GG, Lynch KE, Hill RD, Zapol WM. Bedside measurement of pulmonary capillary pressure in patients with acute respiratory failure. Anesthesiology. 1987;66:614–20.

67. Pinsky MR. Clinical significance of pulmonary artery occlusion pressure. Intensive Care Med. 2003;29:175–8.

68. Lichtwarck-Aschoff M, Beale R, Pfeiffer UJ. Central venous pressure, pulmonary artery occlusion pressure, intrathoracic blood volume, and right ventricular end-diastolic volume as indicators of cardiac preload. J Crit Care. 1996;11:180–8.

69. von Spiegel T, Hoeft A. Transpulmonary indicator methods in intensive medicine. Anaesthesist. 1998;47:220–8.

70. Arfors KE, Malmberg P, Pavek K. Conservation of thermal indicator in lung circulation. Cardiovasc Res. 1971;5:530–4.

71. Tibby SM, Hatherill M, Marsh MJ, Morrison G, Anderson D, Murdoch IA. Clinical validation of cardiac output measurements using femoral artery thermodilution with direct Fick in ventilated children and infants. Intensive Care Med. 1997;23:987–91.

72. Pauli C, Fakler U, Genz T, Hennig M, Lorenz HP, Hess J. Cardiac output determination in children: equivalence of the transpulmonary thermodilution method to the direct Fick principle. Intensive Care Med. 2002;28:947–52.

73. von Spiegel T, Wietasch G, Bursch J, Hoeft A. Cardiac output determination with transpulmonary thermodilution. An alternative to pulmonary catheterization? Anaesthesist. 1996;45:1045–50.

74. Davey-Quinn A, Gedney JA, Whiteley SM, Bellamy MC. Extravascular lung water and acute respiratory distress syndrome–oxygenation and outcome. Anaesth Intensive Care. 1999;27:357–62.

75. Lemson J, van Die LE, Hemelaar AE, van der Hoeven JG. Extravascular lung water index measurement in critically ill children does not correlate with a chest x-ray score of pulmonary edema. Crit Care. 2010;14:R105.

76. Lemson J, Merkus P, van der Hoeven JG. Extravascular lung water index and global end-diastolic volume index should be corrected in children. J Crit Care. 2011;26:432.e7–12.

77. Newman EV, Merrell M, Genecin A, Monge C, Milnor WR, McKeever WP. The dye dilution method for describing the central circulation. An analysis of factors shaping the time-concentration curves. Circulation. 1951;4:735–46.

78. Boehne M, Schmidt F, Witt L, Köditz H, Sasse M, Sümpelmann R, Bertram H, Wessel A, Osthaus WA. Comparison of transpulmonary thermodilution and ultrasound dilution technique: novel insights into volumetric parameters from an animal model. Pediatr Cardiol. 2012;33:625–32.

79. Cecchetti C, Lubrano R, Cristaldi S, Stoppa F, Barbieri MA, Elli M, Masciangelo R, Perrotta D, Travasso E, Raggi C, Marano M, Pirozzi N. Relationship between global end-diastolic volume and cardiac output in critically ill infants and children. Crit Care Med. 2008;36:928–32.

80. Proulx F, Lemson J, Choker G, Tibby SM. Hemodynamic monitoring by transpulmonary thermodilution and pulse contour analysis in critically ill children. Pediatr Crit Care Med. 2011;12:459–66.

81. Krivitski NM, Kislukhin VV, Thuramalla NV. Theory and in vitro validation of a new extracorporeal arteriovenous loop approach for hemodynamic assessment in pediatric and neonatal intensive care unit patients. Pediatr Crit Care Med. 2008;9:423–8.

82. de Boode WP, van Heijst AF, Hopman JC, et al. Cardiac output measurement using an ultrasound dilution method: a validation study in ventilated piglets. Pediatr Crit Care Med. 2010;11:103–8.

83. Nusmeier A, de Boode WP, Hopman JC, Schoof PH, van der Hoeven JG, Lemson J. Cardiac output can be measured with the transpulmonary thermodilution method in a paediatric animal model with a left-to-right shunt. Br J Anaesth. 2011;107:336–43.

84. Vrancken SL, de Boode WP, Hopman JC, Singh SK, Liem KD, van Heijst AF. Cardiac output measurement with transpulmonary ultrasound dilution is feasible in the presence of a left-to-right shunt: a validation study in lambs. Br J Anaesth. 2012;108:409–16.

85. Imai T, Takahashi K, Fukura H, Morishita Y. Measurement of cardiac output by pulse dye densitometry using indocyanine green: a comparison with the thermodilution method. Anesthesiology. 1997;87:816–22.

86. Hillis LD, Firth BG, Winniford MD. Analysis of factors affecting the variability of Fick versus indicator dilution measurements of cardiac output. Am J Cardiol. 1985;56:764–8.

87. Linton RA, Band DM, Haire KM. A new method of measuring cardiac output in man using lithium dilution. Br J Anaesth. 1993;71:262–6.

88. Linton RA, Linton NW, Band DM. A new method of analysing indicator dilution curves. Cardiovasc Res. 1995;30:930–8.

89. Linton RA, Jonas MM, Tibby SM, et al. Cardiac output measured by lithium dilution and transpulmonary thermodilution in patients in a paediatric intensive care unit. Intensive Care Med. 2000;26:1507–11.

90. Fick A. Über die Messung des Blutquantums in den Herzventrikeln. Sitx der Physik-Med ges Wurzburg. 1870;2:16.

91. Fishman AP. Respiratory gases in the regulation of the pulmonary circulation. Physiol Rev. 1961;41:214–79.

92. Takala J, Keinanen O, Vaisanen P, Kari A. Measurement of gas exchange in intensive care: laboratory and clinical validation of a new device. Crit Care Med. 1989;17:1041–7.

93. Weyland W, Weyland A, Fritz U, Redecker K, Ensink FB, Braun U. A new paediatric metabolic monitor. Intensive Care Med. 1994;20:51–7.

94. Chang AC, Kulik TJ, Hickey PR, Wessel DL. Real-time gas-exchange measurement of oxygen consumption in neonates and infants after cardiac surgery. Crit Care Med. 1993;21:1369–75.

95. Wippermann CF, Huth RG, Schmidt FX, Thul J, Betancor M, Schranz D. Continuous measurement of cardiac output by the Fick principle in infants and children: comparison with the thermodilution method. Intensive Care Med. 1996;22:467–71.

96. Behrends M, Kernbach M, Brauer A, Braun U, Peters J, Weyland W. In vitro validation of a metabolic monitor for gas exchange measurements in ventilated neonates. Intensive Care Med. 2001;27:228–35.

97. Rasanen J. Continuous breathing circuit flow and tracheal tube cuff leak: sources of error during pediatric indirect calorimetry. Crit Care Med. 1992;20:1335–40.

98. Chwals WJ, Lally KP, Woolley MM. Indirect calorimetry in mechanically ventilated infants and children: measurement accuracy with absence of audible airleak. Crit Care Med. 1992;20:768–70.

99. Selby AM, McCauley JC, Schell DN, O'Connell A, Gillis J, Gaskin KJ. Indirect calorimetry in mechanically ventilated children: a new technique that overcomes the problem of endotracheal tube leak. Crit Care Med. 1995;23:365–70.

100. Bernstein G, Knodel E, Heldt GP. Airway leak size in neonates and autocycling of three flow-triggered ventilators. Crit Care Med. 1995;23:1739–44.

101. Castle RA, Dunne CJ, Mok Q, Wade AM, Stocks J. Accuracy of displayed values of tidal volume in the pediatric intensive care unit. Crit Care Med. 2002;30:2566–74.

102. Ultman JS, Bursztein S. Analysis of error in the determination of respiratory gas exchange at varying FIO sub 2. J Appl Physiol. 1981;350:210–6.

103. Kalhan SC, Denne SC. Energy consumption in infants with bronchopulmonary dysplasia. J Pediatr. 1990;116(4):662–4.

104. Light RB. Intrapulmonary oxygen consumption in experimental pneumococcal pneumonia. J Appl Physiol. 1988;64:2490–5.

105. Schulze A, Abubakar K, Gill G, Way RC, Sinclair JC. Pulmonary oxygen consumption: a hypothesis to explain the increase in oxygen consumption of low birth weight infants with lung disease. Intensive Care Med. 2001;27:1636–42.

106. Weyland A, Weyland W, Sydow M, Weyland C, Kettler D. Inverse Fick's principle in comparison to measurements of oxygen consumption in respiratory gases. Does intrapulmonary oxygen uptake account for differences shown by different system methods? Anaesthesist. 1994;43:658–66.

107. Wilkinson JL. Haemodynamic calculations in the catheter laboratory. Heart. 2001;85:113–20.

108. Miller HC, Brown DJ, Miller GA. Comparison of formulae used to estimate oxygen saturation of mixed venous blood from caval samples. Br Heart J. 1974;36:446–51.

109. Jaffe MB. Partial CO2 rebreathing cardiac output–operating principles of the NICO system. J Clin Monit Comput. 1999;15:387–401.

110. Haryadi DG, Orr JA, Kuck K, McJames S, Westenskow DR. Partial CO_2 rebreathing indirect Fick technique for non-invasive measurement of cardiac output. J Clin Monit Comput. 2000;16:361–74.

111. Lumb AB. Nunn's applied respiratory physiology. 5th ed. Oxford: Butterworth-Heinemann; 2000.

112. Levy RJ, Chiavacci RM, Nicolson SC, Rome JJ, Lin RJ, Helfaer MA, Nadkarni VM. An evaluation of a noninvasive cardiac output measurement using partial carbon dioxide rebreathing in children. Anesth Analg. 2004;99:1642–7.

113. Tachibana K, Imanaka H, Takeuchi M, Takauchi Y, Miyano H, Nishimura M. Noninvasive cardiac output measurement using partial carbon dioxide rebreathing is less accurate at settings of reduced minute ventilation and when spontaneous breathing is present. Anesthesiology. 2003;98:830–83.

114. Tibby SM. The indirect Fick principle: great idea, but can we use it in critical care? Pediatr Crit Care Med. 2006;7(3):284–5.

115. Franklin DL, Schlegel WA, Rushmer RF. Blood flow measured by Doppler frequency shift of back-scattered ultrasound. Science. 1961;134:564–5.

116. Colan SD. Echocardiography. In: Chang AC, Hanley FL, Wernovsky G, Wessel DL, editors. Pediatric cardiac intensive care. Philadelphia: Lippincott Williams & Wilkins; 1998. p. 431–3.

117. Side CD, Gosling RG. Non-surgical assessment of cardiac function. Nature. 1971;232:335–6.

118. Cholley BP, Singer M. Esophageal Doppler: noninvasive cardiac output monitor. Echocardiography. 2003;20:763–9.

119. Singer M, Clarke J, Bennett ED. Continuous hemodynamic monitoring by esophageal Doppler. Crit Care Med. 1989;17:447–52.

120. Tibballs J. Doppler measurement of cardiac output–a critique. Anaesth Intensive Care. 1988;16:475–7.

121. Tibby SM, Hatherill M, Murdoch IA. Use of transesophageal Doppler ultrasonography in ventilated pediatric patients: derivation of cardiac output. Crit Care Med. 2000;28:2045–50.

122. Wodey E, Senhadji L, Carre F, Ecoffey C. Extrapolation of cardiac index from analysis of the left ventricular outflow velocities in children: implication of the relationship between aortic size and body surface area. Paediatr Anaesth. 2002;12:220–6.

123. Morrow WR, Murphy Jr DJ, Fisher DJ, Huhta JC, Jefferson LS, Smith EO. Continuous wave Doppler cardiac output: use in pediatric patients receiving inotropic support. Pediatr Cardiol. 1988;9:131–6.

124. Rein AJ, Hsieh KS, Elixson M, Colan SD, Lang P, Sanders SP, Castaneda AR. Cardiac output estimates in the pediatric intensive care unit using a continuous-wave Doppler computer: validation and limitations of the technique. Am Heart J. 1986;112:97–103.

125. Lefrant JY, Bruelle P, Aya AG, Saissi G, Dauzat M, de La Coussaye JE, Eledjam JJ. Training is required to improve the reliability of esophageal Doppler to measure cardiac output in critically ill patients. Intensive Care Med. 1998;24:347–52.

126. Murdoch IA, Marsh MJ, Tibby SM, McLuckie A. Continuous hemodynamic monitoring in children: use of transoesophageal Doppler. Acta Paediatr. 1995;84:761–4.

127. Chew MS, Poelaert J. Accuracy and repeatability of pediatric cardiac output measurement using Doppler: 20-year review of the literature. Intensive Care Med. 2003;29:1889–94.

128. Chew MS, Brandberg J, Bjarum S, et al. Pediatric cardiac output measurement using surface integration of velocity vectors: an in vivo validation study. Crit Care Med. 2000;28:3664–71.

129. Chew MS, Brandberg J, Canard P, Sloth E, Ask P, Hasenkam JM. Doppler flow measurement using surface integration of velocity vectors (SIVV): in vitro validation. Ultrasound Med Biol. 2000;26:255–62.

130. Skubas N. Intraoperative Doppler tissue imaging is a valuable addition to cardiac anesthesiologists' armamentarium: a core review. Anesth Analg. 2009;108:48–66.

131. Van de Veire NR, De Sutter J, Bax JJ, Roelandt JR. Technological advances in tissue Doppler imaging echocardiography. Heart. 2008;94:1065–74.

132. Parra DA. New imaging modalities to assess cardiac function: not just pretty pictures. Curr Opin Pediatr. 2012;24:557–64.

133. Dragulescu A, Mertens LL. Developments in echocardiographic techniques for the evaluation of ventricular function in children. Arch Cardiovasc Dis. 2010;103:603–14.

134. Simpson JM, Miller O. Three-dimensional echocardiography in congenital heart disease. Arch Cardiovasc Dis. 2011;104:45–56.

135. Rushmer RF, Crystal DK, Wagner C, Ellis RM. Intracardiac impedance plethysmography. Am J Physiol. 1953;174:171–4.

136. Kubicek WG, Karnegis JN, Patterson RP, Witsoe DA, Mattson RH. Development and evaluation of an impedance cardiac output system. Aerosp Med. 1966;37:1208–12.

137. Stokes K, Bornzin G. The electrode interface: stimulation. In: Barold SS, editor. Modern cardiac pacing. Mount Kisco: Futura Publishing Co Inc; 1985. p. 33–77.

138. Bonjer FH, van den Berg J, Dirken MN. The origin of the variations of body impedance occurring during the cardiac cycle. Circulation. 1952;6:415–20.

139. Patterson RP, Kubicek WG, Witsoe DA, From AH. Studies on the effect of controlled volume change on the thoracic electrical impedance. Med Biol Eng Comput. 1978;16:531–6.

140. Ikegaki J, Goto R, Obara H. Bioimpedance measurement of cardiac output after open heart surgery. J Pediatr. 1990;116:668–9.

141. Tibballs J. Bioimpedance measurement of cardiac output after open heart surgery. J Pediatr. 1990;116:669.

142. Jensen L, Yakimets J, Teo KK. A review of impedance cardiography. Heart Lung. 1995;24:183–93.

143. Fuller HD. The validity of cardiac output measurement by thoracic impedance: a meta-analysis. Clin Invest Med. 1992;15:103–12.

144. Bernstein DP, Lemmens HJM. Stroke volume equation for impedance cardiography. Med Biol Eng Comput. 2005;43:443–50.

145. Norozi K, Beck C, Osthaus WA, Wille I, Wessel A, Bertram H. Electrical velocimetry for measuring cardiac output in children with congenital heart disease. Br J Anaesth. 2008;100:88–94.

146. Grollmuss O, Demontoux S, Capderou A, Serraf A, Belli E. Electrical velocimetry as a tool for measuring cardiac output in small infants after heart surgery. Intensive Care Med. 2012;38:1032–9.

147. Geddes LA, Hoff HE, Mello A. The development and calibration of a method for the continuous measurement of stroke-volume in the experimental animal. Jpn Heart J. 1966;7:556–65.

148. Baan J, van der Velde ET, de Bruin HG, et al. Continuous measurement of left ventricular volume in animals and humans by conductance catheter. Circulation. 1984;70:812–23.

149. Salo RW, Wallner TG, Pederson BD. Measurement of ventricular volume by intracardiac impedance: theoretical and empirical approaches. IEEE Trans Biomed Eng. 1986;33:189–95.

150. Salo RW. Improvement in intracardiac impedance volumes by field extrapolation. Eur Heart J. 1992;13(Suppl E):35–9.

151. Grossman W, Braunwald E, Mann T, McLaurin LP, Green LH. Contractile state of the left ventricle in man as evaluated from end-systolic pressure-volume relations. Circulation. 1977;56:845–52.

152. Sagawa K. The end-systolic pressure-volume relation of the ventricle: definition, modifications and clinical use. Circulation. 1981;63:1223–7.

153. Glower DD, Spratt JA, Snow ND, et al. Linearity of the Frank-Starling relationship in the intact heart: the concept of preload recruitable stroke work. Circulation. 1985;71:994–1009.

154. Little WC, Cheng CP, Mumma M, Igarashi Y, Vinten-Johansen J, Johnston WE. Comparison of measures of left ventricular contractile performance derived from pressure-volume loops in conscious dogs. Circulation. 1989;80:1378–87.

155. Chaturvedi RR, Lincoln C, Gothard J, et al. Left ventricular dysfunction after open repair of simple congenital heart defects. J Thorac Cardiovasc Surg. 1998;116:881–4.

156. Erlanger J, Hooker DR. An experimental study of blood pressure and of pulse pressure in man. Johns Hopkins Hosp Rep. 1904;12:145–378.

157. Rhodes A, Sunderland R. Arterial pulse contour analysis: the LiDCO™ plus system. In: Pinsky MR, Payen D, editors. Functional hemodynamic monitoring, vol. 42. Berlin: Springer; 2005. p. 183–92. Update in Intensive Care and Emergency Medicine.

158. Dart AM, Kingwell BA. Pulse pressure: a review of mechanisms and clinical relevance. J Am Coll Cardiol. 2001;37:975–84.

159. Kouchoukos NT, Sheppard LC, McDonald DA. Estimation of stroke volume in the dog by a pulse contour method. Circ Res. 1970;26:611–23.

160. Remington JW, Nobach CB, Hamilton WF, Gold JJ. Volume elasticity characteristics of the human aorta and the prediction of stroke volume from the pressure pulse. Am J Physiol. 1948;153:198–308.

161. Langewouters GJ, Wesseling KH, Goedhard WJ. The pressure dependent dynamic elasticity of 35 thoracic and 16 abdominal human aortas in vitro described by a five component model. J Biomech. 1985;18:613–20.

162. Langewouters GJ, Wesseling KH, Goedhard WJ. The static elastic properties of 45 human thoracic and 20 abdominal aortas in vitro and the parameters of a new model. J Biomech. 1984;17:425–35.

163. de Vaal JB, de Wilde RB, van den Berg PC, Schreuder JJ, Jansen JR. Less invasive determination of cardiac output from the arterial pressure by aortic diameter-calibrated pulse contour. Br J Anaesth. 2005;95:326–31.

164. Heerman JR, Segers P, Roosens CD, Gasthuys F, Verdonck PR, Poelaert JI. Echocardiographic assessment of aortic elastic properties with automated border detection in an ICU: in vivo application of the arctangent Langewouters model. Am J Physiol Heart Circ Physiol. 2005;288:H2504–11.

165. Linton NWF, Linton RAF. Estimation of changes in cardiac output from the arterial blood pressure waveform in the upper limb. Br J Anaesth. 2001;86:486–96.

166. Jansen JRC, Schreuder JJ, Mulier JP, et al. A comparison of cardiac output derived from the arterial pressure wave against thermodilution in cardiac surgery patients. Br J Anaesth. 2001;87:212–22.

167. Godje O, Hoke K, Goetz AE, et al. Reliability of a new algorithm for continuous cardiac output determination by pulse-contour analysis during hemodynamic instability. Crit Care Med. 2002;30:52–8.

168. Toorop GP, Westerhof N, Elzinga G. Beat-to-beat estimation of peripheral resistance and arterial compliance during pressure transients. Am J Physiol. 1987;252:H1275–83.

169. Wesseling KH, Jansen JR, Settels JJ, Schreuder JJ. Computation of aortic flow from pressure in humans using a nonlinear, three-element model. J Appl Physiol. 1993;74:2566–73.

170. Frank O. Die Grundform des Arteriellen Pulses. Z Biol. 1899;37:483–526.

171. Saxena R, Durward A, Puppala NK, Murdoch IA, Tibby SM. Pressure recording analytical method for measuring cardiac output in critically ill children: a validation study. Br J Anaesth. 2013;110:425–31.

172. Petretta M, Storto G, Ferro A, Cuocolo A. Radionuclide monitoring of left ventricular function. J Nucl Cardiol. 2001;8:606–15.

173. Kaji S, Yang PC, Kerr AB, et al. Rapid evaluation of left ventricular volume and mass without breath-holding using real-time interactive cardiac magnetic resonance imaging system. J Am Coll Cardiol. 2001;38:527–33.

174. Muthurangu V, Taylor A, Andriantsimiavona R, et al. Novel method of quantifying pulmonary vascular resistance by use of simultaneous invasive pressure monitoring and phase-contrast magnetic resonance flow. Circulation. 2004;110:826–34.

175. Shoemaker WC. Diagnosis and treatment of the shock syndromes. In: Shoemaker WC, Ayres SM, Grenvik A, Holbrook PR, editors. Textbook of critical care. 3rd ed. London: WB Saunders and company; 1995. p. 85–102.

176. Leach RM, Treacher DF. The pulmonary physician in critical care 2: oxygen delivery and consumption in the critically ill. Thorax. 2002;57:170–7.

177. Barratt-Boyes BG, Wood EH. The oxygen saturation of blood in the venae cavae, right-heart chambers, and pulmonary vessels of healthy subjects. J Lab Clin Med. 1957;50:93–106.

178. Freed MD, Miettinen OS, Nadas AS. Oximetric detection of intracardiac left-to-right shunts. Br Heart J. 1979;42:690–4.

179. Kandel G, Aberman A. Mixed venous oxygen saturation. Its role in the assessment of the critically ill patient. Arch Intern Med. 1983;143:1400–2.

180. Nelson LD. Continuous venous oximetry in surgical patients. Ann Surg. 1986;203:329–33.

181. Schumacker PT, Cain SM. The concept of a critical oxygen delivery. Intensive Care Med. 1987;13:223–9.

182. Bloos F, Reinhart K. Venous oximetry. Intensive Care Med. 2005;31:911–3.

183. Schulze A, Whyte RK, Way RC, Sinclair JC. Effect of the arterial oxygenation level on cardiac output, oxygen extraction, and oxygen consumption in low birth weight infants receiving mechanical ventilation. J Pediatr. 1995;126:777–84.

184. Buheitel G, Scharf J, Hofbeck M, Singer H. Estimation of cardiac index by means of the arterial and the mixed venous oxygen content and pulmonary oxygen uptake determination in the early post-operative period following surgery of congenital heart disease. Intensive Care Med. 1994;20:500–3.

185. Barnea O, Santamore WP, Rossi A, Salloum E, Chien S, Austin EH. Estimation of oxygen delivery in newborns with a univentricular circulation. Circulation. 1998;98:1407–13.

186. Charpie JR, Dekeon MK, Goldberg CS, Mosca RS, Bove EL, Kulik TJ. Postoperative hemodynamics after Norwood palliation for hypoplastic left heart syndrome. Am J Cardiol. 2001;87:198–202.

187. Whyte RK. Mixed venous oxygen saturation in the newborn. Can we and should we measure it? Scand J Clin Lab Invest. 1990;50(Suppl203):203–11.

188. Finch CA, Lenfant C. Oxygen transport in man. N Engl J Med. 1972;286:407–15.

189. Rasanen J, Peltola K, Leijala M. Superior vena caval and mixed venous oxyhemoglobin saturations in children recovering from open heart surgery. J Clin Monit. 1992;8:44–9.

190. Tibby SM, Sykes K, Durward A, Austin C, Murdoch IA. Utility of mixed venous versus central venous oximetry following cardiac surgery in infants. Crit Care. 2002;6 Suppl 1:P205. abstr.

191. Reinhart K, Kuhn HJ, Hartog C, Bredle DL. Continuous central venous and pulmonary artery oxygen saturation monitoring in the critically ill. Intensive Care Med. 2004;30:1572–8.

192. Scheinman MM, Brown MA, Rapaport E. Critical assessment of use of central venous oxygen saturation as a mirror of mixed venous oxygen in severely ill cardiac patients. Circulation. 1969;40:165–72.

193. Edwards JD, Mayall RM. Importance of the sampling site for measurement of mixed venous oxygen saturation in shock. Crit Care Med. 1998;26:1356–60.

194. Rivers E, Nguyen B, Havstad S, et al. Early goal-directed therapy in the treatment of severe sepsis and septic shock. N Engl J Med. 2001;345:1368–77.

195. de Oliveira CF, de Oliveira DS, Gottschald AF, Moura JD, Costa GA, Ventura AC, Fernandes JC, Vaz FA, Carcillo JA, Rivers EP, Troster EJ. ACCM/PALS hemodynamic support guidelines for paediatric septic shock: an outcomes comparison with and without monitoring central venous oxygen saturation. Intensive Care Med. 2008;34:1065–75.

196. Salim MA, DiSessa TG, Arheart KL, Alpert BS. Contribution of superior vena caval flow to total cardiac output in children. A Doppler echocardiographic study. Circulation. 1995;92:1860–5.

197. Kasman N, Brady K. Cerebral oximetry for pediatric anesthesia: why do intelligent clinicians disagree? Paediatr Anaesth. 2011;21:473–8.

198. Drayna PC, Abramo TJ, Estrada C. Near-infrared spectroscopy in the critical setting. Pediatr Emerg Care. 2011;27:432–9.

199. Moerman A, Vandenplas G, Bové T, Wouters PF, De Hert SG. Relation between mixed venous oxygen saturation and cerebral oxygen saturation measured by absolute and relative near-infrared spectroscopy during off-pump coronary artery bypass grafting. Br J Anaesth. 2013;110:258–65.

200. Davie SN, Grocott HP. Impact of extracranial contamination on regional cerebral oxygen saturation: a comparison of three cerebral oximetry technologies. Anesthesiology. 2012;16:834–40.

201. Hirsch JC, Charpie JR, Ohye RG, Gurney JG. Near-infrared spectroscopy: what we know and what we need to know–a systematic review of the congenital heart disease literature. J Thorac Cardiovasc Surg. 2009;137:154–9.

202. Ghanayem NS, Wernovsky G, Hoffman GM. Near-infrared spectroscopy as a hemodynamic monitor in critical illness. Pediatr Crit Care Med. 2011;12(4 Suppl):S27–32.

203. Mizock BA, Falk JL. Lactic acidosis in critical illness. Crit Care Med. 1992;20:80–93.

204. James JH, Luchette FA, McCarter FD, Fischer JE. Lactate is an unreliable indicator of tissue hypoxia in injury or sepsis. Lancet. 1999;354:505–8.

205. James JH, Fang CH, Schrantz SJ, Hasselgren PO, Paul RJ, Fischer JE. Linkage of aerobic glycolysis to sodium-potassium transport in rat skeletal muscle. Implications for increased muscle lactate production in sepsis. J Clin Invest. 1996;98:2388–97.

206. Bundgaard H, Kjeldsen K, Suarez Krabbe K, et al. Endotoxemia stimulates skeletal muscle Na+–K+–ATPase and raises blood lactate under aerobic conditions in humans. Am J Physiol Heart Circ Physiol. 2003;284:H1028–34.

207. Levy B, Gibot S, Franck P, Cravoisy A, Bollaert PE. Relation between muscle Na+K+ ATPase activity and raised lactate concentrations in septic shock: a prospective study. Lancet. 2005; 365:871–5.

208. Brealey D, Brand M, Hargreaves I, Heales S, Land J, Smolenski R, Davies NA, Cooper CE, Singer M. Association between mitochondrial dysfunction and severity and outcome of septic shock. Lancet. 2002;360(9328):219–23.

209. Gladden LB. Lactate metabolism: a new paradigm for the third millennium. J Physiol. 2004;558:5–30.

210. Hatherill M, Waggie Z, Purves L, Reynolds L, Argent A. Mortality and the nature of metabolic acidosis in children with shock. Intensive Care Med. 2003;29:286–91.

211. Hatherill M, McIntyre AG, Wattie M, Murdoch IA. Early hyperlactataemia in critically ill children. Intensive Care Med. 2000;26:314–8.

212. Munoz R, Laussen PC, Palacio G, Zienko L, Piercey G, Wessel DL. Changes in whole blood lactate levels during cardiopulmonary bypass for surgery for congenital cardiac disease: an early indicator of morbidity and mortality. J Thorac Cardiovasc Surg. 2000;119:155–62.

213. Nguyen HB, Rivers EP, Knoblich BP, et al. Early lactate clearance is associated with improved outcome in severe sepsis and septic shock. Crit Care Med. 2004;32(8):1637–42.

214. Kolkman JJ, Otte JA, Groeneveld AB. Gastrointestinal luminal PCO2 tonometry: an update on physiology, methodology and clinical applications. Br J Anaesth. 2000;84:74–86.

215. Antonsson JB, Haglund UH. Gut intramucosal pH and intraluminal PO2 in a porcine model of peritonitis or haemorrhage. Gut. 1995;37:791–7.

216. Heino A, Hartikainen J, Merasto ME, Alhava E, Takala J. Systemic and regional pCO2 gradients as markers of intestinal ischaemia. Intensive Care Med. 1998;24:599–604.

217. Tang W, Weil MH, Sun S, Noc M, Gazmuri RJ, Bisera J. Gastric intramural PCO2 as monitor of perfusion failure during hemorrhagic and anaphylactic shock. J Appl Physiol. 1994;76:572–7.

218. Calvo C, Ruza F, Lopez-Herce J, Dorao P, Arribas N, Alvarado F. Usefulness of gastric intramucosal pH for monitoring hemodynamic complications in critically ill children. Intensive Care Med. 1997;23:1268–74.

219. Casado-Flores J, Mora E, Perez-Corral F, Martinez-Azagra A, Garcia-Teresa MA, Ruiz-Lopez MJ. Prognostic value of gastric intramucosal pH in critically ill children. Crit Care Med. 1998;26:1123–7.

220. Duke T, Butt W, South M, Shann F. The DCO2 measured by gastric tonometry predicts survival in children receiving extracorporeal life support. Comparison with other hemodynamic and biochemical information. Chest. 1997;111:174–9.

221. Hatherill M, Tibby SM, Evans R, Murdoch IA. Gastric tonometry in septic shock. Arch Dis Child. 1998;78:155–8.

222. Krafte-Jacobs B, Carver J, Wilkinson JD. Comparison of gastric intramucosal pH and standard perfusional measurements in pediatric septic shock. Chest. 1995;108:220–5.

223. Duke TD, Butt W, South M. Predictors of mortality and multiple organ failure in children with sepsis. Intensive Care Med. 1997;23:684–92.

224. Thorburn K, Hatherill M, Roberts PC, Durward A, Tibby SM, Murdoch IA. Evaluation of the 5-French saline paediatric gastric tonometer. Intensive Care Med. 2000;26:973–80.

225. Uusaro A, Lahtinen P, Parviainen I, Takala J. Gastric mucosal end-tidal PCO2 difference as a continuous indicator of splanchnic perfusion. Br J Anaesth. 2000;85:563–9.

226. Odes HS, Hogan DL, Steinbach JH, Ballesteros MA, Koss MA, Isenberg JI. Measurement of gastric bicarbonate secretion in the human stomach: different methods produce discordant results. Scand J Gastroenterol. 1992;27:829–36.

227. Thorburn K, Durward A, Tibby SM, Murdoch IA. Effects of feeding on gastric tonometric measurements in critically ill children. Crit Care Med. 2004;32:246–9.

228. Groeneveld AB, Kolkman JJ. Splanchnic tonometry: a review of physiology, methodology, and clinical applications. J Crit Care. 1994;9:198–210.

229. Marik PE, Bankov A. Sublingual capnometry versus traditional markers of tissue oxygenation in critically ill patients. Crit Care Med. 2003;31:818–22.

230. Weil MH, Nakagawa Y, Tang W, et al. Sublingual capnometry: a new noninvasive measurement for diagnosis and quantitation of severity of circulatory shock. Crit Care Med. 1999;27:1225–9.

231. Schabauer AM, Rooke TW. Cutaneous laser Doppler flowmetry: applications and findings. Mayo Clin Proc. 1994;69:564–74.

232. Lima AP, Beelen P, Bakker J. Use of a peripheral perfusion index derived from the pulse oximetry signal as a noninvasive indicator of perfusion. Crit Care Med. 2002;30:1210–3.

233. De Felice C, Latini G, Vacca P, Kopotic RJ. The pulse oximeter perfusion index as a predictor for high illness severity in neonates. Eur J Pediatr. 2002;161:561–2.

234. Groner W, Winkelman JW, Harris AG, Ince C, Bouma GJ, Messmer K, Nadeau RG. Orthogonal polarization spectral imaging: a new method for study of the microcirculation. Nat Med. 1999;5:1209–12.

235. Skarda DE, Mulier KE, Myers DE, Taylor JH, Beilman GJ. Dynamic near-infrared spectroscopy measurements in patients with severe sepsis. Shock. 2007;27:348–53.

236. Creteur J. Muscle StO2 in critically ill patients. Curr Opin Crit Care. 2008;14:361–6.

237. Saavedra JM, Harris GD, Li S, Finberg L. Capillary refilling (skin turgor) in the assessment of dehydration. Am J Dis Child. 1991;145:296–8.

238. Hoelzer DJ, Brian MB, Balsara VJ, Varner WD, Flynn TC, Miner ME. Selection and nonoperative management of pediatric blunt

trauma patients: the role of quantitative crystalloid resuscitation and abdominal ultrasonography. J Trauma. 1986;26:57–62.

239. Mackenzie A, Barnes G, Shann F. Clinical signs of dehydration in children. Lancet. 1989;2:605–7.

240. Tibby SM, Hatherill M, Murdoch IA. Capillary refill and core-peripheral temperature gap as indicators of haemodynamic status in paediatric intensive care patients. Arch Dis Child. 1999;80:163–6.

241. Schriger DL, Baraff L. Defining normal capillary refill: variation with age, sex and temperature. Ann Emerg Med. 1988;17:932–5.

242. Lobos AT, Lee S, Menon K. Capillary refill time and cardiac output in children undergoing cardiac catheterization. Pediatr Crit Care Med. 2012;13:136–40.

243. Raimer PL, Han YY, Weber MS, Annich GM, Custer JR. A normal capillary refill time of ≤ 2 seconds is associated with superior vena cava oxygen saturations of ≥ 70%. J Pediatr. 2011;158:968–72.

244. Lobos AT, Menon K. A multidisciplinary survey on capillary refill time: inconsistent performance and interpretation of a common clinical test. Pediatr Crit Care Med. 2008;9:386–91.

245. Braunwald E, Sonnenblick EH, Ross J. Mechanisms of cardiac contraction and relaxation. In: Braunwald E, editor. Heart disease. Philadelphia: WB Saunders; 1988. p. 389–425.

246. Guyton AC. Determination of cardiac output by equating venous return curves with cardiac response curves. Physiol Rev. 1955;35:123–9.

247. Michard F, Teboul JL. Predicting fluid responsiveness in ICU patients: a critical analysis of the evidence. Chest. 2002;121:2000–8.

248. Michard F, Reuter DA. Assessing cardiac preload or fluid responsiveness? It depends on the question we want to answer. Intensive Care Med. 2003;29:1396.

249. Axler O, Tousignant C, Thompson CR, et al. Small hemodynamic effect of typical rapid volume infusions in critically ill patients. Crit Care Med. 1997;25:965–70.

250. Wiesenack C, Prasser C, Keyl C, Rodig G. Assessment of intrathoracic blood volume as an indicator of cardiac preload: single transpulmonary thermodilution technique versus assessment of pressure preload parameters derived from a pulmonary artery catheter. J Cardiothorac Vasc Anesth. 2001;15:584–8.

251. Magder S. How to use central venous pressure measurements. Curr Opin Crit Care. 2005;11:264–70.

252. Skinner JR, Milligan DW, Hunter S, Hey EN. Central venous pressure in the ventilated neonate. Arch Dis Child. 1992;67:374–7.

253. Michard F, Alaya S, Zarka V, Bahloul M, Richard C, Teboul JL. Global end-diastolic volume as an indicator of cardiac preload in patients with septic shock. Chest. 2003;124:1900–8.

254. Sinclair S, James S, Singer M. Intraoperative intravascular volume optimisation and length of hospital stay after repair of proximal femoral fracture: randomised controlled trial. BMJ. 1997;315:909–12.

255. Venn R, Steele A, Richardson P, Poloniecki J, Grounds M, Newman P. Randomized controlled trial to investigate influence of the fluid challenge on duration of hospital stay and perioperative morbidity in patients with hip fractures. Br J Anaesth. 2002;88:65–71.

256. McKendry M, McGloin H, Saberi D, Caudwell L, Brady AR, Singer M. Randomised controlled trial assessing the impact of a nurse delivered, flow monitored protocol for optimisation of circulatory status after cardiac surgery. BMJ. 2004;329(7460):258.

257. Colan SD, Trowitzsch E, Wernovsky G, Sholler GF, Sanders SP, Castaneda AR. Myocardial performance after arterial switch operation for transposition of the great arteries with intact ventricular septum. Circulation. 1988;78:132–41.

258. Appleton CP, Hatle LK, Popp RL. Relation of transmitral flow velocity patterns to left ventricular diastolic function: new insights from a combined hemodynamic and Doppler echocardiographic study. J Am Coll Cardiol. 1988;12:426–40.

259. Bendjelid K, Romand JA. Fluid responsiveness in mechanically ventilated patients: a review of indices used in intensive care. Intensive Care Med. 2003;29:352–60.

260. Magder S. Clinical usefulness of respiratory variations in arterial pressure. Am J Respir Crit Care Med. 2004;169:151–5.

261. Michard F, Boussat S, Chemla D, et al. Relation between respiratory changes in arterial pulse pressure and fluid responsiveness in septic patients with acute circulatory failure. Am J Respir Crit Care Med. 2000;162:134–8.

262. Reuter DA, Bayerlein J, Goepfert MS, Weis FC, Kilger E, Lamm P, Goetz AE. Influence of tidal volume on left ventricular stroke volume variation measured by pulse contour analysis in mechanically ventilated patients. Intensive Care Med. 2003;29:476–80.

263. De Backer D, Heenen S, Piagnerelli M, Koch M, Vincent JL. Pulse pressure variations to predict fluid responsiveness: influence of tidal volume. Intensive Care Med. 2005;31:517–23.

264. Lansdorp B, Lemson J, van Putten MJ, de Keijzer A, van der Hoeven JG, Pickkers P. Dynamic indices do not predict volume responsiveness in routine clinical practice. Br J Anaesth. 2012;108:395–401.

265. Colan SD, Borow KM, Neumann A. Left ventricular end-systolic wall stress-velocity of fiber shortening relation: a load-independent index of myocardial contractility. J Am Coll Cardiol. 1984;4:715–24.

266. Feltes TF, Pignatelli R, Kleinert S, Mariscalco MM. Quantitated left ventricular systolic mechanics in children with septic shock utilizing noninvasive wall-stress analysis. Crit Care Med. 1994;22:1647–58.

267. Bryant RM, Shirley RL, Ott DA, Feltes TF. Left ventricular performance following the arterial switch operation: use of noninvasive wall stress analysis in the postoperative period. Crit Care Med. 1998;26:926–32.

268. Vogel M, Cheung MM, Li J, et al. Noninvasive assessment of left ventricular force-frequency relationships using tissue Doppler-derived isovolumic acceleration: validation in an animal model. Circulation. 2003;107:1647–52.

269. Oki T, Tabata T, Yamada H, et al. Clinical application of pulsed Doppler tissue imaging for assessing abnormal left ventricular relaxation. Am J Cardiol. 1997;79:921–8.

270. Gould KL, Lipscomb K, Hamilton GW, Kennedy JW. Relation of left ventricular shape, function and wall stress in man. Am J Cardiol. 1974;34:627–34.

271. Weber KT, Janicki JS. The dynamics of ventricular contraction: force, length, and shortening. Fed Proc. 1980;39:188–95.

272. Lang RM, Borow KM, Neumann A, Janzen D. Systemic vascular resistance: an unreliable index of left ventricular afterload. Circulation. 1986;74:1114–23.

273. Rowland DG, Gutgesell HP. Use of mean arterial pressure for noninvasive determination of left ventricular end-systolic wall stress in infants and children. Am J Cardiol. 1994;74:98–9.

274. Haney MF, Johansson G, Haggmark S, Biber B. Analysis of left ventricular systolic function during elevated external cardiac pressures: an examination of measured transmural left ventricular pressure during pressure-volume analysis. Acta Anaesthesiol Scand. 2001;45:868–74.

275. Groeneveld AB, Nauta JJ, Thijs LG. Peripheral vascular resistance in septic shock: its relation to outcome. Intensive Care Med. 1988;14:141–7.

276. Ceneviva G, Paschall JA, Maffei F, Carcillo JA. Hemodynamic support in fluid-refractory pediatric septic shock. Pediatrics. 1998;102:e19.

277. Wiggers CJ. Studies on the duration of the consecutive phases of the cardiac cycle. 1: the duration of the consecutive phases of the cardiac cycle and criteria for their precise determination. Am J Physiol. 1921;56:415–38.

278. Zile MR, Brutsaert DL. New concepts in diastolic dysfunction and diastolic heart failure: Part I: diagnosis, prognosis, and measurements of diastolic function. Circulation. 2002;105:1387–93.

279. Villars PS, Hamlin SK, Shaw AD, Kanusky JT. Role of diastole in left ventricular function, I: biochemical and biomechanical events. Am J Crit Care. 2004;13:394–403.

280. Bers DM. Calcium fluxes involved in control of cardiac myocyte contraction. Circ Res. 2000;87:275–81.

281. Tanigawa T, Yano M, Kohno M, et al. Mechanism of preserved positive lusitropy by cAMP-dependent drugs in heart failure. Am J Physiol Heart Circ Physiol. 2000;278:H313–20.

282. Yano M, Kohno M, Ohkusa T, et al. Effect of milrinone on left ventricular relaxation and Ca(2+) uptake function of cardiac sarcoplasmic reticulum. Am J Physiol Heart Circ Physiol. 2000;279:H1898–905.

283. Hamlin SK, Villars PS, Kanusky JT, Shaw AD. Role of diastole in left ventricular function, II: diagnosis and treatment. Am J Crit Care. 2004;13:453–66.

284. Quinones MA. Assessment of diastolic function. Prog Cardiovasc Dis. 2005;47:340–55.

285. Perloff WH. Invasive measurements in the PICU. In: Fuhrman BP, Zimmerman JJ, editors. Pediatric critical care. 2nd ed. St. Louis: Mosby; 1998. p. 70–86.

286. Shann F. Drug doses. 8th ed. Melbourne: Collective Pty Ltd; 1994. p. 61.

Neurological Monitoring of the Critically-Ill Child

Elizabeth A. Newell, Bokhary Abdulmohsen, and Michael J. Bell

Abstract

Mortality rates from critical illnesses in children continue to decline and neurological morbidity has become the next frontier of to cross for advancing pediatric critical care. Since neurological injuries from lack of nutrients, inadequate removal of metabolic byproducts and alterations of blood flow can rapidly lead to permanent disabilities, a variety of means to monitor the nervous system have been developed over the years with a goal of determining injuries at the earliest possible time. These systems have been utilized in various brain injuries – either acquired prior to ICU admission or during the critical illness – but none have sufficient reliability to be utilized in all conditions. This chapter will review the various non-invasive (physical examination, electrophysiological, ultrasonographic and serum neuromarkers) and invasive (intracranial pressure monitoring, brain oxygen tension and others) neurological monitors that are currently in use or emerging from clinical research. The purpose of this chapter is to briefly review the monitoring systems that can be used by the pediatric intensivist at this time and to describe newer technologies that might be available in the future.

Keywords

Neurological monitor • Acquired brain injury • Intracranial pressure monitoring • Electrophysiological monitoring

As overall mortality rates from critical illnesses continue to decline – because of advances in quality controls, improvements in guidelines and standard therapies as well as technical advances within the field – the new benchmark for quality improvement processes will move toward improved overall quality of life and well-being. As a result, improvement in the neurological outcome of children with critical illnesses has been increasingly viewed as the next threshold to overcome. Within the pediatric intensive care unit, the overall goal of monitoring the brain is to detect injurious processes at a time when they can be corrected. An ideal neurological monitor would have several properties that would ultimately allow proven interventions that could treat the injury – be available at the bedside for minute-to-minute use, gather data through non-invasive means, use technology that is easily interpreted by the clinician, have high reliability, sensitivity, specificity and accurately predict overall outcomes. Unfortunately, such a monitor does not exist at the present time and our understanding on how to intervene for such injuries remains rudimentary. Instead, a number of monitoring systems can be used and the most commonly used techniques are described below (Table 41.1). The intent of this chapter is to outline how these systems may be utilized in the current PICU environment.

E.A. Newell, MD • M.J. Bell, MD (✉)
Department of Critical Care Medicine, Children's Hospital of Pittsburgh, 400 45th Street, Pittsburgh, PA 15116, USA
e-mail: newellea@upmc.edu; bellmj4@upmc.edu

B. Abdulmohsen, MD
Department of Pediatric Critical Care, Al Hada Armed Forces Hospital, 1347, Tai 21944, Kingdom of Saudi Arabia
e-mail: drbokhary@hotmail.com

D.S. Wheeler et al. (eds.), *Pediatric Critical Care Medicine*,
DOI 10.1007/978-1-4471-6362-6_41, © Springer-Verlag London 2014

Table 41.1 Comparisons of clinically available neuromonitors

Monitor	Physiological process measured	Sampling area	Advantages	Disadvantages
ICP monitor	Intracerebral pressure	Global without localization	Bedside, reliable, therapeutic (intraventricular)	Invasive
EEG	Cerebral activity and metabolism	Global with localization	Bedside, non-invasive, continuous data gathering available	Expertise required
Evoked potentials	Localized cerebral activity after applied stimuli	Global with localization	Bedside, non-invasive	Expertise required
Xenon techniques	Cerebral blood flow	Global with localization	Bedside (Xe-133 only), non-invasive, reliable	Patient transport required (Xe-CT), infrastructure costly, specialized instruments
Transcranial Doppler ultrasonography	Cerebral blood flow velocity of specified arteries	Regional	Bedside, non-invasive	Expertise required
Jugular venous oxygen saturation	Cerebral metabolism	Global without localization	Bedside, ideally reflects blood flow to metabolic demands	Invasive, thrombosis, infection, questionable reliability
Near infrared spectroscopy	Cerebral oxygenation	Regional	Bedside, non-invasive, continuous data gathering	Reliability, standards unclear
Brain tissue oxygen tension	Cerebral oxygenation	Focal	Bedside, continuous data gathering	Invasive, threshold unclear
Cerebral microdialysis	Selected metabolites	Focal	Bedside, continuous data gathering, choice of metabolites for study	Invasive, thresholds unclear
MR spectroscopy	Cerebral metabolism	Focal with many areas available for sampling	Non-invasive, no radiation exposure	Patient transport required, limited number of samples to compare
Neuromarkers	Cellular injury or disruption	Global without localization, although specific cell types may be detected	Bedside, non-invasive, no special equipment needed	Specificity to CNS injury, reliability

Physical Examination

The most critical and fundamental method to monitor the brain of a critically-ill child is by a detailed, focused physical examination. Often, the earliest signs of evolving brain injuries are obvious from the repetitive observations of bedside providers, such as changes in cranial nerve function, muscle tone, strength, sensation and altered levels of consciousness. These "low-tech" assessments can be performed virtually continuously without undue harm to the child and serve as a screening tool for more invasive or costly procedures to document the evolving injury, such as an evolving stroke manifested as unilateral weakness of a limb or a new encephalopathy detected by a decreased level of consciousness.

A standardized tool to assess neurological function in critically ill children is the Glasgow Coma Scale (GCS) score [1] (Table 41.2). Initially developed to assess adults after traumatic brain injury, this simple scale can provide a rapid, objective assessment of a child's level of consciousness (as measured by eye opening, verbal responses and

motor responses) that is reproducible between caregivers [2]. The GCS is an effective predictor of neurological outcome of traumatically injured adults, but its predictive value in children has not been validated. This may be a result of poorer reporting of the GCS by caregivers in children. In the stabilization of traumatically-injured adults or children, the GCS can be used to track significant neurological deterioration. As an example, a decrease of more than 3 points in the scale is often interpreted as an indication of a clinical change that warrants further investigation [3]. Its utility as a quantitative, repeatable assessment of mental status is clear and serves a valuable function as a neurological screening tool.

Intracranial Pressure (ICP) Monitoring

Measurement and management of abnormal increases in intracranial pressure has been a mainstay of medical care of children and adults for decades. Monitoring ICP after traumatic brain injury is likely the most common use of the technology,

Table 41.2 Glasgow Coma Scale (GCS) score

E (Eye)

4 = Opens eyes spontaneously

3 = Opens eyes in response to voice

2 = Opens eyes in response to painful stimulus

1 = Does not open eyes

V (Verbal)

5 = Oriented, converses normally (smiles, orients to sound, follows/tracks)

4 = Confused, disoriented (cries, but consolable)

3 = Utters inappropriate words (moaning)

2 = Incomprehensible sounds (inconsolable, agitated)

1 = Makes no sounds

M (Motor)

6 = Obeys commands (moves spontaneously)

5 = Localizes painful stimuli (withdraws from touch)

4 = Withdraws to painful stimuli (withdraws from pain)

3 = Abnormal flexion to painful stimuli (decorticate posturing)

2 = Abnormal extension to painful stimulu (decerebrate posturing)

1 = Makes no movements

The pediatric version of the GCS is shown in parentheses, where appropriate

Decorticate posturing is present when the arms (elbows, wrists, and fingers) are flexed and bent inward on the chest, the hands are clenched into fists, and the legs are extended and internally rotated

Decerebrate posturing is present when the arms and legs are both extended and internally rotated

but it has been utilized for hypoxic injuries, metabolic disorders (Reye's syndrome and hepatic encephalopathy) and a wide variety of other conditions [4–9]. The main rationales for measuring ICP are (i) detection and treatment of fatal cerebral herniation events and (ii) detection of possible secondary insults related to either increased intracranial pressure or decreased brain perfusion. While the first rationale is obvious, the application of the second rationale has been more difficult. Following TBI, up to 80 % of autopsy specimens from patients demonstrate significant ischemic lesions [10], and it was theorized that episodes of increased ICP represented periods of decreased brain perfusion. Early studies by Gopinath and colleagues demonstrated that episodes of intracranial pressure greater than 20 mmHg correlated with poor neurological outcome in adults after traumatic brain injury [11]. This threshold value has largely been adopted in adult TBI and now transferred into pediatric practice, yet evidence to support this threshold is sparse for children with TBI [12, 13] and is entirely absent for children with other conditions such as meningitis, hydrocephalous or stroke.

Measurement of ICP can be accomplished using monitors in a variety of locations [14]. Currently, ICP monitors are placed either in the brain parenchyma or in the ventricular space. Parenchymal monitors are easy to place (requiring only a reflection of the dura) and are believed to carry a decreased risk for infection. However, intraparenchymal monitors cannot be recalibrated and first-generation intraparenchymal monitors were found to have significant drift [15]. Newer intraparenchymal monitors have corrected this problem. The advantages of intraventricular monitors are the ability to withdraw CSF as a therapy for increased intracranial pressure and the ease of recalibration, which can be accomplished using the same techniques as any intravascular catheter. Intraventricular monitors may be more technically challenging to place (especially when significant cerebral swelling has already occurred) and there have been anecdotal reports of an increased infection risk. No systematic reviews of this complication are available at the time of the writing of this chapter. In selecting monitor location, the underlying disease process needs to be strongly considered. For TBI, we believe that intraventricular monitors should be strongly considered when intracranial hypertension is likely to develop and when the procedure is technically-feasible. In a recent study completed at our institution, the utility of placement of both ventricular and parenchymal monitors demonstrated improved detection of ICP crises [16]. On the other hand, for monitoring brain function during hepatic encephalopathy where profound coagulopathy and bleeding risks are substantial, placement of catheters within the epidural space have been associated with decreased morbidity (3.8 % incidence compared to 20 and 22 % for parechymal and ventricular devices, respectively) and mortality (1 % incidence compared to 5 and 4 %) [17]. Careful considerations should be given to locations based on individual risk/benefit profiles for each patient undergoing this invasive monitoring procedure.

Electrophysiological Monitoring

Electrophysiological monitoring in the ICU has become more common over the last decade with portable digital systems. The various monitoring systems outlined below can serve any of four vital functions (detection of epileptiform activity; monitoring of cerebral metabolic rate as evidenced by depth of sedation or drug-induced coma; early detection of neurological deterioration as in hypoxic-ischemic processes or herniation; prognostication of overall clinical outcome) in critically ill children. In general, electrophysiological monitors have similar strengths and weaknesses. All of the monitors discussed below are non-invasive, can be used effectively at the patient's bedside and can be used serially to follow interval changes in the child's condition. However, most of the monitors require relatively advanced training in interpretation (all except for the Bispectral index monitor) and can be adversely affected by the relatively hostile electrical environment within intensive care units. Nevertheless, electrophysiological monitoring is a mainstay in the care of children with critical neurological disorders.

Bispectral (BIS) Index Monitoring

Since most critically ill children require sedation for procedures (mechanical ventilation, in particular), an objective assessment of the depth of sedation is critical. Several physical examination scores (the COMFORT score, the Ramsey scale) have been used but a more objective measure of sedation depth has been sought [18–20]. The BIS index is derived from two surface EEG electrodes placed over the frontal cortex and generates numerical values that correlate with levels of sedation from a wide variety of anesthetics (0 = isoelectric, 100 = fully awake). The mathematical computations from the EEG signal used to generate the BIS index involve artifact filtering, suppression detection, fast Fourier transformation, and estimation of signal quality. Intraoperative studies have demonstrated that adequate anesthesia, as assessed by movement at incision, correlates well with BIS values <60 [21] and that BIS values of 40–60 are typical during maintenance of general anesthesia [22].

Most relevant to pediatric intensivists, studies suggest that amnesia reliably occurs at BIS values <64–80 [23]. Ideally, medications could be administered to critically ill children and titrated to given BIS scores to maintain an adequate, but not excessive, level of sedation. At present, several small series have attempted to correlate BIS values with both clinical sedation scores and signs of drug withdrawal [18–20, 24]. The correlations have been relatively weak and because of this, the BIS monitor has not yet become standard at this time.

Electroencephalography (EEG)

Electroencephalograms are surface tracings of brain electrical activity. Traces are generated by measuring amplified electrical potential differences between two electrodes (represented as an EEG channel) placed in designated locations on the child's skull using the International 10–20 system (sometimes with modifications). Typically, 16 or 32 EEG channels are recorded in a variety of montages (which can be now be retrospectively montaged with digital machines). Rhythmicity, amplitude and location of waveforms are determined and can be indicative of normal or abnormal function of the relevant brain regions. For instance, alpha waves of 8–13 Hz over the posterior portions of the head occur during wakefulness, while waves of frequencies over 13 Hz (designated as beta activity) can be seen with common ICU medications (i.e. benzodiazepines, phenytoin, and barbiturates). Young children have greater amounts of theta activity (frequencies of 4–7 Hz) but focal or lateralized theta activity is indicative of localizing CNS pathology. Overall, much can be gleaned from careful interpretation of EEG. However, more detailed examination of these waves is beyond the

scope of this chapter (and beyond most pediatric intensivists). A team-based approach to the monitoring and management of these critically ill patients is therefore warranted and highly desired.

EEGs can be performed as a single routine examination (rEEG) or as a continuous recording (cEEG). rEEG monitoring was the most common neurological procedure of a newly formed neurocritical care service (occurring in 152 children of the 373 seen over a 14-month period), with the most common indication to diagnose a suspected seizure [25]. With rEEG, provocative stimuli or commands (eye opening and closing, loud auditory stimuli, induced hyperventilation, photic stimuli) are routinely used to elicit characteristic wave changes or epileptic events. However, with the advent of digital monitors to record and sometimes interpret data, cEEG is becoming a more common neurological monitoring device for the critically-ill child [26]. There is accumulating evidence that non-convulsive status epilepticus (NCS) is underappreciated in critically-ill children with altered (or unable to be assessed) mental status [27, 28]. The incidence of NCS in children with acute encephalopathy ranges between 16 and 47 % and a recent prospective study of the use of cEEG in this patient population led to a change in management in 59 % of cases [29]. Jordan and colleagues applied continuous EEG to 124 consecutive neuroscience intensive care unit patients and recorded seizures in 35 %, of which 76 % were NCS [30]. cEEG is commonly used to monitor the depth of drug-induced coma in children since the duration of burst suppression is highly correlative with tissue concentrations of these agents. In adults, cEEG has also been used to detect impending cerebral ischemia caused by vasospasm after subarachnoid hemorrhage, a less common complication in children. Potential indications for cEEG monitoring include severe traumatic brain injury with GCS less than 13, intracranial hypertension, requirement for neuromuscular blockade in a neurologically-vulnerable child, early or partial seizures, use of hypothermia, treatment of refractory status epilepticus, coma of unknown etiology and global brain ischemia [31–34].

EEG monitoring is non-invasive and provides immediate bedside data, yet improvements in overall patient outcomes have not been demonstrated through large clinical trials. Significant limitations to EEG monitoring include the requirement for trained staff for lead placement, the necessity of frequent expert interpretation of waveforms and the difficulties in obtaining clear signals in an artifact abundant environment. To aid in interpretation, various strategies including compression of waveforms and trending displays have been adopted for clinical practices. The compressed spectral array method displays a pseudo-three dimensional image of the temporal evolution of the EEG frequency distribution and relative amplitude [35]. A fast Fourier transform analysis of the EEG generates a frequency spectrum for a given epoch of time. Serial epochs are then displayed behind each other giving a three-dimensional appearance. The pattern of frequencies over time suggests different states (i.e. predominant low frequencies suggesting sedation or coma and predominant high frequencies suggesting seizures). Amplitude-integrated EEGs were first developed in the 1960s [35, 36] and these allowed for the trending of EEG amplitude over extended time periods on a logarithmic scale. Patterns of amplitude changes were shown to correlate with cerebral states (burst suppression, seizures) but only a small number of recording channels (1 or 2) is generally measured. In the recently completed studies that demonstrated the efficacy of hypothermia for perinatal asphyxia, amplitude-integrated EEGs were likely the most important factor in selecting subjects that would benefit from the experimental therapy [37]. Evolution of EEG technology, both in acquiring signals and in data interpretation, will likely continue for the foreseeable future to determine the state of neurological activity in critically ill children.

Evoked Potentials

Evoked potentials are measurements of electrical activity of relevant brain regions after a peripheral stimulus has been applied. Stimuli are applied to sensory nerves (normally the median or posterior tibial nerve), visual fields or auditory pathways and the conduction of the impulses to the cortex is measured. Characteristic waves are generated and amplitudes and latencies can implicate regions of damage to sensory nerves, pathways or nuclei within the CNS.

Within the intensive care unit, testing for the presence of somatosensory (SSEP), brainstem (BAEP) and visual (VEP) evoked potentials has generally been performed to prognosticate outcomes of subjects with coma, spinal cord and brainstem injury. In adults with coma, several meta-analyses have shown SSEPs to be the best predictor of outcome. In children, the data regarding the prognostic value of SSEPs is less extensive. A recent systematic review of the literature examining the predictive power of SSEPs supported the value of this test [38] while another review identified children who demonstrated absence of cortical SSEPs who survived with only mild neurological deficits [39]. Similarly, BAEP and VEP combined were prognostic of poor outcome in a series of children following hypoxic coma [32]. Abnormal SSEP latencies have been shown to correlate with encephalopathy secondary to sepsis in adults [40]. The main advantage of evoked potentials is that these waveforms are relatively unaffected by sedative medications. The tests are relatively labor intensive, require technical expertise and can only be performed intermittently. These monitoring modalities are less frequently used than conventional EEG, but are useful in select patient populations within the intensive care unit.

Assessments of Blood Flow and/or Metabolism

Because of the brain's large requirement for oxygen and its dependence on aerobic respiration for optimal neuronal functioning, it has been widely accepted that measures of cerebral blood flow, metabolism and oxygenation are useful indicators of local or global cerebral function. A variety of monitors have been developed to assess these parameters either locally or globally and those that are in widespread use are summarized below. Some of the monitors directly measure one or more of these parameters while others use inferences to derive data that can be used by clinicians. Monitoring techniques that are available at specialized centers for research purposes (such as positron emission tomography) will not be discussed in this review.

Xenon Cerebral Blood Flow Determination

Xenon is an inert gas that is taken up by the brain but not metabolized. As such, it can be used in conjunction with a variety of detection devices to estimate both local and global cerebral blood flow by measuring its overall distribution and clearance [41]. Xenon can be administered via inhalation or intravenously. Intravenously-injected, radioactive Xe-133 can be detected within the cranial vault using multiple stationary scintillation detectors around the head. By this method, xenon-133 uptake and elimination can be measured and global cerebral blood flow can be determined. Alternatively, inhalation of xenon gas can be used to estimate blood flow using CT imaging (Xe-CT). Using software and detection methods within the CT scanner, uptake of xenon within the brain can be measured and a cerebral blood flow map can be generated. Cerebral blood flow of individual brain structures (white matter vs. grey matter, structures within the deep brain structures, peritrauma areas and others) can be quantified in ml/100 g tissue/min [41]. This technique has the disadvantage of requiring transportation to the imaging facility, and inhaled Xe currently is only approved from the FDA for use for experimental applications. While Xenon cerebral blood flow techniques could have many clinical applications [42], its use in pediatrics has been quite limited. Adelson and colleagues recently reported a series of over 60 children who had blood flow determinations early after TBI using Xe-CT where they found a relationship between decreased CBF and poor outcome[43]. The future of determinations of CBF using direct imaging techniques may require either a broader application of Xe-based techniques or adaptations of magnetic resonance imaging applications.

Transcranial Doppler Ultrasonography: (TCD)

Transcranial Doppler ultrasonography (TCD) is a non-invasive technique to determine the cerebral blood velocity in large intracranial vessels [44]. The handheld probe can be placed over the temporal bone window, foramen magnum window and/or transorbital window allowing evaluation of anterior cerebral circulation, vertebrobasilar circulation and ophthalmic artery and carotid siphon circulation, respectively. TCD measures mean cerebral blood flow velocity (MCBFV) using the principles of ultrasound and spectral Doppler shift of blood cell flow through these large vessels and can (i) determine the presence or absence of flow, (ii) calculate systolic, diastolic and mean velocities and (iii) determine the direction of flow. With these determinations graphically represented, a pulsatility index (PI) can be calculated (PI = [Peak velocity – diastolic velocity]/mean velocity) that represents downstream resistance to blood flow. The hemispheric index or Lindegaard's ratio of the mean velocity within the middle cerebral artery to that in the internal carotid artery ($MCBFV_{MCA}/MCBFV_{ICA}$) is indicative of cerebral vasospasm when >3 and of hyperemia (edema) <3.

The main clinical indications for TCD in children are determining vessel patency, detecting focal areas of vasospasm, confirmation of the clinical diagnosis of brain death (criteria includes severely diminished $MCBFV_{ICA}$, absent diastolic flow, reverberating flow and severely elevated PI) [45] and determination of cerebral autoregulation. In an elegant series of studies over the past decade or more, Vavilala and colleagues have identified autoregulatory abnormalities in children with traumatic brain injuries and found that these disturbances are associated with overall outcome [46–50]. TCD is readily available at the bedside but requires a relatively high level of technical expertise, yet it appears that the future of this technique may bring about important advances in neurological monitoring.

Jugular Venous Oxygen Saturation: (SjvO₂)

Measurement of the oxygen saturation in the blood leaving the brain ($SjvO_2$) is a global, indirect measure of cerebral blood flow that is contingent upon both blood flow and oxygen metabolism. It assumes that the sampling of blood from a single jugular vein can adequately represent the entire venous return from the entire brain while excluding contributions from extracerebral sources. The saturation of this blood can lead to inferences regarding cerebral blood flow and metabolism. Sub-optimal saturation (usually defined as <50 % saturated), indicates inadequate CBF for metabolic demands, implying that cerebral ischemia may be occurring. Based on these findings, clinical protocols for restoration of $SjvO_2$ can be initiated that may mitigate this potential

secondary insult – including treatment of inadvertent hyperventilation, treatment of unrecognized anemia, restoration of adequate cerebral perfusion or mitigation of intracranial hypertensive crises.

The use of $SjvO_2$ monitoring in children is generally limited to traumatic brain injury and during extracorporeal membrane oxygenation [51–53]. Despite potential advantages of $SjvO_2$ monitoring (ease of placement and interpretation, use of relatively basic technology, and real-time data generation), its use is limited because of its questionable reliability and potential complications. In a series of 32 adults in traumatic coma, both jugular vein saturations were measured simultaneously and a difference of at least 15 % between each monitor was noted in almost half of the patients during the study [54]. Catheter thrombosis and infection have been reported in adults, and the potential for these complications to worsen the outcome of children (with smaller vessel calibers based on development) has also limited the utilization of this monitoring methodology.

Near-Infrared Spectroscopy: NIRS

Near-infrared spectroscopy (NIRS) is a noninvasive tool allowing for detection of changes in regional tissue oxygen saturation (rSO2) and thus provides information on perfusion-metabolism coupling. NIRS devices rely on the principle that one is able to measure the concentration of a substance based on its absorption of light (Beer-Lambert law). NIRS devices thus consist of a light source and detector and use two wavelengths of near-infrared light (730, 810 nm) taking advantage of the differential absorption of light by deoxyhemoglobin and oxyhemoglobin. As deoxygenated hemoglobin absorbs more light below wavelengths of 805 nm, the ratio of absorbance at 810 and 730 nm provides a percentage of oxyhemoglobin. As most hemoglobin in tissue is in the venous circulation, the relative oxygen index measured by the probe is venous weighted. Additionally, data from skin and skull are subtracted to provide a regional oxygen saturation for cerebral tissue 1–2 cm below the skin [55]. While accepted reference ranges exist for rSO_2 values, absolute normal values have not been determined. In healthy term newborns, a recent study reported a median cerebral rSO_2 of 76 %. In a series of critically ill children including those with both systemic and neurologic diseases, a mean cerebral rSO_2 of 68 % was found with 46.7 % being 2SD below the mean and a potential threshold value [56].

NIRS may be a better neuromonitor for children than adults since the quality of the signal will be affected by the density of the bones of the skull. NIRS has been used in small studies to assess cerebral oxygenation in children with coma [57, 58], during heart surgery [59] and in several other assorted conditions. In adults, the inability of the NIRS to detect occult ischemic events (infarctions in subcortical tissue directly under the probe) has been reported. Currently, NIRS is used as a bedside screening tool to rapidly diagnose accumulation of secondary hematomas after trauma (signal is lost as fluid accumulates) [60]. Since NIRS is non-invasive, it can be measured continuously and both trends and absolute values of cerebral oxygenation can be followed. NIRS assumes that other forms of hemoglobin are not present within the blood at significant quantities and would be unreliable in these situations. Furthermore, the penetration of the light from NIRS is limited to several centimeters under normal conditions. Therefore, the calculated oxygenation index will not reflect the deeper structures of the brain in older children. Presently, NIRS is an intriguing clinical tool that needs to be fully evaluated.

Brain Oxygen Monitoring and Cerebral Microdialysis

Clinical use of monitors that directly measure the partial pressure of brain tissue oxygen (PbO$_2$) have increased in recent years. Currently, the most commonly used device relies on a Clark electrode at the end of a catheter that provides a measure of PbO$_2$ in units of tension (mmHg)[61]. Because PbtO$_2$ monitors clearly provide a local measure of oxygen tension, placement of the device in normal or injured tissue can have profound impacts on the values and their interpretation. Many clinical studies place the catheter in normal tissue and measure the effect of global processes on brain oxygenation. Alternatively, as perilesional or penumbral areas may have the highest risk for secondary injury, these locations may ultimately lead to detection of important clinical events. Human and animal studies have attempted to define normal ranges of PbtO$_2$, with the most commonly cited normal values ranging from 20 to 35 [62].

Experience in children is limited but this monitoring technique is gaining acceptance in injured adults [63–66] and it has recently been recommended within the traumatic brain injury guidelines for adult TBI victims [67]. In children, fewer studies regarding the use of PbtO$_2$ monitoring have been conducted. However, in pediatric TBI, there is also evidence that PbtO$_2$ levels below 10–15 mmHg are associated with worse outcome [68, 69]. Moreover, application of PbO$_2$ monitoring to other conditions has been reported [70].

Cerebral microdialysis has been performed the past two decades and serves to measure mediators of interest directly from the brain parenchyma. Microdialysis catheters are constructed with an in-flow port, an out-flow port and a semipermeable membrane. Artificial cerebrospinal fluid is perfused as a dialysate through the in-flow port across the semi-permeable membrane into the brain parenchyma. Solutes from the brain tissue can diffuse across the membrane and are recovered from the out-flow port. The recovery of solutes is dependent upon the dialysate flow rate, the membrane pore size and solute concentrations within the brain. The relative change in dialysate concentration can reflect similar changes within the brain parenchyma. Samples are collected serially and a wide variety of mediators can be measured from the dialysate (including glucose, pyruvate, lactate, glycerol, excitatory amino acids, purines, nitric oxide metabolites and others).

Cerebral microdialysis has become more common over the past several years for a variety of disorders [71–79]. Microdialysis is a relatively invasive measure of local concentrations of metabolites within a small area of brain. For these reasons, extrapolations of this information to larger areas of brain are problematic. Since serial measurements can be obtained, valuable information can be gleaned during the monitoring period regarding the state of the brain and the effect of various therapies, yet its use in children with critical brain injuries remains very limited.

MR Spectroscopy: MRS

Nuclei of atoms, protons or 31P, can be excited by a strong magnetic field. When the field is interrupted, the nuclei resonate in a frequency that can be detected and quantified. Using this method, metabolites of cellular metabolism can be detected with the spatial resolution of MR images. Proton MRS can detect N-acetyl compounds, primarily N-acetylaspartate (NAA), creatine (including phosphocreatine and its precursor, creatine) and choline-containing compounds (including free choline, phosphoryl, and glycerophosphoryl choline). NAA is a neuronal marker, whereas the choline compounds are released as glial membranes are damaged. Proton MRS can determine the concentration of lactate (accumulating from tissue damage) and various neurotransmitters (GABA and glutamate). Concentrations of ATP, phosphocreatine, and some of the other high-energy phosphates involved in cellular energetics can be assessed using 31P-MRS. Spectra can be acquired within 1 h, and changes in intracellular pH and metabolites can be followed.

Proton and 31P-MRS has been used in the localization of epileptic foci, evaluation of the extent of post-traumatic lesions, classification of brain tumors, prediction of outcome after brain trauma and diagnosis of the various mitochondrial disorders, leukodystrophies, and other demyelinating disorders [80, 81]. The ability to non-invasively measure a host of metabolites within the brain is the unique function of MRS. However, scanning times are still prolonged and caution must be taken to ensure patient safety during the time the spectra are being generated. Furthermore, while studies can be repeated, each image reflects the brain milieu at a single time point.

Serum Markers of Neurological Injuries: Neuromarkers

The field of neurological monitoring has generally been hampered by several factors – the need for transportation of a critically-ill child to a machine to detect an injury (such as neurological imaging), the requirement of specialized expertise at the bedside for routine testing (such as with evoked potentials, EEG) or the need for invasive monitoring (such as with ICP or PbO_2). Because of these limitations, the development of serological markers that are associated with CNS injury would be a powerful advance for the field and the evolution of neuromarkers has made great strides in recent years. Currently, several CNS-specific proteins – neuron-specific enolase (NSE) from neurons, $S100\beta$ from astrocytes, myelin-basic protein (MBP) from oligodendrocytes – have been tested in a variety of clinical conditions to detect neurological injuries. The concept underpinning neuromarkers assumes that the detection of these brain-related proteins within the serum (or sometimes urine) necessarily implies the death of brain cells within the CNS and release of these proteins within the systemic circulation. Currently, these markers remain an extremely innovative approach toward detecting neurological injuries after stroke, cardiac arrest, traumatic brain injury or abusive head trauma [82, 83], and their clinical utility remains to be determined.

Conclusion

Clinical neuromonitoring is a rapidly advancing field in pediatric critical care medicine and the present chapter reviews the most commonly used modalities. Currently, no single monitor can effectively perform all of the functions demanded by clinicians caring for critically ill children. Developing the proper combination of techniques appropriate for each child is the challenge of the coming years to improve neurological outcomes.

References

1. Lieberman JD, et al. Use of admission Glasgow Coma Score, pupil size, and pupil reactivity to determine outcome for trauma patients. J Trauma. 2003;55(3):437–42; discussion 442–3.
2. Hooper SR, et al. Caregiver reports of common symptoms in children following a traumatic brain injury. NeuroRehabilitation. 2004;19(3):175–89.
3. Adelson PD, et al. Guidelines for the acute medical management of severe traumatic brain injury in infants, children, and adolescents. Chapter 5. Indications for intracranial pressure monitoring in pediatric patients with severe traumatic brain injury. Pediatr Crit Care Med. 2003;4(3 Suppl):S19–24.
4. Lundberg N, Troupp H, Lorin H. Continuous recording of the ventricular fluid pressure in patients with severe acute traumatic brain injury. J Neurosurg. 1965;22:581–9.
5. Pople IK, et al. Results and complications of intracranial pressure monitoring in 303 children. Pediatr Neurosurg. 1995;23(2):64–7.
6. Le Roux PD, et al. Pediatric intracranial pressure monitoring in hypoxic and nonhypoxic brain injury. Childs Nerv Syst. 1991;7(1):34–9.
7. Jenkins JG, et al. Reye's syndrome: assessment of intracranial monitoring. Br Med J (Clin Res Ed). 1987;294(6568):337–8.
8. Alper G, et al. Outcome of children with cerebral edema caused by fulminant hepatic failure. Pediatr Neurol. 1998;18(4):299–304.
9. Luerssen TG. Intracranial pressure: current status in monitoring and management. Semin Pediatr Neurol. 1997;4(3):146–55.
10. Graham D, Adams J, Doyle D. Ischemic brain damage in fatal, nonmissile head injuries. J Neurol Sci. 1978;39:213–9.
11. Gopinath SP, et al. Jugular venous desaturation and outcome after head injury. J Neurol Neurosurg Psychiatry. 1994;57(6):717–23.
12. Chambers IR, et al. Critical thresholds of intracranial pressure and cerebral perfusion pressure related to age in paediatric head injury. J Neurol Neurosurg Psychiatry. 2006;77(2):234–40.
13. Chambers IR, et al. Age-related differences in intracranial pressure and cerebral perfusion pressure in the first 6 hours of monitoring after children's head injury: association with outcome. Childs Nerv Syst. 2005;21(3):195–9.
14. North B, Reilly P. Comparison among three methods of intracranial pressure recording. Neurosurgery. 1986;18:730–2.
15. Ghajar J. Intracranial pressure monitoring techniques. New Horiz. 1995;3(3):395–9.
16. Exo J, et al. Intracranial pressure-monitoring systems in children with traumatic brain injury: combining therapeutic and diagnostic tools. Pediatr Crit Care Med. 2011;12(5):560–5.
17. Blei AT, et al. Complications of intracranial pressure monitoring in fulminant hepatic failure. Lancet. 1993;341(8838):157–8.
18. Courtman SP, Wardurgh A, Petros AJ. Comparison of the bispectral index monitor with the Comfort score in assessing level of sedation of critically ill children. Intensive Care Med. 2003;29(12):2239–46.
19. Crain N, Slonim A, Pollack MM. Assessing sedation in the pediatric intensive care unit by using BIS and the COMFORT scale. Pediatr Crit Care Med. 2002;3(1):11–4.
20. Grindstaff RJ, Tobias JD. Applications of bispectral index monitoring in the pediatric intensive care unit. J Intensive Care Med. 2004;19(2):111–6.
21. Liu J, Singh H, White PF. Electroencephalographic bispectral index correlates with intraoperative recall and depth of propofol-induced sedation. Anesth Analg. 1997;84(1):185–9.
22. Avramov MN, White PF. Methods for monitoring the level of sedation. Crit Care Clin. 1995;11(4):803–26.
23. Simmons LE, et al. Assessing sedation during intensive care unit mechanical ventilation with the Bispectral Index and the Sedation-Agitation Scale. Crit Care Med. 1999;27(8):1499–504.
24. Tobias JD, Berkenbosch JW. Tolerance during sedation in a pediatric ICU patient: effects on the BIS monitor. J Clin Anesth. 2001;13(2):122–4.
25. Bell MJ, et al. Development of a pediatric neurocritical care service. Neurocrit Care. 2009;10(1):4–10.
26. Procaccio F, et al. Electrophysiologic monitoring in neurointensive care. Curr Opin Crit Care. 2001;7:74–80.
27. Raspall-Chaure M, et al. Outcome of paediatric convulsive status epilepticus: a systematic review. Lancet Neurol. 2006;5(9):769–79.
28. Wirrell E, Farrell K, Whiting S. The epileptic encephalopathies of infancy and childhood. Can J Neurol Sci. 2005;32(4):409–18.
29. Abend NS, et al. Impact of continuous EEG monitoring on clinical management in critically ill children. Neurocrit Care. 2011;15(1):70–5.

30. Jordan K. Continuous EEG and evoked potential monitoring in the neuroscience intensive care unit. J Clin Neurophysiol. 1993;10:445–75.

31. Mandel R, et al. Prediction of outcome after hypoxic-ischemic encephalopathy: a prospective clinical and electrophysiologic study. J Pediatr. 2002;141:45–50.

32. Mewasingh L, et al. Predictive value of electrophysiology in children with hypoxic coma. Pediatr Neurol. 2003;28:178–83.

33. Hosoyaa M, et al. Low-voltage activity in EEG during acute phase of encephalitis predicts unfavorable neurological outcome. Brain Dev. 2002;24:161–5.

34. Vespa P, Nenov V, Nuwer MR. Continuous EEG monitoring in the intensive care unit: early findings and clinical efficacy. J Clin Neurophysiol. 1999;16(1):1–13.

35. Bickford R, et al. The compressed spectral array. A pictorial EEG. Proc San Diego Biomed Symp. 1972;11:365–70.

36. Prior P, Maynard DE, editors. Monitoring cerebral function: long-term monitoring of EEG and evoked potentials. Amsterdam: Elsevier Science Ltd; 1986.

37. Shankaran S, et al. Whole-body hypothermia for neonates with hypoxic-ischemic encephalopathy. N Engl J Med. 2005;353(15):1574–84.

38. Carrai R, et al. Prognostic value of somatosensory evoked potentials in comatose children: a systematic literature review. Intensive Care Med. 2010;36(7):1112–26.

39. Wohlrab G, Boltshauser E, Schmitt B. Neurological outcome in comatose children with bilateral loss of cortical somatosensory evoked potentials. Neuropediatrics. 2001;32(5):271–4.

40. Zauner C, et al. Impaired subcortical and cortical sensory evoked potential pathways in septic patients. Crit Care Med. 2002;30:1136–9.

41. Perez-Arjona E, et al. New techniques in cerebral imaging. Neurol Res. 2002;24:S17–26.

42. Kilpatrick M, et al. CT-Based assessment of acute stroke: CT, CT angiography, and xenon-enhanced CT cerebral blood flow. Stroke. 2001;32:2543–9.

43. Adelson PD, et al. Cerebrovascular response in children following severe traumatic brain injury. Childs Nerv Syst. 2011;27(9):1465–76.

44. Manno E. Transcranial Doppler ultrasonography in the neurocritical care unit. Crit Care Clin. 1997;13:79–104.

45. Hassler W, Steinmetz H, Gawlowski J. Transcranial Doppler ultrasonography in raised intracranial pressure and in intracranial circulatory arrest. J Neurosurg. 1988;68:745–51.

46. Philip S, et al. Cerebrovascular pathophysiology in pediatric traumatic brain injury. J Trauma. 2009;67(2 Suppl):S128–34.

47. Vavilala MS, et al. Hemispheric differences in cerebral autoregulation in children with moderate and severe traumatic brain injury. Neurocrit Care. 2008;9(1):45–54.

48. Vavilala MS, et al. Neurointensive care; impaired cerebral autoregulation in infants and young children early after inflicted traumatic brain injury: a preliminary report. J Neurotrauma. 2007;24(1):87–96.

49. Vavilala MS, Lam AM. Propofol decreases cerebral blood flow velocity in anesthetized children. Can J Anaesth. 2003;50(5):527–8, author reply 528.

50. Vavilala MS, et al. Cerebral autoregulation before and after blood transfusion in a child. J Neurosurg Anesthesiol. 2001;13(3):233–6.

51. Pettignano R, et al. The use of cephalad cannulae to monitor jugular venous oxygen content during extracorporeal membrane oxygenation. Crit Care (Lond). 1997;1(3):95–9.

52. Perez A, et al. Jugular venous oxygen saturation or arteriovenous difference of lactate content and outcome in children with severe traumatic brain injury. Pediatr Crit Care Med. 2003;4(1):33–8.

53. Schneider GH, et al. Continuous monitoring of jugular bulb oxygen saturation in comatose patients–therapeutic implications. Acta Neurochir (Wien). 1995;134(1–2):71–5.

54. Stocchetti N, et al. Cerebral venous oxygen saturation studied with bilateral samples in the internal jugular veins. Neurosurgery. 1994;34(1):38–43; discussion 43–4.

55. Drayna PC, Abramo TJ, Estrada C. Near-infrared spectroscopy in the critical setting. Pediatr Emerg Care. 2011;27(5):432–9, quiz 440–2.

56. Subbaswamy A, et al. Correlation of cerebral Near-infrared spectroscopy (cNIRS) and neurological markers in critically ill children. Neurocrit Care. 2009;10(1):129–35.

57. Wagner BP, Pfenninger J. Dynamic cerebral autoregulatory response to blood pressure rise measured by near-infrared spectroscopy and intracranial pressure. Crit Care Med. 2002;30(9):2014–21.

58. Nagdyman N, et al. Comparison between cerebral tissue oxygenation index measured by near-infrared spectroscopy and venous jugular bulb saturation in children. Intensive Care Med. 2005;31(6):846–50.

59. Hayashida M, et al. Cerebral ischaemia during cardiac surgery in children detected by combined monitoring of BIS and near-infrared spectroscopy. Br J Anaesth. 2004;92(5):662–9.

60. Gopinath S, et al. Near-infrared spectroscopic localization of intracranial hematomas. J Neurosurg. 1993;79:43–7.

61. Maloney-Wilensky E, Le Roux P. The physiology behind direct brain oxygen monitors and practical aspects of their use. Childs Nerv Syst. 2010;26(4):419–30.

62. Maloney-Wilensky E, et al. Brain tissue oxygen and outcome after severe traumatic brain injury: a systematic review. Crit Care Med. 2009;37(6):2057–63.

63. Jodicke A, Hubner F, Boker DK. Monitoring of brain tissue oxygenation during aneurysm surgery: prediction of procedure-related ischemic events. J Neurosurg. 2003;98(3):515–23.

64. Kett-White R, et al. Cerebral oxygen and microdialysis monitoring during aneurysm surgery: effects of blood pressure, cerebrospinal fluid drainage, and temporary clipping on infarction. J Neurosurg. 2002;96(6):1013–9.

65. Sarrafzadeh AS, et al. Cerebral oxygenation in contusioned vs. nonlesioned brain tissue: monitoring of PtiO2 with Licox and Paratrend. Acta Neurochir Suppl. 1998;71:186–9.

66. Valadka AB, et al. Relationship of brain tissue PO2 to outcome after severe head injury. Crit Care Med. 1998;26(9):1576–81.

67. Bratton SL, et al. Guidelines for the management of severe traumatic brain injury. X. Brain oxygen monitoring and thresholds. J Neurotrauma. 2007;24 Suppl 1:S65–70.

68. Figaji AA, et al. Pressure autoregulation, intracranial pressure, and brain tissue oxygenation in children with severe traumatic brain injury. J Neurosurg Pediatr. 2009;4(5):420–8.

69. Figaji AA, et al. Brain tissue oxygen tension monitoring in pediatric severe traumatic brain injury. Part 2: relationship with clinical, physiological, and treatment factors. Childs Nerv Syst. 2009;25(10):1335–43.

70. Allen BB, et al. Continuous brain tissue oxygenation monitoring in the management of pediatric stroke. Neurocrit Care. 2011;15(3):529–36.

71. Vespa P, et al. Metabolic crisis without brain ischemia is common after traumatic brain injury: a combined microdialysis and positron emission tomography study. J Cereb Blood Flow Metab. 2005;25(6):763–74.

72. Parkin M, et al. Dynamic changes in brain glucose and lactate in pericontusional areas of the human cerebral cortex, monitored with rapid sampling on-line microdialysis: relationship with depolarisation-like events. J Cereb Blood Flow Metab. 2005;25(3):402–13.

73. Johnston AJ, et al. Effect of cerebral perfusion pressure augmentation on regional oxygenation and metabolism after head injury. Crit Care Med. 2005;33(1):189–95; discussion 255–7.

74. Nelson DW, et al. Cerebral microdialysis of patients with severe traumatic brain injury exhibits highly individualistic patterns as visualized by cluster analysis with self-organizing maps. Crit Care Med. 2004;32(12):2428–36.

75. Bellander BM, et al. Consensus meeting on microdialysis in neuro-intensive care. Intensive Care Med. 2004;30(12):2166–9.

76. Winter CD, et al. Raised parenchymal interleukin-6 levels correlate with improved outcome after traumatic brain injury. Brain. 2004;127(Pt 2):315–20.

77. Sarrafzadeh AS, et al. Metabolic changes during impending and manifest cerebral hypoxia in traumatic brain injury. Br J Neurosurg. 2003;17(4):340–6.

78. Vespa PM, et al. Persistently low extracellular glucose correlates with poor outcome 6 months after human traumatic brain injury despite a lack of increased lactate: a microdialysis study. J Cereb Blood Flow Metab. 2003;23(7):865–77.

79. Magnoni S, et al. Lack of improvement in cerebral metabolism after hyperoxia in severe head injury: a microdialysis study. J Neurosurg. 2003;98(5):952–8.

80. Shutter L, Tong KA, Holshouser BA. Proton MRS in acute traumatic brain injury: role for glutamate/glutamine and choline for outcome prediction. J Neurotrauma. 2004;21(12):1693–705.

81. Brenner T, et al. Predicting neuropsychologic outcome after traumatic brain injury in children. Pediatr Neurol. 2003;28:104–14.

82. Berger RP, et al. Neuron-specific enolase and S100B in cerebrospinal fluid after severe traumatic brain injury in infants and children. Pediatrics. 2002;109(2):E31.

83. Topjian AA, et al. Neuron-specific enolase and S-100B are associated with neurologic outcome after pediatric cardiac arrest. Pediatr Crit Care Med. 2009;10(4):479–90.

Nutrition Monitoring in the PICU

George Briassoulis

Abstract

The ideal set of variables for nutritional monitoring that may correlate with patient outcomes has not been identified. This is particularly difficult in the PICU patient because many of the standard modes of nutritional monitoring, although well described and available, are fraught with difficulties. Thus, repeated anthropometric and laboratory markers must be jointly analyzed but individually interpreted according to disease and metabolic changes, in order to modify and monitor the nutritional treatment. In addition, isotope techniques are neither clinically feasible nor compatible with the multiple measurements needed to follow progression. On the other hand, indirect alternatives exist but may have pitfalls, of which the clinician must be aware. Risks exist for both overfeeding and underfeeding of PICU patients so that an accurate monitoring of energy expenditure, using targeted indirect calorimetry, is necessary to avoid either extreme. This is very important, since the monitoring of the nutritional status of the critically ill child serves as a guide to early and effective nutritional intervention.

Keywords

Nutrition • Monitoring • PICU • Energy expenditure • Metabolic monitor • Anthropometrics

Introduction

Metabolic demands of critical illness and underfeeding or overfeeding may expose seriously ill children to the threat of malnutrition or metabolic overload (acute metabolic syndrome). In addition, nutritional status itself affects every pediatric patient's response to illness. Reports of poor provision of nutrition in intensive care units, as well as evidence of malnutrition [1] or overfeeding [2] in critically ill patients are still frequent. Recent studies, compared with similar surveys performed up to three decades ago, showed that there has been little improvement in nutritional status in pediatric populations in the interim [3].

Although caloric intake lower than the basic metabolic rate has been associated with higher mortality and morbidity

G. Briassoulis, MD, PhD
PICU, University Hospital, University of Crete,
Voutes Area, Heraklion, Crete 71110, Greece
e-mail: ggbriass@med.uoc.gr

rates [4], critically ill children have been reported to only receive a median 58.8 % of their energy requirements, which could not be optimized until the 10th intensive care day [5]. In another study, patients in the Pediatric Intensive Care Unit (PICU) received a median of 37.7 % (range, 0.2–130.2 %) of their estimated energy requirements [6]. Only 52 % achieved full estimated energy requirements at any time during their admission. Failure to estimate energy requirements accurately [7], barriers to bedside delivery of nutrients, and reluctance to perform regular nutritional assessments are responsible for the persistence and delayed detection of malnutrition in this cohort [8]. At the same time, using targeted indirect calorimetry, a high incidence of unintended overfeeding in critically ill children with a long stay has been recently detected [2]. The predominance of hypometabolism, failure of physicians to correctly predict metabolic state, use of stress factors, and inaccuracy of standard equations all contributed to cumulative energy excess in this cohort [8].

Nutritional monitoring should be an integral part of the care for every pediatric critically ill patient. Despite the realization of its importance and the high incidence of combination of malnutrition and low energy intake, most medical professionals seldom assess and monitor the nutritional status of hospitalized patients [9]. A survey in 111 European PICUs from 24 countries showed that a multidisciplinary nutritional team was available in 73 % of PICUs. Approximately 70 % of PICUs used dedicated software for nutritional support and acknowledged nutritional support as an important aspect of patient care, yet only 17 % of them regularly monitored energy expenditure by indirect calorimetry. In most PICUs daily energy requirements were estimated using weight, age, predictive equations with correction factors, and a wide range of biochemical blood parameters [9].

Assessing Nutritional Status

Subjective Global Nutritional Assessment (SGNA)

The ideal set of variables for nutritional monitoring that may correlate with patient outcomes has not been identified. This is particularly difficult in the PICU patient because many of the standard modes of nutritional monitoring, although well described and available, are fraught with difficulties. Thus, repeated anthropometric and laboratory markers must be jointly analyzed but individually interpreted according to disease and metabolic changes, in order to modify and monitor the nutritional treatment. In addition, isotope techniques are neither clinically feasible nor compatible with the multiple measurements needed to follow progression. On the other hand, indirect alternatives exist but may have pitfalls, of which the clinician must be aware. Overall, among assessment instruments, only 11 original instruments and three modified ones were published with enough information to allow appropriate usage [10]. This is very important, since the monitoring of the nutritional status of the critically ill child serves as a guide to appropriately modify nutritional intervention.

Because of the 24-h 7-day-a-week time requirement for the initial nutrition screen in a PICU, many units use staff nurses to complete the screening at the time of admission. These screens are generally shorter in length than more in depth screens that include laboratory values, but have the advantage that they can be done efficiently and in a timely fashion. Certain components of nutritional assessment have been combined into a clinical tool described as the subjective global nutritional assessment (SGNA) that physicians can use to systematically document and recognize nutritional problems in their hospitalized patients [11]. It provides a systematic method for obtaining essential information about nutritional status from the history and the physical exam, such as the history of weight loss, altered food consumption, gastrointestinal derangements, decreased functional capacity, subcutaneous tissue loss, muscle wasting, and the presence of edema. It demands training but is easily learned, adds little additional effort to a routine admission history and physical examination, and is a powerful predictor of adverse outcomes [12]. Thus, SGNA has been validated by anthropometry and albumin measurement, and predicted morbidity and mortality in severely ill patients [13]. Those patients classified as severely malnourished by the SGNA presented with a consistent worsening of the traditional objective markers, had significantly more complications, remained in the hospital longer and had a higher mortality rate. Additionally, it has been shown that SGNA is a sensitive and specific nutrition assessment tool for assessing nutritional status in children having major thoracic or abdominal surgery and identifying those at higher risk of nutrition-associated complications and prolonged hospitalizations [14]. Therefore, application of the protocol as a complement of standard anthropometric tool in a PICU setting should be considered.

Anthropometrics

In the initial evaluation of nutritional status, only updated national or regional standard growth curves, the most rudimentary of assessment tools, are necessary. The child who suddenly or progressively deviates from an established pattern is at high risk for depletion. The height indexed to the height of the 50th percentile is useful in assessing chronic changes, but its value in acute illness is not clear. Weight is more likely to be affected by acute changes, while deviation from the height curve perhaps reflects long-standing caloric deprivation. The current body weight is often compared with the ideal body weight for height in order to roughly estimate the patient's body habitus versus norms. These measurements can be converted to growth velocities or to height-for-age and weight-for-height Z-scores or percent of expected values to provide a measure of the degree of under- or overnutrition in the child [15]. There are several important caveats, however, in monitoring anthropometries in the critically ill. They suffer from the influence of intra-observer and interobserver errors and are compared with tables derived from healthy populations. Furthermore, the edema and ecchymoses often encountered in the PICU setting interfere with accurate determinations. Monitoring the weight/height/age ratios, therefore, based on the National Center for Health Statistics [16] and the World Health Organization child growth charts [17] can be used as reference but there is a risk of over- and underestimation of malnutrition rates compared with country-specific growth references [18]. For children with specific medical conditions and syndromes, specific growth references should be used for appropriate interpretation of nutritional status [19].

Body mass index (BMI) may also be used to assess nutritional status. This weight-stature index is calculated as weight in kilograms divided by height in meters squared. Although there is no consensus on how to interpret BMI in relation to nutritional status, a BMI of <15 kg/m^2 has been associated with significant increases in morbidity and mortality. In moderately malnourished children, percentage of standard BMI was the best predictor for serum leptin concentrations, which were low not only in severe acute malnutrition, but also in children with mild-to-moderate malnutrition without chronic disease [20]. In adults, it has been suggested that the relationship between BMI and patient outcomes is "U" shaped, with worse outcomes for both underweight (BMI <18.5 kg/m^2) and morbidly obese (>40 kg/m^2) patients [21, 22]. In evaluating more severe changes, chronic and acute nutritional status was defined by interpreting the Waterlow stages for chronic protein-energy malnutrition (CPEM) and acute protein-energy malnutrition (APEM) [23]. Patients classified by these criteria as CPEM or APEM are more than 2 SD from the median (Table 42.1). Another widely used anthropometric classification is the Z score [24]. It may be used for children of any age, and rates lower than −2 Z scores or less than average indicate undernutrition. Children whose rates are lower than −3 Z scores or less than 70 % in relation to average, or those who present with edema provenly due to nutrition, are considered severely undernourished.

Skinfold thickness (TSF) and circumference measurements of the arms, legs and/or trunk may be useful to characterize the changes in peripheral fat depots and muscle mass, respectively. Upper arm TSF and mid-arm circumferences (MAC) represent body-compartment measurements of adipose tissue and muscle. Arm muscle size is been calculated from arm circumference and triceps skinfold and should be useful in monitoring the depletion of lean body mass [25]. In infants, 10 % of body weight should be fat; by 5–10 months of age, this should be up to 20 %. Even in adults, compared with the BMI, the MAC was a better mortality predictor in patients with chronic obstructive pulmonary disease [26]. MAC and cutaneous TSF are determined using Lange skinfold callipers and a tape measure [27]. From these measurements, mid-arm muscle circumference (MMC), mid-arm muscle area (MMA), and mid-arm fat area (MFA) are calculated. Fat stores are assessed by measurements of TSF and MFA; somatic protein stores are assessed by MMC and MMA. Both, fat and protein stores are classified as normal, nutritionally at risk, or deficient, according to Frisancho [28, 29] and Ryan, Martinez [30] or the Standards of the Ten-State Nutritional Survey [31] tables (Table 42.2). Critically ill patients whose arm circumference values are below the fifth percentile have a higher mortality rate [32]. Acute fluid shifts and changes in circulating albumin, however, cannot only influence weight, but also arm circumference and skinfold thickness determinations. In a recent prospective study, however, in which 80 % of children received enteral nutrition, there was no statistically significant change in most anthropometric indicators evaluated in the PICU, suggesting that nutrition probably helped patients maintain their nutrition status [33]. Importantly, in children with cancer, although the weight-for-height values were normal, MAC and TSF values were significantly less than control values [34]. In a prospective PICU study, although weight and all arm anthropometrics decreased, only arm circumference and

Table 42.1 Criteria for relative risk for malnutrition

A. Acute protein energy malnutrition (APEM): weight for height = (actual weight)/(50th percentile weight for subject's height and age)

Waterlow stage[a]			
0	1	2	3
Normal	At risk	Greater risk	Protein-calorie malnutrition
>90 %	80–89 %	70–79 %	<69 %

B. Chronic protein energy malnutrition (CPEM): subject's height/50th percentile height for subject's age

Waterlow stage[a]			
0	1	2	3
Normal	At risk	Greater risk	Growth retarded
>95 %	90–95 %	85–89 %	<85 %

[a]Each Waterlow stage represents approximately 1 SD from the population median; patients are classified by these criteria as APEM or CPEM, if they are 2 SD or more from the median (stages 2–3)

Table 42.2 Anthropometric nutritional status assessment

Somatic protein stores:		
Midarm muscle circumference: MMC (mm) = MAC[a] (mm) − (TSF $[mm]$ × 3.14)		
Midarm muscle area: MMA (mm^2) = (MAC $[mm]$ − [TSF $[mm]$ × 3.14])^2/4π		
Fat stores:		
Triceps skinfold thickness (TSF) $[mm]$		
Midarm fat area (MFA) (mm^2) = MAA[b] − MMA		
Frisancho tables		
Normal	Nutritionally at risk	Deficient
>10 percentile	5–10 percentile	<5 percentile

[a]Midarm circumference = MAC
[b]Midarm area: MAA (mm^2) = π/4 × (MAC/π)^2

triceps skinfold thickness were significantly decreased at day 7 compared with initial measurements [33]. Thus, it has been suggested that arm anthropometry should replace the use of weight-related indices to identify malnutrition in children with co-morbidity [24].

Obesity

The National Health and Nutrition Examination Survey and Pediatric Nutrition Surveillance System report a tripling of the prevalence of BMI at least 95 % (obesity) among US school-age children and adolescents over the past three decades [35]. International data confirm similar upward shifts in pediatric BMI distribution, especially in countries undergoing economic transitions favoring industrialized, western urban lifestyles [24]. Among adults, nearly one-third of ICU patients are obese and nearly 7 % are morbidly obese, frequencies that are predicted to increase as the prevalence of obesity in the general population rises [36]. However, there is a critical lack of research on how obesity may affect complications of critical illness and patient long-term outcomes. Data of 8,813 mechanically ventilated adults >18 years who remained in the ICU for >72 h (multicenter international observational study of ICU nutrition practices that occurred in 355 ICUs in 33 countries during 2007–2009) showed that during critical illness, extreme obesity is not associated with a worse survival advantage compared to normal weight [37]. It showed, however, that among survivors, BMI $\geq$40 kg/m^2 is associated with longer time on mechanical ventilation and in the ICU.

Malnutrition

Adequate nutrient intake is critical for optimal cellular and organ functions, protein synthesis, immunity, repair, and capacity of skeletal, cardiac, and respiratory muscles and tissue repair [38]. Disease related malnutrition, however, frequently occur in infants and children, often with more rapidly obvious and detrimental consequences than in adults. Other factors such as age, social background, congenital heart disease, burn injury, and length of hospital stay also negatively impact nutritional status. The consequences of hospital malnutrition are well described and recognized as causing skeletal-muscle weakness, increased rate of hospital-acquired infection, impaired wound healing, prolonged convalescence, length of hospital stay, increasing mortality [39] and, consequently, the costs of providing health care [40, 41] A number of studies have demonstrated that children with newly diagnosed diseases may already be malnourished [3]. It has also been indicated that malnutrition and nutrient store deficiencies commonly occur early in the course of critical

illnesses in children [42]. In a recent study, 16.7 % of patients were already depleted of protein and 31 % of fat stores upon admission to the PICU [43]. Overall, 16.9 % were at risk for and 4.2 % had already CPEM and 21.1 % were at risk for and 5.6 % had already APEM. In addition, levels of many complement components are reduced and trace mineral and vitamin deficiencies are associated with profound effects on cell-mediated immunity such as impaired lymphocyte stimulation response, decreased CD4+:CD8+ cell number and function, decreased chemotaxis and function of phagocytes, and diminished secretory immunoglobulin A antibody response [44]. These changes are driven by a combination of the counter regulatory hormones and the direct and indirect action of the various inflammatory mediators such as prostaglandin and kallikreins [45], the balance of which may be crucial in regulating the ability to generate an anabolic response [46].

Monitoring Biochemical Markers

Plasma Proteins

Because of the problems associated with anthropometrics, a number of other measurements are used in conjunction both for establishing the initial nutritional status and monitoring changes. Hepatic proteins such as albumin, transthyretin (pre-albumin), transferrin, and retinol binding protein have been used as nutritional markers. Among them, the shorter half-life proteins correlate better with acute changes, and the longer-lived proteins are better for the evaluation of chronic problems. Thus, isolated starvation does not alter plasma protein concentrations reflecting the uniform loss of water and cellular mass until severe depletion is present. On the other hand, critical illness leads to a decrease of protein concentrations without severe loss of body cell mass, mainly reflecting reprioritization of liver protein synthesis.

Serum albumin represents equilibrium between hepatic synthesis and albumin degradation and losses from the body. It is also influenced by intravascular and extravascular albumin compartments and water distribution. About one-third of the albumin pool is in the intravascular compartment, and two-thirds is in the extravascular compartment. Once albumin is released into the plasma, its half-life is about 21 days. Levels of this visceral protein may decline in the setting of acute injury and illness as the liver reprioritizes protein synthesis from visceral proteins to acute-phase reactant proteins and as a consequence of increased degradation, transcapillary losses and fluid replacement [47, 48]. Albumin losses from plasma to the extravascular space increase threefold in patients with septic shock [49]. Albumin might be also altered because of factors other than malnutrition, such as in hepatic disorders, extra protein losses (nephrotic syndromes, in fistula, peritonitis), and in cases of acute infection or inflammation. However, it has been shown that serum albumin correlates very poorly with monitoring of nutritional status based on a patient's history and physical exam [50].

Transthyretin, also referred to as prealbumin, is a transport protein for thyroid hormone. It is synthesized by the liver and partly catabolized by the kidneys. Normal serum transthyretin concentrations range from 16 to 40 mg/dL; values of <16 mg/dL are associated with malnutrition. Levels may be increased in the setting of renal dysfunction, corticosteroid therapy, or dehydration, whereas physiological stress, infection, liver dysfunction, and over-hydration can decrease transthyretin levels. The half-life of transthyretin (2–3 days) is much shorter than that of albumin, making it a more favorable marker of acute change in nutritional status [43].

Transferrin has also been used as a marker of nutritional status. This acute-phase reactant is a transport protein for iron; normal concentrations range from 200 to 360 mg/dL. Transferrin has a relatively long half-life (8–10 days) and is influenced by several factors, including liver disease, fluid status, stress, and illness. Levels decrease in the setting of severe malnutrition, but this marker is unreliable in the assessment of mild malnutrition, and its response to nutrition intervention is unpredictable. Transferrin has not been studied as extensively as albumin and transthyretin in relation to nutritional status, and the test can be expensive. It also suffers from the influence of other non-nutritional situations such as hepatic and renal failure and hormone infusion.

Despite these limitations, it has been shown that transferrin and prealbumin levels improved at the end of a period of early enteral feeding in critically ill children, while survivors had higher prealbumin levels than non-survivors (22.3 versus 15.5 mg/dL) [43]. Similarly, a greater positive trend in levels of prealbumin, transferrin, retinol-binding protein, and total protein has been shown in a protein-enriched diet group [51].

Nutritional Indices

Nutritional indices, such as the Prognostic Nutrition Index, are mathematically derived equations that combine measurements of albumin, triceps skinfold thickness, transferrin, and delayed hypersensitivity skin testing. Each measurement has its own restrictions, as previously mentioned, but, when combined, they have been shown to increase the sensitivity of prediction of major morbidity in surgical patients [52]. Two multi-parameter nutritional status indices, the Maastricht Index (MI) [53] and the Nutritional Risk Index (NRI) [54] were used to assess the nutritional status of patients. Also, acute phase reactants such as C-reactive protein have been used as a marker of metabolic state [55]. By combining nutritional and acute stress markers, a modified form of Prognostic Inflammatory and Nutritional Index (PINI) has

been shown to be significantly correlated with protein intake by the end of early enteral nutrition (EN) and to be negatively correlated to myocardial contractility in critically ill children [43].

Nitrogen Balance

Significant negative nitrogen balance and somatic protein depletion develops in critically ill pediatric patients, especially when they are inadequately fed, develop Multiple Organ System Failure (MOSF), or have previous chronic illness. Thus, an alternative to specific protein determinations is measurement of nitrogen balance. In the human body, only protein is composed of nitrogen, thus measurement of nitrogen excretion is a method for assessing protein metabolism and indirectly assessing metabolic stress and following up nutrition repletion. Achievement of positive protein and energy balance in relation to the basic metabolic rate using an aggressive early EN protocol improved nitrogen balance during the acute phase of stress in two-thirds of critically ill children [56]. The breakdown of muscle proteins has been proved to be sensitive to alterations in nutrient and substrate supply [57]. It has been speculated that ATP is utilized in the process of peptide bond synthesis, for the formation of the tertiary structure of proteins, and for the synthesis of tRNA, mRNA, and the nucleotides from which they are, in turn, found [58]. On the contrary, the oxidation of amino acids in muscle is stimulated by fasting, sepsis, stress, hormonal influence, and other conditions associated with negative NB [59]. It was recently shown that caloric intake and MOSF independently affect substrate utilization [60]. In particular, the incidence of negative NB was 91 % when the caloric intake was less than REE and 9 % when it was equal to or greater than REE. Without MOSF there was a trend toward positive nitrogen balance by day 7 while with MOSF, negative nitrogen balance persisted even by day 7 [51].

Nitrogen balance, in the absence of exogenous support, can he estimated from urinary urea nitrogen excretion over a 24-h period. This will constitute about 93 % of total urinary nitrogen losses. Additionally, it has been suggested that 0.5 g per day of nitrogen be added to the output to account for nitrogen lost through skin [61]. Ideally, urine output should be collected for 24 h measurements of total urinary nitrogen and additional fecal, stoma, drainage fluid, and/or other body fluid losses should be obtained to determine concentrations of daily nitrogen excretion [49]. In critically ill children, nitrogen balance estimated by total urinary nitrogen and justified for other losses differed significantly from the estimated values using urine urea nitrogen or even unjustified total urinary nitrogen (Fig. 42.1). Nitrogen drainages are usually determined by manual micro-Kjeldahl digestion or

Fig. 42.1 Comparison of 24-h nitrogen balance estimations (g/day), using three different calculated methods (based on urine urea nitrogen, unjustified total urinary nitrogen or justified for other losses total urinary nitrogen) in the same population of critically ill patients (p <0.0001) (Courtesy of G. Briassoulis)

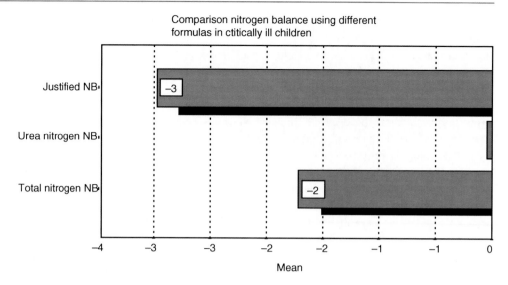

by high-resolution liquid chromatography [62]. Nitrogen balance is then calculated by subtracting output (corrected for daily changes in total-body urea content assuming that urea is uniformly distributed in body water) from input (enteral, parenteral, and non-feeding protein), according to the following formula:

$$\text{Justified for other body fluid losses nitrogen balance}(g/day): N \text{ intake}$$
$$-\left(\text{Total urinary } N + \text{change in BUN}^* + \text{faecal losses} + \text{other body fluid losses} + 0.5g \text{ for cutaneous losses}\right).$$

$$^*\text{Change in BUN } (g) = 0.6 \times \text{weight} \times \text{BUN initial} - \text{BUN final}.$$

Creatinine Height Index- Body Protein Turnover

The creatinine height index may also be used to monitor nutritional status. It is derived from the measurement of 24 h urinary creatinine excretion as follows: (24 h excretion of creatinine/creatinine excretion of normal individuals of same height and sex) × 100. Thus the determined creatinine height index is compared with predicted values based on height and sex and then the somatic protein status may be calculated as follows: <80 % = moderate depletion of somatic protein status, <60 % = severe depletion of somatic protein status [53]. Any factor that might interfere with creatinine excretion, such as age, renal disease, stress or diet, might interfere with its interpretation. In a mixed critically ill pediatric population, 27 % had mild to moderate somatic protein depletion and 5.4 % had severe somatic protein depletion on day 1 [60]. Only the persistence of stress and co-morbidity were associated with the creatinine-height index. Monitoring this index in a prospective study of early EN in a PICU, children who had severe depletion of somatic protein status on stress day 1 reached the normal range of somatic protein status on post-stress day 5 (CHI >80 %) [56].

Although, 3-methylhistidine excretion has been proposed as an index of skeletal muscle degradation and, therefore,

proteolysis associated with stress, at least 25 % of urinary 3-methylhistidine has been also attributed to extra-skeletal sources [63]. Tracer studies of whole body protein turnover underestimate actual protein turnover because intercellular recycling of amino acids occurs, and thus some amino acids may not be in equilibrium with a tracer such as nitrogen.

Monitoring Resting Energy Expenditure

Energy expenditure can be difficult to predict in PICU patients because of the effects of various disease states, therapeutic interventions, stress, and each patient's own inherent metabolic requirements. It was recently shown that there was no relationship between resting energy expenditure (REE) and clinical severity evaluated using the PRISM, PIM2 and PELOD scales or with the anthropometric nutritional status or biochemical alterations [64]. Thus, neither nutritional status nor clinical severity was shown to relate to REE which should be measured individually in each critically ill child at risk, preferably using indirect calorimetry. Risks exist for both overfeeding and underfeeding of PICU patients so that an accurate assessment of energy needs is necessary to avoid either extreme.

Indirect Calorimetry

Indirect calorimetry continues to be the 'gold standard' for measuring energy expenditure in the critically ill child. Unfortunately, indirect calorimetry is expensive and is not available to the majority of PICU clinicians or registered dietitians. Obviously, when a metabolic monitor is available, critically ill children's energy requirements should be based on measured REE as the Food and Agriculture Organization (FAO) and the World Health Organization (WHO) recommend. Traditional components of total energy expenditure (TEE) include REE, diet-induced thermogenesis and physical activity energy expenditure. The TEE is considered the REE plus a 5 % activity factor [65] and plus 15 % for day-to-day variability [66]. The magnitude of the diet-induced thermogenesis depends on the type of substrate provided, the amount of substrate ingested, and the way the body handles the substrate, ranging from 5 to 30 % [67].

Indirect calorimetry is based on the recognition that the body is a chemical furnace and, like all physical entities, must follow the basic laws of thermodynamics. In combustion, the use of energy involves the consumption of oxygen (VO_2) and production of carbon dioxide (VCO_2), nitrogenous waste, and water in a stoichiometric fashion. Further, according to the first law of thermodynamics, energy can be neither consumed nor created, but can merely change forms. When basic nutrients are converted to heat in cells, measurement of VO_2 and VCO_2 would indirectly reflect the basal metabolic expenditure involved. Mean REE and respiratory quotient (RQ) are automatically obtained using an integrated microprocessor. Respiratory quotient is calculated from gas fractions alone, according to the Haldane transformation and REE is calculated according to Weir's equation [68] (Table 42.3).

The RQ reflects whole body substrate use, but is also affected by factors such as body habitus, acid-base disturbances, underlying metabolic conditions, or critical illness. Physiologically, RQ represents an instantaneous summary of the interplay between oxidation and synthesis of various metabolic substrates. The ratio can vary from 0.7 to 1.2. The non-protein RQ is calculated from the measured respiratory quotient (i.e. VO_2/VCO_2) after correction for protein oxidation as measured by urinary nitrogen excretion after correction for changes in serum urea levels. Thus, the non-protein RQ reflects the 'net' metabolism of glucose and lipids. A RQ value greater than 1 indicates that patients have been overfed, especially in excess of carbohydrate calories, which can result in net fat synthesis. Lipogenesis or net fat synthesis is also defined as a non-protein RQ >1. A high carbohydrate intake, defined as a continuous glucose infusion >8 mg*kg^{-1}*min^{-1}, to acutely ill patients may increase CO_2 production by 50–66 %. Overfeeding a respiratory compromised child might increase the RQ to >1, producing

Table 42.3 Measured resting energy expenditure (REE) and Respiratory Quotients (RQ)

According to Haldane transform, which states the relationship between the inspiratory (I) and expiratory (E) volume, **the respiratory quotients (RQ) can be calculated from gas fractions alone**:

$VO_2 = V_I(F_IO_2) - V_E(F_EO_2)$

$VCO_2 = V_I(F_ICO_2) - V_E(F_ECO_2)$

$RQ = VCO_2/VO_2$

Fuels	Respiratory quotients
Carbohydrate	RQ = 1
Fat	RQ = 0.7
Protein	RQ = 0.8

REE can be derived from metabolic cart measurements, using the following formulae:

REE Weir formula:

REE = 5.68 VO_2 + 1.59 VCO_2 – 2.17 Urine N_2

If urine N_2 is not entered, the REE is calculated as follows:

REE = 5.466 VO_2 + 1.748 VCO_2

unnecessary CO_2 that he/she might be unable to eliminate creating difficulty in weaning from mechanical ventilation [69] and prolonging the length of hospitalization [70]. Thus, when there is a need for increasing energy intake, the energy source should be carefully chosen to avoid giving excess carbohydrate calories. In adults on parental nutrition, however, RQ >1.0 was not a specific marker of excessive caloric intake [71] whereas RQ >1.0 was reported in <30 % of all adults who were overfed [72]. Similarly, in critically ill children, a single measurement of RQ had poor sensitivity (21 % for overfeeding) when a specific cutoff of RQ >1.0 was used to classify the degree of overfeeding [73]. Therefore, the best indicator of overfeeding remains the difference between energy intake and energy expenditure as measured by metabolic monitors.

Indirect calorimetry circumvents many of the problems associated with other modes of nutritional assessment. Since the method directly measures the conversion of energy to heat, there is no need to apply age-related, population-based data to individual critically ill children. Alterations in tissue composition also will not obscure the meaning of the data. Patients may be classified as hypermetabolic (as defined by a REE >10 % of the predicted value), normometabolic (REE within the ±10 % prediction range), and hypometabolic (REE <10 % of the prediction range) [62]. Compared with a 'normometabolic' group, hypermetabolic patients show higher fat oxidation suggesting that fat is preferentially oxidized. A high carbohydrate intake is associated with lipogenesis and thus with an increase in thermogenesis [62]. RQ is also strongly affected by the ratio of energy intake/total daily REE and by the cumulative energy balance. Following a patient over time will allow recognition of the nature of the metabolic problem and tailoring of support to meet individual needs. Thus, during the week following PICU admission,

REE was not shown to be different from Schofield's Predicted Basal Metabolic Rate (PBMR), but it was 20 % lower than TEE [74]. During convalescence, for clinically stable patients, adding approximately 20–25 % to the REE might better approximate TEE requirements [75]. From the median nitrogen excretion, optimal daily protein intake has been calculated as 1.9 g/kg, whereas a high protein intake (about 2.8 g/kg per day) has been shown to result in a positive nitrogen balance [62].

Monitoring nutrition of critically ill children, subjects may be divided into three groups, based on the degree of feeding as previously described [76]. Underfed is defined as a subject's actual average energy intake being less than 90 % of total energy requirements. Appropriately fed is defined as a subject's actual average energy intake being within ± 10 % of TEE requirements. In overfed patients the actual average energy intake is larger than 110 % of the TEE requirements. Additionally, careful monitoring with indirect calorimetry and nitrogen balance studies should help prevent inadequate protein or excessive carbohydrate intake. The non-protein RQ and the net substrate (fat, carbohydrate, and protein) oxidation rates are calculated using the Weir formula modified by Frayn [77].

The Standard Metabolic Monitor

The metabolic monitors have been widely validated and tested for accuracy and reproducibility by both in vitro and in vivo means, which enables its clinical use in PICU [78]. They measure the VO_2 and VCO_2 from gas exchange measurements, and calculate the REE and RQ by using the Weir equation [68], ignoring the urinary nitrogen [79]. For most children a single measurement of total daily energy expenditure provides reasonable insight as to the daily energy needs [80]. The mean percentage of between day variations in energy expenditure has been estimated at 21 ± 16 %, [81] but the early phase of stress response is characterized by a greater variability in REE because of the fast biphasic metabolic response to injury in children [82]. In a previous study conducted for validation of the predictive equations in the early post-injury period, no differences with clinical relevance were found in the REE throughout the 24-h post-injury phase [83]. In another study, the within-day variation of REE in ventilated, critically ill children was only 7.2 % [81] also supporting the approach that a single 30-min indirect calorimeter measurement may provide an acceptable guide to set up the nutritional support. Thus, in critically ill, ventilated children energy expenditure can be measured with acceptable accuracy but daily measurements are necessary because of huge between-day variations.

Patients receiving continuous enteral or parenteral infusions are not interrupted during the measurement. The patient is connected via an endotracheal tube to a spirometer filled with 100 % O_2 attached to a kymograph (closed circuit spirometry method). As the patient breathes, the oxygen is consumed and CO_2 is exhaled. The water and CO_2 vapor are mechanically absorbed, so that volume changes in the spirometer are only due to the consumption of oxygen. The oxygen uptake by the lungs is determined from the amount of oxygen consumed from the spirometer. Since the magnitude of tube leakage of mixed expiratory gases cannot be predicted from endotracheal tube diameter, ventilator settings, or infant activity or posture [84], lack of an air leak must be confirmed on clinical examination by absence of an audible air leak during mechanical inspiration, by determining the difference between inspired and expired tidal volumes (<15 %), and/or during testing by the presence of stable minute to minute RQ values. Patients with FiO_2 >0.80, with incompetent endotracheal tube cuffs, leaking chest tubes, bronchopleural fistulas losing expired gases to the environment, on other ventilators (not suitable for REE measurement) [85], or on continuous nitric oxide or CO_2 inhalation may not have reliable measurements. The device permits uninterrupted patient ventilation and provides non-invasive measurement of inspired and exhaled gases. The flowmeter and the CO_2 and O_2 analyzers are automatically calibrated before each measurement and oxygen consumption is measured for at least 30 min each time.

Recent Advances in Monitoring REE in the Critically Ill

With the advent of newer technology, continuous and accurate metabolic monitoring in critically ill children has been possible at the bedside. Two of the most well studied metabolic monitors; the Deltatrac II NMN-200 (Datex-Ohmeda, Helsinki) and the E-COVX (former M-COVX) from Datex-Ohmeda (Helsinki) are systems that use the open circuit technique. The Deltatrac II measures gas volume in a mixing chamber and the E-COVX uses a breath-by-breath method to analyze VO_2 and VCO_2 [86]. The Deltatrac II, validated in different patients in the past but no longer produced, used to require a high level of technical expertise and was time consuming to calibrate. The newer compact E-COVX is able to continuously analyze VO_2 and VCO_2, is cheaper and simpler to use, performs calibration automatically and is much smaller in size [87]. It was suggested, however, that although in adult patients it compared more [87] or less [88] favorably to the Deltatrac II, it might not provide measurement within a clinically accepted range in certain ventilation modes and in non-sedated patients [89].

Extending the previous studies we have recently shown that, despite an immediate decrease in dynamic compliance and expired tidal volume that result in inadequate or inaccurate sidestream respiratory monitoring, pulmonary mechanics and continuous indirect calorimetry monitoring were not influenced after uneventful open endotracheal suctioning in well-sedated children [90]. Especially, when using a compact modular metabolic monitor (E-COVX), attending physicians may be able to reliably record spirometry and metabolic indices as early as 5 min after suctioning at different ventilator modes. In addition, we have shown that the influence of different ventilator modes on VO_2 and VCO_2 measurements in adequately sedated critically ill children is not significant [91]. Thus, new compact metabolic monitors, like the E-COVX metabolic module, are suitable for continuous REE monitoring in well-sedated mechanically ventilated children with stable respiratory patterns using the PRVC, SIMV, or BiVent modes of ventilation.

The Short Douglas Bag Protocol

The Douglas bag method uses the fraction of expiratory CO_2 to determine VCO_2 and calculate energy expenditure through a double in/outlet, separated by a valve, allowing airflow to and from the bag or to outside air by turning a tap. It compared favorably to the metabolic monitor in a study in which predictive equations failed to predict individual energy expenditure [92]. Intra-measurement variability was within 10 % for both methods, which showed significant bias compared to Schofield equations. Considering its low cost, these data render the short and simple Douglas bag method a possible robust measure and a routinely applicable instrument for tailored nutritional assessment in critically ill children.

Alternative Methods Used to Predict Energy Expenditure

Bicarbonate Dilution Kinetics

Energy expenditure can be determined over a period of several days [93] by bicarbonate dilution kinetics if the energy equivalents of carbon dioxide (food quotient) from the diet ingested are known. Accordingly, using this method it is necessary to know the fraction of carbon dioxide produced during the oxidative process but not excreted. By measuring the dilution of ^{13}C infused by metabolically produced carbon dioxide (continuous tracer infusion of $NaH^{13}CO_3$) the rates of $^{13}CO_2$ appearance were estimated in critically ill children [94]. Determining the energy expenditure by this method, it was shown that the 2001 World Health Organization and Schofield predictive equations overestimated and underestimated, respectively, energy requirements compared with those obtained by bicarbonate dilution kinetics [94].

Indirect Estimations of REE

Because protein oxidation represents 8–12 % of the total energy expenditure, it has been speculated that changes in nitrogen balance are associated with changes in REE [95]. Benotti et al. proposed that an estimation of REE could be made from measurement of urea excretion and nitrogen balance [96]. In a study, in which the patients received only 5 % dextrose infusion and no nitrogen, a week correlation between daily nitrogen excretion and REE, has been shown [97]. In patients receiving mixed nutritional regimens, however, we could not find any correlation or independent association of the nitrogen balance with REE [98]. Instead, the efficacy of increased protein and energy intakes to promote protein anabolism and the underlying mechanisms were studied by measuring whole body protein balance (WbPBal) using intravenous-enteral phenylalanine/tyrosine stable isotope method protocol [99].

Predictive Equations

Energy requirements can be predicted with some accuracy. Estimations are based on measurements of energy expenditure in greater reference populations. Conceptually, estimates of energy requirements refer to the mean of groups and not to individuals. Predictive equations based on measurements in a considerable number of individuals have been developed for REE and also for TEE. Most of these equations are valid for adults. Alternatively, since patients in an ICU environment are rarely in a basal state, Kinney et al. have defined REE as the measured energy expenditure in a quiet supine individual. PBMR of assumed (non-measured) REE in ventilated, critically ill children, has usually been calculated using the Talbot's tables, Harris-Benedict, Caldwell-Kennedy, Schofield, Food and Agriculture/World Health Organization/United Nation Union, Maffeis, Fleisch, Kleiber, Dreyer, and Hunter equations, using the actual and ideal weight [100].

The formulae most frequently used in practice (e.g. the FAO/WHO/UNU prediction equations or Schofield's formulae) are based on measurements in considerable numbers of participants (i.e. more than 7,500 3–18-year-old children in the case of the FAO/WHO/UNU who were investigated between 1910 and 1980 in different areas all over the world) [101]. For children and adolescents a sufficient database on REE has only recently been established [102]. Henry et al. developed new equations to estimate REE in children aged 10–15 years [103]. These equations were based on measurements of REE by indirect calorimetry in 195 school children (40 % boys, 60 % girls). Sex, weight, height, puberty stage and skinfolds were used to develop more specific regression equations. In adults, and probably in adolescences, the predicted basal metabolic rate (PBMR) is a function of sex, age, height, and weight and can be calculated using the Harris-Benedict equations [104]. It has been suggested that until more accurate prediction equations are developed, the following should be utilized: Schofield-HW equation [105] for field studies with a mixed population of obese and non-obese children and adolescents; the FAO/WHO/UNU equation in girls; and the Schofield-W equation in non-obese children [106]. Corresponding Predicted Energy Expenditure (PEE) is estimated by PBMR multiplied by stress-related correction factors (Table 42.4). In critically ill children PBMR and PEE are often obtained according to FAO/WHO/UNU, Schofield-HW, and Seashore [107] equations and in adolescents after the Harris-Benedict equations [108].

Lessons Learned From Adult Studies

As shown recently, seven prediction equations applied to critically ill patients were rarely within 10 % of the measured REE [109]. In 34 mechanically ventilated cancer adult patients the Harris-Benedict PBMR *without* added stress and activity factors correlated better with measured REE than did the clinically estimated PEE based on recommendations of the American Society for Parenteral and Enteral Nutrition [110]. Thus indirect calorimetry is now suggested as the method of choice to estimate caloric requirements in critically ill, mechanically ventilated adult patients [111].

Current clinical practice guidelines suggest that an adequate energy goal to be monitored for most ICU patients is approximately equivalent to the measured or estimated REE multiplied by 1.0–1.2 [112]. Although, an alternative method is to initially use 20–25 kcal per kilogram of body weight as the total caloric target range for most adults in the ICU [113], a REE monitoring period of about 12 min for patients on controlled ventilation and 21 min for those on assisted mode was found to be enough for a successful daily REE estimation in the majority of cases (difference between TDEE and REE <5 %) [45]. In addition, it has been shown that indirect calorimetry with 5-min steady state test correlated very well with the 30-min steady state test in both mechanically ventilated and spontaneously breathing patients [114]. A 5-min period of measurement, if variation in that measurement is less than 5 % [115], or multiple short measurement periods (twice 15 min) or a single 20-min measurement have also been shown accurate in approximating TDEE [116]. Later in the period of hospitalization multiple factors influence the REE and due to these factors, there can be a significant variability in the daily REE, ranging from 4 to 56 %. Occasionally, attention to the RQ has been considered important in roughly evaluating substrate utilization and/or nutritional support and in determining overfeeding and underfeeding [117].

The Pediatric Experience

The unreliability of prediction equations to determine caloric requirements in ventilated, critically ill children is well established. Obesity, malnutrition, dehydration, excess body water, or population differences may impose difficulty in accurately monitoring body weight, height or other variables used in the prediction equations [111]. In particular, most of the predictive equations overestimate REE in critically ill children during the early post-injury period [83]. Similarly, recommended daily allowances and energy expenditure predicted by using a stress-related correction to the PEE grossly overestimate REE [98, 100]. In fact, in critically ill mechanically ventilated children, REE is close to PBMR and in many patients it is lower than PBMR and associated with higher morbidity [98]. Since a proportion of children do not become hypermetabolic during the acute phase of critical illness [98], agreement between REE and PEE remains broad [118, 119], confirming therefore that PEE equations are inappropriate for use in critically ill children [120, 121]. Although none of the remaining methods stood out as being more precise, the recommended dietary allowance for energy has been shown to be the least accurate and differed significantly even from the other predictive methods, overestimating energy expenditure in 50 of 52 children [122]. In young children (birth to 3 years) with failure to thrive WHO, Schofield weight-based, and Schofield weight- and height-based equations were all within 10 % accuracy <50 % of the time [123]. Agreement between measured resting energy expenditure and equation-estimated energy expenditure was poor, with mean bias of 72.3 ± 446 kcal/day (limits of agreement −801.9 to +946.5 kcal/day).

Besides disparity between equation-estimated PEE, REE, and TDEE among critically ill children, a high incidence of underfeeding or overfeeding and a wide range of metabolic alterations were also recorded [124], strongly suggesting that nutritional repletion should be ideally based on indirect calorimetry. Hopefully, targeted indirect calorimetry on high-risk patients selected by a dedicated nutrition team may prevent cumulative excesses and deficits in energy balance [124].

Body-Composition Tests

Body-composition methods, such as nuclear magnetic resonance, whole-body conductance and impedance, neutron activation, hydrodensitometry and other techniques, have been evaluated as additional nutritional assessment tools in healthy populations and in athletes [125]. Except for a few studies from investigative centers, very little research has been done to prove the utility of these methods in sick patients. It is extremely difficult to perform these tests in bedridden children, those who are connected to ventilators,

Table 42.4 Equations used to estimate PBMR and PEE

1a. Harris-Benedict equation: (kilocalories/day) (after age 15) [204]	
Males: $66.473 + (13.7516 \times Wt) + (5.0033 \times Ht) - (6.755 \times Age)$	
Females: $665.0955 + (9.5634 \times Wt) + (1.8496 \times Ht) - (4.6756 \times Age)$	
1b. PEE = PBMR × correction factor for stress (1.4–2.0)	
Stress components	**%**
Elevated body temperature (per °C above 37 °C)	12
Severe infection/sepsis	10–30
Recent extensive operation	10–30
Fracture/trauma	10–30
Burn wounds	50–150
ARDS	20
2a. FAO/WHO/UNU equation: (kilocalories/day)	
<3 years:	Boy–$(60.9 \times Wt) - 54$
	Girl–$(61 \times Wt) - 51$
3–10 years:	Boy–$(22.7 \times Wt) + 495$
	Girl–$(22.5 \times Wt) + 499$
10–18 years:	Boy–$(17.5 \times Wt) + 651$
	Girl–$(12.2 \times Wt) + 746$
3a. Schofield – WH [204] equations (MJ/day) (1 kcal = 4.186 kJ)	
<3 years:	Boy–$(0.0007 \times Wt) + (6.349 \times Ht) - 2.584$
	Girl–$(0.068 \times Wt) + (4.281 \times Ht) - 1.730$
3–10 years:	Boy–$(0.082 \times Wt) + (0.545 \times Ht) + 1.736$
	Girl–$(0.071 \times Wt) + (0.677 \times Ht) + 1.553$
10–18 years:	Boy–$(0.068 \times Wt) + (0.574 \times Ht) + 2.157$
	Girl–$(0.035 \times Wt) + (1.948 \times Ht) + 0.837$
2b–3b. Correction factors (% of PBMR added to PBMR)	
Elevated temperature	+12 % per °C above 37°
ARDS	+20 %
Sepsis	+10–30 % depending on severity
Trauma	+10–30 % depending on severity
Surgery	+10–30 % depending on severity

4a–b. Seashore's equation for PBMR and PEE (kilocalories/day) (infants and children up to age 15)

Estimation of energy requirements		Add
PBMR	$[55 - (2 \times Age\ in\ years)] \times Weight\ in\ kg$	
Maintenance:[a]	PBMR + 20 %	
Activity:[b]	PBMR + 0–25 %	
Sepsis:	PBMR + 13 % for each 1 °C above normal	
Simple trauma:	PBMR + 20 %	
Multiple injuries:	PBMR + 40 %	
Burns:	PBMR + 50–100 %	
Growth and anabolism:[c]	PBMR + 50–100 %	

5a. **Henry's regression formulae** for estimating REE (kilojoules per day):	
Boy Wt × 66.9 + 2876	
Girl Wt × 47.9 + 3230	

Ht Height in cm, *Wt* weight in kilograms, *Age* age in years, *°C* degree centigrade, *PBMR* predicted basal metabolic rate, *PEE* Predicted Energy Expenditure, *WHO* Food and Agriculture Organization/World Health Organization/United Nations University equation, *Mj* Megajoules, *kj* kilojoules, *kcal* kilocalorie, *ARDS* Acute Respiratory Distress Syndrome, *F* female, *M* male

[a]Includes specific dynamic action and amount of energy needed for equilibrium in the resting but awake state with minimal muscular movements

[b]0 % for comatose state, 25 % for hospitalized child who ambulates two to three times a day, 50 % for active non-hospitalized child

[c]100 % for growth in infancy and adolescence; 50 % for the years in between

and those who have fluid imbalances. For example, hydrodensitometry, which some consider the 'gold standard' for body-composition analysis, would be impossible to perform in bedridden patients, as it requires total immersion of the child in water.

Dual-Energy X-Ray Absorptiometry

The dual-energy X-ray absorptiometry (DEXA) designed for the diagnosis of osteoporosis provides accurate information about the body compartments (fat, lean mass and bone) and is considered a referential method for this assessment [126]. DEXA has been used in conjunction with gamma in vivo neutron activation analysis, tritiated water dilution, total body potassium and calorimetry to assess body composition and energy expenditure in a small group of patients with blunt trauma [127]. During the first 25 days, a relationship was demonstrated between the changes in body compartments and metabolic requirements.

Bioelectrical Impedance: Magnetic Resonance Spectroscopy

Bioelectrical impedance is a simple, noninvasive, easy and low-cost technique; monitoring results of the body composition in adults and children are consistent [128]. Although it has been showed that bioelectrical impedance is good for clinical studies in patients in intensive-care units, it has not been proved very accurate in individual cases [129]. Especially, this method has been studied in patients on dialysis, because of the difficulty to perform anthropometric and laboratorial nutritional assessment of such patients [130]. However, although it was demonstrated that the electrical bioimpedance was more sensitive to body changes than the anthropometric measurements [131], for many PICU patients, bioelectrical impedance may not be useful as a nutritional monitoring tool because of fluctuation in fluid volumes and changing body weight [132].

Doubly Labeled Water Technique

Another approach to measure TEE is an isotope dilution, the so-called doubly labeled water (DLW) technique. DLW is based on the differences in turnover rates of ^2H_2O and $H_2^{18}O$ in body water. After equilibration, both ^2H and ^{18}O are lost as water whereas only ^{18}O is lost by respiration as carbon dioxide. The difference in the rate of turnover of the two isotopes can be used to calculate the VCO_2. Assuming a mean respiratory quotient (i.e. VO_2/VCO_2) of 0.85, the VO_2 and thus energy expenditure can then be calculated from VO_2 and VCO_2. The DLW technique is validated against indirect calorimetry and is now considered to be a gold standard for measurements of TEE under free-living conditions.

It is clear that ^2H_2O can now be used to address questions related to carbohydrate, lipid, protein and DNA synthesis. Using this novel tracer method, it is thus possible to elucidate new, highly relevant, knowledge regarding health and disease [133]. Especially, the DLW method is most convenient in children because it places low demands on the participant's performance (only drinking a glass of water and the collection of some urine samples). Sources of error are analytical errors in the mass spectrometric determination of isotopic enrichment, biological variations in the isotope enrichment, isotopic fractionation during formation of carbon dioxide and during vaporization of water, the calculation of total body water and the assumption or calculation of the 24 h respiratory quotient.

Whole-Body Counting/Neutron Activation

The elements K, N, P, H, O, C, Na, Cl, and Ca can be measured with a group of techniques referred to as whole-body counting/in vivo neutron activation analysis. Whole-body counting neutron activation methods are important because they provide a means of estimating all major chemical components in vivo. These methods are considered the standard for evaluating the body-composition components of nutritional interest, including body-cell mass, fat, fat-free body mass, skeletal muscle mass, and various fluid volumes [134]. Shielded whole-body counters can count the γ-ray decay of naturally occurring ^{40}K, but there is no experience in critically ill settings.

Miscellaneous Tests Indicating Nutritional Status/Stress Response

This section covers different tools that have been used to assess nutritional status but which have either had their capacity to monitor malnutrition questioned or have been found to be too difficult to perform routinely in a clinical setting [135].

Comparison with Recommended Dietary Allowances

The Recommended Dietary Allowances (RDA) is the most commonly used reference allowances in the pediatric population. These recommended levels for nutrient intake are estimated to meet the nutritional needs of practically all healthy children. Caloric allowances are estimated using the tables proposed by the Food and Nutrition Board of the Institute of Medicine [136], and Dietary Reference Intakes [137]. Although the upper intake level is the appropriate Dietary Reference Intake to use in assessing the proportion of a group at risk of adverse health effects [137], RDA is inappropriate to assess the nutrient adequacy of groups such as the critically ill [98].

Routine Laboratory Tests

The routine electrolyte, mineral (calcium, phosphorus and magnesium) and triglyceride laboratory tests monitoring are not related to anthropometric rates, although they are important to follow nutritional protocols, especially those of parenteral nutrition, and determine specific nutritional deficiencies [138]. Serum cholesterol levels lower than 160 mg/dl have been considered a reflection of low lipoprotein and thus of low visceral protein levels [139]. Hypocholesterolemia, however, seems to occur late in the course of malnutrition, limiting the value of cholesterol as a screening tool.

Selenium, Zinc, Chromium, Iodine, Iron, Copper and vitamin (A, B2, B6, B12, E) deficiencies, which are very common in patients belonging to low socioeconomic class in developing countries, may inhibit T4 to T3 conversion and lead to functional hypothyroidism and severe hypometabolism (extremely low REE) [140].

Glucose Control

Stress-induced hyperglycemia has been well described in the literature in the acutely ill patient population owing to insulin resistance and increase gluconeogenesis [141]. In fact, insulin resistance is an adaptive mechanism that prioritizes utilization of energy for immune response in the presence of infection or injury [142]. In the presence of fatty acids mitochondrial pathogen associated molecular patterns (PAMPs) and danger associated molecular patterns (DAMPs) receptors, acting as nutrient sensors, may induce an inflammatory cascade that affects insulin signaling with development of insulin resistance [142]. In a prospective, observational cohort study in children with meningococcal sepsis and septic shock [143] hyperglycemia (glucose >8.3 mmol/l) was present in 33 % of the children on admission whereas 62 % of the hyperglycemic children had overt insulin resistance (glucose >8.3 mmol/l and homeostasis model assessment (HOMA) [β-cell function <50 %], 17 % had β-cell dysfunction, and 21 % had both insulin resistance and β-cell dysfunction. Normalization of blood glucose levels occurred within 48 h, typically with normal glucose intake and without insulin treatment [143].

In the face of stress-induced hyperglycemia, the provision of dextrose infusion in the form of parenteral nutrition (PN) can further exacerbate hyperglycemia, which can lead to increased infectious complications and increased mortality [144]. Landmark trials in adults by Van den Berghe et al. suggested that targeting normoglycemia (a blood glucose concentration of 80–110 mg/dL [4.4–6.1 mmol/L]) reduced mortality and morbidity [145], but other investigators have not been able to replicate these findings. Recently, the international multicenter Normoglycemia in Intensive Care Evaluation-Survival Using Glucose Algorithm Regulation (NICE-SUGAR) study reported increased mortality with this approach, and recent meta-analyses do not support intensive glucose control for critically ill patients [146]. Although the initial trials in Leuven produced enthusiasm and recommendations for intensive blood glucose control, the results of the NICE-SUGAR study have resulted in the more moderate recommendation to target a blood glucose concentration between 144 and 180 mg/dL (8–10 mmol/L) [146]. Thus, it was recently shown that the incidence of hypoglycemia was significantly higher with intensive insulin therapy (absolute risk increase 23.5 %, number needed to harm 4) [147]. Studies in children also suggest that special consideration should be given to the safety of the youngest patients given their higher risk of hypoglycemia if an investigation of tight glycemic control is performed [148]. Especially high rates of hypo-/hyperglycemia are noted in sicker patients and in those requiring more therapeutic interventions. Adding to this skepticism, it has been recently shown that the current recommended parenteral amino acid intakes are insufficient to maintain protein balance in insulin-resistant patients during tight glucose control [149]. Concerns are raised that high amino acid intakes may exacerbate insulin resistance and favor gluconeogenesis, thereby offsetting their beneficial effects on protein balance by enhancing endogenous glucose production and lipolysis [149].

Cell-Mediated Immunity and Lymphopenia

Total lymphocyte counts and impaired cell-mediated immunity have been correlated with nutritional status. These may be difficult to interpret in children, given the variable response of an immature immune system. Additionally, numerous other factors, including sepsis, cancer, collagen vascular diseases, uremia, hepatic dysfunction, and drug administration may impair cell-mediated immunity. Quantification of T-lymphocyte subpopulations, with particular reference to killer cells, may be more specific [150]. However, in the critically ill child, many factors can alter delayed cutaneous hypersensitivity and render it useless in assessing the state of nutrition. Therefore, immunity is neither a specific indicator of malnutrition nor is it easily studied.

Delayed cutaneous hypersensitivity, which results from the inoculation of antigens such as *Candida* spp., *Trichophyton* spp., or the mumps virus, has been used to measure immunological competence and, indirectly, nutritional status. These tests are influenced by a number of other situations that cause anergy, such as various drugs (especially steroids and antirejection drugs), the presence of infection, malignancy, and burns, among others [151].

Functional Tests of Malnutrition

The use of exercise tolerance by ergometers and measurement of heart rate are useful for population studies but difficult for sick patients with cardiorespiratory impairment and for children in intensive care. Grip strength, respiratory muscle strength, and function by electrical stimulation all demonstrate changes with nutrition. Among them, relaxation rate of single twitches may be a simple, non-invasive, and reproducible way of studying function in sick patients [152].

Clinical Data Impacting Nutrition and Metabolic Response Monitoring

Cytokines

It is generally accepted that the degree of catabolism of the acutely ill child reflects the degree of stress of the individual, since with more stress there is more neurohumoral activation and more muscle proteolysis [153]. It is known that during stress, interleukin-6 increases plasma arginine vasopressin, indicating that this cytokine has a role in the inappropriate secretion of antidiuretic hormone that can occur in patients with infectious or inflammatory diseases or trauma [154].

Counter-Regulatory Stress Hormones

In addition to their short-term effects on the hypothalamus, the inflammatory cytokines can apparently stimulate pituitary corticotrophin and adrenal cortisol secretion directly by interacting with these tissues [155]. Accordingly, it has been shown that hormonal acute stress responses may explain the shift toward fat oxidation and either gluconeogenesis or impaired peripheral carbohydrate uptake, but does not quantitatively affect energy expenditure [156]. Similarly, glucocorticoids may increase nitrogen wasting in head-injured patients without increasing metabolic rate. Although counter-regulatory stress hormones do not cause hypoalbuminemia in healthy volunteers, they do produce protein catabolism [157]. It has been postulated that stress hormones alter the configuration of ribosomes in muscle, decreasing protein synthesis, inducing proteolysis, and fluxing essential amino acids for high priority use in other tissues [158]. Another study has also provided evidence that nutrition intervention may modulate cortisol-binding globulin and the concentration of free circulating cortisol after a severe stress [159]. On the contrary, supplemental insulin may have provided mild improvement in nitrogen utilization, probably related to the insulin effect on the skeletal muscle. This hormone is known to increase protein synthesis in skeletal muscle [160] and decrease degradation in liver and muscle [161].

Drugs Influencing Monitoring

Catecholamines are primary mediators of elevated energy expenditure and tissue catabolism in critically ill patients. Systemic corticosteroids also induce a hypermetabolic response and increase protein catabolism. Long-term beta receptor blockade was capable of decreasing REE and tissue catabolism [162]. This effect was associated with an improvement in both muscle protein balance as well as body cell mass conservation. It was also found that propranolol induced an increase in intracellular recycling of free amino acids. Opiates, muscle relaxants, and barbiturates variably significantly reduce energy expenditure [163, 164].

Critical Illness

Liver dysfunction is common in critically ill patients, caused by shock or hypodynamic circulatory states, intra and extra-abdominal infections, drugs, infectious hepatitis, as well as metabolic and nutritional causes. The metabolic changes induced by critical illness and inadequate nutritional supply foster the development of fatty liver. The increased release of stress hormones, proinflammatory cytokines and other inflammatory mediators, as well as insulin resistance, are hallmarks of the physiological response to injury. Initial assessment of these critically children would probably show characteristic metabolic changes, such as hyperglycemia, increased hepatic glucose production, increased lipolysis and stimulation of the *de novo* lipogenesis pathway.

Excessive fluid therapy has emerged as a new mechanism of gastrointestinal failure in critically ill patients during the past few years [165]. While timely administration of fluids is lifesaving, positive fluid balance after hemodynamic stabilization may affect the PICU course in children who do not receive renal replacement therapy by impacting organ function and negatively influencing important outcomes in critically ill patients [166]. More specifically, excessive fluid administration may harm the abdominal organs, because it increases intra-abdominal pressure and fosters the development of abdominal compartment syndrome. The latter is characterized by high intraabdominal pressure and decreased abdominal perfusion pressure, and is associated with signs of abdominal organ hypoperfusion, multiple organ failure, and decreased survival. Monitoring of patients with major burns or trauma shows that excessive fluid therapy exerts deleterious effects on the gut, delaying the return of gastrointestinal functions and preventing the use of early enteral feeding [167].

Nutrition Monitoring

Early Nutrition Monitoring

Among patients who have protein-energy malnutrition at the time of admission to the ICU and enteral feeding is not possible, the American clinical practice guidelines suggest that PN should be initiated without delay [168]. Although the time frame for initiation of PN to supplement patients who are receiving inadequate EN or no EN is not specified by the A.S.P.E.N. pediatric critical care nutrition guidelines [169], the European Society for Clinical Nutrition and Metabolism (ESPEN) recommends PN in 24–48 h if EN will be contraindicated for 3 days, or after 48 h to supplement insufficient EN in critically ill adults [112]. PN infusion protocols, therefore, should always be in place to assure safe administration and close monitoring for the metabolic complications of refeeding syndrome, tolerance of electrolytes and macronutrients, as well as glucose control is necessary; [170] monitoring of specific micronutrients is crucial in long-term PN usage. Since the use of EN as opposed to PN results in an important decrease in the incidence of infectious complications in the critically ill and is less costly, should be the first choice for nutritional support in the critically ill [171]. Fortunately, most critically ill patients who require specialized nutrition (85–90 %) can be fed enterally through gastric or intestinal tubes [166], whereas increases of caloric intake during the acute phase of a critical illness are well tolerated in children and may approach PBMR by the second day and PEE by the fourth day [4].

The refeeding syndrome is of particular importance to critically ill patients, who can be moved from the starved state to the fed state rapidly via enteral or parenteral nutrition, but is often under-appreciated [172]. There are a variety of risk factors for the development of the refeeding syndrome, but all are tied together by starvation physiology. Complications of the refeeding syndrome can include hypophosphatemia, hypokalemia, hypomagnesemia, rapid fluid shifts, peripheral edema, and sometimes thiamine deficiency, heart failure, respiratory failure, and death [173]. The most commonly seen abnormality is hypophosphatemia, which

should be monitored very closely and replenished as needed to avoid heart failure, arrhythmia, and life-threatening respiratory failure [174]. An initial phosphate depleted state is further exacerbated by the introduction of dextrose infusion. Insulin leads to an increase in cellular uptake of phosphate, as well as increased synthesis of ATP, 2,3DPG, and creatine phosphokinase, all leading to decreased serum phosphorus levels. In addition, accelerated carbohydrate metabolism increases the body's use of thiamine and can precipitate symptoms and signs of thiamine deficiency [175].

The Immunonutrition Question

It is not known if a low plasma glutamine or selenium concentration is an independent prognostic factor for an unfavorable outcome in the PICU, so that their monitoring is not currently recommended. Recently, a reduced adult ICU mortality was observed during intravenous glutamine supplementation in a broad range of ICU patients [176]. However, no change in the SOFA score was recorded and mortality did not differ at 6 months. Similarly, in a randomized, double blinded, factorial, controlled multicenter trial, the primary (intention to treat) analysis showed no effect on new infections or on mortality when PN was supplemented with glutamine or selenium [177]. Only patients who received PN supplemented with the antioxidant selenium for ≥5 days did show a reduction in new infections.

In a blinded, prospective, randomized, controlled clinical trial, nitrogen balance, nutritional indices, antioxidant catalysts, and outcome were compared in critically ill children given an immune-enhancing formula (IE) or conventional early EN (C) [178]. Although it had a favorable effect on nitrogen balance, nutritional indices and antioxidant catalysts, it did not influence outcome hard endpoints. In group IE nitrogen balance became positive by day 5 compared with group C in which the mean nitrogen balance remained negative (p<0.001). Also, early IE nutrition was shown to modulate cytokines in children with septic shock, but again there was no evidence that this immunomodulation has any impact on short-term outcome [179]. On day 5 IL-6 levels were significantly lower and IL-8 significantly higher in the IE than in the C group, whereas after 5 days of nutritional support a significant decrease in IL-6 levels was recorded only in group IE. In another randomized study in children with severe head injury, nitrogen balance became positive in 30.8 % of patients in the C group and in 69.2 % of patients in the IE group by day 5 [180]. It was also shown however, that although it decreased interleukin-8 and gastric colonization, it was not associated with additional advantage over the one demonstrated by regular early enteral nutrition.

Protocols in the Role of Monitoring

To account for alterations in energy metabolism, caloric amounts equal to the measured REE [167, 181] or, if not available, to the PBMR should be provided during the acute metabolic stress period [4]. Especially, targeted indirect calorimetry may allow detection of an altered metabolic state energy imbalance in a subset of critically ill children at a high risk of overfeeding, such as those with existing malnutrition on admission, prolonged stay in the ICU, and those who are unable to wean from mechanical ventilatory support, having therefore a role in optimizing energy intake in the PICU [124]. On the other hand, inadequate nutritional intake in the PICU, often due to fluid restriction, further leads to protein and energy deficits, especially early after admission [182]. Other factors that hinder adequate nutrition are impaired intracellular insulin signaling [183], impaired glucose uptake [184] and reduced mitochondrial capacity during critical illness [185]. These factors are probably the reason why protein-energy malnutrition is observed in 16–24 % of critically ill children and is associated with adverse clinical outcome [43, 186].

Mechanically ventilated subjects are at the highest risk of EN interruptions. It was recently shown that avoidable EN interruption was associated with increased reliance on PN and impaired ability to reach caloric goal [187]. EN interruption, however, is frequently avoidable in critically ill children; knowledge of existing barriers to EN combined with institution of protocolized feeding approach may allow appropriate interventions to optimize nutrition provision in the PICU [184]. In a recent study aimed to assess the impact of enteral feeding protocols on nutritional support practices through a continuous auditing process over a defined period it was found that the time taken to initiate nutrition support was reduced from 15 to 4.5 h [188]. Simultaneously, an increase was documented in the percentage of patients receiving a daily energy provision of up to 70 % of the estimated average requirement, whereas the proportion of patients on parenteral feeds was reduced from 11 to 4 %. In a multicenter adult study, on average, protocolized sites used more EN alone (70.4 % of patients vs 63.6 %, p=0.0036), started EN earlier (41.2 h from admission to ICU vs 57.1, p=0.0003), and used more motility agents in patients with high gastric residual volumes (64.3 % of patients vs 49.0 %, p=0.0028) compared with sites that did not use a feeding protocol [189]. Importantly, in a 7-day prospective before–after study, early EN without residual gastric volume monitoring in mechanically ventilated adult patients improved the delivery of enteral feeding and did not increase vomiting or ventilator associated pneumonia [190]. Awaiting confirmatory studies before removing the residual gastric volume assessment from their ICUs, however, clinicians are advised to take guidance from published evidence-based guidelines [191].

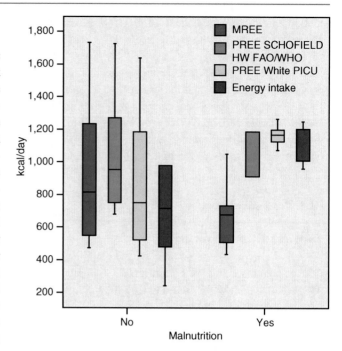

Fig. 42.2 Boxplots of energy intake and resting energy expenditure measured by indirect calorimetry (MREE) or basal metabolic rate (without stress factors) predicted by the SCHOHW or the White equations (Courtesy of G. Briassoulis)

Of equal significance of this therapeutic protocols strategy is also to avoid the provision of calories and nutritional substrates which the patient cannot probably handle in order to maintain the metabolic homeostasis of the acute stress response [2]. An increase of caloric intake during the acute phase of a stress state has been shown to be feasible and well tolerated in non-cardiac critically ill children [5]. Also, increased protein and energy intakes have been recommended in critically ill infants with viral bronchiolitis [99]. However, future studies will need to examine the safety of such protocols and the impact of large cumulative energy excess on patient outcomes. In fact, many chronically ill children with malnutrition would be rather overfed (if their daily energy requirements were calculated based on PEE during acute illness) than underfed (Fig. 42.2 [192]). Monitoring of energy expenditure, therefore, has been used to characterize alterations in metabolism accompanying critical illness and to provide accurate information necessary for appropriate nutritional repletion, including the type and amount of macronutrient substrates that exactly meets the patient's energy requirements and avoids the complications of overfeeding [193]. Accordingly, it has been shown that when caloric intake was less than REE, mean substrate utilization was 48.6 % from lipid, 37.1 % from carbohydrate but, when it was greater than REE, mean substrate utilization was 83.3 % from carbohydrate and 16.7 % from protein [60].

Recent studies have shown that computerized information systems do improve nutritional monitoring (energy delivery and balance, protein and fat delivery), quality of nutrition, glucose control, and reduce nurse workload associated with the multiple balance calculations and ease visualization of events out of planned targets [194]. Overfeeding, particularly carbohydrate overfeeding, increases ventilatory work by increasing CO_2 production, can potentially prolong the need for mechanical ventilation, may increase the risk of infection secondary to hyperglycemia, and can impair liver function by inducing hepatic steatosis and cholestasis [195]. Azotemia can result from overzealous protein infusion, whereas fat-overload syndrome can result from either overall total calorie overfeeding, overfeeding of lipids, or both [196]. Algorithms to control glucose using insulin therapy and alterations in formula administration are intended to prevent hyperglycemia, under close glucose control, and increase synthesis of fatty acids from glucose and other non-lipid precursors in the liver and in peripheral tissues [197]. Parenteral intakes of essential and nonessential amino acids supplied to critically ill children are supplied in lower or higher amounts than the content of mixed muscle proteins or breast milk and are not based on measured requirements to maintain nutrition and functional balance and on knowledge of toxicity [198]. Instead, protocol-driven implementation of nutrition therapy by the third day of admission to the PICU with goal intake achieved by the end of the first week was recently shown to help preserve lean body mass in a group of children with a high prevalence of baseline malnutrition [33].

Monitoring the Metabolic Response

Acute stress may result in a substantial decrease of energy needs. The acute stress may induce a catabolic response that is proportional to the magnitude, nature, and duration of the injury. Increased serum counter-regulatory hormone concentrations induce insulin and growth hormone resistance, resulting in the catabolism of endogenous stores of protein, carbohydrate, and fat to provide essential substrate intermediates and energy necessary to support the ongoing metabolic stress response. During this catabolic response, somatic growth cannot occur and, therefore, the caloric allotment for growth, which is substantial in infancy, should *not* be administered. The intensive care environment is temperature-controlled, and insensible energy losses are substantially reduced and most patients are ventilated with heated, humidified air, thus reducing insensible losses by one third. In addition, children treated in the intensive care setting are frequently sedated and mechanically ventilated, so that their work of breathing and activity level are markedly reduced further lowering energy needs

[199]. Similarly, various pharmacologic agents and the capacity of the patient to respond to the metabolic demands imposed by the injury might further alter the metabolic response [200].

Comparing simultaneous REE and PBMR recordings, patients may be classified as hypermetabolic, normometabolic, and hypometabolic when REE is >110, 90–110 % and, <90 % of the PBMR, respectively. Although sustained hypermetabolism has been reported for weeks after burn injury, REE peak returns to baseline within 12 h after some surgical procedures [201]. More studies in children [2, 118] and adults [202] have now verified results of a pioneer indirect calorimetry study reporting lack of hypermetabolic response during critical illness [4]. Using various equations to predict acute phase energy expenditure in mechanically ventilated children whose REE was continuously monitored through an E-COVX metabolic monitor, the mean REE/PBMR ratio was <1 in all but one (Fig. 42.3, G. Briassoulis et al. University of Crete, unpublished work). In a study examining the metabolic patterns in pediatric patients with critical illness, it was shown that the initial predominance of the hypometabolic pattern (48.6 %) declined within 1 week of acute stress (20 %), and the hypermetabolic patterns dominated only after 2 weeks (60 %) [185]. High IL-10 levels and low measured REE were independently associated with mortality (11.7 %), which was higher in the hypometabolic compared to other metabolic patterns. However, although in SIRS or sepsis the cytokine response was reliably reflected by increases in Nutritional Index and triglycerides, it was different from the metabolic (VO_2, VCO_2) or glucose response [201].

The SIRS elicited by peritonitis in mice was accompanied by mitochondrial energetic metabolism deterioration and reduced peroxisome proliferator-activated receptor gamma coactivator (PGC)-1alpha protein expression [203]. Because ATP production by mitochondrial oxidative phosphorylation accounts for more than 90 % of total oxygen consumption, a severe mitochondrial dysfunction implicating bioenergetic failure during stress might explain both: a predominant hypometabolic pattern and the raised tissue oxygen tensions in septic animals and human beings. Performing skeletal muscle biopsies on 28 critically ill septic patients within 24 h of admission to intensive care, Brealey et al. [204] showed that skeletal muscle ATP concentrations were significantly lower in patients with sepsis who subsequently died than in septic patients who survived and in controls and that complex I respiratory-chain activity had a significant inverse correlation with norepinephrine requirements and a significant positive correlation with concentrations of reduced glutathione and ATP. Electron paramagnetic resonance spectra analysis of the paramagnetic centres in the muscle confirmed that a decreased concentration of mitochondrial Complex I iron-sulfur redox centres is linked to mortality [205].

Fig. 42.3 Boxplots of ratios of resting energy expenditure (*REE*) measured by E-COVX metabolic monitor/basal metabolic rates (*PBMR*) predicted by various equations without stress factors in children during critical illness. Equations used are shown by their names (Courtesy of G. Briassoulis)

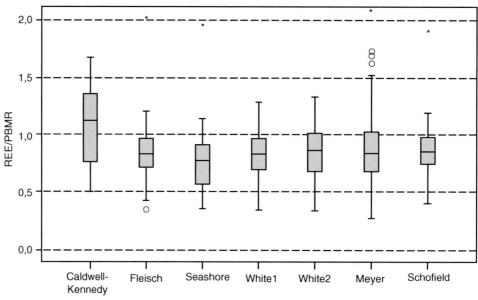

Conclusions

Nutritional monitoring should be an integral part of the care for every pediatric critically ill patient. The nutrition monitoring records the changing nutrition status of the critically ill child and facilitates the development of a nutrition care plan. However, there is little research in the area of pediatric nutrition monitoring upon which to formulate evidence based practice guidelines. A nutrition screen, incorporating objective data such as height, weight, arm circumference, triceps skinfold, primary diagnosis, and presence of co-morbidities should be a component of the initial evaluation of all pediatric patients in an intensive care setting. Following that, repeated anthropometric and laboratory markers must be jointly analyzed, but individually interpreted according to disease and metabolic changes, in order to modify and monitor the nutritional treatment. The recently revised national guidelines for adult and pediatric critical care have emphasized the importance of accurately measured energy expenditure in patients admitted to the intensive care unit. Increases of caloric intake during the acute phase of a critical illness are well tolerated in children and may approach PBMR by the second day and PEE by the fourth day. Over the course of the disease, it seems that the most practical tool is metabolic assessment based on the combination of indirect calorimetry, nitrogen balance, plasma proteins. Since the nutrition monitoring can be viewed as an ongoing process, particularly in the acute care setting, it provides accurate information necessary for appropriate nutritional repletion and helps avoiding the complications of under- and overfeeding. Accordingly, as part of the nutrition care process, the energy expenditure and metabolic monitoring using targeted indirect calorimetry, should be completed and updated at specific intervals, as warranted by metabolic alterations in the patient's needs or condition.

References

1. Joosten KF, Hulst JM. Malnutrition in pediatric hospital patients: current issues. Nutrition. 2011;27(2):133–7.
2. Mehta NM, Bechard LJ, Dolan M, Ariagno K, Jiang H, Duggan C. Energy imbalance and the risk of overfeeding in critically ill children. Pediatr Crit Care Med. 2011;12(4):398–405.
3. Hendricks KM, Duggan C, Gallagher L, Carlin AC, Richardson DS, Collier SB, Simpson W, Lo C. Malnutrition in hospitalized pediatric patients. Arch Pediatr Adolesc Med. 1995;149:1118–22.
4. Briassoulis GC, Zavras NJ, Hatzis TD. Effectiveness and safety of a protocol for promotion of early intragastric feeding in critically ill children. Pediatr Crit Care Med. 2001;2:113–21.
5. Taylor RM, Preedy VR, Baker AJ, Grimble G. Nutritional support in critically ill children. Clin Nutr. 2003;22:365–9.
6. Rogers EJ, Gilbertson HR, Heine RG, Henning R. Barriers to adequate nutrition in critically ill children. Nutrition. 2003;19:865–8.
7. De Wit B, Meyer R, Desai A, Macrae D, Pathan N. Challenge of predicting resting energy expenditure in children undergoing surgery for congenital heart disease. Pediatr Crit Care Med. 2010;11(4):496–501.
8. Mehta NM, Duggan CP. Nutritional deficiencies during critical illness. Pediatr Clin North Am. 2009;56(5):1143–60.
9. Waitzberg DL, Caiaffa WT, Correia MITD. Hospital malnutrition: the Brazilian national survey (IBRANUTRI): a study of 4000 patients. Nutrition. 2001;17:575–80.
10. Jones JM. The methodology of nutritional screening and assessment tools. J Hum Nutr Diet. 2002;15:59–71.
11. Detsky AS, Smalley PS, Chang J. Is this patient malnourished? JAMA. 1994;271:54–8.
12. Detsky AS, McLaughlin JR, Baker JP, Johnston N, Whittaker S, Mendelson RA, Jeejeebhoy KN. What is subjective global assessment of nutritional status? JPEN J Parenter Enteral Nutr. 1987;11:8–13.

13. Fiaccadori E, Lombardi M, Leonardi S, Rotelli CF, Tortorella G, Borghetti A. Prevalence and clinical outcome associated with pre-existing malnutrition in acute renal failure: a prospective cohort study. J Am Soc Nephrol. 1999;10:581–93.

14. Secker DJ, Jeejeebhoy KN. Subjective global nutritional assessment for children. Am J Clin Nutr. 2007;85(4):1083–9.

15. WHO. Physical status: the use and interpretation of anthropometry. Report of a WHO Expert Commitee, WHO Technical Report Series No. 854. Geneva: WHO; 1995.

16. NCHS (National Center for Health Statistic). Growth curves children birth–18. Washington, DC: National Center for Health Statistics; 2000.

17. World Health Organization Multicentre Growth Reference Study Group. WHO child growth standards based on length/height, weight and age. Acta Paediatr Suppl. 2006;450:76S–85.

18. Hermanussen M, Aßmann C, Wöhling H, Zabransky M. Harmonizing national growth references for multi-centre surveys, drug monitoring and international postmarketing surveillance. Acta Paediatr. 2012;101(1):78–84.

19. Brooks J, Day S, Shavelle R, Strauss D. Low weight, morbidity, and mortality in children with cerebral palsy: new clinical growth charts. Pediatrics. 2011;128(2):e299–307.

20. Buyukgebiz B, Ozturk Y, Yilmaz S, Arslan N. Serum leptin concentrations in children with mild-to-moderate protein-energy malnutrition. Pediatr Int. 2003;45:550–4.

21. Finkielman J, Gajic O, Afessa B. Underweight is independently associated with mortality in postoperative and non-operative patients admitted to the intensive care unit: a retrospective study. BMC Emerg Med. 2004;4:1–7.

22. Garrouste-Orgeas M, Troché G, Azoulay E, Caubel A, de Lassence A, Cheval C, Montesino L, Thuong M, Vincent F, Cohen Y, Timsit JF. Body mass index. An additional prognostic factor in ICU patients. Intensive Care Med. 2004;30(3):437–43.

23. Waterlow JC. Classification and definition of protein – calorie malnutrition. Br Med J. 1972;3:566–9.

24. Shoeps DO, de Abreu LC, Valenti VE, Nascimento VG, de Oliveira AG, Gallo PR, Wajnsztejn R, Leone C. Nutritional status of preschool children from low income families. Nutr J. 2011;10:43.

25. Onis M, Yip R, Mei Z. The development of PMB-for-age reference datarecommended by a WHO Expert Committee. Bull World Health Organ. 1997;75:11–8.

26. Soler-Cataluña JJ, Sánchez-Sánchez L, Martínez-García MA, Sánchez PR, Salcedo E, Navarro M. Mid-arm muscle area is a better predictor of mortality than body mass index in COPD. Chest. 2005;128:2108–15.

27. Fomon SJ. Nutritional disorders of children. Prevention, screening, and follow-up. Rockville: Department of Health. Education and Welfare Publication No (HSA); 1974. p. 77–5104.

28. Frisancho AR. Triceps skinfold and upper arm muscle size norms for assessment of nutritional status. Am J Clin Nutr. 1974;27:1052–8.

29. Frisancho AR. New norms of upper limb fat and muscle areas for assessment of nutritional status. Am J Clin Nutr. 1981;34:2540–5.

30. Ryan A, Martinez GA. Physical growth of infants 7 to 13 months of age: results from a national survey. Am J Phys Anthropol. 1987;73:449.

31. Gurney JM, Jelliffe DB. Arm anthropometry in nutritional assessment: nomogram for rapid calculation of muscle circumference and cross-sectional muscle and fat areas. Am J Clin Nutr. 1973;26:912–5.

32. Ravasco P, Camilo ME, Gouveia-Oliveira A, Adam S, Brum G. A critical approach to nutritional assessment in critically ill patients. Clin Nutr. 2002;21:73–7.

33. Zamberlan P, Delgado AF, Leone C, Feferbaum R, Okay TS. Nutrition therapy in a pediatric intensive care unit: indications, monitoring, and complications. JPEN J Parenter Enteral Nutr. 2011;35(4):523–9.

34. Oguz A, Karadeniz C, Pelit M, Hasanoglu A. Arm anthropometry in evaluation of malnutrition in children with cancer. Pediatr Hematol Oncol. 1999;16:35–41.

35. Orsi CM, Hale DE, Lynch JL. Pediatric obesity epidemiology. Curr Opin Endocrinol Diabetes Obes. 2011;18:14–22.

36. Hogue Jr CW, Stearns JD, Colantuoni E, Robinson KA, Stierer T, Mitter N, Pronovost PJ, Needham DM. The impact of obesity on outcomes after critical illness: a meta-analysis. Intensive Care Med. 2009;35:1152–70.

37. Martino JL, Stapleton RD, Wang M, Day AG, Cahill NE, Dixon AE, Suratt BT, Heyland DK. Extreme obesity and outcomes in critically ill patients. Chest. 2011;140(5):1198–206.

38. Ziegler TR. Parenteral nutrition in the critically ill patient. N Engl J Med. 2009;361(11):1088–97.

39. Villet S, Chiolero RL, Bollmann MD, Revelly JP, Cayeux RNMC, Delarue J, Berger MM. Negative impact of hypocaloric feeding and energy balance on clinical outcome in ICU patients. Clin Nutr. 2005;24(4):502–9.

40. Correia MI, Waitzberg DL. The impact of malnutrition on morbidity, mortality, length of hospital stay and costs evaluated through a multivariate model analysis. Clin Nutr. 2003;22:235–9.

41. Waitzberg DL. Efficacy of nutritional support: evidence-based nutrition and cost-effectiveness. Nestle Nutr Workshop Ser Clin Perform Programme. 2002;7:257–71.

42. Pollack MM, Wiley JS, Holbrook PR. Early nutritional depletion in critically ill children. Crit Care Med. 1981;9:580–3.

43. Briassoulis G, Zavras N, Hatzis T. Malnutrition, nutritional indices, and early enteral feeding in critically ill children. Nutrition. 2001;17:548–57.

44. Chandra RK. Nutrition and immunology: from the clinic to cellular biology and back again. Proc Nutr Soc. 1999;58:681–3.

45. Baue AE. Nutrition and metabolism in sepsis and multisystem organ failure. Surg Clin North Am. 1991;71:549–65.

46. Chang HR, Bistrian B. The role of cytokines in the catabolic consequences of infection and injury. JPEN J Parenter Enteral Nutr. 1998;22:156–66.

47. Fleck A, Raines G, Hawker F, Trotter J, Wallace PI, Ledingham IM, Calman KC. Increased vascular permeability: a major cause of hypoalbuminemia in disease and injury. Lancet. 1985;1:781–4.

48. Brugler L, Stankovic A, Bernstein L. The role of visceral protein markers in protein calorie malnutrition. Clin Chem Lab Med. 2002;40:1360–9.

49. Jeejeebhoy KN. Nutritional assessment. Gastroenterol Clin N Am. 1998;27:347–69.

50. Covinsky KE, Covinsky MH, Palmer RM, Sehgal AR. Serum albumin concentration and clinical assessments of nutritional status in hospitalized older people: different sides of different coins? J Am Geriatr Soc. 2002;50:631–7.

51. Botrán M, López-Herce J, Mencía S, Urbano J, Solana MJ, García A. Enteral nutrition in the critically ill child: comparison of standard and protein-enriched diets. J Pediatr. 2011;159(1):27–32.

52. Buzby GP, Mullen JP, Matthews DC. Prognostic nutritional index in gastrointestinal surgery. Am J Surg. 1980;139:160–7.

53. Bistrian BR, Blackburn GL, Sherman M, Scrimsaw NS. Therapeutic index of nutritional depletion in hospitalized patients. Surg Gynecol Obstet. 1975;141:512–6.

54. Hall JC. Use of internal validity in the construct of an index of undernutrition. JPEN J Parenter Enteral Nutr. 1990;14:582–7.

55. Chwals WJ, Letton RW, Jamie A, Charles B. Stratification of injury severity using energy expenditure response in surgical infants. J Pediatr Surg. 1995;30:1161–4.

56. Briassoulis G, Tsorva A, Zavras N, Hatzis T. Influence of an aggressive early enteral nutrition protocol on nitrogen balance in critically ill children. J Nutr Biochem. 2002;13:560–9.

57. Sandstrom R, Hyltander A, Korner U, Lundholm K. The effect on energy and nitrogen metabolism by continuous, bolus, or sequential

infusion formulation in patients after major surgical procedures. JPEN J Parenter Enteral Nutr. 1996;19:333–40.

58. Reeds PJ, Wahle KW, Haggarty P. Energy costs of protein and fatty acid synthesis. Proc Nutr Soc. 1982;41:155–9.

59. Freund H, Gimmon Z, Fischer JE. Nitrogen sparing effects and mechanism of branched chain amino acids in the injured rat. Clin Nutr. 1982;1:137–46.

60. Briassoulis G, VenkataramanS, Thompson A. Nutritional-metabolic factors affecting nitrogen balance and substrate utilization in the critically ill. J Pediatr Intensive Care. 2012;1(2):77–86.

61. Nettleton JA, Hegsted DM. Protein-energy interrelationships during dietary restriction: effects on tissue nitrogen and protein turnover. Nutr Metab. 1975;18:31–40.

62. Coss-Bu JA, Klish WJ, Walding D, Stein F, Smith EO, Jefferson LS. Energy metabolism, nitrogen balance, and substrate utilization in critically ill children. Am J Clin Nutr. 2001;74:664–9.

63. Millward DJ, Bates PC, Grimble GK, Brown JG, Nathan M, Rennie MJ. Quantitative importance of non-skeletal-muscle sources of N-methylhistidine in urine. Biochem J. 1980;190:225–8.

64. Botrán M, López-Herce J, Mencía S, Urbano J, Solana MJ, García A, Carrillo A. Relationship between energy expenditure, nutritional status and clinical severity before starting enteral nutrition in critically ill children. Br J Nutr. 2011;105(5):731–77.

65. Weissman C, Kemper M, Elwyn DH, Askanazi J, Hyman AI, Kinney JM. The energy expenditure of the mechanically ventilated critically ill patient: an analysis. Chest. 1986;89:254–9.

66. Weissman C, Kemper M, Hyman AI. Variation in the resting metabolic rate of mechanically ventilated critically ill patients. Anesth Analg. 1989;68:457–61.

67. Bursztein S, Elwyn DH, Askanazi J. Energy metabolism and indirect calorimetry in critically ill and injured patients. Acute Care. 1988–89;14–15:91–110.

68. Weir JB. New methods for calculating metabolic rate with special reference to protein metabolism. 1949. Nutrition. 1990;6:213–21.

69. Askanazi J, Rosenbaum SH, Hyman AI, Silverberg PA, Milic-Emili J, Kinney JM. Respiratory changes induced by the large glucose loads of total parenteral nutrition. JAMA. 1980;243:1444–7.

70. Covelli HD, Black JW, Olsen MS, Beekman JF. Respiratory failure precipitated by high carbohydrate loads. Ann Intern Med. 1981;95:579–81.

71. Guenst JM, Nelson LD. Predictors of total parenteral nutrition-induced lipogenesis. Chest. 1994;105:553–9.

72. McClave SA, Lowen CC, Kleber MJ, McConnell JW, Jung LY, Goldsmith LJ. Clinical use of the respiratory quotient obtained from indirect calorimetry. JPEN J Parenter Enteral Nutr. 2003;27:21–6.

73. Hulst JM, van Goudoever JB, Zimmermann LJ, Hop WC, Büller HA, Tibboel D, Joosten KF. Adequate feeding and the usefulness of the respiratory quotient in critically ill children. Nutrition. 2005;21:192–8.

74. van der Kuip M, de Meer K, Westerterp KR, Gemke RJ. Physical activity as a determinant of total energy expenditure in critically ill children. Clin Nutr. 2007;26(6):744–51.

75. Swinamer DL, Phang PT, Jones RL, Grace M, King EG. Twenty-four hour energy expenditure in critically ill patients. Crit Care Med. 1987;15:637–43.

76. McClave SA, Lowen CC, Kleber MJ, Nicholson JF, Jimmerson SC, McConnell JW, Jung LY. Are patients fed appropriately according to their caloric requirements? JPEN J Parenter Enteral Nutr. 1998;22:375–81.

77. Frayn KN. Calculation of substrate oxidation rates in vivo from gaseous exchange. J Appl Physiol. 1983;55:628–34.

78. Joosten KF, Jacobs FI, van Klaarwater E, Baartmans MG, Hop WC, Meriläinen PT, Hazelzet JA. Accuracy of an indirect calorimeter for mechanically ventilated infants and children: the influence of low rates of gas exchange and varying FiO2. Crit Care Med. 2000;28:3014–8.

79. Simonson DC, DeFronzo RA. Indirect calorimetry: methodological andinterpretative problems. Am J Physiol. 1990;258:E399–412.

80. de Klerk G, Hop WC, de Hoog M, Joosten KF. Serial measurements of energy expenditure in critically ill children: useful in optimizing nutritional therapy? Intensive Care Med. 2002;28:1781–5.

81. White MS, Shepherd RW, McEniery JA. Energy expenditure measurements inventilated critically ill children: within- and between-day variability. JPEN J Parenter Enteral Nutr. 1999;23:300–4.

82. Imura K, Okada A. Perioperative nutrition and metabolism in pediatric patients. World J Surg. 2000;24:1498–502.

83. Vázquez Martínez JL, Dorao Martínez-Romillo P, Diez Sebastian J, Ruza TF. Predicted versus measured energy expenditure by continuous, on-line indirect calorimetry in ventilated, critically ill children during the early post injury period. Pediatr Crit Care Med. 2004;5:19–27.

84. Knauth A, Baumgart S. Accurate, noninvasive quantitation of expiratory gas leak from uncuffed infant endotracheal tubes. Pediatr Pulmonol. 1990;9:55–60.

85. Branson RD. The measurement of energy expenditure: instrumentation, practical considerations, and clinical application. Respir Care. 1990;35:640–59.

86. Branson RD, Johannigman JA. The measurement of energyexpenditure. Nutr Clin Pract. 2004;19:622–36.

87. McLellan S, Walsh T, Burdess A, Lee A. Comparison between the Datex-Ohmeda M-COVX metabolic monitor and the Deltatrac II in mechanically ventilated patients. Intensive Care Med. 2002;28:870–8.

88. Singer P, Pogrebetsky I, Attal-Singer J, Cohen J. Comparison of metabolic monitors in critically ill, ventilated patients. Nutrition. 2006;22:1077–86.

89. Meyer R, Briassouli E, Briassoulis G, Habibi P. Evaluation of the M-COVX metabolic monitor in mechanically ventilated adult patients. e-SPEN. 2008;3(5):e232–9.

90. Briassoulis G, Briassoulis P, Michaeloudi E, Fitrolaki DM, Spanaki AM, Briassouli E. The effects of endotracheal suctioning on the accuracy of oxygen consumption and carbon dioxide production measurements and pulmonary mechanics calculated by a compact metabolic monitor. Anesth Analg. 2009;109(3):873–9.

91. Briassoulis G, Michaeloudi E, Fitrolaki DM, Spanaki AM, Briassouli E. Influence of different ventilator modes on Vo(2) and Vco(2) measurements using a compact metabolic monitor. Nutrition. 2009;25(11–12):1106–14.

92. van der Kuip M, de Meer K, Oosterveld MJ, Lafeber HN, Gemke RJ. Simple and accurate assessment of energy expenditure in ventilated paediatric intensive care patients. Clin Nutr. 2004;23:657–63.

93. Keshen TH, Miller RG, Jahoor F, Jaksic T. Stable isotopic quantitation of protein metabolism and energy expenditure in neonates on and post extracorporeal life support. J Pediatr Surg. 1997;32:958–63.

94. Sy J, Gourishankar A, Gordon WE, Griffin D, Zurakowski D, Roth RM, Coss-Bu J, Jefferson L, Heird W, Castillo L. Bicarbonate kinetics and predicted energy expenditure in critically ill children. Am J Clin Nutr. 2008;88(2):340–7.

95. Duke Jr JH, Jorgensen SB, Broell JR, Long CL, Kinney JM. Contribution of protein to caloric expenditure following injury. Surgery. 1970;68:168–74.

96. Benotti P, Blackburn GL. Protein and caloric or macronutrient metabolic management of the critically ill patient. Crit Care Med. 1979;12:520–5.

97. Tilden SJ, Watkins S, Tong TK, Jeevanandam M. Measured energy expenditure in pediatric intensive care patients. Am J Dis Child. 1989;143:490–2.

98. Briassoulis G, Venkataraman S, Thompson AE. Energy expenditure in critically ill children. Crit Care Med. 2000; 28:1166–72.

99. de Betue CT, van Waardenburg DA, Deutz NE, van Eijk HM, van Goudoever JB, Luiking YC, Zimmermann LJ, Joosten KF. Increased protein-energy intake promotes anabolism in critically ill infants with viral bronchiolitis: a double-blind randomised controlled trial. Arch Dis Child. 2011;96(9):817–22. Epub 2011 Jun 14.

100. Vazquez Martinez JL, Martinez-Romillo PD, Diez Sebastian J, Ruza Tarrio F. Predicted versus measured energy expenditure by continuous, online indirect calorimetry in ventilated, critically ill children during the early post injury period. Pediatr Crit Care Med. 2004;5:19–27.

101. World Health Organization. Energy and protein requirements. Report of a joint FAO/WHO/UNU expert consultation, WHO Technical Report Series No. 724. Geneva: World Health Organization; 1985.

102. Torun B, Davies PS, Livingstone MB, Paolisso M, Sackett R, Spurr GB. Energy requirements and dietary energy recommendations for children and adolescents. Eur J Clin Nutr. 1996; 50:S37–81.

103. Henry CJK, Dyer S, Ghusein-Choueiri A. New equations to estimate basal metabolic rate in children aged 10–15 years. Eur J Clin Nutr. 1999;3:134–42.

104. Harris JA, Benedict FG. Biometric studies of basal metabolism in man. Washington, DC: Carnegie Institute, publication; 1919. p. 279.

105. Schofield WN. Predicting basal metabolic rate, new standards and review of previous work. Hum Nutr Clin Nutr. 1985;39c:5–42.

106. Rodriguez G, Moreno LA, Sarria A, Fleta J, Bueno M. Resting energy expenditure in children and adolescents: agreement between calorimetry and prediction equations. Clin Nutr. 2002;21:255–60.

107. Seashore JH. Nutritional support of children in the intensive care unit. Yale J Biol Med. 1984;57:111–34.

108. Finan K, Larson DE, Goran MI. Cross-validation of prediction equations for resting energy expenditure in young, healthy children. J Am Diet Assoc. 1997;97:140–5.

109. Walker RN, Heuberger RA. Predictive equations for energy needs for the critically ill. Respir Care. 2009;54(4):509–21.

110. Pirat A, Tucker AM, Taylor KA, Jinnah R, Finch CG, Canada TD, Nates JL. Comparison of measured versus predicted energy requirements in critically ill cancer patients. Respir Care. 2009; 54(4):487–94.

111. McArthur CD. Prediction equations to determine caloric requirements in critically ill patients. Respir Care. 2009;54(4):453–4.

112. Singer P, Berger MM, Van den Berghe G, Biolo G, Calder P, Forbes A, Griffiths R, Kreyman G, Leverve X, Pichard C, ESPEN. ESPEN guidelines on parenteral nutrition: intensive care. Clin Nutr. 2009;28(4):387–400.

113. Kreymann KG, Berger MM, Deutz NE, Hiesmayr M, Jolliet P, Kazandjiev G, Nitenberg G, van den Berghe G, Wernerman J, DGEM (German Society for Nutritional Medicine), Ebner C, Hartl W, Heymann C, Spies C, ESPEN (European Society for Parenteral and Enteral Nutrition). ESPEN guidelines on enteral nutrition: intensive care. Clin Nutr. 2006;25(2):210–23.

114. Petros S, Engelmann L. Validity of an abbreviated indirect calorimetry protocol for measurement of resting energy expenditure in mechanically ventilated and spontaneously breathing critically ill patients. Intensive Care Med. 2001;27(7):1164–8.

115. Cunningham KF, Aeberhardt LE, Wiggs BR, Phang PT. Appropriate interpretation of indirect calorimetry for determining energy expenditure of patients in intensive care units. Am J Surg. 1994;167(5):547–9.

116. van Lanschot JJ, Feenstra BW, Vermeij CG, Bruining HA. Calculation versus measurement of total energy expenditure. Crit Care Med. 1986;14(11):981–5.

117. Joosten KF. Why indirect calorimetry in critically ill patients: what do we want to measure? Intensive Care Med. 2001; 27(7):1107–9.

118. Framson CM, LeLeiko NS, Dallal GE, Roubenoff R, Snelling LK, Dwyer JT. Energy expenditure in critically ill children. Pediatr Crit Care Med. 2007;8:264–7.

119. Verhoeven JJ, Hazelzet JA, van der Voort E, Joosten KF. Comparison of measured and predicted energy expenditure in mechanically ventilated children. Intensive Care Med. 1998;24:464–8.

120. Taylor RM, Cheeseman P, Preedy V, Baker AJ, Grimble G. Can energy expenditure be predicted in critically ill children? Pediatr Crit Care Med. 2003;4(2):176–80.

121. White MS, Shepherd RW, McEniery JA. Energy expenditure in 100 ventilated, critically ill children: improving the accuracy of predictive equations. Crit Care Med. 2000;28:2307–12.

122. Hardy CM, Dwyer J, Snelling LK, Dallal GE, Adelson JW. Pitfalls in predicting resting energy requirements in critically ill children: a comparison of predictive methods to indirect calorimetry. Nutr Clin Pract. 2002;17(3):182–9.

123. Sentongo TA, Tershakovec AM, Mascarenhas MR, Watson MH, Stallings VA. Resting energy expenditure and prediction equations in young children with failure to thrive. J Pediatr. 2000; 136:345–50.

124. Mehta NM, Bechard LJ, Leavitt K, Duggan C. Cumulative energy imbalance in the pediatric intensive care unit: role of targeted indirect calorimetry. JPEN J Parenter Enteral Nutr. 2009;33(3): 336–44.

125. Brodie D, Moscrip C, Hutcheon R. Body composition measurement: a review of hydrodensitometry, anthropometry, and impedance methods. Nutrition. 1998;14:296–309.

126. Woodrow G. Body composition analysis techniques in adult and pediatric patients: how reliable are they? How useful are they clinically? Perit Dial Int. 2007;27 Suppl 2:245–9.

127. Monk DN, Plank LD, Franch-Arcas G, Finn PJ, Streat SJ, Hill GL. Sequential changes in the metabolic response in critically injured patients during the first 25 days after blunt trauma. Ann Surg. 1996;223:395–405.

128. Wright CM, Sherriff A, Ward SC, McColl JH, Reilly JJ, Ness AR. Development of bioelectrical impedance-derived indices of fat and fat-free mass for assessment of nutritional status in childhood. Eur J Clin Nutr. 2008;62:210–7.

129. Chiolero RL, Gay LJ, Cotting J, Gurtner C, Schutz Y. Assessment of changes in body water by bioimpedance in acutely ill surgical patients. Intensive Care Med. 1992;18:322–6.

130. Park J, Yang WS, Kim SB, Park SK, Lee SK, Park JS, Chang JW. Usefulness of segmental bioimpedance ratio to determine dry body weight in new hemodialysis patients: a pilot study. Am J Nephrol. 2009;29:25–30.

131. Edefonti A, Picca M, Damiani B, Garavaglia R, Loi S, Ardissino G, Marra G, Ghio L. Prevalence of malnutrition assessed by biompedance analysis and anthropometrics in children on peritoneal dialysis. Perit Dial Int. 2001;21:172–9.

132. Matarese LE, Steiger E, Seidner DL, Richmond B. Body composition changes in cachectic patients receiving home parenteral nutrition. JPEN J Parenter Enteral Nutr. 2002;26:366–71.

133. Dufner D, Previs SF. Measuring in vivo metabolism using heavy water. Curr Opin Clin Nutr Metab Care. 2003;6:511–7.

134. McNaughton SA, Shepherd RW, Greer RG, Cleghorn GJ, Thomas BJ. Nutritional status of children with cystic fibrosis measured by total body potassium as a marker of body cell mass: lack of sensitivity of anthropometric measures. J Pediatr. 2000;136:188–94.

135. Sermet-Gaudelus I, Poisson-Salomon AS, Colomb V, Brusset MC, Mosser F, Berrier F, Ricour C. Simple pediatric nutritional-risk score to identify children at risk of malnutrition. Am J Clin Nutr. 2000;72:64–70.

136. Zlotkin S. A critical assessment of the upper intake levels for infants and children. J Nutr. 2006;136(2):502S–6.

137. Murphy SP, Poos MI. Dietary reference intakes: summary of applications in dietary assessment. Public Health Nutr. 2002;5(6A):843–9.

138. Hulst JM, van Goudoever JB, Zimmermann LJ, Tibboel D, Joosten KF. The role of initial monitoring of routine biochemical nutritional markers in critically ill children. J Nutr Biochem. 2006;17:57–62.

139. Bistrian BR. Interaction of nutrition and infection in the hospital setting. Am J Clin Nutr. 1977;30:1228–35.

140. Samra T, Sharma S, Pawar M. Metabolic monitors as a diagnostic tool. J Clin Monit Comput. 2011;25(2):149–50.

141. McMahon MM. Management of parenteral nutrition in acutely ill patients with hyperglycemia. Nutr Clin Pract. 2004;19:120–8.

142. Dhar A, Castillo L. Insulin resistance in critical illness. Curr Opin Pediatr. 2011;23(3):269–74.

143. Verhoeven JJ, den Brinker M, Hokken-Koelega AC, Hazelzet JA, Joosten KF. Pathophysiological aspects of hyperglycemia in children with meningococcal sepsis and septic shock: a prospective, observational cohort study. Crit Care. 2011;15(1):R44. Epub 2011 Jan 31.

144. Cheung NW, Napier B, Zaccaria C, Fletcher JP. Hyperglycemia is associated with adverse outcomes in patients receiving total parenteral nutrition. Diabetes Care. 2005;28:2367–71.

145. Ellger B, Debaveye Y, Vanhorebeek I, Langouche L, Giulietti A, Van Etten E, Herijgers P, Mathieu C, Van den Berghe G. Survival benefits of intensive insulin therapy in critical illness: impact of maintaining normoglycemia versus glycemia-independent actions of insulin. Diabetes. 2006;55(4):1096–105.

146. Scurlock C, Raikhelkar J, Mechanick JI. Critique of normoglycemia in intensive care evaluation: survival using glucose algorithm regulation (NICE-SUGAR)–a review of recent 2011 Nov;12(6):e386–90 literature. Curr Opin Clin Nutr Metab Care. 2010;13(2):211–4.

147. Ulate KP. A critical appraisal of Vlasselaers D, Milants I, Desmet L, Wouters PJ, Vanhorebeek I, van den Heuvel I, Mesotten D, Casaer MP, Meyfroidt G, Ingels C, Muller J, Van Cromphaut S, Schetz M, Van den Berghe G. Intensive insulin therapy for patients in paediatric intensive care: a prospective, randomised controlled study. Lancet. 2009;373:547–56.

148. Ognibene KL, Vawdrey DK, Biagas KV. The association of age, illness severity, and glycemic status in a pediatric intensive care unit. Pediatr Crit Care Med. 2011;12(6):e386–90.

149. Verbruggen SC, Coss-Bu J, Wu M, Schierbeek H, Joosten KF, Dhar A, van Goudoever JB, Castillo L. Current recommended parenteral protein intakes do not support protein synthesis in critically ill septic, insulin-resistant adolescents with tight glucose control. Crit Care Med. 2011;39(11):2518–25.

150. Abbott WC, Tayek JA, Bistrian BR, Maki T, Ainsley BM, Reid LA, Blackburn GL. The effect of nutritional support on T-lymphocyte subpopulations in protein calorie malnutrition. J Am Coll Nutr. 1986;5:577–84.

151. Twomey P, Ziegler D, Rombeau J. Utility of skin testing in nutritional assessment: a critical review. JPEN J Parenter Enteral Nutr. 1982;6:50–8.

152. Jeejeebhoy KN. Nutritional assessment. Nutrition. 2000;16:585–9.

153. Alberti KG, Batstone GF, Foster KJ, Johnston DG. Relative role of various hormones in mediating the metabolic response to injury. JPEN J Parenter Enteral Nutr. 1980;4:141–6.

154. Mastorakos G, Weber JS, Magiakou MA, Gunn H, Chrousos GP. Hypothalamic-pituitary-adrenal axis activation and stimulation of systemic vasopressin secretion by recombinant interleukin 6 in humans: potential implications for the syndrome of inappropriate vasopressin secretion. J Clin Endocrinol Metab. 1994;79:934–9.

155. Salas MA, Evans SW, Levell MJ, Whicher JT. Interleukin-6 and ACTH aft synergistically to stimulate the release of corticosterone from adrenal gland cells. Clin Exp Immunol. 1990;79:470–3.

156. Tappy L, Girardet K, Schwaller N, Vollenweider L, Jéquier E, Nicod P, Scherrer U. Metabolic effects of an increase of sympathetic activity in healthy humans. Int J Obes Relat Metab Disord. 1995;19:419–22.

157. Smeets HJ, Kievit J, Harinck HI, Frolich M, Hermans J. Differential effects of counterregulatory stress hormones on serum albumin concentrations and protein catabolism in healthy volunteers. Nutrition. 1995;11:423–7.

158. Wernerman J, Botta D, Hammarqvist F, Thunell S, von der Decken A, Vinnars E. Stress hormones given to healthy volunteers alter the concentration and configuration of ribosomes in skeletal muscle, reflecting changes in protein synthesis. Clin Sci. 1989;77:611–6.

159. Garrel DR, Razi M, Larivière F, Jobin N, Naman N, Emptoz-Bonneton A, Pugeat MM. JPEN J Parenter Enteral Nutr. 1995;19:482–91.

160. Fulks RM, Li JB, Goldberg AL. Effects of insulin, glucose, and amino acids on protein turnover in rat diaphragm. J Biol Chem. 1975;250:290–8.

161. Mortimore GE, Mondon CE. Inhibition by insulin of valine turnover in liver. Evidence for a control of proteolysis. J Biol Chem. 1970;245:2375–83.

162. Herndon DN, Hart DW, Wolf SE, Chinkes DL, Wolfe RR. Reversal of catabolism by beta blockade after severe burns. N Engl J Med. 2001;345:1223–9.

163. Terao Y, Miura K, Saito M, Sekino M, Fukusaki M, Sumikawa K. Quantitative analysis of the relationship between sedation and resting energy expenditure in postoperative patients. Crit Care Med. 2003;31(3):830–3.

164. Vernon DD, Witte MK. Effect of neuromuscular blockade on oxygen consumption and energy expenditure in sedated, mechanically ventilated children. Crit Care Med. 2000;28(5):1569–71.

165. Kudsk KA, Chiolero RL. Current concepts in nutrition – editorial review. Curr Opin Clin Nutr Metab Care. 2005;8:167–70.

166. Arikan AA, Zappitelli M, Goldstein SL, Naipaul A, Jefferson LS, Loftis LL. Fluid overload is associated with impaired oxygenation and morbidity in critically ill children. Pediatr Crit Care Med. 2012;13(3):253–8.

167. Balogh Z, McKinley BA, Holcomb JB, Miller CC, Cocanour CS, Kozar RA, Valdivia A, Ware DN, Moore FA. Both primary and secondary abdominal compartment syndrome can be predicted early and are harbingers of multiple organ failure. J Trauma. 2003;54:848–59.

168. McClave SA, Martindale RG, Vanek VW, McCarthy M, Roberts P, Taylor B, Ochoa JB, Napolitano L, Cresci G, A.S.P.E.N. Board of Directors, American College of Critical Care Medicine, Society of Critical Care Medicine. Guidelines for the provision and assessment of nutrition support therapy in the adult critically ill patient: Society of Critical Care Medicine (SCCM) and American Society for Parenteral and Enteral Nutrition (A.S.P.E.N.). JPEN J Parenter Enteral Nutr. 2009;33(3):277–316.

169. Mehta NM, Compher C. ASPEN: clinical guidelines: nutrition support of the critically ill child. JPEN J Parenter Enteral Nutr. 2009;33:260–76.

170. Peterson S, Chen Y. Systemic approach to parenteral nutrition in the ICU. Curr Drug Saf. 2010;5(1):33–40.

171. Gramlich L, Kichian K, Pinilla J, Rodych NJ, Dhaliwal R, Heyland DK. Does enteral nutrition compared to parenteral nutrition result in better outcomes in critically ill adult patients? A systematic review of the literature. Nutrition. 2004;20(10):843–8.

172. Crook MA, Hally V, Panteli JV. The importance of the refeeding syndrome. Nutrition. 2001;17:632–7.

173. Byrnes MC, Stangenes J. Refeeding in the ICU: an adult and pediatric problem. Curr Opin Clin Nutr Metab Care. 2011; 14(2):186–92.

174. Varsano S, Shapiro M, Taragan R, Bruderman I. Hypophosphatemia as a reversible cause of refractory ventilator failure. Crit Care Med. 1983;11:908–9.

175. Stanga Z, Brunner A, Leuenberger M, Grimble RF, Shenkin A, Allison SP, Lobo DN. Nutrition in clinical practice-the refeeding syndrome: illustrative cases and guidelines for prevention and treatment. Eur J Clin Nutr. 2008;62(6):687–94.

176. Wernerman J, Kirketeig T, Andersson B, Berthelson H, Ersson A, Friberg H, Guttormsen AB, Hendrikx S, Pettilä V, Rossi P, Sjöberg F, Winsö O, For the Scandinavian Critical Care Trials Group. Scandinavian glutamine trial: a pragmatic multi-centrerandomised clinical trial of intensive care unit patients. Acta Anaesthesiol Scand. 2011;55(7):812–8.

177. Andrews PJ, Avenell A, Noble DW, Campbell MK, Croal BL, Simpson WG, Vale LD, Battison CG, Jenkinson DJ, Cook JA, Scottish Intensive Care Glutamine or Selenium Evaluative Trial Trials Group. Randomised trial of glutamine, selenium, or both, to supplement parenteral nutrition for critically ill patients. BMJ. 2011;342:d1542.

178. Briassoulis G, Filippou O, Hatzi E, Papassotiriou I, Hatzis T. Early enteral administration of immunonutrition in critically ill children: results of a blinded randomized controlled clinical trial. Nutrition. 2005;21(7–8):799–807.

179. Briassoulis G, Filippou O, Kanariou M, Hatzis T. Comparative effects of early randomized immune or non-immune-enhancing enteral nutrition on cytokine production in children with septic shock. Intensive Care Med. 2005;31(6):851–8.

180. Briassoulis G, Filippou O, Kanariou M, Papassotiriou I, Hatzis T. Temporal nutritional and inflammatory changes in children with severe head injury fed a regular or an immune-enhancing diet: a randomized, controlled trial. Pediatr Crit Care Med. 2006;7(1):56–62.

181. Martindale RG, McClave SA, Vanek VW, McCarthy M, Roberts P, Taylor B, Ochoa JB, Napolitano L, Cresci G, American College of Critical Care Medicine, A.S.P.E.N. Board of Directors. Guidelines for the provision and assessment of nutrition support therapy in the adult critically ill patient: Society of Critical Care Medicine and American Society for Parenteral and Enteral Nutrition: Executive Summary. Crit Care Med. 2009; 37:1757–61.

182. Hulst JM, van Goudoever JB, Zimmermann LJ, Hop WC, Albers MJ, Tibboel D, Joosten KF. The effect of cumulative energy and protein deficiency on anthropometric parameters in a pediatric ICU population. Clin Nutr. 2004;23:1381–9.

183. Sugita H, Kaneki M, Sugita M, Yasukawa T, Yasuhara S, Martyn JA. Burn injury impairs insulin-stimulated Akt/PKB activation in skeletal muscle. Am J Physiol Endocrinol Metab. 2005; 288(3):E585–91.

184. Vanhorebeek I, Langouche L. Molecular mechanisms behind clinical benefits of intensive insulin therapy during critical illness: glucose versus insulin. Best Pract Res Clin Anaesthesiol. 2009;23(4):449–59.

185. Pollack MM, Ruttimann UE, Wiley JS. Nutritional depletions in critically ill children: associations with physiologic instability and increased quantity of care. JPEN J Parenter Enteral Nutr. 1985;9(3):309–13.

186. Mehta NM, McAleer D, Hamilton S, Naples E, Leavitt K, Mitchell P, Duggan C. Challenges to optimal enteral nutrition in a multidisciplinary pediatric intensive care unit. JPEN J Parenter Enteral Nutr. 2010;34(1):38–45.

187. Meyer R, Harrison S, Sargent S, Ramnarayan P, Habibi P, Labadarios D. The impact of enteral feeding protocols on nutritional support in critically ill children. J Hum Nutr Diet. 2009;22(5):428–36.

188. Heyland DK, Cahill NE, Dhaliwal R, Sun X, Day AG, McClave SA. Impact of enteral feeding protocols on enteral nutrition delivery: results of a multicenter observational study. JPEN J Parenter Enteral Nutr. 2010;34(6):675–84.

189. Poulard F, Dimet J, Martin-Lefevre L, Bontemps F, Fiancette M, Clementi E, Lebert C, Renard B, Reignier J. Impact of not measuring residual gastric volume in mechanically ventilated patients receiving early enteral feeding: a prospective before-after study. JPEN J Parenter Enteral Nutr. 2010;34(2):125–30.

190. Davies AR. Gastric residual volume in the ICU: can we do without measuring it? JPEN J Parenter Enteral Nutr. 2010; 34(2):160–2.

191. Chwals WJ. Energy expenditure in critically ill infants. Pediatr Crit Care Med. 2008;9(1):121–2.

192. Briassoulis G, Briassouli E, Tavladaki T, Ilia S, Fitrolaki DM, Spanaki AM. Unpredictable combination of metabolic and feeding patterns in malnourished critically ill children: the malnutrition-energy assessment question. Intensive Care Med. 2014;40(1):120–2.

193. Berger MM, Que YA. Bioinformatics assistance of metabolic and nutrition management in the ICU. Curr Opin Clin Nutr Metab Care. 2011;14(2):202–8.

194. Chwals WJ. Overfeeding the critically ill child: fact or fantasy? New Horiz. 1994;2:147–55.

195. Klein CJ, Stanek GS, Wiles CE. Overfeeding macronutrients to critically ill adults: metabolic complications. J Am Diet Assoc. 1998;98:795–806.

196. McCowen KC, Bistrian BR. Hyperglycemia and nutrition support: theory and practice. Nutr Clin Pract. 2004;19:235–44.

197. Verbruggen S, Sy J, Arrivillaga A, Joosten K, van Goudoever J, Castillo L. Parenteral amino acid intakes in critically ill children: a matter of convenience. JPEN J Parenter Enteral Nutr. 2010;34(3):329–40.

198. McCall M, Jeejeebhoy K, Pencharz P, Moulton R. Effect of neuromuscular blockade on energy expenditure in patients with severe head injury. JPEN J Parenter Enteral Nutr. 2003;27:27–35.

199. Li J, Zhang G, Herridge J, Holtby H, Humpl T, Redington AN, Van Arsdell GS. Energy expenditure and caloric and protein intake in infants following the Norwood procedure. Pediatr Crit Care Med. 2008;9(1):55–61.

200. Jaksic T, Shew SB, Keshen TH, Dzakovic A, Jahoor F. Do critically ill surgical neonates have increased energy expenditure? J Pediatr Surg. 2001;36:63–7.

201. Finestone HM, Greene-Finestone LS, Foley NC, Woodbury MG. Measuring longitudinally the metabolic demands of stroke patients: resting energy expenditure is not elevated. Stroke. 2003;34:502–7.

202. Briassoulis G, Venkataraman S, Thompson A. Cytokines and metabolic patterns in pediatric patients with critical illness. Clin Dev Immunol. 2010;2010:354047. Epub 2010 May 16.

203. Lancel S, Hassoun SM, Favory R, Decoster B, Motterlini R, Neviere R. Carbon monoxide rescues mice from lethal sepsis by supporting mitochondrial energetic metabolism and activating mitochondrial biogenesis. J Pharmacol Exp Ther. 2009; 329(2):641–8.

204. Brealey D, Brand M, Hargreaves I, Heales S, Land J, Smolenski R, Davies NA, Cooper CE, Singer M. Association between mitochondrial dysfunction and severity and outcome of septic shock. Lancet. 2002;360(9328):219–23.

205. Svistunenko DA, Davies N, Brealey D, Singer M, Cooper CE. Mitochondrial dysfunction in patients with severe sepsis: an EPR interrogation of individual respiratory chain components. Biochim Biophys Acta. 2006;1757(4):262–72.

Monitoring Kidney Function in the Pediatric Intensive Care Unit

43

Catherine D. Krawczeski, Stuart L. Goldstein, Rajit K. Basu, Prasad Devarajan, and Derek S. Wheeler

Abstract

The kidneys play a principle role in homeostatic balance. Acute kidney injury (AKI) carries numerous sequelae both obvious and subtle which, in combination, increase the morbidity and mortality of pediatric patients. Recent standardization of diagnostic criteria has resulted in a heightened awareness of AKI, increased AKI incidence, and recognition of the deleterious impact of AKI. Since no singular therapy for established AKI exists, a determinant of effective AKI therapy is expeditious diagnosis. In critically ill children, these therapies and the institution of concurrent supportive and preventive care depends on the ability to accurately monitor the kidney and specifically detect the presence of kidney dysfunction. Unfortunately, diagnosis of AKI is traditionally reliant on numerous tests and monitors of kidney function which carry different degrees of precision and accuracy. Additionally, delay in AKI diagnosis can render potential AKI therapy ineffective and significantly limit alternative treatment options. In this chapter we will describe the epidemiology of AKI in pediatrics, the classic serum and urinary markers of kidney dysfunction, the impact of fluid overload, the limitations of classic markers of kidney function and several emerging AKI biomarkers, AKI risk stratification using renal angina, and the future of monitoring kidney function. Understanding these concepts is crucial to delivery of effective care for the critically ill child with AKI.

Keywords

Acute kidney injury • Biomarkers • Fluid overload • NGAL • KIM-1 • IL-18 • Cystatin C • Renal angina

C.D. Krawczeski, MD (✉)
Division of Pediatric Cardiology, Stanford University School of Medicine, 750 Welch Rd, Suite 321, Palo Alto, CA 94304, USA
e-mail: ckrawczeski@gmail.com

S.L. Goldstein, MD
Division of Nephrology and Hypertension, Center for Acute Care Nephrology, Cincinnati Children's Hospital Medical Center, 3333 Burnet Avenue, MLC 7022, Cincinnati, OH 45229, USA
e-mail: stuart.goldstein@cchmc.org

R.K. Basu, MD, FAAP
Division of Critical Care Medicine,
Cincinnati Children's Hospital Medical Center,
3333 Burnet Avenue, MLC 2005, Cincinnati, OH 45229, USA
e-mail: rajit.basu@cchmc.org

P. Devarajan, MD
Division of Nephrology and Hypertension,
Cincinnati Children's Hospital Medical Center,
3333 Burnet Avenue, MLC 7022,
Cincinnati, OH 45229-3039, USA
e-mail: prasad.devarajan@cchmc.org

D.S. Wheeler, MD, MMM
Division of Critical Care Medicine, Cincinnati Children's Hospital Medical Center, University of Cincinnati College of Medicine, 3333 Burnet Avenue, Cincinnati, OH 45229-3039, USA
e-mail: derek.wheeler@cchmc.org

D.S. Wheeler et al. (eds.), *Pediatric Critical Care Medicine*,
DOI 10.1007/978-1-4471-6362-6_43, © Springer-Verlag London 2014

Introduction

The kidney plays an integral role in the maintenance of the normal homeostasis in the body, through (1) regulation of both the intracellular and extracellular concentration of water, electrolytes, and metabolic waste-products; (2) regulation of acid-base balance (largely in concert with the respiratory system); (3) regulation of calcium, phosphate, and bone metabolism via secretion of 1,25-dihydroxyvitamin D_3; (4) regulation of red blood cell (RBC) production via synthesis of erythropoietin; (5) regulation of systemic and local vasomotor tone via the production of renin, angiotensin II, endothelin, prostaglandins, and nitric oxide; and (6) regulation of normal glucose metabolism via participation in gluconeogenesis during fasting/starvation states. Derangements in nearly all of these vital functions of the kidney have been observed in critically ill children admitted to the pediatric intensive care unit (PICU). Hence, a very simplistic definition of "kidney dysfunction" or even overt "kidney failure" is based upon the observation of clinically measurable derangements in one or more of these vital processes. By maintaining normal homeostasis, the kidney directly impacts the normal function of other vital organs systems. A normally functioning kidney is therefore central to normal health. Given its role in maintaining homeostasis, monitoring of kidney function in the ICU becomes paramount.

Defining the Problem

Acute kidney injury (AKI), formerly known as acute renal failure, continues to represent a very common and potentially devastating problem in critically ill children and adults [1–5]. Historically, the reported incidence of AKI has varied greatly due to the lack of a standard, consensus definition [6]. For example, Novis et al. [7] performed a systematic review of nearly 30 studies conducted between 1965 and 1989 involving AKI patients undergoing vascular, general, cardiac, or biliary tract surgery. No two studies used the same criteria for AKI. Similarly, a survey of 589 physicians and nurses attending a critical care nephrology meeting noted that nearly 200 different definitions of AKI were used

in everyday clinical practice [8]. Not surprisingly then, the reported incidence of AKI affects anywhere between 5 and 50 % of critically ill children and adults [4, 9–13]. Most of the definitions of AKI that have been previously used in the literature have common elements – usually the diagnosis of AKI is based upon an absolute increase in the serum creatinine and/or a reduction in urine output. While the kidney has numerous functions, these two routinely and easily measured parameters are uniquely linked to kidney function and are thought to reflect glomerular filtration rate (GFR). GFR is perhaps the best and most widely used global index of kidney function in the clinical setting.

In an attempt to standardize the definition of AKI, the Acute Dialysis Quality Initiative (ADQI) group proposed the RIFLE criteria [14]. The RIFLE criteria are based upon either a reduction in GFR or decreased urine output. However, it should be intuitive that very few patients are likely to have GFR directly measured in the clinical setting – hence the use of changes in serum creatinine, or estimated creatinine clearance as a surrogate for GFR. In the absence of a baseline serum creatinine, the ADQI group recommended using the MDRD (modification of diet in renal disease) equation to retrospectively estimate creatinine using a low normal value for GFR (75 mL/min/1.73 m^2 BSA) [14, 15]. The RIFLE consensus definition is essentially a mnemonic for three levels of severity – <u>R</u>isk, <u>I</u>njury, and <u>F</u>ailure – and two outcomes, namely <u>L</u>oss and <u>E</u>nd-stage kidney disease (Table 43.1). These criteria have been validated in several different populations of critically ill adults [16–22] and have been further modified and validated for use in critically ill children (pediatric RIFLE criteria, or pRIFLE) (Table 43.2) [25, 26].

Recent data suggest that even smaller changes in serum creatinine than those defined by the RIFLE criteria are associated with adverse outcome [16, 27–36]. Consequently, the Acute Kidney Injury Network (AKIN) proposed a new, revised classification that defines AKI as an abrupt (within 48 h) reduction in kidney function as measured by an absolute increase in serum creatinine ≥ 0.3 mg/dL, a percentage increase in serum creatinine ≥ 50 %, or documented oliguria (<0.5 mL/kg/h) for more than 6 h [16]. The AKIN criteria represent only a slight modification of the previously

Table 43.1 RIFLE criteria (acute dialysis quality initiative)

Stage	Serum creatinine criteria	GFR criteria	Urine output criteria
R = Risk for renal dysfunction	Increase in serum creatinine $\geq 1.5\times$ baseline	Decrease in GFR ≥ 25 %	<0.5 mL/kg/h for 6 h
I = Injury to the kidney	Increase in serum creatinine $\geq 2.0\times$ baseline	Decrease in GFR ≥ 50 %	<0.5 mL/kg/h for 12 h
F = Failure of kidney function	Increase in serum creatinine $\geq 3.0\times$ baseline OR serum creatinine ≥ 4.0 mg/dL in the setting of an acute rise ≥ 0.5 mg/dL	Decrease in GFR ≥ 75 %	<0.3 mL/kg/h for 24 h or anuria for 12 h
L = Loss of kidney function	Persistent failure >4 weeks		
E = End-stage renal disease (ESRD)	Persistent failure >3 months		

Based on data from Ref. [14]

Table 43.2 The modified pediatric version of the RIFLE criteria (pRIFLE)

Stage	Estimated creatinine clearance (eCCL)	Urine output
R = Risk for renal dysfunction	eCCl decrease by 25 %	<0.5 mL/kg/h for 8 h
I = Injury to the kidney	eCCl decrease by 50 %	<0.5 mL/kg/h for 16 h
F = Failure of kidney function	eCCl decrease by 75 % or eCCl <35 mL/min/1.73 m²	<0.3 mL/kg/h for 24 h or anuria for 12 h
L = Loss of kidney function	Persistent failure >4 weeks	
E = End-stage renal disease (ESRD)	Persistent failure >3 months	

Estimated Creatinine clearance is estimated by the Schwartz formula [23, 24]

eCCl = CL$_{CR}$ = (k × Ht)/Scr, where Ht is height (length) in cm, SCr is the serum creatinine, k is a constant (k = 0.45 in children less than 1 year of age and k = 0.55 in children greater than 1 year of age), and BSA is body surface area

Table 43.3 Comparison of the ADQI RIFLE criteria with the AKIN staging criteria

RIFLE stage	RIFLE criteria	AKIN stage	AKIN criteria
R	≥150 % increase in serum creatinine, or >25 % GFR decrease	I	≥150 % or ≥0.3 mg/dL increase in serum creatinine
I	≥200 % increase in serum creatinine, or >50 % GFR decrease	II	>200 % increase in serum creatinine
F	≥300 % increase in serum creatinine, or serum creatinine of ≥4.0 mg/dL in setting of increase ≥0.5 mg/dL, or >75 % GFR decrease	III	>300 % increase in serum creatinine, or serum creatinine of ≥4.0 mg/dL in setting of increase ≥0.5 mg/dL

The urine output criteria are the same for both RIFLE and AKIN

defined RIFLE criteria (Table 43.3) [37, 38]. The AKIN criteria broadens the "risk" category of RIFLE to include an increase in serum creatinine of at least 0.3 mg/dL in order to increase the sensitivity of RIFLE for detecting AKI at an earlier timepoint. In addition, the AKIN criteria sets a window on first documentation of any criteria to 48 h and categorizes patients in the "failure" category of RIFLE if they are treated with renal replacement therapy, regardless of either changes in creatinine or urine output. Finally, AKIN replaces the three levels of severity R, I, and F with stage 1, 2, and 3.

Bagshaw and colleagues [37] compared the RIFLE and AKIN criteria by interrogating the Australian and New Zealand Intensive Care Society (ANZICS) Adult Patient Database (APD), which included over 120,000 critically ill adults admitted to 57 ICUs over a 5 year period. The differences between the RIFLE and AKIN classification systems were trivial and involved less than 1 % of patients. As expected, based on the change in serum creatinine of at least 0.3 mg/dL, AKIN slightly increased the number of patients classified as Stage I injury (category R in RIFLE) and decreased the number of patients classified as Stage II injury (category I in RIFLE). Similarly, Lopes and colleagues [39] compared RIFLE versus AKIN criteria in critically ill adults admitted to a single center and found that while AKIN criteria improved the sensitivity of AKI diagnosis, there was no difference between RIFLE versus AKIN criteria in predicting outcome. For all intents and purposes then, the AKIN and RIFLE classification systems are essentially the same [38, 40]. To date, there have not been any direct comparisons of AKIN and pRIFLE in critically ill children.

Recent studies in children admitted to the PICU have revealed the incidence of AKI defined by doubling of serum

creatinine at about 5–6 %. This was illustrated by a prospective study from a Canadian PICU that identified 985 cases of AKI for an incidence rate of 4.5 % of all PICU admissions [13]. In the largest study reported to date, 3,396 admissions to a single PICU in the United States were retrospectively analyzed and found that 6 % of children had AKI (by RIFLE) on admission. An additional 10 % of critically ill children developed AKI during their PICU stay [41]. When only children receiving mechanical ventilation and vasopressors are analyzed, the incidence of pRIFLE-positive AKI significantly increases to as high as 82 % [25].

Classic Parameters of Acute Kidney Injury

Glomerular Filtration Rate (GFR)

GFR is perhaps the best known and most widely used global index of kidney function. In fact, decreased GFR (commonly observed in the clinical setting as either a dramatic reduction in urine output or a significant increase in serum creatinine) is central to the definition of AKI in both the RIFLE and AKIN classification systems. GFR may be thought of as the sum of the filtration rates for all of the functioning nephrons in a given patient and is typically measured by calculating the clearance of a filtered marker solute, administered either as a bolus or continuous infusion:

$$\text{GFR}(\text{mL}/\text{min}) = (\text{U}_a \times \text{V})/\text{P}_a \qquad (43.1)$$

where *a* represents the filtered marker solute, U_a is the urinary concentration of the filtered marker solute, *V* is the urine flow rate, and P_a is the serum concentration of the marker solute.

Table 43.4 Reported factors that impact the accuracy of commonly used markers of acute kidney injury (AKI) in the clinical setting

Serum marker	Factor	
Creatinine	**Increase S$_{CR}$**	**Decrease S$_{CR}$**
	Younger age	Older age
	Male gender	Female gender
	Large lean muscle mass	Small lean muscle mass
	High protein diet (meat)	Vegetarian diet
	Strenuous exercise	Neuromuscular disease
	Rhabdomyolysis	Malnutrition
	Drugs (e.g., cimetidine, trimethoprim)	Amputation
		Jaffe reaction (e.g. DKA)
Urea	**Increase BUN**	**Decrease BUN**
	Dehydration	Overhydration
	High protein diet	Vegetarian diet
	Critical illness	Pregnancy
	Gastrointestinal bleeding	Liver disease
	Drugs (e.g., corticosteroids)	
Cystatin C	**Increase cystatin C**	**Decrease cystatin C**
	Older age	Younger age
	Male gender	Female gender
	Large lean muscle mass	Small lean muscle mass
	Inflammation	Immunosuppression
	Hyperthyroidism	Hypothyroidism
	Smoking	

Ideally, the marker solute used to calculate GFR should be water-soluble with minimal protein binding, freely filtered at the glomerulus, and excreted unchanged in the urine (i.e. the marker solute is not secreted, reabsorbed, or metabolized). The marker solute should be stable (not synthesized in the body), non-toxic, and easily measured using inexpensive and widely available assays. Commonly used solute markers for measurement of GFR in the clinical setting include inulin, iohexol, iothalamate, chromium Cr 51-labeled ethylenediaminetetraacetic acid (EDTA) (^{51}Cr-EDTA), and technetium Tc 99 m-labeled diethylene-triamine pentaacetic acid (^{99m}TC-DTPA) [42–44]. Unfortunately, the ideal marker solute, as defined above, does not exist. The measurement of even these commonly used marker solutes can be technically challenging, expensive, and infeasible in the everyday clinical setting.

GFR can be indirectly assessed by measuring the clearance of endogenous marker solutes, such as creatinine or urea. Creatinine clearance may be directly measured or estimated using one of several equations, such as the Cockcroft-Gault equation [45, 46], Modification of Diet in Renal Disease (MDRD) Study equation [47], and the Schwartz formula (for estimating creatinine clearance in children) [23, 24].

Cockcroft-Gault Equation [46]:

$$GFR = \frac{(140 - age) \times Weight}{0.8 \times S_{CR}} \qquad (43.2)$$

The serum creatinine (S$_{CR}$) concentration is multiplied by a factor of 0.8 in males, 0.85 in females.

MDRD Study Equation [47]:

$$GFR = 186.3 \times S_{CR}^{-1.154} \times Age^{-0.203} \times 1.212 (\text{if black}) \times 0.742 (\text{if female}) \qquad (43.3)$$

Schwartz Formula (for children) [23]:

$$GFR = (k \times Ht) / S_{CR} \qquad (43.4)$$

where Ht is height (length) in cm and k is a constant (k = 0.45 in children less than 1 year of age and k = 0.55 in children greater than 1 year of age). Recent investigations have allowed for a simplification of this formula, and have indicated that a single uniform k value of 0.413 provides a good approximation of GFR in children of all ages and both genders [48]. However, it should be emphasized that this simplification was derived in patients with chronic kidney disease, and have not been validated for use in AKI. These equations have been widely used to estimate creatinine clearance from a patient's age, body weight, and serum creatinine, even in critically ill patients admitted to the PICU [15, 49–52]. However, these equations should not be used to estimate GFR in patients with rapidly changing GFR, as would occur in the unstable critically ill patient with AKI.

The use of creatinine clearance for measuring GFR is problematic. For example, the serum creatinine concentration is affected by a multitude of factors, including age, body mass, gender, and dietary intake [53] (Table 43.4). Changes in serum creatinine often lag several days behind the changes in GFR and are not particularly sensitive or specific for small changes in GFR. Creatinine is secreted by the renal tubules, so that creatinine clearance will overestimate GFR. Certain medications can decrease tubular secretion of creatinine, including the oral histamine (H$_2$)-receptor antagonist, cimetidine [54]. While cimetidine administration has been used to improve the accuracy of creatinine clearance [53, 55–57], this particular method requires pre-treatment with cimetidine and is practically not feasible in the PICU setting.

Recent attention has focused on the use of a nonglycosylated, low molecular weight protein called cystatin C as a solute marker for estimating GFR. Cystatin C is synthesized at a relatively stable rate by virtually all nucleated cells in the body and is freely filtered by the glomerulus. It is neither secreted nor reabsorbed in the kidney, though it is almost completely metabolized by the proximal renal tubular epithelial cells [58, 59]. A reduction in GFR therefore correlates with a rise in serum cystatin C, and vice versa. Cystatin C is not significantly affected by age, gender, body mass, or dietary intake (Table 43.4). However, serum albumin, C reactive protein (CRP), and white blood cell (WBC) count have all been shown to affect serum cystatin C levels [60].

Recently, equations based upon serum cystatin C concentration have been used to estimate GFR and appear to function reasonably well in critically ill children [61–63].

Serum Creatinine

Creatinine is an amino acid compound derived from the metabolism of creatine, a protein found in skeletal muscle, as well as dietary protein intake. It is freely filtered by the glomerulus and is not reabsorbed or metabolized by the kidney. Therefore, creatinine clearance is frequently used to estimate the GFR in the clinical setting (see above discussion). There is an inverse relationship between serum creatinine and GFR, such that a reduction in GFR produces an increase in serum creatinine. However, the limitations to the use of serum creatinine as a surrogate marker of AKI are well described. First, the inverse relationship between GFR and serum creatinine is not linear. Second, approximately 10–40 % of creatinine clearance occurs via tubular secretion (see above) in the proximal renal tubules [64]. Serum creatinine may therefore grossly underestimate any reduction in GFR. Third, serum creatinine concentrations typically do not change until approximately 50 % of kidney function has already been lost [65]. As such, serum creatinine does not accurately reflect kidney function until a steady state has been reached, which may require several days following an acute insult [65]. Fourth, serum creatinine is directly affected by a number of factors (Table 43.4) which may lead to either underestimation or overestimation of GFR. For example, differences in age, gender, race, lean muscle mass, and dietary protein intake can result in significant variations in baseline serum creatinine. Similarly, patients with malnutrition or neuromuscular disease generally have lower serum creatinine levels at baseline. Rhabdomyolysis or strenuous exercise may increase serum creatinine through the release of preformed creatinine from damaged muscles [58]. Fifth, several drugs can impair creatinine secretion and elicit a transient, reversible increase in serum creatinine. Finally, other less common factors may impact the serum creatinine concentration. For example, the increased levels of acetoacetate in patients with diabetic ketoacidosis can cause interference with certain assays, resulting in a falsely elevated serum creatinine concentration (known as the Jaffe reaction) [66].

Serum Urea

Urea is a water-soluble, low molecular weight byproduct of normal protein metabolism that is produced by the liver and excreted by the kidney. Azotemia is defined as an increase in the serum concentration of nitrogenous compounds, such as urea – classically, azotemia is classified by the underlying pathophysiology as pre-renal, intrinsic, or post-renal. Similar to creatinine, there is a nonlinear and inverse relationship between serum urea (commonly measured as "blood urea nitrogen" or BUN) and GFR. In contrast to serum creatinine however, large increases in serum urea are potentially toxic. The pathophysiology of the uremic syndrome is well beyond the scope of the present discussion, but suffice it to say that uremic toxins affect almost every organ system to some degree [67–69].

Unfortunately, the use of BUN as a surrogate marker for AKI is even more problematic than the use of serum creatinine. Several factors commonly influence the BUN concentration (Table 43.4). For example, intravascular volume depletion (e.g., dehydration, sepsis, burns) can increase BUN, while intravascular volume expansion (e.g., overly zealous administration of fluids, SIADH) can decrease BUN. Gastrointestinal hemorrhage classically increases BUN, as does the administration of corticosteroids. Chronic liver disease can decrease the production of urea, with a concomitant decrease in BUN. Protein restriction, malnutrition, or decreased lean muscle mass similarly result in decreased production of urea, leading to a lower than expected BUN in the face of even dramatic reductions in GFR.

Nearly half of the filtered urea is passively reabsorbed in the proximal tubule. In addition, a decreased effective intravascular volume results in increased reabsorption of sodium, water, and urea in the proximal tubule. The subsequent increase in BUN occurs out of proportion to any reduction in GFR. As such, the ratio of BUN to creatinine is often used as an index to discriminate between pre-renal and renal azotemia (Table 43.5).

Urine Output

Urine output is one of the more commonly measured parameters of kidney function measured in hospitalized patients. Decreased urine output, or oliguria, is generally defined as urine output less than 400 mL in 24 h in adults, or urine output less than 1 mL/kg/h in children [70–73]. The differential diagnosis of oliguria is broad in scope and is relatively nonspecific for AKI. Oliguria is typically classified according to pre-renal, renal (intrinsic), or post-renal (primarily obstructive) causes (Table 43.6) [70, 71]. The importance of urine output as a marker of kidney function is perhaps best reflected in the inclusion of oliguria in the definition and classification of AKI (Tables 43.1, 43.2, and 43.3) [14, 16, 40, 74]. Oliguria can certainly be an important marker of renal dysfunction and has been associated with increased mortality [75, 76]. However, oliguria in and of itself is neither sensitive nor specific for AKI. There are certain critically ill patients with marked kidney dysfunction as exhibited by significant increases in the serum creatinine or uremic toxins who can

Table 43.5 Pre-renal versus intrinsic or renal AKI

Index	Pre-renal AKI	Intrinsic or renal AKI
Urine color	Dark yellow	Yellow
Urine specific gravity	High (>1.020)	Low (<1.020)
Urine sodium	Low (<10 mmol/L)	High (>20 mmol/L)
Urine sediment	Normal	Epithelial casts
FE_{NA}	<1 %	>1 %
FE_{Urea}	<35 %	>35 %
Urine osmolality	High (>500 mOsm/kg H_2O)	Close to serum (<300 mOsm/kg H_2O)
Urine/plasma osmolality	>1.5	1–1.5
Urine/plasma creatinine ratio	High (>40)	Low (<10)
BUN/creatine ratio	High	Normal
Urine sodium/potassium ratio	Low (<1/4)	High
RFI (renal failure index)	<1	>2

Table 43.6 Differential diagnosis of decreased urine output (oliguria)

Pre-renal causes	Renal (intrinsic) causes	Post-renal causes
Absolute decrease in effective intravascular volume	**Acute glomerulonephritis**	**Upper urinary tract obstruction**
Hemorrhage	Post-streptococcal glomerulonephritis	Ureteral obstruction
Gastrointestinal losses (vomiting, diarrhea, NG suction)	Rapidly progressive glomerulonephritis	
Trauma		
Surgery		
Burns		
Excessive urine output (from diuretics or glucosuria)		
"Third space losses" (pancreatitis, bowel surgery, ascites)		
Decreased po intake		
Fever A		
Relative decrease in effective intravascular volume	**Small vessel vasculitis**	**Lower urinary tract obstruction**
Sepsis	Systemic lupus erythematosus	Bladder-outlet obstruction
Acute liver failure	Scleroderma	
Anaphylaxis	Malignant hypertension	
Vasodilatory drugs	Pre-eclampsis	
Nephrotic syndrome	Polyarteritis nodosa	
	Drug-related	
Absolute or relative decrease in renal blood flow	**Interstitial nephritis**	
Renal-artery or renal-vein occlusion by thrombosis, stenosis, etc.	Drug-related (e.g., penicillin)	
Administration of ACE inhibitors	Infection	
	Cancer	
	Acute tubular necrosis	
	Ischemia-reperfusion injury	
	Nephrotoxic antibiotics	
	Heavy metal poisoning	
	Ethylene glycol poisoning	
	Radiographic contrast	
	Uric acid or oxalate crystals	
	Myoglobinuria/hemoglobinuria	

still maintain a normal (so-called non-oliguric AKI) [77, 78] or even increased urine output (so-called high output AKI). While most studies in the past have suggested that non-oliguric AKI is associated with better outcomes, recent studies have called this into question [58, 71, 78]. For example, higher urine output may be associated with a delay in the initiation of renal replacement therapy, leading to increased mortality [78]. In addition, conversion of oliguric AKI to non-oliguric AKI with the use of loop diuretics [79, 80] has not resulted in significant improvements in mortality [58, 81–83].

Fluid Overload

Fluid overload is also relatively easy to measure in the clinical setting and has been associated with worsening outcome in critically ill children and adults. While fluid balance lacks sensitivity and specificity for the diagnosis of AKI, fluid overload in patients with established AKI may have prognostic value.

$$\% \text{ Fluid Overload} = \left(\frac{\text{Fluid in } [L] - \text{Fluid out } [L]}{\text{ICU admit weight}} \right) \times 100\%$$

(43.5)

For example, a retrospective series of 21 critically ill children receiving continuous renal replacement therapy (CRRT) for AKI suggested that the degree of fluid overload at the initiation of CRRT was significantly lower in survivors compared to non-survivors, independent of the severity of illness [84]. The authors of this study proposed that the earlier initiation of CRRT, defined as 10 % fluid overload vs. 25 % fluid overload, may prevent morbidity and mortality in critically ill children with AKI by allowing earlier administration of nutritional support and necessary blood products. A larger retrospective series involving 113 children with MODS [85] confirmed these results – in this study, the median %fluid overload was significantly lower in survivors compared to non-survivors, independent of severity of illness. In fact, %fluid overload was independently associated with survival in patients with ≥3 organ failures by multivariate analysis. A multi-center, retrospective study by the Prospective Pediatric Continuous Renal Replacement Therapy Registry Group (ppCRRT Registry Group) involving 116 critically ill children concluded that increased fluid administration from the time of admission to the PICU to the time of initiation of CRRT was independently associated with mortality [86]. A follow-up prospective study by the ppCRRT Registry Group confirmed these findings in a study involving 297 critically ill children from 13 centers across the United States [87]. Collectively, these studies strongly suggest that fluid balance is an important marker for worse outcome in critically ill patients with AKI who require CRRT [88, 89]. More importantly, a recent study suggests that fluid overload is an independent risk factor for negative outcomes in critically ill children even in the absence of CRRT [90].

Urinalysis and Microscopy

The urinalysis is a non-invasive, commonly used, readily available test that can yield important diagnostic information. For example, urine is normally clear with a light yellow color. A dark yellow, concentrated urine is usually associated with a pre-renal state, while red urine is associated with hematuria (suggestive of glomerulonephritis), hemoglobinuria, or myoglobinuria. The urine specific gravity (defined as the ratio of the weight of a given solution compared to that of an equal volume of distilled water) is also clinically useful, in that a urine specific gravity ≥1.020 is usually consistent with a pre-renal state or the presence of large macromolecules, such as glucose or radiographic contrast. Similarly, the urine osmolality fluctuates widely in response to changes in serum osmolality (which is tightly regulated between 290 and 290 mOsm/kg) and hydration status. A high urine osmolality is usually consistent with a pre-renal state. The urine pH is not particularly helpful in discerning either pre-renal or intrinsic renal AKI, unless a significant metabolic acidosis is present (i.e. secondary to decreased peripheral perfusion).

Critical illness is frequently associated with endothelial dysfunction with increased capillary leak. Increased capillary leak in the kidney results in proteinuria, a frequent finding in critically ill patients [58, 91, 92]. For example, the presence of microalbuminuria appears to correlate with severity of illness, as well as increased morbidity and mortality in critically ill patients with trauma [93], acute lung injury [94], sepsis [95, 96], multiple organ dysfunction syndrome (MODS) [92, 94, 97–100], and in children following surgery [101]. Gosling observed that the peak in microalbuminuria in critically ill patients occurred up to 2 days before a detectable rise in other markers of inflammation [96]. However, while microalbuminuria has been associated with poor outcome in critically ill adults, there are currently no studies that correlate microalbuminuria with progression or outcome from AKI in critically ill children. Alternatively, urinary α_1-microglobulin has been used as a marker for the need for renal replacement therapy in a small cohort of patients with AKI [102]. Other urinary proteins have also been used as markers of AKI with some limited success, including proteins from the glomerulus (e.g., albumin, transferrin), proximal tubule (e.g., alpha-1-microglobulin, beta-2microglobulin, cathepsin), and distal tubule (e.g., Tamm-Horsfall protein, lactate dehydrogenase) [80, 103–106].

The urinary sediment is yet another relatively simple and readily available test that has been used to differentiate between pre-renal AKI and intrinsic renal AKI [91]. Classically, pre-renal AKI is characterized by hyaline casts or fine granular casts. Conversely, intrinsic renal AKI is characterized by coarse granular casts containing renal tubular epithelial cells. Once again, however, these tests lack sufficient specificity and sensitivity for predicting the early onset of AKI in the critical care setting [91].

Urine Chemistry and Similarly Derived Indices

Several urinary biochemical tests and derived indices have been used in the diagnosis and classification of AKI [107], some of which have already been listed in Table 43.5. While all of these tests are readily available and technically simple to perform, as a group they lack sufficient specificity and sensitivity for the diagnosis of AKI in the clinical setting [58, 59, 71, 108, 109]. Perhaps the best known urinary index of AKI is the fractional excretion of sodium (FE_{Na}) [110]. FENa is calculated by determining the amount of sodium that is excreted in the urine (urine sodium concentration, $Urine_{Na}$ multiplied by the urinary flow rate) as a fraction of how much sodium was filtered by the kidney (plasma sodium concentration, S_{Na} multiplied by the GFR). If creatinine clearance is used as a surrogate for the GFR, the urinary flow rates cancel each other out and the equation for FE_{Na} becomes:

$$FE_{Na} = \frac{Urine_{Na} \times S_{CR}}{S_{Na} \times Urine_{CR}} \times 100 \qquad (43.6)$$

The utility of the FE_{Na} is based upon the principle that filtered sodium is avidly reabsorbed in the proximal renal tubules in the setting of either an absolute or relative reduction in the effective intravascular volume (i.e. pre-renal AKI). Therefore, under these conditions, the FE_{Na} is <1 %. In contrast, in the setting of tubular injury (i.e. renal or intrinsic AKI), the resulting FE_{Na} is >2 % [107, 110, 111]. A FE_{Na} between 1 and 2 % is non-diagnostic. In reality, however, the FE_{Na} lacks sufficient sensitivity and specificity for widespread use in the critical care setting [58, 59, 91, 109, 112–120]. In addition, calculation of the FE_{Na} requires a priori measurement of both urine sodium and creatinine, neither of which are routinely measured. Interpretation of FE_{Na} must take into account any previous fluid administration, diuretic therapy, or any abnormal presence of substances in the urine such as protein, glucose, mannitol, or contrast agents. In neonates, the FE_{Na} is generally higher because of their decreased ability to reabsorb sodium. In neonates, the FE_{Na} is usually below 2.5 % in prerenal AKI and usually greater than 2.5 % in intrinsic AKI. The FE_{Na} can be falsely elevated following administration of loop or distal tubule diuretics, which increase urinary sodium excretion.

The utility of the fractional excretion of urea (FE_{Urea}) has been compared with the FE_{Na} in several clinical studies [121–123].

$$FE_{Urea} = \frac{S_{CR} \times Urine_{Urea}}{BUN \times Urine_{CR}} \times 100 \qquad (43.7)$$

The major limitation to the FE_{Na} is the fact that diuretics are commonly used to enhance urine output in oliguric patients [80]. In addition, the excessive use of diuretics may in fact result in a pre-renal state, though with an increased urinary sodium concentration and hence increased FE_{Na}. Furthermore, the pre-renal state in patients with excessive gastrointestinal losses secondary to nasogastric (NG) suction or vomiting is characterized by volume depletion and increased urinary sodium concentration, resulting in a falsely elevated FE_{Na}. In these cases, the concentration of serum bicarbonate exceeds the bicarbonate reabsorption capacity of the proximal tubule, leading to excretion of sodium bicarbonate and hence an alkaline urine [124]. The purported advantage of FE_{Urea} over FE_{Na} is that it can be used in patients who have received diuretic therapy. Diuretic therapy alters the urinary concentration of sodium, leading to falsely elevated FE_{Na} results, even in the face of pre-renal AKI. In contrast, loop diuretics do not appreciably affect the urinary

concentration of urea [122]. The FE_{Urea} in well-hydrated patients ranges between 50and 65 % [125], while a FE_{Urea} ≤35 % is generally indicative of pre-renal AKI [122, 126]. A FE_{Urea} >50 % in the presence of oliguria is generally indicative of intrinsic renal AKI [122]. Unfortunately, FE_{Urea} appears to be no more sensitive or specific in the diagnosis of AKI than FE_{Na} [123].

Several additional urinary indices deserve mention, primarily for historical reference, but again all of these markers lack sufficient specificity and sensitivity for use in the critical care setting. These include the urinary sodium, urine osmolality, urine/plasma creatinine ratio, BUN/creatinine ratio, and urine/serum urea ratio (Table 43.5) [58, 107, 109, 127]. Additional tests include the urine uric acid/creatinine ratio [109, 128], fractional excretion of uric acid [109, 121, 128], fractional excretion of chloride [109, 121], and the renal failure index (RFI) [107, 109, 121].

$$RFI = \left(U_{Na} / U_{CR} \right) \times S_{CR} \qquad (43.8)$$

A RFI <1 is usually indicative of pre-renal AKI, while RFI >2 is more consistent with intrinsic renal AKI.

The Need for Better Markers of AKI

Animal models have contributed greatly to the mechanistic understanding of AKI and strongly support the concept that early intervention and treatment of AKI is more effective [129]. These intensive research efforts have further resulted in several novel and promising therapeutic approaches for the management of AKI in critically ill patients. Unfortunately, the clinical application of these treatments has heretofore met with limited, if any success [130]. A major reason for this failure is the lack of early markers for AKI, and hence a delay in initiating timely therapy [1, 2, 129–131]. For example, the RIFLE criteria discussed above are based primarily upon changes in either serum creatinine or urine output. Unfortunately, neither of these two classic markers of AKI is particularly sensitive or specific for AKI. Moreover, both a decrease in urine output and an increase in serum creatinine are relatively late signs of AKI. Holding potentially effective treatment until the serum creatinine increases above a threshold level is analogous to initiating definitive treatment in patients with an acute myocardial infarction (AMI) until 48 h after the occlusion of a coronary artery [59]. Perhaps the most crucial aspect of caring for patients presenting with an AMI is the early recognition and diagnosis of AMI based upon validated biomarkers, such as the troponins. A troponin-like biomarker of AKI that is easily measured, unaffected by other biological variables, and capable of both early detection and risk stratification would represent a tremendous advance in the field of critical care medicine [132–137]. The quest for such AKI biomarkers is an area of intense contemporary research. Fortunately, the application of functional genomics and proteomics to human and animal models of the acutely stressed kidney has recently uncovered several novel genes and gene products that are emerging as biomarkers [138]. The most promising of these are discussed further below.

Emerging Biomarkers

The ideal biomarker would be non-invasive, inexpensive, accurate, and rapidly measurable (ideally at the bedside), be sensitive to subclinical disease, and would correlate with disease severity, allowing prognostic information. Optimally, biomarkers should also allow differentiation of AKI etiologies or subtypes (such as ischemic or toxic) and allow monitoring of the course of injury and response to therapy. Conventional urinary biomarkers such as casts and fractional excretion of sodium have been insensitive and nonspecific for the early recognition of AKI [139]. Other traditional urinary biomarkers, such as filtered high molecular weight proteins and tubular proteins or enzymes, have also suffered from lack of specificity and dearth of standardized assays [140]. Fortunately, the application of innovative technologies such as functional genomics and proteomics to human and animal models of AKI has uncovered several novel genes and gene products that are emerging as potential biomarkers for AKI [141, 142]. The most promising of these are neutrophil gelatinase-associated lipocalin (NGAL), cystatin C, interleukin-18 (IL-18), liver fatty acid binding protein (L-FABP), and kidney injury molecure-1 (KIM-1).

NGAL

Human neutrophil gelatinase-associated lipocalin (NGAL) is a 25 kDa protein covalently bound to gelatinase from neutrophils. NGAL is normally expressed at very low levels in several human tissues, including kidney, lungs, stomach, and colon. Released primarily by activated neutrophils in the setting of infection, NGAL also functions as an acute-phase factor indicative of sustained inflammatory injury. The gene for NGAL is significantly up-regulated in the kidney very quickly after ischemic injury, and the protein is over-expressed in distal tubule cells [143]. NGAL has been identified as one of the earliest and most robustly induced genes and proteins in the kidney after ischemic or nephrotoxic injury [141, 143–145] and is easily measured in plasma or urine very early after injury [135, 144, 146]. Multiple studies have validated NGAL as a biomarker of ischemic AKI [144, 147]. Additional studies have demonstrated elevations in NGAL with other forms of kidney injury, including contrast

nephropathy, lupus nephritis, nephrotoxic injury, and delayed graft function in kidney transplants [148–152]. As an iron transporting protein, NGAL may play a primary role in renal tubular survival and recovery, and has been used therapeutically in ischemia-reperfusion injury animal models [153]. NGAL has emerged as the center-stage player in the AKI biomarker field. However, it is acknowledged NGAL appears to be most sensitive and specific in relatively uncomplicated patient populations with AKI [154] and that NGAL measurements may be influenced by a number of coexisting variables, such as preexisting renal disease [155] and systemic or urinary tract infections [156].

Cystatin C

Cystatin C is an endogenous cysteine proteinase inhibitor produced by nucleated cells at a constant rate. It is freely filtered at the glomerulus, reabsorbed and catabolized but is not secreted by the tubules. As blood levels of cystatin C are not significantly affected by age, gender, race, or muscle mass, it is a better predictor of glomerular function than is serum creatinine in patients with chronic kidney disease [157]. Urinary excretion of cystatin C has been shown to predict the requirement for renal replacement therapy in patients with established AKI [102]. Cystatin C has been shown to be predictive of AKI in the intensive care setting [158] and in a recent prospective study of cystatin C in pediatric post-CPB patients, cystatin C levels at 12 h after CPB were strong independent predictors of AKI [159]. Although NGAL outperforms cystatin C at earlier time points, an advantage of cystatin C is the commercial availability of a standardized immunonephelometric assay, which is automated and provides results in minutes. Additionally, routine clinical storage conditions, freeze/thaw cycles, the presence of interfering substances do not affect serum cystatin C measurements.

IL-18

IL-18, a mediator of inflammation, is produced by proximal tubules, and is activated by caspase-1 [160]. The source of urine IL-18 elevation in AKI is in part from injured tubules. It is more specific to ischemic AKI and is not affected by nephrotoxins, CKD or urinary tract infections. In a cross-sectional study, urine IL-18 levels were markedly increased in patients with established AKI but not in subjects with urinary tract infection, chronic kidney disease, nephritic syndrome, or prerenal failure [161]. Urinary NGAL and IL-18 have been shown to represent early, predictive, sequential AKI biomarkers in children undergoing CPB [162]. In patients who developed AKI, urinary NGAL was induced within 2 h and peaked at 6 h, whereas urine IL-18 levels increased around 6 h and peaked at 12 h after CPB. Both NGAL and IL-18 were independently associated with duration of AKI among cases. Urine NGAL and IL-18 have also emerged as predictive biomarkers for delayed graft function following kidney transplantation [163].

KIM-1

KIM-1 is a type 1 trans-membrane protein that is over-expressed in dedifferentiated proximal tubule cells after ischemic or toxic injury and is easily detected in urine [164]. It is specific to ischemic/toxic injury and is not markedly upregulated in contrast induced nephropathy, CKD or urinary tract infections. Urinary KIM-1 has been shown in small studies to be elevated in adult and pediatric patients following CPB [165, 166].

L-FABP

L-FABP is a 14 kDa protein normally expressed in the proximal convoluted and straight tubules. L-FABP binds selectively to free unsaturated fatty acids and lipid peroxidation products, decreasing lipid peroxidation stress and potentially mitigating tissue damage in the setting of ischemia-reperfusion injury. Ischemia induces free fatty acid overload in the proximal tubule which can exacerbate tubulointerstitial disease. L-FABP has been shown to predict AKI after CPB-associated injury [167] and in the intensive care setting [168]. L-FABP correlates with the histologic severity of disease [169].

AKI Biomarker Combinations

Since many pathways are involved in the pathogenesis of AKI, it is believed that combinations of biomarkers with different properties may prove most predictive. In a recent study of biomarker combinations in pediatric cardiopulmonary bypass patients, the addition of a urine biomarker "panel", consisting of NGAL, IL-18, L-FABP, and KIM-1, to a clinical model, enhanced the prediction of AKI at 6–24 h after surgery [170]. In this study, biomarkers rose in a predictable pattern in AKI patients, with significant NGAL elevations at 2 h, IL-18 and L-FABP at 6 h, and KIM-1 at 12 h after cardiopulmonary bypass. The importance of determining the temporal sequence of biomarkers is underscored by the four phases of AKI [171]. In the initiation phase during the ischemic insult, intracellular ATP depletion is profound, and generation of reactive oxygen molecules and labile iron is initiated. Vasodilator, ATP-donor, anti-oxidant, and iron chelation therapies may be especially effective during this

phase, and the appearance of NGAL may be used to trigger such therapies. Prolongation of ischemia followed by reperfusion ushers in the extension phase. Tubules undergo reperfusion-mediated cell death, and the injured endothelial and epithelial cells amplify the inflammatory cascades. This phase probably represents a window of opportunity for early diagnosis with intermediate biomarkers such as L-FABP and IL-18, and active therapeutic intervention with anti-apoptotic and anti-inflammatory strategies. During the maintenance phase, both cell injury and regeneration occur simultaneously. Measures such as growth factors and stem cells that accelerate the endogenous regeneration processes, initiated by later biomarkers with high specificity such as KIM-1, may be most effective during this phase. In the future, the use of "biomarker panels" will likely allow us to pinpoint the timing of injury and assist in selecting appropriately timed therapies.

Renal Angina: Risk Stratification to Optimize AKI Biomarker Utility

The primary limitation of AKI biomarkers is loss of fidelity by capricious use. An apt analogy is seen in troponin-I measurements. Troponin-I would not be expected to function well for prediction of myocardial ischemia in an otherwise healthy 25 year old that experienced chest pain after eating a fatty meal. Likewise, a troponin-I should not be drawn on every 85 year old seen in an emergency room irrespective of the presence of chest pain just because myocardial infarctions are more prevalent in older individuals. In fact, when troponin is tested in critically patients without signs and symptoms of acute coronary syndrome, it loses its diagnostic capacity. Therefore, it seems crucial to identify critically ill patients at-risk for development of AKI [172]. The empiric concept of 'renal angina' seeks to add risk stratification to critically ill patients and to identify patients for whom use of an AKI biomarker (or a panel of markers) would be a "rule-out" test, instead of a generic "rule-in" test (i.e., serum creatinine) [172]. The renal angina construct is a composite of baseline and contextual risk factors (e.g. diabetes, high-risk procedures like cardiopulmonary bypass) and evidence of injury (fluid overload, oliguria, increased SCr). Renal angina (ANG) can be thought of in terms of a simple equation:

$$\text{Renal Angina Threshold} = \text{Risk of AKI} \times \text{Evidence of AKI}$$
$$(43.9)$$

Thus, as the risk of AKI increases (e.g. BMT patient on vasopressors and mechanical ventilation), less initial evidence of AKI is needed (small changes in SCr) to meet the threshold for ANG. Conversely, a patient with few risk factors of AKI (a young child admitted to ICU for bronchiolitis but not intubated) would require more evidence of AKI in order to achieve the ANG threshold. Once patients achieve ANG, then the task of the clinician is to 'rule out AKI', using AKI biomarkers and other clinical investigation. We believe that this diagnostic framework is consistent with other clinical syndromes and provides an approach that non-nephrology clinicians can utilize. In short, renal angina is a clinical guide that identifies patients at high-risk for AKI by integrating baseline, contextual, and clinical evidence of kidney injury. Examples of its potential utility are the following examples: (1) pediatric patients undergoing bone marrow transplantation (BMT) are at high risk for AKI, but there is little utility is measuring biomarkers every 6 h in every patient every day (2) Patients with sub-RIFLE changes in estimated creatinine clearance and increases in fluid overload are at risk for progression to more severe AKI, but many do not progress (3) many patients may present with acutely elevated creatinine levels, which may be easily reversible with hydration ("prerenal azotemia" or fluid responsive AKI). By risk stratification using renal angina, it is theoretically possible to then use an AKI biomarker to identify the patient who actually IS at risk for persistent AKI.

The creation of the pediatric renal angina construct was based on epidemiologic data for AKI risk in critically ill children. The three-tiered clinical risk stratification scheme was based on observed AKI rates (defined as pRIFLE-I, or a 50 % rise in serum creatinine) in a number of pediatric epidemiological studies. For all ICU patients, the AKI rates have been reported as 4–10 % [13, 41], pediatric BMT recipients have a reported AKI rates of 11–21 % [173, 174], and critically ill patients receiving mechanical ventilation have reported AKI rates of 50 % [25, 26]. The strata are deemed moderate, high and very high risk, respectively. Other patients, such as general oncology patients, solid organ transplant recipients, and immunosuppressed patients also carry increased risk for AKI, but were grouped together in the moderate risk groups (ICU admission) for simplicity. With increasing risk strata, the thresholds for the corresponding clinical sign (serum creatinine change or percent fluid accumulation) to fulfill renal angina criteria decreases accordingly. Numerous retrospective pediatric studies have demonstrated the potential negative implication of excessive fluid overload. Based on aggregate analysis of data and consensus opinion within the ppCRRT, an estimated 10–15 % FO at time of initiation of CRRT is associated with increased mortality. Using the 10 % number as a median, initial thresholds for renal angina fluid overload reflect standard intervals above and below based on risk of AKI (e.g., 5, 10, 15 %) [175]. To further relate ANG to the troponin-MI paradigm, if a patient has diabetes, hypertension, and smokes, the amount of chest pain or dyspnea required to raise suspicion of acute coronary syndrome is much less than a thin patient without any of these risk factors. Additionally, the construct was created with the intent that the negative predictive value should be extremely high in patients who do not fulfill the renal angina criteria, thus precluding capricious biomarker testing/assessment in patients who will not likely develop AKI.

The initial studies of the renal angina construct in critically ill children support the idea that risk stratification with secondary use of AKI biomarkers increases predictive precision for persistent AKI. A broad based study of four large PICU cohorts derived and validated the construct; area under curve-receiver operating constructs for angina prediction of severe AKI at 72 h after assessment of 0.72–0.80 and negative predictive values were >95 %. Further, inclusion of AKI biomarkers (NGAL included) increased the precision of the AUC-ROC for angina prediction of AKI . With appropriate risk stratification, renal angina may improve the performance of AKI biomarkers for prediction of AKI – which then would expedite therapy and improve outcomes.

Future Perspectives in AKI Biomarkers

Although recently discovered biomarkers, most notably NGAL, have been validated as a superior mechanism of diagnosing AKI earlier than current modalities, little has been done to demonstrate clinical translation of these studies. Although animal data are abundant, there is currently no study that demonstrates that clinical outcomes can be improved by earlier AKI diagnosis. Prospective studies that demonstrate improved outcomes with early targeted therapy are needed. Additionally, since the majority of pediatric AKI studies have been performed in cardiac surgical patients, it is important to confirm results in populations with other mechanisms of kidney injury.

References

1. Brady H, Singer G. Acute renal failure. Lancet. 1995;346:1533–40.
2. Thadhani R, Bonventre JV. Acute renal failure. N Engl J Med. 1996;334:1448–60.
3. Nolan CR, Anderson RJ. Hospital-acquired acute renal failure. J Am Soc Nephrol. 1998;9:710–8.
4. Hui-Stickle S, Brewer ED, Goldstein SL. Pediatric ARF epidemiology at a tertiary care center from 1999 to 2001. Am J Kidney Dis. 2005;45:96–101.
5. Uchino S. The epidemiology of acute renal failure in the world. Curr Opin Crit Care. 2006;12:538–43.
6. Mehta RL, Chertow GM. Acute renal failure definitions and classification: time for change? J Am Soc Nephrol. 2003;14:2178–87.
7. Novis BK, Roizen MF, Aronson S, Thisted RA. Association of preoperative risk factors with postoperative acute renal failure. Anesth Analg. 1994;78:143–9.
8. Liano F, Junco E, Pacual J, Madero R, Verde E. The spectrum of acute renal failure in the intensive care unit compared with that seen in other settings. The Madrid Acute Renal Failure Study Group. Kidney Int Suppl. 1998;66:S16–24.
9. Wilkins RG, Faragher EB. Acute renal failure in an intensive care unit: incidence, prediction and outcome. Anaesthesia. 1983;38:628–34.

10. Brivet FG, Kleinknecht DJ, Loirat P, et al. Acute renal failure in intensive care units – causes, outcome, and prognostic factors of hospital mortality: a prospective, multicenter study. French Study Group on acute renal failure. Crit Care Med. 1996;24:192–8.

11. de Mendonca A, Vincent JL, Suter PM, et al. Acute renal failure in the ICU: risk factors and outcome evaluated by the SOFA score. Intensive Care Med. 2000;26:915–21.

12. Williams DM, Sreedhar SS, Mickell JS, Chan JCM. Acute kidney failure: a pediatric experience over 20 years. Arch Pediatr Adolesc Med. 2002;156:893–900.

13. Bailey D, Phan V, Litalien C, Ducruet T, Merouani A, Lacroix J, et al. Risk factors of acute renal failure in critically ill children: a prospective descriptive epidemiological study. Pediatr Crit Care Med. 2007;8:29–35.

14. Bellomo R, Ronco C, Kellum JA, et al. Acute renal failure – definition, outcome measures, animal models, fluid therapy, and information technology needs: the second international consensus conference of the Acute Dialysis Quality Initiative (ADQI) Group. Crit Care. 2004;8:R204–12.

15. Bagshaw SM, Uchino S, Cruz D, Bellomo R, Morimatsu H, Morgera S, et al. A comparison of observed versus estimated baseline creatinine for determination of RIFLE class in patients with acute kidney injury. Nephrol Dial Transplant. 2009;24(9):2739–44.

16. Mehta RL, Kellum JA, Shah SV, Molitoris BA, Ronco C, Warnock DG, et al. Acute Kidney Network: report of an initiative to improve outcomes in acute kidney injury. Crit Care. 2007;11:1–8.

17. Uchino S, Bellomo R, Goldsmith D, et al. An assessment of the RIFLE criteria for acute renal failure in hospitalized patients. Crit Care Med. 2006;34:1913–7.

18. Kuitunen A, Vento A, Suojaranta-Ylinen R, Pettila V. Acute renal failure after cardiac surgery: evaluation of the RIFLE classification. Ann Thorac Surg. 2006;81:542–6.

19. Abosaif NY, Tolba YA, Heap M, Russell J, El Nahas AM. The outcome of acute renal failure in the intensive care unit according to RIFLE: model application, sensitivity, and predictability. Am J Kidney Dis. 2005;46:1038–48.

20. Lin CY, Chen YC, Tsai FC, Tian YC, Jeng CC, Fang JT, et al. RIFLE classification is predictive of short-term prognosis in critically ill patients with acute renal failure supported by extracorporeal membrane oxygenation. Nephrol Dial Transplant. 2006;21:2867–73.

21. Hoste EA, Clermont G, Kersten A, Venkataraman R, Angus DC, De Bacquer D, et al. RIFLE criteria for acute kidney injury are associated with hospital mortality in critically ill patients: a cohort analysis. Crit Care. 2006;10:R73.

22. Hoste EA, Kellum JA. RIFLE criteria provide robust assessment of kidney dysfunction and correlate with hospital mortality. Crit Care Med. 2006;34:2016–7.

23. Schwartz GJ, Haycock GB, Edelmann CMJ, Spitzer A. A simple estimate of glomerular filtration rate in children derived from body length and plasma creatinine. Pediatrics. 1976;58:259–63.

24. Schwartz GJ, Haycock GB, Spitzer A. Plasma creatinine and urea concentration in children: normal values for age and sex. J Pediatr. 1976;88:828–30.

25. Akcan-Arikan A, Zappitelli M, Loftis LL, Washburn KK, Jefferson LS, Goldstein SL. Modified RIFLE criteria in critically ill children with acute kidney injury. Kidney Int. 2007;71:1028–35.

26. Plotz FB, Bouma AB, van Wijk JA, Kneyber MC, Bokenkamp A. Pediatric acute kidney injury in the ICU: an independent evaluation of pRIFLE criteria. Intensive Care Med. 2008;34:1713–7.

27. Lassnigg A, Schmidlin D, Mouhieddine M, Bachmann LM, Druml W, Bauer P, et al. Minimal changes of serum creatinine predict prognosis in patients after cardiothoracic surgery: a prospective cohort study. J Am Soc Nephrol. 2004;15:1597–605.

28. Praught ML, Shlipak MG. Are small changes in serum creatinine an important risk factor? Curr Opin Nephrol Hypertens. 2005;14:265–70.

29. Chertow GM, Burdick E, Honour M, Bonventre JV, Bates DW. Acute kidney injury, mortality, length of stay, and costs in hospitalized patients. J Am Soc Nephrol. 2005;16:3365–70.

30. Gruberg L, Mintz GS, Mehran R, Gangas G, Lansky AJ, Kent KM, et al. The prognostic implications of further renal function deterioration within 48 h of interventional coronary procedures in patients with pre-existing chronic renal insufficiency. J Am Coll Cardiol. 2000;36:1542–8.

31. Gottlieb SS, Abraham W, Butler J, Forman DE, Loh E, Massie BM, et al. The prognostic importance of different definitions of worsening renal function in congestive heart failure. J Card Fail. 2002;8:136–41.

32. Smith GL, Vaccarino V, Kosiborod M, Lichtman JH, Cheng S, Watnick SG, et al. Worsening renal function: what is a clinically meaningful change in creatinine during hospitalization with heart failure? J Card Fail. 2003;9:13–25.

33. Levy MM, Macias WL, Vincent JL, Russell JA, Silva E, Trzaskoma B, et al. Early changes in organ function predict eventual survival in severe sepsis. Crit Care Med. 2005;33:2194–201.

34. Samuels J, Ng CS, Nates J, Price K, Finkel K, Salahudeen A, et al. Small increases in serum creatinine are associated with prolonged ICU stay and increased hospital mortality in critically ill patients with cancer. Support Care Cancer. 2011;19:1527–32.

35. Coca SG, Peixoto AJ, Garg AX, Krumholz HM, Parikh CR. The prognostic importance of a small acute decrement in kidney function in hospitalized patients: a systematic review and meta-analysis. Am J Kidney Dis. 2007;50:712–20.

36. Nin N, Lombardi R, Frutos-Vivar F, Esteban A, Lorente JA, Ferguson ND, et al. Early and small changes in serum creatinine concentrations are associated with mortality in mechanically ventilated patients. Shock. 2010;34:109–16.

37. Bagshaw SM, George C, Bellomo R. A comparison of the RIFLE and AKIN criteria for acute kidney injury in critically ill patients. Nephrol Dial Transplant. 2008;23:1569–74.

38. Kellum JA. Defining and classifying AKI: one set of criteria. Nephrol Dial Transplant. 2008;23:1471–2.

39. Lopes JA, Fernandes P, Jorge S, Goncalves S, Alvarez A, Costa e Silva Z, et al. Acute kidney injury in intensive care unit patients: a comparison between the RIFLE and the Acute Kidney Injury Network classifications. Crit Care. 2008;12:R110.

40. Murray PT, Devarajan P, Levey AS, Eckardt KU, Bonventre JV, Lombardi R, et al. A framework and key research questions in AKI diagnosis and staging in different environments. Clin J Am Soc Nephrol. 2008;3:864–8.

41. Schneider J, Khemani R, Grushkin C, Bart R. Serum creatinine as stratified in the RIFLE score for acut kidney injury is associated with mortality and length of stay for children in the pediatric intensive care unit. Crit Care Med. 2010;38:933–9.

42. Gaspari F, Perico N, Remuzzi G. Measurement of glomerular filtration rate. Kidney Int Suppl. 1997;63:S151–4.

43. Rahn KH, Heidenreich S, Bruckner D. How to assess glomerular function and damage in humans. J Hypertens. 1999;17:309–17.

44. Andersen TB, Eskild-Jensen A, Frokiaer J, Brochner-Mortensen J. Measuring glomerular filtration rate in children: can cystatin C replace established methods? A review. Pediatr Nephrol. 2009;24:929–41.

45. Gault MH, Cockcroft DW. Letter: creatinine clearance and age. Lancet. 1975;2:612–3.

46. Cockcroft DW, Gault MH. Prediction of creatinine clearance from serum creatinine. Nephron. 1976;16:31–41.

47. Levey AS, Bosch JP, Lewis JB, Greene T, Rogers N, Roth D. A more accurate method to estimate glomerular filtration rate from serum creatinine: a new prediction equation. Modification of Diet in Renal Disease Study Group. Ann Intern Med. 1999;130:461–70.

48. Schwartz GJ, Munoz A, Schneider MF, Mak RH, Kaskel F, Warady BA, et al. New equations to estimate GFR in children with CKD. J Am Soc Nephrol. 2009;20:629–37.

49. Confil JM, Georges B, Fourcade O, Sequin T, Lavit M, Samii K, et al. Assessment of renal function in clinical practice at the bedside of burn patients. Br J Clin Pharmacol. 2006;63:583–94.

50. Robert S, Zarowitz BJ, Peterson EL, Dumler F. Predictability of creatinine clearance estimates in critically ill patients. Crit Care Med. 1993;21:1487–95.

51. Pesola GR, Akhavan I, Madu A, Shah NK, Carlon GC. Prediction equation estimates of creatinine clearance in the intensive care unit. Intensive Care Med. 1993;19:39–43.

52. Hoste EA, Damen J, Vanholder RC, Lameire NH, Delanghe JR, Van den Hauwe K, et al. Assessment of renal function in recently admitted critically ill patients with normal serum creatinine. Nephrol Dial Transplant. 2005;20:747–53.

53. White CA, Huang D, Akbari A, Garland J, Knoll GA. Performance of creatinine-based estimates of GFR in kidney transplant recipients: a review. Am J Kidney Dis. 2008;51:1005–15.

54. van Acker BA, Koomen GC, Koopman MG, de Waart DR, Arisz L. Creatinine clearance during cimetidine administration for measurement of glomerular filtration rate. Lancet. 1992;340:1326–9.

55. Tangri N, Alam A, Giannetti N, Deedwardes MB, Cantarovich M. Predicting glomerular filtration rate in heart transplant recipients using serum creatinine-based equations with cimetidine. J Heart Lung Transplant. 2008;27:905–9.

56. Kabat-Koperska J, Safranow K, Golembiewska E, Domanski L, Ciechanowski K. Creatinine clearance after cimetidine administration: is it useful in the monitoring of the function of transplanted kidney? Ren Fail. 2007;29:667–72.

57. Kemperman FA, Surachno J, Krediet RT, Arisz L. Cimetidine improves prediction of the glomerular filtration rate by the Cockcroft-Gault formula in renal transplant recipients. Transplantation. 2002;73:770–4.

58. Bagshaw SM, Bellomo R, Kellum JA. Oliguria, volume overload, and loop diuretics. Crit Care Med. 2008;36:S172–8.

59. Bonventre JV. Diagnosis of acute kidney injury: from classic parameters to new biomarkers. Contrib Nephrol. 2007;156:213–9.

60. Stevens LA, Schmid CH, Greene T, Li L, Beck GF, Joffe MM, et al. Factors other than glomerular filtration rate affect serum cystatin C levels. Kidney Int. 2009;75:652–60.

61. Hassinger AB, Backer CL, Lane JC, Haymond S, Wang D, Wald EL. Predictive power of serum cystatin C to detect acute kidney injury and pediatric-modified RIFLE class in children undergoing cardiac surgery. Pediatr Crit Care Med. 2012;13:435–40.

62. Laskin BL, Nehus E, Goebel J, Khoury JC, Davies SM, Jodele S. Cystatin C-estimated glomerular filtration rate in pediatric autologous hematopoietic stem cell transplantation. Biol Blood Marrow Transplant. 2012;18(11):1745–52.

63. Asilioglu N, Acikgoz Y, Paksu MS, Gunaydin M, Ozkaya O. Is serum cystatin C a better marker than serum creatinine for monitoring renal function in pediatric intensive care unit? J Trop Pediatr. 2012;58(6):429–34.

64. Shemesh O, Golbetz H, Kriss JP, Myers BD. Limitations of creatinine as a filtration marker in glomerulopathic patients. Kidney Int. 1985;28:830–8.

65. Moran SM, Myers BD. Course of acute renal failure studied by a model of creatinine kinetics. Kidney Int. 1985;27:928–37.

66. Molitch ME, Rodman E, Hirsch CA, Dubinsky E. Spurious serum creatinine elevations in ketoacidosis. Ann Intern Med. 1980;93:280–1.

67. Vanholder R, Van Laecke S, Glorieux G. What is new in uremic toxicity? Pediatr Nephrol. 2008;23:1211–21.

68. Vanholder R, Argiles A, Baurmeister U, Brunet P, Clark W, Cohen G, et al. Uremic toxicity: present state of the art. Int J Artif Organs. 2001;24:695–725.

69. Boure T, Vanholder R. Biochemical and clinical evidence for uremic toxicity. Artif Organs. 2004;28:248–53.

70. Klahr S, Miller SB. Acute oliguria. N Engl J Med. 1998;338:671–5.

71. Sladen RN. Oliguria in the ICU. Systematic approach to diagnosis and management. Anesthesiol Clin North America. 2000;18:739–52.

72. Subramanian S, Ziedalski TM. Oliguria, volume overload, Na + balance, and diuretics. Crit Care Clin. 2005;21:291–303.

73. Wilson WC, Oliguria AS. A sign of renal success or impending renal failure? Anesthesiol Clin North America. 2001;19:841–83.

74. Himmelfarb J, Ikizler TA. Acute kidney injury: changing lexicography, definitions, and epidemiology. Kidney Int. 2007;71:971–6.

75. Macedo E, Malhotra R, Claure-Del Granado R, Fedullo P, Mehta RL. Defining urine output criterion for acute kidney injury in critically ill patients. Nephrol Dial Transplant. 2011;26:509–15.

76. Macedo E, Malhotra R, Bouchard J, Wynn SK, Mehta RL. Oliguria is an early predictor of higher mortality in critically ill patients. Kidney Int. 2011;80:760–7.

77. Dixon BS, Anderson RJ. Nonoliguric renal failure. Am J Kidney Dis. 1985;6:71–80.

78. Liangos O, Rao M, Balakrishnan VS, Pereira BJ, Jaber BL. Relationship of urine output to dialysis initiation and mortality in acute renal failure. Nephron Clin Pract. 2005;99:c55–60.

79. Majumdar S, Kjellstrand CM. Why do we use diuretics in acute renal failure? Semin Dial. 1996;9:454–9.

80. Bagshaw SM, Langenberg C, Haase M, Wan L, May CN, Bellomo R. Urinary biomarkers in septic acute kidney injury. Intensive Care Med. 2007;33:1285–96.

81. Townsend DR, Bagshaw SM. New insights on intravenous fluids, diuretics, and acute kidney injury. Nephron Clin Pract. 2008;109:c206–16.

82. Bagshaw SM, Delaney A, Haase M, Ghali WA, Bellomo R. Loop diuretics in the management of acute renal failure: a systematic review and meta-analysis. Crit Care Resusc. 2007;9:60–8.

83. Karajala V, Mansour W, Kellum JA. Diuretics in acute kidney injury. Minerva Anestesiol. 2009;75:251–7.

84. Goldstein SL, Currier H, Graf JM, Cosio CC, Brewer ED, Sachdeva R. Outcome in children receiving continuous venovenous hemofiltration. Pediatrics. 2001;107:1309–12.

85. Foland JA, Fortenberry JD, Warshaw BL, Pettignano R, Merritt RK, Heard ML, et al. Fluid overload before continuous hemofiltration and survival in critically ill children: a retrospective analysis. Crit Care Med. 2004;32:1771–6.

86. Goldstein SL, Somers MJG, Baum MA, Symons JM, Brophy PD, Blowey D, et al. Pediatric patients with multi-organ dysfunction syndrome receiving continuous renal replacement therapy. Kidney Int. 2005;67:653–8.

87. Sutherland SM, Zappitelli M, Alexander SR, Chua AN, Brophy PD, Bunchman TE, et al. Fluid overload and mortality in children receiving continuous renal replacement therapy: the prospective pediatric continuous renal replacement therapy registry. Am J Kidney Dis. 2010;55:316–25.

88. Bagshaw SM, Brophy PD, Cruz D, Ronco C. Fluid balance as a biomarker: impact of fluid overload in critically ill patients with acute kidney injury. Crit Care. 2008;12:169.

89. Mehta RL. Fluid balance and acute kidney injury: the missing link for predicting adverse outcomes? Nat Clin Pract Nephrol. 2009;5:10–1.

90. Arikan AA, Zappitelli M, Goldstein SL, Naipaul A, Jefferson LS, Loftis LL. Fluid overload is associated with impaired oxygenation and morbidity in critically ill children. Pediatr Crit Care Med. 2012;13:253–8.

91. Bagshaw SM, Langenberg C, Bellomo R. Urinary biochemistry and microscopy in septic acute renal failure: a systematic review. Am J Kidney Dis. 2006;48:695–705.

92. Gopal S, Carr B, Nelson P. Does microalbuminuria predict illness severity in critically ill patients on the intensive care unit? A systematic review. Crit Care Med. 2006;34:1805–10.

93. De Gaudio AR, Spina R, Di Filippo A, Feri M. Glomerular permeability and trauma: a correlation between microalbuminuria and injury severity score. Crit Care Med. 1999;27:2105–18.

94. Abid O, Sun Q, Sugimoto K, Mercan D, Vincent JL. Predictive value of microalbuminuria in medical ICU patients: results of a pilot study. Chest. 2001;120:1984–8.

95. MacKinnon KL, Molnar Z, Lowe D, Watson ID, Shearer E. Use of microalbuminuria as a predictor of outcome in critically ill patients. Br J Anaesth. 2000;84:239–41.

96. Gosling P. Microalbuminuria: a marker of systemic disease. Br J Hosp Med. 1995;54:285–90.

97. Thorevska N, Sabahi R, Upadya A, Manthous C, Amoateng-Adjepong Y. Microalbuminuria in critically ill medical patients: prevalence, predictors, and prognostic significance. Crit Care Med. 2003;31:1075–81.

98. Koike K, Aiboshi J, Shinozawa Y, Sekine K, Endo T, Yamamoto Y. Correlation of glomerular permeability, endothelial injury, and postoperative multiple organ dysfunction. Surg Today. 2004;34:811–6.

99. Gosling P, Brudney S, McGrath L, Riseboro S, Manji M. Mortality prediction at admission to intensive care: a comparison of microalbuminuria with acute physiology scores after 24 hours. Crit Care Med. 2003;31:98–103.

100. Gosling P, Czyz J, Nightingale P, Manji M. Microalbuminuria in the intensive care unit: clinical correlates and association with outcomes in 431 patients. Crit Care Med. 2006;34:2158–66.

101. Sarti A, De Gaudio AR, Messineo A, Cuttinini M, Ventura A. Glomerular permeability after surgical trauma in children: relationship between microalbuminuria and surgical stress score. Crit Care Physiol. 2001;29:1626–9.

102. Herget-Rosenthal S, Poppen D, Husing J, Marggraf G, Pietruck F, Jakob HG, et al. Prognostic value of tubular proteinuria and enzymuria in nonoliguric acute tubular necrosis. Clin Chem. 2004;50:552–8.

103. Coca SG, Yalavarthy R, Concato J, Parikh CR. Biomarkers for the diagnosis and risk stratification of acute kidney injury: a systematic review. Kidney Int. 2008;73:1008–16.

104. Trof RJ, Di Maggio F, Leemreis J, Groeneveld AB. Biomarkers of acute renal injury and renal failure. Shock. 2006;26:245–53.

105. Herrero-Morin JD, Malaga S, Fernandez N, Rey C, Diequez MA, Solis G, et al. Cystatin C and beta2-microglobulin: markers of glomerular filtration in critically ill children. Crit Care. 2007;11:R59.

106. Filler G, Priem F, Lepage N, Sinha P, Vollmer I, Clark H, et al. Beta-trace protein, cystatin C, beta(2)-microglobulin, and creatinine compared for detecting impaired glomerular filtration rates in children. Clin Chem. 2002;48:729–36.

107. Miller TR, Anderson RJ, Linas SL, Henrich WL, Berns AS, Gabow PA, et al. Urinary diagnostic indices in acute renal failure: a prospective study. Ann Intern Med. 1978;89:47–50.

108. Yalavarthy R, Edelstein CL. Therapeutic and predictive targets of AKI. Clin Nephrol. 2008;70:453–63.

109. Durakovic Z, Durakovic A, Durakovic S. The lack of clinical value of laboratory parameters in predicting outcome in acute renal failure. Ren Fail. 1989–1990;11:213–9.

110. Espinel CH. The FENa test. Use in the differential diagnosis of acute renal failure. JAMA. 1976;236:579–81.

111. Espinel CH, Gregory AW. Differential diagnosis of acute renal failure. Clin Nephrol. 1980;13:73–7.

112. Pru C, Kjellstrand CM. The FENa test is of no prognostic value in acute renal failure. Nephron. 1984;36:20–3.

113. Zarich S, Fang LS, Diamond JR. Fractional excretion of sodium. Exceptions to its diagnostic value. Arch Intern Med. 1985;145:108–12.

114. Corwin HL, Schreiber MJ, Fang LS. Low fractional excretion of sodium. Occurrence with hemoglobinuric- and myoglobinuric-induced acute renal failure. Arch Intern Med. 1984;144:981–2.

115. Fang LS, Sirota RA, Ebert TH, Lichtenstein NS. Low fractional excretion of sodium with contrast media-induced acute renal failure. Arch Intern Med. 1980;140:531–3.

116. Vaz AJ. Low fractional excretion of urine sodium in acute renal failure due to sepsis. Arch Intern Med. 1983;143:738–9.

117. Brosius FC, Lau K. Low fractional excretion of sodium in acute renal failure: role of timing of the test and ischemia. Am J Nephrol. 1986;6:450–7.

118. Diamond JR, Yoburn DC. Nonoliguric acute renal failure with a low fractional excretion of sodium. Ann Intern Med. 1982;96:597–600.

119. Steiner RW. Interpreting the fractional excretion of sodium. Am J Med. 1984;77:699–702.

120. Pru C, Kjellstrand CM. Urinary indices and chemistries in the differential diagnosis of prerenal failure and acute tubular necrosis. Semin Nephrol. 1985;5:224–33.

121. Fushimi K, Shichiri M, Marumo F. Decreased fractional excretion of urate as an indicator of prerenal azotemia. Am J Nephrol. 1990;10:489–94.

122. Carvounis CP, Nisar S, Guro-Razuman S. Significance of the fractional excretion of urea in the differential diagnosis of acute renal failure. Kidney Int. 2002;62:2223–9.

123. Pepin MN, Bouchard J, Legault L, Ethier J. Diagnostic performance of fractional excretion of urea and fractional excretion of sodium in the evaluations of patients with acute kidney injury with or without diuretic treatment. Am J Kidney Dis. 2007;50:566–73.

124. Nanji AJ. Increased fractional excretion of sodium in prerenal azotemia: need for careful interpretation. Clin Chem. 1981;27:1314–5.

125. Dole VP. Back diffusion of urea in the mammalian kidney. Am J Physiol. 1943;139:504–19.

126. Kaplan AA, Kohn OF. Fractional excretion of urea as a guide to renal dysfunction. Am J Nephrol. 1992;12:49–54.

127. Perlmutter M, Grossman SL, Rothenberg S, Dobkin G. Urine serum urea nitrogen ratio: simple test of renal function in acute azotemia and oliguria. JAMA. 1959;170:1533–7.

128. Tungsanga K, Boonwichit D, Lekhakula A, Sitprija V. Urine uric acid and urine creatinine ratio in acute renal failure. Arch Intern Med. 1984;144:934–7.

129. Star RA. Treatment of acute renal failure. Kidney Int. 1998;54:1817–31.

130. Jo SK, Rosner MH, Okusa MD. Pharmacologic treatment of acute kidney injury: why drugs haven't worked and what is on the horizon. Clin J Am Soc Nephrol. 2007;2:356–65.

131. Edelstein CL, Ling H, Schrier R. The nature of renal cell injury. Kidney Int. 1997;51:1341–51.

132. Devarajan P. NGAL in acute kidney injury: from serendipity to utility. Am J Kidney Dis. 2008;52:395–9.

133. Parikh CR, Devarajan P. New biomarkers of acute kidney injury. Crit Care Med. 2008;36:S159–65.

134. Devarajan P. Neutrophil gelatinase-associated lipocaline (NGAL): a new marker of kidney disease. Scand J Clin Lab Invest. 2008;241:89–94.

135. Bennett M, Dent CL, Ma Q, Dastrala S, Grenier F, Workman R, et al. Urine NGAL predicts severity of acute kidney injury after cardiac surgery: a prospective study. Clin J Am Soc Nephrol. 2008;3(3):665–73.

136. Devarajan P. Emerging biomarkers of acute kidney injury. Contrib Nephrol. 2007;156:203–12.

137. Nguyen MT, Devarajan P. Biomarkers for the early detection of acute kidney injury. Pediatr Nephrol. 2008;23:2151–7.

138. Devarajan P, Parikh C, Barasch J. Case 31-2007: a man with abdominal pain and elevated creatinine. N Engl J Med. 2008;358:312.

139. Zhou H, Hewitt SM, Yuen PS, Star RA. Acute kidney injury biomarkers – needs, present status, and future promise. Nephrol Self Assess Program. 2006;5(2):63–71.

140. Han WK, Bonventre JV. Biologic markers for the early detection of acute kidney injury. Curr Opin Crit Care. 2004;10(6):476–82.

141. Devarajan P, Mishra J, Supavekin S, Patterson LT, Potter SS. Gene expression in early ischemic renal injury: clues towards pathogenesis, biomarker discovery, and novel therapeutics. Mol Genet Metab. 2003;80:365–76.

142. Nguyen MT, Ross GF, Dent CL, Devarajan P. Early prediction of acute renal injury using urinary proteomics. Am J Nephrol. 2005;25(4):318–26.

143. Mishra J, Ma Q, Prada A, Mitsnefes M, Zahedi K, Yang J, et al. Identification of neutrophil gelatinase-associated lipocalin as a novel early urinary biomarker for ischemic renal injury. J Am Soc Nephrol. 2003;14(10):2534–43.

144. Mishra J, Dent C, Tarabishi R, Mitsnefes MM, Ma Q, Kelly C, et al. Neutrophil gelatinase-associated lipocalin (NGAL) as a biomarker for acute renal injury after cardiac surgery. Lancet. 2005;365(9466):1231–8.

145. Supavekin S, Zhang W, Kucherlapati R, Kaskel FJ, Moore LC, Devarajan P. Differential gene expression following early renal ischemia/reperfusion. Kidney Int. 2003;63(5):1714–24.

146. Dent CL, Ma Q, Dastrala S, Bennett M, Mitsnefes MM, Barasch J, et al. Plasma neutrophil gelatinase-associated lipocalin predicts acute kidney injury, morbidity and mortality after pediatric cardiac surgery: a prospective uncontrolled cohort study. Crit Care. 2007;11(6):R127.

147. Haase-Fielitz A, Bellomo R, Devarajan P, Story D, Matalanis G, Dragun D, et al. Novel and conventional serum biomarkers predicting acute kidney injury in adult cardiac surgery–a prospective cohort study. Crit Care Med. 2009;37(2):553–60.

148. Hirsch R, Dent C, Pfriem H, Allen J, Beekman 3rd RH, Ma Q, et al. NGAL is an early predictive biomarker of contrast-induced nephropathy in children. Pediatr Nephrol. 2007;22(12):2089–95.

149. Schaub S, Rush D, Wilkins J, Gibson IW, Weiler T, Sangster K, et al. Proteomic-based detection of urine proteins associated with acute renal allograft rejection. J Am Soc Nephrol. 2004;15(1):219–27.

150. Zappitelli M, Washburn KK, Arikan AA, Loftis L, Ma Q, Devarajan P, et al. Urine neutrophil gelatinase-associated lipocalin is an early marker of acute kidney injury in critically ill children: a prospective cohort study. Crit Care. 2007;11(4):R84.

151. Brunner HI, Mueller M, Rutherford C, Passo MH, Witte D, Grom A, et al. Urinary neutrophil gelatinase-associated lipocalin as a biomarker of nephritis in childhood-onset systemic lupus erythematosus. Arthritis Rheum. 2006;54(8):2577–84.

152. Mishra J, Ma Q, Kelly C, Mitsnefes M, Mori K, Barasch J, et al. Kidney NGAL is a novel early marker of acute injury following transplantation. Pediatr Nephrol. 2006;21(6):856–63.

153. Mishra J, Mori K, Ma Q, Kelly C, Barasch J, Devarajan P. Neutrophil gelatinase-associated lipocalin: a novel early urinary biomarker for cisplatin nephrotoxicity. Am J Nephrol. 2004;24(3):307–15.

154. Haase M, Bellomo R, Devarajan P, Schlattmann P, Haase-Fielitz A. Accuracy of neutrophil gelatinase-associated lipocalin (NGAL) in diagnosis and prognosis in acute kidney injury: a systematic review and meta-analysis. Am J Kidney Dis. 2009;54(6):1012–24.

155. Mitsnefes MM, Kathman TS, Mishra J, Kartal J, Khoury PR, Nickolas TL, et al. Serum neutrophil gelatinase-associated lipocalin as a marker of renal function in children with chronic kidney disease. Pediatr Nephrol. 2007;22(1):101–8.

156. Pisitkun T, Johnstone R, Knepper MA. Discovery of urinary biomarkers. Mol Cell Proteomics. 2006;5(10):1760–71.

157. Dharnidharka VR, Kwon C, Stevens G. Serum cystatin C is superior to serum creatinine as a marker of kidney function: a meta-analysis. Am J Kidney Dis. 2002;40(2):221–6.

158. Herget-Rosenthal S, Marggraf G, Husing J, Goring F, Pietruck F, Janssen O, et al. Early detection of acute renal failure by serum cystatin C. Kidney Int. 2004;66(3):1115–22.

159. Krawczeski CD, Vandevoorde RG, Kathman T, Bennett MR, Woo JG, Wang Y, et al. Serum cystatin C is an early predictive biomarker of acute kidney injury after pediatric cardiopulmonary bypass. Clin J Am Soc Nephrol. 2010;5(9):1552–7.

160. Melnikov VY, Faubel S, Siegmund B, Lucia MS, Ljubanovic D, Edelstein CL. Neutrophil-independent mechanisms of caspase-1- and IL-18-mediated ischemic acute tubular necrosis in mice. J Clin Invest. 2002;110(8):1083–91.

161. Parikh CR, Jani A, Melnikov VY, Faubel S, Edelstein CL. Urinary interleukin-18 is a marker of human acute tubular necrosis. Am J Kidney Dis. 2004;43(3):405–14.

162. Parikh CR, Mishra J, Thiessen-Philbrook H, Dursun B, Ma Q, Kelly C, et al. Urinary IL-18 is an early predictive biomarker of acute kidney injury after cardiac surgery. Kidney Int. 2006;70(1):199–203.

163. Parikh CR, Jani A, Mishra J, Ma Q, Kelly C, Barasch J, et al. Urine NGAL and IL-18 are predictive biomarkers for delayed graft function following kidney transplantation. Am J Transplant. 2006;6(7):1639–45.

164. Vaidya VS, Ramirez V, Ichimura T, Bobadilla NA, Bonventre JV. Urinary kidney injury molecule-1: a sensitive quantitative biomarker for early detection of kidney tubular injury. Am J Physiol Renal Physiol. 2006;290(2):F517–29.

165. Han WK, Wagener G, Zhu Y, Wang S, Lee HT. Urinary biomarkers in the early detection of acute kidney injury after cardiac surgery. Clin J Am Soc Nephrol. 2009;4(5):873–82.

166. Han WK, Bailly V, Abichandani R, Thadhani R, Bonventre JV. Kidney Injury Molecule-1 (KIM-1): a novel biomarker for human renal proximal tubule injury. Kidney Int. 2002;62(1):237–44.

167. Portilla D, Dent C, Sugaya T, Nagothu KK, Kundi I, Moore P, et al. Liver fatty acid-binding protein as a biomarker of acute kidney injury after cardiac surgery. Kidney Int. 2008;73(4):465–72.

168. Ferguson MA, Vaidya VS, Waikar SS, Collings FB, Sunderland KE, Gioules CJ, et al. Urinary liver-type fatty acid-binding protein predicts adverse outcomes in acute kidney injury. Kidney Int. 2010;77(8):708–14.

169. Negishi K, Noiri E, Doi K, Maeda-Mamiya R, Sugaya T, Portilla D, et al. Monitoring of urinary L-type fatty acid-binding protein predicts histological severity of acute kidney injury. Am J Pathol. 2009;174(4):1154–9.

170. Krawczeski CD, Goldstein SL, Woo JG, Wang Y, Piyaphanee N, Ma Q, et al. Temporal relationship and predictive value of urinary acute kidney injury biomarkers after pediatric cardiopulmonary bypass. J Am Coll Cardiol. 2011;58(22):2301–9.

171. Devarajan P. Update on mechanisms of ischemic acute kidney injury. J Am Soc Nephrol. 2006;17(6):1503–20.

172. Goldstein SL, Chawla LS. Renal angina. Clin J Am Soc Nephrol. 2010;5(5):943–9.

173. Michael M, Kuehnle I, Goldstein SL. Fluid overload and acute renal failure in pediatric stem cell transplant patients. Pediatr Nephrol. 2004;19(1):91–5.

174. Kist-van Holthe JE, Goedvolk CA, Brand R, van Weel MH, Bredius RG, van Oostayen JA, et al. Prospective study of renal insufficiency after bone marrow transplantation. Pediatr Nephrol. 2002;17(12):1032–7.

175. Goldstein SL. Advances in pediatric renal replacement therapy for acute kidney injury. Semin Dial. 2011;24(2):187–91.

Part V

Special Situations in Pediatric Critical Care Medicine

W. Bradley Poss

Principles of Mass Casualty and Disaster Medicine

David Markenson

Abstract

Hospital and emergency department emergency management is an essential aspect of modern healthcare. If one looks back more than 30 years, it would be almost impossible to find a hospital role called hospital emergency management or even a position for a healthcare emergency manager in a hospital or medical center. Yet, certain aspects of healthcare emergency management responsibilities have always been addressed by hospitals, such as fire safety, backup power, and the ability to handle victims from a mass casualty event. In addition, the public has strong expectations of the roles hospitals should play during times of disaster. Healthcare institutions are expected to provide both emergency care and continuance of the day to day healthcare responsibilities regardless of the volume and demand. The public believes that hospitals will have light, heat, air conditioning, water, food, and communications capabilities, regardless of the fact that the institution may itself be affected by the calamity.

The emergency management activity must be a directed by a multi-disciplinary group that is central to all activities and reports directly to hospital administrative and medical leadership. This planning effort must focus on all phases of disasters, mitigation, preparedness, response and recovery. These activities must be based on an all hazards approach to ensure preparedness for disasters, terrorism events and public health emergencies. Lastly these efforts must be inclusive of the entire populations and assure that the hospital is able to continue to function during any event to serve its critical resource in the community and serve the entire population. In addition to their traditional roles of child expert, advocate for children, community provider, family resource, and a force behind new research, pediatricians must now take on new roles regarding disaster, terrorism and public health emergency preparedness. Information, education and participation are important initial steps for all child health professionals.

Keywords

Emergency preparedness • Emergency management • Disaster • Terrorism • Public health emergency

Introduction

In the more than 10 years that have passed since September 11, 2001, emergency preparedness has taken an increased place in the minds, practice and training of healthcare professions to prepare for several potential scenarios – whether for terrorist attacks (e.g. September 11, 2001 attacks or the

D. Markenson, MD
Sky Ridge Medical Center,
10101 Ridge Gate Drive,
Lone Tree, CO 80124, USA
e-mail: david.markenson@healthonecares.com

Oklahoma City bombing), natural disasters (e.g. Hurricane Katrina or the Alabama tornadoes in 2011), or public health emergencies (e.g. pandemic influenza). Although not a new idea, the notion of "emergency preparedness" has taken on both a new meaning and a new emphasis. Understanding how to adapt and scale up preparedness to enable effective response to natural disasters, potential attacks with chemical, biological, radiological and/or explosive weapons, and public health emergencies has become a major national priority with specific emphasis on healthcare emergency preparedness. Significant funds have been spent on healthcare emergency preparedness, including training health care providers in disaster response and recovery and in conducting hospitals and other healthcare institutions disaster drills and exercises. Despite these efforts, there still remain major gaps in emergency preparedness in the healthcare environment, and additional efforts are needed in education, systems and plans.

Children have long been known as innocent victims of disasters, public health emergencies and terrorist attacks. The literature on natural disasters has also shown that children are particularly vulnerable to injury both during and in the recovery phase of natural disasters. During the actual event, the most common injuries are trauma to which children have unique susceptibilities. During the following recovery phase, children are uniquely susceptible to typical illnesses such as food or waterborne and to injury from unsupervised periods in what are often unsafe areas due to downed trees, power lines and other debris. With regard to public health emergencies, examples such as the recent pandemic influenza have shown that children may be affected differently from adults, such as unique vulnerability, different disease presentations and response to therapy. Lastly the classic thinking in the past of children as innocent and unattended victims of terrorism has been re-evaluated. There is increasing thought being given to the possibility that children could be the primary targets of a group or individual out to undermine morale and destabilize our society. In 2002, for instance, Suleiman Abu Gheith a senior Al-Qaeda planner said "We have not reached parity with [the Americans]. We have the right to kill four million Americans – two million of them children..." [1]. In addition, in 2003 the Singapore government foiled an Al-Qaeda connected plan to attack the American School (in Singapore) with 3,000 American expatriate children [2]. And in late 2004 Chechnean terrorists, presumably with Al Qaeda connections, attacked a strategically unimportant school in Russia.

For decades, emergency planning for natural disasters, workplace accidents, and other calamities has been the responsibility of government agencies on all levels and certain non-government organizations such as the American Red Cross and other international aid organizations. In recent years entirely new approaches to emergency planning are under development for a variety of reasons. Terrorism preparedness is a highly specific component of general emergency preparedness. In addition to the unique pediatric issues involved in general emergency preparedness, terrorism preparedness must consider several additional issues, including the unique vulnerabilities of children to various agents as well as the limited availability of age and weight appropriate antidotes and treatments. While children may respond more rapidly to therapeutic intervention, they are at the same time more susceptible to various agents and conditions and are more likely to deteriorate if not carefully monitored. It is therefore imperative to develop strategies to protect children from any hazard, including the horrific possibility of an intentional attack on our youngest citizens.

In a time of emergency, pediatric critical care providers will not only have to provide direct care to children, but also they will more likely have to orchestrate systems of care for children and advise governmental and non-governmental agencies on the needs of children. In addition, as the experts on the needs of children, they must advocate for the needs of children in emergency planning to ensure that the unique needs of children are satisfactorily addressed in the overall process. As a result, pediatric critical care providers – in addition to the knowledge needed for direct patient care and operation of pediatric critical care units in times of disasters, terrorism and public health emergencies – must also understand the systems of emergency response and the unique needs of children which must be addressed in these systems. To optimally prepare pediatric critical care physicians need to become familiar with some key areas of emergency preparedness:

- Emergency, Public Health and Terrorism preparedness
- Unique aspects of children related to disasters, terrorism and public health emergencies
- Managing family concerns about terrorism and disaster preparedness
- Hospital preparedness including inpatient and pediatric critical care unit preparedness
- Community, government, and public health preparedness

Disaster Types, Preparedness, and Management

The World Association of Disaster Emergency Medicine and the Office of U.S. Foreign Disaster Assistance define a "disaster" as a situation or event that overwhelms local capacity, necessitating a request to national or international level for external assistance, or an unforeseen and often sudden event that causes great damage, destruction, and human suffering. Disasters are usually described as natural (including earthquakes, hurricanes, tornadoes, and floods) or man-made (including fire, mass transportation incidents, environmental toxins, terrorism and civil unrest). More narrowly defined and distinct are "mass casualty incidents"—events that cause large numbers of injuries but do not threaten or harm large segments of the community. The effects of each disaster are different. Considerations are given to the size of the area involved, the extent of damage, and the effect on community resources. The extent of damage includes the physical injury to persons and damage to property, especially destruction of infrastructure (roadways, bridges, and communication lines). The effects on community resources include the absence of electricity, gas, sanitation, and potable water; the necessity for portable shelters; and the potential for recurrence (e.g., earthquakes with aftershocks). The planning for and response to disasters traditionally has been the responsibilities of federal, state, and local governments, usually via an office of emergency management. In the U.S., the Federal Emergency Management Agency (FEMA), a federal agency under the Department of Homeland Security, is involved in declared national emergencies and responsible for the coordination of federal resources. These authorities are responsible for preparedness, response, recovery and conduct these activities through duties which include: (1) hospital damage assessment; (2) allocation, designation, and distribution of casualty collection points; (3) identification, prevention, and elimination of public health hazards; (4) coordination of activities with support departments, agencies, and public utilities; and (5) coordination of requests for mutual aid. In addition to governmental agencies, non-governmental and volunteer organizations, such as the Red Cross and Salvation Army, have key roles in disaster response.

Emergency preparedness is important at many levels – personal, family, community, regional, state, and federal, with the state and federal governments having pivotal roles. The federal government provides significant funding for disaster preparedness and response and also, to a large extent, establishes the framework that is then followed by states, regions, and communities. In disaster response, the funding and planning tends to be from the top down, whereas the response and use of resources tends to be from the bottom up. In other words, as resources are exhausted at the local level, assistance is requested from the next level, such as the state, which then requests federal assistance. A successful response to a disaster requires the interaction of personnel and resources from multiple agencies in an organized and coordinated manner according to a well-formulated plan. Although this planning has increased in recent times, the attention to the unique needs of children and the inclusion of pediatric expertise in the planning phases is still lacking or in many cases nonexistent.

Hospital Emergency Preparedness

The health care facilities responsible for treating pediatric victims in a disaster, terrorism and public health emergency including biological, radiologic, nuclear, chemical, or explosive event could be strained or overwhelmed. In most situations hospital disaster plans provide for alert systems and

call for victims to be triaged in the field and carefully distributed among available resources to prevent any single facility from being overwhelmed. Despite these plans medical facilities can become unexpectedly inundated with patients if large numbers of victims appear without ambulance transport and pre-arrival notification. Along similar lines, victims appearing without full hospital preparation could thwart attempts to isolate contaminated victims from other patients and hospital staff. Large-scale biological, chemical, nuclear, radiologic, or explosive incidents may necessitate the use of alternative health care sites (e.g., auditoriums and arenas), which requires that health care resources be dispersed to areas where victims may not receive optimal care.

Hospitals must ensure that they have adequate plans to handle disasters, terrorism and public health emergencies and that these approaches conform to an all-hazards approach to ensure preparedness for any possible event. These plans must also include an effective incident command system that incorporates those capable of making decisions for the care of pediatric patients. They must also address issues such as surge capacity, decontamination, initial care, secondary transport (if needed), maintenance of hospital function despite regional events (hurricane, floods, etc.), evacuation (if needed) and staff support and protection. Finally these plans must be tested and improved through drills and exercises and staff must be educated.

Community and/or Local Government Emergency Preparedness

Local authorities are the first line of defense in emergencies and are primarily responsible for managing the response to most disasters. The primary responsibility for the protection of citizens belongs to local elected officials such as mayors, city council members, and boards of commissioners. When a local government receives a warning that an emergency could be imminent, its first priorities are to warn citizens and to take whatever actions are needed to minimize damage and protect life and property. If necessary, an evacuation may be ordered. The emergency operations plan is at the center of comprehensive emergency planning. This plan spells out the scope of activities required for community response. It needs to be a living document that accurately describes what the community can realistically do. Unfortunately, these documents have rarely contained any pediatric consideration, and in only the rarest of cases have pediatricians been part of the planning process.

State Government Emergency Preparedness

In the U.S., states have laws that describe the responsibilities of the state government in emergencies and disasters. In other areas of the world there may be county or district levels above the local authority, whose structure and responsibility mirrors the system in the United States. These laws provide governors and state agencies with the authority to plan for and carry out the necessary actions to respond to and recover from emergencies. State emergency management legislation describes the duties and powers of the governor, whose authority includes the power to declare a state of emergency and to decide when to terminate this declaration.

Performing and maintaining the provisions of emergency management legislation is generally the responsibility of the state emergency management offices (some municipalities also have offices of emergency management). These offices are organized in a number of ways and have different names. Emergency managers are responsible for preparing for emergencies and for coordinating the activation and use of resources controlled by the state government when they are needed to help local governments respond to and recover from emergencies and disasters. In its coordinating role, the state emergency management office is involved in virtually all serious emergencies, terrorism, or disasters. Using procedures specified in the state emergency operations plan, the state emergency management organization coordinates deployment of personnel and resources to the affected areas. As noted above, pediatric concerns are rarely considered.

Federal Government Emergency Preparedness

In most countries the ultimate responsibility for disaster response rests at the national level (e.g., the U.S. Department of Homeland Security (USDHS) through FEMA). In addition to the activities of FEMA, one of the other functions of the USDHS is to foster a closer connection between prevention of terrorist attacks and preparedness for events and response after an event. While this organization is a U.S. governmental agency, similar agencies have existed in many other countries for many years. The USDHS and equivalent national agencies in other countries are charged with the review and creation of a National Response Plan (NRP).

One of the major functions physicians will be involved with is the assurance of public health and provision of medical services. For example in the U.S. Plan, this aspect is covered in is Emergency Support Function (ESF) 8, Public Health and Medical Services. The role of the Public Health and Medical Services ESF is to define how the national government provides assistance to supplement state and local resources for public health and medical care needs during a disaster. An example of a national resource which could be deployed locally is a medical response team. In the U.S. these are known as Disaster Medical Assistance Teams (DMATs), which are deployable units of 35 physicians, nurses, technicians, equipment, and supplies for austere medical care.

Another major component of the U.S. national preparedness program that is important to all involved in health care preparedness and exists in a similar form in many other countries is the Strategic National Stockpile (SNS), created by Congress in 1999. The SNS is a national repository of antimicrobials, chemical antidotes, antitoxins, life-support medications, intravenous administration and airway maintenance supplies, and medical/surgical items. The SNS is designed to supplement and resupply state and local public health agencies in the event of a national emergency anywhere and at any time within the U.S. or its territories. The SNS is organized for flexible response. The first line of support lies within the immediate-response 12-h push packages. These are caches of pharmaceuticals, antidotes, and medical supplies designed to provide rapid delivery of a broad spectrum of assets for an ill-defined threat in the early hours of an event. These push packages are positioned in strategically located and secure warehouses ready for immediate deployment to a designated site within 12 h of the federal decision to deploy SNS assets. If the incident requires additional pharmaceuticals and/or medical supplies, follow-up vendor-managed inventory (VMI) supplies will be shipped to arrive within 24–36 h. If the agent is well defined, VMI supplies can be tailored to provide pharmaceuticals, supplies, and/or products specific to the suspected or confirmed agent(s). In this case, VMI supplies could act as the first option for immediate response from the SNS. It is important for Pediatric Hospital Providers to understand the contents of their countries national stockpile of medications and supplies which may be available for hospitals during times of emergencies. This will help them to determine the items and quantities which must be stocked locally and which items in emergency may be available from national assets.

In the past, stockpiles have had limited pediatric capability, but in recent years more pediatric-specific items have been added. Although still not optimal for pediatric care, these national stockpiles in most countries still do not address some key pediatric needs. The reasons for limited pediatric inclusion are varied and may include limited data on usage in children, limited sizing for children, and in some cases bureaucratic barriers. In the U.S. for example, one of the key barriers to pediatric inclusion in the SNS is the restriction that the SNS may stock only FDA-licensed items and only for their FDA-approved indications. With regard to antimicrobial and other therapeutic agents in children, FDA indications are often lacking. In terms of terrorism-related items, this is an even larger issue. As a result, although the stockpile does contain many items for children, such as equipment and certain pharmaceuticals, including the recent addition of medications in suspension preparations, the stockpile does not contain therapeutic agents for all indications for children. Whatever the reasons for lack of pediatric inclusion in national stockpiles, it is imperative that existing agents and those developed in the future have the scientific research conducted to allow for pediatric indications or development of agents appropriate for use in children.

Public Health Emergency Preparedness

When discussing emergency preparedness, we must also recognize the need for public health preparedness, which ensures coordination of individual responding facilities and local communities with the broader response mounted at the district, state, and regional level. This requires the presence of a strong public health system. To allow for rapid and efficient response, this requires central organization, local implementation, and decentralization of some resources such as diagnostic capabilities. Healthcare providers must understand the importance of public health and their relationship to departments of health. This includes their role in public health, reporting requirements and mechanisms, and mechanisms for receiving and soliciting information from departments of health. Recent events such as pandemic influenza have shown the strength of an effective public health system in disease surveillance and detection, infection control, public messaging and management of large scale public health events. Despite these successes, recent events have also highlighted some of the gaps in our public health system of which most significantly are the lack of strong linkages between public health agencies and other healthcare entities such as hospital and primary care primary care providers and public health agencies with sufficient resources as the federal, regional and local levels.

Mass Casulaty Incidents

While not all disasters, terrorism events and public health emergencies may lead to mass numbers of ill or injured individuals, those which lead to mass casualties arriving in a short period of time can be some of the most challenging events for hospitals to handle. There are two distinct phases of care in a mass casualty event [3, 4]. Initially, during casualties' arrival, the full magnitude of the event is unknown and the key element is conservation of limited hospital resources and facilities. Stable patients will temporarily receive only minimal acceptable care and will be transferred to other hospital areas awaiting later definitive care. Only critically – but salvageable – patients will have immediate access to key hospital resources such as imaging techniques and operating rooms.

The element of uncertainty in the first phase becomes even more prominent with the multi-staged tactics practiced by Al Qaeda and associated terror groups. Most recent terror acts were evolving, multi-staged events such as; the attacks

on the Twin Towers, the bombing of the Paradise Hotel in Mombassa, Kenya, the (failed) attempt to hit an Israeli airliner, the train bombings in Spain, the subway and bus bombings in London, or the attacks on tourist resorts in the Sinai peninsula. Such evolving, serial assaults in the same geographical area might disrupt any organized approach to manage MCS, and contingency plans should take this into consideration. To achieve the best results, it is crucial to adhere to the basic principle of prioritization of care to life or organ endangering conditions with postponement of care to less severely wounded patients. The second phase begins after containment of the event and arrival of all casualties. Following secondary triage, a comprehensive, priority-oriented plan for definitive care of all patients can be devised.

Incident Command System (ICS)

All emergency preparedness plans must contain an Incident Command System (ICS). The ICS tries to avoid historical problems related to mass casualty incidents, such as inadequate planning, poor communications, lack of on-scene needs assessment, or triage of patients. In general, besides a command structure, the ICS also implements perimeters and areas to optimize responder safety and patient flow, as well as the preservation of evidence and environment.

The ICS has many potential components and configurations depending on the magnitude, location/terrain, weather, agencies required to be involved, as well as, volunteering groups. For didactic purposes, lists and organizational illustrations may be simplistic, so it is important to keep in mind that these frames are very *elastic*, and should be tailored to the specific needs of the event.

The ICS has eight principles for adequate operation.

1. Common terminology avoids confusion by coordinating terms utilized with different agencies, allowing adequate identification of personnel, areas, equipment and procedures.
2. Modular organization is based upon a "top-down development approach." Starting at the initial phases of the emergency, the Incident Commander will be responsible for the implementation and delegation of duties of the different functional areas as the situation develops.
3. Integrated communications allows the coordination of communications plans, operating procedures, terminology, and common frequencies.
4. Unified command structure (Fig. 44.1) with one Incident Commander or a Unified Command with more than one agency sharing responsibility for the management of the situation. However, the Unity of Command should be followed in which each person reports to one supervisor.
5. Consolidated action plans, verbally or written, ideally follow established strategic goals, objectives, and activities.

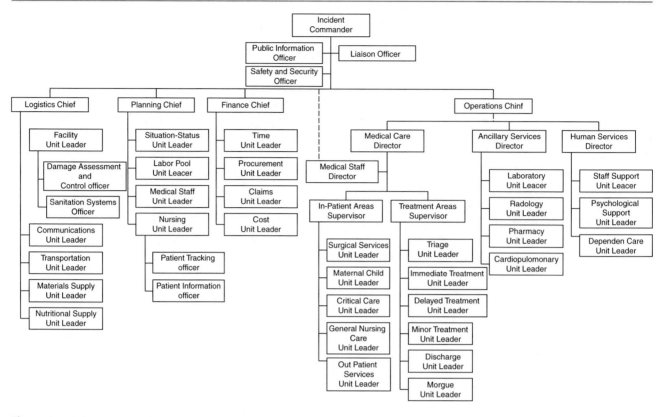

Fig. 44.1 Hospital emergency incident command system organizational chart [14]

6. <u>Manageable span-of-control</u> in which the number of individuals that report to a supervisor is established, ideally 5 with a range of 3–7.
7. <u>Pre-designated incident facilities</u> or zones that clearly indicate areas for command post, search and rescue, staging, decontamination, transport, press, etc.
8. <u>Comprehensive resource management</u> that coordinates and consolidates independent resources, avoiding cluttering of personnel and communications.

The implementation of the Incident Command System within a hospital facility can be done following similar guidelines, as described above. One approach to hospital incident command is called the Hospital Emergency Incident Command System or HEICS. Initially developed in 1993 in California by the County of San Mateo EMS Authority, it has been used more and more nationwide as the basis for the hospital response in these situations. In HEICS, besides the designation of hospital personnel as chiefs and leaders in the different positions, a fourth member serving as the Medical Officer is added to the Command Staff (Information, Liaison and Safety Officers).

Casualties' flow consists typically of three waves. The first wave, shortly after the event, includes casualties – usually with minor injuries – who evacuate themselves or who are brought in by bystanders without previous triage. This wave arrives while the medical facility is still getting organized and most of the casualties arrive in the hospital closest to the scene. This wave can overwhelm any hospital and can practically block its emergency facilities [5–7]. It is therefore vitally important that with first notice, an experienced physician will be positioned in front of the emergency department (ED) to perform primary triage. The second wave consists of casualties with more serious injuries, which were triaged at the scene, may have required extrication and received initial treatment and were evacuated by EMS transportation. The third wave consists of casualties with more minor injuries and of patients with emotional stress. This wave can persist for several hours to days after the initial event.

Casualties' Flow within the Hospital

Rapid, unobstructed casualties' flow within the hospital is crucial. Factors to be considered are the hospital layout, potential bottlenecks and the number of available trauma teams, operating rooms and hospital beds. The basic principle is a one-way, forward flow from the triage area unto the final admitting ward. Therefore, patients proceed in their management track only forwards, with no possibility of backtracking. Backtracking, or slow flow through the ED, while casualty influx continues can have chaotic consequences.

Patient Triage

By definition a mass casualty situation is one in which the number of patients exceeds the available resources. As a result a basic characteristic of the clinical management in MCS is temporary alteration in the standard of care. This often takes the form of a reduction in the individual level of care, giving priority to procedures aimed at saving the largest number of salvageable lives. There is an apparent correlation between triage accuracy and casualty outcome [8]. The triage officer should be a physician experienced in trauma management and knowledgeable in the hospitals emergency preparedness triage system. The triage officer's role is to rapidly identify casualties requiring immediate interventions and who have potentially reversible injuries. To reduce over triage the triage criteria should include physiologic and anatomic indicators rather than only "mechanism of injury" criteria. In most systems casualties are triaged into one of four (or five in some systems) categories. The most commonly recognized categories and the usual colors which are used to designate them include:

Red:	Immediate
Yellow:	Delayed
Green:	Minimal
Grey:	Expectant (used in some systems)
Black:	Deceased (or expectant)

A basic explanation of each color-coded category, with examples, is listed below:

Immediate (Red) – This includes severely injured patients with a high probability for survival. They need procedures of moderately short duration required to prevent death. Casualties with severe but potentially reversible injuries are the focus of medical efforts. Examples of these circumstances are: airway obstructions, accessible hemorrhage, and sometimes emergency amputations.

Delayed (Yellow) – These casualties require operative interventions that may be delayed without compromise of a successful outcome or life endangerment. Temporizing measures include IV fluids, splints, antibiotics, pain management, catheterization or gastric decompression. Some examples are large muscle wounds, major bone fractures, uncomplicated major burns, head or spinal injuries and intra-abdominal and/or thoracic injuries.

Minimal (Green) – This includes patients without serious injuries to vascular structures or nerves. The walking wounded can usually provide self-care or only require minimally trained personnel. The largest number of casualties belongs to this group.

Dead (Black) – This includes patients found to be dead on arrival (DOA) and casualties with non-salvageable injuries who are expected to die. In five category systems

expectant becomes its own category. These receive low treatment priority and are directed to a designated area.

Expectant (Grey) – Casualties who are triaged to the "expectant" category are those who are considered to have a low probability of survival with the currently available medical resources. They will likely die even if all available resources are used to care for them. In a mass casualty setting, such effort is better used on other casualties with higher chances of survival. "Expectant" casualties are therefore placed in the lowest priority for treatment and transport. It is important to remember that casualties assigned to the Expectant category should not simply be ignored. They should receive comfort care or resuscitation should be attempted as soon as sufficient resources become available.

One system for triage which has gained support in the United States is SALT (Fig. 44.2) [9]. The SALT triage methodology was intended, and designed, to be a national guideline for mass casualty triage in the United States. It was designed to be simple to use and easy to remember. It instructs providers to quickly "Sort" casualties by their ability to follow commands, then to individually "Assess" casualties, to rapidly apply "Lifesaving interventions", and assign a priority for "Treatment and/or transport". SALT Triage is intended to allow rapid evaluation and sorting of any age patient injured in any type of event. While applicable to different situations SALT is most suited for scene triage and initial triage of those arriving at the hospital who may not have been triaged.

Step 1: Sort – SALT begins with a global sorting of casualties, prioritizing them into tiers for individual assessment. In this first step, casualties are asked to walk to a designated area. The responder should yell or use a public address system to say "If you can hear my voice and need help please move to _____." Those who walk to the designated area are the last priority for individual assessment, since they are the least likely to have a life threatening condition. Specifically, the ability to walk indicates that they are likely to have an intact airway, breathing, and circulation (they are unlikely to have severe breathing difficulties or a low blood pressure because they are able to walk from the scene) and intact mental status (because they are able to follow commands). Those who remain should be asked to wave (or follow a command) or be observed for purposeful movement (such as trying to free oneself or self-treat an injury). The responder should yell or use a public address system to say "If you can hear my voice and need help please wave your arm or leg." Those who do not move at all, and those with obvious life threats (like major bleeding) are assessed individually first since they are the most likely to need lifesaving interventions. Those who wave are the next to be assessed. Those who walked to the designated location are the last to be assessed. It is important to note that the global sorting process will not be perfect. Therefore, every casualty must be individually assessed, even if they are able to walk.

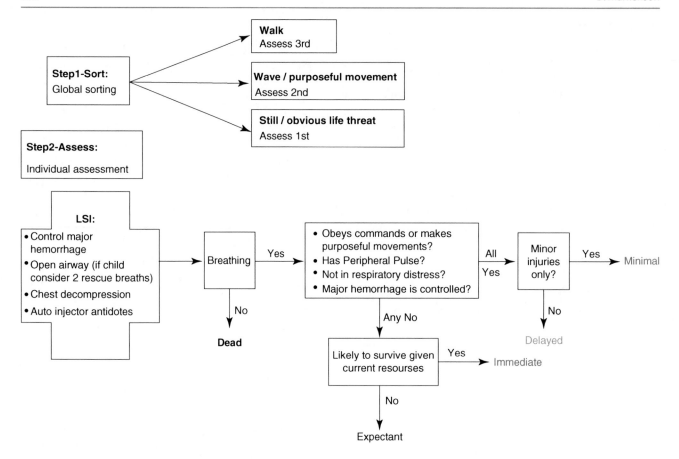

Fig. 44.2 SALT mass casualty triage (Reprinted from Lerner et al. [9])

Step 2: Assess – The second step is individual assessment of each casualty, starting with the first priority tier (patients who could not walk to the designated area and did not wave or have an obvious life threat).

Step 3: Lifesaving Interventions – During individual assessment rapid lifesaving interventions are performed but only if they can be provided quickly, can greatly improve a casualty's likelihood of survival, do not require a care provider to stay with the patient, is within the responder's scope of practice and any equipment that is needed is immediately available. Lifesaving interventions that meet these criteria include the opening of the airway with simple basic airway maneuvers, two rescue breaths in a child, performing needle decompression for casualties with signs of a tension pneumothorax, control of any major hemorrhage using pressure dressing or tourniquet and providing auto-injector antidotes to casualties with known chemical exposure.

Step 4: Treatment/Transport – After any lifesaving interventions are performed, casualties should be prioritized for treatment and/or transport by assigning them to one of the five triage categories described above (Immediate, Delayed, Minimal, Expectant, or Dead). A key point to always remember is that each casualty should be individually assessed as described above no matter what tier, but starting with those

who during global sorting did not move, followed by those who followed the "wave" command, and then those who followed the "walk" command.

Principles of Initial Hospital Management

Treatment priorities in MCS are to save salvageable patients and to prevent complications and future handicaps. Generally, patient management should follow accepted guidelines (i.e. ATLS), though only essential interventions are performed in the first phase and comprehensive treatment of all injuries is postponed. Teamwork is crucial. Teams consisting of a physician and (preferably) two nurses should be pre-assigned to every ED station. The ED director (or other title based on hospital Incident Command System) plays the conductor's role. He coordinates medical teams, oversees specialists' assignments, sets priorities for transfer to the operating room (OR), ICU or ward, decides about further imaging and ensures continuous patient flow through the admitting area. An important task is to prevent overcrowding and excessive commotion in the ED. Personnel not directly participating in patient care should be kept away to avoid havoc.

Use of Radiology

The Radiology Department is a common bottleneck during disasters and should be used judiciously. As a rule, mobile radiography and radiography of the chest, cervical spine and pelvis are not performed on a routine basis. Abdominal sonography (FAST) is fast and beneficial but should be used sensibly, i.e. in unstable patients to confirm or rule out intra-abdominal bleeding. Following the 1988 Armenian earthquake, Sarkisian et al. [10] reported that 4 % of the patients were "operated on solely for physical findings and sonographic data". CT scanning should be reserved for restricted indications and the ED director should make these decisions. Brain CT's are performed only to assist decision-making regarding neurosurgery.

Operating Room

The operating room is also a major bottleneck. Therefore, its immediate use should be reserved for a few "absolute" indications such as compromised airway or control of active bleeding endangering life or limb. Other surgeries are delayed to later phases. Once in surgery, the fundamental approach is "damage control". Basically, this situation demands that surgeons, accustomed to expending enormous resources and time on single patients, reset their priorities and rapidly provide only the minimal acceptable care, moving patients quickly through the mostly needed operative procedures in order to maximize care to as many patients as possible.

Secondary Transport

An important aspect of primary triage at the scene is dividing patient load between available hospitals, taking into consideration "specialty" capabilities such as neurosurgery, burns or pediatric surgery. Secondary transport refers to transfer of casualties between medical facilities. This is indicated when the primary admitting hospital is unable to provide proper care due to lack of essential specialties, overwhelming with patient load, inability to provide needed surgery within a reasonable time period or when the hospital itself is compromised by the event (i.e. nature disaster, hazardous materials event, war/terrorist event).

Re-Assessment Phase

Following the first phases of the event, all casualties should receive definitive, appropriate treatment. To avoid misdiagnoses and overlooking of injuries, designated teams should perform this re-assessment, review every patient's chart and recommend further investigations or interventions. Once again, decision making and planning should be centralized, taking into consideration individual priorities as well as the entire hospital's capabilities.

Communication and Manpower Control

Rapid staff recruitment is crucial and each hospital should have an effective paging system. Insufficient physician's attendance in the ED of a large urban hospital was recorded in the first hours after a major earthquake because physicians were helping their own families and because of lack of communication or transportation [11]. On the other hand, Israeli experience and data from disaster events have repeatedly shown that a large portion of the hospital staff shows up even without being paged. Emergency preparedness plans should allocate a staff waiting area with communication to the event director(s) who will allocate personnel according to needs. An "Emergency Operations Center" should be manned rapidly in a pre-established location and one which has been pre-equipped for this role. Aside from communication within the hospital, communication (preferably radio) with the EMS forces at the scene is critical.

Information Center and Public Relations

A public information center should be opened as soon as possible. Its telephone lines should be designated in advance and their numbers should be announced by the electronic media after the event. The information center should have software for creating database of missing persons in a manner which has been pre-arranged by the hospital and local emergency management and law enforcement agencies. In some cases these agencies may provide staff for this function. As the hospital may be "stormed" by worried relatives, the information center should be located distant from the patient management area.

Personal Protective Equipment

Personal protective equipment (PPE) is a critical component of protection of healthcare workers, regardless of the disaster. It provides a barrier that allows function in a hazardous area or in proximity to patients with infectious agents and must be used properly during all phases of response. In some cases where risk is present for the healthcare worker, casualty care may have to wait until proper PPE is available. In the context of chemical disaster response, PPE is divided into two sub-categories: chemical protective clothing and respiratory protection.

Chemical protective clothing (CPC) refers to the actually protective garment that is worn when performing tasks such as decontamination. CPC is rated based on the duration of time it would take for a chemical to penetrate the garment; the longer the time, the more protective the suit. Also, CPC is designed specifically to keep a worker's clothes clean, protect against liquid chemical agents, or protect against harmful chemical vapors. The highest level of CPC is a fully-encapsulating vapor tight suit. The second highest level of CPC is a fully or partially encapsulating suit, which is resistant to liquid chemicals. The third level of CPC is a hooded coverall, which is typical constructed with a laminated or plasticized Tyvek®-type material. This is designed to keep a worker's clothes clean, but is not designed to be protective against liquid chemicals or vapors. The least level of protection is simply a laboratory apron, or other uniform-type clothing that provides no chemical protection. Chemical protective clothing is typically combined with a corresponding level of respiratory protection to meet the US Environmental Protection Agency (EPA) recommended levels of PPE (A, B, C and D).

For the purposes of chemical disasters there are two types of respiratory protection: air-purifying respirators and supplied air devices. Air-Purifying Respirators (APR): An APR is defined under 29 CFR 1910.134(b) of the Respiratory Protection Standard to be, "…a respirator with an air-purifying filter, cartridge, or canister that removes specific air contaminants by passing ambient air through the air-purifying element." Typically these are either gas mask-type respirators or powered air-purifying respirators (PAPRs). They also are available in half-face models, but these are not suitable for use in emergency response. APRs filter chemical contaminates from breathing air through cartridges or filters resulting in inhaled air which has been purified. In order for APRs to be allowable in a toxic environment, the chemical agent must be known, as well as the concentration of the chemical present in the area work will be performed. The concentration of any chemical must not exceed a level considered to be "immediately dangerous to life and health (IDLH)." An IDLH atmosphere is defined by OSHA to be, "…an atmosphere that poses an immediate threat to life, would cause irreversible adverse health effects, or would impair an individual's ability to escape from a dangerous atmosphere." If the concentration of any chemical exceeded the IDLH level an APR could not be used. Additionally, since the worker is breathing filtered air, he or she must not be working in an oxygen deficient environment, having less than 19.5 % oxygen present. If either of these two conditions exists the workers must breathe supplied air and cannot use an APR.

Supplied air refers to one of two types of respiratory protection devices, the self-contained breathing apparatus (SCBA) or the supplied airline respirator. Both devices provide a full-face mask through which the worker will breathe clean, contaminate-free breathing air, which is either carried in a cylinder on their back (SCBA) or is supplied through a hose which runs to a generator or large breathing air tank in a clean environment. These two levels would be used in environments where the type of chemical present is unknown, environments that are oxygen deficient, or environments that are considered to be IDLH.

OSHA has adopted the EPA "levels of PPE," which are discussed in detail in Appendix B of 29 CFR 1910.120. A brief summary is provided below. Each level is a combination of chemical protective clothing and respiratory protection. OSHA has allowed hospitals to perform on-site decontamination using Level C PPE.

Level A: provides the highest levels of skin, respiratory, and eye protection; it involves:
- Positive pressure, full face-piece self-contained breathing apparatus (SCBA), or positive pressure supplied air respirator with escape SCBA, approved by the National Institute for Occupational Safety and Health (NIOSH).
- Totally-encapsulating chemical-protective suit.
- Gloves, outer, chemical-resistant.
- Gloves, inner, chemical-resistant.
- Boots, chemical-resistant, steel toe and shank.
- Disposable protective suit, gloves and boots (depending on suit construction, may be worn over totally-encapsulating suit).

Level B: provides the highest level of respiratory protection but a lesser level of skin protection; it involves:
- Positive pressure, full-face self-contained breathing apparatus (SCBA), or positive pressure supplied air respirator with escape SCBA (NIOSH approved).
- Hooded chemical-resistant clothing (overalls and long-sleeved jacket; coveralls; one or two-piece chemical-splash suit; disposable chemical-resistant overalls).
- Gloves, outer, chemical-resistant.
- Gloves, inner, chemical-resistant.
- Boots, outer, chemical-resistant steel toe and shank.

Level C: can be worn when the chemical is known, non-oxygen deficient environment, below IDLH; it involves:
- Full-face or half-mask, air purifying respirators (NIOSH approved).
- Hooded chemical-resistant clothing (overalls; two-piece chemical-splash suit; disposable chemical-resistant overalls).
- Gloves, outer, chemical-resistant.
- Gloves, inner, chemical-resistant.

Level D: work uniform affording minimal protection (for nuisance contamination only); it involves:
- Coveralls.
- Boots/shoes, chemical-resistant steel toe and shank.

Hospital Based Decontamination and Pediatric Considerations

For many years, the standard level of preparedness for most hospitals in the case of a patient with a hazardous substance exposure has been the ability to perform a cursory decontamination of the individual in the emergency department. Many hospitals have a dedicated "decon" or "HAZMAT" room, which has a shower and some equipment to perform this function, but it likely serves as an equipment closet or storage area most of the time. Although most hospitals have considered the need to perform emergency decontamination of victims from a hazardous substances incident, many reports have underscored the lack of hospital preparedness for victims from a HAZMAT-related event.

The process of developing the capability to perform single patient or mass casualty decontamination takes time, effort, and funding. It is easier for hospitals to initiate planning for hazardous substances emergencies when a full-time emergency manager is employed by the healthcare organization; however, this is often the exception rather than the rule in healthcare emergency management. It is also important that pediatricians be involved so the specific needs of children in decontamination are included in the hospital plan. The OSHA *Best Practices for Hospital-Based First Receivers of Victims from Mass Casualty Incidents Involving the Release of Hazardous Substances* document discusses elements of decontamination planning which should be include in the decontamination plan as an annex to the hospital's overall emergency operations plan. Engaging community stakeholders during this process can assist in creating a sound operating plan. Community stakeholders include the local hazardous materials response team, the local office of emergency management, the health department, private companies that use toxic industrial chemicals or materials, and others as appropriate.

Essential elements of the decontamination plan should include the following information:

- Notification procedures for staff to implement if information become available that patient decontamination may need to be performed
- How to contact members of the decontamination team and assemble the staff trained to perform decontamination
- Site security procedures to lock down the hospital and secure entrances to ensure that all victims who may present to the hospital are routed to a single entrance to minimize the risk of facility contamination
- Location of decontamination site set-up and appropriate criteria for determining when to set up tents and other equipment
- The appropriate type of personal protective equipment (PPE) and respiratory protection to be used to perform decontamination

- Triage procedures
- Functional roles of team members and relevant Job Action Sheets
- Training requirements of team members and general hospital staff
- Medical surveillance policies and procedures for team members
- Communications procedures
- Staffing configurations and shift rotations for decontamination staff
- Integration of the team Incident Command System (ICS) structure into the overall Hospital Incident Command System (HICS) structure
- Demobilization procedures
- Clean-up and site restoration plans

Initial identification of the hazardous material may be impossible until scene responders contact the hospital with the specific nature of the substance. There are, however, ways to determine the general type of substance, based on the signs and symptoms reported by victims. Chemical agents are usually associated with an acute, or rapid- onset of symptoms consisting of irritation or burning of the eyes, mouth, and nose; dizziness or light-headedness; shortness of breath; altered mental status; or loss of consciousness. The rapidity of symptom onset in these victims is what the key that will usually point to a chemical exposure. Additionally, the history of present illness will give clues to the nature of the exposure, such as what the victim was doing when the symptoms first began. Victims may report they were at work or in a traffic accident when the symptoms began, suggesting an occupational or accidental exposure.

Current mass casualty decontamination procedures designed for adults are risky for children. Children have a higher surface area and a more difficult time with temperature regulation; decontamination with room-temperature or colder water can lead to dangerous hypothermia. Although hypothermia may be a risk, it is less risky than not decontaminating a child. Young children may be unable to understand the concepts of decontamination and will be unable to comprehend why they must be separated from their family and asked to strip down with strangers. Lastly, response personnel should ensure that clothing is available for children after decontamination including diapers for infants.

Many shower systems are not suitable for children, who require systems that use warm water and are high-volume but low-pressure. Shower decontamination units designed for young children and infants must be able to accommodate an adult (parent or caretaker) as well as the child. Specific questions to be addressed for pediatric decontamination are:

- Is the water pressure appropriate? Will it injure a child?
- Is the water temperature acceptable? If water is not warm it may cause hypothermia

- Can the process handle the non-ambulatory child, as well as infants, toddlers, and children with special healthcare needs?
- Does the method and equipment used allow decontamination of a child with a parent or caregiver?
- Will children follow instructions?
- Have mental health concerns been addressed?
- What are the long term effects of such decisions?

Similar to non-ambulatory patients, children will require more time to decontaminate, and require additional staff to assist the child through the decontamination process. Consider the following when decontaminating children:

- Keep children with their families or a care giver whenever possible.
- Have the child go through the decontamination tent with the parent and allow more time to ensure that both the parent and child have been washed for a minimum of 5 min.
- Be conscious of the increased risk for hypothermia in the pediatric population.
- Take steps to ensure that decontamination water is heated when possible and that blankets and heaters are used in the post-decontamination area.
- Attempt (when possible) to have dry pediatric-specific garments (e.g., gowns, diapers) available in various sizes for use at the decontamination location.

Crisis (or Disaster) Standards of Care

An understanding has developed that in order for community healthcare delivery systems to remain viable and effective, community resources changes must occur with respect to the manner in which health care is delivered during disasters, terrorism and public health emergencies. Hence, development of the term, "altered standard of care", emerged. While there is a lack of a standardized definition for the term, the problem is it suggests a degradation of health care which is not the message to be delivered. The term should not be construed to imply a subjective restriction of service or rationing of resources related to clinical care in a subjective fashion due because of the negative connotation coupled with the potential for disparate impact on the population. The more appropriate terms might be either "Crisis Standards of Care", "Disaster Standards of Care", or more simply revert to the term "Standard of Care." As by most definitions the "Standard of Care" is what a prudent person would deliver based on their training, the situation, the environment and the available resources which is precisely what is done in a disaster.

Alternate Care Sites

When planning for surge capacity hospitals often realize that even creative use of existing space may not meet the needs of number of ill or injured patients. A common approach to this problem is the planning for alternate care sites. Alternate care facilities function as an extension to the surge planning process, through selection and utilization of locations to serve as a receiving point for overflow patients or those, for instance, who were impacted by exclusion criteria. This type of facility would likely serve as a holding facility for patients with a lower level of acuity, chronic ailments, and/or those which who require minimal supervised care. The establishment of alternate care facilities incorporates considerations related to the scope of medical care and staffing necessary to support patients using the prescribed standard of care. Alternate Care Facilities are also supported by crisis standards of care due to decreased numbers of clinicians and the resulting increased caregiver/patient ratio which that exceeds recognized standards for example.

Communication and Information Technology Issues

Two key elements cited in all evaluations of disaster, terrorism, and public health emergency events are communication and information technology systems. Telecommunications, including telephone, radio, 2-way radio, video, facsimile, and digital imaging via satellite transmission, have been used in response to disasters. Telemedicine is one technology that can be used not only during the disaster phase but also before and after as a way to educate the community, institute prevention programs, and establish emergency assistance, public health measures, and sanitation services. The use of the Internet and electronic mail can also prove effective. The use of cellular phones is very convenient, but unfortunately, during mass casualty incidents (especially in terror acts) cellular networks tend to collapse due to overcrowding and cannot be relied upon. Radio communication is the preferred mode of communication.

Unique Aspects of Children Related to Terrorism and Disasters

Children are uniquely vulnerable to disasters and terrorism events because of anatomic, physiological, and clinical factors, as well as developmental and psychological concerns [12, 13]. While children may respond more rapidly to therapeutic intervention, they are at the same time more susceptible to various agents and conditions and more likely to deteriorate if not carefully monitored. The general philosophy of children as victims of disasters, terrorism and public health emergencies is:

- Children are more susceptible to certain injuries or environmental insults than adults
- Children with acute injuries or illness are more likely to respond to rapid and efficient medical care than adults
- Since children are not small adults they require equipment and pharmaceuticals designed for their needs

Biologic, Chemical, Radiologic and Trauma Vulnerabilities

The release of chemical or biological toxins would disproportionately affect children through several mechanisms. For example, because children become dehydrated easily and possess minimal reserve, they are at greater risk than adults when exposed to agents that may cause diarrhea or vomiting. Agents that might cause only mild symptoms in an adult could lead to hypovolemic shock in an infant.

Another example involves the unique respiratory physiology of children. Many of the agents used for both chemical and biological attacks are aerosolized (eg, sarin, chlorine, or anthrax). Because children have faster respiratory rates than adults, they are exposed to relatively greater dosages and will suffer the effects of these agents much more rapidly than adults. Children will also potentially absorb more of the substance before it is cleared or diffuses from the respiratory tissues. Many chemical agents, including certain gases such as sarin and chlorine, have a high vapor density and are heavier than air, which means they "settle" close to the ground, in the air space used by children for breathing.

Many biological and chemical agents are absorbed through the skin. Because children have more permeable skin and larger surface area relative to body mass than adults, they receive proportionally higher doses of agents that either affect the skin or are absorbed through the skin. In addition, because the skin of children is poorly keratinized, vesicants and corrosives result in greater injury to children than to adults. A further concern in children because of their relatively large surface area in relation to body mass is that they lose heat quickly when showered. Consequently, skin decontamination with water may result in hypothermia unless heating lamps and other warming equipment are used.

In addition children may present with different symptoms when exposed to the same agent as adults. An example of such a difference is when children are exposed to nerve agents. While adults with organophosphate poisoning usually present with typical muscarinic symptoms, children usually present with rather unspecific central nervous system symptomatology, mainly hard to control seizures and coma.

In terms of radiologic exposures, children are also more vulnerable than adults. First, children have disproportionately higher minute ventilation, leading to greater internal exposure to radioactive gases. Nuclear fallout quickly settles to the ground, resulting in a higher concentration of radioactive material in the space where children live and breathe. Children have a significantly greater risk of developing cancer even when they are exposed to radiation in utero. In addition as radiation has its greatest affects on rapidly growing tissues, children with generally more rapidly developing tissues including bone marrow are particularly vulnerable. Unlike an adult, a young child's central nervous system is still developing which makes it susceptible to damage from even low levels of radiation.

With regard to trauma vulnerabilities, they are well described in chapter on pediatric trauma. Some examples include less rigid thoracic cage providing less protection of internal organs, thinner skull allowing internal injury with less force applied than in an adult, smaller blood volume than an adult allowing the same volume of blood loss to have a larger effect on perfusion and thinner abdominal muscles which provide less protection to internal organs.

Finally, children are particularly vulnerable because of physical developmental limitations. Infants, toddlers, and young children do not have the motor skills to escape from the site of a biological or chemical incident. Even if able to walk, they may not have the cognitive ability to understand the presence of a risk based on a terrorist event and therefore not seek an escape or be able to decide in which direction to flee. Even worse, children may actually migrate toward a disaster event out of curiosity to see the gas, colored agent, or other effects.

Mental Health Vulnerabilities

Disasters and especially terrorist attacks are frightening for adults and can be equally or even more traumatic for children. Feelings of anxiety, sadness, confusion, and fear are all normal reactions. However, if children are anxious, frightened, or confused for long periods of time it can have devastating long-term emotional effects on their well-being. All children are at risk of psychological injury such as anxiety and post-traumatic stress reactions and disorders from experiencing or living under the threat of chemical or biological terrorism. In addition, their emotional responses are heightened by seeing their parents anxious or overwhelmed. Because children often cannot understand what is happening or the steps being taken to mitigate the event, they will often be even more fearful of the event and also of the potential for future events. In a mass casualty incident, children experience or witness injuries and deaths, possibly of their parents, family and friends, which would produce both short- and long-term psychological trauma.

How children understand and react to traumatic events such as sudden death, violence, or terrorism is related to age, developmental status and other factors. A 6-year-old, for example, may react by refusing to separate from parents to attend school. An adolescent, on the other hand, may attempt to hide his or her concern but become sullen, argumentative, unusually irritable, or show a decline in school performance.

Children with Special Health Care Needs

In addition to handling the needs of all children, one needs to also address the unique needs of children with special health care needs. These children will often present to the hospital in times of disasters due to a failure of adequate emergency planning. It is important for physicians to assure prior to discharge guidance to families of children with special health care needs – especially technologically dependant children – regarding:

- Notification of utility companies to provide emergency support during a disaster while also creating contingency plans should the utility company not be able to provide alternative power in the event of power loss;
- Maintenance of medications and equipment should supply be disrupted during a disaster;
- Knowledge of how to obtain additional medications and equipment during times of a disaster;
- Training for family members to assume the role of in-home health care providers who may not be available during a disaster;
- Keeping an up to date emergency information form to provide health care workers with the patient's medical information should the regular care provider be unavailable.

Pediatric Disasters Preparedness

Children have special needs that are rarely considered in disaster planning. A determination of the needs of children and planning for their care is essential, including children at home, school and daycare, in transit, who cannot be reunited with family, or when communication is difficult.

Evaluation of recent natural and man made disasters has highlighted that there are several categories of potential pediatric victims which can be defined:

- Primary victims: those children who sustain emergent physical and mental injuries;
- Secondary victims: those children who lost parents; whose access to health care and resources such as food, shelter, school and health care was compromised; who become injured following the event due to debris and other hazards; illness from issues such as food or water-borne illness; and
- Tertiary victims: those who saw or heard frequent, graphic and explicit scenes of the event but were not directly involved in the incident.

Planning for natural disasters must account for the unique needs of children. A cornerstone of disaster management involves the provision of shelters for those affected. While these will often be established and run by humanitarian or governmental agencies, in certain cases medial professionals may be involved in the design or supervision of these shelters and in certain events hospitals may have to provide shelters for families and worried well. Examples may include medical professional volunteering for disaster relief operations or the need for hospitals to care for victim's families, the worried well or less urgent patients when hospital beds become a scarce resource. Table 44.1 describes the general pediatric requirements for shelters.

In addition to these general requirements, certain pediatric specific supplies should be available in shelters. At a minimum these include:

Table 44.1 Pediatric item requirements for shelters

Nutrition, sleeping arrangements, and recreational and therapeutic activities that are all appropriate for age and stage of development:
Appropriate hygiene/waste disposal resources
Basic health screening to ensure appropriate levels of available care
Safety and supervision of children around frail adults (including preventing access of children to medications)
Security of unattended or unsupervised minors
Availability of medical information resources (computers, posters, phone referral lines, etc.) to aid in appropriate use of medical resources
Standardized health care data collection
Environmental considerations (smoking, alcohol, other drugs, weapons)
Secure transportation within the shelter and the medical care and resources system (transportation of shelter occupants must include appropriate official supervision of and accountability for unattended minors)
Arrangements for children with special health care needs, including providing for patients on long-term medications without affecting local emergency care resources

Based on data from recommendations developed by the Columbia University Mailman School of Public Health National Center for Disaster Preparedness at the Pediatric Disaster and Terrorism National Consensus Conference and published as: Markenson D, Redlener I. Pediatric Disaster and Terrorism National Consensus Conference: Executive Summary. National Center for Disaster Preparedness, 2003

- Formula and baby food
- Age appropriate food for older children
- Diapers and disposal facilities
- Cribs and beds with rails for young children
- Activities for children such as toys and books to help focus children on issues other than the disaster

It is important to remember that the same public health considerations during disasters which apply to adults are even more important to children due to their increased vulnerability. Examples include the need for maintenance of sanitations and clean water supply. In addition it is important to avoid unnecessary prophylactic antibiotics and vaccines but rather return to normal vaccination schedules and well child care.

Lastly pediatric disaster preparedness includes provision of social services for children. An unfortunate but potential reality is that as a result of a disaster, children may temporarily or permanently loose contact with families. Therefore, during – and following – disasters, it is important to ensure that social service agencies and organizations are available to survivors. Rapid reunification of children with parents, or other appropriate relatives is an essential goal.

Epidemics and Pandemics Preparedness

The terms epidemic and pandemic refer to the extent to which an infectious disease spreads in a population. An epidemic is defined by an illness or other health-related issue that occurs in higher numbers than would be expected normally within a country or region. A pandemic is a worldwide epidemic of a disease. Three conditions must be met for a pandemic to occur:

- A new disease emerges to which a population has little or no immunity;
- The disease is infectious for humans; and
- The disease spreads easily among humans.
  Historical examples of pandemics and epidemics are:
- 541–542: the Plague of Justinian (thought to be bubonic plague)
- Fourteenth century: the Black Death (bubonic plague)
- 1855–1950s: bubonic plague: Third Pandemic
- 1918–1920: influenza: Spanish flu: more people were hospitalized in World War I from this epidemic than wounds. Estimates of the dead range from 20 to 100 million worldwide
- 1957–1958: influenza: Asian flu
- 1968–1969: influenza: Hong Kong flu
- 2009–2010: influenza: 2009 H1N1 flu pandemic

Planning requires that health authorities assess possible control measures; drug and vaccine inventories; emergency mechanisms to increase drug and vaccine supplies; legal and liability issues for mass prophylaxis; and research, development, and production capacities for new drugs and vaccines. Although influenza (flu) is a common illness each year, many underestimate the potential public health impact of this disease. Each year, influenza causes respiratory illnesses in thousands of individuals, with severe problems usually occurring in children and the elderly, as well as those with chronic disease such as heart and lung disease, diabetes, and illnesses that weaken the immune system.

In today's world, a communicable disease is no longer a local or even regional event, it can be a national and even global event. As such a communicable disease in one country is a mandated concern for all. This reality forms the basis of the International Health Regulations (IHR; www.who.int/ihr/en/), which gives the World Health Organization (WHO) operational authority to ensure the proper surveillance and control of epidemics and pandemics that threaten the global community. The chapter on pandemic influenza and its potential effect on pediatric critical care covers the topic of pandemics in much greater detail.

Terrorism Preparedness

Terrorism preparedness presents a unique and specific set of emergency preparedness challenges. In addition to the special pediatric issues involved in general emergency preparedness, terrorism preparedness must consider several additional concerns, including the unique vulnerabilities of children to various agents, as well as the limited availability of age and weight appropriate antidotes and treatments.

Conclusion

One of the first steps in addressing emergency preparedness for children is to reinforce the notion that they have unique vulnerabilities and needs which must be integrated in to all levels of planning. But, addressing these particular needs is difficult due to the enormous gaps in the understanding of how disasters and weapons of terror affect children medically and psychologically. A clear research agenda is being developed to examine these and other crucial areas of concern. The fact is that reliable data on children is scant, and planners must often rely on clinical experience and extrapolation from adult studies. These both have significant limitations. While testing of new medications and therapeutics is rarely done in children, it has not been done at all for antidotes or preventive agents for terrorist events. Funding is needed to conduct research that addresses vaccines, resistance, antidotes, pediatric dosing recommendations, resilience, and mental health considerations. Disaster, terrorism and public health emergency preparedness must become an integral part of the scope of academic pediatric activities, including both education and research.

It should also be pointed out that there is significant potential for inequitable distribution of information and resources with respect to terrorism and disaster preparedness. Just as traditional health and public health resources are often relatively unavailable or inaccessible in underserved communities, it would not be unreasonable to expect the same patterns in the distribution of resources for these new challenges. Pediatricians need to be vigilant about such possibilities and be prepared to advocate appropriately for underserved communities, as well as for children in general.

In an age of growing threats of natural disasters, accidental catastrophes and terrorism, emergency preparedness has become increasingly essential. In addition to their traditional roles of child expert, advocate for children, community provider, family resource, and a force behind new research, pediatricians must now take on new roles regarding disaster and terrorism preparedness. Information, education and participation are important initial steps for all child health professionals.

References

1. Center for Islamic Research and Studies. In the Shadow of the Lances. In: Middle East Media Research Institute Special Dispatch Series, No. 388, June 12, 2002.
2. Emerson S. Jihad Incorporated: A Guide to Militant Islam in the US. Prometheus Books, 2006. p 153.
3. Stein M, Hirshberg A. Medical consequences of terrorism. The conventional weapon threat. Surg Clin North Am. 1999;79:1537–52.
4. Holcomb JB, Helling TS, Hirshberg A. Military, civilian, and rural application of the damage control philosophy. Mil Med. 2001;166:490–3.

5. Biancolini CA, Del Bosco CG, Jorge MA. Argentine Jewish community institution bomb explosion. J Trauma. 1999;47:728–32.
6. Caro D. Major disasters. Lancet. 1974;2:1309–10.
7. Rignault DP. Recent progress in surgery for the victims of disaster, terrorism, and war. World J Surg. 1992;16:885–7.
8. Frykberg ER. Medical management of disasters and mass casualties from terrorist bombings: how can we cope? J Trauma. 2002;53:201–12.
9. Lerner EB, Schwartz RB, Coule PL, Weinstein ES, Cone DC, Hunt RC, et al. Mass casualty triage: an evaluation of the data and development of a proposed national guideline. Disaster Med Public Health Prep. 2008;2 Suppl 1:S25–34.
10. Sarkisian AE, Khondkarian RA, Amirbekian NM, et al. Sonographic screening of mass casualties for abdominal and renal injuries following the 1988 Armenian earthquake. J Trauma. 1991;31:247–50.
11. Chen WK, Cheng YC, Ng KC, et al. Were there enough physicians in an emergency department in the affected area after a major earthquake? An analysis of the Taiwan Chi-Chi earthquake in 1999. Ann Emerg Med. 2001;38:556–61.
12. Redlener I, Markenson D. Disaster and terrorism preparedness: what pediatricians need to know. Adv Pediatr. 2003;50:1–37.
13. Chemical-biological terrorism and its impact on children. Pediatrics. 2002;105:662–70.
14. National Center for Injury Prevention and Control. Interim planning guidance for preparedness and response to a mass casualty event resulting from terrorist use of explosives. Atlanta: Centers for Disease Control and Prevention; 2010.

Jennifer S. Storch and Philip C. Spinella

Abstract

Extreme medical conditions often exist in austere settings. The expectations of providers to ensure quality care in these locations is complicated by the short and long-term limitations of medical personnel and equipment. These competing factors are amplified with the care of critically ill children. The over-arching principal for care in the austere setting is to treat those with the best chance of survival, focus on conditions that can be cured, initiate therapies that can be maintained and do the most sustainable good for the largest number people.

Keywords

Austere • Developing countries • Culture • Volunteer opportunities • Non-governmental organizations (NGOs)

Introduction

Medical care is a universal need. An austere environment is one in which access to definitive care is extremely delayed or non-existent. It is in these areas that basic medical care is needed the most. There are many challenges to care delivery in the austere environment. Certain medicines may be unattainable, re-supply of equipment may be infrequent and incomplete, and potable water and sanitation may not be available. Weather conditions can complicate care and the remoteness of some areas can prohibit communication to the outside world. Settings for care of the critically ill child in an austere environment include; natural disasters, war, and remote or underserved areas. Humanitarian responses can be considered in three phases; early or emergency phase, post-emergency or intermediate, and resettlement or long term phase. Each brings their own set of challenges with a variety of rewards for both the patient and the practitioner. Caring for a patient in an austere setting is a strange and complicated mixture of being exciting and challenging while simultaneously being emotionally, mentally and physically demanding. Many healthcare providers gain tremendous personal and career satisfaction by providing care to people in such circumstances, experiencing the culture and customs of a population that they might never have had the opportunity to be exposed to, and developing professional and personal contacts with other individuals that have similar interests.

Provider Opportunities and Readiness

In addition to providing care as a military provider in austere combat-related settings, volunteer opportunities exist for a wide range of provider skill levels and areas of expertise in a variety of organizations. Some groups, like Mercy Ships, have a strong religious component and might require or prefer that volunteers be affiliated with a certain denomination of religion to partici-

J.S. Storch, RN, CNRN, CCRN (✉)
Regional Burn Center ICU, University of California
San Diego Medical Center, 1080 Park Blvd Unit 1518,
San Diego, CA 92101, USA
e-mail: jsstorch@yahoo.com

P.C. Spinella, MD, FCCM
Division of Critical Care, Department of Pediatrics,
Washington University in St. Louis Medical School,
St. Louis Children's Hospital, 8116, One Children's
Place/NWT 10th Fl., St. Louis, MO 63110, USA
e-mail: spinella_p@kids.wustl.edu

Children ensure the survival of society. Adults are entrusted to their well being [1]

D.S. Wheeler et al. (eds.), *Pediatric Critical Care Medicine*,
DOI 10.1007/978-1-4471-6362-6_45, © Springer-Verlag London 2014

pate in their missions. Some organizations require specific knowledge of critical care, a specific patient population like pediatrics, or general humanitarian mission skills. Operation Smile (http://www.operationsmile.org), Physicians for Peace (http://www.physiciansforpeace.org) and Doctors without Borders (http://www.doctorswithoutborders.org) are examples.

Opportunities for volunteering also exist via non-governmental organizations (NGOs) from around the world. In many developing countries, NGOs both indigenous and expatriate provide substantial proportion of health and public healthcare services, often becoming integrated into the very foundations of the local health infrastructure and systems [1]. The social justice principles of NGO operations in the developing world incorporate cultural, ethnic, and religious respect; transparency; human rights; and gender equality [2]. Volunteers should become familiar with the specific goals and objectives of NGO's in the area in which they are practicing in, as well as the people of the particular organization, which will greatly improve their ability to be effective as a health care providers. The U.S. Military and Public Health Service also allow volunteers to assist with certain relief missions. For example, many NGO's and volunteers served on the USS Comfort after the Haiti 2010 earthquake. More information on volunteering with the US Military or public health service can be obtained at http://www.med.navy.mil or http://www.usphs.gov.

In addition to short-term missions, careers can develop and mature while providing care in austere settings. Examples or organizations that allow for long-term experiences include the World Health Organization (http://www.who.int), UNICEF (http://www.unicef.org), United Nations Development Program (http://www.beta.undp.org/undp/en/home.html) and Catholic Medical Mission Board (http://cmmb.org).

One major organization that can be a key resource for international pediatric medicine is the World Federation of Pediatric Intensive and Critical Care Societies (WFPICCS http://wfpiccs.org/). WFPICCS founded in 1997, arose from the vision of several world leaders in the field of Pediatric Critical Care who saw the opportunity to combine international expertise, experience and influence to improve the outcomes of children suffering from life threatening illness and injury. WFPICCS is committed to a global environment in which all children have access to intensive and critical care of the highest standard. It exists to find ways of improving the care of critically ill children throughout the world, and make that knowledge available to those who care for the children.

One major faux pas of humanitarian aid is going where volunteers are not wanted or needed or volunteers being poor guests [3]. It is absolutely necessary to defer to the local officials and to ensure that the goals of the organization are aligned with what they require instead of what the volunteer may perceive to be the need. Local officials must be allowed to develop and execute their plans with foreign teams so as not to have the foreign team viewed as a threat [3].

Preparation is very important prior to volunteering in an austere setting. Obtaining a valid passport is essential.

Table 45.1 Differential diagnosis of common illnesses specific to developing countries according to signs and symptoms

Causes of lethargy, changes in LOC or convulsions:
Cryptococcal meningitis (consider if pt is HIV positive), cerebral malaria, fever, typhoid

Respiratory distress/wheezing:
Malaria, asthma, tuberculosis, pertussis, pneumonia (as a result of a severe systemic viral infection 2nd to measles or flu but can also be bacterial), measles, epiglottitis, diphtheria

Diarrhea:
Cholera, amebic dysentery, giardia, E. coli, typhoid fever

Fever
Dengue or hemorrhagic fever, tuberculosis, typhoid fever

Rash
Dengue or hemorrhagic fever, scabies, rubella, measles, yaws, monkey pox, disseminated intravascular coagulation

Based on data from Eddleston et al. [4]

Table 45.2 WHO criteria for severe malaria

Clinical findings	Laboratory tests
Prostration	Severe anemia
Impaired consciousness	Hypoglycemia
Respiratory distress	Acidosis
Multiple convulsions	Renal impairment
Circulatory collapse	Hyperlactatemia
Pulmonary edema	Hyperparasitaemia
Abnormal bleeding	Blood films
Jaundice	
Hemoglobinuria	

Reprinted from Eddleston et al. [4]. With permission World Health Organization

Becoming familiar with the location of the local embassy, in addition to methods of how to contact it if needed is also highly essential (see information provided at http://www.state.gov/ for more details). Volunteers should inquire about the country's requirements for entrance as well as any additional fees that are required. Volunteers should expect some out of pocket costs related to travel and food. Some organizations require a mandatory donation, which they in turn use to buy supplies for the trip and food for the volunteers. Volunteers should be prepared to have emergency funds available if possible. In addition, volunteers should consider having travel health insurance, which covers evacuations, should the volunteer's own health become compromised.

Knowledge of preventative medicine and of the diseases endemic to the area is very important. The differential diagnosis for signs and symptoms of common endemic diseases in austere settings are listed in Table 45.1. Malaria, tuberculosis, cholera, dengue fever and typhoid are all common throughout parts of the developing world. Table 45.2 describes signs and symptoms of severe malaria, which is common in areas in both Africa and Asia. Standard treatments of common endemic diseases in austere settings are presented in Table 45.3 and a treatment indication score chart for child with suspected TB is displayed in Table 45.4.

Table 45.3 Standard treatment of common conditions in the developing world (Based on data from Eddleston et al. [13])

Disease	Symptoms	Diagnosis	Treatment
Cholera	Varies from mild self-limiting diarrhea to severe watery 'rice water' diarrhea up to 30 l per day. This causes electrolyte imbalances, metabolic acidosis, prostration, and can cause death. Impaired consciousness due to hypovolemic shock and hypoglycemia	If epidemic is occurring diagnosis on clinical grounds alone. In non-epidemic situation acute watery diarrhea. Dark-field microscopy of fecal material shows comma-shaped bacteria darting about	Treatment is rehydration. Start with oral rehydration salts to reduce mortality. If not available sucrose, and rice water based solution are acceptable and successful. In severe cases antibiotics are prescribed. Children-azithromycin 20 mg/kg (max 1 g) PO stat. or erythromycin 12.5 mg/kg PO qday
Dengue fever	Fever, severe headache, retro-orbital pain, and intense myalgia and arthralgia. A blanching rash appears after a few days	Requires special laboratory tests and not available where dengue fever is more prevalent. Dengue viremia correlates well with fever and thus virus can be isolated and confirmed by PCR or viral antigen detection	Supportive symptomatic, avoid aspirin because of bleeding risk
Diptheria	Incubation period is between 2 and 5 days (7 days for cutaneous diptheria). Pt may present with non-specific symptoms; i.e. headache, fever, chills, malaise, sore throat, hoarseness, dysphagia, wheezing, nausea and vomiting	Treat on suspicion, do not wait for confirmation. Arrange for throat swabs, CBC, ECG (look for ectopy, ST segment and T wave changes, RBBB, complete heart block)	Give IM antitoxin as soon as possible. This antitoxin is made from horse serum so be cautious of anaphylaxis
Malaria	Fever, chills, joint pain, vomiting, anemia, renal failure, jaundice, and hepatomegaly, coma **Malaria is a mimic for other diseases with the non-specific symptoms and differential diagnosis must be done to rule out other diseases	Identification of parasites in smears of blood	Multiple medications exist and vary upon the country, and type/severity of malaria. See WHO guidelines www.who.int/malaria/docs/treatmentguidlens2006.pdf
Tuberculosis	Pulmonary TB—majority present with a cough, which is often productive and lasts longer than 3 weeks. Night sweats, malnutrition, large painless lymph nodes (firm soft and in neck, axilla, and groin), hemoptysis, chest pain or breathlessness, fever, tachycardia may be present Pleural TB-yields a straw colored effusion TB lymphadenitis-can involve any site, but cervical lymph nodes are most common, and present initially as rubbery and non-tender becoming matted or fluctuant, and at times discharging spontaneously through the skin Bone TB-Primarily affects the spine (Potts disease). Vertebral collapse may eventually produce a characteristic angular deformity. Some patients will develop features of spinal cord involvement. The presence of angular kyphosis or "gibbus" in a TB-endemic area is virtually diagnostic of spinal TB	Positive TB skin test, no response to malaria treatments. See Table 45.4	Isoniazid, Rifampicin, Pyrazinamide, Streptomycin, Ethambutol, Thiacetazone Doses vary and are weight based

(continued)

Table 45.3 (continued)

Disease	Symptoms	Diagnosis	Treatment
Typhoid	1st week: general malaise, headache, rising remitting fever, with slight cough, constipation 2nd week: Ill-appearing and apathetic; sustained high fever, bradycardia; rose spots distended abdomen; hepatomegaly and or splenomegaly 3rd week: worsening toxicity, persistent high fever, delirium and weakness with weak pulse, tachypnea profuse 'pea soup' diarrhea 4th week: continued fever, if recovering mental status and abdominal distension slowly improve	Culture of bone marrow is gold standard. Blood, stool, or rectal swab may be done	Antibiotics dependent upon country In Africa and the Americas: Chloramphenicol 1 g PO qday for 10–14 days Amoxicillin 500 mg PO TID for 10–14 days Co-trimoxazole 960 mg PO BID for 10–14 days In Asia: Ciprofloxacin 500–750 mg PO BID for 7–14 days, ceftriaxone 60 mg/kg iv od for 7–14 days Azithromycin 500 mg PO OD for 7 days
Yaws	Primary lesion is a papule, which develops in an round 2–5 cm painless, itchy papilloma. It normally heals in 3–6 months. Weeks to years after this lesion resolves, multiple secondary lesions occur in crops on any part of the body and last up to 6 months. They are papules or papillomas of various shapes. They may ulcerate and form yellow-brown scabs. Other lesions include dermatitis or hyperkeratosis or palms and soles, local lymphadenopathy; dactylitis; long bone swelling; after a latent period the disease reappears with nercotic destruction of skin and bones. Hyperkeratosis; palatal destruction and secondary infections; sabre tibia; bursitis	Motile spirochetes can be seen on dark-filed microscopy of lesion exudates. No serological or morphological features that differentiate syphilis-causing T. pallidum from other treponemes	A single dose of benzathine penicillin IM (or erythromycin 250–500 mg PO qid for 15 days)
Yellow fever	Illness onset 3–6 days following a bite of an infected mosquito. Fever, chills, headache, widespread myalgia, conjunctival congestion and relative bradycardia (Faget's sign). Most recover after a few days, if not it will progress into a life threatening illness with increasing fever, jaundice, renal failure, and bleeding. Death is preceded by shock, agitated delirium, stupor, and coma	Confirmed by virus isolation from blood in the first 4 days of illness or by detection of specific IgM	Supportive treatment only, no specific anti-viral therapy exists

Based on data from Eddleston et al. [4]

Table 45.4 Treatment indication score chart for child with suspected TB

Score	0	1	2	3
Length of illness	<2 weeks	2–4 weeks		>4 weeks
Weight for age	>80 %	60–80 %		<60 %
Family TB history (past or present)	None	Reported by family		Diagnosed by sputum
TB skin test				Positive tuberculin skin testing (TST) >5 mm in diameter if patient is HIV positive, and >10 mm in non HIV population. TST isn't the best and most reliable as it is dependent on the fact that cell-mediated hypersensitivity commonly develops within 8 week after infection. 3 sputum smears is the best but more difficult diagnostic tool for adults
Nutritional status				Malnutrition, poor dietary intake, inappropriate weight for height/age not improving after 4 weeks
Additional symptoms			Unexplained fever or night sweats or no response to malaria medications	Large painless lymph nodes in neck, axilla or groin

Adapted from Graham [5]. With permission from Springer Science + Business Media
If the total score is 7 or more treat for TB. If the total score is less than 7 treat if CXR is characteristic of TB or if the child does not respond to two 7 day courses of two different antibiotics

Volunteers in austere settings must also protect themselves from endemic diseases. Pre-travel vaccination is often required and should always be performed if time permits. Vaccination recommendations vary by location with some that are required weeks prior to travel. Vaccination information by region can be found at http://www.who.int. Preparing for anti-malarial prophylaxis if appropriate based on location is also necessary. The CDC is an excellent reference to further research the requirements and recommendations of various countries (http://www.cdc.gov). Maintaining safe eating habits also minimizes the risk of endemic gastrointestinal diseases. Only eating food from sources that have been approved by the organizing entity of the mission is the safest (but not perfect) way to stay healthy. To prevent a parasitic infection, the use of oral anti-parasitic medications, such as mebendazole 500 mg or albendazole 400 mg, just after leaving an austere environment is advisable.

Medical volunteers in austere settings need to be mentally prepared to witness absolute devastation, suffering, and need. The living conditions are often spartan at best and the physical requirements can be as demanding as the mental stress of caring for patients in this setting. The biggest challenge that many volunteers face is the emotional, physical, and mental exhaustion. Most people join the medical field to help others and to reduce pain and suffering. Witnessing continual suffering first hand is difficult and draining. It is vital to proactively address the stress associated with volunteering in these situations. The establishment of a support system of peers and supervisors is necessary to maintain the mental health of the group of providers. Frequent monitoring of the care teams morale and mental health is important to reduce the risk of adverse reactions of being in this high stress environment.

It is necessary for volunteers to be aware of the political climate of the location of their deployment. Developing countries often have political unrest, including civil war, which can increase your risk as a volunteer. Understanding these risks and prospectively developing an exit strategy if the situation becomes too risky is highly recommended. It is also important to be aware of not allowing oneself to be placed in unsafe situations if it can be avoided. Volunteers should leave a copy of their passport back home with someone who knows where they will be traveling. Volunteers should know the resources available within the country that they are traveling. Such resources can include the United Nations, local government, and other NGOs all of can potentially assist with emergency return to your home country.

Providing care in an austere environment is challenging. Volunteering takes individuals away from their comfort level and forces them to see a side of things that they may have been naive too. Confidence and flexibility is necessary since care often needs to be provided in circumstances that the practitioner is not accustomed to providing care within. Providers must be willing to care for young children and elderly patients, as well as for the critically ill versus those with routine illnesses.

Cultural Sensitivity

Understanding the local culture is very important when providing care in austere settings. Volunteers should be particularly sensitive and aware of how they dress, act, eat and drink. Volunteers should embark on their mission with a desire to see a different way to provide care, rather than insisting that their way is the only way [3]. Simple behaviors such as eye contact, a thumbs-up sign or showing the soles of your shoes can be interpreted as offensive. Guidance from people native to the region is very often required to obtain a deeper understanding of what is acceptable behavior and what is not. Some examples of cultural differences include; the presence of the husband for married women requiring a physical examination, prohibition of genital exams, and inquires about sexual practices. Other differences in ethnicity revolve around practical issues such as not keeping appointments, arriving late, or seeking consultation outside of opening hours [6].

Many cultures in austere settings primarily use an elder tribesman as their Medicine Man, Shaman, or Witch Doctor. To gain acceptance it is often required to incorporate or include these individuals in the therapeutic plan, providing it does not increase the risk of harm or adverse effects for the patient. For example, Voodoo medicine is still practiced as the primary source of "medical treatment" for many families in Haiti. The incorporation of bedside prayers or the placement of a significant religious item at the bedside is safe for the patient, allows for the development of trust, and who knows, it might even work. Most organizations ensure translators are present to communicate between the patients and the health care volunteers. That said learning a few useful phrases assist with gaining trust.

Patient Care

There are a few major differences when practicing medicine in austere environments. Triage of patients is not according to who is the most ill, but instead who is most salvageable and whose care can be sustained. Initially, it is difficult to make this paradigm shift, but once the local limitations are recognized it becomes apparent that this approach to triage is appropriate and essential. For patients triaged to not receive care due to low probability of survival or long-term sustainability of treatment, comfort or palliative care is required. In addition to being difficult for providers, it can be initially confusing to the local population that often expects miracles from providers from the developed world. But, if it is explained respectfully that there is nothing that can be done or would be appropriate to do, it is almost always understood and genuinely appreciated that an evaluation was performed and that you cared enough to be there. Table 45.5 lists presenting signs and symptoms that indicate triaging priority.

Recent combat operations in Iraq and Afghanistan have increased the need for pediatric critical care skills for children either injured by combat-related events or for humanitarian aid at military facilities [7–11]. Data collected by the U.S. military indicate that the mean (±standard deviation)

Table 45.5 Children with priority

Children with priority
Any sick child aged <2 months
Visible severe wasting
Fever >38.5
Any respiratory distress
Irritability, restlessness, lethargy
Burns greater than 15 % TBSA
Trauma
Poisoning
Severe pain

Reprinted from Eddleston et al. [4]. With permission World Health Organization

age of children treated in both theaters of war is 10 years (±5) with a mean hospital length of stay of 7 days. Children account for 4–7 % of all admissions to U.S. military hospitals and they account for 10–12 % of all hospital bed days [7, 11]. In Afghanistan, these proportions are increased with children comprising 15 % of all admissions and 25 % of all hospital bed days. Combat casualty care providers will frequently treat children who often sustain severe injuries that are associated with increased mortality compared to adults. In a review of children treated at a Combat Support Hospital (CSH) in Iraq, children less than 8 years of age had an increased severity of injury (as measured by Injury Severity Score) and an increased incidence of death after adjusting for severity of injury as compared to older children and adults [12]. When data from Iraq and Afghanistan are combined, the overall primary causes of death are traumatic brain injury (29 %) and burns (27 %) [13].

Many chronic medical conditions, that can be life threatening in specific circumstances (allergic reactions, asthma, insulin dependent diabetes, and epilepsy) can be successfully treated in the austere environment. It is the long-term management of these conditions that can prove the most challenging due to the inability to maintain a supply of medications and the lack of compliance.

Care in the austere environment presents itself with many unique circumstances that are never encountered in typical settings in modern care facilities. Modern medicine is in an era of medical specialization and few providers' care for patients from start to finish. In the austere environment the complete opposite exists where providers almost always practice outside of their area of expertise and are the sole practitioner for patients. The need for creativity and improvisation with supplies is almost universal in austere settings. One example was recently described in a U.S. military report from the Iraq war [14]. Early in the war patient warming devices were not available. To prevent or treat hypothermia in combat casualties, cardboard boxes that were sent as care packages were cut open and re-secured with duct tape to encase patients below the neck. Hairdryers were then placed into a cut-out hole and a second hole also cut to allow outflow of air was created. This make-shift method of warming patients was very effective and inexpensive. Becoming familiar with supplies not used on a daily basis will be an asset. One such piece of equipment is the intraosseous needle. While all pediatric trained practitioners are well aware of the indications and use of intraosseous needles, adult trained practitioners may not be familiar with pediatric use and technique of insertion. Since children often present in severe hypovolemic shock it is essential that all practitioners caring for children in austere settings be trained on the use of intraosseous needles.

Volunteers should be aware that local myths, religion and beliefs at times cloud the medical knowledge in developing countries and therefore one significant contribution of volunteering is to improve education. There is a large deficiency in the education and knowledge of basic preventative health care in under-developed areas. There is significant need for sexual education to assist with birth control and the spread of sexually transmitted diseases. Basic hygiene practices often need to be taught to decrease the transmission of many infectious diseases. Oral hygiene can be non-existent and dental care sparse, allowing the people to become further susceptible to diseases. Proper education is often appreciated and has significant long-term effects. The risks associated with the lack of potable drinking water often needs to be taught. Villages far from cities in under developed countries suffer the most as some of these remote communities don't have wells to obtain water and epidemics such as cholera are spread quickly through unsanitary living conditions, improper hygiene, and tainted water. Organizations exist that focus on increasing the availability of clean drinking water to remote locations. The water project (www.thewaterproject.org), WaterAid America (www.wateraidamerica.org), and Water for People (www.waterforthepeople.org) are a few of the existing organizations.

The limitation of heroic measures is necessary in austere settings. This at times may be difficult to do since it is common to be very aggressive in the developed world. In this setting it is very important to continually assess that the care being provided is appropriate for the current situation. This requires the assessment of the probable outcome and determining if the local community will be able to sustain care for the child. One major flaw of humanitarian aid is the failure to match available technology with local needs and abilities [3]. Despite what we are accustomed to, a vast part of the world lacks modern electronic equipment, electricity, and drinkable water. It's imperative to resist the urge to bring advanced technology since the local health systems are not built to sustain and maintain such devices.

In the developed world, the value of mental health care is appreciated and becoming more recognized, but in under developed countries mental illness still carries a stigma and is grossly neglected. The sustainability of care for mental illness may not always be feasible in the austere setting, but attention in this area is often needed and it should be focused on when possible. Accounting for how local religion practices view mental disorders is essential in acceptance and efficacy in its treatment.

Returning home to "normal" life is not easy for some. Feelings of guilt regarding the contrast in the level of care provided between the developed and developing world, and concern for the patients left behind may persist for years. In addition, there is often a newfound appreciation for the standard comforts of home that was previously taken for granted. Providing care in austere settings can provide a different perspective on the typical care provided in the developed world and on life in general.

Conclusion

Care for the critically ill child in austere settings is complex. It can be extremely rewarding and challenging and simultaneously can also be depressing, frustrating, and dangerous. Providing care that is appropriate in the local setting requires substantial knowledge of the local culture, medical infrastructure, and capabilities of the population being served. When done well, the indigenous population can benefit significantly. As a secondary benefit, the opportunity to treat critically ill children in austere settings can be very worthy to the practitioner. It provides a perspective that is very valuable for self-growth and provides a unique experience that cannot be replicated elsewhere.

References

1. Wexler ID, Branski D, Kerem E. War and children. JAMA. 2006;296:579–81.
2. Subbarrao I, Wynia MK, Burkle FM. The elephant in the room: collaboration and competition among relief organizations during high profile disasters. J Clin Ethics. 2010;21(4):328–34.
3. Welling DR, Ryan JM, Burris DG, Norman MR. Seven sins of humanitarian medicine. World J Surg. 2010;34:466–70.
4. Eddleston M, Davidson R, Brent A, Wilkinson R. Oxford handbook of tropical medicine. 3rd ed. Oxford: Oxford University Press; 2008.
5. Graham SM. The use of diagnostic systems for tuberculosis in children. Indian J Pediatr. 2011;78(3):334–9.
6. Priebbe S, Sandhu S, Dias S, Gaddini A, et al. Good practice in health care for migrants: views and experiences of care professionals in 16 European countries. BMC Public Health. 2011;11:187.
7. Burnett MW, Spinella PC, Azarow KS, et al. Pediatric care as part of the US Army medical mission in the global war on terrorism in Afghanistan and Iraq, December 2001 to December 2004. Pediatrics. 2008;121(2):261–5.
8. Coppola CP, Leininger BE, Rasmussen TE, et al. Children treated at an expeditionary military hospital in Iraq. Arch Pediatr Adolesc Med. 2006;160(9):972–6.
9. McGuigan R, Spinella PC, Beekley A, et al. Pediatric trauma: experience of a combat support hospital in Iraq. J Pediatr Surg. 2007; 42(1):207–10.

10. Patel TH, Wenner KA, Price SA, et al. A U.S. Army forward surgical team's experience in operation Iraqi freedom. J Trauma. 2004; 57(2):201–7.

11. Spinella PC, Borgman MA, Azarow KS. Pediatric trauma in an austere combat environment. Crit Care Med. 2008;36(7 Suppl):S293–6.

12. Matos RI, Holcomb JB, Callahan C, et al. Increased mortality of young children with traumatic injuries at a US Army combat support hospital in Baghdad, Iraq, 2004. Pediatrics. 2008;122(5):e959–66.

13. Creamer KM, Edwards MJ, Shields CH, et al. Pediatric wartime admissions to US military combat support hospitals in Afghanistan and Iraq: learning from the first 2000 admissions. J Trauma. 2009; 67(4):762–8.

14. Beekley AC, Martin MJ, Spinella PC, Telian SP, Holcomb JB. Predicting resource needs for multiple and mass casualty events in combat: lessons learned from combat support hospital experience in operation Iraqi freedom. J Trauma. 2009;66(4):129–37.

Agents of Biological and Chemical Terrorism

46

Michael T. Meyer, Philip C. Spinella, and Ted Cieslak

Abstract

Children have myriad unique needs compared to adults during all types of disasters. Many of these unique needs emanate from the fundamental differences between adults and children in terms of anatomy and physiology. In the event of a biological or chemical terrorism event, the difficulties which arise from these differences are complicated by a lack of weight-based medication dosing guidelines, a lack of appropriate sized supplies, and a lack of evidence-based practices in children. The risk of biological, chemical, or radiological weapon use has increased as terrorists become more familiar with these agents and their potential for harm. Biological agents are invisible to the eye, odorless, potentially lethal in particulate form; natural organisms are readily available, and can be disguised as natural disasters to spread fear and disease. Chemical agents rapidly attack the body's critical physiological centers, disabling or killing victims. Potential biochemical agents of terrorism include; *Bacillus anthracis* (anthrax), *Yersinia pestis* (plague), tularemia, small pox, botulinum toxin, nerve agents and cyanide. Healthcare providers need to be familiar with clinical presentation and life-saving treatment modalities, as well as the precautions necessary to prevent contamination and transmission to healthcare workers and to proactively plan for the needs of children during a disaster.

Keywords

Biological weapons • Chemical weapons • Nerve agents • Small pox • Category A agents

M.T. Meyer, MD (✉)
Division of Pediatric Critical Care Medicine,
Medical College of Wisconsin,
Children's Hospital of Wisconsin,
9000 West Wisconsin Avenue, M.S. #681,
Milwaukee, WI 53226, USA
e-mail: mtmeyer@mcw.edu

P.C. Spinella, MD, FCCM
Division of Critical Care, Critical Care Translation Research
Program, Washington University in St. Louis Medical School,
St. Louis Children's Hospital, 8116, One Children's Place/NWT
10th Fl., St. Louis, MO 63110, USA
e-mail: spinella_p@kids.wustl.edu

T. Cieslak, MD
Clinical Services Division,
US Army Medical Command, Army Surgeon General,
2050 Worth Road, Bldg 2792, Suite 10,
Fort Sam Houston, TX, 78234, USA
e-mail: theodore.cieslak@amedd.army.mil

Introduction

The risk of biological, chemical, or radiological weapon use has increased as terrorists become more familiar with these agents and their potential for harm. Biological and chemical agents possess desirable qualities as weapons of terror. Biological agents are invisible to the eye, odorless, potentially lethal in particulate form; natural organisms are readily available, and can be disguised as natural disasters to spread fear and disease. Chemical agents rapidly attack the body's critical physiological centers, disabling or killing victims. Biological and chemical weapons also force consumption of vast amounts of response resources, restrict normal activity in the contaminated area, and induce fear and panic [1, 2]. These agents are often referred to as "weapons of mass destruction (WMD)", but from a medical sense

D.S. Wheeler et al. (eds.), *Pediatric Critical Care Medicine*,
DOI 10.1007/978-1-4471-6362-6_46, © Springer-Verlag London 2014

they are weapons of potential mass injury since they may lead to major loss of life in the absence of early life support measures [3].

Compared to military situations, the intentional release of biological or chemical agents into the civilian populace is usually unforeseen; and since detection systems are not widely available, the victim's signs and symptoms are usually the first attack indicators. Confusion and chaos are expected and the provision of prompt and effective care will be challenging. Healthcare providers need to be familiar with clinical presentation and life-saving treatment modalities, as well as the precautions necessary to prevent contamination and transmission to healthcare workers. Providers will face several challenges in caring for victims of biological and chemical terrorism: (1) the agents, treatments and diagnostic tools are unfamiliar; (2) victims may present far removed in time and place from a "release" event due to incubation periods; (3) presenting signs and symptoms will be nonspecific and when disease-specific ones are present, treatment is likely to be ineffective; (4) stockpiles of therapeutic drugs are not readily available, approved for children, routinely prescribed by pediatricians, or available in liquid preparations; and (5) providers lack adequate

training [4]. The epidemiologic clues to a potential terrorist attack are presented in Table 46.1. Prompt notification of local and state public health officials is critical when there is a suspicion of exposure to a biological, chemical or radiological agent. The contact information for the Centers for Disease Control (CDC) and other relevant federal government agencies are listed in Table 46.2. Moreover, an organized, 10-step approach for the management of victims of biological terrorism has been published and could be extended to include victims of chemical warfare (see Table 46.3) [5].

Intentional biologic and chemical exposures are made possible by "weaponization". Each of the biologic or chemical agents discussed in this chapter has been manufactured in dry (powder) and/or wet forms which permit aerosolization. Agent dissemination can occur via explosive, injection or spraying devices. Spray dissemination is the most effective and can be utilized within closed ventilation systems [6]. Secondary transmission of bioweapons occurs because of person-to-person transmission. Treatment regimens for specific biochemical intoxications are listed in Table 46.4. For the purpose of this chapter, we will assume that all patients will receive standard supportive care as well as appropriate emergency and resuscitative therapies as clinically indicated. This chapter will discuss the disease presentations associated with the intentional dissemination of biological and chemical agents, not radioactive agents.

Table 46.1 Epidemiologic clues of a bioterrorist attack

Presence of an unusually large epidemic
High infection rate
Disease limited to a discrete population
Unexpected severity of disease
Evidence of an unusual route of exposure
Disease in an atypical geographic locale
Disease occurring outside normal transmission seasons
Disease occurring in the absence of usual vector
Simultaneous outbreaks of multiple diseases
Simultaneous occurrence of human & zoonotic disease
Unusual organism strains
Unusual antimicrobial sensitivity patterns
Disparity in attack rates among persons indoors & outdoors
Terrorist claims
Intelligence reports
Discovery of unusual munitions

Based on data from Pavlin [4]

Table 46.3 10-steps in managing a potential biochemical event

1. Maintain an index of suspicion
2. Protect thyself
3. Assess the patient (primary survey)
4. Decontaminate as appropriate
5. Establish a diagnosis (secondary survey)
6. Render prompt treatment
7. Practice good infection control
8. Alert the proper authorities
9. Assist in the epidemiological investigation
10. Know and spread the gospel (remain proficient)

Reprinted from Cieslak and Henretig [5]. With permission from Military Medicine: *International Journal of AMSUS*

Table 46.2 Points of contact and training resources

CDC emergency response hotline:	770-488-7100
CDC bioterrorism preparedness & response program:	404-639-0385
CDC emergency preparedness resources:	http://www.bt.cdc.gov
FBI (general point of contact):	202-324-3000
FBI (suspicious package info):	http://www.fbi.gov/pressrel/pressrel01/mail3.pdf
Health Canada (suspicious package info):	http://www.hc-sc.gc.ca/english/epr/packages.html
USAMRIID general information:	http://www.usamriid.army.mil
USAMRICD training materials:	http://ccc.apgea.army.mil
U.S. Army Medical NBC defense information:	http://www.nbc-med.org

Table 46.4 Therapeutic recommendations for specific biological and chemical agent exposure

Condition	Adults	Children	Notes/alternative therapy
Nerve Agents	Atropine 2–5 mg/kg IV, q 5–10 min Pralidoxime 1–2 g IV, q1h	Atropine 0.02–0.05 mg/kg IV, q 5–10 min Pralidoxime 20–50 mg/kg IV, q 1 h	Dose until heart rate > 80 bpm
Cyanide	Sodium nitrate; 300 mg IV THEN Sodium thiosulfate; 12.5 g IV OR Hydroxocobalamin 5 g IV	Sodium nitrate; 0.33 ml/kg, IV THEN Sodium thiosulfate; 400 mg/kg IV OR Hydroxocobalamin 70 mg/kg	Inhaled amyl nitrite 1 ampule (0.2 ml) if IV access not available
Botulism (therapy)	Supportive care; Antitoxin and immunoglobulin may halt the progression, not reverse symptoms.	Supportive care; Antitoxin and immunoglobulin may halt the progression but not reverse symptoms.	
Anthrax-inhalational (therapy[D,E])	Ciprofloxacin[C] 400 mg IV q12h OR Doxycycline 100 mg IV q12h AND Clindamycin[A] 900 mg IV q8h AND Penicillin G[B] 4 mil U IV q4h	Ciprofloxacin[C] 10–15 mg/kg IV q12h OR Doxycycline 2.2 mg/kg IV q12h AND Clindamycin[A] 10–15 mg/kg IV q8h AND Penicillin G[B] 400–600 k U/kg/d IV ÷ q4h	A – Rifampin/Clarithromycin B – Ampicillin, Imepenem, Meropenem, or Chloramphenicol for CSF penetration C – Levofloxacin/Ofloxacin D – After 14 days, switch to oral E – Parenteral therapy preferred, mass casualty/resource constrains may necessitate oral therapy
Anthrax-inhalational	Ciprofloxacin 500 mg PO q12h OR Doxycycline 100 mg PO q12h	Ciprofloxacin 10–15 mg/kg PO q12h OR Doxycycline 2.2 mg/kg PO q12h	60 day therapy course Post-Exposure Prophylaxis--14 days, then switch to oral agent
Plague & tularemia (therapy)	Gentamicin 5 mg/kg IV qd OR Doxycycline 100 mg IV q12h OR Ciprofloxacin 400 mg IV q12h	Gentamicin 2.5 mg/kg IV q8h OR Doxycycline 2.2 mg/kg IV q12h OR Ciprofloxacin 15 mg/kg IV q12h	
Plague Tularemia	Doxycycline 100 mg PO q12h OR Ciprofloxacin 500 mg PO q12h	Doxycycline 2.2 mg/kg PO q12h OR Ciprofloxacin 20 mg/kg PO q12h	Prophylaxis
Smallpox	Supportive care Vaccination may be effective, give within several days of exposure	Supportive care Vaccination may be effective, give within several days of exposure	Therapy Prophylaxis

Based on data from Cieslak et al. [6]

Historical Context of Biological and Chemical Agents

The deployment of biological and chemical agents has been described throughout human history; as early as 400 BC the Persians, Greeks and Romans used various biological toxins during battles [7]. Smallpox-contaminated blankets were used as bioweapons by European soldiers against fifteenth century South American natives and British soldiers initiated a smallpox outbreak during the French and Indian Wars (1754–1767) among American Indians sympathetic to the Americans [8]. Chemical warfare was introduced into modern warfare during World War I; the Germans used chlorine gas against French troops at Ypres, Belgium in 1915 yielding an estimated 5,000 casualties [9].

Chemical and biological weapons have been used against civilian targets in the modern era as well. Saddam Hussein and the Iraqi military used the nerve agent sarin against Kurdish villagers and the Iranian military during the Iraq-Iran War in 1988. Sarin was used in 1995 by the Japanese terror cult Aum Shinrikyo, who released the agent in a Tokyo subway station, killing 12 and injuring 5,500. Notably, many of the injured were unprepared healthcare providers [10].

Finally, there was the well publicized attack in the United States in October 2001, wherein anthrax spores disseminated via contaminated mail resulted in 22 cases of clinical anthrax and five deaths [11].

Pediatric Unique Factors

Children have myriad unique needs compared to adults during all types of disasters. Many of these unique needs emanate from the fundamental differences between adults and children in terms of anatomy and physiology. The difficulties which arise from these differences are complicated by a lack of weight-based medication dosing guidelines, a lack of appropriate sized supplies, and a lack of evidence-based practices in children [12]. These effects are further compounded by the age and developmental stage of the child when it comes to the ability to communicate with responders, the motor and cognitive skills necessary to detect and avoid danger, and the inability to comprehend and to follow instructions [13]. Moreover, the psychological trauma suffered by children will potentially be immense. Children have an incomplete concept of body integrity, ill-defined concept of death, and fear of medical procedures which might cause a child to cry inconsolably, resist decontamination, and attempt to run away from medical assistance. Finally, children are susceptible to both acute and post traumatic stress disorder and to the stresses of family separation and reunification during disaster management [2]. Thus, it is vital to proactively plan for the needs of children during a disaster.

Many factors place children at increased risk of injuries from biological and chemical agents; children are smaller, so the same amount of exposure results in a higher dose per weight and is thus more likely to result in clinical illness. Children have a smaller blood volume, making them more susceptible to agents that cause vomiting and diarrhea, such as staphylococcal enterotoxins or *Vibrio cholerae*. Agents absorbed through the skin (vesicants and nerve agents) pose an increased threat since a child's dermis is thinner, less keratinized and results in increased permeability. Permeability is also increased by the larger body-surface-area-to-volume ratio of children (which also serves to increase the risk for hypothermia associated with wet dressings or decontamination). A child's increased minute ventilation increases the risk of aerosolized agents, radioactive gas, and fallout. Children, given their relative shorter height, have increased exposure to heavier than air biological aerosols since the agents are within the child's "breathing zone". Vaccines such as Anthrax (and a previously-licensed Plague vaccine) are approved for adults, but not for children, adding to the difficulties faced by those caring for pediatric patients. Vaccines such as smallpox have increased adverse effects in children [6]. Similarly, available nerve agent antidote autoinjectors (Pralidoxime, Valium) are unit dosed for adults, not children. Atropine autoinjectors recently became available in pediatric standard doses but are not widely available at this time. Current pediatric expert consensus is that it is better for symptomatic infants and toddlers to receive an overdose of atropine and pralidoxime than to not receive therapy [12]. The bioterrorism agent treatment recommendations presented are a combination of consensus expert opinion, as well as the Centers for Disease Control in the United States (CDC) and the Task Force for Biological and Chemical Agents and Threats in the European Union (BICHAT) clinical guidelines; providers should utilize careful consideration when prescribing for pregnant women and children. Under normal conditions, many of the recommended therapies would entail risk to pregnant women and children or even be contraindicated. However the risk-benefit ratio may change depending on the situation; for example, the risks to children of a transient arthropathy seen with fluoroquinolones or skeletal/teeth abnormalities seen with tetracycline must be balanced with the serious risk of life-threatening infections and likely antibiotic shortages during a crisis [1].

Given the unique needs of children (as well as The Joint Commission's requirements for disaster/emergency management drills for accredited institutions), it is imperative for healthcare organizations and community leaders to work together to develop a systematic approach at local, state and regional levels. Unfortunately, this does not always occur. A 2009 California Hospital Association conference on disaster planning revealed few hospitals include children in their planning, training and drills; there was a lack of system planning related to family reunification and there was limited regional planning and communication systems [13]. A survey of members of the Eastern Association for the Surgery of Trauma demonstrated that the state Level 1 trauma designation did not significantly impact an institution's readiness to handle victims of weapons of mass destruction, and less than 60 % of respondents believed there was an appropriate plan in place [14]. To assist with planning a four-pronged approach to pediatric patient demands during a disaster or emergency has been recommended; Plan, Prepare, Practice and Partner [13].

A final point for consideration during any disaster is patient triage to determine priority for resource utilization. Triage, or "to sort", is based on severity of exposure, amount of staff and resources available, number of casualties involved as well as physiologic and anatomic disturbances. Most triage scales are based on adult experience and pediatric disaster triage tools require validation. When applying a triage process to children, the child's physiologic response to illness and injury as well as the child's psychological and neurologic development level must be accounted for [15]. During military-type triage, victims are categorized as *immediate* (require lifesaving interventions in order to survive), *delayed* (severely injured, but treatment can be postponed without adverse effects), *minimal* (minor injuries), and *expectant* (those not likely to survive). Triage is a dynamic process and the victim's classification can change based on available resources, patients categorized as expectant should be provided comfort care [16].

Specific Chemical and Biological Agents of Terrorism

We will discuss biochemical agents with the greatest potential for use as terroristic weapons; some have been used on the battlefield or on civilians in the past, and others possess properties that theoretically make them potential weapons. Chemical agents are organized based on chemical structure and/or their effects on victims. Four major types of chemical agent classes are typically recognized; *Nerve*, *Pulmonary/Choking*, *Vesicant/Blister*, and *Blood*. For this review, we will discuss *Nerve* and *Blood* agents in depth. The CDC Strategic Planning Group categorized critical biological agents that might be used in a biological attack and thus pose a national security risk. The CDC **Category A Agents**; bacterial and viral agents (as well as Botulinum toxin) are considered high priority agents due to ease of dissemination, person-to-person transmission potential, high mortality rate, and the potential to cause a public panic [17]. Bacteria include *Bacillus anthracis* (anthrax), *Yersinia pestis* (plague) and *Francisella tularensis* (tularemia) [11]. Viral agents include Smallpox and the Viral Hemorrhagic Fevers (VHF's) viruses (Ebola, Marburg, Lassa viruses) [7, 9, 17]. For this review, we will not discuss the VHF's viruses further since aerosol infection in humans has not been proven. But, these viruses deserve special awareness to medical professionals because the former Soviet Union, Russia and the United States have successfully experimented with aerosol infectivity in animal models and the VHF's are highly infective by direct contact with needles, fluids and tissues [17]. Pocket reference dosing cards for pediatric treatment have been developed for both chemical and biological agents [18].

Chemical Agents

Nerve Agents (Tabun (GA), Sarin (GB), Soman (GD), and VX

Mechanism of Action

Nerve agents are organophosphate analogs of common pesticides that are potent inhibitors of the enzyme acetyl cholinesterase. The agents are colorless liquids at room temperature, and most are odorless. The G-agents have the consistency and evaporation characteristics similar to water and are a vapor hazard. VX has the consistency of motor oil and vaporizes at high temperatures [15]. Absorption occurs by ingestion, inhalation, or cutaneous exposure. Acetyl cholinesterase inhibition results in the accumulation of acetylcholine at neural and neuromuscular junctions (Fig. 46.1), causing excess stimulation of both nicotinic and muscarinic receptors (Fig. 46.2).

Signs/Symptoms

Symptom onset and severity depend on concentration, form of the agent, and environmental variables; vapors produce symptoms within seconds, droplet exposure symptoms may take hours to develop. Mild symptoms include flushing, sweating, miosis, blurred vision, profuse lacrimation, watery rhinorrhea, salivation, nausea, vomiting, diarrhea, and abdominal cramps. Mild respiratory symptoms include cough and wheezing with bronchorrhea to severe symptoms of dyspnea, respiratory depression and cyanosis. Severe neuromuscular symptoms include muscle fasciculations, convulsions, ataxia, altered mental status, and coma. Cardiovascular manifestations consist of bradycardia, hypotension, and atrioventricular block. Without prompt intervention, death results from cardiopulmonary arrest within 5–10 min of lethal dose exposure.

Diagnosis

Acutely, the diagnosis of nerve agent intoxication is clinical, based on symptoms and the response to antidotal therapy. Rapid detection devices are also available to detect nerve agents. Definitive diagnosis is established by measuring RBC or plasma acetyl cholinesterase concentrations.

Decontamination/Isolation

Skin decontamination limits absorption and eliminates healthcare worker contamination; this can be accomplished with 0.5 % hypochlorite solutions or large amounts of soap and water after removal of all clothing and jewelry. The skin should be blotted rather than forcefully wiped, aggressive scrubbing can lead to abrasions and increased cutaneous

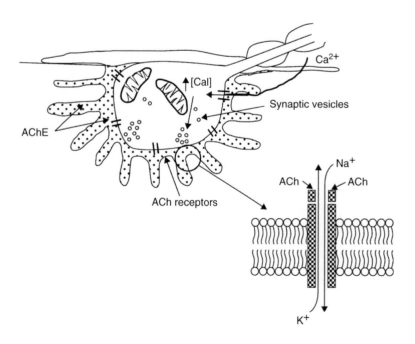

Fig. 46.1 Cholinergic synapse

Fig. 46.2 The peripheral and autonomic nervous systems

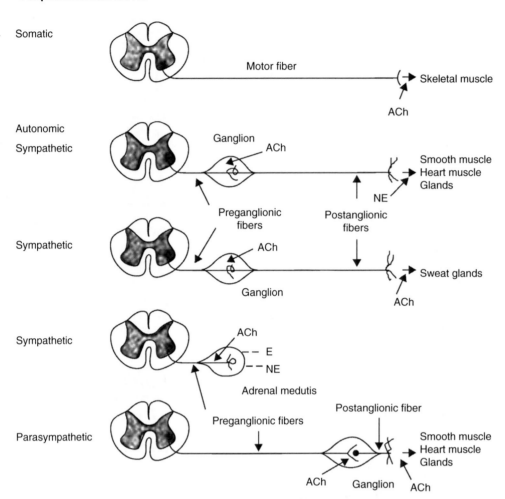

absorption. Isolation is not required after thorough decontamination [19].

Treatment

Atropine is indicated for all signs/symptoms to decrease muscarinic stimulation, pediatric dosage is 0.02–0.05 mg/kg, repeat dosing every 5–10 min until papillary dilation occurs and the heart rate is greater than 80 beats/min [3]. A pediatric intramuscular atropine autoinjector is available (0.5 mg, 1 mg dosages) in addition to the adult autoinjector (2 mg) (Fig. 46.3) [12, 18]. Patients with severe sign/symptoms should additionally be administered pralidoxime chloride (2-PAM) and a benzodiazepine. Atropine is not effective at nicotinic receptors, it does not reverse respiratory muscle paralysis; pralidoxime regenerates cholinesterase systemically (provided enzyme "aging" or inactivation has not occurred) with its predominant effect at the neuromuscular junction. No pediatric 2-PAM autoinjector exists,

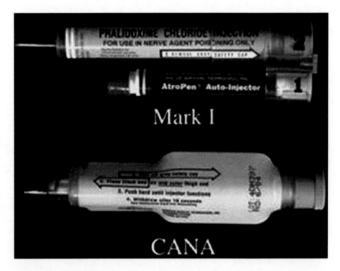

Fig. 46.3 The Mark I auto-injector (2 mg Atropine and 600 mg 2-PAM) and CANA auto-injector (10 mg Diazepam)

the adult injector contains 600 mg of 2-PAM, which could be used in children as young as 1 year of age [12]. Benzodiazepines are indicated to prevent or treat seizure activity.

Cyanide

Mechanism of Action

Cyanide is found in common foods such as lima beans and apple seeds. The paper, plastic and textile industries produce massive quantities yearly, these products release cyanide gas when burned (i.e. house fire). Cyanide disrupts oxidative phosphorylation by inhibiting cytochrome oxidase, causing a state of dissociative shock. Cyanide intoxication can be caused by inhalation, ingestion or transdermal absorption of vapor, solid, and liquid forms.

Signs/Symptoms

The clinical presentation hallmark is hypoxia without cyanosis. Mild symptoms include transient tachypnea, dizziness, nausea, vomiting, headache, and eye irritation. Severe symptoms include seizure within 30 s, respiratory arrest in 2–4 min and cardiac arrest in 4–8 min.

Diagnosis

Cyanide poisoning is suspected by a bitter almond odor on the patient and a cherry red appearance of the skin. Laboratory testing demonstrates a metabolic acidosis (lactate), a narrow arterial-venous difference, and elevated blood cyanide levels (normal <0.5 µg/ml, toxic >2.5–3 µg/ml).

Treatment

Standard decontamination should be performed for cutaneous exposure. Avoid mouth-to-mouth ventilation due to risk of healthcare worker cross contamination. For mild symptoms following low concentration exposure, symptoms resolve quickly with exposure to fresh air [2].

Specific cyanide antidote therapy consists of sodium nitrite, sodium thiosulfate and amyl nitrite (see Table 46.4 for dosing information). The mechanism for nitrite use is not completely understood, but nitrites combine with hemoglobin to form methemoglobin, which has an increased affinity to cyanide compared to cytochrome oxidase. If intravenous access is available, sodium nitrite should rapidly be given over 5–20 min while closely monitoring for hypotension. If IV access not available, one ampule of amyl nitrite should be crushed onto gauze and then inhaled for 30–60 s [9, 19]. Sodium thiosulfate IV provides enzymatic substrate and accelerates cyanide detoxification by the enzyme rhodanese

to water soluble, renally-excreted thiocyanate [3]. The newest therapy is hydroxocobalamin, approved in the United States in 2006 that has an improved safety profile since it does not require the formation of methemoglobin to detoxify cyanide [1].

Biologic Agents

Inhalational Anthrax (Bacillus Anthracis)

Anthrax is considered the most likely agent for a large-scale biological attack; it is relatively easy to acquire, organism growth and sporulation is easy, the spores are stable to degradation by drying, heat, ultraviolet light, and other disinfectants. It can be acquired via the respiratory route and has a high mortality [20]. *Bacillus anthracis* is a Gram-positive spore forming rod, its ability to form a spore enables the anthrax bacillus to survive for long periods in the environment and enhances its ease of weaponization. The agent can be produced in either a dry or wet form and can be delivered as an aerosol. Aerosolized release in a densely populated area could potentially have an impact on human life equivalent to that of a nuclear weapon [11]. Additional details are provided in Table 46.5.

Signs/Symptoms

Inhalational anthrax is a biphasic disease, with early nonspecific signs and symptoms including fever, myalgia, headache, and cough. The absence of rhinorrhea, congestion and coryza differentiates inhalational anthrax from influenza. A brief period of improvement may occur with a rapid deterioration thereafter characterized by; high fever, dyspnea, cyanosis, and shock. Hemorrhagic meningitis, hemorrhagic pleural effusions, transaminitis, and hypoalbuminemia complicate the shock state. Radiographic findings may reveal a widened mediastinum (characteristic finding) and prominent mediastinal lymphadenopathy (Fig. 46.4).

Diagnosis

Anthrax is initially diagnosed clinically and epidemiologically. *Bacillus Anthracis* can be detected by gram stain and culture of infected body fluids.

Infection Control

Standard precautions are recommended. There is no evidence of person-to-person transmission. The Advisory Committee on Immunization Practices (ACIP) recommends 60 days of postexposure prophylaxis (PEP) (see Table 46.4) following inhalation exposure accompanied by a three-dose

Table 46.5 Category a bacterial bioterrorism agents

Disease	Form (attack)	Reservoir	Incubation (days)	Symptoms	Isolation	Transmission	Vaccine	Treated mortality
Anthrax	Gastrointestinal (No)	Soil, herbivores wool	1–2	Ulcers, bleeding	Standard	Direct contact with skin lesions. No person-to-person	Anthrax vaccine adsorbed	Unknown
	Cutaneous (Yes)		3–5	Papule-vesicle-ulcer (eschar)	Contact			<1 %
	Inhalational (Yes)		4–6	Hemorrhagic mediastinitis, pleural effusion, shock	Standard		Military restricted	45 %
Plague	Bubonic (No)	Flea bites, rodents, human-to-human	2–8	Febrile lymphadenitis	Droplet, first 48 h	Pneumonic: droplet aerosols highly contagious	None	<10 %
	1° Septicemia (Yes)		2–4	Sepsis, purpura, acral cyanosis				60 %
	Pneumonic (Yes)		2–4	Fulminant pneumonia				60 %
Tularemia	Ulceroglandular (No)	Arthropods rabbits deer squirrels mice beavers	3–5	Necrotic ulcer, lymph node	Contact	No person-to-person	None	<1 %
	Glandular (No)			Lymph node edema	Standard			
	Oropharyngeal (No)			Severe sore throat				
	Pneumonic (Yes)			Fever, chills, dyspnea, nonproductive cough				
	Typhoidal (Yes)			Fever, chills, non-localizing				

Based on data from Greenfield et al. [11]

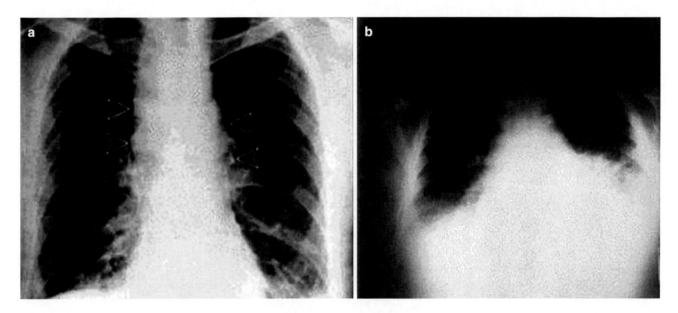

Fig. 46.4 Chest radiograph of a patient with inhalational anthrax demonstrating the characteristic mediastinal widening (**a**, **b**) and pleural effusion (**b**) (Courtesy of Centers for Disease Control and Prevention)

series of Anthrax Vaccine Adsorbed, given at 0, 2, and 4 weeks [21].

Treatment
The fatality rate for inhalational anthrax is 95 % if treatment is not initiated within 48 h of symptoms (see Table 46.4 for antibiotic dosing). Evidence from the 2001 attacks in the United States indicates that aggressive pleural effusion drainage may also improve clinical outcome [20].

Pneumonic Plague (*Yersinia pestis*)

Yersinia pestis is another high-risk potential bioweapon; the human respiratory tract is easily infected, person-to-person spread by respiratory droplet occurs, severe clinical disease with a high attack rate is produced, and medieval references to the 'Black Death' adequately portray the high psychological impact factor associated with Plague (Fig. 46.5) [11]. *Yersinia pestis* is a bipolar-staining, Gram-negative intracellular bacillus that remains viable in water, moist

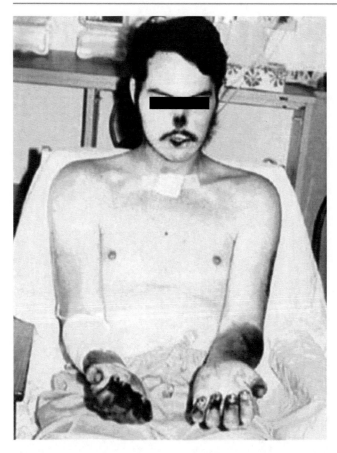

Fig. 46.5 Septicemic plague (Courtesy of Centers for Disease Control and Prevention)

soil, and grains for weeks. It is viable for months at near freezing temperatures, but cannot survive at temperatures >55 °C. Symptoms of pneumonic plague typically begin suddenly after an incubation period of 1–6 days (see Table 46.5).

Signs/Symptoms
Symptom onset is rapid, and disease course is fulminant. High fever, chills, headache, myalgias, and malaise are typically present. Within 24 h, cough (with bloody or purulent sputum) and respiratory distress develop and rapidly progress to pneumonia with respiratory failure, shock and multiorgan failure. Chest radiograph findings are variable but typically reveal bilateral patchy or consolidated infiltrates. Patients may also present with petechiae and purpura and develop fulminant disseminated intravascular coagulation (DIC); meningismus is rare but may occur.

Diagnosis
Presumptive diagnosis can be made by microscopic identification of bipolar-staining, gram-negative intracellular bacilli in body fluids. Immunofluorescent antibody testing is more specific and can be performed on sputum, blood or CSF samples. Definitive diagnosis is obtained via culture of the organism from blood, CSF, sputum or lymph nodes.

Decontamination/Infection Control
Standard decontamination should be performed with soap and water. Strict isolation with respiratory droplet precautions for the initial 48 h required since pneumonic plague is transmissible from person-person. Asymptomatic persons with aerosolized plague exposure or contact with a suspected case of pneumonic plague require PEP with doxycycline (see Table 46.4).

Treatment
The untreated pneumonic plague fatality rate approaches 100 %; therapy must be started within 24 h of symptom onset. Streptomycin or gentamicin is the preferred choice for pneumonic plague. Meningitis necessitates chloramphenicol therapy for CSF penetration.

Tularemia (*Francisella tularensis*)

Six forms of tularemia have been described based on the portal of exposure; cutaneous, pulmonary, gastrointestinal or mucus membrane. The organism is a gram-negative coccobacilli, easily inactivated by heat and disinfectants. The infectious dose is portal of entry dependent; as few as ten organisms inhaled or intradermally injected can cause disease [11]. Pneumonic and typhoidal tularemia are the most common syndromes expected following intentional aerosolization. The incubation period is typically 3–5 days (see Table 46.5).

Signs/Symptoms
Disease spectrum ranges from asymptomatic to a rapidly progressive, fulminant state. Abrupt onset of fever, headache, malaise, and myalgias are classic. Victims with underlying medical conditions present with acute prostration, fulminant disease, and rapid death [11]. Pneumonia is common and has a mortality rate of 35 % in untreated cases. Exudative pharyngitis, hilar adenopathy and pleural effusions are seen with typhoidal tularemia.

Diagnosis
History of exposure and high clinical suspicion are needed to make the diagnosis. Non-specific laboratory findings include leukocystosis with an elevated sedimentation rate. Organism can be cultured from blood, sputum, gastric fluid, or from pharyngeal samples. The organism does not grow well in standard culture mediums and as a result the microbiology staff should be alerted if tularemia is suspected. Serological testing is the diagnostic mainstay.

Infection Control

Standard precautions are adequate. Human-to-human transmission has not been documented. Doxycycline or ciprofloxacin are recommended for PEP within 24 h of exposure.

Treatment

Gentamicin or ciprofloxacin are the antibiotics of choice (see Table 46.4). Historically, streptomycin was the primary antibiotic, but there is limited availability and a fully virulent streptomycin-resistant strain exists [11].

Smallpox (Variola)

Smallpox has a high mortality rate (30 % in non-immune individuals), and a lack of effective antiviral therapy makes this agent a prominent threat; person-to-person droplet transmission could rapidly enlarge an outbreak. A global vaccination program in the 1960–70s effectively eradicated naturally occurring smallpox disease (Fig. 46.6). The only known stockpiles of smallpox virus exist at the CDC in Atlanta, GA, and the Institute of Virus Preparation in Moscow, Russia [7]. Smallpox is caused by variola virus, an *orthopoxvirus*, that is known to only infect humans, incubation period is 7–19 days.

Symptoms/Signs

Few American healthcare providers have seen smallpox; the initial symptoms/signs may be misdiagnosed in a terroristic attack. In the classic form of the disease (90 % of cases, 30 % mortality) the prodromal manifestations are nonspecific and include acute development of high fever, headache, vomiting, and backache. Two to three days later painful ulcerations develop within the oropharynx and on the tongue, and within 24 h an erythematous rash erupts on the hands, forearms and face (Fig. 46.7). The oropharyngeal ulcerations shed large amounts of virus, marking the onset of 3 weeks of infectivity. This rash then spreads centrally to the trunk over the next 3–7 days. The rash morphology changes from erythematous macules to vesicles (day 3–4) followed by umbilicated pustules with a concomitant fever spike (day 7–9) and eventual crusting and scabbing (day 12–13) (Fig. 46.8). The centrifugal distribution of this rash and the non-variability of the stages of the skin lesions are characteristic. Death typically occurred in the second week of illness. One of the most dreaded forms of smallpox, the hemorrhagic type, deserves special notation since it has a predilection for pregnant women and characterized by a shortened, more fulminant course. It occurred in 3 % of cases and was nearly uniformly fatal within 7 days, even before skin manifestations were present [8, 17].

Diagnosis

Prior to eradication, the diagnosis was confirmed by the characteristic skin lesions. Smallpox differential diagnosis

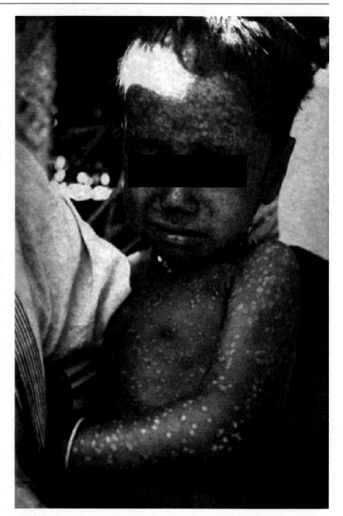

Fig. 46.6 This 1975 photograph depicted a 2 year old female child by the name of Rahima Banu, who was actually the last known case of naturally-occurring of smallpox, or variola major in the world. Her case was reported to public health smallpox eradication team authorities by an 8 year old girl named Bilkisunnessa, who was paid her 250 Taka reward for her diligence. The case occurred in the Bangladesh district of Barisal, in a village named Kuralia, on Bhola Island. The case occurred on October 16, 1975. Note the distribution of the pustules, for their greatest density was found on her face and extremities, which is characteristic of the smallpox maculopapular rash (Courtesy of CDC/World Health Organization; Stanley O. Foster M.D., M.P.H., 1975)

includes varicella and erythema multiforme with bullae. In the case of a suspected case of smallpox, specimens should be collected by public health officials. Presumptive diagnosis of any *poxvirus* can be made by electron microscopy. Definitive diagnosis requires isolation and growth that should only be attempted at the CDC.

Decontamination and Infection Control

One of only a few diseases transmitted by droplet nuclei, strict airborne and contact isolation in a negative pressure room for should be utilized for single cases. In the face of an intentional outbreak, separate hospitals would need to be determined for supportive care for known infected patients as well as home quarantine for exposed contacts. Patients are infectious until all scabs separate. A new vaccine, using a live pox virus called *Vaccinia*, was approved by the FDA in 2007. Almost 200 million doses of this vaccine have been supplied to the U.S. Strategic National Stockpile. This vaccine has multiple contraindications and potential complications that should be reviewed [17].

Treatment

Treatment begins with prompt recognition of the clinical syndrome with immediate notification of public health officials. Cidofovir has in vitro and in vivo activity against smallpox in animal studies but has not been licensed for use against smallpox in humans [17].

Botulinum Toxin

Botulinum toxin is the most poisonous substance per weight known, and experts have estimated that 1 kg of aerosolized toxin could kill 1.5 million people [7, 17]. Botulinum toxin, (there are actually seven distinct types, A-G), is a potent neurotoxin produced by *Clostridium butulinum*, a gram-positive, spore forming anaerobic soil organism found worldwide. Toxin can be absorbed from the gut, lung, or wounds but not through intact skin; aerosolization is considered the prime mechanism for terrorist use. The toxin prevents the release of acetylcholine into the synaptic cleft and causes irreversible inhibition of neuromuscular transmission at the cholinergic muscarinic and nicotinic receptors. Incubation period is 12–72 h for inhalational and food-borne botulism, but varies based on dose of exposure [17]. Recovery requires regeneration of new receptors and may require weeks-to-months.

Symptoms/Signs

Early symptoms include cranial nerve palsies and prominent bulbar signs with ptosis, blurred vision, diplopia, decreased oral secretions, dysphonia and dysphagia. Characteristic presentation is an afebrile, progressive, symmetrical descending flaccid paralysis. Victims remain completely alert.

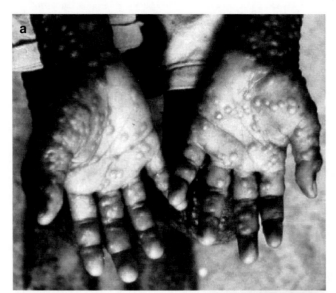

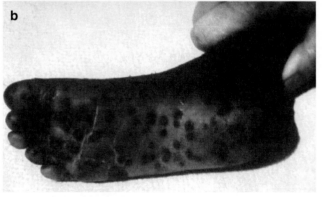

Fig. 46.7 (**a**) This child was infected with the smallpox virus, and on day 8 of the rash, shows the typical lesions on his palms. (**b**) This infant was infected with the smallpox virus, and on day 21 of the rash, shows the typical lesions on the sole of his foot (Courtesy of CDC; Dr Paul B. Dean, 1972)

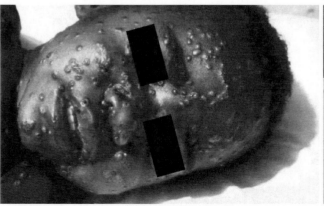

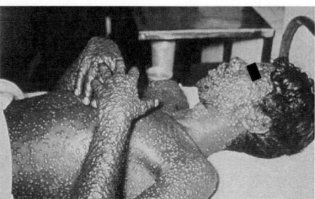

Fig. 46.8 Smallpox (Courtesy of Centers for Disease Control and Prevention)

Diagnosis

Clinical suspicion and epidemiological evidence of multiple patients with descending flaccid paralysis are diagnostic. For isolated cases, the differential includes stroke syndromes, Guillain-Barré syndromes, myasthenia gravis and tick paralysis. Nerve conduction studies and electromyography results can be supportive evidence of exposure. Confirmatory analysis is accomplished by bioassay.

Decontamination/Infection Control

Standard decontamination and precautions are adequate.

Treatment

Supportive therapy, mechanical ventilation and use of anti-toxin are the cornerstones of treatment. Need for mechanical ventilation may be prolonged; one study reported an average of 97 days [22]. Early administration of an equine, tri-valent anti-toxin limits the severity of disease, but does not reverse existing paralysis.

Conclusion

It is imperative that, with increasing worldwide terrorist activity and threats, clinicians are familiar with various biologic and chemical agents that could be used by terror groups. Prompt disease recognition, symptom management, and prevention of transmission are critical. Pediatric patients are at high risk of injury and severe illness from these agents and emergency preparedness plans at the local, state, and federal level must include resource planning for children.

Disclaimer The opinions and assertions contained herein are the private views of the authors and are not to be construed as official or as necessarily reflecting the views of the U.S. Department of Defense, the U.S. Department of Health and Human Services, or their component services, agencies, and institutions.

References

1. Pettineo C, Aitchison R, Leikin SM, Vogel SN, Leikin JB. Biological and chemical weapons of mass destruction: updated clinical therapeutic countermeasures since 2003. Am J Ther. 2009;16(1):35–43.
2. Stokes E, Gilbert-Palmer D, Young C, Persell D. Chemical agents of terrorism: preparing nurse practitioners. Nurs Pract. 2004;29(5):30–9.
3. Baker DJ. Critical care requirements after mass toxic agent release. Crit Care Med. 2005;33(1):S66–74.
4. Pavlin JA. Epidemiology of bioterrorism. Emerg Infect Dis. 1999;5:528–30.
5. Cieslak TJ, Henreitig FM. Medical consequences of biological warfare: the ten commandments of management. Mil Med. 2001;166(S2):11–2.
6. Cieslak TJ, Christopher GW, Eitzen EM. Bioterrorism alert for healthcare workers. In: Fong IW, Alibek K, editors. Bioterrorism and infectious agents: a new dilemma for the 21st century. New York: Springer Science & Business Media Inc; 2005. p. 215–34.
7. Emmad NA, Udeani JC. Biologic toxins. Top Emerg Med. 2002;24(2):72–8.
8. Bronze MS, Huycke MM, Machado LJ, Voskuhl GW, Greenfield RA. Viral agents as biological weapons and agents of bioterrorism. Am J Med Sci. 2002;323(6):316–25.
9. Dang C, Kare J, Shneiderman A, Dang ABC. Chemical warfare agents. Top Emerg Med. 2002;24(2):25–39.
10. American Academy of Pediatrics, Committee on Environmental Health, Committee on Infectious Diseases. Chemical-biological terrorism and its impact on children: a subject review. Pediatrics. 2000;105:662–70.
11. Greenfield RA, Drevets DA, Machado LJ, Voskuhl GW, Cornea P, Bronze MS. Bacterial pathogens as biological weapons and agents of bioterrorism. Am J Med Sci. 2002;323(6):299–315.
12. Foltin G, Tunik M, Curran J, Marshall L, Bove J, van Amerongen R, et al. Pediatric nerve agent poisoning: medical and operational considerations for emergency medical services in a large American city. Pediatr Emerg Care. 2006;22(4):239–44.
13. Gamble MS, Hanners RB, Lackey C, Beaudin CL. Leadership and hospital preparedness: disaster management and emergency services in pediatrics. J Trauma. 2009;67(2):S79–83.
14. Ciraulo DL, Frykberg ER, Feliciano DV, Knuth TE, Richart CM, Westmoreland CD, Williams KA. A survey assessment of the level of preparedness for domestic terrorism and mass casualty incidents among eastern association for the surgery of trauma members. J Trauma. 2004;56(5):1033–41.
15. Lynch EL, Thomas TL. Pediatric considerations in chemical exposures: are we prepared? Pediatr Emerg Care. 2004;20(3):198–208.
16. Kabsai D, Kare J. Prehospital disaster management: implications for weapons of mass destruction. Top Emerg Med. 2002;24(3):37–43.
17. Karwa M, Currie B, Kvetan V. Bioterrorism: preparing for the impossible or the improbable. Crit Care Med. 2005;33(1):S75–95.
18. Montello MJ, Tarosky M, Pincock L, Montello N, Hess WA, Velazquez L, et al. Dosing cards for the treatment of children exposed to weapons of mass destruction. Am J Health Syst Pharm. 2006;63(15):944–9.
19. US Army Medical Research Institute of Chemical Defense. Field management of chemical casualties. 2nd ed. Aberdeen Proving Ground: Chemical Casualty Care Division USAMRICD; 2000. p. 96–135.
20. US Army Medical Research Institute of Infectious Diseases. Medical management of biological casualties handbook. 6th ed. Fort Detrick, Frederick: US Army Medical Research Institute of, Infectious Diseases; 2005. p. 33–48.
21. CDC. Use of anthrax vaccine in response to terrorism: supplemental recommendations of the Advisory Committee on Immunization Practices. MMWR Morb Mortal Wkly Rep. 2002;51:1024–6.
22. Nowara WWS, Samet JM, Rosario PA. Early and late pulmonary complications of botulism. Arch Intern Med. 1983;143:451–6.

Pandemic Influenza

Jill S. Sweney, Eric J. Kasowski, and W. Bradley Poss

Abstract

The Influenza A viruses have been causing pandemics for hundreds of years, but it is only in recent years that the US government has focused on preparation. As national, state, and local governments proposed plans for dealing with an influenza pandemic, many new challenges were faced. In 2009, the world was met with a new influenza A (H1N1) virus that combined genes from human, swine and bird viruses. As few people had immunity to this new strain, it swept the globe in a matter of weeks. This influenza pandemic exemplified the challenges in providing the usual high quality healthcare our country has become accustomed to, when overwhelmed by a surge in critically ill patients. Critical care resources likely to be exhausted during a prolonged pandemic include mechanical ventilators, critical care beds, and personnel. Deciding which patients receive care during a period of limited resources becomes ethically complex. Several groups have incorporated scoring systems into their pandemic plans to help triage patients and allocate resources even though they were not developed for individual use nor have they been validated in children. Further study into appropriate resource allocation is needed to improve our current pandemic influenza plans.

Keywords

Pandemic influenza • Triage • Resource allocation

Introduction

The 2009 influenza pandemic marked the fourth influenza pandemic in 91 years. While difficult to prove for certain, influenza pandemics have likely plagued humans for centuries. The first pandemic to which historians attribute to influenza occurred in 1510 [1]. In that year a respiratory illness causing cough and fever swept Europe, disrupting civil society. It, like the 2009 pandemic, affected children predominantly and resulted in relatively low mortality, overall [2]. Five hundred years and 14 pandemics later, influenza reminded us once more of its potential impact and the importance of preparing for it. Although the 2009 pandemic occurred abruptly, for possibly the first time in history a pandemic arrived with prior preparation. In 2005 the US began preparing officially for a severe influenza pandemic, prompted by the threat of the highly pathogenic avian influenza A (H5N1) virus that has caused an avian epizootic and that emerged among humans in 1997 with high case fatality ratios. With the release of the US National Strategy for Pandemic Influenza [3], the United States Government signaled the importance of preparedness for pandemics.

Due to the unpredictable nature of pandemics, it is important for public health and hospital emergency management professionals to continue to address the challenges of

J.S. Sweney, MD (✉) • W.B. Poss, MD
Department of Pediatric Critical Care,
University of Utah, Salt Lake City, UT, USA
e-mail: jill.sweney@hsc.utah.edu

E.J. Kasowski, DVM, MD, MPH
Global Disease Detection and Emergency Response,
US Centers for Disease Control and Prevention,
Atlanta, GA, USA

D.S. Wheeler et al. (eds.), *Pediatric Critical Care Medicine*,
DOI 10.1007/978-1-4471-6362-6_47, © Springer-Verlag London 2014

pandemic preparedness despite our just having lived through one. As learned from the past influenza outbreaks, patient flow is not only increased in the outpatient setting but in the inpatient wards and intensive care units (ICUs) as well. Here in the United States, healthcare providers have had the luxury of practicing intensive care medicine without the constraints of resource scarcity but with emerging strains of influenza viruses they have been forced to plan for patient care in a setting of potentially limited resources.

This chapter will review the molecular aspects of the influenza virus and how a pandemic virus might emerge. The government planning process and mandates will also be discussed. An overview of the ethics involved in resource allocation including a discussion of tools used for triage will be provided. Finally, we will examine the differences between seasonal and pandemic influenza as well as how they differently affect patients with chronic disease and at various patient ages.

Molecular Description of the Influenza Virus

The influenza viruses are classified into three types: A, B and C, all of which infect man. The type A viruses also occur in a number of wild and domestic animals, especially in swine and birds [4]. The influenza A viruses are further subdivided by their surface hemagglutinin (HA) and neuraminidase (NA) glycoproteins. The inherent genetic lability, combined with the enormous host range in wild avian species and its ability to infect domestic animals, constitute an ideal ecology for the emergence of novel influenza A virus strains with new antigenic properties potentially leading to pandemics. Influenza B and C viruses, in contrast, have not been known to cause pandemics. Influenza viruses are comprised of eight individual strands of RNA coding for 11 recognized gene products. Point mutations in the genome are encouraged by a relatively poor RNA polymerase proofreading mechanism [5]. When these point mutations occur in the HA and/or NA genes causing changes in the two surface antigens primarily responsible for immune recognition, antigenic drift is said to have occurred. These gradual changes in antigenicity, primarily of the HA gene, drive seasonal epidemics and require continued surveillance and annual updating of the influenza vaccine components, and thus annual immunization. Antigenic shift occurs when reassortment results in the swapping of the HA or the HA plus NA genes. The resultant virus's antigenic properties differ radically from most previous viruses and, if efficiently transmitted, can result in a pandemic due to the relative lack of population immunity.

The 2009 influenza pandemic occurred when human, swine and avian genes reassorted to create the Influenza A(H1N1)pdm09 virus (previously known as Influenza A/pH1N1) which had antigenic properties distinct from recent human seasonal influenza A viruses and thus spread with relative ease throughout the population. The 2009 H1N1 virus that emerged from swine can be traced back to the H1N1 virus responsible for the 1918 pandemic. That year, the virus entered both the human and swine populations, remaining relatively stable. In 1957, the human H1N1 virus reassorted with an avian H2N2 virus, combining genes from both and causing the 1957 Asian Influenza A (H2N2) pandemic. It again reassorted with an avian H3 virus in 1968 resulting in the emergence of the H3N2 virus which caused the Hong Kong influenza pandemic that year [6]. This H3N2 virus has continued to circulate in humans as one of the seasonal influenza A strains, just as the 2009 H1N1 virus displaced the previous circulating human H1N1 strain to become the seasonal H1N1 in current circulation.

Government Planning for Pandemic Influenza

The threat of avian influenza led to the development of a variety of governmental, regional, and local response plans around the globe. Although many of the plans are based on the World Health Organization pandemic influenza phases, several of the plans use slightly different terminology and triggers for responses which can lead to confusion. The overarching United States Homeland Security Council plan was released in late 2005 as previously mentioned and was based on three pillars: preparedness and communication, surveillance and detection, and response and containment [3]. Many of the current United States governmental efforts to deal with pandemics were initiated as a result of the Pandemic and All-Hazards Preparedness Act (PAHPA) which was passed in December, 2006. The stated purpose of the Pandemic and All-Hazards Preparedness Act was "to improve the Nation's public health and medical preparedness and response capabilities for emergencies, whether deliberate, accidental, or natural" [7].

As of June 2008, all 50 US states had completed pandemic influenza plans but several governmental reviews that were completed just prior to the 2009 H1N1 influenza pandemic identified "major gaps" in several different aspects of each plan [8, 9]. Among the gaps identified were several critical components including community containment, facilitation of medical surge (adequate treatment of vastly increased numbers of patients under mass-casualty or pandemic conditions), and fatality management.

The concern over H1N1 led to renewed planning at all levels with many of the previous predominantly strategic plans generating new specific tactical plans. A recent Presidential Policy Directive has again placed new emphasis on preparation, mitigation, and recovery from all types of disasters, including acts of terrorism, catastrophic natural disasters, and pandemics [10]. PAHPA (House Resolution. 2405) is being considered at the time of the writing of this chapter in the United States Congress for reauthorization with proposed new language that would add the critical care system to the National Health Security Strategy's medical preparedness goals with a goal of ensuring that critical care is included in federal, state and local planning efforts as well as require the periodic evaluation of medical surge capacity [11].

Critical-Care Planning for Pandemic Influenza

There is a growing body of literature, as well as numerous degree programs, that focus on the field of disaster planning. Much of the current medical literature in this area has focused on an influenza pandemic as a template for hospital resources being quickly overwhelmed. In such a situation, many patients with potentially survivable conditions might not be provided with critical-care services because of limitations in resources such as health-care personnel, ventilators, or other critical resources. Resource scarcity has been demonstrated at both the local and regional level worldwide after a variety of natural disasters as well as after acts of terrorism [12–14]. Although it seems logical that advanced planning and comprehensive mitigation strategies could help maximize critically limited resources during an influenza pandemic, it is also logical that an epidemic, due to either magnitude or duration, could exceed even the strongest plan [15]. Due to space limitations, only an overview of the potential limitations and the strategies to mitigate these will be covered below.

It is estimated that there are approximately 85,000 ICU beds in the United States, with almost 70 % of these capable of supporting a ventilated patient with significant variability in geographic distribution [12, 16]. A 2004 report estimated that there were 350 PICU units but that more than half of them had eight or fewer beds [17]. Many adult and pediatric ICUs operate with high occupancy rates and often practice a modified triage in balancing admissions and transfers with resultant delays in patient transfer and surgeries on a daily basis and cancellations in surgeries and inability to admit additional patients during peak periods. Augmentation of existing critical-care beds can occur by a variety of methods, including cancellation of elective surgeries and provision of critical care in other areas of the hospital would help to temporarily relieve the shortage.

It has been estimated that there are slightly more than 10,000 physicians who identify their practice as critical-care medicine although the number may actually be less due to part-time practice of the specialty [18]. Although there has been an overall increase in critical-care trainees over the past decade, concerns remain about the ability to fill fellowship slots as well as the aging population of current intensivists [19]. Although there are approximately 1,880 board certified pediatric intensivists in the United States [20], it is likely that the demand for pediatric critical-care physicians will exceed the supply during a pandemic. Care of the critically ill patient requires a multidisciplinary team including critical care nurses, respiratory therapists, pharmacists, nutritionists, and other members of the health-care team and shortages of any of component of the healthcare team will have significant impact. Many health-care facilities disasters plans include measures to maximize personnel including adoption of crisis standards of care, canceling vacations, scheduling extra shifts, and requiring the return of administrative personnel to the bedside. Many of these measures will be difficult to sustain over a long period as well as the significant impact of staff members becoming ill or not reporting to work due to concerns over family and personal well-being.

It is difficult to accurately predict the number of patients who will need critical care interventions in a pandemic, including those who will need mechanical ventilation due to respiratory failure. As with other resources, it is highly probable that the number of patients needing mechanical ventilation during a pandemic will outnumber the supply of available ventilators. Several studies have tried to estimate the number of available ventilators in the United States, with results ranging from 17 to 35 ventilators per 100,000 population [12]. A more recent study estimated there were 62,188 full-feature mechanical ventilators available in the United States, a median of 19.7 per 100,000 population with significant interstate variability. Of note, the median number of pediatric-capable full-feature mechanical ventilators was significantly higher at 52.3 per 100,000 pediatric population (<14 years of age). The authors also estimated that there were 98,738 additional respiratory support devices other than full-feature ventilators at all US acute care hospitals [21]. Although the Strategic National Stockpile, a collection of medications and medical supplies maintained by the Centers for Disease Control and Prevention (CDC) for public health emergencies, has a supply of portable ventilators, this is unlikely to match the number of potential patients in need of respiratory support.

Not only will there be a probable deficit of mechanical ventilators in the event of an influenza pandemic but there will also be shortages of other supplies that are routinely used to treat patients who are critically ill from influenza including antivirals. Other expected shortages include antibiotics, vasopressors, sedatives, ventilator tubing, intravenous fluids, and various nutritional therapies. Most hospitals rely on just in time delivery of supplies with some local stockpiles to accommodate minor surges in patients but not to the degree that would be needed in the event of a pandemic.

Pediatric-Specific Issues

Children often represent a disproportionate number of the patients in disaster situations, owing to both their physiologic differences from adults and their innate social vulnerability. The current literature on pediatric disaster medicine planning, although more limited than the adult medical literature, is growing rapidly. Exact morbidity and mortality statistics for pediatric patients in the pandemics previous to the 2009 H1N1 pandemic were lacking but the experience with both H1N1 and avian influenza has demonstrated the fact that children can represent a disproportionate number of the patients affected [22]. Therefore, assurance of appropriate pediatric planning, including age- and weight-appropriate vaccinations antivirals, antibiotics, and containment issues is crucial. Although there has been increased national emphasis for pediatric inclusion in disaster planning it remains vital that pediatricians and pediatric specialists take active roles in community and local health-facility disaster planning [14, 23]. Many emergency-management and disaster plans, including those for pandemics, still fail to fully address the unique needs of children [22, 24]. The proposed PAHPA reauthorization language mentioned earlier in this chapter includes specific language on the need to assess pediatric needs in relation to countermeasures and improve the preparedness and surge capacity of hospitals for pediatric and other at-risk populations [11].

2009 H1N1 Experience

The first cases of the 2009 H1N1 pandemic influenza virus described were from Southern California in mid-April, 2009 although in retrospect, the epidemic in Mexico likely began in February. Because the timing was unusual compared to seasonal influenza outbreaks, other countries began escalating their surveillance systems. Initially cases reported in other countries related to travel to Mexico and the U.S [4]. The World Health Organization reported in January 2010 that greater than 209 countries had reported cases of pandemic influenza H1N1 with approximately 15,000 deaths throughout the world [25].

Here in the United States, the CDC monitored the pandemic utilizing data from traditional systems from the U.S. influenza surveillance system, a collaboration with state, local and territorial health departments, as well as through additional efforts by state and local health departments to track laboratory confirmed hospitalizations and deaths in all age groups. Through this system, epidemiologists were able to monitor influenza activity in the U.S. as the pandemic spread worldwide. Not only did this system provide total number of confirmed cases of pandemic influenza each week, it also provided data on outpatient influenza, hospitalized cases of laboratory confirmed influenza, influenza associated mortality, and information regarding the geographical spread of the virus [26].

As outpatient and emergency waiting rooms began to fill, physicians were faced with the question of which patients to test for influenza A infection and with which method should they be tested. Four modalities are currently available for testing: rapid antigen testing, viral culture, direct fluorescent antibody (DFA) testing, and reverse-transcription polymerase chain reaction (RT-PCR) [27]. Due to the substantial differences among these methods in turn around time, sensitivity, specificity, and unique challenges in testing every symptomatic patient during the pandemic, the CDC recommendations for test interpretation were based on the level of circulating influenza virus levels in the community at the time of analysis.

Rapid Influenza diagnostic tests (RIDTs) are immunoassays that detect influenza antigens in respiratory secretions. They have a fast turnaround time and can be done in both outpatient and inpatient settings. They have poor sensitivity and therefore have the potential for a high number of false negative results. Thus during a time of high community prevalence of influenza an RIDT has a high positive predictive value and a low negative predictive value. Therefore in times of high seasonal influenza circulation, it is recommended to confirm negative results with RT-PCR which also has the ability to characterize the specific influenza subtype [28].

Through the years we have come to understand the impact of seasonal influenza and who will be affected. Seasonal influenza is a leading cause of respiratory infections and has high annual morbidity and mortality. Children contribute significantly to the number of those infected, with the extremes of age and those with co-morbidities being those at greatest risk for influenza complications. Children 5 years and younger usually account for half of all children admitted for influenza and 80 % of those are less than 2 years of age [29]. In contrast, during the 2009 H1N1 pandemic, hospitalized children were older. Morgan et al. conducted a retrospective review of patients hospitalized with 2009 H1N1 as well as patients admitted with seasonal influenza the preceding 3 years. They found that critically ill children hospitalized with the 2009 H1N1 virus to be roughly 3 years older than in the preceding years [30]. Similar differences in ages of children hospitalized in Canada with 2009 H1N1were also found [31].

Although the 2009 H1N1 virus was highly transmissible, particularly in children, the overall proportion of cases with severe disease was low. One study comparing rates of mortality in hospitalized children between previous rates of seasonal influenza and 2009 H1N1, showed no difference [32]. Deaths from 2009 H1N1-associated illness tended to be older and were more likely to have underlying illness, most commonly neurologic disorders (66 %) and non- asthma pulmonary disorders (29 %) [33]. In a study conducted by the CDC Emerging Infections Program, 44 % of children hospitalized with 2009 pandemic influenza versus 32 % of children hospitalized the preceding 8 years of seasonal influenza had a history of asthma. They also found that of these patients, a higher proportion of those asthmatic patients admitted during the 2009 pandemic had pneumonia and required intensive care, although the mortality was the same [34]. Other chronic medical conditions were also found to cause increased hospitalization in children, with one study reporting 60 % of admitted children with 2009 H1N1 had an underlying medical condition compared to the 31–43 % of those hospitalized for seasonal influenza [35]. Global data for the 2009 H1N1 Pandemic is still being published with varying rates of mortality but it should be pointed out that comparing historical rates may be difficult to compare due to likely underreporting in the past [32]. Although the 2009 H1N1 pandemic did not see an overall rise in critically ill patients or deaths in most PICUs in the United States or Canada, it did cause severe strain on critical care resources as the volume of patients admitted occurred over a shorter period of time as compared to normal seasonal influenza or other viral respiratory pathogens effects. In a study looking at 57 pediatric patients admitted to Canadian ICUs, there was a similar proportion of patients with critical illness compared to previous seasonal outbreaks, but these patients were admitted within a 4 week period [32].

Ethics

With the preceding preparation for a potential influenza pandemic as well as analysis of the 2009 experience, increasing emphasis has been put on decision making about allocation of scarce life-sustaining resources. During a peak period of a pandemic, there will be significant stress on hospital supplies, medications, physical hospital space, mechanical ventilators, and staff. Although every effort should be made to provide care that is functionally equal to usual practices, these may be insufficient and crisis standards of care may be needed [36]. A public health emergency creates a need to transition from individual patient-focused clinical care to a population-oriented public health approach intended to provide the best possible outcomes for a large cohort of critical care patients [37]. This is unlike the traditional medical mindset in which the physician is expected to advocate for individual patients [38]. Rationing of care does not coincide with the usual physician-patient relationship, and can cause a feeling of distrust [39].

As seen in seasonal influenza outbreaks and past influenza pandemics, broad spans of ages are affected. When faced with a large patient surge one must have criteria for allocating scarce resources. Age has been proposed as one such criterion. The Ontario Health Plan for an Influenza Pandemic (OHPIP) has adopted age-based criteria with exclusion of patients greater than 85 to receive critical care treatment during periods of resource scarcity but not all triage plans include age as a criterion [40]. This issue is less important in pediatric plans although extreme prematurity should be discussed for potential inclusion in such plans.

In a severe pandemic, when surge capacity has been exceeded, patients should be treated equally, except when unequal treatment can save more lives. Invariably there will be three types of patients presenting for critical care; those who will survive even without treatment, those that will only survive if given treatment, and those that will die even with treatment [36]. Obviously, rationing care to those who will only survive with treatment is the most efficient. Unfortunately, quickly recognizing this population of patients who will only get better if given critical care resources at presentation is problematic.

The ability to objectively distinguish patients by medical severity is essential. The OHPIP chose the Sequential Organ Failure Assessment (SOFA) score to aid in selecting out those most likely to benefit from the use of critical care resources. This score uses physiologic parameters and common laboratory values to produce a score, correlating to mortality rate [41]. This same scoring system was also utilized by the Task Force for Mass Critical Care's plan for resource allocation [12]. The Utah Hospital and Health System Association utilized the modified SOFA score, which includes less laboratory values and equally predicts mortality [42, 43].

Although these scores potentially provide a simple and quick tool in triaging patients, two significant issues remain. These scores are not validated in children and were not developed for use on individual patients. Although pediatric severity of illness scoring systems exist, including the Pediatric Risk of Mortality III and Pediatric Index of Mortality 2, these require extensive variable collection and calculation over the first 1 or 12 h of hospitalization respectively [44, 45]. Other scores under consideration include the Pediatric Risk of Hospital Admission II, Pediatric Early Warning System and Pediatric Logistic Organ Dysfunction scores [46–48]. At this time, none of these scores have been validated for use in critical care triage, nor have they been validated to predict the need for critical care resources. A simple scoring system specific to pediatric patients will need to be researched and validated prior to implementation into any triage system. It is important to note that many concerns exist with the use of severity scores in triage decisions [49, 50].

Conclusion

Although we have come a long way in identification and treatment of influenza since the first pandemic, many challenges still await. Despite extensive preparation, which began in 2005 for a potentially severe pandemic caused by avian influenza, the 2009 H1N1 pandemic created unique challenges. The rapid spread led to large numbers of cases and quickly filled emergency rooms and hospitals., The experience with this virus confirms the need for continued work in all three phases of pandemic influenza planning; preparedness and communication, surveillance and detection, and response and containment.

Disclaimer The findings and conclusions in this textbook chapter are those of the author(s) and do not necessarily represent the views of the Centers for Disease Control and Prevention/the Agency for Toxic Substances and Disease Registry.

References

1. Morens DM, Taubenberger JK, Folkers GK, et al. Pandemic influenza's 500th anniversary. Clin Infect Dis. 2010;51:1442–4.

2. Jhung MA, Swerdlow D, Olsen SJ, et al. Epidemiology of 2009 pandemic influenza A (H1N1) in the United States. Clin Infect Dis. 2011;52(S1):S13–26.

3. US Homeland Security Council. National strategy for pandemic influenza. 2005. http://www.flu.gov/professional/federal/pandemic-influenza.pdf. Accessed 21 Sept 2011.

4. Lagace-Wiens PR, Rubinstein E, Gumel A. Influenza epidemiology-past, present, and future. Crit Care Med. 2010;38:e1–9.

5. Webster RG, Bean WJ, Gorman OT, et al. Evolution and ecology of influenza A viruses. Microbiol Rev. 1992;56:152–79.

6. Taubenberger JK, Kash JC. Influenza virus evolution, host adaptation and pandemic formation. Cell Host Microbe. 2010;7:440–51.

7. Pandemic and All-Hazards Preparedness Act (PAHPA); Public Law No. 109–417. http://www.phe.gov/preparedness/legal/pahpa/pages/default.aspx. Accessed 21 Sept 2011.

8. Levinson DR. State and local pandemic influenza preparedness: medical surge. http://oig.hhs.gov/oei/reports/oei-02-08-00210.pdf. Accessed 21 Sept 2011.

9. Homeland Security Council. Assessment of state's operating plans to combat pandemic influenza. http://www.flu.gov/professional/states/state_assessment.pdf. Accessed 21 Sept 2011.

10. Department of Homeland Security. Presidential Policy Directive/PPD8: National Preparedness. http://www.dhs.gov/xabout/laws/gc_1215444247124.shtm. Accessed 21 Sept 2011.

11. House Resolution. 2405. http://www.gpo.gov/fdsys/pkg/BILLS-112hr2405ih/pdf/BILLS-112hr2405ih.pdf. Accessed 28 Sept 2011.

12. Christian MD, Devereaux AV, Dichter JR, et al. Definitive care for the critically Ill during a disaster: current capabilities and limitations. Chest. 2008;133:8S–17S.

13. Kanter RK, Cooper A. Mass critical care: pediatric considerations in extending and rationing care in public health emergencies. Disaster Med Public Health Prep. 2009;3 Suppl 2:s1–6.

14. Wheeler DS, Poss WB. Mass casualty management in a changing world. Pediatr Ann. 2003;32:98–105.

15. Stiff D, Kumar A, Kisson N, et al. Potential pediatric intensive care unit demand/capacity mismatch due to novel pH1N1 in Canada. Pediatr Crit Care Med. 2011;12:e51–7.

16. Carr BG, Addyson DK, Kahn JM. Variation in critical care beds per capita in the United States: implications for pandemic and disaster planning. JAMA. 2010;303:1371–2.

17. Randolph AG, Gonzales CA, Cortellini L, et al. Growth of pediatric intensive care units in the United States from 1995–2001. J Pediatr. 2004;144:792–8.

18. Krell KE. Critical care medicine growth requires dealing with our "perfect storm" of manpower shortage. Crit Care Med. 2010;38:1613.

19. Chandler E, Langford P. Are there more critical care physician trainees today? SCCM Critical Connections. June 2006.

20. American Board of Pediatrics. Number of diplomate certificates granted through December 2010. https://www.abp.org/abpwebsite/stats/numdips.htm. Accessed 26 Sept 2011.

21. Rubinson L, Vaughn F, Nelson S, et al. Mechanical ventilators in US acute care hospitals. Disaster Med Public Health Prep. 2010;4:199–206.

22. The American Academy of Pediatrics (AAP) and Trust for America's Health (TFAH) report: pandemic influenza: warning, children at-risk. http://healthyamericans.org/reports/fluchildren/. Accessed 26 Sept 2011.

23. National Commission on Children and Disasters report: progress report on children and disasters, 11 May 2010. www.childrenanddisasters.acf.hhs.gov. Accessed 26 Sept 2011.

24. Institute of Medicine. Guidance for establishing crisis standards of care for use in disaster situations: a letter report. 2009. http://www.nap.edu/catalog/12749.html. Accessed 28 Sept 2011.

25. World Health Organization report: Pandemic (H1N1) 2009- update 85. http://www.who.int/csr/don/2010_01_29/en/index.html. Accessed 26 Sept 2011.

26. Centers for Disease Control and Prevention report: overview of influenza surveillance in the United States. http://www.cdc.gov/flu/weekly/overview.htm. Accessed 26 Sept 2011.

27. Boggild AK, McGeer AJ. Laboratory diagnosis of 2009 H1N1 influenza A virus. Crit Care Med. 2010;38:e38–42.

28. Center for Disease Control and Prevention report: guidance for clinicians on the use of rapid influenza diagnostic test for the 2010–2011 influenza season. http://www.cdc.gov/flu/pdf/professionals/diagnosis/clinician_guidance_ridt.pdf. Accessed 26 Sept 2011.

29. Iskander M, Booy R, Lambert S. The burden of influenza in children. Curr Opin Infect Dis. 2007;20:259–63.

30. Morgan CL, Hobson MJ, Seger B, et al. 2009 Pandemic influenza (H1N1) in critically ill children in Cincinnati, Ohio. Pediatr Crit Care Med. 2011;13(3):e140–4.

31. O'Riordan S, Barton M, Yau Y, et al. Risk factors and outcomes among children admitted to hospital with pandemic H1N1 influenza. CMAJ. 2010;182:39–44.

32. Jouvet P, Hutchinson J, Pinto R, et al. Critical illness in children with influenza A/pH1N1 2009 infection in Canada. Pediatr Crit Care Med. 2010;11:603–9.

33. Cox CM, Blanton L, Dhara R, et al. 2009 Pandemic influenza A (H1N1) deaths among children-United States, 2009–2010. CID. 2011;52(S1):S69–74.

34. Dawood FS, Kamimoto L, D'Mello TA, et al. Children with asthma hospitalized with seasonal or pandemic influenza, 2003–2009. Pediatrics. 2011;128:e27–32.

35. Jain S, Kamimoto L, Bramley AM, et al. Hospitalized patients with 2009 H1N1 influenza in the United States, April-June 2009. N Engl J Med. 2009;361:1935–44.

36. Antommaria AH, Sweney J, Poss WB. Critical appraisal of: triaging pediatric critical care resources during a pandemic: ethical and medical considerations. Pediatr Crit Care Med. 2010;11:396–400.

37. Centers for Disease Control and Prevention report: ethical considerations for decision making regarding allocation of mechanical ventilators during a severe influenza pandemic or other public health emergency. http://www.cdc.gov/od/science/integrity/phethics/docs/ethical-considerations-allocation-mechanical-ventilators-in-emergency-201011.pdf. Accessed 26 Sept 2011.

38. Winslow GR. Triage and justice: the ethics of rationing life-saving medical resources. Berkeley: University of California Press; 1982.

39. Powell T, Christ KC, Birkhead GS. Allocation of ventilators in public health disaster. Disaster Med Public Health Prep. 2008;2:20–6.

40. Ontario Health Plan for an Influenza Pandemic August 2008. http://www.health.gov.on.ca/english/providers/program/emu/pan_flu/pan_flu_plan.html. Accessed 26 Sept 2011.

41. Vincent JL, Moreno R, Takala J, et al. The SOFA (Sepsis-related Organ Failure Assessment) score to organ dysfunction/failure. On behalf of the Working Group on Sepsis-Related Problems of the European Society of Intensive Care Medicine. Int Care Med. 1996;227:707–10.

42. Utah Hospitals and Health Systems Association for the Utah Department of Heath: Utah pandemic influenza hospital and ICU triage guidelines. http://www.uha-utah.org/DisasterPrep.htm. Accessed 26 Sept 2011.

43. Grissom CK, Orme JF, Jensen RL, et al. A modified sequential organ failure assessment score for critical care triage. Disaster Med Public Health Prep. 2010;4:277–84.

44. Pollack MM, Patel KM, Ruttimann UE. PRISM III: an updated pediatric risk of mortality score. Crit Care Med. 1996;24:743–52.

45. Slater A, Shann F, Pearson G. PIM2: a revised version of the paediatric index of mortality. Intensive Care Med. 2003;29:278–85.

46. Chamberlain JM, Patel KM, Pollack MM. The pediatric risk of hospital admission score: a second-generation severity of illness score for pediatric emergency patients. Pediatrics. 2005;115:388–95.

47. Duncan H, Hutchison J, Parshuram CS. The pediatric early warning system score: a severity of illness score to predict urgent medical need in hospitalized patients. J Crit Care. 2006;21:271–8.

48. Leteurtre S, Martinot A, Duhamel A, et al. Development of a pediatric multiple organ dysfunction score: use of two strategies. Med Decis Making. 1999;19:399–410.

49. Vincent JL, Opal S, Marshall JC. Ten reasons why we should not use severity scores as entry criteria for clinical trials or in our treatment decisions. Crit Care Med. 2010;38:283–7.

50. Christian MD, Hamielac C, Laza NM, et al. A retrospective cohort pilot study to evaluate a triage tool for use in a pandemic. Crit Care. 2009;13:R170. http://ccforum.com/content/13/5/R170. Accessed 26 Sept 2011.

Pediatric Drowning

48

Jason Coryell and Laura M. Ibsen

Abstract

Drowning is an important cause of childhood morbidity and mortality worldwide, with tremendous discrepancy by demography. The epidemiology, pathoyphysiology, and outcome of drowning in children is reviewed. Evaluation and treatment of the drowning victim at various locations of care is discussed. Prediction of neurologic outcome is often difficult but important for decision making. Various means of predicting outcome, including clinical assessment, radiologic examination, and neurophysiological testing are reviewed.

Keywords

Drowning • Submersion • Hypoxic-ischemic encephalopathy • Cardiac arrest

Introduction

Drowning is an important cause of childhood morbidity and mortality, accounting for thousands of hospitalizations and deaths every year, as well as devastating grief for families. Submersion injury is unique in some respects, but it is a well-studied and common cause of asphyxial injury, and can serve as a model for understanding many of the prognostic, pathophysiologic and therapeutic aspects of all types of asphyxial injury in children. Although attempts at cerebral resuscitation for near drowning victims in the critical care unit have thus far been largely unsuccessful, a thorough understanding of the pathophysiology, effective resuscitation strategies, and data relevant to the prognosis after submersion is key to providing timely, effective, and compassionate care.

Drowning is "the process of experiencing respiratory impairment from submersion/immersion in liquid," as defined by the 2002 World Congress on Drowning and the World Health Organization. The term "near-drowning" is no longer recommended to distinguish survival from non-survival. Instead, drowning outcomes are categorized into "death," "morbidity," or "no morbidity." Those with morbidity may be subcategorized into "moderately disabled," "severely disabled," "vegetative state/coma" and brain death" [1, 2]. Death is due to cardiac arrest as a result of hypoxic-ischemic injury. In those who survive drowning, morbidity results from hypoxic-ischemic injury to the brain.

Epidemiology

Drowning accounts for hundreds of thousands of deaths annually worldwide. However, there is tremendous discrepancy between the death rates due to drowning by region and country income. Generally submersion injuries are more common in warm climates. Ninety-seven percent of drowning deaths occur in low-and-middle income countries. Worldwide, drowning is the third leading cause of death in children 5–14 years of age and the 11th leading cause of death in children 0–4 years of age [3]. In the United States, 4,086 people died due to drowning in 2007 [4]. Of these, 1,033 were 18 years of age or younger, representing 10 % of the deaths due to accidental injury in this age group. Males are more likely to die from drowning compared to females in all age groups (rate per 100,000 population (1.79 vs 0.49). Toddlers

J. Coryell, MD • L.M. Ibsen, MD (✉)
Department of Pediatrics,
Doernbecher Children's Hospital,
Oregon Health and Sciences University,
707 SW Gaines Road, Portland, OR, USA
e-mail: ibsenl@ohsu.edu

D.S. Wheeler et al. (eds.), *Pediatric Critical Care Medicine*,
DOI 10.1007/978-1-4471-6362-6_48, © Springer-Verlag London 2014

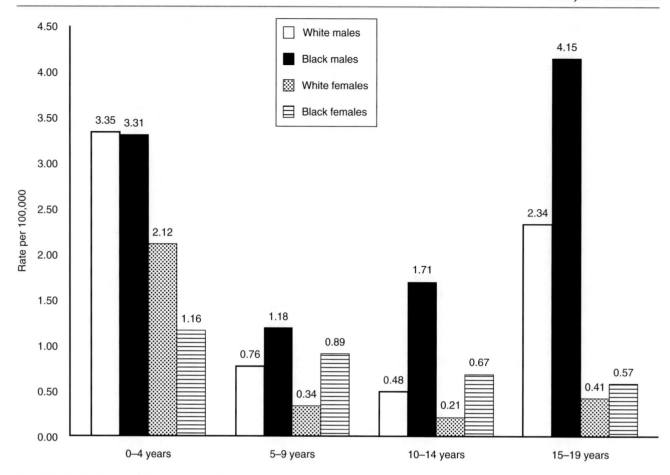

Fig. 48.1 Pediatric drowning rate by age and race

and teenage boys have the greatest risk of drowning. Black males 15–19 years of age have the highest rate of drowning (4.15 per 100,000), followed by white males 0–4 years of age (3.35 per 100,000). The rates for black children over age four was consistently higher than that of white children, while the rate for black and white children 0–4 years of age was nearly identical, possibly reflecting a reduced exposure of young black children to swimming pools [4] (Fig. 48.1).

The majority of submersion events occur in fresh water. The location in which children drown provides some insight into racial and age disparities in drowning rates and may provide information for prevention measures. In 1995, Brenner and colleagues [5] reviewed death certificates of all pediatric victims of unintentional drownings in the US. Among infants, 78 % of drownings were in bathtubs and 20 % occurred in artificial pools or freshwater. Among children 1–4 years, 56 % were in artificial pools and 26 % were in fresh water, while among older children, 63 % of drownings were in bodies of freshwater. Most pool submersions occur at the child's own home, with nearly half occurring within the first 6 months of pool exposure. Isolation fencing of private pools is an important prevention strategy that has been well documented to reduce the risk of drowning [6]. After the age of 5 years, black males had a significantly higher risk

of drowning as compared with white males, with much of the increased risk due to swimming pool events [5]. In low-and-middle income countries, many drownings take place in buckets of water, ponds, tubs, and unprotected wells [3].

Less information is available on the incidence and outcome of drowning survivors. In 2009, the U.S. Centers for Disease Control reported 5,454 (0–18 years) pediatric drowning patients requiring treatment in an emergency department, with 2,273 patients hospitalized or transferred [4]. The World Health Organization reports non-fatal outcomes in terms of disability-adjusted life years (DALYs) which account for life lost from premature death and years of life lived with disability. In 2000, worldwide there were over 1.3 million DALYs lost due to drowning, with over 60 % due to drowning in children less than 15 years of age [3].

Associated Conditions

Associated Medical Conditions

While certain medical illnesses can predispose children to submersion injury, the precise frequency is difficult to determine. Epilepsy has been well documented to increase the risk of drowning [7–9]. Diekama et al. [10], in a population based cohort study of children in King County, WA found that those with epilepsy had a tenfold increased risk of submersion injury even after children with additional handicaps were removed from the analysis. In prospectively following 245 individuals with childhood-onset epilepsy, there was an absolute risk of 2.4 % risk for death from drowning [11]. There have also been reports of drowning victims having previously unknown long QT syndrome, and the suggestion was made that swimming is an arrhythmogenic trigger in some patients with long QT syndrome [12–15]. Although it is reasonable to speculate that certain other conditions, such as paroxysmal cardiac dysrhythmias, might also predispose children to drowning, the contribution of associated medical conditions probably account for a small minority of drowning victims [16]. The possibility of intentional drowning should be considered, especially with young children or infants who nearly drown under suspicious circumstances. For instance, the infant over 12 months of age who sits and rights themselves well should not suffer a submersion injury in a bathtub if unattended for a few minutes.

Associated Injuries

Drowning in older children and adolescents is often associated with boating, diving, or water sport activities. Reports of cervical spine injuries among victims of diving accidents have led some authors to recommend cervical spine stabilization for all drowning victims regardless of whether they have sustained a traumatic injury [17, 18]. There is little data on the frequency of cervical spine injury in strangulation and hanging injuries, but what is available suggest that such injury is rare unless there is significant force involved [19, 20], therefore it seems logical that cervical spine injury would be unlikely with submersion alone. Watson et al. [21] reported a review of submersion victims and found the incidence of cervical spine injury to be low (0.5 %), and all those who sustained c-spine injury had clinical signs of serious injury and a history of high impact trauma prior to submersion. In the event of submersion associated with trauma, cervical spine immobilization and evaluation is warranted. Without a history of trauma, there is little evidence supporting cervical spine immobilization, which can make airway management and warming more difficult.

Because young children often drown in household bodies of water (tubs, buckets, etc.), the composition of that fluid should be considered when evaluating the potential injuries these patients may have sustained. Water that has had bleach or other cleaning solutions may be particularly injurious to the upper airway and esophagus and direct visualization should be considered when the patient's condition has stabilized.

Pathophysiology

Immersion

The physiologic effects of immersion in water itself are applicable to most drowning victims and are not widely appreciated but may have significant impact on the events that occur prior to and during the drowning episode. The series of physiologic events that occur during drowning depends to some extent on the manner of submersion. Head-out immersion in thermo-neutral water results in physiologic alterations in the cardiovascular and respiratory systems that lead to an increase in venous return and hence cardiac output, increase in right to left shunting, movement of the diaphragm, and a significant increase in work of breathing. The increase in venous return results in diuresis, natriuresis, and kaliuresis. Immersion in cold water results in intense vasoconstriction and further increase in right atrial pressure, increased heart rate, increased cardiac output, and enhanced urine output. Respiratory drive is increased and may account for difficulties in swimming even for competent swimmers [22]. Young children or non-swimmers will often not experience the period of time above water that swimmers do, and those who fall into buckets or other unusual containers of water may not experience these phenomena and the effects associated with immersion per se. Those who do experience the immersion phenomena may have a greater degree of dehydration and electrolyte imbalance.

Submersion

The sequence of events occurring after submersion under water was studied extensively in animal models during the 1930s [23, 24] and is thought to be similar to the events that occur with human drowning [25]. During the initial minutes after submersion, there is panic and struggle to surface. Small amounts of fluid are aspirated into the hypopharynx, triggering laryngospasm. The victim then swallows large volumes of water. In 85–90 % of cases, the initial laryngospasm abates and the victim aspirates large volumes of water, in the remainder the laryngospasm continues and there is little aspiration. There may also be vomiting and aspiration of gastric contents. Evolving hypoxemia causes neuronal injury and eventually leads to circulatory collapse with myocardial damage as well as multiple organ system dysfunction, with further ischemic brain injury.

Early work in animal drowning models suggested that drowning induced significant fluid shifts and electrolyte abnormalities that were dependent on the osmolarity of the aspirated fluid [26, 27]. Subsequent studies of human drowning victims have shown that electrolyte abnormalities are minimal [28, 29]. Similarly, hemoglobin concentrations are minimally altered. There may be slight intravascular volume shifts, with increased intravascular volume after fresh water drowning and hypovolemia after salt water drowning, but these are transient and not usually clinically significant. Patients who are in water, struggling, for long periods of time prior to submersion may have more extensive water loss either due to the induced diuresis or insensible losses and may also go on to suffer from complications such as rhabdomyolysis due to overexertion, hypothermia, or shivering [30, 31].

Hypothermia

Hypothermia frequently accompanies submersion injuries and the relatively large surface area to body mass ratio of infants and children puts them at particular risk. Additionally, swallowing or aspiration of cold water may play an important role in the development of core or brain cooling during submersion in cold water [22, 32]. Most organ systems are adversely affected by hypothermia. Moderate hypothermia (32–35 °C) is associated with increased sympathetic tone, shivering, and increased oxygen consumption. Between 32 °C and 28 °C, shivering stops, heart rate and blood pressure decline, and oxygen consumption deceases. A core temperature below 28 °C puts the victim at risk of extreme bradycardia or spontaneous ventricular fibrillation or asystole [30]. Significant hypothermia also leads to clinically significant coagulopathy including prolongation of clotting times and platelet dysfunction, and affects immune cell function [33].

The mammalian "dive reflex" is elicited by contact of the face with cold water and has been postulated by some to explain the seemingly extra-ordinary survival of some victims from prolonged submersion. The reflex consists of breath-holding, intense peripheral vasoconstriction with bradycardia and decreased cardiac output, and increased mean arterial pressure. Selective vasoconstriction and systemic hypertension promotes selective heart and brain perfusion [34]. While the diving reflex clearly benefits aquatic mammals, there is controversy over its role in human submersion [22]. Breath holding is less prominent in children when they are immersed in cold water [35, 36] and the degree of bradycardia is independent of water temperature.

Effects on End-Organs

Respiratory System

All drowning victims are hypoxemic. Those who do not aspirate fluid are hypoxemic initially due to apnea but with time may develop increased permeability of the capillary endothelium and surfactant disruption leading to acute lung injury (ALI) or acute respiratory distress syndrome (ARDS) as a consequence of hypoxia and circulatory inadequacy. Aspiration of freshwater or seawater leads to abnormal surfactant function [37] causing alveolar collapse, atelectasis, intrapulmonary shunting, and ventilation-perfusion mismatch. Aspiration of gastric contents or caustic materials may also contribute to pulmonary injury and contribute to the development of ALI or ARDS. Victims who drown in water contaminated with bacteria or fungi may go on to develop pneumonia or other systemic infections [38, 39], while victims who drown in sterile water but require mechanical ventilation may be at risk for the development of ventilator associated pneumonia. Prophylactic antibiotics do not appear to affect outcome however, and are not recommended [40–42].

Cardiovascular System

The cardiovascular system in drowning survivors is initially characterized by low cardiac index, elevated right and left heart filling pressures, and elevated systemic and pulmonary vascular resistance [43]. Studies in animals show that the detrimental effect on the heart and cardiovascular system from submersion injury is primarily due to hypoxia rather than due to hemodilution or hypo or hypervolemia [44, 45]. Associated hypothermia may lead to bradycardia, asystole, or ventricular fibrillation. The degree to which such cardiovascular dysfunction is reversible after initial resuscitation is related to the length of the anoxic insult as well as the effects of hypothermia and the effectiveness of resuscitation. Examination of the hearts of patients who died due to drowning revealed pathologic changes suggestive of coronary arterial spasm and focal myocyte injury [46], but permanent myocardial dysfunction is rare in survivors.

Central Nervous System

The global hypoxic-ischemic brain injury that can occur in drowning survivors is the most devastating morbidity. During the first minutes, the brain is deprived of oxygen. As the cardiovascular system fails, cerebral blood flow decreases and ischemic injury ensues. Experimentally, hypoxia and ischemia have different effects on the brain. Ischemia leads to an elevation in extracellular glutamate concentrations, which is thought to be directly related to neuronal damage. However, severe hypoxia without ischemia does not lead to elevated extracellular glutamate levels [47] or pathologic changes [47, 48]. This may explain some of he variability in outcomes among victims who suffer near fatal drowning episodes.

Metabolic activity and selective vulnerability to hypoxic-ischemic injury within the brain varies between regions, white matter and gray matter, and is also a function of age. Areas of greatest susceptibility to ischemic injury are usually in vascular end-zones leading to so-called "watershed" infarctions, as well as hippocampus, insular cortex, and basal ganglia. Even within the hippocampus, important for memory and learning, there are widely varying vulnerabilities to hypoxic-ischemia damage [49]. With greater severity of hypoxia-ischemia, more extensive and global neocortical damage will occur.

Clinical Evaluation and Decision Making

Many attempts to define clinical, epidemiological, or laboratory variables that predict which victims of submersion injury should be resuscitated and treated, either at the scene of the injury, in the emergency department, or in the intensive care unit have been evaluated. While there is general agreement that attempts at resuscitation at the scene are nearly always appropriate unless the victim is clearly dead, the degree to which aggressive resuscitation should be pursued and how long it should be continues is an ongoing source of debate. At all times, the potential for loss of patients with unpredictable good outcomes must be weighed against the risk of prolonging death or of survival with devastating neurologic outcome. For emergency departments that are not located in tertiary pediatric facilities, the financial and emotional burdens of transporting patients who clearly will have a very poor outcome to tertiary care centers at some distance must be weighted against the need for both caregivers and family to feel that everything possible has been done to ensure the best possible outcome for the victim.

Numerous reports and case series have documented the intact survival of some children who receive successful cardiopulmonary resuscitation (CPR) in the field, particularly those children who are submerged in cold water [50, 51]. Although reports of survival without neurologic sequelae after prolonged submersion in icy water are dramatic [50, 52–54], in most children hypothermia is a poor prognostic sign [55–57]. Hypothermic protection is dependent on slowing cerebral metabolism before irreversible hypoxic-ischemic injury has occurred and is thought to occur only in the most frigid water. Generally victims have fallen through ice or have remained above water for a time while being cooled.

Small children have a large surface area to mass ratio and will cool more quickly than adults, so they may become hypothermic in more moderate waters. Additionally, temperature variability in various regions should be considered, as there are some reports of intact survival after prolonged submersion in usually temperate climates [58]. Given the

difficulty of predicting outcome of hypothermic victims in the field, most authors recommend attempting resuscitation of all victims of drowning despite initial presentation unless they are clearly dead.

Various attempts at defining which children should be further resuscitated in the emergency department have failed to clearly discriminate intact survivors from non-survivors and severely impaired survivors [59, 60]. Demographic characteristics (age and gender), historical factors (duration of submersion, time to resuscitation, CPR at scene), and clinical parameters (Glasgow Coma Score, arterial pH, serum glucose, need for continued CPR or cardiotonic medications) have been examined as possible factors that might discriminate those children who will survive with a good outcome from those who will be severely neurologically damaged or dead. The presence of coma or fixed and dilated pupils in the emergency department has been suggested by some to accurately discriminate those patients who died or had severe neurologic injury from intact survivors [61, 62], but this finding has proven unreliable in other studies and case reports [51, 58, 63]. Similarly, although the Glasgow Coma Score (GCS) assigned in the emergency department is low in patients who do poorly, it does not reliably discriminate between intact survivors and those with poor outcome [51, 58, 64]. The need for continued CPR in the emergency department was reported to accurately predict poor neurologic outcome [62, 65], but other series document intact survival in some patients who receive CPR in the emergency department [51, 63]. The need for continued CPR after warm water submersion is associated with a higher likelihood of poor neurologic outcome than is the need for CPR after icy coldwater submersion [51, 56, 61, 62].

Orlowski described a scoring system which combined age, submersion time, time to resuscitation, coma on admission to the ED, and pH, and found it could reasonably predict a group of patients who would do well and a group who would do poorly [59, 66]. The score relied on knowledge of length of submersion and time to resuscitation, historical factors which are frequently not accurately known. In a large retrospective review of data from the emergency department of 274 near drowning patients, Christensen et al. [67] constructed a clinical classification system comprised of a physical exam score (apnea and coma), need for CPR in the ED, and pH (<7.0) which had a 93 % overall accuracy. However, no combination of variables they examined could accurately discriminate all intact survivors from all those with poor outcomes.

Extrapolating from studies of pediatric out-of-hospital cardiac arrests, there is increased survival observed when CPR is not needed after arrival to the hospital, no atropine is needed, three or fewer doses of epinephrine are used, and shorter duration of CPR [57, 68]. Among all children with HIE-related arrest, the PPV for poor neurologic outcome with initial CPR > 10 min has been reported as high as 91 % [68]. Because there is no one factor or combination of factors which have been identified to reliably predict good versus poor outcome with a high degree of certainty, some have advocated that resuscitation be attempted, at least briefly, in all patients who arrive in the emergency department after submersion injury [51, 63, 69]. All known clinical variables should be taken into account when deciding how aggressively to resuscitate. It is generally recommended that resuscitation be continued until the victim has been rewarmed to 33–35 °C.

Treatment

Scene

At the scene, mouth-to-mouth breathing of an apneic victim should be attempted even while the victim is in the water, and the victim should be removed from the water as quickly as possible. If possible, victims should be removed from the water in a horizontal position [22]. No attempts to drain water from the lungs should be made before pulmonary resuscitation begins. The Heimlich maneuver should not be performed except where airway obstruction is suspected [70]. Once the victim is on solid ground, chest compressions should be begun if there is no palpable pulse. Because of the intense vasoconstriction that may be present in the hypothermic victim, the carotid pulse should be sought. Further advanced life support measures such as tracheal intubation, defibrillation, or intravenous or intraosseous medications or fluids should be undertaken as indicated if personnel capable of performing such interventions are present. In the presence of core temperature <28 °C defibrillation may not be effective. Further heat loss should be avoided en route to a hospital and all equipment and fluids in contact with the victim should be warmed. Severely hypothermic victims (temperature <32 °C) should not be placed in a warm shower or bath in attempts to re-warm them.

Emergency Department

In the emergency department, standard airway, ventilatory, and cardiovascular resuscitative measures should be instituted as indicated, and particular attention paid in the near drowning patient to the possibility of trauma and to re-warming if necessary. As the patient is being re-warmed, close attention should be paid to acid-base status, electrolytes, and cardiac rhythm and overall cardiovascular status. Hypothermic patients who are hemodynamically stable may be re-warmed slowly via external means—warmed humidified inspired gas, warmed intravenous fluids (40–42 °C), and

warm cloth blankets or convective or radiant warming systems.

Hypothermic patients in cardiac arrest or with an otherwise unstable cardiovascular system should be warmed more aggressively. Such methods include bladder irrigation, gastric lavage, pleural lavage, or peritoneal lavage with warmed isotonic fluid. Extracorporeal re-warming (cardiopulmonary bypass or extra-corporeal membrane oxygenation) may be performed and there are several reports of extra-ordinary survival after near drowning using such a strategy [50, 54, 71, 72].

There are large case series of severely hypothermic patients being re-warmed with cardiopulmonary bypass with a survival of 45–60 % [73] and generally favorable neurologic outcome [73, 74]. Although these large series represent a heterogeneous group of patients, most of them adults who were the victims of exposure hypothermia, near drowning victims had a similar outcome to the overall group and the data thus suggest that extracorporeal re-warming may be a valuable strategy in certain circumstances.

If high impact trauma is suspected, cervical spine immobilization should be instituted as quickly as possible in the field or the emergency department. Assessment of neurologic status during therapy, including brainstem reflexes, Glasgow Coma Score, and a detailed examination if possible may aid in delineating the individual patients prognosis and will serve as a reference later in the course of care.

The clinical course of the drowning victim is determined primarily by the duration of hypoxic-ischemic injury and by the adequacy of initial resuscitation. Some children with brief submersions will begin breathing as soon as they are removed from the water or after brief positive pressure ventilation, and arrive in the Emergency Department alert and awake. Others will require more aggressive intervention. Children who appear well but who have sustained significant submersion and possible aspiration should be observed closely for at least 6–12 h for respiratory distress. Those discharged from the emergency department should be instructed to return if they develop respiratory distress, cough, or fever as some may develop bronchospasm or pneumonia.

Intensive Care Unit

Children who are admitted to the ICU should be monitored for the presence or development of lung injury or cardiovascular instability. Pulmonary dysfunction in the immediate post-injury period is the result ventilation-perfusion (V/Q) mismatch due to atelectasis, aspiration, or pulmonary edema. Pulmonary edema may result from increased capillary permeability, aspiration, massive fluid overload, or myocardial failure. Increasing inspired oxygen concentration alone may not resolve hypoxemia if significant V/Q mismatch is present, and prolonged use of high inspired oxygen concentrations may worsen pulmonary injury. Children who are alert and ventilating adequately may benefit from mask continuous positive airway pressure (CPAP) with a nasogastric tube to prevent gastric distention. Ongoing hypoxemia or impaired ventilation requires endotracheal intubation and mechanical ventilation. Pulmonary sequelae of near drowning may include bronchospasm, fulminant but transient pulmonary edema, aspiration or infectious pneumonia, or acute respiratory distress syndrome (ARDS), alone or in combination. Although there is general concordance between the severity of the lung injury with the severity of the neurologic injury sustained in many patients, victims may develop significant pulmonary pathology and not have suffered neurologic injury.

Ventilation strategies that are used in the setting of traumatic brain injury may be detrimental to those with hypoxic-ischemic brain injury. Hypercapnia may be avoided in potentially brain-injured children, though there is not evidence to suggest that mild or moderate hyperventilation improves neurologic outcome after hypoxic-ischemic brain injury. Since most evidence suggests that the neurologic insult after hypoxic-ischemic injury is primarily determined by the initial primary insult and that increased ICP after hypoxic-ischemic injury is uncommon but ominous, the strategy of mechanical ventilation should focus on preventing ventilator induced lung injury.

In the ICU, cardiovascular instability may be the result of impaired myocardial contractility due to the hypoxic-ischemic event; ongoing hypoxemia, hypothermia, or acidosis; low intravascular volume, or electrolyte abnormalities. Fluid resuscitation and inotropic or pressor agents may be required to restore adequate tissue perfusion. Invasive monitoring, such as an arterial catheter, central venous catheter, or echocardiography should be tailored to the needs of the individual patient.

The majority of long-term morbidity and mortality after drowning is due to hypoxic-ischemic brain injury. Neuro-resuscitative strategies that have been applied to victims of hypoxic-ixchemic brain injury have included ICP monitoring and management, barbiturates, hypothermia, calcium channel blockers, free-radical scavengers, and others.

Conn [75] proposed a therapy based on observations that submersion victims were hyperhydrated, hyperventilating, hyperexcitable, and hyper rigid. HYPER therapy included fluid restriction, hyperventilation, hypothermia, barbiturate coma, glucocorticoids, muscle paralysis, and monitoring and treatment of elevated ICP. Subsequent reviews or prospective evaluations of hypothermia and barbiturate therapy in drowning failed to show improvement in outcome with these therapies [76, 77].

Despite early animal data supporting the use of barbiturates in global ischemia [78], the use of barbiturates after out of hospital cardiac arrest has not been beneficial in humans [79]. Corticosteroids were advocated in the past to treat cerebral edema after submersion injury [28, 75] but subsequent data in both humans and animals failed to demonstrate any benefit of steroids in hypoxic ischemic brain injury but did suggest an increased incidence of infection [40, 69].

Despite early enthusiasm for its use, intracranial pressure (ICP) monitoring and aggressive treatment of intracranial hypertension has proven not to be of benefit to victims of drowning [63, 76, 80–82]. While prognostically, high ICP correlates with poor neurologic outcome or death, initial ICPs of less than 20 do not indicate good outcome [63, 80] and ICP monitoring has fallen out of favor for victims of hypoxic-ischemic brain injury. Connors et al. [83] extended monitoring to include global cerebral blood flow, cross-brain oxygen content difference (CBO_2D), cerebral metabolic rate for oxygen ($CMRO_2$), ICP, and cerebral perfusion pressure (CPP) and evaluated the relationship of these parameters to outcome in 12 nearly drowned children. They found no differences in global CBF, ICP, or CPP between normal survivors and those who died or were severely affected. Those who survived with functional neurologic outcome had higher CBO_2D at 24 h and higher $CMRO_2$ at 48 h, though neither measurement completely discriminated between those with good and those with poor outcome.

Recent data on the therapeutic benefit of mild hypothermia on adult victims of cardiac arrest [84, 85] has renewed interest in the potential benefits of this therapy. In two prominent studies, patients who had been successfully resuscitated from ventricular fibrillation were randomly assigned to undergo therapeutic hypothermia (target 32–34 °C) or standard treatment. The treatment was associated with higher survival to hospital discharge and improved neurologic outcome. An earlier trial of hypothermia after traumatic brain injury did not demonstrated any benefit [86], but there were some methodological concerns regarding this trial, and a trial of therapeutic hypothermia after cardiac arrest in pediatric patients is currently in progress. Current temperature management of pediatric patients with severe submersion injury includes avoidance of hyperthermia, however, use of therapeutic hypothermia not currently standard of care and there are theoretical potential risks associated with its use, including infection and coagulopathy.

In summary, the precise outcome for victims of a significant drowning event may be difficult to determine in the first hours of treatment, although prolonged cardiopulmonary resuscitation, fixed and dilated pupils, and GCS of 3 suggest a poor outcome. Attention to general supportive measures, including adequacy of oxygenation with optimal ventilator strategies to minimize lung injury, cardiovascular support, and avoidance of iatrogenic complications may help to minimize secondary brain injury. Attempts at management of intracranial pressure or specific neuro-resuscitative strategies have been unsuccessful in improving outcomes. Therapeutic hypothermia may be beneficial but as yet we have no data that is specific to hypoxic-ischemic brain injury in the pediatric population.

Predicting Long-Term Outcome

Prediction of the long-term neurologic outcome of drowning victims is a common and often difficult problem in the intensive care unit. Prediction of functional independence versus death or severe disability becomes more reliable with time as the child is treated and recovery or response or lack of response to therapy is observed. The key sources of information for prognostication come from clinical exam findings, radiographic data, and neurophysiologic studies. No individual piece of data has sufficient positive predictive value or specificity to warrant decision-making without consideration of other contextual information.

The neurologic examination, including pupillary response, best motor response, and GCS, often provides very reliable information to predict neurologic outcome within the first 24–72 h. In general, these clinical features have greater positive predictive value for poor neurologic outcomes (typically defined as death, persistent vegetative state, or disability requiring significant dependence). The absence of these findings does not necessarily predict good neurologic outcome. Much of the current information regarding neurologic prognostication in children with severe brain injury is derived from heterogeneous studies, where hypoxic-ischemic encephalopathy (HIE) (including drowning) may make up only one third to one half of the study population. Study findings are only included in this chapter if there were no identifiable differences in subset evaluation between HIE-related brain injury and other causes (most notably traumatic brain injury).

Clinical Neurologic Examination

Absent pupillary response at 24 h portends a poor prognosis in adults, and this is the earliest clinical feature included in the American Academy of Neurology's Practice Parameter [87] for prognostication after post-cardiac arrest coma. While absent pupillary response has not been validated across different age groups within pediatrics, smaller prospective studies suggest that this may be a predictive sign. Absent pupillary response has a predictive value ranging from 96 % to 100 %, although the time point at which it is reported varies (range 24 h–9 days post-injury) [68, 88]. A bilaterally absent, pupillary response is helpful to the clinician when it is observed; however, this finding is not as common as an abnormal motor response.

Absent motor response or extensor posturing to noxious stimuli at 72 h has been well demonstrated to predict poor outcome in adults, and is one of the clinical criteria used by the AAN for prognostication of comatose survivors [87]. In a retrospective series of 44 warm-water near drowning victims admitted to a PICU, all survivors with good neurologic outcome had spontaneous, purposeful movement within 24 h after submersion [64]. All children without spontaneous, purposeful movements within 24 h had severe neurologic deficits or died. Additional studies are less definitive. In additional pediatric studies of brain injury from multiple causes, the finding of absent motor response to noxious stimuli at 24 h or later had PPV ranging from 80 % to 100 % [88, 89]. A best motor response of flexor or extensor posturing is more nebulous, and there is insufficient data about the predictive value of this finding.

While a number of investigators have noted that a GCS ≤5 on presentation to the ED identified patients at high risk for poor outcome [51, 63–65], that observation may not be sufficiently discriminatory to support the decision to withhold or withdraw treatment. Lavelle [51] and Allman [63] noted that GCS ≤5 on arrival in the PICU was more predictive of poor neurologic outcome than was GCS in the emergency department, though again perhaps still not sufficiently discriminatory to withhold or withdraw treatment. Lavelle noted 3 of 20 patients with a GCS of 5 on arrival in the ICU had a good outcome (no patients with GCS of 3 or 4 had good outcome), and Allman noted that while no patients admitted to the ICU with a GCS of 3 had a good outcome, 12 of 24 patients with a GCS or 4 or 5 survived neurologically intact. The GCS has been reported to have its highest positive predictive value at 24 h after admission in a single prospective study of children with HIE-related coma, with scores of <5 having a PPV of 100 % for poor neurologic outcome [68]. A GCS of greater than 5 on arrival in the ED or ICU is highly predictive of good neurologic outcome [51, 63–65]. Children who sustain significant pulmonary injury and require mechanical ventilation and significant sedation or muscle relaxation pose a difficult challenge. Interpretation of clinical information can be limited while patients remain on these medications. Additional neurophysiologic testing or imaging may be appropriate if decisions regarding continuation or withdrawal of treatment are being considered.

Neuroradiology

Neuroimaging may aid in prognostication in the ICU setting. While computed tomography (CT) of the brain and neck is indicated in the ED or ICU if there is a history or suggestion of trauma, the role of CT in the early evaluation of hypoxic-ischemic injury in the drowning victim is limited. In a study of CT among children admitted to the ICU after drowning,

18 % were noted to have abnormal CT scans within the first 24 h, mostly consisting of diffuse absence of cortical grey-white differentiation, basal ganglia edema, or basal ganglia infarct. All of these patients had a GCS of 3 and subsequently died [90]. Edema related to hypoxic-ischemic damage may not be initially present and abnormalities may only emerge on subsequent imaging. A normal CT scan within the first 24 h does not have predictive value. Although abnormal CT may identify some of those who have sustained severe injury, the majority of patients will initially have normal studies regardless of outcome [91, 92].

Magnetic Resonance Imaging (MRI) may be more useful than CT in predicting prognosis [93, 94] though it must be used in conjunction with clinical and physiologic data [87]. The use of diffusion weighted imaging (DWI) sequences along with standard T2-weighted images, has become a standard for early evaluation of infarction (hours after injury until 7–10 days post-anoxia). Regions of vulnerability to ischemic damage include the watershed regions and basal ganglia. The watershed lesions occur mainly in the arterial border zones of major cerebral arteries, generally in vessel end zones in the depth of the sulci. Lesions appear hyperintense on T2-weighted imaging. Besides obvious signal change, other radiographic features include basal ganglia edema and indistinct margins of the grey matter, which may be better seen on T1-weighted images. In the chronic phase (> 2 weeks from initial injury), MRI may show other morphologic changes, including parenchymal atrophy, laminar necrosis, ventriculomegaly, and enlargement of the cisterns and sulci. Dubowitz et al. [94] performed serial brain MRI on 22 children admitted to the ICU after drowning, and Christophe et al. [95] studied MRI in 40 comatose children with any non-traumatic brain injury. Both found a high positive predictive value (92–100 %) for poor outcome when there were radiographically definite signs of watershed and/or basal ganglia infarct in both the acute (day1–3) or subacute (day 4–7) periods. There were fewer false negatives with MRI when imaging was performed on day 4 or later [95]. MRI retained high predictive value in the subgroup of infants. Infants additionally were more likely to also have edema and necrosis of white matter, suggesting a particular vulnerability of areas still undergoing active myelination. Magnetic resonance spectroscopy (MRS) can show an increased lactate or glutatamine/glutamate peak or decreased NAA or creatine peak after significant ischemic damage. MRS showed good correlation with the above MR findings [94] when completed at least 3 days after injury, although it has not been demonstrated that MRS enhances the overall accuracy compared to MRI alone.

In summary, routine MRI with diffusion weighted imaging is the preferred radiologic modality to help with prognostication. The presence of abnormal findings in the first 3 days has significant predictive value, but deferring MRI until 4 days after injury will decrease the likelihood of falsely reassuring families.

Neurophysiology

The early role of EEG is often limited due to use of sedatives, analgesics, and muscle relaxants during resuscitation and early treatment, especially if there is significant pulmonary injury. A single EEG lacks specificity and needs to be interpreted within the full clinical context. While a flat, severely attenuated EEG or burst suppression record is often a poor prognostic indicator, during the initial 24 h it more commonly reflects the initial insult and resuscitation. Repeating an EEG after 24–48 h, or performing an extended study, may help to establish the persistence of abnormal findings and help determine if favorable features, such as normal environmental reactivity and sleep-wake changes emerge. Persistent burst suppression, severe attenuation, or electrocerebral silence are predictive of a poor neurologic prognosis [96]. Additionally, the finding of discontinuity (alternating pattern of severe background attenuation with periods of relatively preserved activity) and lack of reactivity are predictive of poor outcome [68, 97]. Discontinuous activity and loss of reactivity on sequential EEGs had high predictive value for poor outcome (96–100 %) [68]; however, this has not been replicated and the sensitivity of these diagnostic findings are relatively low. There is significant intra-study variability about the predictive value of various EEG findings for poor outcome, ranging from 50 % to 100 % [98]. This likely reflects differences in timing of EEG, intervals between repeated EEGs, and differences in subjective interpretation. Additional obstacles to the interpretation of EEG include scalp edema or subdural collections, particularly when trauma has been associated with drowning.

Somatosensory evoked potentials (SEPs) may be more accurate in predicting outcome in children who have suffered hypoxic-ischemic brain injury [99, 100]. SEP interpretation is not affected by co-administration of sedating or analgesic agents, which offers a potential advantage to relying on clinical exam findings, EEG, or other evoked potentials. The finding of a bilaterally absent N20 peak on SEP has shown high predictive value (83–100 %) for poor outcome in children with severe brain injury of all causes. The predictive value of SEPs increases on subsequent studies (PPV 92–100 % on final study) [68, 88, 89], although the PPV has been demonstrated to be >80 % within the first 2 days. Normal SEPs also show good predictive value (93–100 %) for favorable outcome at any time point [88, 89]. Absent N20 was more sensitive than absent motor response or pupillary response for predicting poor outcome [88]. Intermediate results of SEP (increased latency of N20, unilateral absence of N20 peak) do not have predictive value. False positive results from SEP have resulted from structural barriers to electrical recording, such as subdural fluid collections or following decompressive craniotomy. A normal N13 peak must be confirmed to exclude that the possibility that an absent signal results from a peripheral lesion.

The use of brainstem auditory-evoked response (BAER) in hypoxic-ischemic brain injury remains controversial. BAER testing has been investigated as a method of quantifying global cerebral injury after drowning [101] as well as pediatric coma from any cause [68], but the predictive value is limited. While it may be useful in differentiating survival from death, it is less useful in predicting poor neurocognitive outcome among survivors. There are reported cases of children with eventual persistent vegetative state who had normal BAER with bilaterally absent N20 on SEP. Furthermore, BAER can be altered by both central and peripheral auditory disorders and there is some evidence that BAERs are particularly vulnerable to hypoxia in young patients [102].

One of the greatest challenges in caring for the drowning victim is identifying reliable early predictors of either good or poor neurologic prognosis to aid in clinical decision making. Serial neurologic examination remains one of the most accurate and reproducible methods available for assessment. There is an inherent dichotomy between finding the earliest clinical predictors and the most accurate ones, sometimes necessitating additional time and further reassessment. When the clinical course is uncertain by clinical examination alone, adjunctive tests are often helpful. MRI, and when available, SEP can be particularly useful to clinicians when the physical examination is inconsistent or obscured by medication effect.

References

1. Van Beeck EF, Branche CM, Szpilman D, Modell JH, Bierens JJ. A new definition of drowning: towards documentation and prevention of a global public health problem. Bull WHO. 2005;83(11):853–6.
2. Idris AH, Berg RA, Bierens J, American Heart Association, et al. Recommended guidelines for uniform reporting of data from drowning: the "Utstein" style. Circulation. 2003;108(20):2565–74.
3. Peden MM, McGee K. The epidemiology of drowning worldwide. Inj Control Saf Promot. 2003;10:195–9.
4. Centers for Disease Control, National Center for Injury Prevention and Control: WISQARS. http://www.cdc.gov/injury/wisqars/index.html. Accessed July 2011.
5. Brenner RQ, Trumble AC, Smith GS, Kessler EP, et al. Where children drown. Pediatrics. 2001;108:85–9.
6. Thompson DC, Rivara FP. Pool fencing for preventing drowning in children. Cochrane Database Syst Rev. 2000;2, CD001047.
7. Pearn J, Bart R, Yamaoka R. Drowning risks to epileptic children: a study from Hawaii. BMJ. 1978;2:1284–5.
8. Kurokawa T, Fung KC, Hanai T, Goya N. Mortality and clinical features in cases of death among epileptic children. Brain Dev. 1982;4:321–5.
9. Orlowski JP, Rothner AD, Lueders H. Submersion accidents in children with epilepsy. Am J Dis Child. 1982;136:777–80.
10. Diekema D, Quan L, Holt V. Epilepsy as a risk factor for submersion injury in children. Pediatrics. 1993;91:612–6.
11. Sillanpää M, Jalava M, Kaleva O, Shinnar S. Long-term prognosis of seizures with onset in childhood. N Engl J Med. 1998;338:1715–22.
12. Ackerman MJ, Schroeder JJ, Berry R, Schaid DJ, et al. A novel mutation in KVLQT1 is the molecular basis of inherited long QT syndrome in a near-drowning patient's family. Pediatr Res. 1988;44:148–53.
13. Ackerman MJ, Tester DJ, Porter CJ. Swimming, a gene-specific arrhythmogenic trigger for inherited long QT syndrome. Mayo Clin Proc. 1999;74:1088–94.
14. Ackerman MJ, Tester DJ, Porter CJ, Edwards WD. Molecular diagnosis of the inherited Long-QT syndrome in a woman who died after near-drowning. N Engl J Med. 1999;34:1121–5.
15. Lunetta P, Levo A, Laitinen PJ, et al. Molecular screening of selected long QT syndrome (LQTS) mutations in 165 consecutive bodies found in water. Int J Legal Med. 2003;117:115–7.
16. Mulligan-Smith D, Pepe PE, Branche CM. A seven-year, statewide study of the epidemiology of pediatric drowning deaths. Acad Emerg Med. 2002;9:488–9.
17. Fields AI. Near-drowning in the pediatric population. Crit Care Clin. 1992;8:113–29.
18. Fiser DH. Near-drowning. Pediatr Rev. 1993;14:148–51.
19. Vander Krol L, Wolfe R. The emergency department management of near-hanging victims. J Emerg Med. 1994;12:285–92.
20. Aufderheide TP, Aprahamian C, Mateer JR, Rudnick E, and others. Emergency airway management in hanging victims. Ann Emerg Med. 1994;24:879–884.
21. Watson RS, Cummings P, Quan L, Bratton S. Cervical spine injuries among submersion victims. J Trauma. 2001;51:658–62.
22. Golden F, Tipton MJ, Scott RC. Immersion, near-drowning and drowning. Br J Anaesth. 1997;79:214–25.
23. Karpovich PV. Water in the lungs of drowned animals. Arch Pathol. 1933;15:828–33.
24. Lougheed DW. Physiological studies in experimental asphyxia and drowning. Can Med Assoc J. 1939;40:423–8.
25. Orlowski JP. Drowning, near-drowning, and ice-water submersions. Pediatr Clin North Am. 1987;34:75–92.
26. Swan HG, Brucer M, Moore C, et al. Fresh water and sea water drowning: a study of the terminal cardiac and biochemical events. Tex Rep Biol Med. 1947;5:423–37.
27. Swan HG, Spafford NR. Body salt and water changes during fresh and sea water drowning. Tex Rep Biol Med. 1951;9:356–82.
28. Modell JH, Davis JH, Giammona ST, et al. Blood gas and electrolyte changes in human near-drowning victims. JAMA. 1968;203:99–105.
29. Modell JH, Davis JH. Electrolyte changes in human drowning victims. Anesthesiology. 1969;30:414–20.
30. Bonnor R, Siddiqui M, Ahuja TS. Rhabdomyolysis: a late complication of near-drowning [Case Reports]. Am J Med Sci. 1999;318:201.
31. Lester JL. Rhabdomyolysis: a late complication of near-drowning [Case Review]. J Emerg Nurs. 2002;28:280–3.
32. Conn AW, Miyasaka M, Katayama M, et al. A canine study of cold water drowning in fresh versus salt water. Crit Care Med. 1995;23:2029–37.
33. Biggar W, Bohn DJ, Kent F. Neutrophil circulation and release from bone marrow during hypothermia. Infect Immun. 1983;40:708–12.
34. Giesbrecht GG. Cold stress, near drowning and accidental hypothermia: a review. Aviat Space Environ Med. 2000;71:733–51.
35. Steinman AM. Cardiopulmonary resuscitation and hypothermia. Circulation. 1986;74:VI29–32.
36. Hayward JS, Hay C, Matthews BR, Overweel CH, et al. Temperature effect on the human dive response in relation to cold water near-drowning. J Appl Physiol. 1984;56:202–6.

37. Giammona ST, Modell JH. Drowning by total immersion: effects on pulmonary surfactant of distilled water, isotonic saline, and sea water. Am J Dis Child. 1967;114:612–6.

38. Kowacs PA, Monteiro de Almeida S, Pinheiro RL, et al. Central nervous system *Aspergillus fumigatus* infection after near drowning. J Clin Pathol. 2004;57:202–4.

39. Kowacs PA, Soares-Silverado CE, Monteiro de Almeida S, et al. Infection of the CNS by Scedosporium apiospermum after near drowning: report of a fatal case and analysis of its confounding factors. J Clin Pathol. 2004;57:205–7.

40. Modell JH, Graves SA, Ketovar A. Clinical course of 91 consecutive near-drowning victims. Chest. 1976;70:231–8.

41. Ender PT, Dolan MJ. Pneumonia associated with near-drowning. Clin Infect Dis. 1997;25:896–907.

42. van Berkel M, Bierens JJL, Lie RLK, de Rooy TP, et al. Pulmonary oedema, pneumonia and mortality in submersion victims: a retrospective study in 125 patients. Intensive Care Med. 1996;22:101–7.

43. Lucking SE, Pollack MM, Fields AI. Shock following generalized hypoxic-ischemic injury in previously healthy infants and children. J Pediatr. 1986;108:359–64.

44. Orlowski JP, Abulleil MM, Phillips JM. Effect of tonicities of saline solutions on pulmonary injury in drowning. Crit Care Med. 1987;15:126–30.

45. Orlowski JP, Abulleil MM, Phillips JM. The hemodynamic and cardiovascular effects of near-drowning in hypotonic, isotonic, or hypertonic solutions. Ann Emerg Med. 1989;18:1044–9.

46. Lunt DW, Rose AG. Pathology of the human heart in drowning. Arch Pathol Lab Med. 1987;111:939–42.

47. Pearigen P, Ryder G, Simon RP. The effects in vivo of hypoxia on brain injury. Brain Res. 1996;725:184–91.

48. Miyamoto O, Auer RN. Hypoxia, hyperoxia, ischemia, and brain necrosis. Neurology. 2000;54:362–71.

49. Kreisman NR, Soliman S, Gozal D. Regional differences in hypoxic depolarization and swelling in hippocampal slices. J Neurophysiol. 2000;83:1031–8.

50. Bolte RG, Black PG, Bowers RS, Thorne JK, et al. The use of extracorporeal rewarming in a child submerged for 66 minutes. JAMA. 1988;260:377–9.

51. Lavelle JM, Shaw KN. Near drowning: is emergency department cardiopulmonary resuscitation or intensive care unit cerebral resuscitation indicated? Crit Care Med. 1993;21:368–73.

52. Siebke J, Breivik H, Rod T, et al. Survival after 40 minutes submersion without cerebral sequelae. Lancet. 1975;1:1275.

53. Corneli HM. Accidental hypothermia. J Pediatr. 1992;120:671–9.

54. Thalmann M, Trampitsch E, Haberfellner N, Eisendle E, et al. Resuscitation in near drowning with extracorporeal membrane oxygenation. Ann Thorac Surg. 2001;71:607–8.

55. Biggart MJ, Bohn DJ. Effect of hypothermia and cardiac arrest on outcome of near-drowning accidents in children. J Pediatr. 1990;117:179–83.

56. Quan L, Wentz KR, Gore EJ, Copass MK. Outcome and predictors of outcome in pediatric submersion victims receiving pre-hospital care in King County, Washington. Pediatrics. 1990;86:586–93.

57. Moler FW, Donaldson AE, Dean JM, Pediatric Emergency Care Applied Research Network, et al. Multicenter cohort study of out-of-hospital pediatric cardiac arrest. Crit Care Med. 2011;39(1):141–9.

58. Modell JH, Idris AH, Pineda JA, Silverstein JH. Survival after prolonged submersion in freshwater in Florida. Chest. 2004;125:1948–51.

59. Orlowski JP. Prognostic factors in pediatric cases of drowning and near-drowning. JACEP. 1979;8:176–9.

60. Conn AW, Montes JE, Barker GA, Edmonds JF. Cerebral salvage in near-drowning following neurological classification by triage. Can Anaesth Soc J. 1980;27:201–10.

61. Frates Jr RC. Analysis of predictive factors in the assessment of warm-water near drowning in children. Am J Dis Child. 1981;135:1006–8.

62. Nichter MA, Perry EB. Childhood near-drowning: is cardiopulmonary resuscitation always indicated? Crit Care Med. 1989;17:993–5.

63. Allman FD, Nelson WB, Pacentine GA, McComb G, et al. Outcome following cardiopulmonary resuscitation in severe pediatric near drowning. Am J Dis Child. 1986;140:571–5.

64. Bratton SL, Jardine DS, Morray JP. Serial neurologic examinations after near drowning and outcome. Arch Pediatr Adolesc Med. 1994;148:167–70.

65. Petersen B. Morbidity of childhood near-drowning. Pediatrics. 1977;59:364–70.

66. Dean JM, Kaufman ND. Prognostic indicators in pediatric near-drowning: the Glasgow Coma Scale. Crit Care Med. 1981;9:536–9.

67. Christensen DW, Jansen P, Perken RM. Outcome and acute care hospital costs after warm water near drowning in children. Pediatrics. 1997;99:715–21.

68. Mandel R, Martinot A, Delepoulle F, Lamblin M, Laureau e, Vallee L, Leclerc F. Prediction of outcome after hypoxic-ischemic encephalopathy: a prospective clinical and electrophysiologic study. J Pediatr. 2002;141(1):45–50.

69. Oakes DD, Sherck JP, Maloney JR, Charters 3 AC. Prognosis and management of victims of near drowning. J Trauma. 1982;22:544–9.

70. Rosen P, Stoto M, Harley J. The use of the Heimlich maneuver in near drowning: institute of medicine report. J Emerg Med. 1995;13:397–405.

71. Kumle B, Doring B, Mertes H, Posival H. Resuscitation of a near-drowning patient by the use of a portable extracorporeal circulation device [German]. Anasthesiol Intensivmed Notfallmed Schmerzther. 1997;32:754–6.

72. Wollenek G, Honarwar N, Golej J, Marx M. Cold water submersion and cardiac arrest in treatment of severe hypothermia with cardiopulmonary bypass. Resuscitation. 2002;52:255–63.

73. Vretenar DF, Urschel JD, Parrott JCW, Unruth HW. Cardiopulmonary bypass resuscitation for accidental hypothermia. Ann Thorac Surg. 1994;58:895–8.

74. Letsou GV, Kopf GS, Elefteriades JA, et al. Is cardiopulmonary bypass effective for treatment of hypothermic arrest due to drowning or exposure? Arch Surg. 1992;127:525–8.

75. Conn AW, Edmonds JF, Barker GA. Cerebral resuscitation in near-drowning. Pediatr Clin North Am. 1979;26:691–701.

76. Bohn DJ, Biggar WD, Smith CR, Conn AW, et al. Influence of hypothermia, barbituate therapy, and intracranial pressure monitoring on morbidity and mortality after near-drowning. Crit Care Med. 1986;14:529–34.

77. Nussbaum E, Maggi JC. Pentobarbitol therapy does not improve neurologic outcome in nearly drowned, flaccid-comatose children. Pediatrics. 1988;81:630–4.

78. Bleyaert AL, Nemoto EM, Safar P, Stezoski SM, et al. Thiopental amelioration of brain damage after global ischemia in monkeys. Anesthesiology. 1978;49:390–8.

79. Randomized clinical study of thiopental loading in comatose survivors of cardiac arrest, brain resuscitation clinical trial I study group. N Engl J Med. 1986;314:397–403.

80. Nussbaum E, Gallant SP. Intracranial pressure monitoring as a guide to prognosis in the nearly drowned, severely comatose child. J Pediatr. 1983;102:215–8.

81. Sarniak AP, Preston G, Lieh-Lai M, Eisenbrey AB. Intracranial pressure and cerebral perfusion pressure in near-drowning. Crit Care Med. 1985;13:224–7.

82. Frewen TC, Sumabat WO, Han VK, Amacher AL, et al. Cerebral resuscitation therapy in pediatric near-drowning. J Pediatr. 1985;106:615–7.

83. Connors R, Frewen TC, Kissoon N, Kronick J, et al. Relationship of cross-brain oxygen content difference, cerebral blood flow, and metabolic rate to neurologic outcome after near-drowning. J Pediatr. 1992;121:839–44.

84. Holzer M, Cerchiari E, Martens P, Group The Hypothermia after Cardiac Arrest Study. Mild therapeutic hypothermia to improve the neurologic outcome after cardiac arrest. N Engl J Med. 2002; 346:549–56.

85. Bernard, Stephen A, Gray Timothy W, Buist Michael D, et al. Treatment of comatose survivors of out-of-hospital cardiac arrest with induced hypothermia. N Engl J Med. 2002;346:557–63.

86. Clifton GL, Miller ER, Choi SC, et al. Lack of effect of induction of hypothermia after acute brain injury. N Engl J Med. 2001;344: 556–63.

87. Wijdicks EFM, Hijdra A, Young GB, Bassetti CL, Wiebe S. Practice parameter: prediction of outcome in comatose survivors after cardiopulmonary resuscitation (an evidence-based review): report of the quality standards subcommittee of the American Academy of Neurology. Neurology. 2006;67:203–10.

88. Carter BG, Butt W. A prospective study of outcome predictors after severe brain injury. Intensive Care Med. 2005;31:840–5.

89. Beca J, Cox PN, Taylor MJ, Bohn D, Butt W, Logan WJ, Rutka JT, Barker G. Somatosensory evoked potentials for prediction of outcome in acute severe brain injury. J Pediatr. 1995;126(1):44–9.

90. Rafaat KT, Spear RM, Kuelbs C, Parsapour K, Peterson B. Computed tomographic findings in a large group of children with drowning: diagnostic, prognostic, and forensic implications. Pediatr Crit Care Med. 2008;9:567–72.

91. Romano C, Brown T, Frewen TC. Assessment of pediatric near-drowning victims: is there a role for cranial CT? Pediatr Radiol. 1993;23:261–3.

92. Taylor SB, Quencer RM, Holzman BH, Naidich TP. Central nervous system anoxic-ischemic insult in children due to near-drowning. Radiology. 1985;156:641–6.

93. Kreis R, Arcinue E, Ernst T, Shonk TK, et al. Hypoxic encephalopathy after near-drowning studied by quantitative 1H-magnetic resonance spectroscopy. J Clin Invest. 1996;97:1142–54.

94. Dubowitz DJ, Bluml S, Arcinue E, Dietrich RB. MR of hypoxic encephalopathy in children after near drowning: correlation with quantitative proton MR spectroscopy and clinical outcome. Am J Neuroradiol. 1998;19:1617–27.

95. Christophe C, Fonteyne C, Ziereisen F, Christiaens F, Deltenre P, De Maertelaer V, Dan B. Value of MR imaging of the brain in children with hypoxic coma. Am J Neuroradiol. 2002;23: 716–23.

96. Kruus S, Bergstrom L, Suutarinen T, Hyvonen R. The prognosis of near-drowned children. Acta Paediatr Scand. 1979;68: 315–22.

97. Ramachandrannair R, Sharma R, Weiss SK, Cortez MA. Reactive EEG patterns in pediatric coma. Pediatr Neurol. 2005;33: 345–59.

98. Abend NS, Licht DJ. Predicting outcome in children with encephalopathy. Pediatr Crit Care Med. 2008;9(1):32–9.

99. De Meirleir LJ, Taylor MJ. Prognostic utility of SEPs in comatose children. Pediatr Neurol. 1987;3:78–82.

100. Taylor MJ, Farrell EJ. Comparison of the prognostic utility of VEPs and SEPs in comatose children. Pediatr Neurol. 1989;5: 145–50.

101. Fisher B, Peterson B, Hicks G. Use of brain-stem auditory-evoked response testing to assess neurologic outcome following near drowning in children. Crit Care Med. 1992;20:578–85.

102. Jacinto SJ, Gieron-Korthals M, Ferreira JA. Predicting outcome in hypoxic-ischemic brain injury. Pediatr Clin North Am. 2001;48: 647–60.

Heat Illness and Hypothermia

49

Luke A. Zabrocki, David K. Shellington,
and Susan L. Bratton

Abstract

Children have impaired ability for effective thermoregulation. Environmental exposures and impaired intrinsic thermoregulation can lead to the catastrophic consequences from heat and cold injuries. The most severe form of heat related injury, heat stroke, involves extreme hyperthermia, neurologic impairment and progression to systemic inflammation, disseminated intravascular coagulation and multiple organ dysfunction syndrome (MODS). The mechanism of injury involves the inflammatory cascade, heat shock proteins, gut endotoxin translocation, and the systemic effects of direct thermal injury. Immediate rapid cooling and support of organ function are the mainstays of treatment. Accidental cold injuries commonly present with associated trauma. Regional frostbite and systemic deterioration are progressive with prolonged exposures. Predictable clinical sequelae including neurologic depression and eventual cardiopulmonary arrest occur if uninterrupted. Aggressive rewarming techniques including extracorporeal methods have the potential for excellent neurologic outcomes even in severe cases.

Keywords

Heat stroke • Hypothermia • Hyperthermia • Heat injury • Cold injury

Thermoregulation

The human body has the remarkable ability to maintain a constant internal temperature despite wide and often extreme variations in environmental temperatures. Humans have tolerated brief exposure to extreme heat (documented temperatures ranging from 220 °F to 260 °F) [1] yet cultured mammalian cells show cellular destruction at 107 °F after only a few minutes [2–4]. The clinical consequences of thermoregulatory failure are often dramatic and catastrophic. Individual heat waves have caused over 10,000 deaths in brief periods overwhelming available medical resources, and children left in enclosed automobiles for even brief periods are found with organ necrosis at autopsy.

Effective thermoregulation requires balancing heat production (thermogenesis) and heat absorption with heat loss. Thermogenesis is the sum of exothermic metabolic reactions and mechanical heat generation through muscle activity. Variations in metabolic activity occur through changes in the basal cellular metabolic rate; thyroxine, adrenaline and growth hormone induced cellular metabolism; cellular sympathetic stimulation; temperature-induced changes in chemical activity; and the thermogenic effects of food [5]. This heat gain is balanced with heat loss by varying the temperature gradient from the body core to the skin, regulating the quantity and content of sweat production, and modifying behaviors that alter energy transfer to the surrounding

L.A. Zabrocki, MD (✉)
Division of Pediatric Critical Care,
Naval Medical Center San Diego, San Diego, CA, USA
e-mail: luke.zabrocki@med.navy.mil

D.K. Shellington
Division of Pediatric Critical Care,
University of California, San Diego, San Diego, CA, USA

S.L. Bratton
Department of Pediatrics,
Primary Children's Medical Center, Salt Lake City, UT, USA

D.S. Wheeler et al. (eds.), *Pediatric Critical Care Medicine*,
DOI 10.1007/978-1-4471-6362-6_49, © Springer-Verlag London 2014

environment. Anatomic and physiologic adaptations have evolved to allow regulation of all of the above variables in a finely tuned process to maintain strict internal body temperature [6].

Thermoregulatory inputs include surface skin temperature sensation through the transient receptor potential (TRP) family of ion channels that are located on free nerve endings in dorsal root ganglia (DRG) sensory neurons as well as in keratinocytes [7, 8]. Deep body temperature is sensed in the spinal cord, abdominal viscera, and around the great veins in the abdomen and thorax. Nerve conduction is sent through the DRG by A-delta and C fibers to cross at the level of the spinal cord to the lateral spinothalamic tract and to the ventroposterolateral (VPL) nucleus and eventually to the hypothalamus [9]. Processing of afferent inputs occur in the thalamus, hypothalamus, cortex and parts of the limbic system (Fig. 49.1).

Core body temperature is detected separately by receptors located in the preoptic/ anterior hypothalamus which contains an 'internal thermostat' that initiates the physiologic responses required for normothermia. Normal individual body temperatures range from 36 to 38 °C. As body temperature increases over 37 °C sweat production begins, peripheral vasodilatation increases and arteriovenous (AV) shunts are maximally contracted to optimize heat loss [10]. A drop in core and skin temperature by only 0.2 °C below 37 °C initiates vasoconstriction and AV shunting and eventually shivering to drive body temperature back up to its set point. The threshold from sweating to shivering is only 1.4 +/− 0.6 °C, reflecting the body's tight thermoregulatory control [11, 12].

The efferent limb of this thermoregulatory feedback loop includes cutaneous blood vessels innervated by sympathetic vasodilator and vasoconstrictor nerves responding to core temperature sensation. Sensory afferent nerves in the skin respond to local temperature changes and combined with temperature dependent releases of nitric oxide are responsible for regional variations in blood flow. Sympathetic vasoconstriction utilizes release of norepinephrine and neuropeptide Y while sympathetic vasodilator nerves use an as of yet unidentified neurotransmitter that appears to be responsible for 80–90 % of cutaneous vasodilatation during heat stress. Sensory afferent nerves release a calcitonin gene-related peptide, substance P and neurokinin A for vasodilatation [10]. The above vasoregulation varies the amount of body heat transferred to the skin and available for transfer to the environment.

Heat transfer with the environment relies on conduction, convection, radiation, and evaporation. *Conduction* is the direct transfer of heat between two objects in contact and is of primary importance during water immersion. *Convection* describes the dissipation of heat from the movement of air or liquid across the surface of an object as seen with increased heat loss during windy conditions. *Radiant heat* is

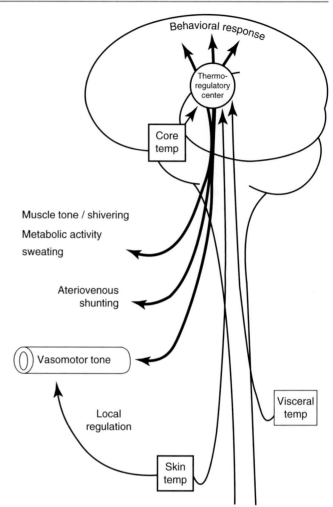

Fig. 49.1 Thermoregulation. Temperature sensation occurs peripherally from receptors located in skin keratinocytes, in deep receptors of the deep viscera and spinal cord, and centrally in hypothalamic core temperature receptors. Signals from skin and visceral receptors travel through A-delta and C fibers to the thermoregulatory center located in the thalamus, hypothalamus and limbic system. Inputs are processed with signals from the hypothalamic 'thermostat' to trigger the efferent response. Surface skin reception primarily affects behavioral responses while deep visceral inputs have a greater effect on physiologic responses. Temperature sensation above the hypothalamic set point triggers sweating, vasodilatation, and decreased arteriovenous shunting. Low temperatures trigger increases in muscle tone leading to shivering, increased metabolic activity, peripheral vasoconstriction and AV shunting. Regional vasomotor tone is also regulated directly by local skin temperature sensation

electromagnetic waves conducting heat away from an object or absorbed from the environment. *Evaporative heat loss* relates to energy consumption from the conversion of liquid water to a gas state and is the primary means of heat loss during conditions of high ambient temperature and low humidity.

All of the mechanisms of heat transfer with the exception of evaporation require ambient temperature be lower than body temperature to provide cooling. Once this criterion is no longer met, as is usually the case with environmental heat injuries, evaporation is the only available method for heat loss. Excessive clothing and high relative humidity impair effective heat loss via evaporation. Guidelines for heat injury prevention therefore are based on heat index or wet bulb globe temperatures (WBGT), which combine air temperature with humidity and in the case of WBGT, wind speed and solar radiation [13].

Children are considered at higher risk for heat illness because of a greater body surface area to mass ratio, lower cardiac output per mass, and a diminished sweating capacity. The actual contribution of these factors to heat illness is uncertain. Infants are known to have a lower concentration of salts in sweat than adults but can have perspiration rates around 50 mL/kg/day [14]. Increased risk of thermal injuries is also related to immature behavioral defenses and lower energy required to heat a smaller mass [15].

Neuronal pathways process afferent inputs in a manner similar to the primitive behavioral responses to pain, thirst, hunger and suffocation, reflecting the fact that behavioral defenses against thermal changes have a much greater effect on temperature regulation than do physiologic defenses [16]. The anatomical basis for this finding is that surface skin temperature receptors have a greater effect on the perception of temperature and trigger a greater behavioral response than temperature sensed at core receptors. Conversely, core temperature sensation has between 3 and 20-fold greater effect on physiologic changes than do skin receptors. Thus, initial changes in temperature are sensed in the skin and lead to early behavioral changes while more severe temperature changes affecting core temperature trigger autonomic responses such as sweating or shivering [17]. Despite developmental limitations, primitive behavioral changes are even seen in infants where exposure to elevated environmental temperatures lead to an increased preference for water intake over milk and a tendency to hold a more open exposed body posture [18, 19]. Failure of behavioral defenses lead to heat stroke as seen in infants that are left in overheated automobiles, over wrapped during febrile illness or not supplied adequate fluid intake. The failure of the above thermoregulatory mechanisms leads to the pathophysiologic events of thermal illness.

Heat Illnesses

Classification

Clinical syndromes of heat related illnesses include mild forms of heat edema, prickly heat, heat cramps, and heat syncope as well as the more severe forms of heat exhaustion and heat stroke. Heat exhaustion presents with a core body temperature between 38 and 40 °C, mild mental status changes including confusion, dizziness and fatigue and

varying findings of headaches, cramps, chills, and emesis. Tachycardia, tachypnea and postural hypotension are typical findings and patients usually have flushed skin with active sweating. Effective treatment includes preventing further excessive heat exposure, aggressive rehydration and correction of electrolyte abnormalities. These are key steps to prevent progression to heat stroke. The transition from heat exhaustion to heat stroke is poorly understood and there may be genetic predispositions for development of heat stroke due to impaired thermoregulation [20, 21].

Heat stroke is defined as a core body temperature over 40 °C with an altered mental status and a history of heat exposure or significant exertion. It is differentiated from heat exhaustion based on more severe alterations of mental status including lethargy, obtundation, seizure activity, and/or coma with a temperature elevation above 40 °C. Additional symptomatology can be quite variable and severe cases progress to multi organ failure. Evidence of hyperthermia, although considered essential to the diagnosis may be absent at the time of presentation, likely because of incorrect or delayed measurements. Based on a better understanding of the natural history and pathophysiology of heat stroke, a definition of "a form of hyperthermia associated with a systemic inflammatory response leading to a syndrome of multiorgan dysfunction in which encephalopathy predominates" may be more accurate [22].

Pathophysiology

The pathophysiologic basis of heat illness/injury involves biochemical, cellular, and systemic alterations, which lead to progressive systemic inflammation, disseminated intravascular coagulation (DIC), and multi-organ failure.

Biochemical and Cellular Alterations

Heat stress causes activation of endothelial, epithelial, local and circulating immune cells and triggers release of cytokines and acute phase proteins [23]. Anti-inflammatory Th2 cytokines are also increased in heat illness, likely as a counter-regulatory mechanism. As the balance of this acute phase system tips to favor progressive inflammation, the pathological sequela of a systemic inflammatory response develops. Increased levels of proinflammatory, Th1 cytokines and chemokines appear to be related to disease severity [24, 25].

Contributing to this inflammatory response are elevated levels of lipopolysaccharide and other endotoxins. Likely translocated from an impaired gut integrity, increases endotoxin levels occur in humans during strenuous exercise and in animal models during heat stress [26–28]. Impaired hemodynamics and severe hypovolemia during heat illness likely further exacerbate impaired gut integrity [29]. Evidence for this endotoxin model has been demonstrated in many studies including evidence that anti-endotoxin antibodies improve outcomes in animal models of heat stroke [26].

Heat shock proteins (HSP) are highly conserved proteins thought to act as chaperones to stabilize cellular proteins and attenuate their propensity to denature under thermal stress. A 72 kD protein, HSP-72, is increased in moderate and severe heat illness in baboons. Its extracellular release correlated with other markers of cellular injury and was found to be statistically higher in non-survivors [22]. The HSP response appears to be protective as transgenic mice that over express HSP-72 confer protection against heat stress induced hyperthermia, circulatory shock, and cerebral ischemia [30]. Details of the protein alterations found in the HSP response, endotoxin release and inflammatory response can be found in several reviews [31].

Direct thermal injury also contributes to tissue and organ dysfunction heat illness. Cellular injury occurs at or above a critical thermal maximum, initially through apoptosis followed by protein denaturation. In humans, this occurs at temperature exposure of 41.6–42 °C for between 8 and 45 min [4]. Central nervous system (CNS) injury is often severe in severe heat illnesses, such as heat stroke, likely a reflection of neurons sensitivity to direct thermal injury. Autopsy findings of infants and children with heat stroke reveal liver necrosis among those that survived at least 6 h potentially as result of prolonged direct thermal exposure of an organ with its own high heat generation [32]. Evidence of elevated circulating inter-cellular adhesion molecule 1 (ICAM-1), endothelin, and von Willebrand factor-antigen in heat stroke victims suggest a possible pathophysiologic link between direct thermal endothelial injury and the triggered systemic inflammatory response and progression to DIC [33].

Systemic Alterations

On a systemic level, peripheral vasodilatation and altered AV shunting as a response to hyperthermia lead to an increase in venous capacitance and decreased systemic venous resistance (SVR) with increases in cutaneous blood flow up to 16-fold [34, 35]. As fluid losses from sweating and increased insensible losses increase, volume depletion leads to hypotension and reflexive peripheral vasoconstriction. An increase in cardiac work load combined with increasing afterload leads to impaired myocardial function, potentially compounded by direct thermal injury to the myocardium [36, 37]. Experiments with healthy children exposed to heat stress show a drop in diastolic blood pressure within 10 min, primarily diastolic. Cardiac output was shown to increase except in children under 5 years old who had a drop in stroke volume [38]. Hemodynamic measurements of critically ill children with heat stroke are not well described.

Changes to regional circulation, systemic hypotension, and altered perfusion can lead to multi-organ injury from inadequate oxygen delivery and clearance of metabolic byproducts. These hemodynamic changes, systemic inflammation, DIC and direct cellular injury lead to progressive multisystem organ dysfunction. Finally, exertional heat stroke victims are further affected by skeletal muscle injury and rhabdomyolysis with resulting renal injury and electrolyte derangements.

Epidemiology

Heat illnesses encompasses a continuum of disorders that range in severity from very mild entities such as *heat cramps* and *heat exhaustion* to the more serious and potentially life-threatening entity known as *heat stroke*. In the pediatric population, exertional heat stroke (EHS) is primarily seen in teenagers involved in athletics or recreation. Cases outside of this population can occur with illicit drug use, a confounding effect of medications such as anticholinergics, or impaired sweat production [39–46]. Most classical heat stroke (CHS) in children occurs in infants or incapacitated patients often because care-givers fail to provide the necessary behavioral adaptations to environmental exposure necessary for thermoregulation such as infants left in automobiles or improperly cared for during heat waves. Heat related injuries have also been described in infants that were over wrapped, placed under electric blankets, and in conditions such as familial dysautonomia and cystic fibrosis.

Hemorrhagic shock encephalopathy syndrome (HSES) is a separately described entity that has a presentation nearly identical to heat stroke but without evidence of an apparent environmental exposure. Patients are typically found in the morning during winter months occasionally with a history of being over wrapped. The classification of HSES and classic heat stroke as separate entities has been hotly debated but it appears that they have a common pathological endpoint with some form of failed thermoregulation leading to systemic injury [42, 47–52].

The true incidence of heat stroke is not known as there is no current tracking database. Epidemiologic data is derived from case series and public safety databases that gather information from news stories and police reports. Heat related illnesses show temporal and geographical variation. The incidence of heat stroke range from 17.6 to 26.5 per 100,000 with about 250 deaths per year in the United States [53–57]. Up to tenfold higher rates are reported in countries with more extreme climates [58]. The increase in heat-related illnesses during heat waves is substantial [59–64]. A 2003 heat wave in France reportedly caused 14,800 excess deaths which overwhelmed medical resources [65]. Most cases of CHS involve the elderly or disabled, especially during heat waves, although infants are also considered at higher risk. A survey of emergency room visits estimated about 26,000 cases of exertional heat-related injuries in patients ≤19 years of age with an incidence of 4.3 cases per 100,000 [66] although less than 10 % of these required hospitalization and less than 2 % were diagnosed with heat stroke. Participation in football accounted for almost half of male cases.

Despite the relatively low incidence of pediatric heat stroke, mortality is high, most cases completely preventable and extremely tragic. There are about 30 deaths per year in the United States from EHS in children [67]. A survey of media reports from 1995 to 2002 found 171 childhood fatalities in the US related to being unattended in automobiles [68]. More than half involved caregivers that had unintentionally left the child in the car, 27 % were reported as intentional accidents where the caregiver was unaware of the inherent risks. The Centers for Disease Control (CDC) reported an annual death rate in children between 0.1 and 0.5/1,000,000 [69]. Tracking by the Department of Geosciences at San Francisco State University found an average annual rate of 38 deaths in the United States from hyperthermia in motor vehicles [64].

Clinical Manifestations

Details of the clinical presentation of pediatric heat stroke are primarily from case series or case reports [70–79]. Most patients with heat stroke have a core temperature over 40 °C, although this is not a universal finding, which may lead to delays in diagnosis and treatment [72, 80–83]. Higher core temperatures appear to correlate with the severity of neurologic symptoms at presentation in adults although this may not be appreciated in infants [72, 80]. Peak temperatures in infants suffering from CHS and HSES can exceed 42.3 °C [72, 84].

CNS Manifestations
The sensitivity of the brain to hyperthermia is apparent in the universal presence of CNS dysfunction in heat stroke, which can range from agitation to confusion or coma. For infants with CHS, mental status may be more related to the initial state of dehydration than to hyperpyrexia [72]. Many cases show improvement in mental status shortly after initial treatment of shock and hyperpyrexia. About 40 % of patients with heat stroke have seizure activity, often severe. Seizures are also very commonly described in patients diagnosed with HSES. Pupillary response is often sluggish and may range from pinpoint to fixed and dilated [85]. Evidence of cerebral edema may be present at the time of admission in severe cases although many rapidly fatal cases of CHS did not have cerebral edema when autopsied [72, 86].

Cardiovascular Manifestations
Varying degrees of dehydration are present in nearly all cases of heat stroke and are related to any combination of increased insensible losses, gastrointestinal losses and poor intake. Children with CHS have required between 80 and 260 mL/kg fluid resuscitation in the first 12 h [72]. Depending on the severity of hyperthermia and dehydration, patients present with a range of findings from bounding pulses and flash capillary refill to weak pulses and poor peripheral perfusion. Hemodynamic studies in adults show a presentation ranging from an elevated cardiac index with low SVR to a hypodynamic state with a low cardiac index and elevated SVR. Patients with HSES are commonly described with relatively normal blood pressure on presentation with hypotension developing within the first 24 h. While cardiac conduction disturbances are reported in adult patients this is not reported in children independent of electrolyte abnormalities [87, 88].

Respiratory Manifestations
Acute respiratory failure is common and can be related to hyperthermia, CNS injury, increased ventilatory demands, acute respiratory distress syndrome (ARDS), or aspiration. Tachypnea is a common response to hyperthermia and elevated carbon dioxide production/acidosis, thus a hyperthermic patient with normal or slowed respirations may be an ominous finding. Metabolic oxygen demands are elevated and low arterial oxygen saturations may be due to an inadequate compensation, primary respiratory disease or may be spurious from poor peripheral perfusion. Signs of a viral upper respiratory illness are often present in HSES.

Skin Manifestations
Infants with CHS typically have poor peripheral circulation and warm 'doughy' skin.

Many patients with EHS present with flush, warm dry skin implying a state of dehydration resulting from an exhaustion of skin sweating capabilities. The presence of dry skin is commonly mistaken as a necessary feature of EHS, yet patients often have active sweating at presentation [89].

Gastrointestinal Manifestations
Emesis and/or watery diarrhea are common in CHS and HSES and the onset of vomiting may precede a rapid deterioration. Hepatomegaly is present in more than half of patients with HSES [84]. Most patients have transaminitis with mild to moderate impairments in liver function. This typically worsens over several days and resolves in 1–2 weeks. About 5 % of adults cases develop acute liver failure although this may be under-estimated [90–96].

Renal Manifestations
Oliguria or anuria is common in heat stroke. It usually reflects a state of dehydration although progression to renal failure is

observed in 25–30 % of patients with EHS from hypoperfusion, rhabdomyolysis and/or direct thermal injury but is also common with CHS [97–100]. Patients with EHS and some patients with HSES have rhabdomyolysis with myoglobinuria. Most patients have improvement in renal function within 1–2 days.

Diagnosis and Clinical Evaluation

Diagnosis is usually straightforward with presenting history and examination although in unclear cases other conditions must be considered (Table 49.1). Metabolic acidosis is typical in HSES. Patients with heat stroke most commonly have metabolic acidosis but often present with respiratory alkalosis or mixed acid base disturbances. Metabolic acidosis severity at presentation is often related to the severity of hyperthermia. Elevated lactate levels are common and often increase early during treatment with prolonged elevation for several days (Table 49.2).

Salt losses from prolonged heat exposure lead to electrolyte derangements – typically hyponatremia and hypochloremia. Hyperkalemia may be present with EHS likely in relation to rhabdomyolysis [70, 101]. Development of hyperkalemia later in the course of illness often is related to acute renal failure. Alterations of other electrolytes are typically mild and quite variable although the presence of hypophosphatemia (<0.5 mmol/L) with liver dysfunction has been shown to be an independent predictor of developing acute liver failure.

Patients that suffer from EHS typically have laboratory findings of rhabdomyolysis including increased CPK, myoglobinuria, AST, ALT, and bilirubin. Elevations in CPK and liver enzymes are also common in patients with HSES and CHS, showing a consistent pattern of initial worsening then rapid improvement [84]. Most blood counts are normal at the time of presentation although moderate to significant anemia, thrombocytopenia and profound DIC can be expected within the first 24 h, which should be taken into consideration when planning invasive procedures. Peripheral smears may reveal neutrophils with radially hypersegmented nuclei (botryoid neutrophils) early in the disease course [102]. C reactive protein is relatively normal in heat stroke at the initial presentation and any more than modest elevations should warrant an evaluation for infection. Although gut integrity is typically impaired with heat stroke this has not been reported as a source of bacteremia.

Treatment

The most severe victims of heat stroke require treatment of shock with support of the airway, ventilation and restoration of a perfusing cardiac rhythm in accordance with basic life saving measures. Elective tracheal intubation for severe pediatric cases may be prudent as this will facilitate tolerance of cooling methods. Care must be taken in the administration of electrical cardioversion to patients with profuse sweating or those undergoing active treatment of hyperthermia with residual surface moisture. Remaining care should focus on early rapid cooling, support of active or impending organ dysfunction and monitoring/preventing complications.

Cooling

Out of hospital providers and transport teams should be instructed to focus on rapid cooling by any means available once life-saving measures have been addressed. Prolonged transport without addressing cooling measures may lead to poor outcomes despite adequate in-hospital care. Patients should be fully exposed, core temperature documented, intravenous access obtained and oxygen administered. Attention to the transport environment is necessary as humid enclosed vehicles impair efficiency of evaporative cooling. Immersion therapy is impractical during transport and conductive methods such as application of ice packs may be the best option. If not completed in the pre-hospital environment patients must be emergently cooled on arrival as time to adequate cooling directly impacts development of multi-organ failure, length of hospitalization and survival [103]. Although limited data exists for children, several reports of adult patients support this finding. A review of 39 adult patients with CHS showed a trend towards improved survival in patients that were cooled to below 38.9 °C within 60 min of presentation [104]. Case reports of military members with heat stroke suggest improved outcome in those cooled in <40 min and worse outcome in those not cooled within 3 h [88, 105, 106].

Table 49.1 Differential diagnosis of heat stroke in children

Meningitis/encephalitis
Sepsis
Hypothalamic infarction, hemorrhage or infection
Neurogenic fever from traumatic brain injury
Status epilepticus
Thyroid storm
Drug overdose or toxicity
Anticholinergics, cocaine, PCP, amphetamines, MDMA, salicylates
Serotonin syndrome
Malignant hyperthermia
Neuroleptic malignant syndrome
N-methyl-D-aspartate receptor antibody-associated encephalitis

Abbreviations: *PCP* Phencyclidine, *MDMA* 3,4-Methylenedioxymethamphetamine

Table 49.2 Laboratory findings in heat stroke

Laboratory test	Findings	Comments
Blood gas	Respiratory alkalosis alone in mild cases	Increased acidosis with higher body temperatures
	Metabolic acidosis typical in HSES	
	Mixed metabolic acidosis and respiratory alkalosis common	
	Low PaO_2 with development of ARDS	
WBC	Normal to modest elevations	Botryoid nuclei commonly seen early
Hemoglobin	Normal to mildly low	Rapid decline in 24–48 h especially with HSES
Platelets	Normal to low at presentation	Expected decrease over 18–36 h
Lactate	Usually normal in CHS	May be slow to resolve
	Moderate to severe elevations in EHS and HSES	
Glucose	Commonly elevated	
Sodium	Variable with level of dehydration and salt depletion	
Potassium	Normal or low in CHS	
	Progressive elevation in EHS with rhabdomyolysis	
Calcium	Normal to low	Aggressive replacement in EHS may lead to muscle deposition
Phosphate	Variable	Hypophosphatemia may predict acute liver failure
Urea nitrogen	Moderate to severe elevation	Usually resolves in 24–48 h
Creatinine	Elevated in about 50 % of CHS	Usually resolves in 24–48 h
	Usually elevated in EHS	
	Normal to mild elevations in HSES	
Creatinine kinase	Mild elevations in CHS	Prolonged elevations in EHS, peaks in 1–2 days in HSES
	Marked elevations in EHS and HSES	
Myoglobin	Usually absent in CHS	Prolonged elevations in EHS
	Commonly present in EHS and HSES	
Uric acid	Mild elevation in CHS	
	Marked elevation with EHS	
AST/ALT	Mild to moderate elevations	Worsens over 48–72 h with resolution 1–2 weeks
Bilirubin	Mild to moderate elevations	
Ammonia	Normal	Late elevations seen with hepatic injury
DIC Panel	Mild to moderately elevated at presentation	Worsens over 48–72 h. Clinical bleeding uncommon
CSF WBC	Normal	
CRP	Normal to mild elevations	Significant elevations may suggest infection

Abbreviations: *CHS* Classic heat stroke, *EHS* Exertional heat stroke, *HSES* Hemorrhagic shock and encephalopathy syndrome, *ARDS* Acute respiratory distress syndrome, *PaO2* Partial pressure of arterial oxygen, *DIC* Disseminated intravascular coagulation, *AST* Aspartate aminotransferase, *ALT* Alanine aminotransferase, *CSF* Cerebral spinal fluid, *WBC* White blood cell count, *CRP* C-Reactive protein

The optimal method for in-hospital cooling will vary based on available resources, environment, and patient's clinical condition. Commonly used methods include ice-water immersion, evaporative cooling with various wetting and fanning methods, ice-pack application, and administration of cooled intravenous fluids (Table 49.3). Ice or cool water immersion and evaporative methods have shown the most consistent results for cooling [107–109]. Although the most efficient method is a subject of continued debate, no randomized studies comparing methods have been performed to date. Whichever cooling method is selected, accurate continuous or frequent intermittent temperature measurements is essential and any patient with an inadequate response requires more aggressive therapy. Evaporative cooling is an attractive option for cooling pediatric patients as it requires equipment that is often readily available and can be easily adapted. Application of fluids to the skin can be done using misting, poured water, moist gauze or sheets. Care must be taken that administered fluids are not ice-cold which will slow the rate of evaporation and may cause local vasoconstriction. Optimizing heat loss requires warm, dry air, large amounts of airflow, and maximal involvement of body surface area [110]. Immersion therapy has proven to be effect and is considered the gold standard by many. Criticisms of this method have included impaired access to the patient, potential for impaired cooling if significant vasoconstriction occurs, and potentially unsanitary conditions especially in pediatric patients who often have diarrhea [111].

Table 49.3 Cooling techniques for heat stroke

Technique	Cooling rate (°C/min)	Advantages	Disadvantages	References
Evaporative	0.07–0.31	Readily available Non invasive Easy patient access Rapid cooling	Labor intensive	[108, 110, 112, 181–185]
Immersion	0.11–0.35	Non invasive Rapid cooling	Difficult patient access Patient discomfort More frequent shivering	[107, 108, 110, 112, 186–190]
Partial immersion	0.11–0.16	Improved patient access	Slower cooling	[186, 191]
Ice packing	0.028–0.11	Non invasive Readily available Easy patient access	Patient discomfort Slower cooling Risk of frostbite	[182, 192]
Wet towels	0.11	Minimal resources needed Readily available Easy patient access	Slower cooling	[112]
Peritoneal lavage	0.11	Combine with other methods Easy patient access	Invasive Slower cooling Minimally researched	[193]
Cold water and ice massage	0.14	Easy patient access	Slower cooling Labor intensive Minimally researched	[108]
Cold intravenous fluids	0.04–0.076	Minimal resources needed Fluid replacement Combine with other methods Easy patient access	Invasive Limited by fluid load Electrolyte disturbances Minimally researched	[105, 194]
Intravascular cooling device	0.01	Combine with other methods Volume exchange	Minimally researched Expensive Invasive	[114]
Gastric lavage	0.018	Minimal resources Combine with other methods Patient access	Invasive Slower cooling Minimally researched	[105]
Cold hemodialysis	0.012	Potentially rapid cooling rates Concurrent therapy for MODS	Invasive Delays in initiation Expensive Minimally researched	[195]

Abbreviations: *MODS* Multiple organ dysfunction syndrome

A non-randomized trial of ice-water immersion cooling versus ambient air exposure with wet towels for the field treatment of EHS in long distance runners showed that both cooling methods had statistically similar cooling rates [112]. Cooling in cold water vs. temperate water is slightly more effective [113]. Endovascular cooling using temperature exchange catheters have been reported for use in adult patients but available catheter sizes limit their use in infants and children [114, 115]. Other methods to reduce body temperature have been proposed. Antipyretics are ineffective and potentially harmful as severely affected patients at high risk of hepatic and renal injury and coagulation abnormalities. Dantrolene is used in malignant hyperthermia to attenuate hyperthermia related to calcium induced muscle contraction but it has not been shown to have consistent benefit in heat stroke [116, 117]. A randomized, prospective double-blinded, placebo controlled study in adults showed no change in cooling time or hospital stay with 2 mg/kg of intravenous dantrolene [118].

End-Organ Support

Assessment should be made as to the patient's hemodynamic and fluid status. Many patients will show some degree of hypovolemia, although fluid resuscitation should be monitored closely as excessive fluids in patients with multi-organ failure complicate management. Fluid resuscitation with isotonic saline or lactated ringers is appropriate although clinicians should be mindful of significant hepatic impairment and renal failure when using fluids with added lactate and potassium. Patients that present with impaired cardiac function or severely altered vascular tone may require vasoactive medication support. Administration of alpha-adrenergic agents early during cooling may theoretically delay cooling. Respiratory care is supportive, about 25 % of adult patients will go on to develop ARDS [119]. Evidence of a focal pneumonia at presentation may be related to aspiration.

Initial treatment of seizure activity should include initial administration of benzodiazepines followed by a longer acting antiepileptic drug chosen in part by organ dysfunction. Ineffective core temperature reduction can contribute to refractory cases and patients with refractory seizures may benefit from continued cooling to mild hypothermia [72]. Although clinicians should beware of shivering during cooling therapy being confused with seizures, benzodiazepines may be effective in treating shivering as well and preventing a rebound hyperthermia [12].

Development of cerebral edema is quite variable in heat stroke. It is seen more common in HSES than CHS and EHS. Evidence of cerebral edema may be present clinically or radiographically and treatment should provide normothermia and avoid hyponatremia, hypercarbia and hemodynamic instability. However, there is no evidence for efficacy of intracranial monitoring devices to direct therapies to lower intracranial pressure or elevate cerebral perfusion pressure, although this has not been adequately studied. Severe cases of heat stroke likely will have neuronal injury from direct thermal injury in which case cerebral edema will likely be severe and refractory.

Renal failure is a common finding in severe heat stroke patients [120]. Patients with EHS or prolonged status epilepticus may develop rhabdomyolysis. Maintaining adequate renal perfusion and urine output is essential. Case reports document successful treatment of hyperuricemia from heat stroke related rhabdomyolsis in two pediatric patients using rasburicase [121]. Most patients with HSES show quickly resolving renal dysfunction with supportive care. Many patients present with a moderate transaminitis with rare progression to fulminate liver failure. Medical management of hepatic dysfunction appears to be prudent. Transplantation should only be considered in patients who are cognitively intact after heat stroke, published outcomes are poor.

Animal studies have shown no benefit of glucocorticoids [122]. It is unclear if steroids or IVIG in human cases are of benefit although they have been used in reported cases [123]. Animal studies of administration of activated protein C in heat stroke showed a cytoprotective effect but no antithrombotic effect and no change in survival [124].

Prognosis

As stated above, reported mortality rates for pediatric heat stroke are high and vary from 10 % to 34 % with some reported rates as high as 70 % [106, 125–127]. Mortality rates for patients with HSES are reported between 35 % and 82 % with only 10–20 % surviving without neurologic sequelae [49, 128–130]. Studies in adults report temperatures

above 40–42 °C, elevated troponin I over 1.5 ng/ml, hypotension requiring vasoactive medications, altered coagulation studies, GCS <12, and the need for intubation are associated with increased risk of mortality [104, 106, 125, 131–133]. Seizures may be associated with mortality in children [72].

Cold Injury

Injury due to cold exposure presents with both systemic manifestations of hypothermia, and regional frostbite. Though induced hypothermia as a therapeutic modality has been studied extensively in vitro and in vivo, accidental cold injury remains less well understood. In uncontrolled cooling, core body temperature may decrease at rates greater than 6 °C per hour and shivering is uncontrolled [134]. Lactic acidosis develops as circulatory collapse ensues and oxygen delivery becomes inadequate to sustain metabolic demands of tissue [135]. Biochemical derangements occur as thermoregulatory mechanisms fail [136].

Classification

Hypothermia is defined as an abnormally low core body temperature, typically less than 35 °C. The degree of hypothermia is somewhat arbitrarily qualified as mild 32–35 °C, moderate 28–31.9 °C, or severe <28 °C based on core body temperature; however the numeric thresholds for each level vary between different studies [135]. Frostbite, also known as *congelatio,* is injury to skin occurring secondary to cold exposure as water freezes in tissue. Frostbite may be classified as superficial or deep, or may be classified by degrees of injury, similar to burn injury. Superficial frostbite affects only skin and subcutaneous tissue. Deep frostbite involved bones, joints, and connective tissues [137]. "Afterdrop" defines a drop in temperature that occurs after application of warming therapies that may be due to reperfusion of cold extremities as cardiac output improves [138]. "Rewarming collapse" describes a constellation of decreased cardiac output and hypotension that occurs after application of warming therapies.

Pathophysiology

Molecular and Cellular Alterations
As temperature decreases metabolism slows with corresponding decreased oxygen utilization and changes in redox state. Cellular stresses develop including (1) protein denaturation, (2) slowing of cell division, (3) inhibition of transcription and translation, (4) disruption of the cellular cytoskeleton, and (5)

changes in cellular permeability to cations [139]. Additional cellular stress and increased expression of HSP, occurs upon rewarming [140]. Depending on the severity of injury, cells may survive, enter apoptosis, or die by necrosis.

DNA microarray analysis reveals alterations in gene expression across a number of functional categories including cell growth and differentiation, growth factors, immune function, membrane transport, metabolism, post-translational processing, protein degradation, and signal transduction. Changes in gene expression occur via several mechanisms. Cold directly inhibits transcription and translation, as well as slows RNA degradation in some species. Conversely, increases in transcription may be mediated by cold-shock proteins, such as the cold-inducible RNA-binding proteins [141]. RNA binding motif 3 can mediate enhanced efficiency of translation for some proteins at lower temperatures [142]. Changes in enzyme function and ATP generation and utilization have also been reported in vitro.

Systemic Alterations

Animal models enhance our understanding of the physiologic changes that occur during accidental hypothermia and rewarming. Multiple animal models describe low cardiac output due to depression of myocardial contractility after severe hypothermia. In dogs, left ventricular systolic pressure, aortic pressure, heart rate, and cardiac output decreased significantly at 25 °C [143]. The effects of hypothermia mediated cardiac dysfunction are a systolic phenomenon caused by disruption of excitation-contraction coupling and the effects on actin-myosin interaction [144]. With the exception of heart rate, these changes continued after rewarming.

Hypothermia also produces changes in tissue vascular beds as well as decreased cardiac output. Peripheral vasoconstriction occurs in response to sympathetic activation, causing depressed tissue blood flow during hypothermia. After rewarming, blood flow to skeletal muscle is restored before perfusion to internal organs. Plasma volume decreases and capillary leak occurs in the context of altered regional blood flow. These changes may further contribute to circulatory collapse after hypothermia [145]. In trauma, the effects of hypothermia on the microcirculation may be augmented. Changes in red blood cell rheology may exacerbate microcirculatory dysfunction at these temperatures [146].

Cerebral metabolic oxygen consumption ($CMRO_2$) is commonly thought to decrease by approximately 6–10 % for each 1 °C decrease in temperature, though studies show this relationship is more complicated than often portrayed [135, 147]. In addition, hypothermia shifts the oxyhemoglobin-dissociation curve towards the left, maintaining greater oxygen content in arterial blood [148]. The combination of increased arterial oxygen content with decreased $CMRO_2$ may provide the cerebral protection that accounts for some dramatic unexpected good outcomes.

Hypothermia produces a brisk diuresis that complicates the microvascular dysfunction previously noted. In rats, glomerular filtration rate decreases despite significantly increased urine output and decreased urine osmolality. This was associated with decreased endogenous vasopressin secretion as well as a loss of the renal medullary concentration gradient [149]. This occurs as peripheral vasoconstriction mobilizes fluid back to the central vasculature, augmenting cardiac preload and initially improving renal perfusion. This process, with microvascular dysfunction, is responsible for rewarming shock after prolonged periods of hypothermia [141].

Epidemiology

The incidence of accidental cold injury in the pediatric population is not well documented. In the United States, hypothermia plays a role in approximately 600 deaths per year, or 0.23 deaths per 100,000 persons [150]. Cold injuries occur most commonly in the northern latitudes, with Alaska and Montana having the highest risk of hypothermic associated mortality in the United States [139]. Both rural and urban populations can be affected. Though the association between age >65 and hypothermia-related mortality has been statistically validated, an association with young age has not been consistently demonstrated in the United States. Other factors associated with environmental cold injury include substance abuse, ingestion, altered mental status, and immersion [151]. Adolescents engaging in outdoor activities, such as skiing and snowboarding, are also more commonly affected. Though infants and children are physiologically predisposed to hypothermia due to their relatively large body surface area, and inability to secure shelter if accidentally subjected to cold exposure they comprise a minority of patients affected by isolated hypothermia [152].

Although hypothermia as an isolated mechanism of injury may be uncommon in pediatrics, its impact on trauma outcomes should be appreciated. A review of pediatric trauma patients admitted to a rural, tertiary medical center revealed that 182 of 1,629 (11.1 %) patients admitted also had an admission temperature <36 °C. In this cohort, hypothermia on admission was associated with mortality [153].

Clinical Manifestations

CNS Manifestations

As core body temperature falls below 35 °C, patients become confused, may experience mild amnesia, and dysarthria [154]. Continued decreases in temperature lead to apathy and impaired judgment such as inappropriately removing clothing despite the extreme environmental conditions.

Though shivering initially occurs as the body attempts to maintain thermogenesis, this response is lost between 24 °C and 35 °C. Unconsciousness typically ensues between 28 °C and 30 °C. Deep tendon reflexes become diminished, then absent. As temperature continues to decline in severe hypothermia, EEG amplitudes decrease until activity is absent at approximately 20 °C [151]. At this time, ocular reflexes are lost. Patients with severe hypothermia have stiffened joints and muscles and appear in a death-like state.

Cardiovascular Manifestations

Mild hypothermia initially produces an adrenergic response with increased heart rate and blood pressure. Peripheral vasoconstriction occurs, decreasing capillary refill and making the skin cool to touch [154]. Cardiac output initially increases but as moderate hypothermia occurs, atrial bradycardia develops leading to a drop in cardiac output. Though cooling may initially cause increased myocardial contractility in mild hypothermia, this compensation fails in the moderate hypothermia range.

Cardiac rhythm abnormalities develop with falling temperatures. Repolarization abnormalities appear initially, as demonstrated by the appearance of a "J" or "Osborn" wave on the ECG (Fig. 49.2), occurring most commonly in the lateral precordial leads [155]. As the temperature falls further, conduction delays develop. The PR interval becomes prolonged and second or third-degree atrioventricular block may occur with lower temperatures. Heart rates decrease with falling temperature. In severe hypothermia, at temperatures <28 °C, ventricular fibrillation may occur spontaneously, followed by asystole at temperatures <24 °C [156].

Respiratory Manifestations

Stress in the setting of mild hypothermia causes adrenergic stimulation and results in an increase in minute ventilation and pulmonary vasodilatation that theoretically can hasten cooling. Both cold induced depression of the respiratory centers and depressed cerebral oxygen utilization slow minute ventilation [157]. Apnea typically occurs around 24 °C. Bronchospasm and bronchorrhea also occurs with a resulting decrease in mucosal function. In severe hypothermia, severe lung endothelial injury from cold may cause pulmonary edema [158].

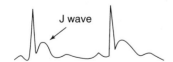

Fig. 49.2 J-Wave (*arrow*). Identified by a prominent bulge at the take-off point of the ST segment from the QRS complex. Also called an Osborn wave, this early ECG finding in hypothermia is due to differences in epicardial and endocardial repolarization. Amplitude and duration appear to be inversely related to the degree of hypothermia

Renal Manifestations

As described above, peripheral vasoconstriction from sympathetic nervous system stimulation redistributes blood volume to the central vasculature increasing renal blood flow with a resultant diuresis. As body temperature falls, renal tubules become resistant to vasopressin, which maintains inappropriate urine output. This cold-induced diuresis causes both volume and electrolyte loss. As hypovolemia ensues in the context of decreased cardiac output, glomerular filtration decreases and oliguria develops.

Hematologic Manifestations

Cold-induced hypovolemia leads to hemoconcentration and increased blood viscosity [159]. Platelet count and white blood cell counts may decrease in moderate to severe hypothermia [160]. The most clinically concerning hematologic derangements are coagulopathies, particularly with co-existing trauma. Hypothermia causes direct inhibition of the clotting-cascade. Careful regard must be given to the temperature at which lab work is performed as coagulation studies from a coagulopathic, hypothermic patient may be falsely normal if the blood is warmed to room temperature prior to assessment.

Diagnosis and Clinical Evaluation

Measurement of a true core body temperature in the hypothermic patient, essential to initiate and guide therapy, may be challenging due to technical limitations of available equipment. A core body temperature should be obtained with placement of rectal or esophageal temperature probes. Measurement of skin temperature should obviously be avoided.

Laboratory studies should include an arterial blood gas to document initial acid-base status, oxygenation, and ventilation. Of note, two different paradigms for interpretation of arterial blood gasses in the setting of hypothermia exist. As temperature decreases, pH naturally rises. At a temperature of 20 °C, the pH of neutrality is 7.70. The alpha-stat strategy focuses on maintaining a neutral pH at the patient temperature. In pH-stat management, the $PaCO_2$ is allowed to rise, compensating for the alkalosis of temperature with a respiratory acidosis to maintain a pH appropriate for 37 °C. Controlled ventilation guided by pH-stat measurements leads to higher arterial $PaCO_2$ and leads to significantly higher cerebral blood flows at hypothermic temperatures.

The two management strategies are used during cardiopulmonary bypass without a clearly preferred method. A recent meta-analysis noted among pediatric patients pH-stat management was superior, while alpha-stat management was preferred for adult bypass, which uses less extreme hypothermia [161].

Treatment

Aggressive treatment of accidental hypothermia has resulted in good outcomes at body core temperatures as low as 13.7 °C in an adult and 14.7 °C in a child, even in the setting of circulatory arrest [162]. Due to the infrequency of hypothermia as an isolated injury and the variety of available treatments, only anecdotal evidence is available to support the administration of one warming therapy over another. A single center study reported 14 different rewarming techniques applied to 84 patients with a variety of warming rates and complications [163]. Current treatment guidelines are based largely on expert opinion [164].

The initial treatment of the hypothermic patient is focused on stabilization of the airway, breathing, and circulation with cardiopulmonary resuscitation administered to arrested patients. Intravenous or intraosseous access should be rapidly attained and fluid expansion with isotonic crystalloid initiated. In concert with stabilization, measures to prevent further hypothermia should begin. Passive external rewarming, removal of cold, wet clothing and placement of dry blankets around the patient, is first tier of therapy. These initial measures can rewarm at a rate of 0.5–4 °C per hour [165]. Particular attention must be provided to insulating the head, which can account for 75 % of heat loss at −15 °C. [141, 159] In mild hypothermia, patients have intact shivering mechanisms and passive external rewarming may be sufficient.

The degree to which an unstable hypothermic patient should be rewarmed in the pre-hospital setting remains controversial. Though prevention of further heat loss via passive external rewarming is generally accepted, more aggressive measures may precipitate circulatory collapse prior to the availability of cardiopulmonary bypass or extracorporeal membrane oxygenation (ECMO). External active rewarming, including warming blankets, radiant heat lamps, and forced air rewarming, may be delayed until arrival at a tertiary care center where equipment for active internal rewarming is available, at the treatment team's discretion.

Modalities for active internal rewarming for accidental hypothermia include administration of warmed intravenous fluids, gastric lavage, pleural lavage, peritoneal lavage, hemodialysis, and cardiopulmonary bypass or ECMO. Choice of rewarming method may depend on availability of equipment at the treating hospital. Generally, rewarming is performed as quickly as possible. Faster rates of rewarming using invasive rewarming catheters are associated with lower early mortality compared to traditional non-invasive warming methods in one study [166].

At centers that frequently manage patients who present in circulatory arrest from severe hypothermia, cardiopulmonary bypass followed by ECMO is often used [164]. Cardiopulmonary bypass has the advantage of restoring cardiac output simultaneously with rewarming. Rewarming after therapeutic hypothermia is commonly done at a slow, controlled rate, but little evidence to support this practice exists in the setting of accidental hypothermia. Cardiopulmonary bypass followed by ECMO provides additional support for patients with cardiorespiratory failure developing during resuscitation. Numerous case series document the potential for survival of the post-arrest or hemodynamically unstable accidental hypothermia victim. A large, single-center study examining outcomes of cardiopulmonary bypass as treatment for circulatory arrest after accidental hypothermia reported long-term survival of 15 out of 46 patients, who had good quality of life on long-term follow-up [167, 168].

Portable, percutaneous catheters for cardiopulmonary bypass have been used in the last decade at some centers with faster rewarming and a shorter time to reaching 34 °C than conventional rewarming methods [169]. In addition, the percutaneous cardiopulmonary bypass system was associated with a lower rate of ventricular fibrillation during rewarming. The use of endovascular rewarming catheters and percutaneous cardiopulmonary bypass catheters in the pediatric population is limited by the availability of appropriate catheter size.

In settings where CPB and ECMO are unavailable, continuous venovenous hemodialysis (CVVHD) may provide a safe, effective rewarming method for both pediatric and adult patients. Rewarming rates of 1–3 °C per hour have been reported [170, 171]. Use of intermittent hemodialysis for rewarming has been described in case reports of adult patients [172]. Peritoneal dialysis and peritoneal lavage with warmed dialysate remains a standard method for rewarming in the setting of accidental hypothermia [173]. Though case reports have used gastric lavage, this technique should be used with caution in the pediatric patient due to the risk of vomiting and aspiration. If concomitant ingestion is suspected, warmed fluids may be used with gastric lavage to facilitate rewarming [174].

Despite the recent emphasis on cardiopulmonary bypass and ECMO, a number of studies have demonstrated success with active, external rewarming alone [175–177]. These studies have used humidified, heated air via ventilator and forced air delivery systems (Bair Hugger devices) together in patients with profound hypothermia. In addition, isotonic crystalloids warmed to 40 °C will both expand intravascular volume and warm the patient.

Prognosis

Mortality of accidental hypothermia varies widely between different series, ranging between 12 % and 80 % [178]. In 1987, a party of 13 mountain climbers (three adults, ten adolescents) became victims of severe hypothermia on Mt. Hood, OR. In this group, no survivor had a temperature less than 20 °C, [179] though reports of survivors with temperatures as low as 13.6 °C have been subsequently reported. In this group, all patients underwent aggressive rewarming. A serum potassium >10 mEq/dL was predictive of mortality. Although arrhythmias and hyperkalemia have documented associations with increased mortality, it is difficult to predict outcomes based on individual characteristics at the time of admission. Good outcomes have been documented, in both adults and children, with periods of asystole as long as 3 h and CPR as long as 4 h [180].

References

1. Blagden C. Further experiments and observations in an heated room. By Charles Blagden, MDFRS. Philos Trans (1683–1775) 1775.
2. Buckley IK. A light and electron microscopic study of thermally injured cultured cells. Lab Invest. 1972;26(2):201–9.
3. Sakaguchi Y, Stephens LC, Makino M, et al. Apoptosis in tumors and normal tissues induced by whole body hyperthermia in rats. Cancer Res. 1995;55(22):5459–64.
4. Pandolf KB, Bynum GD, Schuette WH, et al. Induced hyperthermia in sedated humans and the concept of critical thermal maximum. Am J Physiol. 1978;235(5):R228–36.
5. Guyton AC. Body temperature, temperature regulation, and fever. In: Guyton AC, editor. Textbook of medical physiology. 8th ed. Philadelphia: W.B. Saunders; 1991. p. 889–90.
6. Hammel HT. Neurons and temperature regulation. In: Yamamoto WS, Brobeck JR, editors. Physiological controls and regulations. Philadelphia: W.B. Saunders; 1965. p. 71–97.
7. Brauchi S, Orio P, Latorre R. Clues to understanding cold sensation: thermodynamics and electrophysiological analysis of the cold receptor TRPM8. Proc Natl Acad Sci U S A. 2004;101(43): 15494–9.
8. Moqrich A, Hwang SW, Earley TJ, et al. Impaired thermosensation in mice lacking TRPV3, a heat and camphor sensor in the skin. Science. 2005;307(5714):1468–72.
9. Mendoza JE, Foundas AL. The somatosensory systems. In: Clinical neuroanatomy: a neurobehavioral approach. New York: Springer; 2008. p. 23–47.
10. Charkoudian N. Skin blood flow in adult human thermoregulation: how it works, when it does not, and why. Mayo Clin Proc. 2003;78(5):603–12.
11. Lopez M, Sessler DI, Walter K, et al. Rate and gender dependence of the sweating, vasoconstriction, and shivering thresholds in humans. Anesthesiology. 1994;80(4):780–8.
12. Sessler DI. Thermoregulatory defense mechanisms. Crit Care Med. 2009;37(7 Suppl):S203–10.
13. Steadman R. The assessment of sultriness. Part I: a temperature-humidity index based on human physiology and clothing science. J Appl Meteorol. 1979;18(7):861–73.
14. Cooke RE, Pratt EL, Darrow EC. The metabolic response of infants to heat stress. Yale J Biol Med. 1950;22(3):227–49.
15. Rowland T. Thermoregulation during exercise in the heat in children: old concepts revisited. J Appl Physiol. 2008;105(2):718–24.
16. Egan GF, Johnson J, Farrell M, et al. Cortical, thalamic, and hypothalamic responses to cooling and warming the skin in awake humans: a positron-emission tomography study. Proc Natl Acad Sci U S A. 2005;102(14):5262–7.

17. Frank SM, Raja SN, Bulcao CF, et al. Relative contribution of core and cutaneous temperatures to thermal comfort and autonomic responses in humans. J Appl Physiol. 1999;86(5):1588–93.
18. Lee DHK. A basis for the study of man's reaction to tropical climates. University of Queensland Papers. 1940;1(5).
19. Cooke RE. The behavioural response of infants to heat stress. Yale J Biol Med. 1952;24(4):334–40.
20. Tobin JR, Jason DR, Challa VR, et al. Malignant hyperthermia and apparent heat stroke. JAMA. 2001;286(2):168–9.
21. Howorth PJ. The biochemistry of heat illness. J R Army Med Corps. 1995;141(1):40–1.
22. Dehbi M, Baturcam E, Eldali A, et al. Hsp-72, a candidate prognostic indicator of heatstroke. Cell Stress Chaperones. 2010;15(5):593–603.
23. Gabay C, Kushner I. Acute-phase proteins and other systemic responses to inflammation. N Engl J Med. 1999;340:448–54 [Erratum, N Engl J Med 1999;340:1376.].
24. Lu KC, Wang JY, Lin SH, et al. Role of circulating cytokines and chemokines in exertional heatstroke. Crit Care Med. 2004;32(2):399–403.
25. Bouchama A, Hammami MM, Al Shail E, et al. Differential effects of in vitro and in vivo hyperthermia on the production of interleukin-10. Intensive Care Med. 2000;26(11):1646–51.
26. Gathiram P, Wells MT, Brock-Utne JG, et al. Antilipopolysaccharide improves survival in primates subjected to heat stroke. Circ Shock. 1987;23(3):157–64.
27. Bosenberg AT, Brock-Utne JG, Gaffin SL, et al. Strenuous exercise causes systemic endotoxemia. J Appl Physiol. 1988;65(1):106–8.
28. Pedersen BK, Toft AD. Effects of exercise on lymphocytes and cytokines. Br J Sports Med. 2000;34(4):246–51.
29. Pals KL, Chang RT, Ryan AJ, et al. Effect of running intensity on intestinal permeability. J Appl Physiol. 1997;82(2):571–6.
30. Lee WC, Wen HC, Chang CP, et al. Heat shock protein 72 overexpression protects against hyperthermia, circulatory shock, and cerebral ischemia during heatstroke. J Appl Physiol. 2006;100(6): 2073–82.
31. Bouchama A, Knochel JP. Heat stroke. N Engl J Med. 2002;346(25):1978–88.
32. Krous HF, Nadeau JM, Fukumoto RI, et al. Environmental hyperthermic infant and early childhood death: circumstances, pathologic changes, and manner of death. Am J Forensic Med Pathol. 2001;22(4):374–82.
33. Bouchama A, Hammami MM, Haq A, et al. Evidence for endothelial cell activation/injury in heatstroke. Crit Care Med. 1996;24(7):1173–8.
34. Rowell LB. Cardiovascular aspects of human thermoregulation. Circ Res. 1983;52:367–79.
35. Drinkwater BL, Kupprat IC, Denton JE, et al. Response of prepubertal girls and college women to work in the heat. J Appl Physiol. 1977;43(6):1046–53.
36. O'Donnell TF, Clowes GH. The circulatory abnormalities of heat stroke. N Engl J Med. 1972;287:734–7.
37. Sprung CL. Hemodynamic alterations of heat stroke in the elderly. Chest. 1979;75:362–266.
38. Jokinen E, Välimäki I, K A, et al. Children in sauna: cardiovascular adjustment. Pediatrics. 1990;86(2):282–8.
39. Kessler WR, Andersen DH. Heat prostration in fibrocystic disease of the pancreas and other conditions. Pediatrics. 1951;8(5): 648–56.
40. Feldman KW, Mazor S. Ecstasy ingestion causing heatstroke-like, multiorgan injury in a toddler. Pediatr Emerg Care. 2007;23(10): 725–6.
41. Shimizu T, Yamashita Y, Satoi M, et al. Heat stroke-like episode in a child caused by zonisamide. Brain Dev. 1997;19(5):366–8.
42. Baugnon T, Duracher-Gout C, Blanot S, et al. Hemorrhagic shock and encephalopathy syndrome in a quadriplegic child: an argument

for the triggering role of impaired thermoregulatory response. Spine. 2010;35(15):E730–2.

43. Tirosh I, Hoffer V, Finkelstein Y, Garty BZ. Heat stroke in familial dysautonomia. Pediatr Neurol. 2003;29(2):164–6.

44. Iwanaga R, Matsuishi T, Ohnishi A, et al. Serial magnetic resonance images in a patient with congenital sensory neuropathy with anhidrosis and complications resembling heat stroke. J Neurol Sci. 1996;142(1–2):79–84.

45. Jafferany M, Lowry J. Case report of olanzapine-associated elevation of serum creatine kinase in a 16-year-old boy with heat stroke. Prim Care Companion J Clin Psychiatry. 2008;10(3):250–2.

46. Kew MC, Hopp M, Rothberg A. Fatal heat-stroke in a child taking appetite-suppressant drugs. S Afr Med J. 1982;62(24):905–6.

47. Bacon CJ, Hall SM. Haemorrhagic shock encephalopathy syndrome in the British Isles. Arch Dis Child. 1992;67(8):985–93.

48. Lafeber HN, vd Voort E, de Groot R. Hemorrhagic shock and encephalopathy syndrome. Lancet. 1983;2(8353):795.

49. Levin M, Hjelm M, Kay JD, et al. Haemorrhagic shock and encephalopathy: a new syndrome with a high mortality in young children. Lancet. 1983;2(8341):64–7.

50. Conway EE, Varlotta L, Singer LP, Caspe WB. Hemorrhagic shock and encephalopathy: is it really a new entity? Pediatr Emerg Care. 1990;6(2):131–4.

51. Bass M. The fallacy of the hemorrhagic shock and encephalopathy syndrome. Am J Dis Child. 1991;145(7):718.

52. Sofer S, Phillip M, Hershkowits J, Bennett H. Hemorrhagic shock and encephalopathy syndrome. Its association with hyperthermia. Am J Dis Child. 1986;140(12):1252–4.

53. Jones TS, Liang AP, Kilbourne EM, et al. Morbidity and mortality associated with the July 1980 heat wave in St Louis and Kansas City, Mo. JAMA. 1982;247(24):3327–31.

54. Moore R, Mallonee S, Sabogal RI, Centers for Disease Control and Prevention, et al. Heat-related deaths-four states, July-August 2001, and United States, 1979–1999. JAMA. 2002;288(8):950–1.

55. Centers for Disease Control and Prevention. Heat-related illnesses and deaths-United States, 1994–1995. JAMA. 1995;274(3):209–10.

56. Centers for Disease Control and Prevention. Heat-related illnesses and deaths—Chicago, Illinois, 1996–2001, and United States, 1979–1999. MMWR Morb Mortal Wkly Rep. 2003;52:610–3.

57. Centers for Disease Control and Prevention. Heat-related deaths-United States, 1999–2003. MMWR Morb Mortal Wkly Rep. 2006;55(29):796–8.

58. Ghaznawi HI, Ibrahim MA. Heat stroke and heat exhaustion in pilgrims performing the Haj (annual pilgrimage) in Saudi Arabia. Ann Saudi Med. 1987;7:323–6.

59. Nitschke M, Tucker GR, Bi P. Morbidity and mortality during heat-waves in metropolitan Adelaide. Med J Aust. 2007;187(11–12):662–5.

60. Mayner L, Arbon P, Usher K. Emergency department patient presentations during the 2009 heatwaves in Adelaide. Collegian. 2010;17(4):175–82.

61. Center for disease control: impact of heat waves on mortality – Rome, June-August 2003. MMWR Morb Mortal Wkly Rep. 2004;53:369–71.

62. Ledrans M, Pirard P, Tillaut H, et al. The heat wave of August 2003: what happened? Rev Prat. 2004;54:1289–97.

63. Schuman SH. Patterns of urban heat-wave deaths and implications for prevention: data from New York and St. Louis during July, 1966. Environ Res. 1972;5(1):59–75.

64. Semenza JC, Rubin CH, Falter KH, et al. Heat-related deaths during the July 1995 heat wave in Chicago. N Engl J Med. 1996;335(2):84–90.

65. Fouillet A, Rey G, Laurent F, et al. Excess mortality related to the August 2003 heat wave in France. Int Arch Occup Environ Health. 2006;80(1):16–24.

66. Nelson N, Collins C, Comstock R, Mckenzie L. Exertional heat-related injuries treated in emergency departments in the U.S., 1997–2006. AMEPRE. 2011;40(1):54–60.

67. Hyperthermia deaths of children in vehicles. http://ggweather.com/heat/index.htm. Accessed 6 July 2011.

68. Guard A, Gallagher SS. Heat related deaths to young children in parked cars: an analysis of 171 fatalities in the United States, 1995–2002. Inj Prev. 2005;11(1):33–7.

69. Heat-related deaths – fours states, July-August 2001, and United States, 1979–1999 MMWR. 51(26):567–70.

70. Shibolet S, Coll R, Gilat T, Sohar E. Heatstroke: its clinical picture and mechanism in 36 cases. Q J Med. 1967;36(144):525–48.

71. Malamud N, Haymaker W, Custer RP. Heat stroke; a clinico-pathologic study of 125 fatal cases. Mil Surg. 1946;99(5):397–449.

72. Danks DM, Webb DW, Allen J. Heat illness in infants and young children: a study of 47 cases. 1962. Wilderness Environ Med. 2005;15(4):293–300.

73. Kaszás T. Sun-stroke syndrome in childhood (analysis of 33 cases). Orv Hetil. 1987;128(31):1609–13.

74. Sudhakar PJ, Al-Hashimi H. Bilateral hippocampal hyperintensities: a new finding in MR imaging of heat stroke. Pediatr Radiol. 2007;37(12):1289–91.

75. Nugent SK. Pediatric heatstroke: a case report. Indiana Med. 1987;80(3):235–7.

76. Jeune M, Bertrand J, Potton F. Acute tubular nephritis caused by a heat stroke in infant. Minerva Pediatr. 1956;8(16):594–7.

77. Tham MK, Cheng J, Fock KM. Heat stroke: a clinical review of 27 cases. Singapore Med J. 1989;30(2):137–40.

78. Chesney ML. Pediatric exertional heatstroke. Air Med J. 2003;22(6):6–8.

79. Pitt DC, Kriel RL, Wagner NC, Krach LE. Kluver-Bucy syndrome following heat stroke in a 12-year-old girl. Pediatr Neurol. 1995;13(1):73–6.

80. Ferris EB, Blankenhorn MA, Robinson HW, Cullen GE. Heat stroke: clinical and chemical observations on 44 cases. J Clin Invest. 1938;17(3):249–62.

81. Kark JA, Gardner JW, Ward F. Reducing exercise-related sudden cardiac death rates among recruits by prevention of exertional heat illness. J Am Coll Cardiol. 1998;31(Suppl A):A133–4.

82. Knochel JP. Heat stroke and related heat stress disorders. Dis Mon. 1989;35:301–78.

83. Sutton JR. Heatstroke from running. JAMA. 1980;243:1896.

84. Jardine DS, Bratton SL. Using characteristic changes in laboratory values to assist in the diagnosis of hemorrhagic shock and encephalopathy syndrome. Pediatrics. 1995;96(6):1126–31.

85. Yaqub BA. Neurologic manifestations of heatstroke at the Mecca pilgrimage. Neurology. 1987;37(6):1004–6.

86. Rinka H, Yoshida T, Kobuta T, et al. Hemorrhagic shock and encephalopathy syndrome–the markers for an early HSES diagnosis. BMC Pediatr. 2008;8:43.

87. Akhtar MJ, al-Nozha M, al-Harthi S, Nouh MS. Electrocardiographic abnormalities in patients with heat stroke. Chest. 1993;104(2):411–4.

88. Costrini AM, Pitt HA, Gustafson AB, Uddin DE. Cardiovascular and metabolic manifestations of heat stroke and severe heat exhaustion. Am J Med. 1979;66(2):296–302.

89. Smith L, Kark JA, Gardner JW, Ward F. Unrecognized exertional heat illness as a risk factor for exercise-related sudden cardiac death among young adults. J Am Coll Cardiol. 1997;29(Suppl A):447–8.

90. Weigand K, Riediger C, Stremmel W, et al. Are heat stroke and physical exhaustion underestimated causes of acute hepatic failure? World J Gastroenterol. 2007;13(2):306–9.

91. Hassanein T, Razack A, Gavaler JS, Van Thiel DH. Heatstroke: its clinical and pathological presentation, with particular attention to the liver. Am J Gastroenterol. 1992;87(10):1382–9.

92. Garcin JM, Bronstein JA, Cremades S, et al. Acute liver failure is frequent during heat stroke. World J Gastroenterol. 2008;14(1):158–9.

93. Saissy JM. Liver transplantation in a case of fulminant liver failure after exertion. Intensive Care Med. 1996;22(8):831.

94. Benois A, Coton J, Peycru T, et al. Acute liver failure and severe exertional heat stroke: uneasy management in Africa. Med Trop (Mars). 2009;69(3):289–92.

95. Pardo Cabello AJ, Benticuaga Martínez MN, Martín Moreno A, et al. Acute liver failure following heat stroke. An Med Interna. 2005;22(9):429–30.

96. Lubanda H, Novák F, Trunecka P, et al. Acute liver failure related to the syndrome of exertional heatstroke. Cas Lek Cesk. 2004;143(5):336–8.

97. Knochel JP, Beisel WR, Herndon EG, et al. The renal, cardiovascular, hematologic and serum electrolyte abnormalities of heat stroke. Am J Med. 1961;30:299–309.

98. Raju SF, Robinson GH, Bower JD. The pathogenesis of acute renal failure in heat stroke. South Med J. 1973;66(3):330–3.

99. Vertel RM, Knochel JP. Acute renal failure due to heat injury. An analysis of ten cases associated with a high incidence of myoglobinuria. Am J Med. 1967;43(3):435–51.

100. Pattison ME, Logan JL, Lee SM, Ogden DA. Exertional heat stroke and acute renal failure in a young woman. Am J Kidney Dis. 1988;11(2):184–7.

101. Shapiro Y, Cristal N. Hyperthermia and heat stroke: effects on acid-base balance, blood electrolytes and hepato-renal function. In: Hales JRS, Richards D, editors. Heat stress: physical exertion and enviornment. New York: Elsevier; 1987. p. 289–96.

102. Kitazawa K, Honda A, Maemoto T, et al. Botryoid neutrophils in unexpected heat stroke. Arch Dis Child. 1999;81(2):189.

103. Zeller L, Novack V, Barski L, et al. Exertional heatstroke: clinical characteristics, diagnostic and therapeutic considerations. Eur J Intern Med. 2011;22(3):296–9.

104. Vicario SJ, Okabajue R, Haltom T. Rapid cooling in classic heatstroke: effect on mortality rates. Am J Emerg Med. 1986;4(5):394–8.

105. Heled Y, Rav-Acha M, Shani Y, et al. The "golden hour" for heatstroke treatment. Mil Med. 2004;169(3):184–6.

106. Dematte J, O'Mara K, Buescher J, et al. Near-fatal heatstroke during the 1995 heat wave in Chicago. Ann Intern Med. 1998;129:173.

107. Bouchama A, Dehbi M, Chaves-Carballo E. Cooling and hemodynamic management in heatstroke: practical recommendations. Crit Care (Lond, Engl). 2007;11(3):R54.

108. McDermott BP, Casa DJ, Ganio MS, et al. Acute whole-body cooling for exercise-induced hyperthermia: a systematic review. J Athl Train. 2009;44(1):84–93.

109. Costrini A. Emergency treatment of exertional heatstroke and comparison of whole body cooling techniques. Med Sci Sports Exerc. 1990;22(1):15–8.

110. Weiner JS, Khogali M. A physiological body-cooling unit for treatment of heat stroke. Lancet. 1980;1:507–9.

111. Gaffin SL, Gardner JW, Flinn SD. Cooling methods for heatstroke victims. Ann Intern Med. 2000;132(8):678.

112. Armstrong LE, Crago AE, Adams R, et al. Whole-body cooling of hyperthermic runners: comparison of two field therapies. Am J Emerg Med. 1996;14(4):355–8.

113. Taylor NA, Caldwell JN, Van den Heuvel AM, Patterson MJ. To cool, but not too cool: that is the question–immersion cooling for hyperthermia. Med Sci Sports Exerc. 2008;40(11):1962–9.

114. Broessner G, Beer R, Franz G, et al. Case report: severe heat stroke with multiple organ dysfunction – a novel intravascular treatment approach. Crit Care (Lond Engl). 2005;9(5):R498–501.

115. Megarbane B, Resiere D, Delahaye A, Baud FJ. Endovascular hypothermia for heat stroke: a case report. Intensive Care Med. 2004;30:140.

116. Larner AJ. Dantrolene for exertional heat stroke. Lancet. 1992;339:182.

117. Hadad E, Cohen-Sivan Y, Heled Y, Epstein Y. Clinical review: treatment of heat stroke: should dantrolene be considered? Crit Care (Lond, Engl). 2005;9(1):86–91.

118. Bouchama A, Cafege A, Devol EB, et al. Ineffectiveness of dantrolene sodium in the treatment of heatstroke. Crit Care Med. 1991;19(2):176–80.

119. el-Kassimi FA, Al-Mashhadani S, Abdullah AK, Akhtar J. Adult respiratory distress syndrome and disseminated intravascular coagulation complicating heat stroke. Chest. 1986;90(4):571–4.

120. Wang AY, Li PK, Lui SF, Lai KN. Renal failure and heatstroke. Ren Fail. 1995;17(2):171–9.

121. Lin PY, Lin CC, Liu HC, et al. Rasburicase improves hyperuricemia in patients with acute kidney injury secondary to rhabdomyolysis caused by ecstasy intoxication and exertional heat stroke. Pediatr Crit Care Med. 2011;12(6):e424–7.

122. Bouchama A, Kwaasi A, Dehbi M, et al. Glucocorticoids do not protect against the lethal effects of experimental heatstroke in baboons. Shock. 2007;27(5):578–83.

123. Trujillo MH, Bellorin-Font E, Fragachan CF, Perret-Gentil R. Multiple organ failure following near fatal exertional heat stroke. J Intensive Care Med. 2009;24(1):72–8.

124. Bouchama A, Kunzelmann C, Dehbi M, et al. Recombinant activated protein C attenuates endothelial injury and inhibits procoagulant microparticles release in baboon heatstroke. Arterioscler Thromb Vasc Biol. 2008;28(7):1318–25.

125. Argaud L, Ferry T, Le QH, et al. Short- and long-term outcomes of heatstroke following the 2003 heat wave in Lyon, France. Arch Intern Med. 2007;167(20):2177–83.

126. Misset B, De Jonghe B, Bastuji-Garin S, et al. Mortality of patients with heatstroke admitted to intensive care units during the 2003 heat wave in France: a national multiple-center risk-factor study. Crit Care Med. 2006;34(4):1087–92.

127. Pease S, Bouadma L, Kermarrec N, et al. Early organ dysfunction course, cooling time and outcome in classic heatstroke. Intensive Care Med. 2009;35(8):1454–8.

128. Little D, Wilkins B. Hemorrhagic shock and encephalopathy syndrome. An unusual cause of sudden death in children. Am J Forensic Med Pathol. 1997;18(1):79–83.

129. David TJ, Mughal MZ. Haemorrhagic shock and encephalopathy syndrome: epidemic of a new disease. J R Soc Med. 1984;77(9):721–2.

130. Weibley RE, Pimentel B, Ackerman NB. Hemorrhagic shock and encephalopathy syndrome of infants and children. Crit Care Med. 1989;17(4):335–8.

131. Hausfater P, Doumenc B, Chopin S, et al. Elevation of cardiac troponin I during non-exertional heat-related illnesses in the context of a heatwave. Crit Care (Lond, Engl). 2010;14(3):R99.

132. Hausfater P, Megarbane B, Dautheville S, et al. Prognostic factors in non-exertional heatstroke. Intensive Care Med. 2010;36(2):272–80.

133. LoVecchio F, Pizon AF, Berrett C, Balls A. Outcomes after environmental hyperthermia. Am J Emerg Med. 2007;25(4):442–4.

134. Putzer G, Schmid S, Braun P, et al. Cooling of six centigrades in an hour during avalanche burial. Resuscitation. 2010;81(8):1043–4.

135. Wong KC. Physiology and pharmacology of hypothermia. West J Med. 1983;138(2):227–32.

136. Tisherman SA, Rodriguez A, Safar P. Therapeutic hypothermia in traumatology. Surg Clin North Am. 1999;79(6):1269–89.

137. Biem J, Koehncke N, Classen D, Dosman J. Out of the cold: management of hypothermia and frostbite. CMAJ. 2003;168(3):305–11.

138. Epstein E, Anna K. Accidental hypothermia. BMJ. 2006;332(7543):706–9.

139. Sonna LA, Fujita J, Gaffin SL, Lilly CM. Invited review: effects of heat and cold stress on mammalian gene expression. J Appl Physiol. 2002;92(4):1725–42.

140. Sonna LA, Kuhlmeier MM, Khatri P, et al. A microarray analysis of the effects of moderate hypothermia and rewarming on gene expression by human hepatocytes (HepG2). Cell Stress and Chaperones. 2010;15(5):687–702.

141. Nishiyama H, Higashitsuji H, Yokoi H, et al. Cloning and characterization of human CIRP (cold-inducible RNA-binding protein) cDNA and chromosomal assignment of the gene. Gene. 1997;204(1–2):115–20.

142. Danno S, Nishiyama H, Higashitsuji H, et al. Increased transcript level of RBM3, a member of the glycine-rich RNA-binding protein family, in human cells in response to cold stress. Biochem Biophys Res Commun. 1997;236(3):804–7.

143. Tveita T, Mortensen E, Hevrøy O, et al. Experimental hypothermia: effects of core cooling and rewarming on hemodynamics, coronary blood flow, and myocardial metabolism in dogs. Anesth Analg. 1994;79(2):212–8.

144. Tveita T, Ytrehus K, Myhre ES, Hevrøy O. Left ventricular dysfunction following rewarming from experimental hypothermia. J Appl Physiol. 1998;85(6):2135–9.

145. Tveita T, Ytrehus K, Skandfer M, et al. Changes in blood flow distribution and capillary function after deep hypothermia in rat. Can J Physiol Pharmacol. 1996;74(4):376–81.

146. Knappe T, Mittlmeier T, Eipel C, et al. Effect of systemic hypothermia on local soft tissue trauma-induced microcirculatory and cellular dysfunction in mice. Crit Care Med. 2005;33(8):1805–13.

147. Steen PA, Newberg L, Milde JH, Michenfelder JD. Hypothermia and barbiturates: individual and combined effects on canine cerebral oxygen consumption. Anesthesiology. 1983;58(6):527–32.

148. Carlsson C, Hägerdal M, Siesjö BK. Protective effect of hypothermia in cerebral oxygen deficiency caused by arterial hypoxia. Anesthesiology. 1976;44(1):27–35.

149. Broman M, Källskog O, Nygren K, Wolgast M. The role of antidiuretic hormone in cold-induced diuresis in the anaesthetized rat. Acta Physiol Scand. 1998;162(4):475–80.

150. Centers for Disease Control and Prevention (CDC). Hypothermia-related mortality-Montana, 1999–2004. MMWR Morb Mortal Wkly Rep. 2007;56(15):367–8.

151. Centers for Disease Control and Prevention (CDC). Hypothermia-related deaths-United States, 2003–2004. MMWR Morb Mortal Wkly Rep. 2005;54(7):173–5.

152. Corneli HM. Accidental hypothermia. J Pediatr. 1992;120(5):671–9. http://www.sciencedirect.com/science/article/pii/S0022347605802264. Accessed 2 Nov 2011.

153. Waibel BH, Durham CA, Newell MA, et al. Impact of hypothermia in the rural, pediatric trauma patient. Pediatr Crit Care Med. 2010;11(2):199–204.

154. Mallet ML. Pathophysiology of accidental hypothermia. QJM. 2002;95(12):775–85.

155. Noda T, Shimizu W, Tanaka K, Chayama K. Prominent J wave and ST segment elevation: serial electrocardiographic changes in accidental hypothermia. J Cardiovasc Electrophysiol. 2003;14(2):223.

156. Aslam A, Aslam A, Vasavada B, Khan I. Hypothermia: evaluation, electrocardiographic manifestations, and management. Am J Med. 2006;119(4):297–301.

157. Osborn JJ. Experimental hypothermia; respiratory and blood pH changes in relation to cardiac function. Am J Physiol. 1953;175(3):389–98.

158. Morales C, Strollo P. Noncardiogenic pulmonary edema associated with accidental hypothermia. Chest. 1993;103(3):971–3.

159. Granberg PO. Human physiology under cold exposure. Arctic Med Res. 1991;50 Suppl 6:23–7.

160. Villalobos TJ, Adelson E, Riley PA, Crosby WH. A cause of the thrombocytopenia and leukopenia that occur in dogs during deep hypothermia. J Clin Invest. 1958;37(1):1–7.

161. Abdul Aziz KA, Meduoye A. Is pH-stat or alpha-stat the best technique to follow in patients undergoing deep hypothermic circulatory arrest? Interact Cardiovasc Thorac Surg. 2010;10(2):271–82.

162. Gilbert M, Busund R, Skagseth A, et al. Resuscitation from accidental hypothermia of 13•7°C with circulatory arrest. Lancet. 2000;355(9201):375–6.

163. van der Ploeg G-J, Goslings JC, Walpoth BH, Bierens JJLM. Accidental hypothermia: rewarming treatments, complications and outcomes from one University Medical Centre. Resuscitation. 2010;81(11):1550–5.

164. Monika BM, Martin D, Balthasar E, et al. The Bernese hypothermia algorithm: a consensus paper on in-hospital decision-making and treatment of patients in hypothermic cardiac arrest at an alpine level 1 trauma centre. Injury. 2011;42(5):539–43.

165. Kempainen RR, Brunette DD. The evaluation and management of accidental hypothermia. Respir Care. 2004;49(2):192–205.

166. Gentilello LM, Jurkovich GJ, Stark MS, et al. Is hypothermia in the victim of major trauma protective or harmful? A randomized, prospective study. Ann Surg. 1997;226(4):439–47. discussion 447–9.

167. Kelly KJ, Glaeser P, Rice TB, Wendelberger KJ. Profound accidental hypothermia and freeze injury of the extremities in a child. Crit Care Med. 1990;18(6):679–80.

168. Walpoth BH, Walpoth-Aslan BN, Mattle HP, et al. Outcome of survivors of accidental deep hypothermia and circulatory arrest treated with extracorporeal blood warming. N Engl J Med. 1997;337(21):1500–5.

169. Morita S, Inokuchi S, Yamagiwa T, et al. Efficacy of portable and percutaneous cardiopulmonary bypass rewarming versus that of conventional internal rewarming for patients with accidental deep hypothermia. Crit Care Med. 2011;39(5):1064–8.

170. Hughes A, Riou P, Day C. Full neurological recovery from profound (18.0 C) acute accidental hypothermia: successful resuscitation using active invasive rewarming techniques. Emerg Med J. 2007;24(7):511–2.

171. Komatsu S, Shimomatsuya T, Kobuchi T, et al. Severe accidental hypothermia successfully treated by rewarming strategy using continuous venovenous hemodiafiltration system. J Trauma Inj Infect Crit Care. 2007;62(3):775–6.

172. Sultan N, Theakston KD, Butler R, Suri RS. Treatment of severe accidental hypothermia with intermittent hemodialysis. CJEM. 2009;11(2):174–7.

173. Mehrotra R. Peritoneal dialysis in adult patients without end-stage renal disease. Adv Perit Dial. 2000;16:67–72.

174. Adler P, Lynch M, Katz K, et al. Hypothermia: an unusual indication for gastric lavage. J Emerg Med. 2011;40(2):176–8.

175. de Caen A. Management of profound hypothermia in children without the use of extracorporeal life support therapy. Lancet. 2002;360(9343):1394–5.

176. Ledingham IM, Mone JG. Treatment of accidental hypothermia: a prospective clinical study. Br Med J. 1980;280(6222):1102–5.

177. Balagna R, Abbo D, Ferrero F, et al. Accidental hypothermia in a child. Paediatr Anaesth. 1999;9(4):342–4.

178. Vassal T, Benoit-Gonin B, Carrat F, et al. Severe accidental hypothermia treated in an ICU: prognosis and outcome. Chest. 2001;120(6):1998–2003.

179. Hauty MG, Esrig BC, Hill JG, Long WB. Prognostic factors in severe accidental hypothermia: experience from the Mt. Hood tragedy. J Trauma Inj Infect Crit Care. 1987;27(10):1107–12.

180. Corneli HM. Accidental hypothermia. J Pediatr. 1992;120(5):671–9.

181. Poulton TJ, Walker RA. Helicopter cooling of heatstroke victims. Aviat Space Environ Med. 1987;58(4):358–61.

182. Kielblock AJ, Van Rensburg JP, Franz RM. Body cooling as a method for reducing hyperthermia. An evaluation of techniques. S Afr Med J. 1986;69(6):378–80.

183. Wyndham CH, Strydom NB, Cooke HM, et al. Methods of cooling subjects with hyperpyrexia. J Appl Physiol. 1959;14:771–6.

184. Hadad E, Rav-Acha M, Heled Y, et al. Heat stroke: a review of cooling methods. Sports Med. 2004;34(8):501–11.

185. Barner HB, Wettach GE, Masar M, Wright DW. Field evaluation of a new simplified method for cooling of heat casualties in the desert. Mil Med. 1984;149(2):95–7.

186. Clements JM, Casa DJ, Knight J, et al. Ice-water immersion and cold-water immersion provide similar cooling rates in runners with exercise-induced hyperthermia. J Athl Train. 2002;37(2):146–50.

187. Proulx CI, Ducharme MB, Kenny GP. Safe cooling limits from exercise-induced hyperthermia. Eur J Appl Physiol. 2006;96(4):434–45.

188. Proulx CI, Ducharme MB, Kenny GP. Effect of water temperature on cooling efficiency during hyperthermia in humans. J Appl Physiol. 2003;94(4):1317–23.

189. Scott CG, Ducharme MB, Haman F, Kenny GP. Warming by immersion or exercise affects initial cooling rate during subsequent cold water immersion. Aviat Space Environ Med. 2004;75(11):956–63.

190. Gagnon D, Lemire BB, Casa DJ, Kenny GP. Cold-water immersion and the treatment of hyperthermia: using 38.6°C as a safe rectal temperature cooling limit. J Athl Train. 2010;45(5):439–44.

191. Clapp AJ, Bishop PA, Muir I, Walker JL. Rapid cooling techniques in joggers experiencing heat strain. J Sci Med Sport. 2001;4(2):160–7.

192. Tobalem M, Modarressi A, Elias B, et al. Frostbite complicating therapeutic surface cooling after heat stroke. Intensive Care Med. 2010;36(9):1614–5. Epub 2010 May 4.

193. Horowitz BZ. The golden hour in heat stroke: use of iced peritoneal lavage. Am J Emerg Med. 1989;7(6):616–9.

194. Richards CC. The use of body cooling in pediatrics. Clin Pediatr. 1963;2:55–60.

195. Wakino S, Hori S, Mimura T, et al. Heat stroke with multiple organ failure treated with cold hemodialysis and cold continuous hemodiafiltration: a case report. Ther Apher Dial. 2005;9(5):423–8.

Janice E. Sullivan and Mark J. McDonald

Abstract

Despite the public's heightened awareness of potential toxin exposures in children, poisonings continue to occur and pose a significant challenge to the pediatric intensivist. In 2009, the United States Poison Control centers reported 1,613,272 toxin exposures in children less than 20 years of age which represented 65 % of all reported human exposures. Children younger than 3 years were involved in 38.9 % and children younger than 6 years accounted for just over half of all human exposures (51.9 %). The three most common exposures in children age 5 years or younger were cosmetics/personal care products (13.0 %), analgesics (9.7 %), and household cleaning substances (9.3 %). Despite the majority of human exposures being in the pediatric age group, only 79 (6.8 %) of the 1,158 human deaths were in those less than 20 years of age. As expected, unintentional toxin exposures were more prevalent in children younger than 13 years of age (99.2 %) compared to teenagers (47 %). The intensivist must be prepared to care for children who have serious and sometimes life-threatening exposures. Supportive care is the mainstay of therapy because many poisons have no specific antidote. Much of the current clinical practices for treating the poisoned patient are based on anecdotal reports because there are limited evidenced-based clinical trials that provide guidance for treatment, safety, and outcome.

Keywords

Toxins • Toxidromes • Antidotes • Overdose • Poisoning • Decontamination • Activated • Charcoal

Introduction

Even with public heightened awareness for potential home toxin exposures, poisonings continue to occur and pose a significant challenge to the pediatric intensivist. In 2009, United States Poison Control centers reported 1,613,272 toxin exposures in children less than 20 years of age [1]. This represented 65 % of all reported human exposures. Children younger than 3 years were involved in 38.9 % of exposures and children younger than 6 years accounted for just over half of all human exposures (51.9 %). The three most common exposures in children age 5 years or younger were cosmetics/personal care products (13.0 %), analgesics (9.7 %), and household cleaning substances (9.3 %). Despite the majority of human exposures being in the pediatric age group, only 79 (6.8 %) of the 1,158 human deaths were in those less than 20 years of age. As expected, unintentional toxin exposures were more prevalent in children younger than 13 years of age (99.2 %) compared to teenagers (47 %) [1]. The intensivist must be prepared to care for the children who have serious and sometimes life-threatening exposures.

J.E. Sullivan, MD (✉)
Department of Pediatrics and Pharmacology and Toxicology, University of Louisville, KCPCRU, 231 E. Chestnut, N-97, Louisville, KY 40202, USA
e-mail: sully@louisville.edu

M.J. McDonald, MD
Department of Pediatrics, University of Louisville, 571 S. Floyd St., Suite 332, Louisville, KY 40202, USA
e-mail: mjmcdo01@louisville.edu

D.S. Wheeler et al. (eds.), *Pediatric Critical Care Medicine*,
DOI 10.1007/978-1-4471-6362-6_50, © Springer-Verlag London 2014

Table 50.1 Toxidromes based on physical examination findings

Physical examination	Drug association
Miosis	Opioids, cholinergics, organophosphates, clonidine, phenothiazines
Mydriasis	Sympathomimetics, anticholinergics, antihistamines
Bradycardia	Opioids, β (beta)-blockers, calcium channel blockers, clonidine, cholinergics, digoxin
Tachycardia	Amphetamines, dextromethorphan, "bath salts," anticholinergics, antihistamines, caffeine, cocaine, tricylclic antidepressants (TCAs), phencyclidine (PCP), ketamine, theophylline, carbon monoxide, sympathomimetics
Bradypnea	Benzodiazepines, barbiturates, opioids, gamma-hydroxybutyrate, ethanol
Tachypnea	Methanol, ethylene glycol, salicylates, ketamine, PCP, sympathomimetics, iron, theophylline, cholinergics, carbon monoxide, cyanide, ethanol, cocaine, amphetamines
Hypertension	Cocaine, amphetamines, PCP, ketamine, sympathomimetics, pseudoephedrine, clonidine, dextromethorphan
Hypotension	β-blockers, calcium channel blockers, clonidine, gamma-hydroxybutyrate, TCAs, opioids, benzodiazepines, antiepileptic sodium channel blockers, iron, nitrates, barbiturates, theophylline, diuretics, angiotensin converting enzyme inhibitors, cholinergics, iron, cyanide
Hyperthermia	Amphetamines, anticholinergics, antihistamines, "bath salts," cocaine, TCAs, ketamine, PCP, salicylates, dextromethorphan, theophylline
Hypothermia	Opioids, benzodiazepines, ethanol

Much of the current clinical practices for treating the poisoned patient are based on anecdotal reports because there are limited evidenced-based clinical trials that provide guidance for treatment, safety, and outcome.

Evaluation

Initial history of the ingestion can provide valuable information to direct treatment. The toxin, quantity, and time ingested are vital pieces of information. Caregivers can frequently provide this information in ingestions involving young children as well as a list of possible toxins available to the child at the place of ingestion. Teenagers are less reliable historians, especially if their mental status is altered. In this case, the physician must rely on physical examination findings, the history, and laboratory results to guide treatment.

The physical examination always begins with an initial assessment of airway, breathing and circulation. Mental status, pupillary response and vital signs are invaluable in a poisoned pediatric patient. Altered mental status or coma are often clues to an ingestion, although head trauma, cerebrovascular accident, diabetic ketoacidosis, hyperammonemia, central nervous system (CNS) infection, hypoxia, hypoglycemia, and renal failure must all be considered. Evaluation and treatment for hypoxia and hypoglycemia in the altered mental status patient is essential to prevent CNS injury. Many toxic ingestions alter the autonomic nervous system and provide clues to the potential toxin through abnormalities or changes in vital signs, physical examination and pupillary responses (so-called "toxidromes") (Table 50.1).

Antidotes

Antidotes are chemical or physiological antagonists that prevent or reverse the toxic effects of specific toxins and are principle in treatment of the exposed patients. Specific antidotes may be indicated when there is an ingestion of a toxin that may be life-threatening or a toxin that has serious adverse effects [2–4]. There may be significant risks associated with some antidotes, therefore the healthcare provider must consider the risk versus benefit of therapy on an individual basis. Supportive care may be insufficient in some patients, thus antidote administration may be indicated and life-saving. Antidotes for specific toxins are addressed in Table 50.2 and in latter discussion of the individual toxin.

Ingestion of certain products may produce "toxidromes" which are clinical syndromes consistently associated with the same clinical signs and symptoms after toxin exposure (Table 50.3). Recognition of a toxidrome can help narrow the potential toxic exposure and guide therapy. The treatment for the specific toxidromes is discussed in later sections but the anticholinergic toxidrome bears mentioning because of its frequent occurrence in toxic ingestions. Anticholinergic toxicity may occur alone (jimson weed) or be associated with multiple toxicities (Tricyclic Antidepressants (TCAs)). Anticholinergic treatment focuses on supportive care. Benzodiazepines are effective for CNS effects including seizures and help control the cardiovascular side effects. Physostigmine, an acetylcholinesterase inhibitor, has historically been an antidote for anticholinergic syndrome. However, the toxicities of physostigmine administration can be significant including induction of a cholinergic syndrome, seizures, and cardiac toxicity [5]. The authors recommend avoiding physostigmine if possible, but especially in patients with TCA ingestions, seizures or abnormal electrocardiograms (ECGs).

Laboratory evaluation and point-of-care testing can help direct treatment in the poisoned patient. Essential studies in most poisoned patients include blood chemistries, bedside glucose, pulse oximetry, 12-lead ECG, serum osmolality, urine and serum drug screens, and female pregnancy testing when the patient is of child bearing age. Optional tests that may provide further information depending on the

Table 50.2 Antidotes for selected toxins

Toxin	Antidote
Acetaminophen	N-Acetylcysteine (NAC)
Anticholinergics	Physostigmine salicylate-not generally recommended
Arsenic	Dimercaprol
Benzodiazepines	Flumazenil (use with caution as it may lower the seizure threshold)
β-blockers	Glucagon
Botulism (infantile)	Botulism immune globulin (Baby BIG)
Calcium channel blockers	Calcium chloride, glucagon, dextrose, insulin
Carbon monoxide	Oxygen, Hyperbaric oxygen
Cyanide	Hydroxocobalamin (Cyanokit®) or Amyl nitrite, Sodium nitrite, and Sodium Thiosulfite (Cyanide Antidote Kit)
Digoxin	Digoxin Immune Fab
Ethylene glycol	Fomepizole or ethanol
Fluoride	Calcium chloride
Heparin	Protamine sulfate
Iron	Desferoxamine mesylate
Isoniazid, hydrazine and derivatives	Pyridoxime hydrochloride
Lead	Dimercaprol, Calcium Disodium EDTA, Succimer
Lidocaine, bupivacaine (local anesthetic systemic toxicity)	Intravenous lipid emulsion
Mercury	Dimercaprol
Methanol	Fomepizole or ethanol
Nitrites/Nitrates (Methemoglobinemia)	Methylene blue
Opiates	Naloxone hydrochloride
Organophosphate and N-methyl carbamate insecticides	Atropine sulfate
Organophosphorus insecticides	Pralidoxime hydrochloride
Snake envenomation	Crotalidae Polyvalent immune Fab
Sulfonylurea-induced hypoglycemia	Octreotide acetate
Thyroid radioiodine protection	Potassium iodide
Tricyclic antidepressants	Sodium bicarbonate
Warfarin	Vitamin K

Table 50.3 Toxidromes based on signs and symptoms

Toxidrome	Drug or toxin	Signs and symptoms
Anticholinergic	Antihistamines, atropine, scopolamine, TCAs, belladonna alkaloids, jimson weed, phenothiazines, mushrooms	Tachycardia, hypertension, hyperthermia, mydriasis, altered mental status, confusion, seizures, coma, dry mucous membranes, flushing, urine retention
Cholinergic (muscarinic and nicotinic)	Organophosphates, carbamates, insecticides	SLU**DD**GE BBB (salivation, lacrimation, urination, defecation, diaphoresis, gastric emesis, bronchorrhea, bradycardia, bronchoconstriction), or **DDUMBBB**ELS (defecation, diaphoresis, urination, miosis, bronchorrhea, bradycardia, bronchoconstriction, emesis, lacrimation, salivation). Also may include agitation, confusion, coma, seizures, muscle weakness, muscle fasiculations
Opioid	Heroin, morphine, methadone, fentanyl, meperidine, oxycodone, codeine, hydrocodone	Bradycardia, hypotension, miosis, respiratory depression, confusion, lethargy, coma, ataxia, pulmonary edema
Sedative-hypnotic	Barbiturates, benzodiazepines, ethanol	Bradycardia, hypotension, confusion, stupor, coma, respiratory depression, hypothermia
Sympathomimetic	Amphetamines, cocaine, caffeine, ephedrine, methamphetamines	Tachycardia, hypertension, tachypnea, hyperthermia, mydriasis, excitation, agitation, seizures, diaphoresis
Serotonin	Methamphetamines, selective serotonin reuptake inhibitors, dextromethorphan, lithium, TCAs, monamine oxidase (MAO) inhibitors	Tachycardia, hypertension, tachypnea, hyperthermia, mydriasis, trismus, myoclonus, diaphoresis, confusion, seizures, agitation, coma

toxin and clinical findings include complete blood count, hepatic enzymes, blood gas analysis, prothrombin time (PT), Computerized Tomography (CT) scan of the head, chest or abdominal x-rays, and toxicologic blood levels. When the overdose substance is unknown, blood ethanol, salicylate, and acetaminophen levels should routinely be measured. Note that serum and urine drug testing is not universally similar, therefore healthcare providers need to familiarize themselves with the drug testing that is available at their institution and if there are known products that may

Table 50.4 Urine and serum tests for drugs and toxins

Serum drug tests	Urine drug tests
Acetaminophen	Amphetamines
Carbamazepine	Barbiturates
Carboxyhemoglobin level	Benzodiazepines
Digoxin	Cocaine
Ethanol	Cannabinoids
Ethylene glycol	Opiates
Iron	Phencyclidine
Lithium	Tricyclic antidepressants
Methanol	
Methemoglobin level	
Phenobarbitol	
Phenytoin	
Salicylates	
Theophylline	
Tricyclic antidepressants	
Valproic acid	

cross react and give a false positive test for a substance. Table 50.4 lists common urine and blood toxin levels that may be ordered if available.

The osmolal and anion gaps should be calculated for all unknown ingestions and in the presence of metabolic acidosis. One commonly used mnemonic for remembering the causes of anion gap metabolic acidosis is CUT DIMPLES (cyanide, uremia, toluene, diabetic ketoacidosis, isoniazid/iron, methanol, propylene glycol, lactic acidosis, ethylene glycol, salicylates). The osmolal gap is a rapid approximation of the unmeasured, osmotically active constituents in the serum based on the difference between the measured osmolality and the calculated osmolarity [6]. A normal osmolal gap is less than or equal to 10 mOsm/kg. Osmolarity is calculated using the formula: $[(2 \times Na^+) + (BUN/2.8) + (Glucose/18)]$. Common toxins that may increase the osmolal gap include ethanol, methanol, acetone, isopropyl alcohol, ethanol and propylene glycol. Mannitol and medications containing propylene glycol may also increase serum osmolality.

Decontamination

Indications for decontamination are determined by the type of exposure and may include skin, ocular or gastrointestinal contamination. Decontamination is usually initiated prior to a child being transferred to the PICU but frequently continuation of this process is necessary. There are ongoing discussions about the indications and best methods of decontamination as there is very little evidenced-based research on which to base current recommendations. The healthcare practitioner must determine the toxic agent, its potential toxicity, the status of the patient and the risk-benefit ratio of the

intervention for resolution of signs/symptoms and improved patient outcome. If indicated, healthcare providers should wear protective gear including gowns, gloves, mask and eyewear to protect themselves from toxic exposure.

Surface Decontamination

Both skin and ocular exposure require surface decontamination. Immediate removal of clothing and irrigation with copious amounts of water are essential to prevent corrosive agents from injuring the skin and to minimize systemic absorption and exposure. Following irrigation, a thorough cleansing with soap and water to all exposed areas including behind the ears, under nails and in skin folds is critical to prevent ongoing skin injury and absorption with subsequent systemic exposure. Neutralization of a substance is generally not recommended because heat may be generated from chemical neutralization resulting in additional injury to the skin.

Ocular contamination is an emergency. The cornea is especially sensitive to corrosive agents and hydrocarbon solvents that may lead to corneal damage and permanent scarring. Irrigation should begin immediately with copious amounts of normal saline with a minimum of 1 L to each exposed eye. Instillation of a topical anesthetic agent may minimize discomfort and facilitate irrigation. The pH of the eye should be checked after irrigation if the exposure is an acid or a base. Irrigation should continue until the pH is normal (7.5–8.0). Contact lenses should be removed if present. Ophthalmology should be consulted to assess corneal injury and recommend treatment if use of fluorescein suggests corneal injury.

Gastric Decontamination

Historically syrup of ipecac, activated charcoal (AC), gastric lavage and cathartics have been used for gastric contamination, however syrup of ipecac has not been recommended for over a decade [7]. Gastric lavage is also considered ineffective unless it occurs within 60 min of ingestion. In addition, even with placement of an Ewald tube (40 Fr) in an adult sized patient, it is very difficult to lavage tablets or capsules from the stomach. There is even less of a role for gastric lavage in the pediatric patient. Exceptions may include ingestion of highly toxic agents, drugs or substances not adsorbed to activated charcoal, massive amounts of drugs, corrosive liquids, and sustained release or enteric coated products. Patients who are obtunded or at risk for becoming obtunded should be tracheally intubated with a cuffed endotracheal tube to protect their airway prior to performing gastric lavage.

Activated Charcoal (AC)

Administration of an aqueous preparation of AC is the most utilized and probably most effective method of gastric decontamination, however there is no clinical evidence that it improves clinical outcome [8]. AC is an insoluble, nonabsorbable, fine carbon powder that is made through distillation (exposure to oxidizing gases) of wood pulp and decomposed organic material. One gram of AC has a surface area of 950–2,000 m^2 that will adsorb organic products. AC is indicated only in those patients that have ingested a potentially toxic amount of medication and should be administered within 60 min of ingestion [8]. Although historically the initial dose of AC was administered using the combination product with the cathartic sorbitol, the current recommendation is that AC without sorbitol be administered. The most common method of administration is having the patient take it orally, however if the patient has an altered state of consciousness or is unable to take it orally, placement of a nasogastric tube for administration may be necessary. Patients who are obtunded, or at risk for becoming obtunded, should be tracheally intubated with a cuffed endotracheal tube to protect their airway prior to the performance of nasogastric tube placement and administration of AC. Radiographic verification of correct placement of the nasogastric tube prior to AC administration is recommended. The dose of AC is 1 g/kg with a maximum single dose of 100 g. A recent meta-analysis suggests that the optimal ratio of activated charcoal to drug may be closer to 40:1 (dose of AC:amount of drug ingested) rather than the current accepted ratio of 10:1, particularly for ingestions with greater toxic effect [9, 10]. Repeated doses of AC may be utilized following ingestion of certain substances such as carbamazepine, phenobarbital, phenytoin, salicylates, TCAs, and theophylline for enhanced elimination through enterohepatic and enterogastric circulations. The usual dose is 0.5–1 g/kg up to 50–100 g every 3–4 h with no more than a dose equivalent to 6.25 g/h in children less than 13 years of age and 12.5 g/h for children 13 years and older. An antiemetic may be administered if the patient experiences nausea or vomiting. The dose of AC should be reduced or discontinued if the patient is vomiting. It is advised that the healthcare provider contact the regional poison control center for current recommendations for repeated doses of AC. There are few adverse events reported in the literature, however aspiration pneumonitis, bezoar formation and bowel obstruction are the primary concerns. Aspiration pneumonitis and chronic lung disease have been reported [11]. With repeated doses of AC there may be fluid and electrolyte abnormalities due to diarrhea and fluid shifts. Products that are not adsorbed by charcoal include lithium, alcohols, malathion, petroleum distillates, iron, heavy metals, strong acids/alkalis, boric acid, inorganic salts, and cyanide although AC is usually administered with cyanide ingestions as it will adsorb a sufficient amount of cyanide and decrease the risk of cyanide poisoning if it is administered early following exposure.

Whole Bowel Irrigation (WBI)

WBI has been utilized with increased frequency to enhance gastrointestinal elimination. A nonabsorbable polyethylene glycol in a balanced electrolyte solution (PEG-ES) may be taken orally or administered via a nasogastric tube. Indications for WBI include large ingestions of drugs/substances poorly adsorbed to AC, sustained-release or enteric-coated tablets, drug-filled packet/condoms (e.g. body packers) or ingestion of large amounts of potentially toxic agents. The PEG-ES dose is 20–40 mL/kg/h with a maximum of 500 mL/h in children. It is administered until the rectal effluent is clear or the drug-filled packets are passed which usually takes 4–8 h. Patients who are obtunded or at risk for becoming obtunded should be tracheally intubated with a cuffed endotracheal tube to protect their airway prior to the performance of nasogastric tube placement and administration of PEG-ES. The head of the bed should be elevated to decrease the risk of vomiting and aspiration. Should vomiting occur, the rate of administration of PEG-ES should be decreased. The patient should be monitored for signs of intolerance which may include nausea, vomiting, bloating or signs of an ileus. WBI is contraindicated if there is evidence of a bowel obstruction.

Cathartics

The use of cathartics is generally not recommended although the first dose of AC is frequently administered as a combination product with sorbitol in many institutions. Cathartics such as 10 % magnesium citrate (4 mL/kg up to 250 mL) or 70 % sorbitol (1–2 mL/kg) have been used but generally have no role in gut decontamination. The most commonly associated adverse effects of cathartics are dehydration, hypernatremia and hypermagnesemia.

Enhanced Elimination

Although rapid elimination of potential toxins is desirable, there is little evidence that this practice improves the outcome of patients or that it is feasible and safe. Methods of enhanced elimination include forced diuresis, urine alkalinization, hemodialysis and hemoperfusion. One's approach must begin with determining if the patient will benefit from enhanced elimination and if the toxin is able to be removed through enhanced elimination. Factors to consider are the volume of distribution, protein binding and the molecular size of the toxin. Drugs that have a large volume of distribution or that are highly protein bound are not amenable to enhanced elimination.

Table 50.5 Indications for hemodialysis for applicable toxins and drugs

Toxin	Indication for hemodialysis
Carbamazepine	Seizures, severe cardiotoxicity; serum level>60 mg/L
Ethylene glycol	Intractable acidosis, serum level>50 mg/dL
Lithium	Severe symptoms; level>4 mEq/L more than 12 h after last dose. Note: dialysis of uncertain value; CVVHD may be preferable; consult with medical toxicologist
Methanol	Intractable acidosis, serum level>50 mg/dL
Phenobarbital	Intractable hypotension, acidosis despite maximal supportive care
Salicylate	Severe acidosis, CNS symptoms, level>100 mg/dL (acute overdose) or >60 mg/dL (chronic intoxication)
Theophylline	Serum level>90–100 mg/L (acute) or seizures and serum level>40–60 mg/L (chronic)
Valproic acid	Serum level>900–1,000 mg/L or deep coma, severe acidosis

Forced Diuresis

Renal clearance must be the primary route of elimination for the toxin if this methodology is to be of potential benefit. The goal is to produce volumes of urine up to 1 L/h through the administration of a large volume of fluid and osmotic or loop diuretics. There is no evidence that this practice is effective, therefore forced diuresis is generally not recommended [12].

Urine Alkalinization

Urine alkalinization (ion trapping) through the administration of intravenous fluids containing sodium bicarbonate increases the elimination of certain toxins by increasing and maintaining the urine $pH \geq 7.5$. This applies to drugs that have significant renal clearance. Most drugs exist partly as undissociated molecules at a physiologic pH. The extent of dissociation is a function of the ionization constant (Ka) of the drug and the pH of the fluid in which it is dissolved. The ionization constants are expressed by pKa (form of their negative logarithms) therefore the stronger an acid, the lower its pKa. When pH=pKa, the concentrations of ionized and non-ionized drug are equal. Cell membranes are more permeable to substances that are lipid soluble and in the non-ionized form. By increasing the urine pH, the ionized form of an acidic drug increases, therefore the rate of diffusion from the renal tubular lumen back into the blood is decreased and renal excretion of that drug is increased. Because pKa is a logarithmic function, a small change in urine pH may result in a disproportionally larger effect on renal clearance. Urinary alkalinization is indicated in patients with moderate to severe salicylate poisoning and methotrexate ingestions. Although urine alkalinization is effective in phenobarbital toxicity, AC is preferred because it is much more efficacious. For patients with salicylate poisoning, urine alkalinization in addition to dialysis may shorten the half-life of the drug. The most common complication associated with urine alkalinization is hypokalemia requiring potassium supplementation. Alkalemia may occur, but serious adverse effects from short term therapy have not been reported. The primary contraindication is existing or impending renal failure [12].

Hemodialysis

Patients with ingestions that have significant toxicity or are potentially fatal may be candidates for hemodialysis. Substances effectively removed by hemodialysis are relatively small (<500 Da), water soluble, and have low protein binding. Poison clearance through dialysis is dependent on the flow rate achieved, therefore the higher the flow rate, the higher the clearance. Hemodialysis should be considered in patients with methanol, ethylene glycol, salicylate, theophylline, carbamazepine, phenobarbital, valproic acid and lithium poisonings (Table 50.5). Fluid status and electrolytes should be monitored closely with supplementation as indicated to avoid adverse events. Anticoagulation is required with hemodialysis which may place the patient at risk for bleeding events. Peritoneal dialysis is less effective due to poor extraction ratios and lower flow rates, therefore it has limited use in patients with significant toxic exposure.

Hemoperfusion

Hemoperfusion is a process similar to hemodialysis however the blood is pumped directly through a column containing an adsorbent material (charcoal or Amberlite™). Drug size, water solubility and protein binding have less impact on toxin removal because the drug or toxin becomes in direct contact with the adsorbent material. Systemic anticoagulation is required. Complications include the risk of bleeding secondary to anticoagulation and thrombocytopenia. Although hemoperfusion may be indicated in patients who are toxic from phenobarbital, theophylline, phenytoin and carbamazepine, it is rarely performed because many centers do not have the required equipment.

Intravenous Lipid Emulsion (ILE)

Multiple effective animal studies have led to local anesthetic systemic toxicity being successfully treated with ILE. ILE has been used to treat human cardiac and CNS toxicity in multiple case reports after toxicity associated with local anesthetic administration [13]. Possible mechanisms of action include creating a "lipid sink" where equilibration pulls the lipophilic medication out of tissue, overcoming mitochondrial carnitine acyltransferase inhibition, and increased myocardial calcium levels from fatty acids which may improve inotropy [13–15]. In the lipid sink theory, not only does the newly formed lipid sink sequester lipophilic drugs, but also renders the drug inactive [15]. Successful treatment of local anesthetic toxicity has led to the use of ILE with other lipophilic drug ingestions. Potential targets include calcium channel blockers, β (beta)-blockers, barbiturates, TCAs, antipsychotics and amiodarone [16]. The optimal amount of ILE, rate of infusion, and time elapsed following ingestion to have effect are unknown. A typical treatment dose is 1.5 mL/kg bolus of ILE 20 % followed by a drip at 0.25–0.5 mL/kg/h for 30–60 min with additional boluses as needed [14, 17]. The literature supports the use of ILE use for local anesthetic systemic and cardiac toxicity. However, there is a paucity of data on the risk of adverse effects in humans. The authors recommend a trial of ILE be considered in life threatening lipophilic ingestions after basic management of ingestions with cardiac toxicity [14].

Specific Toxic Ingestions

Recreational Drugs

The recreational use of drugs continues to be a potential cause of morbidity and mortality in the teenage population. Cocaine and "ecstasy" are still abused but are now the older recreational drugs. Newer recreational drugs such as "bath salts" and phenethylamines continue to emerge being newly produced and thus evading illegal status. Users continue to modify the molecule of existing recreational drugs to produce less expensive, readily available and legal designer drugs [18].

Cocaine

Cocaine, still used as a medical local anesthetic, is a powerful stimulant that has remained a drug of abuse for decades. It is commonly sold as a fine white powder that can be abused intranasally, orally, intravenously, or through inhalation. "Crack" cocaine is the solid freebase form of cocaine produced for the purpose of inhalation when heated. Cocaine can produce a sense of euphoria, increased energy, well-being, sociability, anxiety, and paranoia. Clinical CNS effects occur from altered monoamine reuptake. Peak effect from intravenous or inhaled cocaine use occurs between 5 and 11 min while nasal use requires 30–60 min for effect [19]. Elimination half-life ranges between 40 and 60 min [19]. Cocaine testing is routinely available on urine drug screens. Cocaine and multiple cocaine metabolites cause hypertension and vasoconstriction [19]. Significant complications may result with the use of cocaine including a sympathomimetic toxidrome, myocardial infarction, hypertension, dysrhythmias, sudden cardiac death, seizures, rhabdomyolysis,

renal failure, pulmonary edema, and multiple pulmonary complications. Complications can be severe as a result of packet rupture in "body packers."

Cardiac toxicity results from the α₁ receptor stimulation from norepinephrine release, endothelin-1 release and the effect of cocaine metabolites [19]. Resulting tachycardia, hypertension and vasoconstriction of the heart vasculature increases myocardial oxygen demand, limits myocardial blood flow and puts the patient at risk for myocardial infarction. Cocaine also blocks sodium channels, inhibits potassium channels and enhances calcium channel activity which all increase the likelihood of a cardiac dysrhythmia [19]. Sudden cardiac death from cocaine can occur and may be related to cocaine toxicity coupled with existing medical conditions. Seizures, usually generalized tonic-clonic in nature, are rare but may occur with cocaine abuse [20]. The exact mechanism is unknown, but may be related to hypertension, hyperthermia, or altered monoamine levels in the CNS. Increased activity, dehydration and vasoconstriction may lead to varying degrees of hyperthermia, rhabdomyolysis, and renal failure [21]. A wide variety of pulmonary complications have been described and include barotrauma, acute respiratory distress syndrome, cardiogenic or noncardiogenic pulmonary edema, pulmonary hemorrhage, pneumonia and pulmonary hypertension [22]. Noncardiogenic pulmonary edema may be secondary to increased permeability in damaged pulmonary capillaries [22].

Treatment of cocaine toxicity starts with evaluation of airway, breathing, and circulation. Respiratory symptoms should be addressed with supplemental oxygen and additional interventions if necessary. Respiratory distress warrants radiographic imaging and appropriate intervention. ECG, electrolytes and cardiac enzymes are indicated for evaluation of cardiac abnormalities. Hypertension should be addressed first with benzodiazepines to control agitation. If hypertension persists, calcium channel blockers or vasodilators such as nitroprusside may be used, but exclusive β-blockade should be avoided because of the subsequent unopposed α₁-receptor vasoconstriction. If a β-blocker must be used, labetolol, a combined α and β-blocker, would be a reasonable choice. There is no specific treatment for cocaine induced dysrhythmias, but class Ia (sodium channel inhibitors) and class III antiarrhythmics should be avoided because of the prolonged QT interval experienced in cocaine ingestions [19]. Tachycardia may be controlled with benzodiazepines or calcium channel blockers if needed. Ventricular tachydysrythmias have been treated successfully with sodium bicarbonate and lidocaine, a class Ib antiarrythmic [19]. Amiodarone cannot be recommended for cocaine cardiotoxicity at this time. Activated charcoal will bind cocaine and should be administered if they present early after ingestion. For body packers, whole bowel irrigation has been successfully utilized. Seizures are best treated with benzodiazepines. Hyperthermia should be treated with benzodiazepines, cooling techniques, and evaluation of myoglobin and creatine phosphokinase (CPK).

Gamma-hydroxybutyrate (GHB)

GHB is a naturally occurring breakdown product from gamma-hydroxybutyric acid (GABA) that was first manufactured for use as a potential anesthetic agent over 35 years ago [23, 24]. It became popular in health food stores in the United States in the 1980s. It was marketed as a dietary supplement and was used by bodybuilders for its anabolic properties related to growth hormone release. Subsequently, it became a recreational drug because of reported euphoric and sexual effects [25, 26]. The FDA banned over-the-counter sales in 1990 and made GHB a schedule I illegal narcotic in 2000 with the passage of Hillory J. Farias and Samantha Reid Date-Rape Drug Prohibition Act of 1999 [27]. However, GHB has been difficult to police because of the existence of the precursors 1, 4-butanediol (1,4-BD) and gamma-butyrolactone (GBL). These are available in industrial solvents, chemical laboratories, cleaning products, and through internet suppliers. GHB is also available as an FDA approved sleep aid under the name sodium oxybate (Xyrem®) with the indication for narcolepsy with cataplexy [28]. 1,4-BD is metabolized to GHB in the liver in a two-step process including the enzyme alcohol dehydrogenase [23]. This conversion may be competitively inhibited with ethanol or fomepizole. GBL is metabolized by serum lactonases to GHB [23]. GHB usually exists in a liquid form but is also available as a powder. Generally, the liquid is clear, tasteless and odorless. These properties have prompted the use of GHB as a date rape drug and have led to accidental lethal ingestions when the drug is mistaken for water [29]. Once a popular drug of choice at rave and dance parties, poison center reports of GHB exposures in the pediatric population have decreased by 50 % from 2005 [1, 30, 31].

Evidence suggests that most of the physiologic and pharmacologic effects of systemically administered GHB are mediated by the $GABA_B$ receptor [24]. In addition, evidence exists of effects on other pathways including alterations of dopamine levels, serotonin levels, acetylcholine levels and N-methyl-D-aspartate (NMDA) receptor binding [24]. The onset of effects is usually between 10 and 20 min with a peak plasma concentration at 30–90 min. Average elimination half-life is 30–50 min [29]. Resolution of symptoms depends on the dose ingested. Sedation may result from as little as 25 mg/kg and coma from 60 mg/kg of GHB. Exact levels can be measured by gas chromatography or mass spectroscopy [29]. GHB is not detected on routine toxicology tests.

Clinical symptoms include CNS depression, altered mental status, seizures, hypotonia, myoclonic jerking, respiratory depression, bradycardia, hypotension, incontinence,

vomiting, and death [26]. CNS depression can be severe with a Glasgow Coma Scale (GCS) as low as 3 [23, 29]. Care of the patient with an acute GHB ingestion is largely supportive. Treatment includes cardiorespiratory monitoring, vasoactive support and mechanical ventilation if necessary for airway protection or respiratory insufficiency. Mortality from GHB exposure is frequently due to unrecognized respiratory failure and subsequent cardiorespiratory arrest [29]. Physostigmine, flumazenil, and naloxone are not effective antidotes [32–34]. Because of the rapid absorption of GHB, activated charcoal is usually reserved for suspected co-ingestions.

3,4-Methylenedioxymethamphetamine (MDMA)

MDMA is a hallucinogenic, synthetic methamphetamine commonly referred to as "ecstasy." Other psychedelic methamphetamines include 3,4-methylenedioxyamphetamine (MDA) and 3,4-methylenedioxy-N-ethylamphetamine (MDEA). MDMA is a releaser and reuptake inhibitor of serotonin, dopamine and norepinephrine [35]. Users of MDMA report euphoria, well-being, happiness, sociability, mild visual perception alteration, a sense of "closeness," increased empathy, and occasional visual hallucinations. Other effects include mydriasis, dry mouth, bruxism, tachycardia, hypertension and a sympathomimetic toxidrome [35, 36]. Maximum effect occurs within 2 h of exposure and the elimination half-life is 8–9 h [35, 37]. Ecstasy is usually ingested orally with tablet forms revealing a personalized insignia of the manufacturer. Ecstasy can also be crushed and used nasally, intravenously or by inhalation through smoking. Because ecstasy is produced in an uncontrolled environment, the end product is often not MDMA [38]. Only 26 % of ecstasy tablets tested in 2010 contained 100 % MDMA whereas 54 % were completely devoid of MDMA and contained other combinations of inexpensive medications, usually stimulants [39]. Toxicological screens will frequently be positive for amphetamines, however this is not specific to MDMA and gas chromatography or mass spectroscopy must be utilized to determine the presence and concentration of MDMA.

In general, treatment is supportive. Although there is rapid GI absorption, activated charcoal may be considered for patients who present less than 1 h after ingestion and for those suspected of co-ingestions. Severe intoxication or overdose from MDMA can cause multi-system organ dysfunction. MDMA ingestions may cause CNS, cardiac, and hepatic dysfunction as well as hyperthermia. Intense physical activity and dehydration combined with amphetamine use predispose users to hyperthermia. This toxicity resembles that seen with heat stroke and includes rhabdomyolysis, myoglobinemia, renal failure, liver damage and disseminated intravascular coagulopathy [37]. Because of the similarity to heat stroke, MDMA hyperthermia has been treated with dantrolene. A review of 71 cases of MDMA related hyperpyrexia indicates dantrolene may be beneficial in treating hyperthermia secondary to MDMA [40]. The patient should be aggressively cooled and provided supportive care as indicated by organ dysfunction.

MDMA CNS effects include headache, mydriasis, blurred vision, dizziness, seizures, coma, and cerebral edema [41–43]. Hyponatremia secondary to SIADH has been associated with MDMA use [42]. Seizures should be treated aggressively with benzodiazepines. If present, hyponatremia and hyperthermia need to be identified early and addressed to avoid complications. Cerebral imaging should be considered in the patient with altered mental status.

Cardiac toxicity from MDMA ingestion may include chest discomfort, ST elevation, cardiac enzyme elevation, and cardiac dysfunction [44, 45]. The exact mechanism of injury is unknown although animal studies indicate decreased contractility from MDMA and two MDMA metabolites [46]. Dysrhythmias, myocardial infarction, and cardiomyopathy may occur in severe MDMA ingestions [47].

The mechanism of hepatotoxicity is unclear, but ischemia from hyperthermia and drug hypersensitivity have been entertained. Eosinophilia has been identified from the portal tract biopsies which would support the latter [48]. Recovery from acute liver failure with or without hyperthermia is variable ranging from full recovery to the need for transplant [49]. Clinically, patient symptoms mimic viral hepatitis and conservative treatment is usually effective.

"Bath Salts"

"Bath salts" are a relatively new synthetic cathinone drug of abuse. The designer drugs are currently purchased legally via the Internet or through smoke houses, gas stations and convenience stores. They are frequently marketed as bath salts, plant food, or insect repellants, but not intended for such use. Recreational manufacturers continue to produce cathinone derivatives, which evade the illegal status of specific methamphetamines. There appears to be a rapid increase in the use of bath salts. There were 302 calls to poison centers in 2010 about these products, however over 2,200 calls had already been reported in the first trimester of 2011 [50]. In September of 2011, the Drug Enforcement Agency took emergency federal action and made bath salts illegal to sell or possess in the United States.

Cathinones contain a ketone group on the β carbon which causes decreased CNS penetration and less potency, which may lead to overdose or increased adverse effects [18]. These products usually contain either methylenedioxypyrovalerone (MDPV) or 4-methylmethcathinone (mephedrone) which release and inhibit the reuptake of serotonin, dopamine and norepinephrine [51]. The substances are taken orally, nasally or intravenously [52]. Cathinone chemical relatives differ in their receptor activities with mephedrone, showing similar release of serotonin but increased dopamine release in rats when compared to MDMA [53]. Clinical effects mimic drugs that are structurally similar to methamphetamines and thus produce a sympathomimetic toxidrome. Symptoms include euphoria, empathy, bruxism, agitation, tachycardia, delusions, increased sexual desire, panic and hallucinations [52, 54].

Patients who have ingested bath salts should be treated using the same approach as patients with toxic MDMA exposure [51]. Activated charcoal may be considered for patients who present less than one hour after ingestion and for those suspected of co-ingestions. Specific treatment may be necessary for hyperthermia, cardiac toxicity, liver toxicity and changes in CNS status. Hyponatremia secondary to SIADH can also occur [55]. Benzodiazepines are useful to calm these patients and for treatment of seizures [56].

Ketamine

Ketamine is an arylcyclohexylamine similar to phencyclidine (PCP) used for sedation and anesthesia, but also abused as a recreational drug. Street use of ketamine (K, cat tranquilizer, super K, special K, vitamin K) has existed since the 1970s. Ketamine is available in a liquid or powder and is snorted, smoked, ingested or injected. Ketamine, a NMDA receptor antagonist, has less binding affinity to the receptor and a shorter duration of action than PCP [57]. Users describe a floating feeling, a dreamy state, hallucinations, a sense of detachment from the body, and sometimes severe dissociation with reality referred to as a "k-hole" [57, 58]. Ketamine is metabolized by hepatic cytochrome P-450 isoenzymes and has an elimination half-life of 2.1 h [59]. Toxicology testing for ketamine and its major metabolites is not routinely available, however, quantitative results can be obtained by gas chromatography, mass spectroscopy, or high-performance liquid chromatography [60].

GI decontamination is usually not indicated because most illicit methods of ingestion do not involve the GI tract and if orally ingested, absorption is usually complete by the time of presentation. Activated charcoal should be considered if co-ingestion is suspected.

Supportive care is the primary treatment for ketamine ingestions with particular attention to maintaining adequate respiratory status, circulation and temperature control. Clinical symptoms may include abdominal pain, chest pain, dizziness, vomiting, and dysuria [61, 62]. Physical findings may include agitation, tachycardia, altered mental status, slurred speech, hallucinations, hypertension, anxiety, abdominal tenderness and nystagmus [61, 62]. Potential risk exists for liver injury, hyperthermia and/or rhabdomyolysis [61]. Adverse cardiovascular effects and hypertension may require intervention. Respiratory deterioration and other complications may occur from co-ingestions. If severe lower urinary tract symptoms occur, interstitial cystitis treatment methods seem to be effective [63]. Conservative treatment, benzodiazepines for sedation and IV hydration have been effective in the treatment of symptomatic patients following ketamine ingestions [62].

Dextromethorphan

Dextromethorphan, an antitussive ingredient in over-the-counter medications, continues to cause frequent poison control center consultations with a prevalence of abuse in the teen population [1, 64, 65]. Slang names include triple C, CCC, skittles, dex, red hots, sheets and robo [64, 65]. Dextromethorphan is the D-isomer of the codeine analogue levorphanol. It is metabolized by cytochrome CYP2D6 which has great variability due to genetic polymorphisms resulting in fast or slow metabolizers. Approximately 15 % of the population are slow metabolizers and may need to ingest larger amounts to achieve the same desired "high." The active metabolite dextrophan binds to NMDA and opioid σ (sigma)-receptors. Dextromethorphan is also a serotonin re-uptake inhibitor [66]. NMDA receptor stimulation causes ketamine and PCP-like dissociative effects. High doses bind to the opioid σ receptor specifically avoiding μ (mu)-receptor effects such as respiratory depression [67, 68].

Dextromethorphan is ingested by liquid, gel caps or tablets. Abusers prefer the pill form because of the increased dextromethorphan content and avoidance of the unpalatable taste of the syrups [68]. Because over-the-counter dextromethorphan formulations include other medications, physicians should consider co-ingestions such as acetaminophen, aspirin, phenylephrine, pseudoephedrine and antihistamines [64]. The combination of dextromethorphan with serotonergic drugs may result in a serotonin toxidrome [69]. Neurobehavioral effects begin at 30–60 min post-exposure and last up to 6 h. There are several 'plateaus' of effect based on ingested dose. Ingestions of 1.5–2.5 mg/kg give a mild euphoric effect while 2.5–7.5 mg/kg produce mild hallucinations and an intoxicated phase. Amounts of 7.5–15 mg/kg create an 'out-of-body' state and a full dissociative experience occurs with doses over 15 mg/kg [65, 70].

Testing for dextromethorphan is not routinely available and dextromethorphan does not cross react with opiate screening. False-positive testing for phenylcyclidine from high dose dextromethorphan has been reported but limited data exist to support this [71]. Quantitative levels may be obtained through gas chromatography or high pressure liquid chromatography. Clinical symptoms include GI symptoms, altered mental status, tachycardia, hypertension, diaphoresis, hyperthermia, dizziness, lethargy, hallucinations, seizures, dystonic reactions, complete CNS dissociation and coma [67, 72]. Other symptoms may occur if there are co-ingestions and may include anticholinergic symptoms (anti-histamines) or serotonin syndrome (MDMA, MAO inhibitors, SSRIs, lithium, TCAs, and meperidine) [66, 73]. Acetaminophen

and aspirin concentrations should be determined depending on what dextromethorphan preparation was ingested.

Supportive care is generally the mainstay of therapy. Activated charcoal should be administered within 1 h of ingestion and strongly considered especially if co-ingestions have occurred. Anticholinergic and serotonin symptoms may improve with benzodiazepine administration. Hypertension, tachycardia and hyperthermia may require interventional treatment. Naloxone should be considered if coma and respiratory depression are present, however, there are conflicting reports on its effectiveness [74].

2-C Phenethylamines

The 2-C phenethylamines are hallucinogenic designer drug analogues of the hallucinogen 3,4,5-trimethoxy-phenethylamine (mescaline). The 2C synthetic drugs share the 2,5 dimethoxy-phenethylamine building block which allows the common binding to serotonin receptors [75]. Slight alterations to the additional branch of the 2,5 dimethoxyphenethylamine compound help manufactures evade the legal system. Common 2cs include 4-bromo-2,5-dimethoxyphenethylamine (2C-B), 4-iodo-2,5-dimethoxyphenethylamine (2C-I), 4-methyl-2,5-dimethoxyphenethylamine (2C-D), 4-ethyl-2,5-dimethoxyphenethylamine (2C-E), 4-ethylthio-2,5-dimethoxyphenethylamine (2C-T-2), and 4-(n)-propylthio-2,5-dimethoxyphenethylamine (2C-T-7) although numerous other analogues exist. Although closely related to amphetamines, the 2Cs are not picked up on routine drug screens. Quantitative analysis is typically obtained by gas chromatography and mass spectrometry. The 2C series exist in tablet and powder form and may be ingested or insufflated. The 2C series are catabolized by deamination through MAO A and B making patients susceptible to greater 2-C effects when exposed to MAO inhibitors [76]. Duration of effect is 4 to over 24 h, depending on the amount ingested and which 2C phenethylamine is involved. Clinical effects include euphoria, sociability, mydriasis, strong visual hallucinations, altered mental status, dizziness, paranoia, anxiety, insomnia, nausea and vomiting [77]. Supportive care is the mainstay of treatment. Activated charcoal should be administered within 1 h of ingestion and strongly considered if co-ingestions are suspected.

Alcohols

Ethylene Glycol

Ethylene glycol (EG) is a sweet tasting alcohol that continues to remain a cause of morbidity and mortality in the pediatric age group with over 1,000 exposures reported to poison centers in 2009 [1]. EG is most commonly found in antifreeze and de-icing solutions. It is metabolized by alcohol dehydrogenase (ADH) and aldehyde dehydrogenase leading to production of toxic metabolites including glycoaldehyde, glycolic acid, glyoxylic acid and oxalic acid [78]. Animal studies have led to a quoted minimum lethal dose of 1–1.5 mL/kg, although patients ingesting over 1 liter have survived with immediate treatment [78]. The most clinically significant toxins are glycolic acid and oxalic acid. Glycolic acid is responsible for the metabolic acidosis following EG ingestion. Oxalic acid readily binds to calcium producing calcium oxalate crystals. Deposition of these crystals occur throughout the body including the kidney, brain, liver, lungs, and spleen [78–80].

Clinical presentation, ensuing EG ingestion, follows three stages. The neurological stage occurs less than 12 h following ingestion and consists of initial inebriation similar to ethanol ingestion. As EG metabolism progresses, neurological symptoms can progress to altered mental status, ataxia, nystagmus, seizures, hypotonia, coma, and cerebral edema [78]. EG alone is a gastric irritant and may cause vomiting which puts the patient with altered mental status at risk for aspiration. Stage 2 occurs 12–24 h following ingestion and involves cardiopulmonary toxicity with potential development of tachycardia, hypertension, compensatory hyperventilation, hypoxia from aspiration, congestive heart failure and acute respiratory distress syndrome (ARDS) [78]. The last stage, occurring 24–72 h following ingestion, involves the kidneys and is characterized by oliguria, renal failure from acute tubular necrosis, anuria and the need for hemodialysis [78]. Demonstration of calcium oxalate crystals in the urine with a Wood's lamp helps confirm the presence of EG. Acute tubular necrosis occurs as a result of accumulation of calcium oxalate monohydrate (COM) crystals [81]. Laboratory studies are significant for an anion gap metabolic acidosis, an osmolal gap, and renal failure. Hypocalcemia may occur from chelation by oxalate. An EG level should be obtained, but treatment should not be delayed for suspected or known ingestions. Head CT and brain MRI may be helpful in evaluating suspected cerebral edema and sudden neurological changes. Increased ICP secondary to EG ingestion has been described, but data supporting ICP monitoring does not exist at this time [82].

Initial management focuses on airway, breathing and circulation. Competitive inhibition of ADH should be the initial focus of treatment. Historically, ethanol was used to inhibit breakdown of EG by ADH, but 4-methylpyrazole (fomepizole) is now the antidote of choice for EG toxicity [83]. Fomepizole has an affinity for ADH 500–1,000 times greater than ethanol and its use is associated with less medication errors when compared to ethanol [84, 85]. Fomepizole should be given as soon as possible following toxic EG ingestions because prognosis will depend on the amount of toxic metabolites already accumulated. Fomepizole may obviate the need for hemodialysis in EG ingestions if given to patients with normal renal function at the time of presentation [86–88]. Fomepizole also appears to be safe in children [83, 87, 89]. If ingestion occurred less than 1 h prior

to presentation, gastric aspiration and lavage may be considered. Activated charcoal may be considered if a toxic co-ingestion is suspected.

Hemodialysis is useful in severe ingestions. Indications for hemodialysis include severe acidosis, acidosis despite bicarbonate therapy, renal failure, EG concentration > 50 mg/dL, and hemodynamic instability [84]. During hemodialysis, it is important to continue fomepizole at a shortened dosing interval to maintain plasma levels to continue ADH inhibition. Thiamine and pyridoxime can be given in an attempt to prevent oxalic acid formation, however, data supporting this is lacking [78]. Thiamine facilitates the conversion of glyoxylic acid to harmless α hydroxy-β ketoadipic acid and pyridoxime converts glyoxylic acid to glycine, which is non-toxic [90].

Methanol

With nearly 300 pediatric exposures reported to US poison control centers in 2009, methanol continues to pose a risk to children because it is generally readily accessible [1]. Methanol ingestion results from household availability of windshield wiper fluid, cleaning solutions, paint removers, some antifreeze agents, fuel additives, and "moonshine." Methanol is metabolized by ADH to formaldehyde, then rapidly to formic acid. Levels of formic acid correlate with arterial pH, toxicity and clinical outcome [91]. Formic acid may cause hypoxia by effecting cytochrome oxidase activity in mitochondria [6, 92]. Metabolic acidosis results directly from formic acid as well as a lactic acidosis. Neurotoxicity may occur from either formic acid itself or secondary hypoxic injury targeting the basal ganglia and specifically the putamen [6]. Formic acid also causes direct ocular toxicity [6].

Clinical presentation usually involves the CNS, gastrointestinal (GI) tract, kidneys and eyes. CNS involvement can produce headache, altered mental status, seizures, coma and signs of cerebral edema. GI symptoms include vomiting and abdominal pain. Renal dysfunction results in oliguria, anuria, and renal failure. Vision dysfunction manifests as blurred vision, decreased acuity, or even blindness. Laboratory evaluation should include evaluation of electrolytes, anion gap, osmolal gap, renal function, pancreatic enzymes, liver enzymes, and a methanol level [6]. Treatment should not be delayed for methanol level results. Head CT and brain MRI may be used to evaluate possible cerebral edema, sudden neurological changes, and basal ganglia involvement. Data supporting ICP monitoring does not exist at this time.

Airway, breathing and circulation should be assessed and addressed initially. Focus then should be directed toward the likelihood and quantity ingested because a minimum lethal dose is 1.2 mL/kg [84]. Activated charcoal may be considered for toxic co-ingestions. Acidosis of a pH < 7.30 should be treated with sodium bicarbonate which will help reduce the effect on cytochrome oxidase activity [6]. A methanol level>20 mg/dL indicates a need for further treatment. If a level is not immediately obtainable, known methanol ingestion with an osmolal gap>10 mOsm/L is sufficient to start treatment. Otherwise, treatment may ensue for clinical suspicion of methanol ingestion with two of the following criteria: pH≤7.3, serum bicarbonate<20 mmol/L, and osmolal gap>10 mOsm/L [6, 83]. Fomepizole is the drug of choice for methanol poisoning and should be given as soon as possible to stop formic acid production. Early administration of fomepizole to patients without metabolic acidosis may obviate the need for hemodialysis [92]. Folinic acid is a safe drug that enhances formic acid metabolism and may be considered in the methanol poisoned patient [6].

Hemodialysis still plays an important role in methanol poisoning because of the slow elimination of formic acid. Indications for hemodialysis include severe metabolic acidosis (base deficit>−15 mM), vision disturbance, renal failure, hemodynamic instability and a methanol level>50 mg/dL [6, 92]. Lack of a methanol level should not delay treatment because the degree of acidosis correlates better with prognosis and permanent visual impairment [6]. During hemodialysis, it is important to continue fomepizole at a shortened dosing interval to maintain plasma levels to continue ADH inhibition. Hemodialysis is continued with a goal to resolve acidosis and achieve methanol levels<25 mg/dL [6]. Following redistribution, methanol levels may rebound within 36 h and repeat hemodialysis may be needed. Therefore, pH, osmolal gap, electrolytes, and methanol levels should be monitored 36 h following cessation of hemodialysis [6].

Isopropyl Alcohol (Isopropanol)

Isopropanol is a bitter alcohol used in automotive and cleaning products as well as being the solvent in rubbing alcohol. It is metabolized to acetone in the liver. Toxic effects are secondary to isopropanol, not acetone. The minimal lethal dose for children has not been described, but approximately 100 mL may be lethal in an adult [93]. Levels are not routinely available, but can be useful. Levels>400 mg/dL indicate a need for hemodialysis [93, 94]. Hemodialysis should also be considered for isopropanol levels>200 mg/dL, especially when hypotension and coma exist [95]. Isopropanol is absorbed rapidly and elimination half-life is 3–7 h [96]. Clinical signs of isopropanol may include a fruity order, altered mental status, coma, vomiting, abdominal pain, hematemesis, and hypotension. Isopropanol should be strongly suspected when laboratory studies show an elevated osmolal gap and a positive serum acetone test accompanied without a metabolic acidosis. Other clues to the diagnosis include the presence of urine ketones, renal failure and hypoglycemia [93]. Activated charcoal may be considered for toxic co-ingestions. Supportive treatment is usually sufficient if coma and hypotension are not present.

Ethanol

Ethanol exposures accounted for over 3,500 calls to American poison centers in 2009 [1]. Alcoholic beverages, mouthwashes containing ethanol, aftershaves, colognes, and perfumes allow children access to ethanol in the home [97]. Oxidation of ethanol in the liver by alcohol dehydrogenase produces acetaldehyde which leads to the production of ketone bodies [95]. Ethanol ingestion may produce intoxication, altered mental status, coma, vomiting and hypothermia. Metabolic acidosis, ketosis, hypoglycemia, hypokalemia, hypernatremia, hypochloremia, and osmolal gap may also occur [98]. Ethanol is rapidly absorbed and activated charcoal should be reserved for toxic co-ingestions. Ethanol levels are readily available and supportive care is the mainstay of treatment. Management should focus on maintenance of airway, breathing and circulation. Vomiting with aspiration pneumonitis may occur. Hypoglycemia and hypotension should be appropriately addressed. Treatment usually includes volume replacement and dextrose containing fluids until the patient returns to baseline. Currently, a threshold on when to perform hemodialysis does not exist for the severely intoxicated ethanol patient.

Psychoactive Drugs

Antipsychotics

Small amounts of antipsychotics can cause significant toxicity in children. The antipsychotics exert their effects over a large number of different receptors: serotonin, dopamine, histamine, α-adrenergic, and muscarinic. Classes of antipsychotics include the phenothiazines, butyrophenones, and the newer atypical antipsychotics. An aliphatic phenothiazine, chlorpromazine, produces CNS depression, profound sedation, and miosis in overdose. Extrapyramidal symptoms (EPS), neuroleptic malignant syndrome (NMS), dystonic reactions, and seizures may also occur. Thioridazine, a piperidine phenothiazine, is the most cardiotoxic antipsychotic in overdose in adults. Strong sedation effects, miosis and QT prolongation have been seen with pediatric ingestions. Trifluoperazine, perphenazine and fluphenazine are piperazine phenothiazines and cause dystonic reactions, EPS, and CNS depression following overdose. The most widely used butyrophenone antipsychotic is haloperidol. Drowsiness, tremor, dystonic reactions, and EPS are found most commonly with overdose. Olanzapine is an atypical antipsychotic classified as a thienobenzodiazepine. CNS depression, tachycardia and agitation are common, but EPS, miosis, hypersalivation and anticholinergic effects also occur. The atypical antipsychotic risperidone in overdose may cause altered mental status, EPS, tachycardia and hypotension [99]. Ziprasidone is another atypical antipsychotic that usually causes drowsiness, lethargy and tachycardia. Rarely,

QTc prolongation may be seen [100, 101]. Aripiprazole, an atypical antidepressant and antipsychotic, causes CNS depression, vomiting, tachycardia and hypotension in overdose. And finally pimozide, an antipsychotic drug with a special indication to treat tics and Tourette syndrome, may cause seizures, EPS, dystonic reactions, CNS depression and hypotension with overdoses.

Symptomatic care is the mainstay of treatment for all antipsychotic overdoses. Severe CNS depression may necessitate the need for intubation. Hypotension usually resolves with fluid administration. Activated charcoal should be administered within 1 h to the non-sedated patient. Benzatropine or diphenhydramine should be administered to patients with dystonic reactions or EPS. Antipsychotic EPS may require days of treatment before resolving [99]. The combination of fever, tachycardia, muscle rigidity and altered mental status in patients exposed to atypical antipsychotics requires CPK evaluation and NMS consideration. Of note, children and adolescents with atypical antipsychotic NMS had a shorter duration of illness when treated with bromocriptine when compared to dantrolene [102].

Selective Serotonin Reuptake Inhibitors (SSRIs)

Increased use of SSRIs in depression can be traced to less toxicity following overdoses and an improved adverse effect profile in comparison to TCAs [103]. Commonly used SSRIs include sertraline, paroxetine, fluvoxamine, fluoxetine, and citalopram. SSRIs take approximately 4 h to reach peak serum concentration after ingestion [104]. In general, SSRI ingestions are well tolerated in children [105]. There is potential for a clinical serotonin syndrome to occur consisting of tachycardia, hyperthermia, mydriasis, myoclonus, hyperreflexia, shivering, diaphoresis, diarrhea, muscle rigidity, delirium, and agitation [69]. Activated charcoal is indicated for the non-sedated patient following ingestion. Serotonin toxidromes are generally treated with supportive care. Do not confuse serotonin syndrome with NMS. NMS will lack mydriasis, will show lead pipe rigidity and have a history of exposure to neuroleptics. Nonspecific serotonin receptor antagonists (β-blockers, cyproheptadine, methysergide, and chlorpromazine) have been studied in animals, but routine use in humans cannot be recommended at this time [106]. However, a case using cyproheptadine in a 24 month old for a SSRI induced serotonin syndrome has been reported [107].

Tricyclic Antidepressants (TCAs)

TCAs continue to be widely available because of continued clinical use treating a wide variety of disorders including depression, anxiety, chronic pain, headache, and attention deficit hyperactivity disorder. TCAs include amitriptyline, clomipramine, desipramine, dosulepin, doxepin, imipramine, lofepramine, nortriptyline, protriptyline and trimipramine. A dose of 5 mg/kg for all TCAs is a significant ingestion warranting evaluation. Desipramine, nortriptyline, and trimipramine may cause toxicity with 2.5 mg/kg and a dose of 1 mg/kg of protriptyline warrants evaluation for toxicity [108]. TCAs exert their toxicity through anticholinergic effects, antagonism of peripheral α_1 receptors, blockade of cardiac and CNS sodium channels, and by blocking CNS monoamine reuptake. Within 6 h of ingestion, the presence of hypotension, respiratory depression, altered mental status, seizures, cardiac dysrhythmias, or a QRS duration > 100 milliseconds (ms) puts the patient at high risk for complications [109].

Cardiac toxicity from TCA poisoning results from blockade of cardiac sodium channels. ECG changes include widened QRS interval, prolonged PR and QT intervals, right axis deviation, abnormal T waves and ST segments, and atrioventricular (AV) block. Sinus tachycardia is the most common rhythm observed, although supraventricular tachycardia, ventricular tachycardia, and bradydysrhythmias associated with AV block can also occur. Torsades de pointes is uncommon. A QRS duration > 100 ms and right axis deviation appear to be the strongest predictors of cardiac toxicity. A QRS > 160 ms should prompt immediate attention to prevent a ventricular dysrhythmia. ECG changes usually occur within the first 6 h and may last for days. Serious cardiac complications most commonly occur within 24 h of ingestion and rapid deterioration can be common [109].

Hypotension from TCA ingestion may occur because of cardiac toxicity as well as α_1 adrenergic receptor blockade. Systemic anticholinergic effects are often present. Norepinephrine and serotonin reuptake blockade, sodium channel inhibition, anticholinergic effects, and hypotension may all have direct effects on the CNS. Agitation, altered mental status, seizures and coma can all result from TCA poisoning and are signs of a significant TCA ingestion. Glasgow Coma Scale (GCS) levels < 8 predict serious complications [110].

Initial treatment of the TCA poisoned patient should focus on airway, breathing, circulation and neurological status. Gastric decontamination should be performed with activated charcoal. Enterohepatic recirculation accounts for 15 % of TCA elimination [111]. Because activated charcoal is well tolerated, the authors recommend multiple dose activated charcoal for TCA poisonings. However, intubation with a cuffed endotracheal tube should be considered prior to the administration of activated charcoal if the patient has altered mental status and may not be able to protect their airway. Gastric lavage, hemodialysis and charcoal hemoperfusion are not indicated. Again, QRS duration of >100 ms, right axis deviation and abnormal heart rhythm on ECG indicate potential cardiac toxicity. TCA toxicity seems to be worsened by acidosis. Treatment centers on sodium loading and alkalinization by the administration of sodium bicarbonate with a goal blood pH of 7.5–7.55. Hyperventilation may be used to alkalinize the patient in the short term if bicarbonate alkalinization is delayed. Alkalinization increases the proportion of nonionized drug because TCAs are weak bases. This may decrease the cardiac toxic effects. Hypotension is treated with fluid resuscitation and the addition of α_1 adrenergic agonists (norepinephrine, phenylephrine) when necessary [112].

Anticholinergic effects are managed symptomatically. Benzodiazepines may be used to control agitation. Seizures may be treated with benzodiazepines or barbiturates. Sodium channel blockers should theoretically be avoided because of the potential to worsen cardiac and CNS toxicity, although both lidocaine and phenytoin have been used for TCA seizure treatment and have lower cardiac sodium channel blocking activity being class 1B antiarrhythmic agents.

Antihypertensives

Calcium Channel Blockers (CCBs)

CCBs are prescribed for multiple conditions including hypertension, migraine headaches and adult angina. Extended and immediate release preparations exist. The type of CCB ingested is important since CCBs are classified as dihydropyridines and nondihydropyridines. The dihydropyridines cause more vascular vasodilatation and less myocardial contractility effect and include amlodipine, isradipine, felodipine, nicardipine, and nifedipine [113]. The nondihydropyridines, including verapamil and diltiazem, decrease myocardial contractility to a greater degree, affect myocardial conduction, and are weak vasodilators [113].

Management of the CCB poisoned patient should initially focus on airway, breathing, and circulation. Activated charcoal is indicated and multiple doses may be considered if sustained release preparations have been ingested [114]. An ECG should be obtained in all ingestions. Significant ingestions may have hypotension and bradycardia; isotonic fluid resuscitation should be attempted but may not be effective. Atropine can be given for severe bradycardia but may also be ineffective [115]. Calcium gluconate or calcium chloride can be given IV as a bolus or drip to overload the calcium channel and increase contractility and blood pressure [116]. Serum ionized calcium levels should be monitored frequently when using a calcium drip. If ineffective, glucagon may be administered intravenously. Glucagon increases c-AMP in the myocardial cell which can increase contractility. The half-life of glucagon is extremely short so, if effective, a glucagon drip should also be administered. High dose insulin with dextrose can also be given as a bolus or a continuous drip. Insulin affects several intracellular mechanisms in the myocardial cell that contribute to inotropy [117]. If hypotension still exists, vasopressors should be initiated. Epinephrine and norepinephrine are good choices secondary

to their vasoconstrictive and inotropic effects and should be titrated to effect. ILE infusions have shown benefit in animal and human case reports in CCB overdoses [17]. ILE therapy may be considered in life threatening situations. A phosphodiesterase inhibitor may increase contractility but may also cause unwanted vasodilatation. Levosimendan has been used in CCB overdose after conventional therapy failed with improvement of bradycardia but continued hypotension [118]. Temporary cardiac pacing has produced varying outcomes [114]. ECMO has been used with success in refractory cases [119].

Beta-blockers (β-blockers)

β-blockers are available treatment options for a wide range of medical disorders. Their prevalence and toxic potential make β-blocker poisoning a significant cause of morbidity and mortality. In general, children less than 6 years of age, who usually do not ingest a large quantity of pills, do not develop toxicity from β-blocker ingestions [120]. Most patients will develop symptoms of β-blocker toxicity within 6 h of ingestion [121]. Potential toxicity from β-blockers include hypotension, bradycardia, bronchospasm and hypoglycemia [122]. Significant ingestions may cause cardiogenic shock, seizures, altered mental status, respiratory depression, ventricular arrhythmias and asystole [123, 124]. ECG changes include widening of the QRS interval and prolonged PR and QTc intervals [125].

Management of β-blocker toxicity begins with airway, breathing and circulation assessment. ECG and blood glucose are mandatory in any β-blocker ingestion. Activated charcoal, unless contraindicated, should be given to all β-blocker ingestions within 1–2 h of ingestion. Hypotension may be treated with fluids and atropine may treat symptomatic bradycardia. If an artificial airway is needed, atropine should be administered prior to intubation. Benzodiazepines should be used to treat seizures if present. If cardiovascular instability continues despite fluids and atropine, additional treatment includes glucagon, IV calcium, vasopressors, and high dose insulin and glucose. Other therapies supported by case reports and animal studies include a phosphodiesterase inhibitor infusion, sodium bicarbonate, levosimendan, ILE, temporary pacing, and ECMO. Glucagon increases c-AMP in the myocardial cell which can increase contractility. Glucagon therapy in β-blocker poisoning stems from multiple animal studies showing increased cardiac function and human case reports [126]. Again, the half-life of glucagon is extremely short. Therefore, if effective, a glucagon drip should be administered. Case reports have shown cardiovascular improvement with both calcium gluconate and calcium chloride infusions [127]. If a response is seen, a calcium drip can be continued. Serum ionized calcium levels should be monitored frequently when using a calcium drip. If cardiac function does not improve, vasopressor therapy should be started. An epinephrine infusion should be titrated to effect based on desired blood pressure. Insulin affects several intracellular mechanisms in the myocardial cell that contribute to inotropy [117]. High dose insulin with dextrose can also be given as a bolus or a continuous drip. A phosphodiesterase inhibitor can be considered and may increase contractility by also increasing c-AMP in the myocardial cell [128]. Sodium bicarbonate may restore cardiac output and narrow the QRS complex [129]. Levosimendan improved cardiac function and survival from propranolol intoxication in an animal model [130]. ILE has been beneficial in a case report and may be considered following routine therapy [124]. When all else fails, temporary pacing may be attempted and ECMO has previously been life-saving [131].

Clonidine

Clonidine hydrochloride stimulates the imidazoline receptor and the presynaptic α-2 receptor in the brain leading to inhibition of norepinephrine release. This decrease in sympathetic outflow results in decreased peripheral resistance, renal vascular resistance, heart rate and blood pressure. Clonidine is approved for the management of hypertension, however off-label uses in children for opioid withdrawal, management of attention-deficit/hyperactivity disorder (ADHD) and Tourette syndrome has resulted in increased availability of this agent in homes with children. Although most children with clonidine exposure have minimal toxicity, a number of children have serious toxicity and very rarely death has occurred [132]. Toxicity can occur with ingestion of just 0.1 mg or one tablet [133]. Clonidine is available in pill or patch formulations. The patch is changed weekly, therefore significant exposure can occur if a child ingests a patch.

Absorption of clonidine occurs rapidly and peak levels occur within 1–3 h and the majority of patients develop symptoms within 4–6 h of ingestion. Clonidine is renally excreted and has no active metabolites. Patients who have ingested clonidine are at risk for abrupt changes in mental status, therefore caution should be used in treating them with activated charcoal unless it is early after exposure. Whole bowel irrigation may be of benefit if a clonidine patch is ingested.

Transient hypertension is seen due to stimulation of peripheral α-1 receptors. Subsequent altered mental status, hypotension, bradycardia, respiratory depression, hyporeflexia, and hypotonia occurs due to stimulation of central α-2 receptors resulting in decreased sympathetic outflow. Hypertension is usually not treated because it is transient and frequently is followed by prolonged hypotension. Hypotension should be treated with fluid followed by norepinephrine if needed. Bradycardia does not usually require treatment other than stimulation, but if it is significant and persistent, atropine may be indicated. Naloxone as a bolus dose or continuous infusion has been utilized with variable success for central nervous system depression and respiratory depression [133, 134]. If the patient does not respond to a bolus dose of naloxone, then no further doses should be given. Patients with significant CNS depression and respiratory depression require intubation. Supportive care is usually effective therapy.

Analgesics, Analgesics, Sedatives, and Antipyretics

Opioids

Opioids produce analgesia and anxiolysis as pain relievers and can also be found in cough suppressants and antidiarrheals. They are abused for their euphoric properties. Opioids react with μ (mu), κ (kappa), σ (sigma) and δ (delta)-receptors throughout the nervous system and gastrointestinal tract. Opioids commonly encountered include, but are not limited to, codeine, morphine, fentanyl, methadone, heroin, hydrocodone, oxycodone and meperidine. Opioids continue to be a major drug abuse problem and a cause of significant morbidity and mortality. Opioids may be used intravenously, subcutaneously, intramuscularly, transdermally, orally, nasally or inhaled. Transdermal administration of opioids in opioid naïve patients has resulted in significant morbidity and out-of-hospital deaths. Length of clinical effects varies depending on the half-life of the opioid ingested with methadone lasting the longest and fentanyl the shortest. An opioid toxidrome is characterized by bradycardia, hypotension, miosis, respiratory depression, confusion, lethargy, ataxia, and coma (Table 50.3). Opioid induced respiratory depression occurs as a result of opioids decreasing central and peripheral chemoreceptor activity [135]. Noncardiogenic pulmonary edema can also occur with uncertain etiology, but may be related to inspiration against an obstructed airway and disruption of the endothelial-alveolar barrier [136]. The noncardiogenic pulmonary edema usually resolves rapidly over hours to 1–2 days with supportive care [137]. Respiratory depression from μ_2-receptor stimulation can eventually lead to apnea, respiratory arrest and death. Urine toxicology screening for opioids should be positive.

Initial treatment is supportive focusing on airway, breathing and circulation. Respiratory compromise may be treated with naloxone or bag-mask ventilation and intubation. Naloxone is a short acting opioid antagonist with a long history of use in narcotic overdoses both for treatment and diagnostic purposes. If IV access is not available, naloxone should be administered intramuscularly. However, naloxone administration is not without risk. The half-life of naloxone is very short and if used as a reversal agent, opioid toxidrome symptoms may recur once naloxone disappears if the offending agent has a long half-life. An acute withdrawal syndrome can be induced with naloxone in the opioid-dependent patient. And lastly, naloxone may induce severe pain in patients receiving narcotics for acute pain [138]. In this situation, nalbuphrine, an opioid agonist-antagonist, would be a good drug choice to reverse the μ_2 respiratory depression while preserving κ and σ narcotic receptor stimulation [139]. Nalmefene is a long-acting opioid antagonist with a half-life of 8–9 h that has been used in the pediatric population [140]. This could be of benefit in acute opioid ingestions when narcotic dependence and acute pain issues do not exist. Initial hypotension should be addressed with fluid boluses as needed. Activated charcoal should be given unless contraindicated. Activated charcoal is also very valuable in sustained-release, long-acting, and delayed absorption (dephenoxylate-atropine) opiates.

Atypical opioids may also produce toxicity. Tramadol is a weak μ-receptor agonist while also causing inhibition of serotonin and norepinephrine in the CNS. Toxicity can result in CNS depression, respiratory depression, miosis, and even seizure activity [135, 141]. Benzodiazepines can be used to treat seizures, otherwise symptomatic care and activated charcoal administration is the mainstay of treatment. Buprenorphine is an opioid partial agonist, meaning that it still binds to opioid receptors. Clinically, in the correct dosing, it may produce decreased opioid effects. But in overdose, presentation and treatment should proceed as any other opioid ingestion. Buprenorphine/naloxone is a drug used to treat withdrawal symptoms but can still produce the typical CNS and respiratory opioid effects in overdose [142]. Again, treatment should be the same as any opioid ingestion.

Benzodiazepines

The prevalence of benzodiazepines stems from their wide use in treatment for seizures, anxiety, hyperactivity, insomnia, and drug withdrawal. The benzodiazepines exert their effect in the CNS by binding to the $GABA_A$ chloride channel complex. This potentiates the action of GABA which causes the movement of chloride into the cell causing hyperpolarization [143]. Numerous benzodiazepines exist including diazepam, lorazepam, midazolam, flunitrazepam, alprazolam, chlordiazepoxide, and zolpidem. While some act faster than others, all tend to have peak effect within 2 h but differ in their duration of action. Clinical toxicity produces the sedative-hypnotic toxidrome including bradycardia, hypotension, respiratory depression, hypothermia, confusion, stupor, and coma (Table 50.1). Sertraline and oxaprozin (nonsteroidal anti-inflammatory drug) may cause a false positive benzodiazepine urine drug screen [144]. Some evidence suggests that benzodiazepines with differing chemical structure, such as midazolam, chlordiazepoxide, and flunitrazepam, are not detected in many assays causing a false negative result on urine drug screening [144].

Initial treatment is supportive with attention to airway breathing and circulation. Intubation may be necessary depending on the degree of respiratory depression. Fluid boluses are indicated for hypotension. Flumazenil, a competitive antagonist at the $GABA_A$ receptor complex, can be used for diagnosis or treatment but its use remains controversial due to its association with a number of adverse events. Numerous studies report seizures and cardiac dysrhythmias following flumazenil use, especially when associated with TCAs and chloral hydrate [145–147]. Chronic benzodiazepine use prior to flumazenil exposure may precipitate seizure activity. It should be noted that flumazenil is short-acting, therefore, caution and close patient observation should be exercised if flumazenil is given for a long-acting benzodiazepine ingestion. Activated charcoal should be given unless contraindicated. It should be noted that propylene glycol is a diluent in diazepam and lorazepam and may cause adverse effects if taken in large quantities.

Acetaminophen

Acetaminophen (N-acetyl-p-aminophenol; APAP; paracetamol) accounts for a significant proportion of accidental and intentional toxic exposures in pediatric patients which can lead to irreversible hepatotoxicity and death. The American Association of Poison Control Centers in 2009 received 170 reports of death associated with APAP alone and 240 deaths when APAP combination drugs were ingested [1]. More than 600 over-the-counter and prescription products contain APAP. Most patients present early in the course following APAP ingestion and do not require critical care unless they have signs of hepatoxicity, have co-ingested other potentially toxic agents, are symptomatic, or have other significant medical problems that place them at risk. Activated charcoal should be given within 1–2 h of ingestion as it does not interfere significantly with the oral antidote N-acetylcysteine [9].

Federal regulations in 2011 resulted in new recommended maximum therapeutic doses of acetaminophen for children and adults [148]. The infant formulation of 80 mg/mL is no longer available, therefore only the pediatric formulation of 160 mg/5 mL liquid exists and it must come with a measuring device. The therapeutic dose of APAP for children under 12 years of age is 10–15 mg/kg/dose every 4–6 h with a maximum recommended dose from the manufacturer of 75 mg/kg/day. For adults the maximal single dose was reduced to 650 mg with a maximum daily dose of 3,250 mg. These changes in formulations and dosing recommendations are aimed at decreasing unintentional and intentional overdose leading to liver injury from acetaminophen containing products [148]. In 2011 the AAP published a clinical report related to the use of antipyretics that discourages treating fever unless the child is uncomfortable or the child does not tolerate the increased metabolic demands caused by the fever due to an underlying disease process [149]. If healthcare providers and parents implement this practice, fewer children may be at risk for acetaminophen overdoses with subsequent hepatotoxicity.

Normally, more than 90 % of APAP is conjugated with glucuronide or sulfate to form nontoxic renally excreted metabolites. Approximately 2 % is renally excreted and 5 % is metabolized by the hepatic cytochrome p450 mixed-function oxidase enzyme (CYP2E1) to the toxic metabolite N-acetyl-p-benzoquinoneimine (NAPQI) which is then rapidly detoxified by conjugation to intracellular glutathione (GSH) forming a nontoxic conjugate (APAP-GSH). When the conjugation pathways in the liver are overwhelmed in APAP overdose, metabolism of APAP is shunted to the cytochrome p450 pathway which results in an increased production of the toxic metabolite NAPQI and depletion of glutathione [150, 151]. The exact mechanism of hepatocyte death is still not completely elucidated, however it does correlate with the activity of the catalyzing enzyme systems and GSH availability. When GSH stores are reduced by 70–80 %, the detoxification capacity of the liver is exceeded and NAPQI accumulates subsequently destroying hepatocytes and other cells. In the absence of GSH, covalent binding of NAPQI to the cysteine groups on hepatocyte macromolecules occurs forming NAPQI-protein adducts [152]. This process is the initial and irreversible step in development of cell injury. NAPQI binds to critical cellular targets such as mitochondrial proteins. The hepatocytic cellular necrosis occurs due to mitochondrial dysfunction with ATP depletion, DNA damage, alterations in calcium homeostasis and modifications of intracellular proteins. Newer data suggest that inflammatory mediators trigger the innate immune system with subsequent propagation of hepatocyte injury [151, 153].

Although not definitive, factors that may influence the risk for development of hepatotoxicity include age (younger being protective), chronic alcohol ingestion, poor nutritional status, tobacco use and concomitant use of drugs that induce the CYP2E1 system. Infants and children process APAP predominantly through sulfation at a younger age with glucuronidation increasing with age. Children less than 5 years of age appear less susceptible to APAP hepatoxicity which may be due to a lower production of NAPQI and conjugation as the predominant metabolic pathway [151, 153]. Acute ingestions of greater than 200 mg/kg in children and 8–10 g in an adult may result in hepatotoxicity.

Initial signs (first 24 h) of acetaminophen are generally mild and the patient may have nonspecific gastrointestinal symptoms of nausea, vomiting, abdominal pain, anorexia, and malaise. Laboratory tests are usually normal at this time, however hypoglycemia may occur and reflects impaired hepatic gluconeogenesis, inability to mobilize hepatic glycogen stores and elevated levels of circulating insulin [153]. Over the next 24–72 h, the patient may have improvement of clinical symptoms but still have the onset of subclinical

hepatotoxicity with rising aminotransferases, PT and total bilirubin. Metabolic acidosis occurs in approximately 50 % of patients and may reflect inhibition of uptake and metabolism of lactic acid by the liver and impaired hepatic clearance [153]. Patients may develop right upper quadrant pain during this time. Between 72 and 96 h the patient has signs of overt hepatocellular necrosis with marked elevations of aminotransferases, PT and total bilirubin. Signs and symptoms are variable depending on the extent of hepatic injury but many patients experience anorexia, nausea, vomiting, abdominal pain, malaise and may develop hepatic encephalopathy. Patients who develop acute liver failure may develop cerebral edema with increased intracranial pressure and fatal uncal herniation. Renal insufficiency may occur secondary to APAP-induced acute tubular necrosis and dehydration. The degree of hypophosphatemia reflects the severity of the overdose. A rising PT and bilirubin beyond 96 h is ominous. Approximately 70 % of patients survive acute liver failure and recover over 4 days to 2 weeks following ingestion. If there are significant signs of worsening of severe hepatotoxicity, early evaluation for liver transplant should be initiated [151, 153]. Mahadevan et al. identified the following poor prognostic indicators and the potential need for a liver transplant based on a retrospective review of APAP-induced hepatotoxicity in pediatric patients: (1) delayed presentation to the emergency department; (2) delay in treatment; (3) PT greater than 100 s; (4) serum creatinine greater than 2.3 mg/dL; (5) hypoglycemia; (6) metabolic acidosis; and (7) hepatic encephalopathy grade III or higher. According to this review, markedly elevated hepatic transaminase levels were not predictive of a poor outcome [154].

Initial therapy for APAP ingestions includes supportive care and obtaining serum APAP levels approximately 4 h post-acute ingestion. This result is plotted on the Rumack-Matthew nomogram (Fig. 50.1). If the APAP level falls above the "possible toxicity" line, therapy with oral, nasogastric or intravenous (IV) NAC should be initiated. Although the cost for the IV formulation is significantly higher than oral NAC, shorter hospitalization stays and less laboratory testing should ultimately reduce overall costs [2, 156]. The normal half-life of APAP is 2–4 h, but it may be prolonged in APAP overdose or co-ingestion with other substances, particularly those that delay gastric emptying. The nomogram cannot be used for prediction of risk for patients who have chronic ingestion of APAP or have taken extended-release products [157]. For these patients, NAC is usually administered if they have elevated liver enzymes or they are at risk for hepatotoxicity. A second APAP level may be obtained 4–6 h after the first level if the time of ingestion is unclear to determine if the level is rising or declining.

N-acetylcysteine (NAC), the antidote for APAP toxicity, replenishes glutathione stores in the liver. It is very effective at preventing significant hepatic injury if it is initiated within

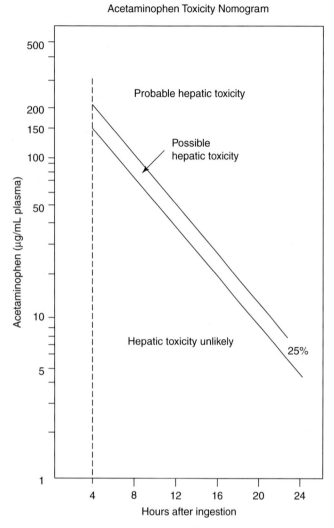

Fig. 50.1 The Rumack-Matthew nomogram, relating expected severity or live toxicity to serum acetaminophen concentrations (Reprinted from Smilkstein et al. [155]. With permission from Elsevier.)

8–10 h of ingestion. However, many clinicians will institute NAC therapy if the patient presents within 16–24 h of ingestion and is at risk for severe hepatotoxicity. Historically, NAC was administered orally with a loading dose of 140 mg/kg followed by 17 doses of 70 mg/kg every 4 h. However, intravenous NAC (Acetadote®) is now available. For adult IV dosing, the loading dose is 150 mg/kg in 200 mL of 5 % dextrose for 60 min, followed by 50 mg/kg in 500 mL of 5 % dextrose for 4 h, and 100 mg/kg in 1,000 mL of 5 % dextrose for 16 h. For children, standard IV dosing can cause hyponatremia and secondary seizures due to the free water load. Therefore, the resolution is to dilute 20 % NAC to a final concentration of 40 mg/mL (Table 50.6). The final mg/kg dosing (loading dose, 150 mg/kg; 50 mg/kg for 4 h and 100 mg/kg for 16 h) is the same, but the free water is less than in the adult schedule. Adverse reactions to IV NAC include anaphylactoid reactions including rash, urticaria,

pruritis, hypotension, tachycardia, bronchospasm and respiratory distress, which most commonly occur during the initial loading dose and may occur in up to 10 % of patients [2, 158]. Due to these adverse events, it has been recommended to use a maximum ceiling weight of 110 kg when calculating the dose [158]. The following laboratory tests should be collected at baseline and at 48–72 h if on oral NAC and at the end of the 21 h treatment regimen if on IV NAC: alanine aminotransferase, aspartate aminotransferase, blood urea nitrogen, creatinine, electrolytes, complete blood count, prothrombin (PT)/International Normalized Ratio (INR). If the liver or coagulation laboratory results are abnormal and the patient is on IV NAC, therapy should be continued at a rate of 6.3 mg/kg/h until these laboratory values improve.

Salicylates

The association of aspirin with the occurrence of Reye's syndrome in the early 1980s resulted in a marked decrease in the use of salicylate products in children. However, although salicylates are not recommended for children, there continues to be a number of exposures and even deaths in pediatric patients. Salicylates are used for their analgesic, antipyretic, anti-inflammatory and antiplatelet effects. They are in many over-the-counter oral and topical formulations as a single agent or combination product. Products that may include salicylates include aspirin, antidiarrheal preparations (e.g. Pepto-Bismol®, Kaopectate®, etc.), analgesics (in combination with codeine, opiates or caffeine), antihistamines, cough/cold combination products with aspirin and acetaminophen, topical wart removers, and oil of wintergreen (methyl salicylate). Pure oil of wintergreen, used as a food flavoring agent, contains 7 g of salicylate in 1 teaspoon, which may be fatal. Many liniments and ointments contain methyl salicylate and are used as rubifacients. Dermal absorption of topical preparations can be significant, particularly after repeated applications. Sustained release and enteric coated products are also available.

Salicylates are rapidly absorbed in the proximal GI tract, however in overdose the absorption may be delayed, bezoars may form and levels may continue to rise for hours, particularly with enteric coated products. Peak serum concentrations are achieved within 1 h of ingestion unless it is an extended release product, which extends the peak level to 4–14 h. The half-life at therapeutic dose is about 2–4 h but can be as long as 18–36 h in an overdose. Peak levels are achieved within 0.5–2 h with therapeutic doses. With therapeutic doses, 80–90 % of salicylate remains intravascular and protein bound which is evident by the small volume of distribution of 0.1–0.3 L/kg. However, the volume of distribution of salicylates increases with the dose, due to saturation of plasma protein binding [159, 160].

Salicylates undergo first order kinetics with serum concentrations proportional to dose concentrations. Hepatic metabolism is via glucuronidation, oxidation and glycine

Table 50.6 N-acetylcysteine dosage guidelines

N-acetylcysteine dosage guidelines: Acetadote® 20 % (200 mg/mL)
Note: The 3 doses are administered sequentially for a continuous 21 h infusion
Dosage calculator available at http://www.acetadote.net/dosecalc.php

Weight	Loading dose (over 60 min)			Second dose (over 4 h)			Third dose (over 16 h)		
	Acetadote® (mL)		5 % Dextrose	Acetadote® (mL)		5 % Dextrose	Acetadote® (mL)		5 % Dextrose
kg	mg	mL	(mL)	mg	mL	(mL)	mg	mL	(mL)
5	750	3.75	15	250	1.25	35	500	2.5	70
10	1,500	7.5	30	500	2.5	70	1,000	5	140
15	2,250	11.25	45	750	3.75	105	1,500	7.5	210
20	3,000	15	60	1,000	5	140	2,000	10	280
25	3,750	18.75	100	1,250	6.25	250	2,500	12.5	500
30	4,500	22.5	100	1,500	7.5	250	3,000	15	500
35	5,250	26.25	100	1,750	8.75	250	3,500	17.5	500
40	6,000	30	200	2,000	10	500	4,000	20	1,000
50	7,500	37.5	200	2,500	12.5	500	5,000	25	1,000
60	9,000	45	200	3,000	15	500	6,000	30	1,000
70	10,500	52.5	200	3,500	17.5	500	7,000	35	1,000
75	11,250	56.25	200	3,750	18.75	500	7,500	37.5	1,000
80	12,000	60	200	4,000	20	500	8,000	40	1,000
85	12,750	63.75	200	4,250	21.25	500	8,500	42.5	1,000
90	13,500	67.5	200	4,500	22.50	500	9,000	45	1,000
95	14,250	71.25	200	4,750	23.75	500	9,500	47.5	1,000
≥100	15,000	75	200	5,000	25	500	10,000	50	1,000

Acetadote® is hyperosmolar (2,600 MOsm/L) and is compatible with 5 % dextrose, 0.5 normal saline (0.45 % sodium chloride injection), and water for injection

(Adapted from Package insert, Acetadote®, Cumberland Pharmaceuticals.)

conjugation. However, in overdose, the enzyme systems become saturated at salicylate concentrations of 20–30 mg/dL and elimination changes from first-order to zero order (Michaelis-Menton) kinetics resulting in exponential increases in serum concentrations. Salicylate serum concentrations should be obtained at least 4 h following ingestion. Acute toxicity is defined as exposure of less than 8 h, whereas chronic toxicity is defined as exposure longer than this duration. For acute exposure, serum concentrations above 90 mg/dL are associated with severe toxicity and for chronic exposure, levels above 60 mg/dL are associated with significant toxicity. The Done nomogram is not useful for management of salicylate toxicity. Mild toxicity occurs with ingestions of 150–200 mg/kg. Severe toxicity following 300–500 mg/kg and more than 500 mg/kg may be fatal. Patients with more severe poisoning usually have a large anion gap metabolic acidosis and altered mental status. Clinical decisions should be based on overall clinical signs and symptoms of salicylism and not on the salicylate level alone as they do not reflect the severity of toxicity [159, 160].

Symptoms associated with salicylate poisoning are dose-related. Symptoms from mild toxicity include nausea, vomiting, tinnitus, tachypnea, and respiratory alkalosis. Symptoms from severe toxicity include nausea, vomiting, diarrhea, tinnitus, vertigo, metabolic acidosis, hyperpnea, hyperventilation, diaphoresis, hyperthermia, altered mental status, seizures, coma, cerebral edema, hypotension, dysrhythmias, noncardiogenic pulmonary edema and death. Cerebral edema is a common autopsy finding. Pancreatitis is a rare complication. PT prolongation is fairly common. Chronic overdoses present more insidiously and cause more severe toxicity than acute ingestions. Symptoms with chronic exposure may consist primarily of neurologic manifestations such as confusion, delirium, and agitation. Onset of clinical toxicity and peak serum levels may be delayed in patients with ingestion of sustained release or enteric coated aspirin or if a bezoar develops. If the patient requires intubation, respiratory alkalosis from pre-intubation self-hyperventilation must be maintained by achieving pre-intubation minute ventilation through mechanical ventilation. If not, abrupt decompensation may occur due to worsening acidemia increasing the salicylate concentration in the brain [160, 161]. It is suggested that if the patient requires intubation, hemodialysis should start simultaneously [160].

Salicylates are metabolic poisons. In toxic concentrations, they stimulate the respiratory center in the brainstem (medulla), interfere with the Krebs cycle (limiting ATP production), uncouple oxidative phosphorylation (causing accumulation of pyruvic and lactic acid and heat production), and increase fatty acid metabolism (generating ketone bodies) [159, 160]. The net result is a mixed respiratory alkalosis and metabolic acidosis. Respiratory alkalosis develops early and may be the only acid base disturbance with mild salicylism. A primary respiratory alkalosis with compensatory metabolic acidosis develops in most adults with moderate intoxication. A primary metabolic acidosis and compensatory respiratory alkalosis develops in severe overdose and is associated with a higher rate of complications and death. Patients with marked metabolic acidosis are at risk for cerebral and pulmonary edema. Myocardial depression, hypotension, and central nervous system toxicity may precede cardiopulmonary arrest. Respiratory alkalosis may be brief or not occur at all in infants and young children who primarily develop a primary metabolic acidosis. Hypoglycemia may also develop and is more common in children [159–161].

Salicylate-induced pulmonary edema is a known complication associated with acute or chronic salicylate overdoses. Salicylate toxicity should be considered in patients presenting with non-cardiogenic pulmonary edema and neurological changes, anion-gap metabolic acidosis, or presumed sepsis. The biochemical cause of pulmonary edema may be related to an increase in permeability within the capillaries of the lung leading to "protein leakage" and transudation of fluid in pulmonary tissue [161].

Initial therapy includes monitoring a patient's mental status, vital signs and administering intravenous fluids to correct hypovolemia. Serial salicylate levels should be obtained every 1–2 h until levels have peaked and are declining and the patient's clinical symptoms have improved. Single determinations of salicylate levels are not sufficient because absorption may be delayed and erratic. Activated charcoal should be administered to patients with large ingestions even if after 2 h of ingestion because salicylate absorption can be delayed and erratic. A second dose of activated charcoal may be administered if salicylate levels continue to rise despite urine alkalinization. Whole bowel irrigation with polyethylene glycol should be considered in patients with large ingestions of enteric coated products if their airway is protected. Electrolytes should be monitored every 2 h and corrected as clinically indicated until the patient is clinically improved. Arterial or venous blood gases should be monitored for patients with moderate to severe toxicity and in all patients undergoing serum and urinary alkalinization. In patients with moderate to severe toxicity, a complete blood count, liver enzymes, electrolytes, blood urea nitrogen, creatinine, INR and partial thromboplastin time (PTT) should be obtained at baseline and periodically as indicated. A CT of the head may be indicated for patients with altered mental status as they may have cerebral edema and may require mannitol therapy [159, 160].

Administration of intravenous sodium bicarbonate and initial hyperventilation of intubated patients is used to maintain a goal target arterial pH for serum alkalinization of 7.50–7.55. Urine alkalinization to a urine pH greater than 7.5 facilitates urinary excretion of unbound salicylate. Urine alkalinization also promotes salicylate mobilization from the tissues to the plasma. If the initial serum salicylate concentration is greater than 30 mg/dL and rising, serum and urine alkalinization should be initiated by administering 1–2 mEq/kg sodium bicarbonate by intravenous bolus followed by a continuous infusion of sodium bicarbonate containing intravenous fluids. Sodium bicarbonate (150 mEq or 3 ampules) in 1 l of 5 % dextrose with 20–40 mEq/L of potassium chloride will create an isotonic fluid and should be infused at 2–3 mL/kg/h. Alkalosis decreases the amount of non-ionized salicylate in the blood which should decrease penetration across the blood brain barrier and into other tissues [159–161]. Urine output should be monitored hourly. Blood gases and urinary pH should be monitored every 2 h and used to titrate the sodium bicarbonate infusion rate. Alkalinization may cause hypokalemia, hypocalcemia, hypernatremia, and dysrhythmias. Hypokalemia should be corrected because it causes increased bicarbonate absorption in the renal tubules which decreases the effectiveness of urinary alkalinization.

Patients who should be considered for hemodialysis include those with renal failure, refractory or severe acidosis, progressive clinical deterioration despite appropriate fluid therapy and urinary alkalinization, inability to maintain appropriate respiratory alkalosis, altered mental status, seizures, evidence of cerebral edema, or rising serum concentrations despite adequate therapy (above 90–100 mg/dL for acute exposure and 50–60 mg/dL for chronic exposure). A declining salicylate concentration in a patient who is not improving or is clinically deteriorating requires immediate interventions including dialysis to reverse the process. In addition, a patient who appears clinically stable but has increasing salicylate concentrations may have ongoing absorption and is at risk of decompensation. Hemodialysis may improve acid-base balance and help correct electrolyte abnormalities [159–161].

Nonsteroidal Anti-Inflammatory Drugs (NSAIDs)

NSAIDs are used as analgesics, antipyretics and anti-inflammatory drugs. These drugs inhibit cyclooxygenase enzymes (COX-1 and COX-2) which results in decreased prostaglandin production and decreased pain and inflammation. Severe overdose, although very rare, may result in a significant metabolic acidosis that may be related to the formation of acidic metabolites, however death is almost non-existent [162, 163]. Other signs and symptoms of severe toxicity include seizures, delirium, coma, hypotension, tachycardia, renal failure, hepatic dysfunction, hypoprothrombinemia, gastrointestinal bleeding and hyperkalemia. Most symptoms are manifested within the first 4 h after ingestions. There have been several case reports of children who presented with severe toxicity [164–168]. Furthermore, there have been several reported cases of severe hypokalemia secondary to ibuprofen induced renal tubular acidosis which resolved with discontinuation of ibuprofen [169]. Serum electrolytes, blood urea nitrogen, creatinine and acid-base status should be determined in severe overdose. Intubation may be needed in patients with central nervous system depression or recurrent seizures. Hypotension responds well to intravenous fluids. Supportive care is generally effective and further interventions are usually not required. Anaphylactoid reactions have been reported with some NSAIDs [162].

Organophosphates and Carbamates

Organophosphates and carbamates are insecticides that are usually used in rural areas. These products are readily absorbed through the skin, lungs, mucous membranes and gastrointestinal tract. Organophosphates induce a competitive and irreversible inhibition of pseudocholinesterase and acetylcholinesterase (AChE) whereas carbamates have competitive but reversible inhibition (transient) as they spontaneously hydrolyze within 48 h. Organophosphates phosphorylate the serine hydroxyl group of AChE preventing hydrolysis and inactivation of AChE. This leads to accumulation of AChE at the cholinergic synapses leading to dysfunction of the sympathetic, parasympathetic, peripheral and CNS [170, 171]. Clinical signs of cholinergic excess develop. Serious toxicity is rare in the United States now, but is more common in developing countries. The onset, duration and extent of effect depend on the agent, rate of absorption, amount of exposure, and rate of metabolic breakdown. The diagnosis is based on the clinical signs and symptoms although a history of known exposure is helpful. Most patients develop symptoms within 6 h of exposure although lipophilic organophosphates may have subtle early signs that progress to severe toxicity over many hours. Some organophosphates undergo "aging", a process by which the bond of the organophosphate to AChE becomes stronger and cannot be reversed by oximes (pralidoxime in the USA; obidoxime in some other countries). For these agents, early administration of an oxime may prevent aging and shorten clinical manifestations of toxicity. There continues to be ongoing debate about the efficacy of oximes for organophosphate poisoning [172].

Muscarinic effects include bronchorrhea, bronchospasm, salivation, lacrimation, diaphoresis, vomiting, diarrhea, urination and miosis (Table 50.3). Nicotinic effects include tachycardia, hypertension, mydriasis, muscle fasiculations and cramps, weakness, and respiratory failure (Table 50.3). CNS effects include depression, agitation, confusion, delirium, coma and seizures. Children may have fewer muscarinic and nicotinic signs compared to adults [171, 173].

Other clinical effects may include hypotension, ventricular dysrhythmias, heart block, metabolic acidosis, pancreatitis and hyperglycemia. Delayed effects include intermediate syndrome which is characterized by paralysis of respiratory, cranial motor, neck flexor and proximal limb muscles. This can occur 1–4 days after apparent recovery from cholinergic toxicity and prior to development of delayed peripheral neuropathy. Recovery usually requires months, however some deficits may only partially recover. Chemical pneumonitis may also occur due to exposure to the hydrocarbon component of the product.

Initial therapy includes immediate decontamination of the skin, continuous monitoring of vital signs and cardiac rhythm, and monitoring neurological status. Healthcare workers must protect themselves to avoid contamination. Serial electrocardiograms should be performed to identify prolongation of the QTc and premature ventricular contractions. Red blood cell cholinesterase activity should be measured if available as it can help predict the degree of toxicity as it is a reflection of the activity in the brain and neuromuscular junction. Greater than 50 % reduction of RBC cholinesterase activity is associated with severe poisoning. Plasma cholinesterase levels are usually available and are a marker of exposure. However, they do not correlate with the degree of toxicity. Therefore many times these are not measured because the clinical symptoms are classic. Serum electrolytes and lipase should be obtained at baseline and monitored periodically. Negative inspiratory force (NIF) may be used to monitor for signs of impending respiratory failure and the need for intubation. Many children may require intubation and mechanical ventilation.

Administration of the antidotes atropine and pralidoxime (an oxime) should be initiated immediately to reverse the muscarinic and nicotinic effects, respectively, because earlier intervention results in better efficacy [171–175]. Atropine dosing should be titrated to decrease bronchorrhea, however the patient should be monitored closely for cholinergic effects or atropine toxicity. Tachycardia is not a contraindication to atropine therapy. The initial intravenous atropine dose is 0.02 mg/kg (adult dose 1–3 mg). If the response is inadequate in 3–5 min the dose should be doubled. The intravenous dose can be increased and given every 3–5 min as needed to dry pulmonary secretions. Once secretions are dried, a maintenance infusion at 10–20 % of the loading dose may be given every hour. Pralidoxime is generally started on any patient who requires atropine therapy and is continued for at least 12 h. A loading dose of 25–50 mg/kg followed by a repetitive administration or a continuous infusion of 10–20 mg/kg per hour is administered until muscle weakness and fasiculations resolve. Pralidoxime does not cross the blood-brain barrier to reverse CNS effects. Inhaled ipratropium or glycopyrrolate may reduce bronchospasm. Fluid resuscitation and vasoactive agents may be needed if

Table 50.7 Clinical stages of iron poisoning

Clinical stages of iron poisoning		
Stage or phase	Symptoms	Time from ingestion[a]
1	Vomiting, diarrhea, gastrointestinal blood and fluid loss, abdominal pain, hematemesis, hematochezia, lethargy, shock, acidosis, coagulopathy	0–6 h
2	Transient resolution of gastrointestinal symptoms; subtle signs	6–24 h
3	Recurrence of gastrointestinal symptoms, severe metabolic acidosis, profound shock, acute respiratory syndrome, hypotension, CNS depression, hypovolemia	12–48 h
4	Hepatotoxicity to recovery; may develop acute lung injury	48–96 h
5	Vomiting, gastric outlet obstruction, strictures	2–4 weeks

(Adapted from Madiwale and Liebelt [179]. With permission from Lippincott Williams & Wilkins)
[a]Note: There may be variability in duration of the stages and symptoms

the patient develops hypotension. Organophosphate-induced seizures should be treated with benzodiazepines. There has been a single study that showed that adding magnesium sulfate to conventional therapy reduced hospital length of stay and decreased mortality [176]. There is a single case report of improved cholinesterase levels following plasmaphoresis for sepsis in a patient who had organophosphate poisoning [177]. Patients should be monitored closely for 48 h after discontinuation of atropine and pralidoxime for signs of recurrent toxicity or development of intermediate syndrome.

Iron

Iron exposure continues to be a significant problem in children, particularly younger children. In 2009 there were over 20,000 exposures in children reported to the American Association of Poison Control Centers but no reported deaths. The youngest reported patient with iron toxicity was a 7 week old ex-28 week infant who was given an accidental overdose which was recognized early and she survived without sequelae [178]. Because ion products are available in multiple formulations, it is important to obtain a good history of the product ingested as the elemental iron content varies by product, but it is the standard for determining risk of toxicity. Ingestion of 40–60 mg/kg of elemental iron in children places them at risk for significant toxicity.

Under normal circumstances, damage from free radicals does not occur because of transport and storage proteins such as transferrin and ferritin [179]. In iron overdose, however, these protective mechanisms become overwhelmed and free radicals are produced which poison mitochondria, uncouple oxidative phosphorylation and inhibit the Kreb's cycle [179]. Poisoning with iron salts produces five classic stages (Table 50.7) which may not occur in all cases but include: (1) gastrointestinal toxicity which occurs within a few hours after ingestion and is due to the corrosive effects of iron; it is characterized by vomiting and diarrhea which varies from mild to bloody and severe; gastrointestinal hemorrhagic necrosis may result in large fluid losses; anion gap metabolic acidosis and shock may occur in this stage; (2) apparent stability for up to 24 h, however this stage may

not be present in patients with severe toxicity; (3) shock and acidosis occurring 12–48 h after exposure caused by free iron depositing in tissues and disrupting cellular function; coma, seizures, respiratory distress and renal dysfunction may occur in severe poisoning; distributive shock as a result of hypovolemia and cardiogenic shock as a result of direct iron toxicity on the myocardium; (4) hepatotoxicity; and 5) gastrointestinal scarring and strictures which occurs 2–4 weeks after exposure. Most deaths are due to circulatory collapse. Postmortem examinations of fatal cases show corrosive injury to the gastrointestinal tract, hepatic necrosis, renal tubular necrosis, and deposition of iron in cardiac muscle and the brain [178–180].

Initial management includes treating hypovolemia, metabolic acidosis and shock. Some patients may require tracheal intubation. Useful laboratory tests include electrolytes, blood urea nitrogen, creatinine, liver function tests, coagulation tests (PT and PTT) and blood gas analysis. Significant elevations of aminotransferases, lactate dehydrogenase and bilirubin may occur 1–4 days post-ingestion in severe poisoning. Total iron binding capacity (TIBC) is unreliable in iron overdose. A serum iron concentration should be obtained between 2 and 6 h after ingestion if possible and interpreted based on the history and clinical signs and symptoms. Peak concentration usually occurs between 4 and 6 h post-ingestion. Patients with serum iron levels between 300 and 500 µg/dL are either asymptomatic or have mild symptoms. Moderate to severe toxicity occurs in patients with levels between 500 and 1,000 µg/dL. Patients that have levels greater than 1,000 µg/dL usually have serious toxicity and have the highest mortality risk. The serum iron level may be lower than expected if chelation therapy was initiated prior to the level. An elevated white blood cell count of $15 \times 10^3/mm^3$ and a serum glucose level of 150 mg/dL have only a 50 % sensitivity to identify patients with serum iron levels greater than 300 µg/dL, therefore they are not a predictor of toxicity [179]. An abdominal radiograph is considered standard for pure iron ingestions, however the pills may not always be visualized radiographically due to differing concentrations or if absorption was complete prior to the radiograph. The number of pills seen on the radiograph may not correlate with toxicity.

Iron absorption increases during an overdose because of disruption of GI mucosa as well as increased passive absorption across a larger concentration gradient. Gastric lavage, including the use of complexing and chelating agents in lavage fluid, is not indicated. Formation of an iron bezoar could cause a slower rate of absorption with delayed clinical effects. PEG-ES may be given orally or by nasogastric tube. The dose for children 6–12 years is 1,000 mL/h, children 9 months to 6 years is 500 mL/h and adolescents 1.5–2 L/h. This should be continued until rectal effluent is clear and there is no radiographic evidence of iron in the gastrointestinal tract. There is a case report of laparoscopic-assisted gastrotomy for the treatment of an iron bezoar in an adolescent who ingested a potentially lethal dose [181].

Chelation therapy with deferoxamine should be initiated if there is evidence of hypovolemia, shock, lethargy, persistent vomiting, diarrhea, positive anion gap metabolic acidosis, large number of pills on abdominal radiograph, or a serum iron level > 500 µg/dL. Deferoxamine works by binding the ferric form of iron (Fe3+) and forms the water-soluble complex ferrioxamine, which is then excreted in the urine and is responsible for the brick-orange 'vin-rosé' urine color. Vin-rosé colored urine occurs in about one-third of patients. Deferoxamine is most effective when given as a continuous intravenous infusion. The starting dose is 15 mg/kg per hour and is titrated up to a maximum of 35 mg/kg per hour based on the severity of clinical symptoms. The most frequent side effect is hypotension, therefore it is essential to adequately volume resuscitate the patient prior to starting deferoxamine. If hypotension develops, the rate of deferoxamine infusion may need to be decreased. Deferoxamine therapy is usually stopped when clinical signs and symptoms of systemic iron poisoning resolve, radio-opaque iron pills on abdominal radiographs are gone, and return of normal urine color if vin-rosé colored urine was present. Sometimes deferoxamine will be continued until the serum iron level is below 150–300 µg/dL. Following discontinuation, the patient should continue to be monitored closely and deferoxamine infusion may be resumed if clinical deterioration occurs. If deferoxamine infusion continues longer than 24–48 h, there may be a risk of developing acute respiratory distress syndrome. Other chelation therapies are being investigated but are not currently recommended [182, 183].

Hydrocarbons and Inhalation Abuse

Hydrocarbons are a diverse group of organic compounds that include gasoline, kerosene, lamp oils, diesel fuels, mineral oils, naphtha, lighter fluids, carbon tetrachloride, mineral spirits, turpentine, lubricating oils and many other products commercially available. In 2009 there were over 43,000 single substance exposures to hydrocarbons reported to the American Association of Poison Control Centers with nearly half of those in infants, children and adolescents [1]. Usually,

in young children, it is an accidental ingestion or aspiration, however in older children and adolescents, it may be due to inhalation abuse or intentional ingestion. Two key factors that increase the risks related to hydrocarbon exposures are their viscosity and surface tension properties. Low viscosity hydrocarbons that are absorbed systemically have the highest potential for toxicity [184].

Aspiration with subsequent pneumonitis, respiratory failure and acute respiratory distress syndrome are the most common adverse effects seen following hydrocarbon exposure. The aspiration risk is highest with those substances that have high volatility and low viscosity and surface tension. Surfactant is solubilized leading to atelectasis, interstitial inflammation and formation of hyaline membranes. Patients may have signs of a systemic inflammatory response. The chest radiograph may initially appear normal, but by 12–24 h post-aspiration significant changes are usually seen. Patients with significant aspiration will usually have a history of coughing, choking, respiratory distress and possibly vomiting. Clinical signs may include tachypnea, dyspnea, retractions, cyanosis and anxiety. Pulmonary auscultation may reveal rales, rhonchi or decreased breath sounds. Antibiotics and corticosteroids are not indicated. Oxygen and positive pressure ventilation may be indicated based on the clinical examination and blood gas results. Surfactant may be considered, however there is limited data on its benefits. Extracorporeal membrane oxygenation has been used successfully in patients who failed conventional ventilation therapy.

Halogenated and aromatic hydrocarbons are readily absorbed through the skin, respiratory and gastrointestinal systems which can result in systemic toxicity including CNS depression, seizures and cardiac dysrhythmias (Table 50.8). These patients may also have nausea, vomiting and diarrhea. Rarely, renal dysfunction or failure will occur following an acute exposure to hydrocarbons. Gastric decontamination may be indicated, but only with very large ingestions or ingestion of certain halogenated, aromatic or substituted hydrocarbons (Table 50.8). Prior to emptying the stomach and gastric lavage, the airway must be protected with a cuffed endotracheal tube, sedation and possible paralysis should occur to minimize the risk of vomiting and aspiration.

Inhalation abuse is the intentional inhalation of a volatile substance for the purpose of achieving a euphoric state or "high". It is known as sniffing, huffing, snorting, solvent abuse, volatile substance abuse, bagging, and other names [185]. It is an under-recognized entity with more than 2.1 million children in the United States experimenting annually with approximately 20 % of middle and high schoolers having experimented. The peak age of abuse is 13–15 years and males experiment more than females. The substances abused are volatile, capable of producing a pleasurable sensory experience, readily available, legal, and may be region specific. Many of the products are hydrocarbons and contain

Table 50.8 Hydrocarbons with potential adverse effects on CNS, cardiac, hepatic, renal and pulmonary systems

Aromatic hydrocarbons	Halogenated (with chlorine, bromine or fluoride)	Petroleum distillates and other substituted hydrocarbons
Benzene	Chloroform	Hydrocarbon with toxic additives
Xylene	Carbon tetrachlorize	Insecticides
Toluene	Trichloroethylene	Nitrobenzene
	Carbon tetrachloride	Aniline
	Ethylene dichloride	Heavy metals
	Tetrachloroethane	Kerosene[a]
	Fluorocarbons	Gasoline[a]
	Brominated hydrocarbons	Furniture polish[a]
	Vinyl trichloride (1,1,2-trichloroethane)	Mineral spirits[a]
	Methylene chloride	Lighter fluid[a]

[a]Primary risks are chemical pneumonitis and ARDS associated with aspiration

propellants and solvents. The vapors are readily absorbed from the lungs and reach high concentrations in the CNS due to their lipid solubility. Inhalants are depressants, however the user is initially stimulated, uninhibited, prone to impulsive behavior, and may appear "drunk." The most common cause of death is "sudden sniffing death syndrome." This is thought to be a result of hydrocarbon induced myocardial sensitivity to epinephrine, hypercarbia and hypoxia. Other adverse effects, depending on the product abused, include laryngospasm, respiratory distress, chemical pneumonitis, seizures, altered mental status and renal failure. Rarely methemoglobinemia may occur. Patients should have an initial electrocardiogram followed by continuous cardiopulmonary monitoring. Laboratory studies should include a complete blood count, comprehensive chemistry panel and blood gases if indicated. A chest radiograph may be indicated if respiratory symptoms are present. Supportive care and specific treatment for seizures and dysrhythmias are the primary interventions [186].

Caustic Agents

Caustic agents are readily available and include products such as drain cleaners, household cleaners, hair relaxers and automatic dishwasher soaps. Alkaline agents are more common than acidic agents but both can cause significant mucosal injury and long-term sequelae. Exposures in young children are usually accidental and involve small volumes, however exposures in adolescents and adults may be intentional with larger volumes ingested and greater risk of significant injury.

Alkaline corrosives cause liquefaction necrosis. They destroy the cell and allow deep penetration into mucosal tissue which may result in perforation. The initial inflammation is followed by tissue necrosis, granulation and eventually stricture formation. Acids cause coagulation necrosis with eschar formation which is usually limited in depth compared to alkaline necrosis. Inflammation follows necrosis with development

of vascular thrombosis, granulation tissue, fibrogenesis and strictures. The risk of perforation is increased during the time granulation tissue forms. Determinants of the extent of injury with both alkaline and acidic products include the concentration, pH, viscosity, the amount ingested and the duration of contact with the tissue [187].

Ingestions may result in burns to the lips, mouth, pharynx, esophagus, stomach and even airway. Esophageal burns result in the most serious complications. Patients with mild ingestions may only develop irritation, edema, erythema and are classified as Grade I burns. Patients with moderate toxicity may develop Grade II (a or b) burns (superficial blisters and ulcerations) and are at risk for subsequent stricture formation. Patients with severe exposure may develop deep circumferential burns, necrosis, and even perforation of the gastrointestinal mucosa [Grade III (a or b)]. Other complications include fistula formation (tracheoesophageal), gastrointestinal bleeding and later stricture formation. Hypotension, tachycardia, tachypnea and fever may develop but usually occur later due to severe gastrointestinal bleeding or necrosis. Young children are at risk for life threatening upper airway edema even with less severe ingestions. Fortunately, severe toxicity is generally limited to deliberate ingestions in adults because alkaline products available in the home are generally of low concentration. Spontaneous vomiting may occur and may worsen the exposure. The absence of visible oral burns does NOT exclude the presence of esophageal or gastric burns. More serious esophageal injury should be considered in patients with stridor, vomiting, drooling, and abdominal pain. Dysphagia is the most common symptom of significant esophageal injury. Patients with hypotension, a rigid abdomen or radiographic evidence of intraperitoneal or mediastinal air may require surgical intervention. Dermal exposure may result in skin irritation and partial thickness burns. Prolonged exposure or products with high concentrations can cause full thickness burns. Ocular exposure can produce severe conjunctival irritation, corneal injury, or permanent visual loss. An ophthalmologist should be consulted early in the course.

Supportive therapy should be initiated and should include administration of anti-emetics if needed to decrease the risk of vomiting. Neutralizing agents results in heat production increasing tissue injury and should be avoided. Corticosteroids and antibiotics are generally not recommended. Endoscopy should be performed within 12–24 h of ingestion in patients with stridor, vomiting, drooling, significant oral burns, difficulty swallowing or abdominal pain. The earlier it is performed, the less risk there is of perforation with the examination. The grade of mucosal injury at the initial endoscopy is the best predictive factor for development of esophageal and gastrointestinal complications and mortality. A nasogastric tube should be placed under direct visualization if there are extensive burns and a gastrostomy tube may be indicated. If there are Grade II or III burns, then a barium swallow should be performed in several weeks and endoscopy repeated. Children with strictures are at risk for obstruction in the future. Esophageal dilation can be performed once the tissues have granulated. The length of the esophageal stricture may indicate those who can successfully be treated with dilation. However, if extensive strictures are present, a gastrostomy tube may be indicated. Stent placement or esophagectomy and colonic interposition grafts may be necessary [187–190].

Smoke Exposure, Cyanide (CN) and Carbon Monoxide (CO)

Smoke exposure may result is a range of signs and symptoms based on the type and length of exposure. Important information includes if the exposure was in an open or enclosed space, length of exposure, type of burning material, presence of fire or explosion, loss of consciousness, status of other victims, and the amount, color, and odor of smoke. The preliminary evaluation should include arterial blood gases with co-oximetry to determine presence of carboxyhemoglobin (COHb), chest radiograph, cyanide level, electrocardiogram (ECG), comprehensive chemistry panel, and indirect laryngoscopy if the patient is not tracheally intubated. Symptoms are usually related to the effects of the irritants and asphyxiants in the smoke. Neurological symptoms may be related to chemical exposure or to hypoxemia. CN poisoning is initially manifested as transient hyperpnea and tachycardia accompanied by headache, dizziness, nausea and vomiting. Hypoxia leads to hypoventilation, hypotension, myocardial depression, cardiac dysrhythmias, stupor, coma, and seizures. Cardiorespiratory arrest and death may occur. The breath of some patients may have a bitter, almond-like odor, however this is not always present. The symptoms of carbon monoxide poisoning are similar to CN. The cherry-red discoloration of the skin and mucus membranes is not commonly found. Other clinical findings from smoke inhalation include a nonproductive cough, eye irritation, lacrimation, confusion, anxiety, vertigo, respiratory distress, and trauma. Acute pulmonary edema and lactic acidosis may be seen.

Intubation and mechanical ventilation with higher PEEP may be required to maintain adequate oxygenation in patients with smoke inhalation. ARDS may occur and should be treated accordingly. Good pulmonary toilet should be maintained regularly. Fluid resuscitation will be required if burns of the skin are present. Bronchodilators such as albuterol and ipratropium may be used to treat bronchospasm.

Cyanide

Combustion of many plastics and fabrics produces hydrocyanic acid (HCN) gas which is one of the leading causes of death in patients with smoke exposure and the most common cause of CN toxicity [191–193]. HCN may be inhaled or absorbed through the skin. It is a rapidly fatal asphyxiant that causes cellular hypoxia by formation of a stable complex with cytochrome oxidase leading to disruption of the mitochondrial electron transport chain. The cells switch from aerobic to anaerobic metabolism which results in decreased availability of adenosine triphosphate (ATP) and increased production of byproducts such as lactic acid [193–195]. The heart, brain and liver are primary targets because of their oxygen requirement [193–195]. CN toxicity is a medical emergency because from the time of onset of symptoms to death can be short depending on the exposure. Another potential exposure to cyanide is the highly toxic acetonitrile-containing cosmetics, particularly false-fingernail removers, which may be confused with the less-toxic acetone-containing fingernail-polish removers [193].

Two treatment options are approved in many countries and include the Cyanide Antidote Kit (amyl nitrite pearls, sodium nitrite and sodium thiosulfate) and the Cyanokit® (hydroxocobalamin). Both the nitrite/thiosulfate combination and hydroxocobalamin are effective antidotes, however hydroxocobalamin appears to offer an improved safety profile, especially for children, pregnant women and victims of smoke inhalation [195–197]. Therapy should be administered emergently to any patient with signs and symptoms of CN poisoning. This includes those patients who present with coma, severe metabolic acidosis, severe cardiac dysrhythmias, and COHb level greater than 15 %. Hydroxocobalamin combines with cyanide to form cyanocobalamin which is a nontoxic, water soluble metabolite that is eliminated in the urine. Sodium thiosulfate may also be administered with hydroxocobalamin in the critically ill patient, but it is not part of the kit [197]. The main adverse effects from hydroxocobalamin, which itself is red, is red discoloration of the mucous membranes, skin, urine, and serum, but this is thought to be benign [191, 198]. Allergic reactions and transient hypertension also have been rarely reported [195]. Hydroxocobalamin can also interfere with many colorimetric based tests and has also been shown to interfere with tests for carboxyhemoglobin, metHb, and oxyhemoglobin, all potentially pertinent tests for victims of smoke inhalation or cyanide poisoning [199]. The standard adult dose of hydroxocobalamin is 5 g intravenously over 15 min. A second 5 g dose can be given in patients with severe toxicity. For pediatric patients, 70 mg/kg (maximum of 5 g) has been administered, but there are only case reports but no prospective trials evaluating this therapy in children [195, 200, 201]. It can be followed by a repeat dose of 35 mg/kg if needed [195].

If hydroxocobalamin is not available, amyl nitrite is administered first to stabilize the patient and is inhaled or held close to the patient's nose or mouth with 1.00 FiO_2 for 30 s of each minute until intravenous access is established. It is followed by intravenous sodium nitrite (pediatrics: 10 mg/kg IV/adults 300 mg IV over 3–5 min) and finally sodium thiosulfate (pediatrics: 400 mg/kg IV; adults: 12.5 g IV). The goal of both amyl nitrite and sodium nitrite treatment is to produce methemoglobin by oxidizing iron in hemoglobin from the ferrous (Fe^{2+}) to ferric form (Fe^{3+}). The ferric form rapidly removes cyanide from cytochrome oxidase forming cyanomethemoglobin and subsequent restoration of cellular respiration. Cyanomethemoglobin then reacts with sodium thiosulfate to form thiocyante which is renally excreted leaving methemoglobin free to bind to more cyanide. Patients with renal failure may require hemodialysis to eliminate thiocyanate. Seizures that occur secondary to thiocyanate accumulation are effectively treated with a benzodiazepine. Blood methemoglobin levels should be monitored for 30–60 min following the infusion to prevent severe toxicity. If the methemoglobin concentration is greater than 30 %, methylene blue 1 % should be administered. The components of the cyanide antidote kit have potentially serious toxicity. Nitrites may cause significant vasodilation and hypotension which may require treatment with fluids or vasoactive agents. Nitrite-induced methemoglobinemia reduces the oxygen-carrying capacity of the blood which may already be compromised if the patient has carbon monoxide toxicity or shock. In children, if an immediate hemoglobin measurement is unavailable, nitrites should be avoided because hemoglobin kinetics vary with age. Therefore, methemoglobinemia associated with nitrite-based antidotes, may be excessive and result in death [4, 191, 193].

Carbon Monoxide

Carbon monoxide exposure most commonly occurs due to faulty furnaces, automobile fumes, space heaters, portable generators, or from smoke exposure in a fire. CO rapidly crosses the pulmonary capillary membrane and combines with hemoglobin at 200–250 times the affinity of oxygen, binds at the same site and shifts the oxyhemoglobin curve to the left resulting in hypoxia (Fig. 50.2) [170, 202]. In addition

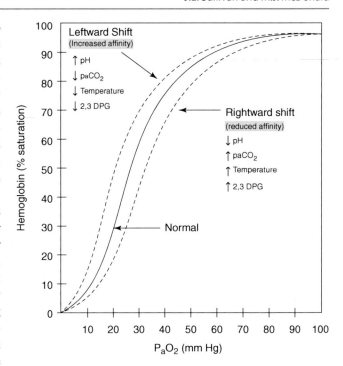

Fig. 50.2 Oxyhemoglobin dissociation curve

to generating carboxyhemoglobin, other mechanisms of toxicity include direct disruption of cellular oxidative processes by binding to myoglobin and cytochromes. During recovery, there may be marked oxidative stress and inflammatory responses [202]. Patients with carboxyhemoglobin levels less than 10 % are usually asymptomatic, levels of 20 % or greater usually have a headache, dyspnea, and difficulty in concentrating, and those with levels of 30–40 % have irritability, nausea, confusion, tachypnea, chest pain, ST segment depression, AV conduction block and ventricular dysrhythmias. Patients with levels of 40–60 % may experience seizures, coma, and death [170]. Other complications that rarely occur (2–10 %) and may be delayed for days to several weeks after the initial hypoxic insult include diffuse cerebral demyelination resulting in gradual neurological deterioration with apathy, apraxia, gait disturbances, incontinence, movement disorders (parkinsonism, choreoathetosis), hallucinations, seizures, cortical blindness, dementia and coma [170, 202].

Unconscious patients should be intubated and ventilated with 100 % oxygen. The elimination half-life of carboxyhemoglobin decreases from 350 to 90 min when the patient breathes 100 % oxygen and increases when normocarbia is maintained [170]. Oxygen supplementation should continue until CO is <5 % [202]. Hyperbaric oxygen at twice atmospheric pressure (2 atm) decreases the elimination half-life further to 30 min and is often used for patients who were initially unconscious, which is usually associated with an initial carbon monoxide level greater than 40 %. The use of hyperbaric oxygen for cyanide toxicity and smoke inhalation remains controversial although it is frequently utilized if available [202–205]. Myocardial injury may exist in children with CO poisoning, therefore electrocardiogram and cardiac enzymes should be obtained. If abnormal, a cardiac echocardiogram should be obtained [206].

Antihistamines

Overdose with antihistamines are rarely serious. Severe adverse effects may include agitation, delirium, psychosis, seizures, coma, dysrhythmias including torsades de pointe and anticholinergic effects (Table 50.3). Other medications that undergo hepatic metabolism may complicate the course of delirium, either by competing for the same metabolizing isoenzymes or by directly inhibiting their functional capacity [207]. Administration of other medications with anticholinergic properties should be avoided. Supportive care is generally all that is required however death has resulted from seizures and dysrhythmias [208–210].

Anticonvulsants

There have several new anticonvulsants added to the pharmaceutical armamentarium in the last 10 years which has decreased pediatric exposures to some of the older anticonvulsant drugs and their toxicities. Both old and newer drugs have the potential for CNS effects including significant CNS depression. Supportive care is still the mainstay of therapy. However, monitoring for seizures and signs of cardiac and other organ toxicities is critical with the newer drugs on the market.

Barbiturates

There has been a decrease in the use of barbiturates with the introduction of the newer anticonvulsants, however patients are still seen with barbiturate toxicity. The presentation is variable based on the onset and duration of action of the particular barbiturate ingested. Barbiturate overdose manifests as sedation, while severe poisoning results in coma, areflexia, apnea, respiratory failure, hypotension, myocardial depression, and hypothermia [211]. An ECG should be obtained in patients with severe toxicity. Laboratory tests may include a barbiturate level, complete metabolic profile, blood gases (if indicated), and creatinine phosphokinase in patients with prolonged immobilization due to coma. Mortality is low from barbiturate poisoning with supportive care alone. Supportive care is the mainstay of therapy, however enhanced elimination may be indicated in some patients. Fluids and vasopressors may be used to treat hypotension. The main aim of enhanced elimination is to reduce the duration of admission or to minimize complications of a prolonged intubation [211]. Multiple dose activated charcoal may be used for enhanced elimina-

tion in severe phenobarbital poisoning. Hemoperfusion or hemodialysis can be used in patients who have ingested a longer acting barbiturate and exhibit signs of severe poisoning or in patients remaining hypotensive despite maximal supportive care [211]. These patients must be monitored for rebound toxicity and barbiturate withdrawal post-dialysis, particularly for short acting barbiturates and in those who take barbituates regularly [211].

Phenytoin

Phenytoin and its prodrug fosphenytoin are less commonly prescribed to children than they have been historically, nevertheless there are still children who present with toxicity. Phenytoin is extensively bound to serum proteins (approximately 90 %), especially albumin. It has a large volume of distribution (0.6–0.7 L/kg) and freely diffuses into all tissues including the CNS with higher CNS than serum concentrations. Therefore, serum levels may underestimate the CNS drug concentration. Phenytoin is metabolized by hepatic microsomal enzymes to inactive metabolites, undergoes enterohepatic recycling, and is excreted in the urine. The mean plasma half-life is approximately 22 h, but it is variable and dose-dependent. Metabolism of phenytoin changes from first-order to zero-order kinetics in overdose because the oxidative metabolic pathway is saturable in the upper therapeutic range resulting in a constant rate, rather than a linear rate of metabolism and excretion. Cardiovascular toxicity is the major adverse effect seen with rapid intravenous administration of phenytoin and this can result in hypotension, prolonged QT interval, and cardiac dysrhythmias. CNS dysfunction is the major toxicity after oral ingestion and includes nystagmus, ataxia, sedation, altered mental status and coma [212]. Tracheal intubation should be performed for significant respiratory decompensation or a persistently decreased conscious state. Fluids and vasopressors may be required to treat hypotension. Toxicity after an acute ingestion is reversible and correlates well with serum levels. Free phenytoin blood levels (therapeutic range = 1–2 mg/L, toxicity usual when >5 mg/L) most accurately reflect clinical effects, however they are not always available. Total phenytoin levels of >30 mg/L result in evidence of neurotoxicity. Death from overdose is a rare complication. Supportive care is the mainstay of treatment. AC is often recommended in the initial treatment and there is some evidence that multiple-dose AC reduces half-life and enhances elimination of phenytoin, but does not alter outcome. Whole-bowel irrigation with large doses of PEG-ES by nasogastric tube until a clear rectal effluent is obtained may be useful in the patient with an overdose of sustained-release phenytoin or in those patients whose serum phenytoin levels continue to rise after 24 h in the setting of a large overdose. The airway should be protected prior to administering activated charcoal or PEG-ES if the patient has an altered state of consciousness [213].

Valproic Acid (VPA)

VPA toxicity is usually mild, self-limiting and may require supportive care although CNS depression, serious toxicity, and even death may occur [214]. CNS depression, the most common sign of toxicity, ranges from mild drowsiness to profound coma and fatal cerebral edema [214]. An exact mechanism for the action of the drug has yet to be determined. The net result of the actions of the drug is thought to be an increase in brain concentrations of γ-aminobutyric acid (GABA). VPA is also thought to inhibit neuronal firing by prolonging recovery from inactivation of voltage-sensitive sodium channels and to reduce the flow of calcium ions through T-type calcium channels, thus reducing neuronal pacemaker current [215]. Respiratory and multiorgan failure may occur in those patients with significant toxicity. Plasma valproic acid concentrations do not correlate with the severity of CNS toxicity [214]. Patients who ingest more than 200 mg/kg VPA or have plasma concentrations greater than 450 mg/L usually develop severe CNS depression. Other signs and symptoms include respiratory depression, nausea, vomiting, diarrhea, hypothermia or fever, hypotension, tachycardia, miosis, agitation, hallucinations, tremors, myoclonus, and seizures. Rarely, heart block, pancreatitis, acute renal failure or acute respiratory distress syndrome will develop. Hyperammonemia, anion gap metabolic acidosis, hyperosmolality, hypernatremia, and hypocalcaemia may also develop [214]. Administration of AC is recommended.

Other interventions may involve blood pressure support with intravenous fluids and vasopressors, correction of electrolyte abnormalities such as hypernatremia or anion gap metabolic acidosis. Because valproic acid depletes carnitine stores, supplementation with L-carnitine may attenuate some of these adverse effects and reverse hyperammonemia. Severely toxic patients who have renal dysfunction, refractory hypotension, severe metabolic abnormalities, recurrent seizures, persistent coma or levels greater than 1,000 mg/L may benefit from hemodialysis although there are no controlled trials that demonstrate improved outcome [214, 216–218].

Carbamazepine

Toxicity related to carbamazepine is due to its anticholinergic activity, sodium channel blockade, and CNS and myocardial depression effects. Signs of severe toxicity include coma, seizures, respiratory depression, pulmonary edema, poor myocardial contractility, hypotension, tachycardia, and dysrhythmias with conduction delays that may include PR, QRS and QTc prolongation [219]. Mydriasis and nystagmus are common clinical signs, but may also be present in therapeutic doses [220]. Children may manifest signs of overdose at lower concentrations than adults. Neurologic symptoms and tachycardia are the most common presentation in children [220, 221]. Laboratory tests should include a comprehensive metabolic panel, complete blood count, and arterial blood gas if indicated. Carbamazepine levels should be collected every 4 h until they have peaked and are declining. Levels of 20 μg/mL or greater may be associated with significant toxicity [222]. Diphenhydramine may be administered if the patient develops a dystonic reaction. Interventional treatment for seizures, respiratory depression and cardiac dysrhythmias may be necessary. The airway will need to be protected in those patients with severe toxicity prior to nasogastric tube placement for AC administration. There is no evidence that multiple doses of AC improves clinical outcome although it is frequently administered. Carbamazepine induced bowel hypomotility may increase the risks associated with multiple dose activated charcoal [219]. Whole bowel irrigation is effective for patients who have ingested a large amount of the sustained release product.

Oxcarbazepine

Oxcarbazepine has a similar profile to carbamazepine but has lower toxicity and is better tolerated. Overdose data is limited. Hyponatremia has been reported which may lead to seizures and coma [223]. Other adverse effects include bradycardia, hypotension, tinnitus, vertigo and lethargy for which supportive care is usually sufficient. Administration of AC is recommended.

Levetiracetam

This drug is newer to the market, therefore the toxicologic data is limited. Awaad reported an overdose of 4 and 10 times the recommended daily dosage in two children without significant adverse effects [224]. Vomiting, drowsiness, coma and respiratory depression have been reported [225]. Treatment for the patient with a toxic ingestion is supportive and directed at the presenting symptoms. Discretion should be used regarding administration of AC due to the potential for deterioration of the patient's mental status.

Methemoglobinemia

Methemoglobinemia is rare, but the intensivist must recognize and treat it promptly. Methemoglobinemia results from exposure to chemicals that oxidize the ferrous iron ($Fe2+$) in hemoglobin to the ferric state ($Fe3+$) and the rate of methemoglobin production exceeds the rate of reduction [226]. The oxygen-dissociation curve shifts to the left resulting in tissue hypoxia due to reduced-oxygen carrying capacity (Fig. 50.2). Causes of methemoglobinemia include but are not limited to local anesthetic agents, dapsone, nitrites, nitrates, sulfonamides, aniline dyes, contaminated well-water, naphthalene and nitrous gases.

Nonspecific findings that help clinicians differentiate methemoglobin from other life-threatening conditions include persistent cyanosis, tachypnea, low pulse oximetry and a lack of response despite therapy with 100 % oxygen therapy. Additional confirmation is provided by the results of the arterial blood gas accompanied by the classic chocolate-brown color appearance of the arterial blood sample. The diagnosis should be confirmed by at least one of the following: methemoglobin measurement, positive co-oximetry result, or confirmation of the oxygen saturation gap. Co-oximetry cannot be repeated after the administration of methylene blue because it will be read as methemoglobin. Methemoglobin levels of 10–25 % are associated with cyanosis. Headache, fatigue, dizziness, and dyspnea occur at levels of 35–40 % and levels of 60 % may cause arrhythmias, seizures, lethargy, and stupor. Levels greater than 70 % may result in vascular collapse and death [226, 227].

Administration of oxygen and removal of the offending agent should be done immediately. Therapy with methylene blue 1 % is directed at restoration of adequate oxygen-carrying capacity by the reduction of methemoglobin if the patient is symptomatic or has a level above 20 %. Methylene blue is the co-factor that acts as an electron acceptor for the hexose monophosphate shunt pathway (NADPH) within erythrocytes resulting in ferric to be reduced to ferrous. It is given intravenously at a dose of 1–2 mg/kg over 5 min. The dose may be repeated 30–60 min later if the patient remains cyanotic. At high doses, methylene blue can actually cause methemoglobinemia. Patients with G6PD deficiency should not be given methylene blue because they cannot generate sufficient NADPH, therefore it will cause a severe oxidant hemolysis [226]. Patients should be monitored for an additional 24 h following treatment due to the risk of rebound methemoglobinemia.

References

1. Bronstein AC, et al. 2009 Annual report of the American Association of Poison Control Centers' National Poison Data System (NPDS): 27th annual report. Clin Toxicol (Phila). 2010;48(10):979–1178.
2. White ML, Liebelt EL. Update on antidotes for pediatric poisoning. Pediatr Emerg Care. 2006;22(11):740–6. quiz 747–9.
3. Dart RC, et al. Expert consensus guidelines for stocking of antidotes in hospitals that provide emergency care. Ann Emerg Med. 2009;54(3):386–94. e1.
4. Betten DP, et al. Antidote use in the critically ill poisoned patient. J Intensive Care Med. 2006;21(5):255–77.
5. Frascogna N. Physostigmine: is there a role for this antidote in pediatric poisonings? Curr Opin Pediatr. 2007;19(2):201–5.
6. Barceloux DG, et al. American Academy of Clinical Toxicology practice guidelines on the treatment of methanol poisoning. J Toxicol Clin Toxicol. 2002;40(4):415–46.
7. American Academy of Pediatrics Committee on Injury, Violence, and Poison Prevention. Poison treatment in the home. Pediatrics. 2003;112(5):1182–5.
8. Chyka PA, et al. Position paper: single-dose activated charcoal. Clin Toxicol (Phila). 2005;43(2):61–87.
9. Olson KR. Activated charcoal for acute poisoning: one toxicologist's journey. J Med Toxicol. 2010;6(2):190–8.
10. Jurgens G, Hoegberg LC, Graudal NA. The effect of activated charcoal on drug exposure in healthy volunteers: a meta-analysis. Clin Pharmacol Ther. 2009;85(5):501–5.
11. Graff GR, et al. Chronic lung disease after activated charcoal aspiration. Pediatrics. 2002;109(5):959–61.
12. Proudfoot AT, Krenzelok EP, Vale JA. Position paper on urine alkalinization. J Toxicol Clin Toxicol. 2004;42(1):1–26.
13. Rothschild L, et al. Intravenous lipid emulsion in clinical toxicology. Scand J Trauma Resusc Emerg Med. 2010;18:51.
14. Cave G, Harvey M. Intravenous lipid emulsion as antidote beyond local anesthetic toxicity: a systematic review. Acad Emerg Med. 2009;16(9):815–24.
15. Samuels TL, Uncles DR, Willers JW. Intravenous lipid emulsion treatment for propranolol toxicity: another piece in the lipid sink jigsaw fits. Clin Toxicol (Phila). 2011;49(8):769.
16. Cave G, Harvey M. Intravenous lipid emulsion as antidote: how should we chew the fat in 2011? Crit Care Med. 2011;39(4):919–20.
17. Jamaty C, et al. Lipid emulsions in the treatment of acute poisoning: a systematic review of human and animal studies. Clin Toxicol (Phila). 2010;48(1):1–27.
18. Hill SL, Thomas SH. Clinical toxicology of newer recreational drugs. Clin Toxicol (Phila). 2011;49(8):705–19.
19. Phillips K, et al. Cocaine cardiotoxicity: a review of the pathophysiology, pathology, and treatment options. Am J Cardiovasc Drugs. 2009;9(3):177–96.
20. Winbery S, et al. Multiple cocaine-induced seizures and corresponding cocaine and metabolite concentrations. Am J Emerg Med. 1998;16(5):529–33.
21. Horowitz BZ, Panacek EA, Jouriles NJ. Severe rhabdomyolysis with renal failure after intranasal cocaine use. J Emerg Med. 1997;15(6):833–7.
22. Restrepo CS, et al. Pulmonary complications from cocaine and cocaine-based substances: imaging manifestations. Radiographics. 2007;27(4):941–56.
23. Wood DM, Brailsford AD, Dargan PI. Acute toxicity and withdrawal syndromes related to gamma-hydroxybutyrate (GHB) and its analogues gamma-butyrolactone (GBL) and 1,4-butanediol (1,4-BD). Drug Test Anal. 2011;3(7–8):417–25.
24. Snead 3rd OC, Gibson KM. Gamma-hydroxybutyric acid. N Engl J Med. 2005;352(26):2721–32.
25. Takahara J, et al. Stimulatory effects of gamma-hydroxybutyric acid on growth hormone and prolactin release in humans. J Clin Endocrinol Metab. 1977;44(5):1014–7.
26. Zvosec DL, et al. Adverse events, including death, associated with the use of 1,4-butanediol. N Engl J Med. 2001;344(2):87–94.
27. Placement of gamma-butyrolactone in List I of the Controlled Substances Act (21 U.S.C. 802(34)). Drug Enforcement Administration, Justice. Final rule. Fed Regist. 2000;65(79):21645–7.
28. Fuller DE, Hornfeldt CS. From club drug to orphan drug: sodium oxybate (Xyrem) for the treatment of cataplexy. Pharmacotherapy. 2003;23(9):1205–9.
29. Zvosec DL, et al. Case series of 226 gamma-hydroxybutyrate-associated deaths: lethal toxicity and trauma. Am J Emerg Med. 2011;29(3):319–32.
30. Lai MW, et al. 2005 Annual report of the American Association of Poison Control Centers' national poisoning and exposure database. Clin Toxicol (Phila). 2006;44(6–7):803–932.
31. Krul J, Girbes AR. Gamma-hydroxybutyrate: experience of 9 years of gamma-hydroxybutyrate (GHB)-related incidents during rave parties in The Netherlands. Clin Toxicol (Phila). 2011;49(4):311–5.
32. Zvosec DL, et al. Physostigmine for gamma-hydroxybutyrate coma: inefficacy, adverse events, and review. Clin Toxicol (Phila). 2007;45(3):261–5.
33. Li J, Stokes SA, Woeckener A. A tale of novel intoxication: seven cases of gamma-hydroxybutyric acid overdose. Ann Emerg Med. 1998;31(6):723–8.

34. Miro O, et al. Trends in illicit drug emergencies: the emerging role of gamma-hydroxybutyrate. J Toxicol Clin Toxicol. 2002;40(2):129–35.

35. de la Torre R, et al. Human pharmacology of MDMA: pharmacokinetics, metabolism, and disposition. Ther Drug Monit. 2004;26(2):137–44.

36. Peroutka SJ, Newman H, Harris H. Subjective effects of 3,4-methylenedioxymethamphetamine in recreational users. Neuropsychopharmacology. 1988;1(4):273–7.

37. Kalant H. The pharmacology and toxicology of "ecstasy" (MDMA) and related drugs. CMAJ. 2001;165(7):917–28.

38. Centers for Disease Control and Prevention (CDC). Ecstasy overdoses at a New Year's Eve rave–Los Angeles, California, 2010. MMWR Morb Mortal Wkly Rep. 2010;59(22):677–81.

39. Ecstasy test result statistics: summary data. Available from: http://www.ecstasydata.org/stats.php. Accessed 24 June 2011.

40. Grunau BE, Wiens MO, Greidanus M. Dantrolene for the treatment of MDMA toxicity. CJEM. 2010;12(5):457–9.

41. Halpern P, et al. Morbidity associated with MDMA (ecstasy) abuse: a survey of emergency department admissions. Hum Exp Toxicol. 2011;30(4):259–66.

42. Hartung TK, et al. Hyponatraemic states following 3,4-methylenedioxymethamphetamine (MDMA, 'ecstasy') ingestion. QJM. 2002;95(7):431–7.

43. Kaye S, Darke S, Duflou J. Methylenedioxymethamphetamine (MDMA)-related fatalities in Australia: demographics, circumstances, toxicology and major organ pathology. Drug Alcohol Depend. 2009;104(3):254–61.

44. Sano R, et al. A fatal case of myocardial damage due to misuse of the "designer drug" MDMA. Leg Med (Tokyo). 2009;11(6):294–7.

45. Moller M, et al. Ecstasy-induced myocardial infarction in a teenager: rare complication of a widely used illicit drug. Clin Res Cardiol. 2010;99(12):849–51.

46. Shenouda SK, et al. Metabolites of MDMA induce oxidative stress and contractile dysfunction in adult rat left ventricular myocytes. Cardiovasc Toxicol. 2009;9(1):30–8.

47. Madhok A, Boxer R, Chowdhury D. Atrial fibrillation in an adolescent–the agony of ecstasy. Pediatr Emerg Care. 2003;19(5):348–9.

48. Andreu V, et al. Ecstasy: a common cause of severe acute hepatotoxicity. J Hepatol. 1998;29(3):394–7.

49. Ellis AJ, et al. Acute liver damage and ecstasy ingestion. Gut. 1996;38(3):454–8.

50. Wehrman J. U.S. Poison Centers raise alarm about toxic substance marketed as bath salts; states begin taking action. 2011.

51. Schifano F, et al. Mephedrone (4-methylmethcathinone; 'meow meow'): chemical, pharmacological and clinical issues. Psychopharmacology (Berl). 2011;214(3):593–602.

52. Centers for Disease Control and Prevention (CDC). Emergency department visits after use of a drug sold as "bath salts" — Michigan, November 13, 2010–March 31, 2011. MMWR Morb Mortal Wkly Rep. 2011;60(19):624–7.

53. Kehr J, et al. Mephedrone, compared to MDMA (ecstasy) and amphetamine, rapidly increases both dopamine and serotonin levels in nucleus accumbens of awake rats. Br J Pharmacol. 2011;164(8):1949–58.

54. Winstock A, et al. Mephedrone: use, subjective effects and health risks. Addiction. 2011;106(11):1991–6.

55. Wood DM, et al. Case series of individuals with analytically confirmed acute mephedrone toxicity. Clin Toxicol (Phila). 2010;48(9):924–7.

56. Wood DM, et al. Recreational use of mephedrone (4-methylmethcathinone, 4-MMC) with associated sympathomimetic toxicity. J Med Toxicol. 2010;6(3):327–30.

57. Muetzelfeldt L, et al. Journey through the K-hole: phenomenological aspects of ketamine use. Drug Alcohol Depend. 2008;95(3):219–29.

58. Ring K. Life at death: a scientific investigation of the near-death experience. New York: Coward, McCann & Geoghegan; 1980.

59. Reich DL, Silvay G. Ketamine: an update on the first twenty-five years of clinical experience. Can J Anaesth. 1989;36(2):186–97.

60. Wolff K, Winstock AR. Ketamine : from medicine to misuse. CNS Drugs. 2006;20(3):199–218.

61. Ng SH, et al. Emergency department presentation of ketamine abusers in Hong Kong: a review of 233 cases. Hong Kong Med J. 2010;16(1):6–11.

62. Weiner AL, et al. Ketamine abusers presenting to the emergency department: a case series. J Emerg Med. 2000;18(4):447–51.

63. Middela S, Pearce I. Ketamine-induced vesicopathy: a literature review. Int J Clin Pract. 2011;65(1):27–30.

64. Bryner JK, et al. Dextromethorphan abuse in adolescence: an increasing trend: 1999–2004. Arch Pediatr Adolesc Med. 2006;160(12):1217–22.

65. Levine DA. "Pharming": the abuse of prescription and over-the-counter drugs in teens. Curr Opin Pediatr. 2007;19(3):270–4.

66. Ganetsky M, Babu KM, Boyer EW. Serotonin syndrome in dextromethorphan ingestion responsive to propofol therapy. Pediatr Emerg Care. 2007;23(11):829–31.

67. Boyer EW. Dextromethorphan abuse. Pediatr Emerg Care. 2004;20(12):858–63.

68. Carr BC. Efficacy, abuse, and toxicity of over-the-counter cough and cold medicines in the pediatric population. Curr Opin Pediatr. 2006;18(2):184–8.

69. Boyer EW, Shannon M. The serotonin syndrome. N Engl J Med. 2005;352(11):1112–20.

70. Erowid. DXM. http://www.erowid.org/chemicals/dxm/. Accessed 28 June 2011.

71. Schier J. Avoid unfavorable consequences: dextromethorpan can bring about a false-positive phencyclidine urine drug screen. J Emerg Med. 2000;18(3):379–81.

72. Banerji S, Anderson IB. Abuse of Coricidin HBP cough & cold tablets: episodes recorded by a poison center. Am J Health Syst Pharm. 2001;58(19):1811–4.

73. Schwartz AR, Pizon AF, Brooks DE. Dextromethorphan-induced serotonin syndrome. Clin Toxicol (Phila). 2008;46(8):771–3.

74. Chyka PA, et al. Dextromethorphan poisoning: an evidence-based consensus guideline for out-of-hospital management. Clin Toxicol (Phila). 2007;45(6):662–77.

75. de Boer D, Bosman I. A new trend in drugs-of-abuse; the 2C-series of phenethylamine designer drugs. Pharm World Sci. 2004;26(2):110–3.

76. Meyer MR, Maurer HH. Metabolism of designer drugs of abuse: an updated review. Curr Drug Metab. 2010;11(5):468–82.

77. Erowid. Psychoactive chemicals – 2Cs. http://www.erowid.org/chemicals/. Accessed 11 July 2011.

78. Barceloux DG, et al. American Academy of Clinical Toxicology practice guidelines on the treatment of ethylene glycol poisoning. Ad Hoc Committee. J Toxicol Clin Toxicol. 1999;37(5):537–60.

79. Wollersen H, et al. Oxalate-crystals in different tissues following intoxication with ethylene glycol: three case reports. Leg Med (Tokyo). 2009;11 Suppl 1:S488–90.

80. Bowen DA, Minty PS, Sengupta A. Two fatal cases of ethylene glycol poisoning. Med Sci Law. 1978;18(2):101–7.

81. Guo C, McMartin KE. The cytotoxicity of oxalate, metabolite of ethylene glycol, is due to calcium oxalate monohydrate formation. Toxicology. 2005;208(3):347–55.

82. Bobbitt WH, Williams RM, Freed CR. Severe ethylene glycol intoxication with multisystem failure. West J Med. 1986;144(2):225–8.

83. Brent J. Fomepizole for ethylene glycol and methanol poisoning. N Engl J Med. 2009;360(21):2216–23.

84. Megarbane B, Borron SW, Baud FJ. Current recommendations for treatment of severe toxic alcohol poisonings. Intensive Care Med. 2005;31(2):189–95.

85. Lepik KJ, et al. Medication errors associated with the use of ethanol and fomepizole as antidotes for methanol and ethylene glycol poisoning. Clin Toxicol (Phila). 2011;49(5):391–401.

86. Buchanan JA, et al. Massive ethylene glycol ingestion treated with fomepizole alone-a viable therapeutic option. J Med Toxicol. 2010;6(2):131–4.

87. Detaille T, et al. Fomepizole alone for severe infant ethylene glycol poisoning. Pediatr Crit Care Med. 2004;5(5):490–1.

88. Moreau CL, et al. Glycolate kinetics and hemodialysis clearance in ethylene glycol poisoning. META Study Group. J Toxicol Clin Toxicol. 1998;36(7):659–66.

89. Boyer EW, et al. Severe ethylene glycol ingestion treated without hemodialysis. Pediatrics. 2001;107(1):172–3.

90. Brent J. Current management of ethylene glycol poisoning. Drugs. 2001;61(7):979–88.

91. Brent J, et al. Fomepizole for the treatment of methanol poisoning. N Engl J Med. 2001;344(6):424–9.

92. Hovda KE, Jacobsen D. Expert opinion: fomepizole may ameliorate the need for hemodialysis in methanol poisoning. Hum Exp Toxicol. 2008;27(7):539–46.

93. Abramson S, Singh AK. Treatment of the alcohol intoxications: ethylene glycol, methanol and isopropanol. Curr Opin Nephrol Hypertens. 2000;9(6):695–701.

94. Jammalamadaka D, Raissi S. Ethylene glycol, methanol and isopropyl alcohol intoxication. Am J Med Sci. 2010;339(3):276–81.

95. Kraut JA, Kurtz I. Toxic alcohol ingestions: clinical features, diagnosis, and management. Clin J Am Soc Nephrol. 2008;3(1):208–25.

96. Zaman F, Pervez A, Abreo K. Isopropyl alcohol intoxication: a diagnostic challenge. Am J Kidney Dis. 2002;40(3):E12.

97. Vogel C, et al. Alcohol intoxication in young children. J Toxicol Clin Toxicol. 1995;33(1):25–33.

98. Bouthoorn SH, et al. Alcohol intoxication among Dutch adolescents: acute medical complications in the years 2000–2010. Clin Pediatr (Phila). 2011;50(3):244–51.

99. Isbister GK, Balit CR, Kilham HA. Antipsychotic poisoning in young children: a systematic review. Drug Saf. 2005;28(11):1029–44.

100. Klein-Schwartz W, et al. Prospective observational multi-poison center study of ziprasidone exposures. Clin Toxicol (Phila). 2007;45(7):782–6.

101. Gresham C, Ruha AM. Respiratory failure following isolated ziprasidone ingestion in a toddler. J Med Toxicol. 2010;6(1):41–3.

102. Neuhut R, Lindenmayer JP, Silva R. Neuroleptic malignant syndrome in children and adolescents on atypical antipsychotic medication: a review. J Child Adolesc Psychopharmacol. 2009;19(4):415–22.

103. Isbister GK, et al. Relative toxicity of Selective Serotonin Reuptake Inhibitors (SSRIs) in overdose. J Toxicol Clin Toxicol. 2004;42(3):277–85.

104. Nelson LS, et al. Selective serotonin reuptake inhibitor poisoning: an evidence-based consensus guideline for out-of-hospital management. Clin Toxicol (Phila). 2007;45(4):315–32.

105. Baker SD, Morgan DL. Fluoxetine exposures: are they safe for children? Am J Emerg Med. 2004;22(3):211–3.

106. Martin TG. Serotonin syndrome. Ann Emerg Med. 1996;28(5):520–6.

107. Horowitz BZ, Mullins ME. Cyproheptadine for serotonin syndrome in an accidental pediatric sertraline ingestion. Pediatr Emerg Care. 1999;15(5):325–7.

108. Woolf AD, et al. Tricyclic antidepressant poisoning: an evidence-based consensus guideline for out-of-hospital management. Clin Toxicol (Phila). 2007;45(3):203–33.

109. Thanacoody HK, Thomas SH. Tricyclic antidepressant poisoning : cardiovascular toxicity. Toxicol Rev. 2005;24(3):205–14.

110. Bateman DN. Tricyclic antidepressant poisoning: central nervous system effects and management. Toxicol Rev. 2005;24(3):181–6.

111. Dargan PI, Colbridge MG, Jones AL. The management of tricyclic antidepressant poisoning: the role of gut decontamination, extracorporeal procedures and fab antibody fragments. Toxicol Rev. 2005;24(3):187–94.

112. Bradberry SM, et al. Management of the cardiovascular complications of tricyclic antidepressant poisoning: role of sodium bicarbonate. Toxicol Rev. 2005;24(3):195–204.

113. Eisenberg MJ, Brox A, Bestawros AN. Calcium channel blockers: an update. Am J Med. 2004;116(1):35–43.

114. Salhanick SD, Shannon MW. Management of calcium channel antagonist overdose. Drug Saf. 2003;26(2):65–79.

115. Proano L, Chiang WK, Wang RY. Calcium channel blocker overdose. Am J Emerg Med. 1995;13(4):444–50.

116. Lam YM, Tse HF, Lau CP. Continuous calcium chloride infusion for massive nifedipine overdose. Chest. 2001;119(4):1280–2.

117. Engebretsen KM, et al. High-dose insulin therapy in beta-blocker and calcium channel-blocker poisoning. Clin Toxicol (Phila). 2011;49(4):277–83.

118. Osthoff M, et al. Levosimendan as treatment option in severe verapamil intoxication: a case report and review of the literature. Case Report Med. 2010;2010:546904.

119. Durward A, et al. Massive diltiazem overdose treated with extracorporeal membrane oxygenation. Pediatr Crit Care Med. 2003;4(3):372–6.

120. Love JN, et al. Lack of toxicity from pediatric beta-blocker exposures. Hum Exp Toxicol. 2006;25(6):341–6.

121. Love JN, et al. Acute beta blocker overdose: factors associated with the development of cardiovascular morbidity. J Toxicol Clin Toxicol. 2000;38(3):275–81.

122. Love JN, Sikka N. Are 1-2 tablets dangerous? Beta-blocker exposure in toddlers. J Emerg Med. 2004;26(3):309–14.

123. Love JN, et al. Characterization of fatal beta blocker ingestion: a review of the American Association of Poison Control Centers data from 1985 to 1995. J Toxicol Clin Toxicol. 1997;35(4):353–9.

124. Jovic-Stosic J, et al. Severe propranolol and ethanol overdose with wide complex tachycardia treated with intravenous lipid emulsion: a case report. Clin Toxicol (Phila). 2011;49(5):426–30.

125. Love JN, et al. Electrocardiographic changes associated with beta-blocker toxicity. Ann Emerg Med. 2002;40(6):603–10.

126. Bailey B. Glucagon in beta-blocker and calcium channel blocker overdoses: a systematic review. J Toxicol Clin Toxicol. 2003;41(5):595–602.

127. Brimacombe JR, Scully M, Swainston R. Propranolol overdose-a dramatic response to calcium chloride. Med J Aust. 1991;155(4):267–8.

128. Hoeper MM, Boeker KH. Overdose of metoprolol treated with enoximone. N Engl J Med. 1996;335(20):1538.

129. Shanker UR, Webb J, Kotze A. Sodium bicarbonate to treat massive beta blocker overdose. Emerg Med J. 2003;20(4):393.

130. Leppikangas H, et al. Levosimendan as a rescue drug in experimental propranolol-induced myocardial depression: a randomized study. Ann Emerg Med. 2009;54(6):811–7. e1-3.

131. De Rita F, et al. Rescue extracorporeal life support for acute verapamil and propranolol toxicity in a neonate. Artif Organs. 2011;35(4):416–20.

132. Klein-Schwartz W. Trends and toxic effects from pediatric clonidine exposures. Arch Pediatr Adolesc Med. 2002;156(4):392–6.

133. Matteucci MJ. One pill can kill: assessing the potential for fatal poisonings in children. Pediatr Ann. 2005;34(12):964–8.

134. Eddy O, Howell JM. Are one or two dangerous? Clonidine and topical imidazolines exposure in toddlers. J Emerg Med. 2003;25(3):297–302.

135. Pattinson KT. Opioids and the control of respiration. Br J Anaesth. 2008;100(6):747–58.

136. Daugherty LE. Extracorporeal membrane oxygenation as rescue therapy for methadone-induced pulmonary edema. Pediatr Emerg Care. 2011;27(7):633–4.

137. Sporer KA, Dorn E. Heroin-related noncardiogenic pulmonary edema: a case series. Chest. 2001;120(5):1628–32.

138. van Dorp EL, Yassen A, Dahan A. Naloxone treatment in opioid addiction: the risks and benefits. Expert Opin Drug Saf. 2007;6(2):125–32.

139. Wang JJ, Ho ST, Tzeng JI. Comparison of intravenous nalbuphine infusion versus naloxone in the prevention of epidural morphine-related side effects. Reg Anesth Pain Med. 1998;23(5):479–84.

140. Chumpa A, et al. Nalmefene for elective reversal of procedural sedation in children. Am J Emerg Med. 2001;19(7):545–8.

141. Mazor SS, et al. Pediatric tramadol ingestion resulting in seizure-like activity: a case series. Pediatr Emerg Care. 2008;24(6):380–1.

142. Pedapati EV, Bateman ST. Toddlers requiring pediatric intensive care unit admission following at-home exposure to buprenorphine/naloxone. Pediatr Crit Care Med. 2011;12(2):e102–7.

143. Seger DL. Flumazenil–treatment or toxin. J Toxicol Clin Toxicol. 2004;42(2):209–16.

144. Moeller KE, Lee KC, Kissack JC. Urine drug screening: practical guide for clinicians. Mayo Clin Proc. 2008;83(1):66–76.

145. Perry HE, Shannon MW. Diagnosis and management of opioid- and benzodiazepine-induced comatose overdose in children. Curr Opin Pediatr. 1996;8(3):243–7.

146. McDuffee AT, Tobias JD. Seizure after flumazenil administration in a pediatric patient. Pediatr Emerg Care. 1995;11(3):186–7.

147. Weinbroum AA, et al. A risk-benefit assessment of flumazenil in the management of benzodiazepine overdose. Drug Saf. 1997; 17(3):181–96.

148. Acetaminophen information. http://www.fda.gov/drugs/drugsafety/informationbydrugclass/ucm165107.htm. Accessed 18 Sept 2011.

149. Sullivan JE, Farrar HC. Fever and antipyretic use in children. Pediatrics. 2011;127(3):580–7.

150. Rowden AK, et al. Updates on acetaminophen toxicity. Med Clin North Am. 2005;89(6):1145–59.

151. Larson AM. Acetaminophen hepatotoxicity. Clin Liver Dis. 2007;11(3):525–48. vi.

152. James LP, et al. Acetaminophen-associated hepatic injury: evaluation of acetaminophen protein adducts in children and adolescents with acetaminophen overdose. Clin Pharmacol Ther. 2008;84(6):684–90.

153. Chun LJ, et al. Acetaminophen hepatotoxicity and acute liver failure. J Clin Gastroenterol. 2009;43(4):342–9.

154. Mahadevan SB, et al. Paracetamol induced hepatotoxicity. Arch Dis Child. 2006;91(7):598–603.

155. Smilkstein MJ, Bronstein AC, Linden C, et al. Acetaminophen overdose: a 48-hour intravenous N-Acetylcysteine treatment protocol. Ann Emerg Med. 1991;20(10):1058.

156. Martello JL, Pummer TL, Krenzelok EP. Cost minimization analysis comparing enteral N-acetylcysteine to intravenous acetylcysteine in the management of acute acetaminophen toxicity. Clin Toxicol (Phila). 2010;48(1):79–83.

157. Heard KJ. Acetylcysteine for acetaminophen poisoning. N Engl J Med. 2008;359(3):285–92.

158. Duncan R, Cantlay G, Paterson B. New recommendation for N-acetylcystiene dosing may reduce incidence of adverse effects. Emerg Med J. 2006;23(7):584.

159. Chyka PA, et al. Salicylate poisoning: an evidence-based consensus guideline for out-of-hospital management. Clin Toxicol (Phila). 2007;45(2):95–131.

160. O'Malley GF. Emergency department management of the salicylate-poisoned patient. Emerg Med Clin North Am. 2007;25(2):333–46. abstract viii.

161. Glisson JK, Vesa TS, Bowling MR. Current management of salicylate-induced pulmonary edema. South Med J. 2011; 104(3):225–32.

162. Volans G, Monaghan J, Colbridge M. Ibuprofen overdose. Int J Clin Pract Suppl. 2003;135:54–60.

163. Wood DM, et al. Fatality after deliberate ingestion of sustained-release ibuprofen: a case report. Crit Care. 2006;10(2):R44.

164. Kim J, et al. Acute renal insufficiency in ibuprofen overdose. Pediatr Emerg Care. 1995;11(2):107–8.

165. Zuckerman GB, Uy CC. Shock, metabolic acidosis, and coma following ibuprofen overdose in a child. Ann Pharmacother. 1995;29(9):869–71.

166. al-Harbi NN, Domrongkitchaiporn S, Lirenman DS. Hypocalcemia and hypomagnesemia after ibuprofen overdose. Ann Pharmacother. 1997;31(4):432–4.

167. Oker EE, et al. Serious toxicity in a young child due to ibuprofen. Acad Emerg Med. 2000;7(7):821–3.

168. Linden CH, Townsend PL. Metabolic acidosis after acute ibuprofen overdosage. J Pediatr. 1987;111(6 Pt 1):922–5.

169. Ng JL, et al. Life-threatening hypokalaemia associated with ibuprofen-induced renal tubular acidosis. Med J Aust. 2011; 194(6):313–6.

170. Worthley LI. Clinical toxicology: part II. Diagnosis and management of uncommon poisonings. Crit Care Resusc. 2002;4(3): 216–30.

171. van Heel W, Hachimi-Idrissi S. Accidental organophosphate insecticide intoxication in children: a reminder. Int J Emerg Med. 2011;4(1):32.

172. Buckley NA, et al. Oximes for acute organophosphate pesticide poisoning. Cochrane Database Syst Rev. 2011;2:CD005085.

173. El-Naggar Ael R, et al. Clinical findings and cholinesterase levels in children of organophosphates and carbamates poisoning. Eur J Pediatr. 2009;168(8):951–6.

174. Peter JV, Moran JL, Graham PL. Advances in the management of organophosphate poisoning. Expert Opin Pharmacother. 2007; 8(10):1451–64.

175. Farrar HC, Wells TG, Kearns GL. Use of continuous infusion of pralidoxime for treatment of organophosphate poisoning in children. J Pediatr. 1990;116(4):658–61.

176. Pajoumand A, et al. Benefits of magnesium sulfate in the management of acute human poisoning by organophosphorus insecticides. Hum Exp Toxicol. 2004;23(12):565–9.

177. Guven M, Sungur M, Eser B. The effect of plasmapheresis on plasma cholinesterase levels in a patient with organophosphate poisoning. Hum Exp Toxicol. 2004;23(7):365–8.

178. Valentine K, Mastropietro C, Sarnaik AP. Infantile iron poisoning: challenges in diagnosis and management. Pediatr Crit Care Med. 2009;10(3):e31–3.

179. Madiwale T, Liebelt E. Iron: not a benign therapeutic drug. Curr Opin Pediatr. 2006;18(2):174–9.

180. Manoguerra AS, et al. Iron ingestion: an evidence-based consensus guideline for out-of-hospital management. Clin Toxicol (Phila). 2005;43(6):553–70.

181. Haider F, et al. Emergency laparoscopic-assisted gastrotomy for the treatment of an iron bezoar. J Laparoendosc Adv Surg Tech A. 2009;19 Suppl 1:S141–3.

182. Porter JB, et al. Ethical issues and risk/benefit assessment of iron chelation therapy: advances with deferiprone/deferoxamine combinations and concerns about the safety, efficacy and costs of deferasirox [Kontoghiorghes GJ, Hemoglobin 2008; 32(1-2):1-15.]. Hemoglobin. 2008;32(6):601–7.

183. Kontoghiorghes GJ. Ethical issues and risk/benefit assessment of iron chelation therapy: advances with deferiprone/deferoxamine combinations and concerns about the safety, efficacy and costs of deferasirox. Hemoglobin. 2008;32(1–2):1–15.

184. Cobaugh DJ, Seger DL, Krenzelok EP. Hydrocarbon toxicity: an analysis of AAPCC TESS data. Przegl Lek. 2007;64(4–5):194–6.

185. McGarvey EL, et al. Adolescent inhalant abuse: environments of use. Am J Drug Alcohol Abuse. 1999;25(4):731–41.

186. Research report series: inhalant abuse. H.a.H. Services, editor. National Institute of Drug Abuse; 2010.

187. Abaskharoun RD, Depew WT, Hookey LC. Nonsurgical management of severe esophageal and gastric injury following alkali ingestion. Can J Gastroenterol. 2007;21(11):757–60.

188. Bicakci U, et al. Minimally invasive management of children with caustic ingestion: less pain for patients. Pediatr Surg Int. 2010;26(3):251–5.

189. Erdogan E, et al. Management of esophagogastric corrosive injuries in children. Eur J Pediatr Surg. 2003;13(5):289–93.

190. Thirlwall AS, et al. Caustic soda ingestion – a case presentation and review of the literature. Int J Pediatr Otorhinolaryngol. 2001;59(2):129–35.

191. Dart RC. Hydroxocobalamin for acute cyanide poisoning: new data from preclinical and clinical studies; new results from the prehospital emergency setting. Clin Toxicol (Phila). 2006;44 Suppl 1:1–3.

192. Eckstein M, Maniscalco PM. Focus on smoke inhalation–the most common cause of acute cyanide poisoning. Prehosp Disaster Med. 2006;21(2):s49–55.

193. Geller RJ, et al. Pediatric cyanide poisoning: causes, manifestations, management, and unmet needs. Pediatrics. 2006;118(5):2146–58.

194. Guidotti T. Acute cyanide poisoning in prehospital care: new challenges, new tools for intervention. Prehosp Disaster Med. 2006;21(2):s40–8.

195. Shepherd G, Velez LI. Role of hydroxocobalamin in acute cyanide poisoning. Ann Pharmacother. 2008;42(5):661–9.

196. Hall AH, Saiers J, Baud F. Which cyanide antidote? Crit Rev Toxicol. 2009;39(7):541–52.

197. Borron SW, et al. Hydroxocobalamin for severe acute cyanide poisoning by ingestion or inhalation. Am J Emerg Med. 2007;25(5):551–8.

198. Uhl W, et al. Safety of hydroxocobalamin in healthy volunteers in a randomized, placebo-controlled study. Clin Toxicol (Phila). 2006;44 Suppl 1:17–28.

199. Lee J, et al. Potential interference by hydroxocobalamin on cooximetry hemoglobin measurements during cyanide and smoke inhalation treatments. Ann Emerg Med. 2007;49(6):802–5.

200. Haouach H, Fortin JL, LaPostolle F. Prehospital use of hydroxocobalamin in children exposed to fire smoke. Ann Emerg Med. 2005;46:S30.

201. Espinoza OB, Perez M, Ramirez MS. Bitter cassava poisoning in eight children: a case report. Vet Hum Toxicol. 1992;34(1):65.

202. Weaver LK. Clinical practice. Carbon monoxide poisoning. N Engl J Med. 2009;360(12):1217–25.

203. Lo Vecchio F, Gerkin RD, Curry SC. CO poisoning and hyperbaric oxygen therapy: more studies need to be done. Am J Respir Crit Care Med. 2008;178(3):314. author reply 314-5.

204. Hampson NB, Hauff NM. Risk factors for short-term mortality from carbon monoxide poisoning treated with hyperbaric oxygen. Crit Care Med. 2008;36(9):2523–7.

205. Buckley NA, et al. Hyperbaric oxygen for carbon monoxide poisoning. Cochrane Database Syst Rev. 2011;4:CD002041.

206. Teksam O, et al. Acute cardiac effects of carbon monoxide poisoning in children. Eur J Emerg Med. 2010;17(4):192–6.

207. Scott J, et al. Prolonged anticholinergic delirium following antihistamine overdose. Australas Psychiatry. 2007;15(3):242–4.

208. Jang DH, et al. Status epilepticus and wide-complex tachycardia secondary to diphenhydramine overdose. Clin Toxicol (Phila). 2010;48(9):945–8.

209. Benson BE, et al. Diphenhydramine dose-response: a novel approach to determine triage thresholds. Clin Toxicol (Phila). 2010;48(8):820–31.

210. Scharman EJ, et al. Diphenhydramine and dimenhydrinate poisoning: an evidence-based consensus guideline for out-of-hospital management. Clin Toxicol (Phila). 2006;44(3):205–23.

211. Roberts DM, Buckley NA. Enhanced elimination in acute barbiturate poisoning – a systematic review. Clin Toxicol (Phila). 2011;49(1):2–12.

212. Index of suspicion. Pediatr Rev. 2002;23(7):249–53.

213. Craig S. Phenytoin poisoning. Neurocrit Care. 2005;3(2):161–70.

214. Eyer F, et al. Acute valproate poisoning: pharmacokinetics, alteration in fatty acid metabolism, and changes during therapy. J Clin Psychopharmacol. 2005;25(4):376–80.

215. Manoguerra AS, et al. Valproic acid poisoning: an evidence-based consensus guideline for out-of-hospital management. Clin Toxicol (Phila). 2008;46(7):661–76.

216. Lheureux PE, Hantson P. Carnitine in the treatment of valproic acid-induced toxicity. Clin Toxicol (Phila). 2009;47(2):101–11.

217. Hicks LK, McFarlane PA. Valproic acid overdose and haemodialysis. Nephrol Dial Transplant. 2001;16(7):1483–6.

218. Sztajnkrycer MD. Valproic acid toxicity: overview and management. J Toxicol Clin Toxicol. 2002;40(6):789–801.

219. Spiller HA. Management of carbamazepine overdose. Pediatr Emerg Care. 2001;17(6):452–6.

220. Lifshitz M, Gavrilov V, Sofer S. Signs and symptoms of carbamazepine overdose in young children. Pediatr Emerg Care. 2000;16(1):26–7.

221. Perez A, Wiley JF. Pediatric carbamazepine suspension overdose-clinical manifestations and toxicokinetics. Pediatr Emerg Care. 2005;21(4):252–4.

222. Montgomery VL, et al. Severity and carbamazepine level at time of initial poison center contact correlate with outcome in carbamazepine poisoning. J Toxicol Clin Toxicol. 1995;33(4):311–23.

223. Wade JF, et al. Emergent complications of the newer anticonvulsants. J Emerg Med. 2010;38(2):231–7.

224. Awaad Y. Accidental overdosage of levetiracetam in two children caused no side effects. Epilepsy Behav. 2007;11(2):247.

225. Barrueto Jr F, et al. A case of levetiracetam (Keppra) poisoning with clinical and toxicokinetic data. J Toxicol Clin Toxicol. 2002;40(7):881–4.

226. El-Husseini A, Azarov N. Is threshold for treatment of methemoglobinemia the same for all? A case report and literature review. Am J Emerg Med. 2010;28(6):748 e5–748 e10.

227. Alapat PM, Zimmerman JL. Toxicology in the critical care unit. Chest. 2008;133(4):1006–13.

Envenomations

51

James Tibballs, Christopher P. Holstege, and Derek S. Wheeler

Abstract

This chapter discusses the type, incidence and management of envenomation caused by a wide variety of terrestrial and marine creatures in North America and Australia including snakes, spiders, scorpions, bees, wasps, ants, jellyfish, octopuses, stinging fish and cone shells. Death from snake bite and scorpion stings world-wide are respectively estimated at 20,000–94,000 and 3,000 per year. While few deaths from envenomation by snakes and other creatures occur in North America and other developed countries such as Australia, serious injury and hospitalizations are not infrequent. Principles of management of snake bite include first-aid, administration of antivenom (antivenin) and intensive supportive treatment. Spider bites are the most frequent type of envenomation, but deaths are rare with the availability of antivenoms. Important spider species in North America are widow spiders and the brown recluse spider, while in Australia important species are funnel-web spiders and the red-back spider. Mortality from anaphylactic reactions to bee, wasp and ant stings in developed countries equals or exceeds that from snake bite. Envenomation by jellyfish is frequent world-wide but mortality is very low except after envenomation by chirodropid species common in the Indo-Pacific region. Immunological responses to jellyfish stings are a relatively unrecognized phenomenon. Injury from species of stinging fish account for many hospitalizations while envenomations by specific octopuses and cone shells occur sporadically.

Keywords

Envenomation • Snake • Spider • Scorpion • Bee • Wasp • Ant • Jellyfish • Stinging fish

J. Tibballs, MBBS, MEd, MBA, MD (✉)
Paediatric Intensive Care Unit,
Royal Children's Hospital,
50 Flemington Road, Parkville, Melbourne, Victoria, Australia
e-mail: james.tibballs@rch.org.au

C.P. Holstege, MD
Department of Emergency Medicine,
University of Virginia Health System,
Room 4601, 4th Floor Poison Center Suite,
Charlottesville, VA, USA
e-mail: ch2xf@virginia.edu

D.S. Wheeler, MD, MMM
Division of Critical Care Medicine, Cincinnati Children's Hospital
Medical Center, University of Cincinnati College of Medicine,
3333 Burnet Avenue, Cincinnati, OH 45229-3039, USA
e-mail: derek.wheeler@cchmc.org

Introduction

The specialty of pediatric critical care medicine crosses both the boundaries separating several different medical disciplines as well as the geographical boundaries that separate different regions around the world. In the past, textbook chapters dealing with the recognition and management of bites and stings by venomous animals have dealt almost exclusively with those species found within the continental United States and Canada, often with only a passing reference to species found outside North America. As pediatric critical care medicine is a global specialty, this chapter will emphasize the recognition and management of bites and stings by venomous animals found within and outside North

D.S. Wheeler et al. (eds.), *Pediatric Critical Care Medicine*,
DOI 10.1007/978-1-4471-6362-6_51, © Springer-Verlag London 2014

America, in the latter case using Australia as a reference, though the principles are applicable universally. This is particularly pertinent to all pediatric critical care clinicians as amateur collection of non-endemic, exotic species is a growing problem in the United States and other countries, and therefore envenomations by non-endemic species will be mentioned briefly as well. A large proportion of the injuries that result from such *exotic* bites and stings frequently involve the pediatric age group, many of which are often severe enough to necessitate admission to the pediatric intensive care unit (PICU). Advice on management of envenomation by Australian venomous creatures may be obtained from the Australian Venom Research Unit (AVRU) advisory service on their 24-h telephone number: 1300 760 451. Advice on management of envenomation in the United States may be obtained through the regional Poison Control Center (which may be accessed through the national hotline at 1 800 222 1222).

Venomous Snakes

There are over 2,500-3,000 species of snakes worldwide, of which approximately 375 species are considered venomous, belonging to one of five families (i) the Viperidae family (Old World Vipers), including adders and asps; (ii) the Crotalidae family (pit vipers), including several species found in North America such as the copperhead, rattlesnake, and cottonmouth; (iii) the Elapidae family, including the coral snake (North America), cobra, krait, mamba, brown snake (Australia), and black snake (Australia); (iv) the family Colubridae, including the boomslang; and (v) the family Hydrophiidae (sea snakes).

In Australia, of approximately 130 species of terrestrial and marine snakes (all of which are found in either the Elapidae or Hydrophiidae family), the majority are venomous and more than 20 species are dangerous to humans. The terrestrial species belong to genera *Pseudonaja* (brown snakes), *Notechis* (tiger snakes), *Oxyuranus* (taipans), *Pseudechis* (black snakes), and *Acanthophis* (death adders). All are elapids, including death adders. The last group, belonging to the Hydrophiidae family are the sea snakes. Nearly 2,000 people require hospitalization after a snake bite in Australia each year [1], and of these at least 300 require treatment with antivenom. The mean death rate from snake bite in Australia from 1981 to 1999 was 2.6 deaths per year (approximately 0.14 cases/one million population) [2].

Several venomous snake species are found in North America as well, and with the exception of the coral snake (Elapidae family), all are found exclusively in the Crotalidae (pit-viper) family [3]. The pit-vipers are so-named because of small,

heat-sensitive pits between the eye and nostril that allow these snakes to sense their prey. These snakes can regulate the amount of venom they inject during a bite based upon their ability to sense the size of their prey with the aid of these specialized pits, though the amount of venom injected in a defensive bites are often less controlled. The pit vipers are further distinguished from other species by the presence of a triangular-shaped head with an elliptical pupil, a single row of subcaudal scales (as opposed to a double row in nonvenomous snakes), and a venom apparatus consisting of two glands situated in the maxilla, two ducts, and two hollow maxillary teeth or fangs. These fangs are long and retract posteriorly when the mouth is closed. Several pairs of replacement fangs (usually at least three pairs) in various stages of development lie posterior to these fangs and move forward to replace shed or broken fangs. At least one indigenous species of venomous snake has been identified in every state but Alaska, Maine, and Hawaii [4]. Coral snakes account for only 1-2 % of all venomous snakebites in the United States and belong to the genus' *Micruroides* and *Micrurus*. They are not overly aggressive and rarely bite unless provoked – these snakes transfer their venom by chewing rather than injecting. Coral snakes are indigenous to the Southwestern and Southeastern United States. The pit vipers (family Crotalidae) include several species of rattlesnakes (genus *Crotalus* and *Sistrurus*) (Fig. 51.1), copperheads (genus *Agkistrodon*) (Fig. 51.2), and cottonmouths (genus *Agkistrodon*). Because of their widespread distribution, rattlesnakes are responsible for the majority of fatalities from snakebites in North America – the eastern diamondback and western diamondback varieties, in fact, account for almost 95 % of these deaths [3, 5, 6]. Copperheads are common to the eastern United States and require less utilization of antivenom therapy due to a modestly potent venom and neglible fatality rate. Cottonmouths, also known as water moccasins, are highly aggressive, semi-aquatic snakes found primarily in the southeastern United States. These snakes are so-named from the distinctive white color of their open mouths.

The American Association of Poison Control Centers reports almost 6,000 snakebites in the United States each year, of which at least 2,000 involve venomous snakes [5]. The true incidence of snakebites is probably vastly underestimated, as reporting is not mandatory and most snakebites probably go unreported. Experts estimate that the number of venomous snakebites in the United States is probably closer to 7,000–8,000 per year, resulting in 5–6 deaths per year [6]. For example, 57 deaths from snakebites were reported during the period between 1991 and 2001, yielding an annual rate of 0.019 cases/one million population [7]. Worldwide, it is estimated that as many as 5.5 million snake bites occur on an annual basis, with between 0.42 and 1.84 million envenomations and between 20,000 and 94,000 deaths every year, most of which

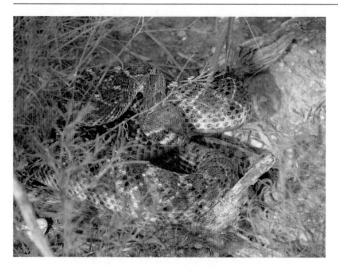

Fig. 51.1 Western diamond-back rattlesnake (Used with permission of Christopher P. Holstege, MD, University of Virginia, Charlottesville, Virginia)

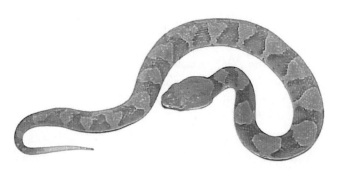

Fig. 51.2 Copperhead (Used with permission of Christopher P. Holstege, MD, University of Virginia, Charlottesville, Virginia)

occur in South Asia, Southeast asia and sub-Saharan Africa [8]. Snake envenomations are therefore a global problem that result in significant morbidity and mortality.

The typical victims in most cases, at least in North America and Australia, are males between 17 and 27 years of age [3, 4, 8–10]. The vast majority of bites affect the hands or arms and result from deliberate attempts to handle or harm the snake. Not surprisingly, alcohol intoxication is a factor in a large percentage of these envenomations [3, 4, 8–10]. Children are also unwitting victims due to their natural inquisitiveness and adventurous spirits. In most cases involving young children, snake bites are *accidental*, as when a snake is trodden upon or suddenly disturbed. In such cases, the lower extremities are more commonly affected.

The management of snake bite in young children poses additional problems. Diagnosis of envenomation is difficult when a bite has not been observed by an adult. The symptoms of early envenomation may pass unsuspected or misinterpreted and early neurological signs are difficult to elicit.

Bite marks may resemble everyday minor limb trauma. Due to higher venom to body mass ratio, the onset of envenomation is more rapid and more severe than in adults. Equally, parents often bring their child to medical attention when they fear or suspect snake bite after seeing a snake in the child's vicinity but saw no contact. The question then is whether the child has been bitten, and if so, has he or she been envenomated.

Finally, herpetologists and amateur snake collectors are also prone to snake bite – it is merely a question of time until they sustain a bite. Herpetologists sustain on average 4–5 bites in their working life and a life-threatening bite every 10 years [11]. Persons who are repeatedly bitten have a risk of developing allergic reactions to venoms and to the antivenoms used in their treatment. Amateur snake collectors endanger themselves and others who share their environments and may not know the true identity of captive specimens.

Snake Venoms and Toxins

Death and critical illness after snake bite is usually due to (i) respiratory failure secondary to neuromuscular paralysis, (ii) hypotension secondary to hemorrhage, or (iii) renal failure occurring secondarily to rhabdomyolysis, disseminated intravascular coagulation (DIC), hypotension, hemolysis, or to their combinations. Rapid collapse, not accompanied by respiratory failure, within minutes after a snake bite may be due to anaphylaxis to venom or possibly due to the myocardial ischemia [12] secondary to effects of DIC. Snake venoms are complex mixtures of proteins ranging from 6 to 100 kDa, many of which have enzymatic properties, e.g. phospholipases (especially phospholipase A2), proteases, collagenases, hyaluronidases, acetylcholinesterase, metalloproteinases, lactate dehydrogenase, thrombin-like enzymes, etc. Inorganic substances, such as zinc and magnesium are variably present as well and may serve as cofactors for the aforementioned enzymes. Histamine-like factors are also present, which increase capillary permeability and lead to local tissue edema. Many of the toxins are specific to a given species, with the quantity, composition, and lethality varying with the species, geographic location, and the time of the year [10, 13]. It is probably inaccurate to classify any one particular venom as a *neurotoxin, hemotoxin, myotoxin, cardiotoxin*, etc., as venom exerts its effect on multiple organ systems [13, 14].

The main toxins in venoms of Australian snake genera cause paralysis, coagulopathy (disordered coagulation), rhabdomyolysis, and hemolysis (Table 51.1). Local tissue destruction is not usually a feature. There is variation of effects within a genus – for example, the venom of the Eastern brown snake (*Pseudonaja textilis*) causes paralysis

Table 51.1 Main components of venoms and their effects in poisonous snakes found in North American and Australia

Neurotoxins (brown snakes[a], tiger snakes, taipans, death adders, black snakes, coral snakes, mojave rattlesnake)

Presynaptic and postsynaptic neuromuscular blockers cause paralysis

Postsynaptic blockers readily reversed by antivenom

Presynaptic blockers are more difficult to reverse, particularly if treatment is delayed

Some presynaptic blockers are also rhabdomyolysins

Prothrombin activators (brown snakes, tiger snakes, taipans, crotalids)

Cause disseminated intravascular coagulation with consumption of clotting factors including fibrinogen

Intrinsic fibrin(ogen)lysis generates fibrin(ogen) degradation products

Significant risk of haemorrhage

Anticoagulants (black snakes, death adders, crotalids)

Present in a relatively small number of dangerous species

Prevent blood clotting without consumption of clotting factors

Rhabdomyolysins (taipans, black snakes, sea snakes, crotalids)

Some presynaptic neurotoxins also cause lysis of skeletal and cardiac muscle

Myoglobinuria may cause renal failure

Hemolysins

Present in a few species

Rarely a serious clinical effect

[a]Some species of brown snakes do not contain neurotoxins

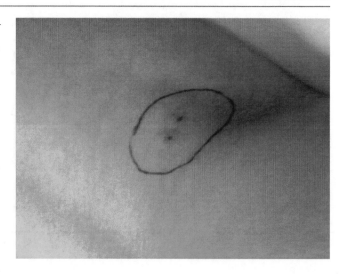

Fig. 51.3 Snake envenomation site – *dry bite* (Used with permission of Christopher P. Holstege, MD, University of Virginia, Charlottesville, Virginia)

[17, 18]. Myotoxin A is found in several species and produces direct necrosis of skeletal muscle tissue [19]. The venom of the Mojave rattlesnake (*Crotalus scutulatus scutulatus*) contains several neurotoxins as well as hemotoxins and toxins that cause tissue necrosis (myotoxins) [20–23]. Coral snake venom, also contains several neurotoxins, hemotoxins, and myotoxins [24–26].

Clinical Manifestations of Envenomation

Bites are usually observed by the victim but are relatively painless and occasionally go unnoticed, especially in cases associated with alcohol intoxication. Paired fang marks surrounded by inflammation or bruising are usually evident but sometimes only scratches or single puncture wounds are found (Fig. 51.3). Infrequently, when the snake strikes a second time, there will be two sets of paired fang marks. The bite-site may continue to bleed slightly. In some venomous snake bites, there will also be a second row of smaller teeth marks (which can occasionally be mistaken for a nonvenomous snakebite). Australian snake venoms do not cause extensive damage to local tissues, though occasionally the viability of a digit may be threatened or a small skin graft required. This contrasts markedly with bites by the North American pit vipers, where massive local reaction, hemorrhage, and tissue necrosis are often major features of envenomation and frequently threaten the viability of the affected limb (Figs. 51.4 and 51.5). Envenomation does not always accompany a bite (a so-called *dry bite*) – in several studies the incidence of clinical envenomation after observed snake bite was approximately 25–50 % [2, 10, 13, 15, 26], presumably because no or very little venom was injected.

whereas the Western brown snake (*Pseudonaja nuchalis*) does not, while the dugite (*Pseudonaja affinis*) has weak paralytic activity. Coagulopathy is often due to a procoagulation effect of prothrombin activators (Factor Xa-like enzymes). This process consumes clotting factors (*consumption coagulopathy*) forming fibrin which undergoes endogenous fibrinolysis to generate fibrin degradation products. Australian snake venoms, in contrast to some exotic venoms, do not cause primary fibrinolysis. The appearance of fibrin degradation products is therefore evidence that procoagulation has occurred. However, in a limited number of species coagulopathy is due to a direct anti-coagulant effect which does not generate fibrin degradation products.

Pit viper venoms also affect almost every major organ system (Table 51.1). In contrast to the Australian snake genera, pit viper venoms contain toxins that cause local tissue damage, thereby allowing the venom to penetrate deeper into the tissues. Hemotoxins directly damage the vascular endothelium, resulting in third-spacing of fluids and extravasation of erythrocytes [15], clinically manifest as edema, ecchymosis, and bleb formation. Pit-viper venoms, in particular, contain several hemostatically active components, some of which have been used in preclinical trials as anticoagulants [16]. Venom metalloproteinases cleave pro-tumor necrosis factor (TNF)-α, and the subsequent release of activated TNF-α leads to further inflammation and tissue destruction

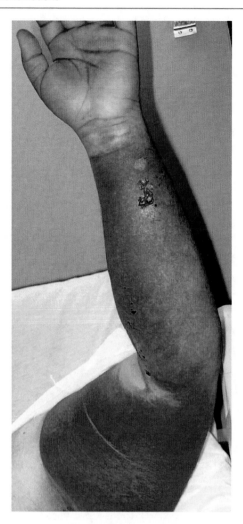

Fig. 51.4 Marked arm ecchymosis following timber rattlesnake (*Crotalus horridus horridus*) envenomation (Used with permission of Alexander B. Baer, MD, University of Virginia, Charlottesville, Virginia)

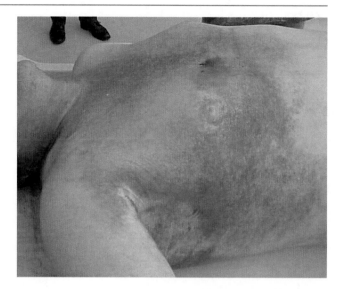

Fig. 51.5 Chest wall ecchymosis and death following timber rattlesnake (*Crotalus horridus horridus*) envenomation with the bite site noted in the mid thorax (Used with permission of Christopher P. Holstege, MD, University of Virginia, Charlottesville, Virginia)

Table 51.2 Onset of major systemic symptoms and signs of envenomation (Elapids)

<1 h after bite
Headache
Nausea, vomiting, abdominal pain transient hypotension associated with confusion or loss of consciousness
Coagulopathy (laboratory testing)
Regional lymphadenitis
1–3 h after bite
Paresis/paralysis of cranial nerves, e.g. ptosis, double vision, external ophthalmoplegia, dysphonia, dysphagia, myopathic facies
Hemorrhage from mucosal surfaces and needle punctures
Tachycardia, hypotension
Tachypnea, shallow tidal volume
>3 h after bite
Paresis/paralysis of truncal and limb muscles
Paresis/paralysis of respiratory muscles (respiratory failure)
Peripheral circulatory failure (shock), hypoxemia, cyanosis
Rhabdomyolysis
Dark urine (due to myoglobinuria or hemoglobin)
Renal failure

In massive envenomation or in a child, a critical illness may develop in minutes rather than hours

The time course of symptoms and signs after effective envenomation is somewhat predictable (Tables 51.2 and 51.3), but sometimes one symptom or sign may predominate or may wax and wane. These phenomena may be explained by variations in venom toxins of the same species in different geographical areas, or by variable absorption rates of different toxins. The fear associated with the snakebite itself may lead to symptoms of nausea, vomiting, diarrhea, syncope, and tachycardia almost immediately. These signs and symptoms must be differentiated from systemic signs and symptoms of envenomation (see below), though this may at times be quite difficult. As stated above, local findings such as pain, edema, erythema, or ecchymosis commonly emerge at the site of the bite and surrounding areas within 30–60 min following pit-viper envenomation. Bullae (containing either serous fluid or hemorrhage), lymphangitis, and tender, swollen regional lymph nodes soon follow (Fig. 51.6). Regional lymphadenitis also occurs

with bites by mildly venomous snakes in the absence of serious systemic illness. Localized pain is almost immediate and occurs in more than 90 % of cases associated with pit viper envenomation, though a bite by the Mojave rattlesnake may produce numbness without pain. Similarly, coral snake envenomation produces little pain, but occasionally may produce tremors, marked salivation, and altered mental status. Local tissue injury, especially when it affects an

Table 51.3 Onset of major systemic symptoms and signs of envenomation (crotalids)

<1 h after bite

Sense of impending doom (fear, anxiety)

Nausea, vomiting, abdominal pain (secondary to the above)

Pain at the bite site (often described as burning in nature)

  Local tissue edema proximal and distal to the bite site (usually 10–30 min after the bite)

  Bullae formation (either serous or hemorrhagic)

  Regional lymphadenitis

1–3 h after bite

Ecchymosis at the bite site

Coagulopathy (laboratory testing)

  Hemorrhage from mucosal surfaces and needle punctures

Nausea, vomiting

  Perioral paresthesias

  Paresthesias of the fingertips and toes

  Rubbery, minty or metallic taste in the mouth

  Tachycardia, hypotension

Tachypnea, shallow tidal volume

>3 h after bite

Peripheral circulatory failure (shock), hypoxemia, cyanosis

DIC

  Rhabdomyolysis

Dark urine (due to myoglobinuria or hemoglobinuria)

Acute renal failure

In massive envenomation or in a child, a critical illness may develop in minutes rather than hours

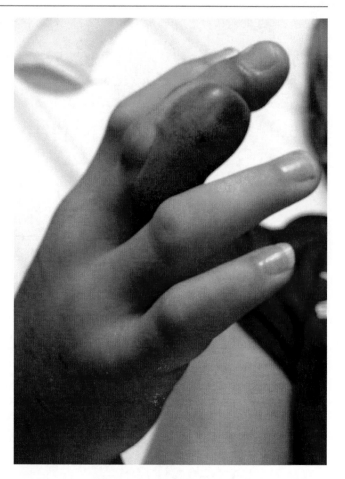

Fig. 51.6 Hemorrhagic bullae of the finger following copperhead (*Agkistrodon contortrix*) envenomation (Used with permission of Christopher P. Holstege, MD, University of Virginia, Charlottesville, Virginia)

extremity, may result in compartment syndrome, rarely necessitating fasciotomy. Australian species are less commonly associated with local tissue injury.

Neurotoxic effects (i.e. coral snake, most of the Australian species, Mojave rattlesnake, and occasionally the eastern diamonback rattlesnake) include headache, nausea, vomiting, and cranial nerve palsies – these are manifest by ptosis, dysarthria, dysphagia, and dyspnea. Gross muscle weakness usually occurs over several hours, eventually culminating in neuromuscular respiratory failure. Coagulopathy, determined by laboratory tests (see below), is likely to be present within 15 min after envenomation by a coagulopathy-producing species. Venom-induced thrombocytopenia, fibrinolysis, and DIC have all been reported and may clinically manifest as epistaxis, hemoptysis, mucosal bleeding, bleeding from the wound itself, or petechiae (Fig. 51.7) [27]. Massive envenomation may cause rapid cardiovascular collapse, though this occurs in less than 7 % of pit viper envenomations [28] and contrary to popular belief, pit viper bites are usually not immediately fatal (unless the venom enters a blood vessel directly).

The cause of transient hypotension not accompanied by respiratory failure or hemorrhage within 30 min after envenomation, is obscure but it may be related to intravascular coagulation since prothrombin activators gain access to the circulation within a number of minutes after subcutaneous

injection and this effect is prevented experimentally by heparin [29–32]. Third space loss of fluids may also lead to hypotension and shock. Tachycardia and relatively minor electrocardiogram abnormalities are common. Direct myocardial toxicity may occur in species causing rhabdomyolysis, but this does not explain rapid cardiovascular collapse.

Other sequelae are less common. Coagulopathy-induced intracranial hemorrhage may occur. General rhabdomyolysis is caused by some species but even so is not common unless massive envenomation has occurred or delayed, inadequate or incorrect antivenom (antivenin) has been given. Rhabdomyolysis involves all skeletal musculature and sometimes cardiac muscle. Myoglobinuria (secondary to cell lysis and extravasation of erythrocytes) may cause acute renal failure. The etiology of nephrotoxicity is mutifactorial. A high intake of alcohol by adults before snake-bite is common, and may complicate management such as delay in presentation and multiple bites. Pre-existing anticoagulant therapy or ulcerative gastro-intestinal tract disease may also complicate coagulopathy management.

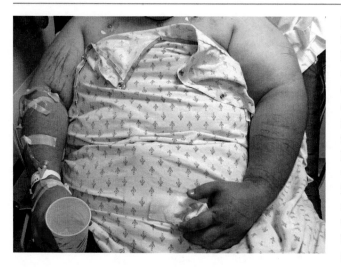

Fig. 51.7 Marked thrombocytopenia, left arm ecchymosis and edema following timber rattlesnake (*Crotalus horridus horridus*) envenomation of the left hand. Note the petechaie of the right upper arm following blood pressure cuff insufflation (Used with permission of Alexander B. Baer, MD, University of Virginia, Charlottesville, Virginia)

Identification of the Snake

Identification of the snake stipulates the selection of antivenin, if needed, and forewarns the doctor of characteristic clinical problems. Although physical identification of the species is helpful, it is not usually mandatory for good management. Misidentification of the species may lead to administration of an antivenin which has little or no venom neutralizing capability and may, in fact, produce untoward and potentially dangerous adverse effects (see below). Finally, safety should always be the main priority, and no attempt should be made to capture or kill the snake. Even if the snake is dead, it should not be picked up with the hands as envenomation by reflex biting after death of the snake has been reported [33]. Physicians in North America are quite fortunate in that all of the pit viper envenomations are treated with the same antivenin. Coral snake envenomation requires a different antivenin, but the clinical features of this envenomation are usually easily distinguished from a pit viper envenomation.

A venom detection kit (VDK; CSL [Commonwealth Serum Laboratories Ltd]) is available in Australia that is designed for bedside use – the kit indicates which genus of snake is involved and which antivenin is appropriate. It is an in vitro enzyme immunoassay test for detection and identification of snake venom swabbed from the bite site or in the urine, blood, or other tissue of the victim of snake bite in Australia and Papua New Guinea. The kit is widely available. It is a bank of test wells containing specific rabbit antibodies to the venoms of the main genera of snakes. By a series of reactions with chromogen and peroxide solutions a positive reaction with venom antigen and venom antibody is indicated within 25 min by a color change, thereby indicating the type of antivenin to be administered, if required. The kit detects venoms from tiger, brown, black, death adder, and taipan genera. It does not identify an individual species of snake and several genera may yield a positive result in a specified well. The sensitivity and specificity of the test is unknown, but are generally regarded as high. The test is able to detect venom in very low concentration (<10 ng/mL). Despite the result of the test, the decision to administer antivenin, or not, is a clinical decision. If a test of urine or blood is positive in the absence of clinical signs or abnormal coagulation studies, then antivenin should not be administered. On the other hand, a very high concentration of venom in a biological sample or bite site swab may overwhelm the test and give a false negative result (so-called *Hook effect*). If that possibility exists, say in the case of an obviously clinically envenomated victim, a diluted sample should be tested. A positive VDK test of a bite site swab per se does not likewise indicate that the victim has been envenomated since snakes may leave venom on the skin but not envenomate. If the snake cannot be identified physically or a VDK test is not practical, a monovalent antivenin, or a combination of monovalent antivenins or polyvalent antivenin able to neutralize venoms of all snakes in the geographical region (Australia) should be administered on a contingency basis (see below).

The appearance of a bite site cannot be used to reliably identify the snake. Although each species of snake has characteristic toxins, the clinical signs of envenomation are common to numerous species. Unless the snake is identified by an expert, morphological identification can be misleading and is not generally recommended. Most snakes, with few exceptions, are fast moving and usually quickly depart the scene of encounter with a victim. Consequently, snakes are not often observed clearly by the victim or witnesses. In this circumstance and even when the snake is under close observation, it is dangerous in Australia for example to assume that a brown-colored snake belongs to the brown snake genus, a black-colored snake belongs to the black snake genus, or a banded snake belongs to the Tiger snake genus. Similarly, with respect to North American snakes, relying on eyewitness accounts for identification may be fraught with error and is usually not necessary. For example, many texts commonly cite the phrase *Red on yellow, kill a fellow*; *Red on black, venom lack* in order to differentiate a coral snake from a non-venomous snake. It is difficult to remember this phrase in the best of circumstances, let alone when confronted with a snake. Rather, the more prudent decision when confronted with an unconfirmed, but nevertheless suspected coral snake envenomation is to monitor the victim in an inpatient setting for a period of up to 12–24 h and initiate antivenin if signs and symptoms of envenomation develop [10, 13, 15, 27].

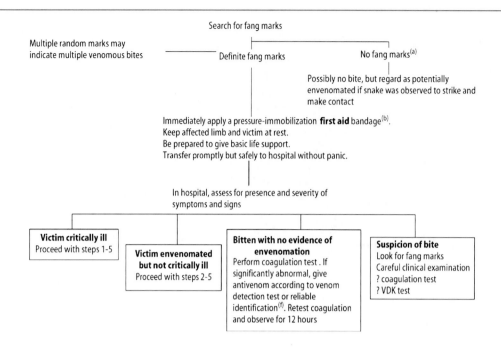

Fig. 51.8 Management plan for snake envenomation

1. **Resuscitate** (treat hypoxemia and shock). Be prepared to intubate and mechanically ventilate. Admit to intensive care.
2. **Apply pressure immobilization bandage. Do not remove if already applied.**[b]
3. **Give antivenom intravenously.**[c,d,e,f,g]
   - Give monovalent if species reliably known or appropriate antivenom indicated by venom detection test.
   - For critically ill victim, do not wait for venom test result or if species cannot be determined; give according to geographic location:
     Victoria: brown and tiger snake
     Tasmania: tiger snake
     Other states and territories: polyvalent
   - Titrate antivenom against clinical and coagulation status (*Note:* Death adders do not cause significant coagulopathy).
4. **Perform investigations.**
   - Bite site swab for venom detection. (First-aid bandage may be cut to expose bite site and then reinforced.)
   - Blood for venom detection, coagulation, type and cross-match (if bleeding), fibrin degradation products, full blood examination, enzymes, electrolytes, urea, creatinine.
   - Urine for venom detection, red blood cells, hemoglobin, myoglobin.
5. **Examine frequently** to detect slow onset of paralysis,[h] coagulopathy, rhabdomyolysis and renal failure.

Dangers and mistakes in management:
a. Fang marks not visible to naked eye.
b. Premature release of bandage may result in sudden systemic envenomation. Leave in situ until victim reaches full medical facilities. If clinically envenomated, remove only after antivenom given.
c. Erroneous identification of snake may cause wrong antivenom to be given. If any doubt, treat as unidentified.
d. Antivenom without premedication. Anaphylaxis is not rare and may not respond to treatment.
e. Insufficient antivenom. Titrate dose against clinical and coagulation status.
f. Blood and coagulation factors (fresh frozen plasma, cryoprecipitate) not preceded by antivenom will worsen coagulopathy.
g. Antivenom given without clinical or laboratory evidence of envenomation.
h. Delayed onset of paralysis may be missed. Victim must be examined at least hourly.

Initial Management: Resuscitation and Stabilization (Fig. 51.8)

The key features of emergency management of envenomation are common to any scenario and include securing and maintaining a patent airway (*A = Airway*), assuring adequate oxygenation and ventilation (*B = Breathing*), and establishing vascular access and reversing shock (*C = Circulation*). Additional keys to management include the application of a pressure-immobilization bandage, as well as the administration of antivenin (antivenom). All jewelry (especially watches, rings, bracelets) and other constrictive clothing should be removed. The overwhelming majority of snake bites occur on the victims' arms or legs which can be treated with Sutherland's pressure-immobilization technique [34] for elapid snake bite. The efficacy of this technique has been shown experimentally in coral snake (*Micrurus fulvius fulvius*) [35], Eastern diamondback rattlesnake (*Crotalus adamanteus*) [36], Western diamondback rattlesnake (*Crotalus atrox*) [37, 38], and Indian cobra (*Naja naja*)

[39] envenomation. The technique is recommended by the American Heart Association and the American Red Cross [40]. With this technique (Figs. 51.9), a bandage of elasticized material (preferred) [41], crêpe or crêpe-like material is applied from the fingers or toes up the limb as far as possible, completely covering the bite site. This applies pressure and immobilizes the limb – a pressure-immobilization bandage (PIB). The PIB should be as applied as firmly as required for a sprained ankle. Additional immobilization of the limb is achieved with a rigid splint, with the aim of immobilizing the joints on both sides side of the bite site.

The rationale of the technique is simple. Venom is deposited subcutaneously and access to the systemic circulation is dependent on its absorption and transport by lymphatics [42] or the small blood vessels. Lymph flow is dependent at least in part by surrounding muscle action. Application of pressure to the bite site combined with immobilization of the limb effectively prevents lymph flow and delays the access of venom to the blood circulation [34]. The technique was designed for use in the field, but it should also be part of initial management in hospital since it is likely to impede further access of venom to the circulation. Some experimental [1] and anecdotal evidence with death adder bites [43] suggests that the technique allows inactivation of venom at the bite site but this has not been subjected to a controlled study. Premature removal of the PIB may permit a sudden elevation in blood concentration of venom with subsequent collapse of the victim and should be avoided. Its removal therefore should be dictated by the circumstances. When an asymptomatic snake-bite victim reaches hospital with a PIB in place, it should not be disturbed until antivenin, appropriate staff, and equipment have been assembled. If the victim is symptomatic and antivenin is indicated, the PIB should not be removed until after antivenin has been administered, and

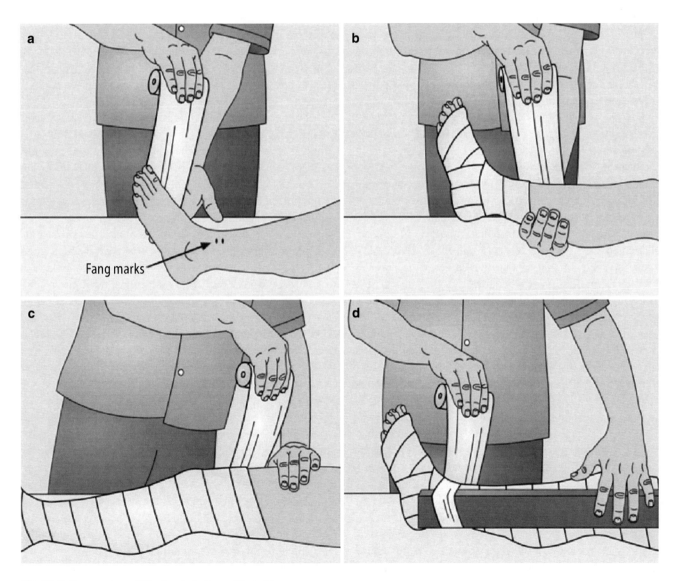

Fig. 51.9 Pressure-immobilization technique of first-aid

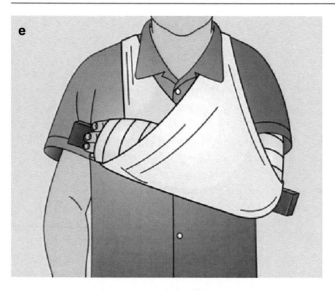

Fig. 51.9 (continued)

re-applied if the victim's condition deteriorates. If a swab of the bite site is needed, it may be obtained by removing the splint temporarily and cutting a window in the bandage. The PIB should then be made good and the splint re-applied.

Previously recommended measures such as incision, application of suction devices to the wound, tourniquets, cryotherapy, electric shock therapy, and application of heat or cold in the field are no longer advocated [3, 10, 13–15, 27, 32]. Instead, focus should be directed towards timely transfer to a medical facility. From a clinical point of view, one of the four following situations usually arises after snake bite.

Victim envenomated and critically ill: Initial emphasis is on resuscitation and stabilization in the Emergency Department (ED) with the re-establishment of airway, ventilation, oxygenation, and adequate organ perfusion pressure. Intravenous fluids are usually required and sometimes inotropic agents. A PIB, if not already applied, should be applied to the bite site and should not be removed until antivenin has been administered. The bitten extremity should be immobilized and elevated to a level above the heart (though this is debated – some authorities recommend keeping the bitten extremity below the level of the heart to hypothetically impede lymphatic flow – there is no definitive evidence one way or another, and we prefer elevation). Intravenous access should be obtained and antivenin administered intravenously according to the identity of the snake, if known. Antivenin must not be delayed, however, and can often be administered even if the snake has not been identified with 100 % certainty (see below). After stabilization, admission to the PICU is required.

Victim envenomated but not critically ill: More time is available when the envenomated victim is not critically ill to identify the snake by investigations and subsequently administer specific antivenin. If not already in place, a PIB should be applied, and not removed until after antivenin administration.

The bitten extremity should be elevated to a level above the heart – this may result in proximal progression of swelling and discoloration, though this does not represent progression of toxicity if swelling distal to the bite subsides [32]. After initial treatment, admission to either the PICU or hospital ward may be needed according to local resources and capabilities.

Victim bitten but does not appear envenomated: A victim bitten by a snake but showing no symptoms or signs of envenomation should have initial investigations performed in the ED, with subsequent consideration of observational or hospital ward admission. Close observation and re-examination is potentially needed for up to 12–24 h in the case of a child depending upon the type of snake found within the region of envenomation, though perhaps less time is required for an adult [3, 10, 13–15, 27, 32]. An asymptomatic child, regardless of age, bitten by a North American copperhead and other non-venomous snakes, however probably does not need 12 h of observation.

The syndrome of envenomation may be very slow in onset over numerous hours with a symptom free initial period. An initial test of coagulation should be considered in most snake envenomations (again, depending upon the region and species of snake; e.g., copperhead envenomations rarely, if ever, cause coagulopathy). If a coagulopathy is present, specific antivenin should be administered after identification of the species or as indicated by a VDK test. If only a mild coagulopathy is present it may be acceptable to withhold antivenin in the hope of spontaneous resolution but coagulation should be checked at intervals and the victim maintained under surveillance until coagulation is normal.

Suspicion of bite: If snake bite is suspected but was not observed, a careful search should be made for fang marks and a careful clinical examination performed. The question of investigations is dictated by the degree of suspicion and the presence or absence of any appropriate symptoms and signs. If there is no progression of local signs on the affected extremity and no coagulopathy is documented after an appropriate clinical observation time period, a reliable patient can be sent home.

Management: Antivenom (Antivenin) Therapy

After initial resuscitation and stabilization, the next most important step in the aforementioned scenarios involves deciding when to administer antivenin therapy. For Australian envenomations, CSL Ltd. produces highly purified equine monovalent antivenins against the venoms of the main terrestrial snake genera, including the tiger snake, brown snake, black snake, death adder, and taipan. A polyvalent antivenin consisting of a mixture of aliquots of all the monovalent antivenins described above is also available. CSL Ltd also produces a sea snake antivenin from horses immunized with

Table 51.4 Antivenin and *initial* dosages when snake identified (Australian species)

Snake	Antivenom	Dose (units)
Common brown snake	Brown snake	4,000–6,000
Chappell island tiger snake	Tiger snake	12,000
Copperheads	Tiger snake	3,000–6,000
Death adders	Death adder	6,000
Dugite	Brown snake	4,000–6,000
Gwardar	Brown snake	4,000–6,000
Mulga (king brown) snake	Black snake	18,000
Papuan black snake	Black snake	18,000
Red-bellied black snake	Tiger snake or	3,000
	Black snake[a]	18,000
Rough-scaled (clarence river) snake	Tiger snake	3,000
Sea-snakes	Sea-snake or	1,000
	Tiger snake	3,000
Small-scaled (fierce) snake	Taipan	12,000
Taipan	Taipan	12,000
Tasmanian tiger snake	Tiger snake	6,000
Tiger snake	Tiger snake	3,000

[a]Smaller protein mass tiger snake antivenom preferable. Antivenom units per ampule: brown snake 1,000; tiger snake 3,000; black snake 18,000; taipan 12,000; death adder 6,000; polyvalent 40,000

Table 51.5 Antivenin and *initial* dosages when identity of snake uncertain (Australian species)

State	Antivenom	Dose (units)
Tasmania	Tiger snake	6,000
Victoria	Tiger snake	3,000
	and	
	Brown snake	4,000–6,000
New South Wales	Polyvalent	40,000
Australian capital territory		
Queensland		
South Australia		
Western Australia		
Northern Territory		
Papua New Guinea	Polyvalent	40,000

Note: (1) If the victim on presentation is critically-ill, 2–3 times these amounts should be given initially; (2) additional antivenom may be required in the course of management since absorption of venom may be delayed

beaked sea snake (*Enhydrina schistosa*) and tiger snake venoms (Tables 51.4 and 51.5).

Two crotalid antivenins are available for clinical use in North America – a polyvalent crotalid antivenin of equine origin (Antivenin Crotalidae Polyvalent, ACP; Wyeth-Ayerst Laboratories, Philadelphia, PA) (Table 51.6) and a purified ovine polyvalent Fab immunoglobulin fragment product (CroFab; Protherics, Brentwood, TN) (Table 51.7). However, the equine-based ACP is associated with a high incidence of immediate hypersensitivity reactions, which may pose an even greater risk to the patient than the envenomation itself [reviewed in 3, 10, 13–15, 27, 32, 44, 45]. CroFab appears to be safer in this regard with a lower incidence of adverse effects, but its widespread use is relatively limited due its expense. However, as more experience with CroFab accrues, use of ACP will become less common in the United States [32]. Historically, copperhead envenomations were rarely considered severe enough to warrant the risks associated with the equine antivenin, though CroFab may be more commonly considered as experience accrues [46]. Wyeth-Ayerst also manufactures antivenin for coral snake envenomations, *Micrurus fulvius* Antivenin (Wyeth-Ayerst Laboratories, Philadelphia, PA), though Wyeth has stated that they will discontinue production of all snake antivenins in the near future. Generally, three to five vials of *Micrurus fulvius* antivenin should be administered immediately, and if systemic manifestations are present, the dose should be increased to six to ten vials. A ovine polyvalent Fab immunoglobulin for coral snake envenomations is currently undergoing clinical testing and will hopefully be available in the near future.

The decision to administer antivenin must be based on clinical criteria of envenomation. If the victim is significantly envenomated, antivenin must be administered as soon as possible (preferably within 4 h of the snake bite, but with pit viper envenomation, antivenin may have some efficacy as far out as 24 h following the snake bite) as there is no other effective treatment. However, several situations may justify withholding antivenin therapy, e.g., if envenomation is so mild that spontaneous recovery could occur or if the consequences of antivenin administration are likely to outweigh the benefit to be gained. Because of the multiple species of venomous snakes, definitive indications for antivenin administration following pit viper envenomation are not clear and will probably continue to evolve as physicians gain more experience with CroFab. However, general guidelines include rapid progression of swelling, significant coagulopathy, neuromuscular paralysis with respiratory failure, and shock [3, 10, 13–15, 27, 32]. Snake antivenins must be administered by the intravenous route, though in dire circumstances when vascular access cannot be readily achieved, antivenin may be administered by the intraosseous route. The intramuscular route is ineffective because of the large volume of fluid and the slow absorption of protein antibodies.

Skin testing has no predictive value for determining whether or not the victim will develop an allergic reaction to the antivenin and is probably a waste of precious time in most situations [13–15, 27, 47]. Instead, some Australian authorities recommend premedication with subcutaneous epinephrine at a dose of approximately 0.25 mg for an adult and 0.005–0.01 mg/kg for a child about 5–10 min before commencement of the antivenin infusion, especially for the Australian envenomations or exotic envenomations. Anaphylaxis associated with CroFab administration is rare,

Table 51.6 Antivenin administration (North America)

Antivenin (crotalidae) polyvalent, ACP (Wyeth-Ayerst)
1. Reconstitute by injecting 10 ml of sterile water diluent into each vial and swirl to mix (do not shake)
2. Dilute the reconstituted antivenin in 500 ml of normal saline or 5 % dextrose. An alternative method is to reconstitute 10 vials of antivenin in 1 l of normal saline
3. Administer trial dose of 5–10 ml intravenously over 5 min. If no reaction occurs, adjust the rate to administer dose (based upon the degree of envenomation[a]) over the next 60 min. Do not administer into a finger or toe
4. Additional doses of antivenin are based on clinical response to the initial dose. If swelling continues to progress, symptoms increase in severity, hypotension occurs, or decrease in hematocrit appears, additional treatment with 10–50 ml of the reconstituted antivenin should be administered
5. Pre-medication recommended: diphenhydramine (1–2 mg/kg IV)
6. Manufacturer recommends performing a skin test prior to administration of antivenin, though the predictive value of skin testing is quite poor and should not delay treatment
7. initial dose should be administered within 4 h of the bite, though antivenin may have some efficacy up to 24 h following the bite

Mild envenomation (Administration of five vials – some experts suggest that the potential risks of the antivenin outweigh the benefit in these cases and recommend supportive care only). Defined by localized pain, tenderness, edema at the site of the bite; no systemic symptoms, with the possible exception of a metallic taste in the mouth or perioral paresthesias
Moderate envenomation (Administration of ten vials). Defined by pain, tenderness, edema beyond the area adjacent to the bite, often with systemic signs of mild coagulopathy
Severe envenomation (Administration of 15–20 vials). Defined by intense pain and swelling of the entire extremity, often with severe systemic signs and symptoms and laboratory evidence of coagulopathy
Life-threatening envenomation (Administration of 25 vials). Defined by the presence of shock, acute respiratory failure in addition to the signs and symptoms listed above
[a]The degree of envenomation is estimated by the following recommended grading scale

Table 51.7 CroFab administration (North America)

Crotalidae polyvalent immune fab (ovine), CroFab
1. The initial dose of antivenin should be administered as soon as possible (within 6 h after the crotalid snakebite). Skin testing prior to administering antivenin is not required
2. Reconstitute by injecting 10 ml of sterile water diluent into each vial and swirl to mix (do not shake). Further dilute the number of vials needed for total dose (4–6 vials) in 250 ml NS and continue to mix by gently swirling
3. Infuse slowly over the first 10 min at 25–50 ml/h and monitor closely for any allergic reaction; if no reaction occurs, may increase to 250 ml/h until total dose is infused
4. Observe patient for 1 h following the completion of the first dose. If initial control is not achieved after the first dose, an additional 4–6 vials may be repeated until initial control of the envenomation syndrome has been achieved
5. After initial control has been established: 2 vials every 6 h for up to 18 h (3 doses); an additional 2 vial dose may be administered if deemed necessary based on clinical response

though it is prudent to monitor for signs and symptoms of hypersensitivity and treat appropriately in these cases as well. In the moribund or critically ill victim, when it is essential to administer antivenin quickly, the epinephrine may be administered intramuscularly or even intravenously in smaller doses. However, in general, epinephrine is not recommended by intravenous or intramuscular routes because of the risk of intracerebral hemorrhage occasioned by the combination of possible epinephrine-induced hypertension and venom-induced coagulopathy. Although intracerebral hemorrhage has been recorded in the past in association with premedication, all such cases were accompanied by intravenous epinephrine, none with subcutaneous epinephrine [48]. On the other hand, many authorities believe that the incidence of adverse reactions (8–13 %) to polyvalent crotalid antivenin of equine origin is sufficient to warrant premedication with epinephrine, which is the only medication proven effective in reducing the incidence of antivenom induced reactions to snake antivenoms and their severity [49]. At a minimum, resuscitation medications and equipment (airway equipment, oxygen source, bag-valve-mask ventilation, suction catheters, etc.) should be immediately available. It is not prudent to forgo premedication and elect to treat anaphylaxis if it occurs. Antivenom has caused fatal anaphylaxis [2, 50]. Iatrogenic anaphylaxis has a high mortality despite vigorous and expert resuscitation [51]. Repeated doses of epinephrine before each dose of antivenin are not required unless allergy has already been established. If an adverse reaction to the first ampule of antivenin has not occurred, subsequent ampules do not need to be preceded by epinephrine premedication. The adverse reaction rate to polyvalent antivenins is higher than to monovalent antivenins and should not be used when a monovalent antivenin or combinations would suffice. The antihistamine, promethazine, is not recommended as a premedication for snake antivenin – it does not reduce the adverse reaction rate [52] and may cause obtundation and hypotension which may both exacerbate and confound a state of envenomation. Other drugs, including corticosteroids and aminophylline are also not useful in preventing anaphylaxis because their actions, apart from being unproven, are too slow in onset.

Administration of antivenin should always be administered in a location equipped and staffed by personnel capable of managing anaphylaxis – most authorities recommend the PICU or ED. Management of anaphylaxis is discussed elsewhere in this textbook, but suffice it to say that if anaphylaxis occurs during administration of antivenin, the infusion should be discontinued temporarily and re-started when the victim's condition is stable. Further treatment includes diphenhydramine (1.25 mg/kg IV every 6 h) and subcutaneous epinephrine (0.01 mg/kg, or 0.01 mL/kg/dose of 1:1,000 solution). Less severe adverse reactions consisting of headache, chest discomfort, fine rash, arthralgia, myalgia, nausea, abdominal pain, vomiting, and pyrexia may be managed by temporary cessation of the infusion followed by administration of corticosteroids and diphenhydramine before re-commencement.

A delayed hypersensitivity reaction, *serum sickness*, should be anticipated and patients warned of the symptoms and signs which usually appear several days to 2 weeks after antivenin administration. Severity ranges from a faint rash and pyrexia to serious multi-system disease including lymphadenitis, polyarthralgia, urticaria, nephritis, neuropathy, and vasculitis. The treatment is a course of corticosteroids, e.g. methylprednisolone 2 mg/kg per day tapered over 5–7 days. The incidence of serum sickness appears to be greater with use of multiple doses of monovalent antivenin and with polyvalent antivenin and thus should be prevented with a restricted course of corticosteroids for 3–5 days.

Monitoring

Laboratory tests are essential and should be performed regularly, interpreted quickly, and treated promptly to counter venom effects and its complications. Serial coagulation tests and tests of renal function are especially important. Absorption of venom from the bite site is a continuing process and management must anticipate unabsorbed venom. Apart from regular monitoring of vital signs and oxygenation, the following are specifically recommended. In Australia, a swab of the bite site for venom testing should be done. It has the highest likelihood of detecting venom provided the site has not been washed. If the site has been washed, it may be squeezed to yield venom if no other suitable biological sample can be acquired. Aside from cleaning the wound to prevent secondary infection, there is no clinical value in washing a site to remove venom. Venom may be detectable in the urine, this may be especially helpful when venom in blood has been bound by antivenin and is therefore undetectable in the blood. Urine should also be tested for blood and protein. Pigmentation of urine may be due to either hemoglinuria or myoglobinuria – distinction is not possible with rapid bedside tests. Recording urine output is essential. Coagulation tests should include prothrombin time, activated thromboplastin time, serum fibrinogen, and fibrin degradation products. If these are not possible, a bedside whole blood clotting time or bleeding time are helpful in establishing a diagnosis. A full blood examination and blood film seeking haemoglobin level, evidence of haemolysis and platelet count. A mild elevation in white cell count is expected. Thrombocytopenia may occur in association with DIC. Electrolytes, blood urea nitrogen, creatinine, calcium, creatine phosphokinase (isoenzymes), and troponin are useful to monitor rhabdomyolysis and possible renal dysfunction. Electrocardiogram abnormalities including sinus tachycardia, ventricular ectopy, and ST segment and T-wave changes may occur. These effects may be the result of victim stress response, venom toxins or from electrolyte disturbances induced by rhabdomyolysis or renal failure.

Secondary Management and Follow-Up Care

The bites of Australian elapid snakes do not cause severe pain. However, the extensive tissue necrosis produced by North American pit viper envenomation can be associated with significant discomfort. In these cases, liberal use of narcotics is recommended for the relief of pain – aspirin and non-steroidal anti-inflammatory agents are contraindicated due to their inhibitory effects on platelets and therefore hemostasis. The incidence of infection following snake bit is surprisingly low given the abundance of microorganisms found in the mouth of snakes (*Enterobacter*, *Pseudomonas*, *Aerobacter*, *Proteus*, gram-positive cocci, *Clostridium*, Salmonella and others) [53–57]. Prophylactic antibiotics are therefore unnecessary and not routinely required. Tetanus prophylaxis, however, should be reviewed.

Coagulopathy often resolves after several doses of antivenin, but antivenin per se does not restore coagulation – it permits newly released or manufactured coagulation factors to act unopposed by venom. If coagulation is not restored after several doses of antivenin over several hours or if there is hemodynamically significant bleeding, replacement of coagulation factors with fresh frozen plasma is indicated. Because regeneration of depleted coagulation factors takes many hours, treatment with antivenin alone while waiting for their regeneration exposes the patient to serious hemorrhage. On the other hand, fresh frozen plasma should not be administered unnecessarily. Administration of fresh frozen plasma or cryoprecipitate should be preceded by antivenin in order to neutralize any circulating venom prothrombin activator. Platelet transfusion may be required as well.

After acute resuscitation, intravenous fluids in sufficient volume to maintain urine output at about 40 mL/kg per day in an adult or 1–2 mL/kg per hour in a child are required to prevent acute tubular necrosis as a consequence of rhabdomyolysis. Life-threatening hyperkalemia and hypocalcemia may develop with rhabdomyolysis, and in these cases hemofiltration or dialysis may be required. Heparin has prevented the action of prothrombin activators in animal models of envenomation, but it does not improve established DIC [31] and is therefore not recommended following snake envenomation. Recovery is expected after appropriate treatment but it may be slow, taking many weeks or months particularly after severe envenomation or after delayed presentation with neurotoxicity, marked tissue necrosis, rhabdomyolysis or renal failure. Isolated neurological or ophthalmic signs may persist. Long-term loss of taste or smell occurs occasionally.

Severe crotalid envenomations may be complicated by compartment syndrome. Neurovascular checks are an important part of the ongoing assessment and management of any snake bite. Compartment syndrome (generally defined as a compartment pressure > 30 mmHg) should be managed with mannitol (1–2 g/kg IV), elevation of the affected extremity, and administration of four to six vials of CroFab over 1 h [10, 32]. Compartment syndrome arises in part from the extensive tissue necrosis produced by the crotalid venom, hence the justification for additional antivenin to neutralize the venom and hopefully reduce compartment pressures. Fasciotomy is required if these measures fail to relieve the compartment syndrome, or if there is neurologic or circulatory compromise.

Sea-Snake Bite

The venoms of some sea-snakes cause widespread rhabdomyolysis, neuromuscular paralysis, and direct renal damage. Many species of sea-snakes exist in northern Australian waters but are rare in southern waters. Many have not been researched. The principles of treatment are essentially the same as for envenomation by terrestrial snakes. The venoms of significant species are neutralized adequately with CSL Ltd beaked sea-snake (*Enhydrina schistosa*) antivenom. If that preparation is not available, tiger snake or polyvalent antivenin should be used. Sea-snake bites are rare in Australia waters but common among fishermen of nearby Asian countries.

Uncommon and Exotic Snake Bites

Zoo personnel, herpetologists, and amateur collectors who catch, maintain, and breed species of uncommon or exotic snakes or who import or breed exotic (overseas) snakes are at risk. Illegal importation sometimes endangers customs services personnel. Minton reported that he consulted on 54

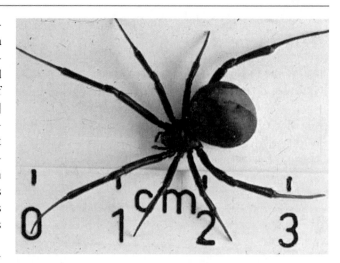

Fig. 51.10 Red-back spider (*Latrodectus hasselti*)

cases of bites from at least 29 different exotic, venomous species between 1977 and 1995 [58]. The most common species was the cobra, which was involved in 40 % of the cases [58]. Assistance with these exotic envenomations (cobra, mamba, etc.) is available either through the American Association of Poison Control Centers (800 222 1222), the American Zoo and Aquarium Association (301 562 0777), or the Australian Venom Research Unit (AVRU) (1300 760 451).

Spiders

Although several thousand species of spiders exist in Australia, only funnel-web spiders (genera *Atrax* and *Hadronyche*) and the red-back spider (*Latrodectus hasselti*) (Fig. 51.10) have caused death or significant illness. In North America, the arthropods of medical importance include the black widow spider (genus *Lactrodectus*) (Fig. 51.11), brown recluse spider (genus *Loxosceles*) (Fig. 51.12), and scorpions. All spiders have venom but although some are capable of causing local injury and necrosis [59], the necrotic effects of these spider bites have been over-rated [60]. In the interest of space, the present discussion will concentrate on the most common spider envenomations in Australia and North America and briefly consider scorpion envenomations. The interested reader is directed to other sources for additional information [2, 13, 15, 27, 61].

Funnel-Web Spiders

Numerous species of the genera *Atrax* and *Hadronyche* inhabit the Australian states of New South Wales and Queensland. Several species cause significant illness and are

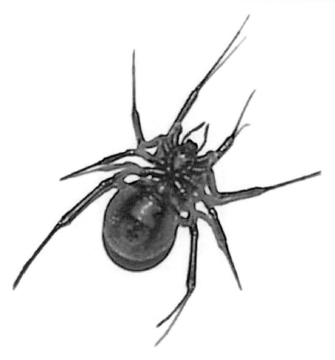

Fig. 51.11 Black widow spider (*Latrodectus mactans*) (Used with permission of Christopher P. Holstege, MD, University of Virginia, Charlottesville, Virginia)

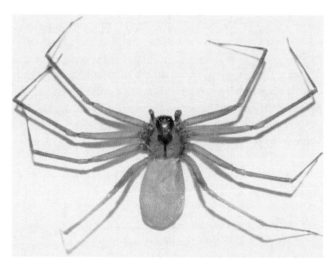

Fig. 51.12 Brown recluse spider (*Loxosceles reclusa*) (Used with permission of Sue Kell, PhD, University of Virginia Health System, Charlottesville, Virginia)

potentially lethal. *Atrax robustus* (Sydney Funnel-web Spider) is a large aggressive spider inhabiting an area within an approximate 160 km radius of Sydney. It has caused more than a dozen deaths. The male spider is more dangerous than the female, in contrast to other species, and is inclined to roam after rainfall. In doing so, it may enter houses and seek shelter among clothes or bedding. Its bite is painful and it may be difficult to dislodge. Bites do not always result in envenomation, but envenomation may be rapidly fatal. The

venom contains polypeptides which stimulate the release of acetylcholine at neuromuscular junctions and within the autonomic nervous system, and release catecholamines. The early features of the envenomation syndrome include nausea, vomiting, profuse sweating, salivation, and abdominal pain. Life threatening features of envenomation are usually preceded by the onset of muscle fasciculation at the bite site, which quickly involves distant muscle groups. Hypertension, tachyarrhythmias, vasoconstriction, hypersalivation and bronchorrhoea quickly follow. The victim may lapse into coma, develop central hypoventilation and have difficulty maintaining an airway free of secretions. Finally, respiratory failure, pulmonary oedema and severe hypotension culminate in death. The syndrome usually develops within several hours but it may be more rapid. Several children have died within 90 min of envenomation, and one died within 15 min.

First aid treatment is application of a pressure-immobilization bandage which delays the onset of the envenomation syndrome and appears to enable some inactivation of venom at the bite site [2]. Definitive treatment is intravenous administration of antivenom and support of vital functions, which may include airway support and mechanical ventilation. No deaths or serious morbidity have been reported since the introduction of antivenom in 1981.

Red-Back Spider

This spider (*Latrodectus hasselti*) is distributed throughout Australia where it is found outdoors in household gardens in suburban and rural areas. Related species occur in many parts of the world (e.g., black widow spider in North America). All produce a similar syndrome of envenomation – *Latrodectism*. Red-back spider bite is the most common cause for antivenom administration in Australia at 300–400/annum and responsible for 2,300 of 11,600 (20 %) of annual hospital admissions for envenomation [1]. The adult female spider is identified easily – its body is about 1 cm in size and has a distinct red or orange dorsal stripe over its abdomen.

The hallmark of envenomation is severe local and distal pain. The spider gives a *pin prick-like* bite. The site quickly becomes inflamed. During the following minutes to several hours, severe pain, exacerbated by movement, commences locally and may extend up the limb or radiate elsewhere. Pain may be accompanied by profuse sweating, headache, nausea, vomiting, abdominal pain, fever, hypertension, paraesthesias, and rashes. Historically, in a small percentage of cases progressive muscle paralysis occurred over many hours, requiring mechanical ventilation. If untreated or treated inadequately, muscle weakness, spasm and arthralgia may persist for months after the bite. In this circumstance, antivenom treatment is still beneficial. No fatalities have occurred since introduction of an antivenom in 1956. If the effects of a bite are minor and confined to the bite site, antivenom may be withheld but otherwise, antivenom should be given intramuscularly. Several doses or intravenous administration may be required.

The rate of anaphylaxis to antivenom is low (<0.5 %). A premedication with promethazine is recommended and adrenaline should be at hand. In contrast to a bite from a snake or funnel-web spider, a bite from a red-back spider is not immediately life-threatening. There is no effective first aid, but application of a cold pack or iced-water may help relieve pain. Bites by *Steatoda* spp (cupboard spiders) may cause a similar syndrome and can be treated effectively with Red-back Spider antivenom. The antivenom is also experimentally effective against the venoms of black widow spiders of North America and Europe [62].

Black Widow Spiders

As discussed above, the widow spider (genus *Latrodectus*) and closely related spiders (including the red-back spider in Australia) are found throughout the world, though the most common species found in North America is the black widow spider (Fig. 51.11). The female black widow spider is characterized by its shiny black color and a red hourglass shape – essentially two triangles arranged apex to apex – of variable size found on the ventral surface of the abdomen. These spiders are generally not very aggressive and bite only in self-defense. Bites are more common during the summer months when the spider is more active.

The principal toxin in *Latrodectus* venom is α-latrotoxin and is generally considered to be one of the more potent toxins found in North America. The toxin binds to multiple sites to open calcium channels, resulting in the uncontrolled release of acetylcholine at the neuromuscular junction and pre-ganglionic and post-ganglionic synapses of the autonomic nervous system (producing characteristic cholinergic and sympathomimetic effects).

Most black widow spider bites probably go unnoticed, though there may be a slight *pin prick-like* sensation at the site of the bite. The systemic reaction is often delayed from 30 min to several hours and is usually heralded by the onset of cramping pain in the chest, abdomen, and back. Additional manifestations include diaphoresis, hypersalivation, lacrimation, and increased bronchial secretions (classic cholinergic symptoms), followed soon by nausea, vomiting, and muscle rigidity. Acute neuromuscular respiratory failure and/or convulsions may occur. These signs and symptoms generally respond to the combination of an antispasmodic agent such as diazepam and an opioid analgesic. antivenin (see above). *Latrodectus mactans* antivenom (equine-derived) is rapidly effective at relieving the clinical effects associated with toxicity. However, its use is limited to those patients manifesting significant toxicity not relieved by conventional therapy or those with health problems that place them at increased risk for complications. The antivenom has an associated risk of anaphylaxis and, if utilized, should be administered in a hospitalized setting with full resuscitation capabilities.

Brown Recluse Spiders

The brown recluse spider, also commonly known as the violin or fiddleback spider due to the violin-shaped coloring on its back, is found throughout the United States (Fig. 51.12). These spiders live both indoors and outdoors and range in size from 1 to 4 cm from leg to leg. The venom of the brown recluse contains several different toxins, including sphingomyelinase D2, which is believed to be the most significant [27]. Envenomation ranges from a mild, local skin reaction to a severe systemic illness characterized by fever, chills, nausea, vomiting, arthralgia, rash, and convulsions. Patients rarely develop haemolytic anemia, DIC, thrombocytopenia, and acute renal failure [27, 61]. The diagnosis of brown recluse spider bite is overused for necrotic skin wounds of uncertain etiology and misdiagnosis is not uncommon [63].

Initially, the bite is painless, but over the next few hours, the patient will develop localized pain, erythema, and pruritus at the site of the bite. A small blister surrounded by a ring of erythema commonly develops, and over the course of the next 2–3 days, the blister may enlarge and become necrotic. An escar develops that may slough off and leave an ulcer – which occasionally is severe enough to warrant skin grafting [27, 61]. Treatment largely is supportive and includes good wound care, tetanus prophylaxis, and antibiotics. Currently, there is no proven antivenin available in the United States.

Scorpions

Stings by scorpions are the second largest cause of envenomation world-wide. Approximately 1.2 million stings lead to more than 3,250 deaths annually [64]. Of the known 1,500 species, about 30 are dangerous to humans and include those in the genera of *Tityus*, *Centruroides*, *Leiurus*, *Androctonus*, *Buthus*, *Parabuthus*, *Mesobuthus*, *Hottenta* and *Hemiscorpius*. Generally, scorpions inhabit hot dry regions. Regions with a high burden of stings are north Saharan Africa, Sahelian Africa, South Africa, Near and Middle-East, South India, Mexico and South Latin America east of the Andes.

In United States, scorpion stings occur principally in Texas, Arizona and California where *Centruroides sculpturatus* exists. Most stings do not required hospitalisation and mortality is very low. Australia does not have significant scorpion species.

Scorpion toxins are neurotoxic peptides which act on sodium and other ionic channels of cell membranes of excitable cells causing release of synaptic neurotransmitters resulting in an "autonomic storm" and signs of catecholamine release. Characteristic severe clinical effects are initial severe pain followed after several hours by fever, systemic muscarinic effects (sweating, epigastric pain, vomiting, colic, diarrhoea, priapism, hypotensioin, bradycardia) and pulmonary effects (bronchial hypersecretion, pulmonary oedema and bronchospasm). In addition, hypertension, cardiac arrhythmias and signs of myocardial ischaemia may end with fatal hypotension. The syndrome may evolve rapidly over several hours. Management consists of intravenous antivenom therapy, pain relief and supportive invasive cardiorespiratory care including control of hypertension.

Bees, Wasps, and Ants

Fatal anaphylactic reactions to bee, wasp and ant stings are a major cause of envenomation deaths in every country [65–69]. The common European Honey Bee (*Apis mellifera*) is largely responsible. The red imported fire ant (*Solenopsis invicta*), a native of South America is also a common cause of anaphylaxis in the United States and has also become established in the Brisbane region of Australia where it has caused anaphylaxis [70]. Persons who develop reactions to insect bites should seek immunotherapy and always carry and use injectable epinephrine. Management of anaphylaxis from bee, wasp, and ants was discussed in the chapter on anaphylaxis.

Venomous Marine Animals

There are more than 80,000 miles of coastline in the United States, and with the increasing popularity of recreational water sports (e.g., scuba diving, ocean kayaking, snorkelling, surfing, etc.), encounters with potentially dangerous marine animals are becoming more commonplace. Numerous species of venomous marine animals inhabit Australian waters as well – in fact, some of the most dangerous animals known to man inhabit this region. Some of these marine envenomations will be reviewed briefly here, though the reader is also referred to other references in the literature for additional information [27, 71–81].

Jellyfish

Marine invertebrates that are dangerous to humans include the coelenterates (e.g., jellyfish). The coelenterates comprise three classes – Hydrozoa (hydroids, fire coral, Portugese man-of-war, bluebottle), Scyphozoa (true jellyfish), and Anthozoa (sea anemones). Envenomation by fire corals and sea anemones is rarely life-threatening and will not be discussed further here. Jellyfish and related species are found throughout the world. These invertebrate marine animals have stinging cells, called nematoblasts, which incorporate an explosive cystic organelle (nematocyst) containing an eversible spine-laden tubule carrying venom. When a jellyfish tentacle comes into contact with an unsuspecting swimmer, thousands of nematocysts discharge their tubules simultaneously, thereby releasing venom and causing a *jellyfish sting*. Importantly, these nematocysts can still discharge even if the tentacle is detached from the jellyfish! Stings not only inject venom but also deposit tubules which are composed of immunologically active substances, particularly chitin, which may cause immediate and long-term allergic responses [82].

Several Scyphozoa species are found in North America, including the sea nettle (*Chrysaora quinquecirrha*) and several species of true jellyfish. The box jellyfish (*Chironex fleckeri*) is reputedly the most dangerous jellyfish in the world (see below) and is common around northern Australia and in the South Pacific. A related species, *Chiropsalmus quadrumanus* caused a lethal envenomation in a 4 year-old child in Galveston Island, Texas in 1990 [77]. The Portuguese man-of-war (*Physalia physalis*) is the most dangerous Hydrozoan and can produce life-threatening envenomation [78, 79, 83, 84].

Jellyfish envenomation produces immediate pain commonly described as a *burning* or *stinging* pain, which is followed by an erythematous rash – the rash usually reflects the pattern of the tentacle at the contact site but may occur distally as well. For the majority of jellyfish stings, the rash evolves over the next 24 h and then slowly subsides with no sequelae. However, more severe envenomations (i.e. by one of the species described below) produce signs and symptoms that affect several organ systems, with possible death usually resulting from anaphylaxis, direct cardiotoxicity, or neuromuscular respiratory failure. Management of jellyfish envenomation includes removal of attached tentacles (the rescuer should not use the bare hands!) after decontamination with 5 % acetic acid (or vinegar), which inactivates undischarged nematocysts, analgesia, and attention to airway/breathing/circulation. Topical corticosteroids, antihistamines, and systemic corticosteroids may alleviate anaphylaxis and other immunological sequelae. Further species-specific management is discussed below.

Box Jellyfish: The box jellyfish, *Chironex fleckeri*, is probably the most venomous marine animal in the world. It has caused numerous deaths in the waters of northern Australian [71]. It has a cuboid bell up to 30 cm in diameter. Numerous tentacles arise from the four corners of the bell and trail several meters. It is semi-transparent and difficult to see by a person wading or swimming in shallow water. The tentacles are armed with millions of nematocysts, which on contact, discharge threaded barbs, which pierce subcutaneous tissue, including small blood vessels. The victim may die within minutes. The precise mode of action of the venom is unknown but its toxins appear to be proteins which induce pore formation in cell membranes. The clinical effects are both neurotoxic (principally causing apnea) and cardiotoxic. In mechanically ventilated animals, fatal hypotension occurs rapidly upon envenomation. Although controversial, calcium channel blockade worsens the outcome of experimental envenomation and is not recommended for human envenomation [81]. Contact with the tentacles causes severe pain and the skin which sustains the injury heals with disfiguring scars.

Management of severe envenomation consists of first aid, cardiopulmonary resuscitation, and administration of an ovine-derived antivenin (CSL Ltd) but which is of moderate efficacy The victim may need to be rescued from the water. First-aid consists of dousing the skin with 5 % acetic acid (vinegar) which inactivates undischarged nematocysts, preventing further envenomation. Prevention of stings is of paramount importance. Water must not be entered during the *stinger season* (October – May) except at beaches protected by nets. Wet suits, clothing and *stinger suits* offer some protection. Other similar deadly chirodropid jellyfish which exist in Australian tropical waters (*Chiropsalmus* sp.) also inhabit many other oceans and seas [71]. A similar chirodropid, *Chiropsalmus quadrumanus*, inhabits the Gulf of Mexico and has caused at least one fatal envenomation (see above) [85].

Irukandji: Stings by the Irukandji jellyfish, *Carukia barnesi* and other related carybdeid jellyfish cause a syndrome known as the *Irukandji syndrome*. An Irukandji-like syndrome has occurred in divers in South Florida [86]. *Carukia barnesi* is a small cubozoan jellyfish with a squarish bell up to several centimetres in diameter and with single tentacles trailing from its four corners. It is barely visible in ocean water. The sting is mild, sometimes unnoticed, and marked only by a small area of cutaneous erythema. However, severe general symptoms may follow which include abdominal cramps, hypertension, back pain, nausea and vomiting, limb cramps, chest tightness and marked distress [87]. Occasionally, cardiogenic pulmonary edema has necessitated mechanical ventilation and inotropic therapy [88]. The mechanism of heart failure is uncertain but experimental studies in animals have shown that the venom causes a massive release of catecholamines [89] which explains in part the clinical syndrome. However, the cause of acute heart failure is unclear.

Physalia: Although regarded as jellyfish, each animal is in fact a hydrozoan colony. Two species, the Pacific *Physalia physalis* (Portuguese man-o'-war) and *Physalia utriculus* (Bluebottle) are present in Australian waters but have caused no deaths. However, the smaller (Bluebottle), causing a mild-moderate sting, is the most common cause of stings in Australian waters, up to 10,000 annually [90]. Deaths elsewhere in the world have been caused by the Atlantic *Physalia physalis*.

Blue-Ringed Octopus

Several species of *Hapalochlaena* inhabit the Australian coastline. When handled, these octopuses bite and inject tetrodotoxin – a neurotoxin, found in many different species of marine animals (including the puffer fish), which causes flaccid paralysis. Several deaths amongst a dozen serious envenomations are recorded [2]. The required treatment is immediate cardiopulmonary resuscitation and mechanical ventilation until spontaneous recovery occurs usually after several hours.

Stinging Fish

Venomous marine vertebrates include stingrays, scorpionfish, lionfish, stonefish, and catfish (Figs. 51.13 and 51.14). These stinging fish are dangerous because they produce direct trauma, pain and swelling from venom, and eventually tissue necrosis and secondary infection, if left untreated. Wound debridement and removal of spine fragments may be needed. The stingray is the most common cause of marine envenomation in the United States – these stinging fish produce a constellation of systemic signs and symptoms that rarely results in death. However, serious or fatal chest injury caused by a stingray barb may be sustained when an unwary diver swims too close or when an occupant of an open vessel is struck by an airborne stingray [2].

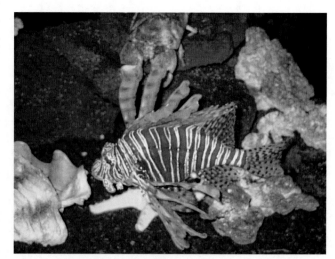

Fig. 51.13 Lionfish (*Scorpaenidae*) (Used with permission of Stephen Dobmeier, CSPI, University of Virginia Health System, Charlottesville, Virginia)

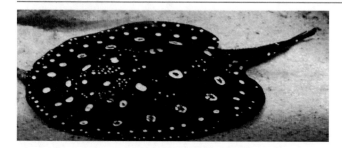

Fig. 51.14 Stingray (*Dasyatidae*) (Used with permission of Christopher P. Holstege, MD, University of Virginia, Charlottesville, Virginia)

Numerous Australian marine and fresh-water fish have spines with attached venom glands, including the scorpion-fish (*Scorpaena*), lionfish (*Pterosis*), and stonefish (*Synanceia*). The most dangerous is the stonefish which is found throughout the Indo-Pacific region. When trodden upon, venom is injected. The immediate effect is extreme pain. Several deaths have been recorded, probably due to the depressive effects of its toxins on cardiovascular and neuro-muscular function, and myotoxicity [2]. An antivenom is available (CSL Ltd). Local or regional nerve blockade may be required for pain relief. Other stinging fish, such as the Australian freshwater bullrout (*Notesthes robusta*) also cause excruciating pain when their spines are contacted. An effec-tive first-aid technique for pain relief of fish stings is immer-sion of the affected limb in warm-to-hot water.

Venomous Cone Shells

Many gastropod molluscs (cone shells) fire a venom-laden harpoon to almost instantaneously immobilize and kill fish prey. The numerous conotoxins, short proteins, stimulate or block neuronal and neuromuscular receptors [2]. A handful of human deaths have been recorded after the attractive shells have been carelessly or unwittingly handled. There is no antivenin. Expired air resuscitation ("mouth to mouth") and subsequent mechanical ventilation would be required until spontaneous recovery occurs.

Shark Attacks

Shark attacks generate significant public and media inter-est – they are mentioned here briefly, even though they do not involve envenomation per se. Shark attacks are relatively rare, especially when compared with the incidence of snake, arthropod, insect, and marine envenomations discussed above. Of the more than 350 described species of sharks, only 32 have been documented to attack humans (The International Shark Attack File at www.flmnh.ufl.edu/fish/sharks). There is

between 70 and 100 shark attacks annually worldwide which result in approximately 5–15 deaths every year [91, 92]. More importantly, although the numbers of sharks are declin-ing, the incidence of shark attacks appears to be on the rise. Again, it should be emphasized, however, that shark attacks are exceedingly rare – some authors suggest that one is more likely to die in an automobile accident while driving to the beach than by a shark attack while swimming at the beach [93]. Shark attacks produce significant soft tissue, vascular, and musculoskeletal trauma which result in a high incidence of secondary infections. Management is consistent with the management of any other traumatic injury.

References

1. Bradley C. Australian Institute of Health and Welfare: venomous bites and stings in Australia to 2005. Injury research and statistics series number 40. Cat no. INJCAT 110. Adelaide: 2008.
2. Sutherland SK, Tibballs J. Australian animal toxins. 2nd ed. Melbourne: Oxford University Press; 2001.
3. Gold BS, Barish RA, Dart RC. North American snake envenom-ation: diagnosis, treatment, and management. Emerg Med Clin North Am. 2004;22:423–43.
4. Parrish HM. Incidence of treated snakebites in the United States. Public Health Rep. 1966;81:269–76.
5. Litovitz TL, Klein-Schwartz W, White S, et al. 1999 annual report of the American Association of Poison Control Centers Toxic Exposure Surveillance System. Am J Emerg Med. 2000;18:517–74.
6. Langley RL, Morrow WE. Deaths resulting from animal attacks in the United States. Wilderness Environ Med. 1997;8:8–16.
7. Langley RL. Animal-related fatalities in the United States – an update. Wilderness Environ Med. 2005;16:67–74.
8. Kasturiratne A, Wickremasinge AR, de Silva N, et al. The global burden of snakebite: a literature analysis and modelling based on regional estimates of envenoming and deaths. PloS Med. 2008;5:1591–604.
9. Wingert WA, Chan L. Rattlesnake bites in southern California and rationale for recommended treatment. West J Med. 1988;148:37–44.
10. Gold BS, Dart RC, Barish RA. Bites of venomous snakes. N Engl J Med. 2002;347:347–56.
11. Pearn JH, Covacevich J, Charles N, et al. Snakebite in herpetolo-gists. Med J Aust. 1994;161:706–8.
12. Johnston MA, Fatovich DM, Haig AD, et al. Successful resuscita-tion after cardiac arrest following massive brown snake envenom-ation. Med J Aust. 2002;177:646–9.
13. Banner Jr W. Bites and stings in the pediatric patient. Curr Probl Pediatr. 1988;18:8–69.
14. Russell FE. Snake venom poisoning in the United States. Annu Rev Med. 1980;31:247–59.
15. Walter FG, Bilden EF, Gibly RL. Envenomations. Crit Care Clin. 1999;15:353–86.
16. Markland FS. Snake venoms and the hemostatic system. Toxicon. 1998;36:1749–800.
17. Laing GD, Clissa PB, Theakston RD, Moura-da-Silva AM, Taylor MJ. Inflammatory pathogenesis of snake venom metalloproteinase-induced skin necrosis. Eur J Immunol. 2003;33:3458–63.
18. Moura-da-Silva AM, Laing GD, Paine MJ, et al. Processing of pro-tumor necrosis factor-alpha by venom metalloproteinases: a hypothesis explaining local tissue damage following snake bite. Eur J Immunol. 1996;26:2000–5.

19. Ownby CL, Colberg TR, White SP. Isolation, characterization, and crystallization of a phospholipase A2 myotoxin from the venom of the prairie rattlesnake (*Crotalus viridis viridis*). Toxicon. 1997;35:111–24.

20. Jansen PW, Perkin RM, Van Stralen D. Mojave rattlesnake envenomation: prolonged neurotoxicity and rhabdomyolysis. Ann Emerg Med. 1992;21:322–5.

21. Farstad D, Thomas T, Chow T, Bush S, Stiegler P. Mojave rattlesnake envenomation in southern California: a review of suspected cases. Wilderness Environ Med. 1997;8:89–93.

22. Bush SP, Cardwell MD. Mojave rattlesnake (Crotalus scutulatus scutulatus) identification. Wilderness Environ Med. 1999;10:6–9.

23. Clark RF, Williams SR, Nordt SP, Boyer-Hassen LV. Successful treatment of crotalid-induced neurotoxicity with a new polyspecific crotalid Fab antivenom. Ann Emerg Med. 1997;30:54–7.

24. Serafim FG, Reali M, Cruz-Hofling MA, Fontana MD. Action of *Mucrurus dumerilii carinicauda* coral snake venom on the mammalian neuromuscular junction. Toxicon. 2002;40:167–74.

25. Alape-Giron A, Stiles B, Schmidt J, et al. Characterization of multiple nicotinic acetylcholine receptor-binding proteins and phospholipases A2 from the venom of the coral snake *Micrurus nigrocinctus*. FEBS Lett. 1996;380:29–32.

26. Kitchens CS, Van Mierop LHS. Envenomation by the eastern coral snake (*Micrurus fulvius fulvius*): a study of 39 victims. JAMA. 1987;258:1615–8.

27. Singletart EM, Rochman AS, Camilo J, Bodmer A, Holstege CP. Envenomations. Med Clin N Am. 2005;89:1195–224.

28. Litovitz TL, Klein-Schwartz W, Dyer KS, Shannon M, Lee S, Powers M. 1997 annual report of the American Association of Poison Control Centers Toxic Exposure Surveillance System. Am J Emerg Med. 1998;16:443–97.

29. Tibballs J, Sutherland S, Kerr S. Studies on Australian snake venoms. Part I: the haemodynamic effects of brown snake (*Pseudonaja*) species in the dog. Anaesth Intensive Care. 1989;17:466–9.

30. Tibballs J. The cardiovascular, coagulation and haematological effects of tiger snake (*Notechis scutatus*) venom. Anaesth Intensive Care. 1998;26:529–35.

31. Tibballs J, Sutherland SK. The efficacy of heparin in the treatment of common brown snake (*Pseudonaja textilis*) envenomation. Anaesth Intensive Care. 1992;20:33–7.

32. Gold BS, Barish BA. Venomous snakebites: current concepts in diagnosis, treatment, and management. Emerg Med Clin North Am. 1992;10:249–67.

33. Suchard JR, LoVecchio F. Envenomations by rattlesnakes thought to be dead. N Engl J Med. 1999;340:1930.

34. Sutherland SK, Coulter AR, Harris RD. Rationalization of first-aid measures for elapid snakebite. Lancet. 1979;1:183–6.

35. German BT, Hack JB, Brewer K, et al. Pressure-immobilization bandages delay toxicity in a porcine model of Eastern coral snake (*Micrurus fulvius fulvius*) envenomation. Ann Emerg Med. 2005;45:603–8.

36. Sutherland SK, Coulter AR. Early management of bites by the Eastern diamondback rattlesnake (*Crotalus adamanteus*): studies in monkeys (*Macaca fascicularis*). Am J Trop Med Hyg. 1981;30:497–500.

37. Bush SP, Green SM, Laack TA, et al. Pressure immobilization delays mortality and increases intracompartmental pressure after artificial intramuscular rattlesnake envenomation in a porcine model. Ann Emerg Med. 2004;44:599–604.

38. Meggs WJ, Courtney C, O'Rourke D, Brewer KL. Pilot studies of pressure-immobilization bandages for rattlesnake envenomations. Clin Toxicol. 2010;48:61–3.

39. Sutherland SK, Harris RD, Coulter AR, et al. First aid for cobra (*Naja naja*) bites. Indian J Med Res. 1981;73:266–8.

40. Markenson D, Ferguson JD, Chameides L, et al. 2010 American Heart Association and American Red Cross guidelines for first aid. Circulation. 2010;122:S934–46.

41. Canale E, Isbister GK, Currie BJ. Investigating pressure bandaging for snakebite in a simulated setting: bandage type, training and the effect of transport. Emerg Med Aust. 2009;21:184–90.

42. Howarth DM, Southee AE, Whyte IM. Lymphatic flow rates and first-aid in simulated peripheral snake or spider envenomation. Med J Aust. 1994;161:695–700.

43. Oakley J. Managing death adder bite with prolonged pressure bandaging. 6th Asia-Pacific Congress on Animal, Plant and Microbial Toxins & 11th Annual Scientific Meeting of the Australasian College of Tropical Medicine, 8–12th. Cairns; 2002. p. 29.

44. Jurkovich GJ, Luterman A, McCullar K, Ramenofsky ML, Curreri PW. Complications of crotalidae antivenin therapy. J Trauma. 1988;28:1032–7.

45. Dart RC, McNally J. Efficacy, safety, and use of snake antivenoms in the United States. Ann Emerg Med. 2001;37:181–8.

46. Levonas EJ. Initial experience with crotalidae polyvalent immune Fab (ovine) antivenom in the treatment of copperhead snakebite. Ann Emerg Med. 2004;43:200–6.

47. Malasit P, Warrell DA, Chanthavanich P, et al. Prediction, prevention, and mechanism of early (anaphylactic) antivenom reactions in victims of snake bites. Br Med J. 1986;292:17–20.

48. Tibballs J. Premedication for snake antivenom. Med J Aust. 1994;160:4–7.

49. Premawardhena AP, de Silva CE, Fonseka M, et al. Low dose subcutaneous adrenaline to prevent acute adverse reactions to antivenom serum in people bitten by snakes: randomised, placebo controlled trial. Br Med J. 1999;318:1041–3.

50. Williams DJ, Jensen SD, Nimorakiotakis B, Müller R, Winkel KD. Antivenom use, premedication and early adverse reactions in the management of snake bites in rural Papua New Guinea. Toxicon. 2007;49:780–92.

51. Pumphrey RS. Lessons for management of anaphylaxis from a study of fatal reactions. Clin Exp Allergy. 2000;30:1144–50.

52. Fan HW, Marcopito LF, Cardoso JL, et al. A Sequential randomised and double blind trial of promethazine prophylaxis against early anaphylactic reactions to antivenom for *Bothrops* snake bites. Br Med J. 1999;318:1451–3.

53. Clark RF, Selden BS, Furbee B. The incidence of wound infection following crotalid envenomation. J Emerg Med. 1993;11:583–6.

54. Weed HG. Nonvenomous snakebite in Massachusetts: prophylactic antibiotics are unnecessary. Ann Emerg Med. 1993;22:220–4.

55. Blaylock RS. Antibiotic use and infection in snakebite victims. S Afr Med J. 1999;89:874–6.

56. Kerrigan KR, Mertz BL, Nelson SJ, Dye JD. Antibiotic prophylaxis for pit viper envenomation: prospective, controlled trial. World J Surg. 1997;21:369–73.

57. LoVecchio F, Klemens J, Welch S, Rodriguez R. Antibiotics after rattlesnake envenomation. J Emerg Med. 2002;23:327–8.

58. Minton Jr SA. Bites by non-native venomous snakes in the United States. Wild Environ Med. 1996;4:297–303.

59. Pincus SJ, Winkel KD, Hawdon GM, et al. Acute and recurrent skin ulceration after spider bite. Med J Aust. 1999;17:99–102.

60. Isbister GK. Necrotic arachnidism: the mythology of a modern plague. Lancet. 2004;364:549–53.

61. Saucier JR. Arachnid envenomation. Emerg Med Clin North Am. 2004;22:405–22.

62. Graudins A, Padula M, Broady K, et al. Red-back spider (*Latrodectus hasselti*) antivenom prevents the toxicity of widow spider venoms. Ann Emerg Med. 2001;37:154–60.

63. Vetter RS, Bush SP. The diagnosis of brown recluse spider bite is overused for dermonecrotic wounds of uncertain etiology. Ann Emerg Med. 2002;39:544–6.

64. Chippaux JP, Goyffon M. Epidemiology of scorpionism: a global appraisal. Acta Trop. 2008;107:71–9.
65. Stawiski MA. Insect bites and stings. Emerg Med Clin North Am. 1985;3:785–808.
66. Jerrard DA. ED management of insect stings. Am J Emerg Med. 1996;14:429–33.
67. Holve S. Treatment of snake, insect, scorpion, and spider bites in the pediatric emergency department. Curr Opin Pediatr. 1996;8: 256–60.
68. Moffitt JE. Allergic reactions to insect stings and bites. South Med J. 2003;96:1073–9.
69. Levick NR, Schmidt JO, Harrison J, et al. Review of bee and wasp sting injuries in Australia and the USA. In: Austin AD, Dowton M, editors. Hymenoptera. Melbourne: CSIRO Publishing; 2000.
70. Solley GO, Vanderwoude C, Knight GK. Anaphylaxis due to red imported fire ant sting. Med J Aust. 2002;176:521–3.
71. Williamson JA, Fenner PJ, Burnett JW, et al. Venomous and poisonous marine animals. Sydney: University of New South Wales Press; 1996.
72. Nimorakiotakis B, Winkel KD. Marine envenomations. Part 1 – jellyfish. Aust Fam Physician. 2003;32:969–74.
73. Nimorakiotakis B, Winkel KD. Marine envenomations. Part 2 – other marine envenomations. Aust Fam Physician. 2003;32:975–9.
74. Hawdon GM, Winkel KD. Venomous marine creatures. Aust Fam Physician. 1997;26:1369–74.
75. Schwartz S, Meinking T. Venomous marine animals of Florida: morphology, behavior, health hazards. J Fla Med Assoc. 1997;84: 433–40.
76. Pearn J. The sea, stingers, and surgeons: the surgeon's role in prevention, first aid, and management of marine envenomations. J Pediatr Surg. 1995;30:105–10.
77. Brown CK, Shepherd SM. Marine trauma, envenomations, and intoxications. Emerg Med Clin North Am. 1992;10:385–408.
78. McGoldrick J, Marx JA. Marine envenomations; Part 1: vertebrates. J Emerg Med. 1991;9:497–502.
79. McGoldrick J, Marx JA. Marine envenomations; Part 2: invertebrates. J Emerg Med. 1992;10:71–7.
80. Auerbach PS. Marine envenomations. N Engl J Med. 1991;325: 486–93.
81. Tibballs J. Australian venomous jellyfish, envenomation syndromes, toxins and therapy. Toxicon. 2006;48:830–59.
82. Tibballs J, Yanagihara AA, Turner HC, Winkel K. Immunological and toxinological responses to jellyfish stings. Inflamm Allergy Drug Targets. 2011;10:438–46.
83. Burnett JW, Gable WD. A fatal jellyfish envenomation by the Portugese man-of-war. Toxicon. 1989;27:823–4.
84. Stein MR, Marraccini JV, Rothschild NE, et al. Fatal Portugese man-of-war (Physalia physalis) envenomation. Ann Emerg Med. 1989;18:312–5.
85. Bengston K, Nichols MM, Schnadig V, et al. Sudden death in a child following jellyfish envenomation by Chiropsalmus quadrumanus. JAMA. 1991;266:1404–6.
86. Grady JD, Burnett JW. Irukandji-like syndrome in South Florida divers. Ann Emerg Med. 2003;42:763–6.
87. Little M, Mulcahy RF. A year's experience of Irukandji envenomation in far north Queensland. Med J Aust. 1998;169:638–41.
88. Little M, Mulcahy RF, Wenck DJ. Life-threatening cardiac failure in a healthy young female with Irukandji syndrome. Anaesth Intensive Care. 2001;29:178–80.
89. Winkel KD, Tibballs J, Molenaar P, et al. The cardiovascular actions of the venom from the Irukandji (Carukia barnesi) jellyfish: effects in human, rat and guinea pig tissues in vitro, and in pigs in vivo. Clin Exp Pharmacol Physiol. 2005;32: 777–88.
90. Fenner PJ, Williamson JA. Worldwide deaths and severe envenomation from jellyfish stings. Med J Aust. 1996;165: 658–61.
91. Woolgar JD, Cliff G, Nair R, Hafez H, Robbs JV. Shark attack: review of 86 cases. J Trauma. 2001;50:887–91.
92. Caldicott DGE, Mahajani R, Kuhn M. The anatomy of a shark attack: a case report and review of the literature. Injury. 2001;32:445–53.
93. Manire CA, Gruber SH. Anatomy of a shark attack. J Wilderness Med. 1992;3:4–8.

Index

R

Radiant heat, 678
Radionuclide angiography, for brain death, 489
Range ambiguity, 550
Rapid influenza diagnostic tests (RIDTs), 660
Rapid sequence intubation (RSI), 319–320, 420
Reactive nitrogen species (RNS), 239–240
    antioxidants, 240
    critical illness
        sepsis, 242–244
        TBI, 245–246
    immune responses, 241
    mitochondrial respiration regulation, 241–242
    physiologic function, 241
    redox homeostasis, 241
    sources
        anti-oxidant mechanisms, 258
        mitochondrial production, 256
        nitric oxide, 257–258
        nitrosative stress, 257–258
        oxidative burst from infiltrated neutrophil, 257
        xanthine oxidase, 256–257
Reactive oxygen species (ROS), 239–240
    antioxidants, 240
    critical illness
        sepsis, 242–244
        TBI, 245–246
    immune responses, 241
    mitochondrial respiration regulation, 241–242
    physiologic function, 241
    redox homeostasis, 241
    sources
        anti-oxidant mechanisms, 258
        mitochondrial production, 256
        nitric oxide, 257–258
        nitrosative stress, 257–258
        oxidative burst from infiltrated neutrophil, 257
        xanthine oxidase, 256–257
Realistic evaluation model, 89
    classic research vs., 90
Recommended Dietary Allowances (RDA), 590–591
Redox homeostasis, 240
    and physiologic function, 241
Refeeding syndrome, 593
Regional lymphadenitis, 733
Regulators of signal transduction, 224
    epigenetics as, 225
    phosphatases as, 224–225
Renal angina, emerging biomarkers, 612–613
Reperfusion injury, 251
    ALI and ARDS, 274
    cellular and molecular defense mechanisms, 262
        autophagy, 263–264
        endogenous hydrogen sulfide production, 264
        heat shock response, 263
        hypoxia-inducible factor-1, 263
        ischemic preconditioning response, 264–265
        RISK pathway, 263
    complement activation, 260–261
    damage associated molecular patterns, 261–262
    endothelial dysfunction, 258–260
    ischemia and (see Ischemia)
    MMP, 262
    multiple trauma and, 417
    neutrophil infiltration, 258–260
    oxidative and nitrosative stress, 253–256
    post-cardiac arrest syndrome, 272–273
    ROS and RNS, 256–258
    toll-like receptors, 261–262
Reperfusion injury salvage kinase (RISK) pathway, 263
Resident and nurse education in PICU, 117–118
    ACGME guidelines, 119–120
    computer assisted learning, 118–119, 122
    didactics, 118
    educating, 121–122
    evaluation, 121
    experiential learning, 122
    factors impacting, 120
    FOPE, 119
    interpersonal and communication skills, 121
    learner-centered teaching, 122
    medical knowledge, 121
    patient care, 121
    practice-based learning and improvement, 121
    problem based learning, 118
    professionalism, 121
    simulators in medical education, 122–123
    system-based practice, 121
    team-based learning, 119
    training and education, 118–119
    unique learning environments, 118
Respiratory alkalosis, 714
Respiratory care, interfacility transport, 452–453
Respiratory depression, 709
Respiratory failure, 521, 522, 525
    acute (see Acute respiratory failure)
    genetic polymorphisms in, 184–187
Respiratory monitoring
    arterial blood gas, 522–525
        analysis, 529
    end-tidal CO_2 monitoring, 529–531
    gas exchange, 522
    loops, 535
        flow-volume, 537–539
        pressure-volume, 536
    mechanical ventilation, 533
    mechanics of, 532–533
    monitoring ventilation, 528
    pulmonary overdistention, 537
    pulse oximetry, 525–528
    recruitment/derecruitment, 537
    scalars, 532
        flow-time, 533–535
        pressure-time, 535
        volume-time, 535
    transcutaneous CO_2 measurements, 531–532
Respiratory muscle insufficiency, 405–406
Respiratory system
    acute lung injury, 668
    acute respiratory distress syndrome, 668
    post-resuscitation care, 273–275
Respiratory therapy, 36
Resting energy expenditure (REE), monitoring
    advances in, 586–587
    energy intake and, 594
    indirect calorimetry, 585–586
    indirect estimations of, 587
    ratios of, 596
    short Douglas bag protocol, 587
    standard metabolic monitor, 586
Resuscitation Outcomes Consortium (ROC), 272
Return of spontaneous circulation (ROSC), 271, 273, 283

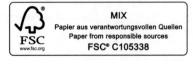

Printed by Books on Demand, Germany